D0753265

Handbook of
Community Psychology

Handbook of Community Psychology

Edited by

Julian Rappaport
University of Illinois at Urbana-Champaign
Urbana, Illinois

and

Edward Seidman
New York University
New York, New York

Kluwer Academic / Plenum Publishers
New York • Boston • Dordrecht • London • Moscow

Library of Congress Cataloging-in-Publication Data

Handbook of community psychology/edited by Julian Rappaport & Edward Seidman.
p. cm.
Includes bibliographical references and index.
ISBN 0-306-46160-9
1. Community psychology—Handbooks, manuals, etc. I. Rappaport, Julian. II. Seidman, Edward.

RA790.55 .H36 1999
362.2—dc21 99-049482

ISBN 0-306-46160-9

233 Spring Street, New York, N.Y. 10013

http://www.wkap.nl/

10 9 8 7 6 5 4 3

A C.I.P. record for this book is available from the Library of Congress

Printed in the United States of America

For our children and our grandchildren

May you always live in a loving community
where justice matters,
where fairness and authenticity abounds
and where the streets are filled
with the joys of life, of learning, and of laughing.

Contributors

LaRue Allen, Department of Applied Psychology, New York University, New York, New York 10003

B. Eileen Altman, 1156 High Street, Santa Cruz, California 95064

Bruce Ambuel, Waukesha Family Practice Center, #201, 210 N. W. Barstow, Waukesha, Wisconsin 53045

Kenneth B. Bachrach, Tarzana Treatment Center, Tarzana, California 91356

Charles Barone, 3003 Van Ness Street N. W., #W1129, Washington, D.C. 20008

Manuel Barrera Jr., Psychology Department, Arizona State University, Tempe, Arizona 85287

G. Ann Bogat, Department of Psychology, Michigan State University, East Lansing, Michigan 48824

Bill Berkowitz, Department of Psychology, University of Massachusetts Lowell, Lowell, Massachusetts 01854

Sanford Braver, Department of Psychology, Arizona State University, Tempe, Arizona 85287

Julia Green Brody, Silent Spring Institute, 29 Crafts Street, Newton, Massachusetts 02458

Geoffrey Carr, Department of Psychology, Simon Fraser University, Burnaby, British Columbia V5A 156, Canada

David M. Chavis, Association for the Study and Development of Community, Gaithersburg, Maryland 20877

Cary Cherniss, Graduate School of Applied and Professional Psychology, Rutgers University, Piscataway, New Jersey 08854

Emory L. Cowen, Center for Community Study, University of Rochester, Rochester, New York 14620

Anthony R. D'Augelli, Department of Human Development and Family Studies, The Pennsylvania State University, University Park, Pennsylvania 16802

William S. Davidson II, Department of Psychology, Michigan State University, East Lansing, Michigan 48824-1117

GENE DEEGAN, Graduate School of Applied and Professional Psychology, Department of Psychology, Rutgers University, Piscataway, New Jersey 08854

CHRISTINA DOUGLAS, Center for Creative Leadership, Greensboro, North Carolina 27438

STEPHEN B. FAWCETT, Department of Human Development and Family Life, University of Kansas, Lawrence, Kansas 66045

ROBERT D. FELNER, School of Education and the National Center on Public Education and Social Policy, University of Rhode Island, Kingston, Rhode Island 02881

TWEETY YATES FELNER, Department of Special Education, University of Illinois, Champaign, Illinois 61820

PAUL FLORIN, Department of Psychology, University of Rhode Island, Kingston, Rhode Island 02881

CARRIE S. FRIED, Department of Psychology, University of Virginia, Charlottesville, Virginia 22903

LEAH GENSHEIMER, Department of Psychology, University of Missouri-Kansas City, Kansas City, Missouri 64110

JOSE ANTONIO GARCIA GONZALEZ, Universidad Central de Venezuela, Caracas 1010-A, Venezuela

MICHELLE GOYETTE-EWING, Child Study Center, Yale University, New Haven, Connecticut 06511

KATHERINE GRADY, Department of Psychiatry, Yale University School of Medicine, New Haven, Connecticut 06511

KENNETH HELLER, Department of Psychology, Indiana University, Bloomington, Indiana 47405

ROBERT HUGHES JR., College of Human Environmental Sciences, University of Missouri, Columbia, Missouri 65211

LEONARD A. JASON, Department of Psychology, De Paul University, Chicago, Illinois 60614

RICHARD A. JENKINS, National Center for HIV, STD, and TB Prevention, Centers for Disease Control and Prevention, Atlanta, Georgia 30333

JAMES G. KELLY, Department of Psychology, University of California, Davis, Davis, California 95616

KATHERINE J. KLEIN, Department of Psychology, University of Maryland, College Park, Maryland 20742

JANE KNITZER, National Center for Children in Poverty, School of Public Health, Columbia University, New York, New York 10032

LEON H. LEVY, Department of Psychology, Virginia Commonwealth University, Richmond, Virginia 23229

RAMSAY LIEM, Department of Psychology, Boston College, Chestnut Hill, Massachusetts 02167

Jean Ann Linney, Department of Psychology, Barnwell College, University of South Carolina, Columbia, South Carolina 29208

Alfred McAlister, School of Public Health, University of Texas, Houston, Texas 77225

Miriam Martinez, Department of Psychiatry, University of California at San Francisco, San Francisco General Hospital, San Francisco, California 94110

Kenneth I. Maton, Department of Psychology, University of Maryland Baltimore County, Catonsville, Maryland 21250

Jeffrey P. Mayer, Department of Community Health, School of Public Health, St. Louis University, St. Louis, Missouri 63108

Gary B. Melton, Institute on Family and Neighborhood and Family Life, Clemson University, Clemson, South Carolina 29634

Judith C. Meyers, Child Health and Development Institute of Connecticut, Inc., Farmington, Connecticut 06032

John R. Morgan, Director of Clinical and Prevention Services, Chesterfield Mental Health–Mental Retardation Department, Chesterfield, Virginia 23832

Anne Morris, Center for Mental Health Services Research, University of California, Berkeley, California 94720

J. R. Newbrough, Department of Psychology, Peabody College of Vanderbilt University, Nashville, Tennessee 37203

Patrick O'Neill, Department of Psychology, Acadia University, Wolfville, Nova Scotia B0P 1X0, Canada

Diana Oxley, Department of Special Education and Community Resources, University of Oregon, Eugene, Oregon 97403-1235

Kenneth I. Pargament, Department of Psychology, Bowling Green State University, Bowling Grccn, Ohio 43402

Dennis N. T. Perkins, The Syncretics Group, Branford, Connecticut 06505

Deborah A. Phillips, Institute of Medicine, National Research Council, Washington, D.C. 20418

Richard H. Price, Department of Psychology, University of Michigan, Ann Arbor, Michigan 48106

R. Scott Ralls, Vice President, Economic and Workforce Development, The North Carolina Community College System, Raleigh, North Carolina 27603

Bruce D. Rapkin, Memorial Sloan-Kettering Cancer Hospital, New York, New York 10021

N. Dickon Reppucci, Department of Psychology, University of Virginia, Charlottesville, Virginia 22903

Tracey A. Revenson, Department of Social-Personality and Health Psychology, CUNY Graduate Center, New York, New York 10016

Jean E. Rhodes, Department of Psychology, University of Illinois, Champaign, Illinois 61820

Ronald Roesch, Department of Psychology, Simon Fraser University, Burnaby, British Columbia V5A 1S6, Canada

Ann Marie Ryan, Department of Psychology, Michigan State University, East Lansing, Michigan 48824

Irwin N. Sandler, Department of Psychology, Arizona State University, Tempe, Arizona 85287

Seymour B. Sarason, Department of Psychology, Yale University, New Haven, Connecticut 06520

Ruth Schelkun, Late of Washtenaw County Community Mental Health Center, Washtenaw County, Michigan

Kathleen M. Schiaffino, Department of Psychology, Fordham University, New York, New York 10458

Irma Serrano-Garcia, Department of Psychology, University of Puerto Rico, Rio Piedras, Puerto Rico 00826

Morton M. Silverman, Department of Psychiatry, University of Chicago, Chicago, Illinois 60615

Marybeth Shinn, Center for Community Research and Action, Department of Psychology, New York University, New York, New York 10003

Virginia Smith-Major, Department of Psychology, University of Maryland at College Park, College Park, Maryland 20742

David L. Snow, The Consultation Center, Department of Psychiatry, Yale University, New Haven, Connecticut 06511

Lonnie R. Snowden, Center for Mental Health Service Research and School of Social Welfare, University of California, Berkeley, California 94720

Ann M. Steffen, Department of Psychology, University of Missouri–St. Louis, St Louis, Missouri 63121

Stephen P. Stelzner, Department of Psychology, College of St. Benedict, St. Joseph, Minnesota 56374

Eric Stewart, Department of Psychology, University of Illinois, Champaign, Illinois 61820

Carolyn F. Swift, 1102 Hilltop Drive, Lawrence, Kansas 66044

Ralph W. Swindle Jr., Health Services Research and Development, VA Medical Center, Indianapolis, Indiana 46202

J. S. Tanaka, Late of the Departments of Educational Psychology and Psychology, University of Illinois at Urban-Champaign, Champaign, Illinois 61820

Edison J. Trickett, Department of Psychology, University of Maryland, College Park, Maryland 20742

Collin van Uchelen, Cross Cultural Psychiatric Program, Department of Psychiatry, University of British Columbia, Vancouver, British Columbia V6T 2A1, Canada

ABRAHAM WANDERSMAN, Department of Psychology, University of South Carolina, Columbia, South Carolina 29208

RODERICK WATTS, Department of Psychology, De Paul University, Chicago, Illinois 60614

GLENN W. WHITE, Department of Human Development and Family Life, University of Kansas, Lawrence, Kansas 66045

SABINE WINGENFELD, School of Psychological Sciences, La Trobe University, Bundoora, VIC 3083, Australia

THOMAS WOLFF, Community Development, Massachusetts Statewide Area Health Education Centers, University of Massachusetts Health Center, Amherst, Massachusetts 01002

JENNIFER L. WOOLARD, Department of Psychology, University of Florida, Gainesville, Florida 32611

ALEX J. ZAUTRA, Department of Psychology, Arizona State University, Tempe, Arizona 85287-1104

MARC A. ZIMMERMAN, Department of Health Behavior and Health Education, School of Public Health, University of Michigan, Ann Arbor, Michigan 48109-2029

Preface

As a field progresses, people write about their own work in journals, chapters, and books; but periodically the work needs to be collected and organized. It needs to be brought together in a format that can both introduce new members to the field and reacquaint continuing members with the work of their colleagues. Such a collection also affords an opportunity for the growing number of people with particular expertise to provide a reference for others whose work is related, but differs in focus.

This is the first *Handbook of Community Psychology*. It contains contributions from 106 different authors, in addition to our editorial introductions. Its thirty-eight chapters (including two that are divided into multiple, individually authored parts) are concerned with conceptual frameworks, empirically grounded constructs, intervention strategies and tactics, social systems, design, assessment and analysis, cross-cutting professional issues, and contemporary intersections with community psychology.

Although interrelated, each chapter stands on its own as a statement about a particular part of the field, and the volume can serve as a reference for those who may want to explore an area about which they are not yet familiar. To some extent community psychologists eschew the distinction between researcher and practitioner; and regardless of one's primary work environment (university, small college, practice setting, government, or grassroots organization), there is something of interest for anyone who wants to explore the community psychology approach.

To say that all the work of importance to the field is presented here would be to promise more than anyone could deliver given the rapid growth, comprehensive development, and broad scope of this field. However, as we suggest in our editorial introductions to each section, we do offer here the overarching narratives that tell the community psychology story and many of the maps that have pointed community psychologists in new directions. We think this volume should be of interest to both graduate students and professionals; and much (if not all of it) is written in a way that makes it accessible to advanced—albeit sophisticated—undergraduates as well, especially those who want to grasp the scope of the field.

Each chapter stands on the shoulders of considerable work, much of which has not previously been brought together in any single place. The volume as a whole has many historical roots. In 1966, Sarason, Levine, Goldenberg, Cherlin, and Bennett published a book describing their work at the Yale Psycho Educational Clinic. In 1967, Emory L. Cowen, Elmer A. Gardner, and Melvin Zax edited an influential book called *Emergent Approaches to Mental Health Problems*. This was shortly followed by Ira Goldenberg's *Build Me a Mountain* (1971), Seymour Sarason's *The Psychological Sense of Community* (1974), and the Austin Conference on the training of community psychologists (Iscoe, Bloom, & Spielberger, 1977). In 1972,

Stewart Golann and Carl Eisdorfer edited a *Handbook of Community Mental Health*. In some ways that ambitious volume is the forerunner of this one, inasmuch as it brought together a wide range of authors and ideas within its focal themes, many of which predated the development of community psychology as distinct from community mental health.

Those early volumes, along with the intellectual, professional, historical, and political events that accompanied the founding of the Division of Community Psychology of the American Psychological Association in 1966 (now organized as the Society for Community Research and Action) and of the *American Journal of Community Psychology* (in 1973), as well as the *Journal of Community Psychology* and more recently the (British) *Journal of Community and Applied Social Psychology*, moved the field to a more prominent place among both the academic and the practice communities.

In the past thirty years, many textbooks on community psychology and community mental health, from various theoretical perspectives, some suitable for undergraduates, some for graduate students, have appeared: Murrell (1973); Zax and Spector (1974); Neitzel, MacDonald, Davidson, and Winett (1977); Bloom (1977, 1984); Heller and Monahan (1977); Mann (1978); Gibbs, Lachenmeyer, and Sigal (1980); Glenwick and Jason (1980); Jeger and Slotnik (1982); Heller, Price, Reinharz, Riger, and Wandersman (1984); Orford (1992); Levine and Perkins (1987, 1997). Many of these remain worth reading today as ways to organize and energize the field.

Our own contributions to codification of the growing literature included a textbook, *Community Psychology: Values, Research, and Action* (Rappaport, 1977); *Handbook of Social Intervention* (Seidman, 1983); and a book of readings, *Redefining Social Problems* (Seidman & Rappaport, 1986). In this volume we resist the temptation to review the history of the field, since many such accounts are available in the works mentioned above. But the time is ripe for community psychology to take another account of itself in the form of a reference work. We do so here with the hope that current researchers and practitioners, as well as newly interested students and colleagues, will find that the spirit of community work, inspired by the values, research, and action that has engaged us in careers linking the personal with the intellectual, and research with practice, will find it both a convenient compendium and a spark for their own ideas and interests.

References

Bloom, B. L. (1977/1984). *Community mental health: A general introduction* (2nd ed.). Monterey, CA: Brooks/Cole.

Cowen, E. L., Gardner, E. A., & Zax, M. (eds.). (1967). *Emergent approaches to mental health problems*. New York: Appleton-Century-Crofts.

Gibbs, M. S., Lachenmeyer, J. R., & Sigal, J. (eds.). (1980). *Community psychology: Theoretical and empirical approaches*. New York: Gardner.

Glenwick, D. S., & Jason, L. A. (Eds.). (1980). *Behavioral community psychology: Progress and prospects*. New York: Praeger.

Golann, S. E., & Eisdorfer, C. (Eds.). (1972). *Handbook of community mental health*. New York: Appleton-Century-Crofts.

Goldenberg, I. I. (1971). *Build me a mountain: Youth, poverty, and the creation of new settings*. Cambridge, MA: MIT Press.

Heller, K., & Monahan, J. (1977). *Psychology and community change*. Homewood, IL: Dorsey.

Heller, K., Price, R. H., Reinharz, S., Riger, S., & Wandersman, A. (1984). *Psychology and community change*. Pacific Grove, CA: Brooks/Cole.

Iscoe, I., Bloom, B. L., & Spielberger, C. D. (Eds.). (1977). *Community psychology in transition*. Washington, D.C.: Hemisphere.

Jeger, A. M., & Slotnick, R. S. (Eds.). (1982). *Community mental health and behavioral ecology: A handbook of theory, research, and practice.* New York: Plenum.

Levine, M., & Perkins, D. V. (1987/1997). *Principles of community psychology: Perspectives and applications* (2nd ed.). New York: Oxford University Press.

Mann, P. (1978). *Community psychology: Concepts and applications.* New York: Free Press.

Murrell, S. A. (1973). *Community psychology and social systems.* New York: Behavioral Publications.

Nietzel, M. T., Winett, R. A., MacDonald, M. L., & Davidson, W. S. (1977). *Behavioral approaches to community psychology.* New York: Pergamon.

Orford, J. (1992). *Community psychology: Theory and practice.* Chichester, England: Wiley.

Rappaport, J. (1977). *Community psychology: Values, research, and action.* New York: Holt, Rinehart, & Winston.

Sarason, S. B. (1974). *The psychological sense of community: Prospects for a community psychology.* San Francisco, CA: Jossey-Bass.

Sarason, S. B., Levine, M., Goldenberg, I. I., Cherlin, D. L., & Bennett, E. M. (1966). *Psychology in community settings: Clinical, educational, vocational, social aspects.* New York: Wiley.

Seidman, E. (Ed.). (1983). *Handbook of social intervention.* Beverly Hills, CA: Sage.

Seidman, E., & Rappaport, J. (Eds.). (1986). *Redefining social problems.* New York: Plenum.

Zax, M., & Spector, G. A. (1974). *An introduction to community psychology,* New York: Wiley.

Contents

Handbook of Community Psychology

PART I

CONCEPTS, FRAMEWORKS, STORIES, AND MAPS

Every field requires a narrative about itself—a vision of its possibilities, a story that explains why it studies what it deems to be important. Those who work in the field also require maps—pictures that show the lay of the land, interesting places, and the ways to get there from here. These narratives and maps are written and drawn by people who care about theory and define concepts. Although the classical model of theory-guided discovery is an idealized version of the way scientists actually work, it remains accurate to say that questions asked by researchers and scholars are guided by either implicit or explicit theoretical ideas about what is important to understand and how that area of the world works.

The questions "what?" and "how?" are the province of theoretical statements and concepts designed to capture our vision. The chapters in this section discuss ways to look at the world in order to ask questions about how it works and what is important in it. Such questions are intimately tied to understanding change and creating interventions, activities that have occupied community psychology since its inception. They tell us what empirical work is important, what systems to look at, how to design research, and what roles to assume in the world.

None of the authors of these chapters would say, "Here, I have presented a classical theory of the sort that is a string of logically consistent statements and corollaries. Out of this, a program of research directly follows so precisely that everyone who understands the theory knows what the next study should be." Few community psychologists believe that such theories are helpful in a rapidly changing, open system, multivariate, iterative social world. Nor can these chapters be read as complete statements of their points of view. Each one refers to a bibliography of related materials that support the underpinnings of the chapter. For these reasons it is perhaps best to see these introductory narratives as frameworks, rather than theories. Yet community psychologists do make theoretical statements, and these statements are thought to be both appropriate and important. They point us in certain directions. The ways pointed to here are among those that most often have served to orient community psychologists. In this sense, they may also be thought of as maps.

Maps are usually drawn for a specific purpose. If one wants to drive from Chicago to New York by the quickest route, a highway map is very helpful. The location of various geographical features that are hospitable to different forms of wildlife is not of interest. A bird-watcher may find a highway map useless. She may be more interested in a topographical map that can help her to predict where certain kinds of birds are likely to be found. A family on a tour of the United States may want a map that details important historical landmarks. A geologist will require yet a different map. A visiting official from the Vatican may need a map showing all the

Catholic dioceses and churches in a given region. Each of these maps, and many others, will present "reality," or point to what exists in some specified space. Yet they are differentially useful depending on one's purposes. It may also be the case that a traveler who heads from Chicago to New York, intent on getting there quickly, could discover a map of historical places and decide that the purpose of his trip should be revised. Maps serve the purpose of helping those who set out on a journey; they also inspire journeys, showing the possibilities for discovery by suggesting what might be seen and how to get there.

The maps that the authors in this section provide are not intended to be detailed so much as orienting and inspiring. They each refer to other maps with more detail. They do intend to orient and inspire the reader to the time and space of community psychology. In that sense they need to be used in conjunction with other maps, depending on one's purposes. One way these maps could be used is to keep them in mind as other sections of this volume are read. One could read each of the other sections (many of which will be both more narrow and more detailed) with these orientations in mind. Together they provide both orientation and detail, weaving a complex story about community psychology.

This section opens with Felner, Felner, and Silverman's map for a science and practice of prevention. It is an approach that makes an explicit conceptual break with the traditional public health framework that has served as a bridge from clinical to community models in the field of mental health. The traditional (blended) view of treatment and prevention (in which degrees of prevention—primary, secondary, and tertiary—are acknowledged) is eschewed in favor of a more explicit distinction between individual clinical work and mass-oriented or population-focused prevention, which aims to modify processes and mediating conditions that create a risk for problems in living.

Important in this view is that the concept of "risk" is recognized to be an actuarial statement about social contexts (as opposed to people). There are no "high-risk" individuals. These authors make the case for a developmental and ecological model that sees people as learning to adapt to their actual environments. They call this a "transactional approach," and repeatedly emphasize the importance of social context as necessary to understand both developmental trajectories and behaviors. Later chapters in this section (see especially the chapter by Kelly and colleagues) and other sections of this handbook will also emphasize social context in both intervention (see, for example, Trickett, Barone, and Watts in Part III) and assessment (Linney in Part V). Indeed, an attempt to understand the transactions of people in their own social contexts (as opposed to people as diagnoses or "problems") may be assumed to underlie much of the field.

Not all behavior is bidirectional, in which there is a simple mutual influence between person and proximal environment. Some behavior is a function of the more distal social regularities of the sort that ties our work as psychologists to larger social systems, including culture, traditions, organizations, and institutionalized beliefs and practices (see Part IV on social systems). Many of these social regularities (Seidman, 1988) are outside the direct control of individuals. It is often the case that change in social contexts requires the concerted effort of many people in positions of power—both scientific and professional. The first chapter of this section provides a map for such concerted effort by telling us where to look and what to look for if we want to influence the social contexts that set developmental pathways for children and youth; but the implications for research and intervention apply to a much wider range of target populations and social issues.

The second and third chapters in this section, Zimmerman's multilevel analysis of empowerment as both value and theory leading to substantive research questions, and van Uchelen's discussion of collectivism as a counter to North American psychology's individualistic bias, are best read together and in the context of Felner, Felner, and Silverman's approach to prevention science, as well as Cowen's chapter, which follows. While both of these chapters about empowerment are entirely compatible with the preceding chapter, they call to our attention and emphasize certain underlying, often implicit, elements in the field of community psychology. Because the idea of prevention has its roots in medicine, and because it is now so widely accepted as a goal for a variety of psychological, developmental, legal, educational, medical, and social interventions, many programs labeled "prevention" are carried out in ways that can be both disempowering and person-blaming (Albee, 1996). From the community-psychology perspective, prevention programs must be empowering rather than disempowering. A simple example would be a crime-prevention program that is based on neighborhood citizen participation or youth-oriented programs, as opposed to one that "prevents" crime by building more prisons in order to keep young offenders in jail for longer sentences. Both kinds of prevention programs might produce the desired result of less crime in a given neighborhood during a given time period; however, it is not only a reduction in the number of crimes with which we are concerned, but also how that result is accomplished.

Such arguments, both critiquing and linking prevention and empowerment, have been developed in more detail elsewhere (Rappaport, 1981, 1987, 1990; Perkins and Zimmerman, 1995). Here, the chapter by Zimmerman emphasizes both the values of empowerment in community psychology and the multilevel analysis necessary for research and intervention consistent with those values. The emphasis on role relationships, participation, and access to resources introduces themes that underlie many of the social concerns of community psychologists, whether they are explicitly referred to as "empowerment" or not. The idea of empowerment is both implicit and explicit in many of the chapters in this volume. It is clearly an underlying issue for the work of many community psychologists. Empowerment concerns are discussed here, however, not simply in terms of values, but also in terms of research questions at the individual, organizational, and community levels with respect to understanding the *processes* of empowerment. In Zimmerman's chapter, empowerment processes are themselves presented as the phenomena of interest. He suggests various research questions that may be addressed when the understanding of the processes of empowerment is itself the point of the research.

Although addressing the issue of multiple levels, or kinds, of empowerment (individual psychological, organizational, and community) the notion of psychological empowerment is most well developed in Zimmerman's chapter. The chapter by van Uchelen attempts to push empowerment thinking a step further. In a sense, his chapter is a critique of empowerment as simply a concern with the development of an individual sense of personal control. He calls on us to expand our notions of empowerment into contexts where the group or collectivity is the overarching social context. It is a chapter that is more about personal identity in collectivist contexts than about power, be it of an individual or a group. But it also may be understood as a reinterpretation of the meaning of power (see, for example, Miller, 1986, on empowerment and women; Sampson, 1993, on ensembled individualism) as a collective, rather than simply a personal, matter.

In the view of Felner, Felner, and Silverman, much of what has been called pathology, particularly among youth, may be understood to be realistic coping with detrimental environments. This is a view that seems to accommodate an empowerment-driven reading of social context, rather than an individual or a public health perspective. They argue, for example, that the exact form of the behavior (what is termed delinquency or mental illness) is less a function of specific disease processes, and more the result of a transaction between efforts to make sense of one's immediate world and the environmental (including official agents) responses to the person. What are the implications of this view if our overarching concern is prevention of illness and promotion of health? What questions does this view raise for someone interested in understanding more about the development of "wellness" as defined by Cowen? Does this map lead us to different places if we overlay it with a concern for empowerment? Can the same data speak to both the wellness and the empowerment orientation, or do they suggest different studies based on different concerns? Would this work be read differently if one's goal were to understand the processes or increase the likelihood of "empowerment," as portrayed by Zimmerman? How do these two ways of construal—wellness and empowerment—relate to social action and social policy? Does the van Uchelen map, moving our concerns from individual motivation, cognition, and behavior to the social processes in collectives, change one's reading of other chapters in this volume? Does it point to new areas of research in those domains that have traditionally concerned the field?

Cowen's chapter is both a counter to empowerment as the central metaphor for community psychology and a call to return to a health-focused metaphor, albeit one that abandons a preoccupation with illness in favor of wellness as the guiding rationale for the field. In many ways it represents both the best of community psychology's impact on the field of human services and our preoccupation with biological, or natural science, metaphors, as opposed to socio-political metaphors. The implications of a system driven by a concern for wellness as opposed to illness, for the roles we assume, and for the research we conduct, are as enormous as the emphasis on prevention and community that moved us from a preoccupation with clinical treatments conducted in our offices. This approach is as radically different from a clinical psychology based on the *Diagnostic and Statistical Manual of Mental Disorders* as public health is from clinical medicine. Cowen's critique of so-called "prevention science" for its trivializing of health promotion is a serious departure from the conventional wisdom of mental health policy. Like the Felner, Felner, & Silverman chapter, it is consistent with an empowerment critique of social policy. Nevertheless, the wellness metaphor also makes a case for retention of psychology's central identity as a health-care profession.

There is something worthwhile and important in examining the tensions between seeing ourselves as health-care professionals, rather than as concerned with understanding and changing socio-political contexts that define power, poverty, social influence, and community (see, for example, Albee, Joffe, & Dusenbury, 1988). Using these different maps, as well as their associated stories about community psychology in the context of building a prevention science, will lead us to make some common and some unique stops along the road to discovery and intervention. The routes we travel may be similar, but where we pause to reflect, and how and when we intervene, may be quite different. One senses that community psychology can embrace the use of both kinds of maps. In this volume, Bogat and Jason do not present the theoretical position of behaviorism, which is by now well known and easy to find in both textbooks and articles. Rather, they suggest that behaviorism and community psychology should be natural allies, and they point to a variety of reasons why, in their view, this has been less the case than it might be otherwise. Is a focus on small wins, characteristic of this field, necessarily a contradiction to the large problems community psychologists worry about? Does Sarason's (1978) view of social problem-solving as different from problem-solving in the natural sciences mean that behaviorism and community psychology are incompatible? Is it contradictory to think that behavioral technology applied to social problems (an optimistic enterprise) can be embraced by a field that sees no social problems as ever perfectly solved because they always have unintended side effects and because the nature of the problems change with time? How do the strategies and tactics of behaviorism fit with the community organizing and social policy strategies described by others (see Part III)?

Some of these and other questions have been addressed optimistically by Rappaport and Chinsky (1974); Rappaport, Seidman, & Davidson (1979), and more particularly by Fawcett,

Mathews, & Fletcher (1980); Nietzel, Winett, MacDonald, & Davidson (1977); and others (Glenwick & Jason, 1980; Jason & Glenwick, 1984). Here Bogat and Jason invite us to reconsider the place of behavioral technology in community psychology, particularly as a way to break down social problems to a manageable size and to develop practicable skills to implement policy or to assist others in obtaining their own goals.

Theoretically, behavioral maps point us to an understanding of how to change individual behavior. It is useful to recognize that the individual behavior of key people in particular social contexts can have a multiplicative effect. The behavior of opinion leaders and people in power will often influence others. It is also useful to keep in mind that public opinion and large-scale behavioral change can be accomplished by the accumulation of individual change using mass communication informed by behavioral technology (see, for example, the chapter by McAllister in Part III), and that all complex tasks can be broken down into specific skills, including those needed for community organizing (see the chapter by Berkowitz in Part III).

One way to think about behavioral techniques is as just that—as techniques. These may be used in the interest of either social control or social change. To some extent, how one uses them will be a matter of policy. Part of the policy decision will be with whom to collaborate; it will be value driven. There is no inherent reason why behavioral technology cannot be used to work for the goals of grass-roots people, workers, managers, corporation executives, or government officials, depending on the policy one seeks to implement (see Chapters by Klein, Ralls, & Douglas, Part II; Phillips, Part III; and Shinn & Perkins, Part IV).

In his chapter on cognition in social context, Patrick O'Neill suggests that a major contribution of community psychology may be its "ability to integrate several levels of analysis to produce a comprehensive understanding of social phenomena." O'Neill's chapter, although concerned with individual beliefs, moves the focus to social and community issues as the content for individual concerns. He links individual, interpersonal, and community levels of analysis by addressing some of the classical concerns of social psychology—stereotyping and intergroup relations—in the context of community psychology concerns with justice and social change. He introduces the importance of group identification and an analysis of the conditions under which people will engage in social action. In the discussion of stereotyping, the author suggests that rather than trying to change the process, community psychologists and our collaborators might make efforts to mediate the content, an approach consistent with recent interest in stories as a cultural resource (see, for example, Belenky, Bond, & Weinstock, 1997; Rappaport, 1995, 1998).

In juxtaposing O'Neill with Bogat and Jason, we confront a longstanding argument among psychologists concerned with the problem of change: Is it more efficient to change behavior directly (albiet in small steps) and wait for attitudes to follow, or does attitude change (or consciousness-raising) lead to more lasting behavior change? Perhaps not surprisingly, both of these strategies may be useful in the world of social action (see, for example, the chapters on social intervention in Part III), and it may be important to have available strategies that can be used at different times depending on the circumstances.

The final chapter in this section, Kelly, Ryan, Altman, and Stelzner's ecological framework for understanding and changing social systems provides a map for the analysis of social context. It calls to our attention a set of concepts that are quite different than variables drawn from individual psychology and applied to groups and organizations by aggregation. These are concepts that directly assess organizational properties. For an assessment-oriented discussion of aggregation as opposed to direct assessment of organizational or system properties, see the chapter by Shinn and Rapkin in Part V.

Because the chapter by Kelly and associates orients us to structures, processes, and interrelationships, it is both abstract and applicable to many different content systems. It may apply to schools, work settings, government or private sector organizations, as well as to neighborhoods and both larger and smaller geographical areas. This is perhaps the chapter that is most structured like a systematic theoretical statement. It discusses four concepts of social structure (the "what" of a system): personal resource potential, social system resources, social settings, and system boundaries. Processes (the "how" of a system) are discussed as reciprocity, networking, boundary spanning, and adaptation. Each of these four structures and four processes are grounded in concrete examples; however, the examples do not define the limits of the framework. The chapter is a map that can be used as an overlay onto a wide variety of settings. As community psychologists engage a social system, they are looking for these processes and structures in a particular system, along with an analysis of its norms, roles, and values, and asking questions about entry, socialization, and development. This fosters a system analysis that enables the community psychologist to escape the temptation of using only concepts derived from individual psychology, and the fallacy of using individual psychology to explain complex social systems. However, this chapter is also about people and how to work with them in collaborative and respectful ways.

The intention of the authors is to provide us with an ecological analysis of social context that can encourage the development of preventive interventions. The theory suggests that the best way to do this is to foster social structures that connect people with the system they are a part of in such a way as to encourage processes that allow members of a setting to have meaningful influence on the system. The goal is to make it more likely that systems provide opportunities for individuals to develop personal and social resources. Here again, this is an approach that is quite compatible with the aims of an empowerment point of view that takes seriously both the social constraints and the personal lives, interests, values, and ideas of individuals who are viewed as able to participate in the creation and recreation of their own settings. It may be useful to read it together with the chapter on consultation by Trickett and Barone in Part III.

What questions do Kelly, Ryan, Altman, and Stelzner's ecological orientation force us to ask about the specific domains of inquiry that have engaged the field? How can the dynamic theoretical concepts of an ecological point of view be integrated with the more traditional static research methods dominant in the field (see also the chapters in Part V, which address issues of assessment, design, and measurement, as well as Sarason's chapter in Part VI). How does this systems view enable researchers to pose new researchable questions? How does it help us to reinterpret what we already know? What are the implications for our role relationships with the people we study and those we try to assist? These are the kinds of questions that come to mind as one is oriented to the field of community psychology by the maps, stories, frameworks, and concepts presented in this section of the handbook.

REFERENCES

Albee, G. W. (1996). Revolutions and counterrevolutions in prevention. *American Psychologist, 51,* 1130–1133.

Albee, G. W., Joffe, J. M., & Dusenbury, L. (Eds.). (1988). *Prevention, powerlessness, and politics.* Beverly Hills: Sage.

Belenky, M. F., Bond, L. A., & Weinstock, J. S. (1997). *A tradition that has no name: Nurturing the development of people, families, and communities.* New York: Basic Books.

Fawcett, S. B., Mathews, R. M., & Fletcher, R. F. (1980). Some promising dimensions for behavioral community technology. *Journal of Applied Behavior Analysis, 7,* 1–9.

Glenwick, D. S., & Jason, L. A. (Eds.). (1980). *Behavioral community psychology: Progress and prospects.* New York: Praeger.

Jason, L. A., & Glenwick, D. S. (1984). Behavioral community psychology: A review of recent research and applications. In M. Hersen, R. M. Eisler, & P. M. Miller (Eds.), *Progress in behavior modification, Vol. 18* (pp. 85–121). New York: Academic.

Miller, J. B. (1986). *Toward a new psychology of women* (2nd edition). Boston: Beacon.

Nietzel, M. T., Winett, R. A., MacDonald, M. L., & Davidson, W. S. (1977). *Behavioral approaches to community psychology*. New York: Pergamon.

Perkins, D. D., & Zimmerman, M. A. (1995). Empowerment theory, research, and application. *American Journal of Community Psychology, 23*, 569–579.

Rappaport, J. (1981). In praise of paradox: A social policy of empowerment over prevention. *American Journal of Community Psychology, 9*, 1–25.

Rappaport, J. (1987). Terms of empowerment/exemplars of prevention: Toward a theory for community psychology. *American Journal of Community Psychology, 15*, 117–148.

Rappaport, J. (1990). Research methods and the empowerment social agenda. In P. Tolan, C. Keys, F. Chertok, & L. Jason (Eds.), *Researching community psychology: Integrating theories and methodologies*. Washington, D.C.: American Psychological Association.

Rappaport, J. (1995). Empowerment meets narrative: Listening to stories and creating settings. *American Journal of Community Psychology, 23*. 795–807.

Rappaport, J. (1998). The art of social change: Community narratives as resources for individual and collective identity. In X. B. Arriaga, & S. Oskamp (Eds.), *Addressing community problems: Research and intervention*. Thousand Oaks, CA: Sage.

Rappaport, J., & Chinsky, J. M. (1974). Models for delivery of service: An historical and conceptual perspective. *Professional Psychology, 5*, 42–50.

Rappaport, J., Seidman, E., & Davidson, W. S. (1979). Demonstration research and manifest versus true adoption: The natural history of a research project to divert adolescents from the legal system. In R. F. Muñoz, L. R. Snowden, & J. G. Kelly (Eds.), *Social and psychological research in community settings*. San Francisco: Jossey-Bass.

Sampson, E. E. (1993). Identity politics. *American Psychologist, 48*, 1219–1230.

Sarason, S. B. (1978). The nature of social problem solving in social action. *American Psychologist, 33*, 370–380.

Seidman, E. (1988). Back to the future, community psychology: Unfolding the theory of social intervention. *American Journal of Community Psychology, 16*, 3–24.

CHAPTER 1

Prevention in Mental Health and Social Intervention

Conceptual and Methodological Issues in the Evolution of the Science and Practice of Prevention

ROBERT D. FELNER, TWEETY YATES FELNER, AND MORTON M. SILVERMAN

Prevention has become a central goal among those concerned with a wide array of human conditions (Cowen, this volume; Felner, Jason, Moritsugu, & Farber, 1983). Illustratively, the Secretary of Health and Human Services has labeled prevention as the nation's number one health and social priority for the 1990s (Department of Health and Human Services, 1990). The reasons for prevention's emergence as a central priority on the national health agenda are quite clear. Simply put, after-the-fact, reconstructive approaches have proven to be inadequate to the task of reducing the crushing levels of social and health problems confronting the nation.

There are several reasons for this failure. Primary among these is the scope of the problems we confront. Most estimates are that 15–20% of all children and families, or approximately 35–50 million people in the United States, are in need of intensive mental health services (Joint Commission on Mental Health and Mental Disabilities, 1961; President's Commission on Mental Health, 1978). Social ills are also at epidemic levels. Current levels of AIDS, "crack babies," births to unmarried teenaged mothers, substance abuse, children living in poverty, suicide, and homicide, are but a few of the social problems where rates are at historic levels. There will never be adequate levels of economic or human resources to address these overwhelming levels of need if we rely on reconstructive and individually focused

---

ROBERT D. FELNER • School of Education and the National Center on Public Education and Social Policy, University of Rhode Island, Kingston, Rhode Island 02881. TWEETY YATES FELNER • Department of Special Education, University of Illinois, Champaign, Illinois 61820. MORTON M. SILVERMAN • Department of Psychiatry, University of Chicago, Chicago, Illinois 60615.

Handbook of Community Psychology, edited by Julian Rappaport and Edward Seidman. Kluwer Academic / Plenum Publishers, New York, 2000.

models of intervention (cf. Albee, 1959; Sarason, 1981). Strategies that are to have a realistic hope of combating these problems must include efforts to reduce the incidence of new cases of dysfunction. As Albee (1982) reminds us, no epidemic was ever successfully eliminated or brought under control by treating those already affected.

Preventive interventions have shown their potential to be both far more effective and cost efficient than those that attempt to reverse existing dysfunction (cf. Schorr, 1988; The Committee for Economic Development, 1991). Studies have shown that for every dollar spent on prevention, cost savings of between $3 and $10 may be realized in reduced demand for after-the-fact service. Adding to the cost efficacy of prevention is that, beyond providing for cost savings, prevention programs also yield additional tax revenues. For example, the Committee on Economic Development (1991), a group led by executives in the private sector, has shown that the prevention of school failure and drop-out would ultimately result in significantly higher levels of taxes paid by those students who avoid these outcomes. These new revenues would far exceed the costs that any prevention programming might require. This understanding answers the critical policy question: "Who will pay for these new prevention services?" The answer is that these services will pay for themselves, many times over, through both cost savings and new revenues! This combination of prevention's cost efficacy and the enormous societal needs we confront constitutes a clarion call for an emphasis on prevention. Unfortunately, the actions of policy-makers and human service providers have not reflected this understanding.

One factor contributing to this puzzling state of affairs may be that there is an implicit level of "acceptable casualties" that the nation is willing to absorb. There are alarming levels of highway deaths, homicides, substance abuse, infant deaths, child abuse, homelessness, school failure, preventable illnesses, unemployment, and other social problems that currently do not have crisis levels of resources allocated to them. This state of affairs supports the view that, as a society, we operate from a core assumption that there is an acceptable or necessary level of casualties. This assumption appears particularly manifest when we view the levels of resources being directed to persons who have racial, socioeconomic level, gender, or other qualities that set them apart and that increase the likelihood of "victim blaming" (Albee, 1982, 1986).

This pernicious assumption is a critical requirement of a reformulated social policy that embraces prevention as a central priority. A fundamental tenet that we, the authors, believe must guide all social, educational, and human service policies is that there are no acceptable levels of "acceptable casualties." When we adopt this position, the litmus test of any social policy becomes the degree to which it reduces the gap between current or projected rates of human casualties and losses and the goal of zero casualties. Embracing this position makes explicit that an adequate framework for prevention must be consistent with the values of empowerment and inconsistent with interventions in which "blaming the victim" is either an implicit or explicit element (cf. Rappaport, 1987).

Several other factors may also contribute to prevention's failure to be fully embraced as a critical element of educational and social policy. The professional socialization experiences of most human service and educational professionals, with their focus on the individual and disorder, often limit the ways in which prevention is understood or conceptualized (Sarason, 1981). Given such socialization, no matter how much discussions may note the importance of context in contributing to disorder and failure, the tropism of professionals will be in the direction of solutions that attempt to assess and change individuals or, at best, families.

The scarce resource context of human services also leads to issues of "turf." Here, treatment and prevention have often been set up, however inappropriately, as competitors.

What is not understood is that if prevention efforts succeed there will be a decrease in demand for treatment such that extant levels of treatment resources may be more effective. Thus, prevention is not a competitor to treatment, but an important ally. Finally, a full embrace of prevention has been slowed by critics who argue that prevention has yet to prove its efficacy (Klitzner, 1987; Lamb & Zusman, 1979).

For prevention to fulfill its promise and to be fully incorporated into the fabric of social policy requires that we reexamine and rethink the guiding frameworks for solving social problems that have been used in the past (Seidman & Rappaport, 1986). A central goal of this chapter is to move us closer to the attainment of a science of prevention. This science of prevention must be built on a conceptual framework that enables us to overcome inefficient, ineffective, victim-blaming models of service delivery. It must also provide for the evolution of more effective means for solving the complex social problems we confront.

In the pages that follow we attempt the further articulation of this framework. Perhaps the best place to start is with what appears to be a very innocent question. This is, what do we mean by the concept of "prevention," and in what ways is it distinct, with unique features and foci, vis-à-vis other forms of intervention? We next consider the ways in which a developmental perspective provides a sound basis for addressing the issues of concern in prevention. Of particular concern is the articulation of the ways in which the design of prevention efforts must be guided by understandings of developmental processes and directly targeted to the modification of critical elements of developmental pathways (e.g., conditions of risk, acquisition of vulnerabilities). We then present a more specific model of development, the transactional-ecological framework, that we propose as especially well-suited to the needs of a unique science of prevention. In a final section, we consider the ways in which we may move from these conceptual considerations and related literatures to applications at both policy and programmatic levels. Here, we consider what we have learned from field trials about the characteristics of effective prevention efforts and the ways in which these understandings are congruent with the theoretical perspectives we have offered.

PREVENTION: DEFINITIONAL ISSUES AND THE QUESTION OF UNIQUENESS

Intentionality and Prevention as a Science

Cowen (1980) argues that a defining characteristic of sound prevention programs is that they are intentional. Intentionality implies that, in prevention efforts, the strategies selected and the targets of change should follow directly from theory and research concerning "pathways" to disorder and adaptation (Felner & Felner, 1989). In prevention, the immediate goal and focus of intervention is the modification of those processes that lead to the emergence of maladaptation so as to reduce the onset of the target problem(s) (Felner & Lorion, 1985; Lorion, Price, & Eaton, 1989). To meet the criteria of intentionality, those involved in the design of a program must first specify those causal processes that are to be changed. Intervention strategies should then be selected that will influence the levels of these processes in ways that first reduce risk or promote resilience and, ultimately, reduce the onset of disorder.

Put otherwise, good prevention is good science. A program that meets the criteria of intentionality can be viewed as a test of hypotheses about etiologically significant pathways to disorder. Systematically mounted prevention programs are the only acceptable and ecologically valid experimental tests of such hypotheses. Consider that there are only two experimental ways to test hypotheses about the causes of disorder (Felner, Silverman, & Adan, 1989, 1992; Mednick, Griffith, & Mednick, 1981). One is to attempt to create conditions in the lives of people to induce disorder. This option is obviously unacceptable. The other option is to locate people who are naturally exposed to those conditions we hypothesize to contribute to disorder. We can then systematically modify these conditions in desired directions to show that when such changes are made the desired reductions in dysfunction follow. The latter approach is synonymous with prevention.

If we accept that prevention efforts must meet the standards of intentionality, we must now ask what we mean by prevention vis-à-vis other forms of intervention. Of central concern is the question of whether conceptual distinctions between prevention and other forms of intervention are necessary and warranted. If they are warranted, we must also clarify the nature of those distinctions that need to be made.

Blended and Unique Prevention Models

Currently, there are two quite different views concerning whether prevention is a unique intervention approach. One position reflects a *blended approach* view of prevention. It holds that prevention is merely an extension of other types of intervention. This position emphasizes the commonalities and downplays the distinctions among prevention and other forms of intervention. By contrast, the second, the *unique approach* stance, holds that prevention is a distinct element of the continuum of care.

The Blended Model

Blended views of prevention trace their roots to the public health model. In this model the term prevention encompasses the full range of traditional medical and human-service interventions. Tertiary prevention focuses on individuals already displaying serious disorder. Its goals are the reduction of the associated disruption both for the target individual and their "significant others." Secondary prevention focuses on those persons showing early signs of disorder, with the goals of reducing the intensity, severity, and duration of dysfunction. Such interventions seek to identify specific individuals who are at risk due to their showing preclinical manifestations of the focal disorder(s) (Lorion et al., 1989). Primary prevention, by contrast, seeks to reduce the incidence of new cases of disorder. It is targeted to entire populations, not to particular individuals (Cowen, 1983).

Proponents of the blended position (e.g., Lorion et al., 1989; Sameroff and Fiese, 1989) argue that the overlap among these prevention types, especially primary and secondary prevention, should be embraced. Illustratively, Lorion et al. (1989) state, "rather than emphasizing the theoretical distinctions between primary (i.e., incidence-focused) and secondary (i.e., prevalence-focused) preventive efforts ... their overlapping value for emotional and behavioral disorders [should] be appreciated." (p. 64).

This argument stems from the observation that the public health model reflects a linear view of the evolution of dysfunction and that such a view does not appear warranted based on research. In a linear model, disorders are seen to move sequentially from onset through clinical syndrome such that the timing of the onset of dysfunction is something that can be readily identified. Sameroff and Fiese (1989) note that current data does not support this linear view of onset for most socioemotional disorders. Rather, they note that early forms of developmental functioning have been linked to a variety of outcomes, depending on the contexts in which they occur (cf. Sameroff, Seifer, Barocas, Zax, & Greenspan, 1987). Thus, conditions that in a linear model are used to mark onset relate in actuality to the ultimate emergence of specific dysfunction only in a probabilistic and non-specific way.

The Unique Model

By contrast to the blended position, others argue that such blending obscures important distinctions among intervention types and perpetuates old problems under new labels. Cowen (1983) states, "To lump such diversity under a unified banner of "prevention" is sheer sleight of hand ... Calling such things prevention ... only dilutes and obscures a set of conceptually attractive alternatives to past ineffectual mental health ways. It perpetuates what we have always done, in a slightly altered technical guise" (p. 12). Similarly, Seidman (1987) argues that overly broad definitional efforts have resulted in the circumstance that the concept of prevention is often "at best, ill defined and misused" (p. 2). This is not an argument for assigning lesser importance to other forms of intervention. Rather, the development of a sound knowledge basis for both prevention and these other forms of intervention will be hindered by inadequate attention to their differences.

To develop the precision necessary for a science of prevention, a fundamental shift must occur in our language. We, along with others (cf. Seidman, 1987), recommended the abandonment of the traditional public-health phraseology. Instead, what is required are terms that are more descriptive and conceptually suited to the approaches being implemented. Adopting this perspective, tertiary prevention becomes treatment, secondary prevention is called early intervention, and primary prevention assumes the sole mantle of prevention.

Beyond the greater conceptual clarity that will accrue, there are several additional bases for assigning a unique status to prevention. First, onset is not the sole distinguishing feature of "true" prevention. It is but one of a defining set of features that hold co-equal status with prevention's "before-the-fact" nature. A second defining feature of particular import is the level of analysis to which prevention is targeted. Prevention efforts are, by definition, mass- or population-focused.

This does not mean that prevention efforts must target all persons in the population at large. Gordon (1983) has proposed a framework for the organization of prevention trials that may be especially helpful here. This organization is based on how the target groups are selected. "Universal" interventions are those that are designed for all segments of a population. "Selected" interventions are targeted to subpopulations that are characterized by shared exposure to some epidemiologically established risk factor(s). Groups of individuals exposed to "risky situations" (Price, 1980), such as the children of teenaged mothers or of parents with serious social/emotional problems, and persons experiencing major life transitions or other conditions of risk are among the populations to which selected interventions would be targeted. By contrast to universal and selected interventions, "indicated" interventions are targeted to specific individuals who are already displaying preclinical levels of disorder and who have been identified through screening procedures.

In a reformulated model of prevention, both universal and selected interventions would continue to be included under the rubric of prevention. In this chapter, when we refer to population-level interventions we include those that would be subsumed under both of these categories; however, indicated interventions would not continue to be included under the flag of prevention. Instead, such efforts are now more clearly and appropriately labeled as early intervention.

A third defining feature of prevention concerns the focus of change efforts. In treatment or early intervention, change efforts center directly on reversal or amelioration of conditions that have already emerged in specific individuals. By contrast, since prevention is before the fact, it cannot have as its first-order targets of change the disorders it seeks to reduce. Instead, prevention applies to the enhancement, disruption, or modification, as appropriate, of the unfolding process [and conditions] that lead to well-being or to serious mental health or social problems. That is, "... a preventive intervention involves the systematic alteration and modification of processes related to the development of adaptation and well-being or disorder, with the goals of increasing or decreasing, respectively, the rate or level with which these occur in the [target] population" (Felner & Lorion, 1985, p. 93).

The above brings with it a fourth defining feature of prevention. That is, integral to prevention programming are efforts to promote strengths, well-being, and positive developmental outcomes (Cowen, this volume). Such promotion-focused efforts are central to prevention, as they lead to significant reduction in the degree to which conditions of risk may precipitate the onset of disorder. The positive developmental outcomes that promotion-focused efforts yield are also important in their own right. It should be understood that throughout the remainder of this chapter, whenever the term prevention appears, we mean prevention and promotion. The framework that we discuss in the remainder of this chapter is predicated on these joint goals.

These defining elements are consistent with the view of Seidman (1987) who states: "All loci of preventive interventions are before the fact, mass-oriented, and ultimately aimed at averting disorder and/or promoting wellness in individuals. Individuals are the immediate target of intervention only when they constitute a group or population of interest" (p. 9). Given these views, an adequate framework for a science of prevention must enable us to develop interventions that are consistent with these defining features and values. More specifically, it must: (1) enable "preventionists" (Price, 1983) to address the evolution of dysfunction in a more differentiated fashion than is provided for by linear models; (2) facilitate the understanding of target problems and "disorders" in ways that do not require personal-level explanations for the cause or maintenance of the disorders and social problems we seek to reduce; (3) allow for identification of conditions to be changed that impact entire sectors of the population; and (4) guide the systematic targeting of conditions that may be developmentally and temporally quite distant from the actual onset of disorder among members of the target population. We now turn to these elements of our framework.

DEVELOPMENTAL PERSPECTIVES ON ADAPTATION AND PREVENTION

A developmental perspective is best suited for explicating pathways to disorder that are congruent with prevention's tasks, assumptions, and defining characteristics (Felner& Felner, 1989; Lorion et al., 1989; Sameroff & Fiese, 1989; Seidman, 1987). This view is built upon emerging research that suggests that the principles of "healthy or normal" development are also useful for understanding the emergence of disorder (Sroufe and Rutter, 1984). Now the prime targets of prevention efforts are deviations in normal developmental processes, experienced by the target population, that lead to the outcomes of concern.

Applying this developmental view to preventive efforts, we can identify a critical set of tasks that must be addressed in their design. These tasks are:

1. assessment of the ways in which normal developmental processes have been disrupted in the target population;

2. identification of those conditions that lead to these disruptions and distortions in developmental processes;
3. design and implementation of interventions whose goals are to modify and "correct" these disrupted processes until they closely approximate those that lead to healthy development and outcomes.

Hence, developmentally based prevention efforts start by identifying those developmental processes that relate to healthy forms of the outcomes of concern (e.g., academic success instead of academic failure). They then consider the differences between the desirable processes and those that are being experienced by the population of concern. Preventive interventions are aimed at closing this gap in the desired direction. Critically for prevention, the outcomes of concern are now seen as predictable and even "normal" results of the deviations in developmental conditions since the mechanisms and processes that lead to problematic developmental outcomes are the same as those that lead to positive ones. It is only the levels and forms of these processes that differ when problematic outcomes emerge. Thus, a guiding assumption of a developmentally based prevention model is that any healthy child, youth, or adult, if exposed to the problematic developmental process of concern, is likely to show similar problematic outcomes.

Adopting the broad developmental approach is a useful step toward clarification of some required features of prevention efforts. But it must also be recognized that such a broadly stated developmental perspective does not possess sufficient specificity concerning the conditions and processes that shape "wellness" (Cowen, this volume), resilience, empowerment (Zimmerman, this volume), and the emergence of one specific outcome over another, for scientifically sound prevention efforts to be built upon it. To attain such specificity we need greater precision and agreement in our definitions of the central concepts that mark potential points for intervention in developmental pathways to disorder. Of particular concern are the ways in which we define risk, vulnerability, resilience, protective conditions, and onset, as the failure to draw clear distinctions among these concepts may lead to ambiguity and confusion, hampering the systematic accumulation of a body of knowledge for prevention science.

Points of Intervention in Developmental Pathways: Disentangling Vulnerability, Risk, Protective Factors, and Onset

Most current perspectives on disorder start with a fundamental "diathesis-stress" perspective. This model holds that individuals may have either genetically based or otherwise acquired vulnerabilities to the onset of disorder. These vulnerabilities are the diathesis side of the equation. They "set" the person's threshold of susceptibility to environmental conditions (e.g., stress) or hazards (e.g., high levels of disorganization, restrictive opportunity structures, or danger) that may precipitate the onset of disorder.

For the purposes of prevention, the concept of risk is defined epidemiologically. It is a conditional statement about the probability that any member of a given population or subpopulation will develop later disorder. Often overlooked in discussions of risk is that the designation of being a member of an "at risk" group says little about any specific member of that group other than that they have been exposed to the condition(s) of risk under consideration. If the conditional probabilities of disorder in a population are "X," it is not that all members of that group possess X levels of predisposition or "riskness" for disorder (Richters & Weintraub, 1990). Many of the members of the risk group will be free of all signs of difficulties, while others will develop significant adaptive difficulties. A risk designation is no more than an actuarial statement about the member of a selected group. Thus, assessment efforts to guide the targeting of a prevention program are based on knowledge of the probabilistic ways in which conditions of risk disrupt developmental processes in the lives of all persons in a cohort. There is no need to know the extent to which these processes have been disrupted for specific individuals. It is more accurate to speak of conditions of risk or populations at risk, rather than of high-risk individuals. Unfortunately, the term "risk" has been frequently applied to individual characteristics and/or to imply that all individuals in a high-risk group are somehow more fragile or vulnerable than all of those in lower risk groups.

Why has this conceptual slippage occurred? Certainly part of the problem stems from the practice of individual-level variables, especially when aggregated for a population or group, being spoken of as risk markers (cf. Hawkins, Catalano, & Miller, 1992). For example, children who are shy, show signs of behavioral problems in the classroom, or have lower levels of self-esteem are often designated "at risk." We feel that this terminology creep is simply unwise and often confusing. Actuarial statements cannot be made about particular individuals, even those who have characteristics that, at the population level, do relate to probability statements.

To address this slippage, there are several corollaries of our definition of risk that may be helpful. First, conditions of risk are primarily environmental in nature (although being part of a population group that may have some genetic risk characteristics would also qualify, so long as we remember we are talking about a population-level attribute). Second, environmental conditions can have two quite distinct roles—as predisposing conditions and as precipitating/compensatory conditions. When environmental conditions act in a predisposing fashion, *vulnerabilities*, which in our definition are always *person-level variables*, are acquired. Their acquisition may stem either from problematic interactions with environmental conditions that are present, or the lack of exposure to important developmentally promoting conditions and resources (Rutter, 1981). For example, poor early parent–child interactions may lead to the development of vulnerabilities and delays in a number of areas of child functioning. Strengths and *personal competencies* may also be acquired from positive developmental contexts and are again person-level variables. Failure to accurately understand that these person-level characteristics are, in fact, "first-order" developmental *outcomes* (i.e., acquired vulnerabilities and competencies/strengths) has, in the past, led to their being incorrectly labeled as individual-level risk conditions or as early signs of onset of specific disorders. Competencies, strengths, and vulnerabilities will influence the probability that an individual will be resilient in the face of stress and other risk conditions. But, as we have seen, they are not markers of individual risk, nor are they typically direct and inevitable markers of the onset of disorder. We must pause here to also note that to talk about building resiliencies in individuals also muddies these concepts. *Resilience* is an outcome, defined by a person or population's response to challenge and stress. Discussions of building "resiliencies" lose this essential defining element and obscure important differences between such outcomes and aspects of developmental pathways that produce them (e.g., strengths, vulnerabilities, environmental resources).

When environmental circumstances act as precipitating conditions, rather than predisposing ones, they interact with existing vulnerabilities and competencies to trigger the onset of more serious dysfunction. Similarly, protective conditions in the environment may act in a compensatory fashion, reducing the likelihood that existing vulnerabilities will be "activated" when the person experiences conditions of risk. Illustratively, acquired vulnerabilities may make an individual susceptible to the development of disorder during major life changes. But if these changes occur in a context in which the person receives additional support and external coping resources, such difficulties may still not be triggered, even if the person brings relatively high levels of acquired vulnerabilities to the situation.

Implicit in this view of unfolding pathways to disorder is that exposure to conditions of risk or the acquisition of vulnerabilities is not synonymous with the onset of disorder (see Table 1). Neither is exposure to protective factors or the acquisition of competencies synonymous with health and resilience. Rather, these are the sequential and interactive elements of *developmental trajectories* to dysfunction and well-being (Cowen, this volume) that are the appropriate direct targets for change by prevention programming. Framed this way, prevention initiatives may include several strategies that target root causes and contributing factors to dysfunction, all of which would qualify as before-the-fact. They include attempts at: (1) reducing levels of conditions of risk or increasing levels of protective factors; (2) efforts to directly, or indirectly through the previous step, reduce the incidence rates of person-level vulnerabilities or the enhancement of personal competencies and strengths; and (3) altering levels of conditions of risk and of protective factors that have been shown to interact with acquired vulnerabilities and strengths to trigger the onset of more serious disorder, or to produce resilience in the face of serious challenge.

This conceptualization of developmental pathways has direct implications for the evaluation of prevention programs. The initial assessments of the efficacy of prevention efforts may take place far sooner than is often thought possible. Illustratively, for some prevention efforts, especially those dealing with children, it may be a number of years before the primary conditions and disorders we seek to reduce are likely to develop. Thus, it has been argued that any clear evaluation of such prevention efforts will require very long follow-up periods. This may be true in order to fully understand the effects of a program. But by adopting a perspective based on the above understandings of developmental pathways, it is possible to obtain relatively rapid assessments of the degree to which the program and its effects are "on course" and show support for having the desired long-term effects. This can be done by assessing the degree to which the initiative has produced changes in the desired directions in key conditions that are earlier in the developmental pathway, even when they are far distant from the time when we might expect the onset of dysfunction.

For example, our first assessments of program impact would focus on the degree to which levels of risk have been reduced and levels of enhancing conditions have been increased. Next we would assess the degree to which the incidence and prevalence of vulnerabilities and competencies in the population have been changed. Finally, as population members experience identifiable conditions that have been shown to have a high likelihood to act as precipitants (e.g., school transitions), and/or move through developmental periods when maximum onset is expected, we would examine differential rates of the occurrence of adaptive difficulties. To the degree to which desired differences emerge between those receiving the prevention trial and the non-participating comparison groups, at each of these points in the developmental course, we can argue with some assurance that the intervention has shown evidence of being on course for attaining its longer-term, central goals. In this way, throughout the period from program involvement until the population reaches the age when they are most likely to experience the onset of the focal problems, we can continuously evaluate the success of the efforts.

Mediating Conditions

A further issue requires attention in considering those elements of developmental pathways that may be targeted by prevention efforts. This is the issue of the way in which

TABLE 1. Developmental Pathways to Wellness and Disorder and Prevention Targeting

Population/selected population-level variables →	Acquired individual characteristics ↔	Ecological and transactional processes →	Developmental outcomes
First-order, direct targets of change; intermediate outcomes	Intermediate outcomes	Second-order targets of change	Longer-term intermediate and focal outcomes. Not direct targets of change but the results of modification in developmental pathways
1. Conditions of risk Developmentally hazardous contents and settings Genetic predispositions of population (e.g., illnesses)	1. Vulnerabilities	1. Interactions between person-level characteristics and setting/context level-protective and hazardous conditions (macrosystem interactions, macrosystem effects)	1. Resilience 2. Disorganization and dysfunction
2. Protective and developmentally enhancing settings and conditions	2. Competencies and strengths	2. Interactions between personal strengths/competencies and demands of the multiple settings in which population members function (macrosystem interactions, macrosystem effects)	3. Adaptation to disordered contexts 4. Health/wellness 5. Sociopathology disorders

prevention effort should focus on *mediating conditions* (cf. Pillow, Sandler, Braver, Wolchik, & Gersten, 1991; Lorion, 1991). Mediating conditions are a subset of the conditions of risk we have discussed above. They are those proximal circumstances in a person's environment that most directly shape daily experience. For example, when children experience parental divorce it is not necessarily the divorce per se that leads to the psychological problems that have often been found to be associated with it. Rather, it is the associated changes in the conditions of the child's life that are actually responsible for the impacts that have been observed (Felner, Farber, & Primavera, 1980, 1983). Changes in parenting patterns, parental depression, and intraparental conflict are but a few of the mediating conditions that have been influential in shaping the post-divorce outcomes of children. These conditions can function as either predisposing and/or precipitating conditions, depending on the child's functioning at the time of the separation/divorce. From this perspective, divorce and other life transitions, stressors, and developmentally hazardous circumstances (e.g., poverty, maternal depression) are seen as markers of the potentially higher levels of these more proximal changes and mediating conditions in the person's developmental context (Felner et al., 1983). In the model we have proposed here the direct focus of intervention would be on reducing the levels of these negative mediators (conditions of risk) as experienced by the entire population. In this way, a focus on identifying and modifying conditions that may mediate the outcomes of stress and transition is a critical element of the approach to prevention we have advocated.

Several authors (cf. Pillow et al., 1991) have taken this position a step further and argued that to increase the statistical power and cost effectiveness of prevention efforts, we should employ interventions that are based on the screening of specific individuals for heightened levels of problematic mediating conditions. This screening would employ a double-gated assessment strategy. As in population-level approaches to mediator-focused preventive interventions, the potential target population would first be selected based on the presence of marker variables (e.g., social and economic disadvantage, major life transitions) that are associated with a probability of experiencing heightened levels of more proximal negative mediators. Additionally, under a double-gated strategy, screenings of those in this broader population would then be carried out in order to identify specific persons who are experiencing heightened levels of these risk mediators, rather than targeting the entire selected population.

This use of mediational variables to identifying targeted groups for prevention would bring selected interventions back under prevention's flag. It brings with it the concerns we have raised about such intervention approaches for prevention. Most critically, it violates the basic tenet of prevention's population focus. It may also be the start of an argument that is a slippery slope back to clinical interventions as the preferred modality. If we accept that identifying those individuals who show the mediators of concern will enable "preventive" interventions to be maximally cost effective, based on the argument that these persons have the highest probability of developing disorder (Pillow et al., 1991), it is a short leap to the view that we should simply wait until actual signs of disorder are present to be even more cost effective in our targeting. This circumstance is both inconsistent with the rationales for preventive efforts as presented above and with an overall human service strategy that is maximally cost effective.

It is also the case that individual screenings are not required to identify those who have a high probability of experiencing certain mediating conditions. Based on epidemiological data, preventive interventions can be focused accurately on entire populations whose members have a high probability of experiencing the critical mediators. Consider the case of poverty. As Lamb (1992) has noted, poverty is an economic, not a psychological, variable. Its implication for preventive interventions lies in its association with the ways these economic conditions relate to altered societal, community, material, and psychological conditions of risk that mediate or translate the economic conditions to direct daily experiences (Felner, 1992). Based on epidemiological data, we can predict, with a high degree of certainty, that children in economically distressed neighborhoods will be exposed to substandard schooling, high levels of environmental stresses, a paucity of local conditions that lead to high expectations and aspirations, and literally dozens of other negative mediators (Wilson, 1987). Such an understanding underscores the importance of mediationally focused population-targeted preventive interventions for those in poverty.

Preventive efforts that address these and other risk or developmentally promoting conditions, for all children living in such neighborhoods, will be far more cost effective and efficient in reaching our target group than screening-based efforts that seek to target only some children and families (Felner, 1992). Illustratively, to screen all of the children in just one public housing community in a city like Chicago for the presence of conditions that may mediate the development of problem social and emotional outcomes would be incredibly costly. It would require all of the dollars that are available for any intervention and then some! Instead, employing selected interventions that target mediators of concern for the entire population, we could, for example, provide to all children and families strong preschool programs, high-quality educational environments, safe neighborhoods, the removal of policies that create disincentives for family success, and access to quality employment opportunities. Put otherwise, Zigler (1990) succinctly summarizes the prospects and problems of early intervention programs, and underscores the importance of efforts that target entire contexts by noting, "No amount of counseling, early childhood curricula, or home visits will ever take the place of jobs that provide decent incomes, affordable housing, appropriate health care, optimal family configurations, or integrated neighborhoods where children encounter positive role models" (p. xiii).

Although poverty may be an extreme example, we can see the same possibilities for mediationally focused selected interventions reflected in the cases of transitional events and/or risky situations, such as divorce. Consider that parental mental health is an important mediator of child divorce outcomes (Felner et al., 1980). In turn, parental mental health is mediated by the level of stress that parents experience, while adequate, affordable child care is a critical mediator of such stress in single parents. We can now easily see that one appropriate selected divorce intervention would be to provide appropriate child-care conditions for all single parents. Indeed, given the number of families where all of the adults work outside the home, and the demonstrated relationship of "latchkey" status to family stress and a wide array of problematic developmental outcomes (cf. Ross, Saavedra, Shur, Winters, Scaramuzzo, & Felner, 1992), the development of quality and affordable child care for all families would be a major step forward in national prevention efforts. Within developmentally based prevention efforts we agree strongly with Pillow et al. (1991) and others (Felner et al., 1981, 1983) that a major focus of such efforts should be on the modification of those conditions that may mediate negative outcomes and enhance positive ones. However, we can do this with both a high degree of accuracy and far more cost effectively at the population-level than at the individual-level.

Summary

In the model we have proposed thus far, the first-order, direct or "immediate" targets of change in prevention efforts will typically be non-individual level elements of developmental trajectories to adaptation and disorder. Prevention strategies will focus on direct efforts to increase or decrease, as appropriate, the levels of conditions of risk, protective factors, and developmentally enhancing experiences to which a population is exposed. Changes in levels of these first-order elements of the developmental pathways of populations will, in turn, radiate to impact the degree to which second-order changes are accomplished. These second-order elements of developmental pathways should show changes and movement in desired directions relatively soon after the attainment of the first-order changes. These early intermediate outcomes provide preliminary evidence that the preventive strategy is on course for being effective in achieving its long-term goals. Second-order targets of change in developmental pathways include levels of acquired vulnerabilities, as well as resilience-related strengths and competencies. Preventive initiatives will thus involve systematic actions aimed at modifying the reciprocal and interactive influences of conditions of risk, strengths, vulnerabilities, and resources, and in shaping trajectories to the developmental outcomes of concern (cf. Table 1).

Given these understandings about those aspects of developmental pathways that are the direct and indirect, intermediate, targets of change, we turn to the question: What are the appropriate long-term goals of prevention? The answer we select for this question is critical, as it defines those specific conditions earlier in developmental pathways with which we will be concerned. For example, it answers the question: Conditions of risk for what? Vulnerability to the development of what? It is to these concerns that we now turn.

Intervention Goals, Outcome Specificity, and Pathways to Disorder

Outcome Specificity

When we consider the question of what the appropriate goals for prevention are, a critical issue is whether a given prevention program should have as its goal(s) the reduction of highly specific disorders, or whether it should be focused on multiple outcomes.

Historically, a major dimension on which most prevention efforts can be categorized reflects two quite different assumptions about the specificity and uniqueness of developmental pathways. Single-outcome-focused programs, such as those targeted to substance abuse, delinquency, school failure, depression, teen suicide, and teen pregnancy reflect a specific disease prevention model that rests heavily on classic medical paradigms of disorder. These paradigms hold that dysfunction is caused by specifiable disease agents or germs that interact with individual vulnerabilities, which also can be specified.

A contrasting perspective to this position is one that holds that there is a need for a comprehensive, multicausal and nonspecific developmental pathways/root causes focused approach (cf. Felner & Felner, 1989). This model recognizes that: (1) most of the disorders we seek to prevent have a large number of common risk factors; (2) conditions that protect against one disorder generally also protect against many others; and (3) there are nonspecific personal vulnerabilities that increase a person's susceptibility to the onset of a wide array of dysfunction. The pathways to most of the social, emotional, and adaptive difficulties with which we are concerned are generally complex and shared by more than one disorder. Hence, for a wide range of developmental outcomes and sociopathologies, it appears that efforts to identify specific and unique etiological "causal" agents are not appropriate.

Current data are highly supportive of this view and come from a number of converging research traditions. Studies of the adaptive impact of a wide array of developmental circumstances have shown that there are common developmental antecedents, such as family resources and interaction patterns, economic and social deprivation, other life stresses, powerlessness, and an array of non-specific protective resiliency factors (e.g., social support, sense of self-efficacy, hope), that all relate to the probability that persons in a population will develop an extraordinary assortment of mental and physical disorders (Felner et al., 1983; Kellam & Brown, 1982; Kellam, Brown, Rubin, & Ensminger, 1983; Sameroff & Fiese, 1989; Silverman, 1989). Converging with this developmental evidence, other authors who have focused on epidemiology of serious disorders (cf. Dryfoos, 1990; Cantwell & Baker, 1989; Jessor & Jessor, 1977; Kellam et al., 1983; Rutter, 1989) have pointed to the high levels of co-morbidity among such disorders, and further underscored the fact that they appear to share a common constellation of antecedent developmental experiences and root causes in their emergent pathways.

The nonlinear and overlapping nature of pathways to disorder is further underscored by a third set of studies on the stability of the developmental course of such difficulties. Cantwell and Baker (1989), for example, examined the "stability" of clinical levels of disorder in childhood and adolescence and found that for some disorders 100% of those who were diagnosed as previously showing clinical levels of dysfunction were symptom-free for years after the time of initial diagnosis. Additionally, among those children who had an initial diagnosis and who still had a diagnosable condition at the follow-up, across all diagnoses only 30–50% were still found to have the original condition, while the remainder manifested quite different clinical conditions than had been originally diagnosed.

Summarizing the findings pertaining to high levels of co-morbidity of disorder, Rutter (1989) reviewed recent studies of child psychiatric epidemiology and concluded, "Perhaps the most striking finding to emerge from all developmental epidemiological studies undertaken up to now has been the extremely high levels of comorbidity" (p. 645). Similarly, in discussing commonalities across root causes and the need to consider broadly focused prevention approaches rather than that focus on specific outcomes, Sameroff and Fiese (1989) state that, "Whereas clear linkages have been found between some "germs" and specific biological disorders, this has not been true for behavioral disorders ..." (p. 24). Less technically, but more succinctly, Lisbeth Schorr (1988) has summarized the interconnectedness among social problems by noting "rotten outcomes cluster," and that children from high-risk environments encounter developmental experiences that are so severe as to increase the rates of morbidity they will develop across the full spectrum of human social, emotional, and health problems.

To this point we have emphasized in our discussions sets of interrelated, but still discreet, issues and understandings that need to be woven together in the creation of a science of prevention. These include the developmentally complex and nonlinear processes that shape the outcomes with which we are concerned, the understandings we have developed about the discrete elements that comprise these unfolding developmental pathways, and that fact that the goals of prevention efforts are to intentionally and systematically modify these processes and pathway elements in directions that influence the incidence of disorder and wellness in desired directions. What is now required is an integrative theoretical framework that allows us to accomplish this weaving. It is to a presentation of that framework we turn next.

TRANSACTIONAL–ECOLOGICAL MODELS FOR PREVENTION

The *transactional–ecological* model is a framework that these authors (Felner & Felner, 1989; Felner, Silverman, & Adix, 1991; Felner et al., 1992) and others (Seidman, 1987, 1990) have argued contains the requisite levels of comprehensiveness to address the range of issues raised above, while also providing for the degree of specificity required by intentionality. This transactional–ecological (T–E) model is obtained from a conceptual synthesis of two other highly complementary frameworks, the transactional (cf. Sameroff & Fiese, 1989) and ecological (cf. Bronfenbrenner, 1979) models of development. Full discussion of each of these approaches is beyond the parameters of this chapter, but we will attempt to capture the key features of each for prevention.

The transactional model has been articulated by Sameroff and colleagues (Sameroff & Chandler, 1975; Sameroff & Fiese, 1989) and others (Lorion et al., 1989) as a guide for preventive efforts. The model emphasizes the dynamic, reciprocal interactions between the individual and their context, with bidirectional influence being a fundamental element (Sarason & Doris, 1979). For example, the interactions between an infant and his parents, or between a youth and her peers, are thought to be a result of the child's influence on the parent or group and the reciprocal effect of the environmental influence on the child. In discussing the need for a transactional perspective, Sameroff & Fiese (1989) state that "to complete the predictive equation [of etiology] one needs to add the effects of context—the child's social and family environment—that foster or impede the continuing positive developmental course of the child. In short, prevention programs cannot be successful if changes are made only in the individual child" (p. 27).

A transactional perspective then is one element of a science of prevention that has as its focal targets for change those developmental processes that lead to disorder. Yet, it is not sufficient for addressing the full range of conditions that must be considered by preventive interventions. The transactional model is still at best dyadic (Seidman, 1987). It can only deal with those proximal environments in which the person directly participates. Further, since the transactional model always views the sources of influence as bidirectional (Sarason & Doris, 1979), there are some proximal contexts on which individual behavior has little influence (e.g., schools) and for which it is not well suited for providing directions for intervention. To address these limitations and provide for a comprehensive model of prevention, several authors (Felner & Felner, 1989; Felner, Silverman, & Adan, 1992; Seidman, 1987, 1990) have advocated joining an ecological model of development (Barker, 1968; Bronfenbrenner, 1979; Lewin, 1951) to the transactional one.

Combining the ecological and transactional perspectives to create a transactional–ecological (T–E) model broadens the focus of each in some ways that are important for prevention. Consistent with transactional perspectives, an ecological view holds that developmental trajectories are shaped by, "Progressive, mutual accommodation between an active, growing human being and the changing properties of the settings in which the developing person lives" (Bronfenbrenner, 1979, p. 21). But an ecological framework also provides for the consideration of critical additional elements of human contexts. It offers a comprehensive and integrative means of viewing the interactions between the various parts of total ecological and psychological systems, rather than only between individuals and their proximal environments. Thus, it better allows for the design of setting- and population-focused interventions. In particular, the ecological perspective allows for the consideration of influences that shape the dynamic relationships between systems, and the ways in which being part of these multiple systems influence human development.

There are at least three important ways in which the synthesis of ecological and transactional models enables us to address these concerns. First, it enables us to consider the etiological significance of conditions with which the person comes into direct contact, but on which their behavior does not have a significant bidirectional influence. Included in this category of conditions are broader "social regularities" (Seidman, 1988, 1990), or "social structural conditions," such as the density and distribution of poverty and social disadvantage (Jencks & Peterson, 1991; Schorr, 1988; Wilson, 1987), shifting economic conditions that influence motivation (W. T. Grant Foundation, 1988), and the regularities or structures of primary developmental contexts such as schools (Sarason, 1982).

Of particular interest for prevention are those systemwide conditions that distort, in pathogenic ways, all of the dyadic transactions that take place within their reach. These conditions may occur at several different system levels. The smallest system level of this type is what has been termed the microsystem (Bronfenbrenner, 1979), or the settings level (Seidman, 1987) system. These systems are the primary developmental contexts in which people live. They include such contexts as schools, religious congregations, the family, the worksite, and peer groups. The regularities of these settings may be only influenced slowly, if at all, by the dyadic interactions that take place within them (Britt, 1991; Sarason, 1982). For example, the overwhelming flux and disorganization that accompanies the transition to a high school "fed" by multiple middle schools create a condition that may seriously disrupt many of the dyadic patterns that are taking place within the school and peer groups. Similarly, the social regularities of a school or workplace, its resource patterns, and other formal system regularities may go far to shape the nature of the interpersonal interactions that take place within it. However, in neither case will the dyadic interactions rapidly or necessarily impact the system regularities that are shaping them.

At the level of macrosystems (i.e., social structural conditions and regularities) (Bronfenbrenner, 1979), there are again conditions on which the individual's behavior has little effect. But, as before, these conditions have significant adaptive implications for individual behavior, both directly and through their impact on the other system relationships that a person experiences. For example, due to societal changes, the earning potential of a high school graduate has dropped over 40% in the past two decades (W. T. Grant Foundation, 1988). This is a structural condition over which the individual has little control, but this shift may have profound effects on the nature of those behaviors students view as adaptive. When this condition is coupled, for example, with others that indicate to youth that they have little hope of attending college, even if they complete high school, this fundamental shift in the economic meaning of graduation may make alternative, societally undesirable behaviors, such as early school departure, early parenthood, and/or involvement in illicit activities to earn money, appear to be intelligent and attractive choices.

A second enhancement for prevention that derives from joining ecological views to transactional ones is that this synthesis allows for consideration of the ways in which interactions between individuals and any specific setting are influenced by differences and similarities between that setting and others that make up their life context (i.e., it allows for consideration of transcontextual effects). These relationships between microsystems have been labeled mesosystems (Bronfenbrenner, 1979). The need to consider transcontextual influences rests on the understanding that persons have a number of primary settings that comprise the ecological map of their life context. Each of these settings has unique demands that shape the nature of the transactions required by them. The solutions, skills, and abilities required by one context may, when applied in other settings, be complimentary, antagonistic, and/or irrelevant. Illustratively, the skills and interaction styles required to be adaptive in an inner-city environment may, when applied to a school setting, be maladaptive or irrelevant. Such conditions may result in children from inner-city environments being mislabeled as lacking in social competence or other abilities when, in fact, the actual problem is not that these children are deficient; rather, there is a poor match in the skills required among the different developmental contexts that make up their lives (e.g., Eccles & Midgley, 1989).

These mesosystemic relationships also add to our efforts to design effective prevention programs in another way. In particular, they bring attention to conditions surrounding prevention programs that may require change in order for particular prevention efforts to be fully effective. Such conditions may play a limiting role in the impact of a prevention program and, if not adequately considered, may lead to false conclusions that a program effort is ineffective when, in fact, it is a necessary, but not sufficient, element of a more complete prevention strategy.

There are a number of instances where this may occur. For example, the impact of a preventively focused life-skills curriculum will certainly be attenuated if the school context of which it is part does not provide adequate academic experiences to enable the students to develop necessary skills in those related areas. Even with the best decision-making skills, the choices available and the motivation to make prosocial decisions will be limited by a student's inability to read. Similarly, programs to develop self-sufficiency skills for families who need them may fail if they do not consider that other systems impacting these families, such as the social welfare system, may provide disincentives for participation. Likewise, parent-training programs may enable parents to gain important knowledge and skills, but the degree to which they apply this new knowledge in their interactions with children may be influenced by conditions in other systems in their lives. As the most highly trained developmental psychologists can tell you, when it has been a "bad day" outside the home, the quality of the parenting may be sharply diminished. Such bad days are, unfortunately, the stark day-to-day reality for single parents with few economic resources, those in negative job surroundings, those in poverty, and other groups with chronic stressors. These conditions will all certainly reduce the degree to which newly acquired parenting skills are translated to action. Thus, an ecological analysis of the interrelated systems of the lives of those we seek to impact is critical for ensuring that change efforts are adequately comprehensive, and that research on them does not lead to the incorrect conclusion that prevention elements that may be necessary, but not sufficient, do not have utility for prevention of disorder.

Third, a comprehensive prevention model must provide for consideration of the impact on individuals of settings with which they do not come into direct contact. Bronfenbrenner (1979) has referred to these as exosystems. For instance, a child may never have direct contact with the neighborhoods and conditions in which their parents or grandparents were raised, or with the workplaces of their parents. But traumas suffered in these earlier developmental contexts (Garbarino, 1990), values learned in them (Sarason, 1981), or conditions within the workplaces must all be part of a broader analysis of influences that contribute to the nature of the parent–infant interactions that occur (Seidman, 1983). T–E based prevention initiatives would seek to understand developmental transactions by attempting to identify the presence of variables in the work settings of concern that have been linked to parent–child and familial difficulties (e.g., poor supervisor/worker communications; high stress levels; high levels of job instability and underemployment). These setting-level regularities would then be directly targeted by introducing systemwide conditions (e.g., improved supervisor relationships; on-site child-care centers that promote parent involvement; linking parents to appropriate employment opportunities) that reduce workers' stresses and enhance well-being and family support resources. These changes would then be expected to radiate to the family/microsystem level interactions of all workers in the setting.

To briefly summarize, joining an ecological perspective to a transactional one to create a T–E model expands our focus to include the ways in which person–setting interactions are impacted by relationships between settings, as well as the broader, macrosystemic contexts in which they may be nested. Equal weight is given to understanding dyadic transactions and to the analysis of the impact of, and interactions among, various settings, mesosystems, and macrosystems that may significantly influence developmental pathways. Such understandings will enable preventive interventions to move closer to the view of Seidman (1987), who states that, in prevention, "At both the setting and mesosystem level, the direct targets are the behavioral regularities and or relationships characterizing each respective level; individual effects are only an indirect result of the intervention" (p. 9).

There is an important corollary of the above features of the T–E model that makes it particularly useful for generating interventions that are congruent with the values and goals that we have set out for prevention, as well as that expand the ways we can conceptualize possible approaches to intervention. The T–E model affords us the ability to view the behaviors that are to be prevented in ways that do not require the assumption that there are deficits or defects in the persons/population targeted—a core factor in victim-blaming—for a condition to be targeted. Clinical-individual models require that we define target behaviors in terms of the existence of pathology and disorder in the individual. At transactional levels of analysis, the person is still, at least in part, seen as responsible for problematic transactions and disorder. Neither of these theoretical frameworks allows us to consider the ways in which the target "disorders" may, in fact, be adaptive solutions to contextual conditions that are disordered. However, by utilizing the lens of a T–E perspective, many of the target conditions with which we are concerned can be seen to be the result of highly appropriate and adaptive efforts in disordered contexts. To state otherwise,

> what might appear to be deviant outcomes may be those that any healthy child [or person] would exhibit in the environments and systems that define their lives ... what might have been seen as disorder or disease may be better understood as a result of the child's appropriate, predictable, and highly adaptive attempts to adjust to contexts and conditions that require responses which are incompatible with those in other contexts inch they live. That is, ... what might have been seen as a disorder or disease may be better understood as the [person's] appropriate, predictable, and highly adaptive attempts to adjust to contexts and conditions ... [that are developmentally inappropriate or disordered] (Felner & Felner, 1989, p. 21).

Applying this view to prevention programs, the first, fundamental questions that must be asked in the design of any prevention effort are: "In what ways were the conditions (e.g., behavior, belief system, etc.) that we wish to prevent adaptive at the time they developed?" "Are there factors that are being experienced by the population that make the condition continue to be adaptive?" A basic assumption of this model is that any adaptive pattern, however problematic, originated as an attempt to positively adapt to conditions that existed at the time. Given this assumption, efforts to understand or change any developmental pathway or outcome must take place independent of a consideration of the full set of historical, familial, economic, social, and political contexts that provide meaning to a person's life experiences. Such an approach will allow us to see that many of the problems we seek to reduce through preventive efforts are simply intelligent, effective attempts at adaptive solutions to disordered contexts. Illustratively, social welfare policies that punish recipients for earning income, acquiring savings, and attempting to accumulate equity (Moynihan, 1986), may lead recipients to behave in ways that society views as inappropriate (e.g., not saving, not seeking employment). Instead, the recipients are actually showing intelligent and adaptive problem-solutions in the face of disordered contextual demands. To avoid the confusion that places the locus of such difficulties inside the person, we might better refer to these and other positive adaptations to disordered contexts, which are dysfunctional in later or other developmental settings, as *sociopathology* rather than psychopathology, with the latter's inherent individual focus. This view further sharpens our focus on the characteristics of contexts that systematically distort normal developmental pathways to produce what appear to be deviant outcomes but which are, in fact, better understood as positive adaptive efforts to dysfunctional contexts when considered in their full ecological–developmental context.

Given our model and its central features, let us now consider its application to current prevention efforts and to the building of next-generation prevention models.

From Theory to Practice

Until now our focus has been on prevention theory, as well as theory and research relating to the evolution of sociopathologies and other problems of human well-being. Before closing, let us turn to an examination of what we know about proven prevention efforts and the ways in which they expand upon, illustrate, and otherwise guide the further translation of the issues discussed above to concrete application.

It is beyond the scope of this chapter to review the full range of prevention efforts that have been shown to be effective. Recent reviews of research on prevention programs (cf. Bond & Wagner, 1988; Dryfoos, 1990; Felner & Felner, 1989; Felner, DuBois, & Adan, 1991; Price, Cowen, Lorion, & Ramos-McKay, 1988) point to a number of features that are common to prevention efforts that have been found to have strong empirical support. These elements are summarized in Table 2. As should be apparent, they are highly consistent with the perspective on prevention that we have offered above.

Given the general characteristics of effective prevention programs, let us next consider

Table 2. Characteristics of Effective Prevention Initiatives

1. Comprehensive rather than narrowly focused; comprised of an integrative "package" of approaches; based on multicausal/complex pathway understandings of developmental outcomes and reflecting multisystem–multilevel perspectives
   Corollary: Recognize that many problematic developmental outcomes/social and emotional problems are interrelated in their pathways and emergence (comorbidity and common antecedents).
2. Combine enhancement/promotion and prevention/risk reduction approaches
3. Based on ecological/developmental analysis of target problems and issues; start with understandings of pathways to normal and healthy development, and analysis of how processes that lead to target conditions differ; context is key to understanding of meaning of targeted outcomes. First-order targets of change are risk reduction and protective-factor enhancement; second-order targets are reduction of acquired vulnerabilities and enhancement of competencies/strengths.
4. Recognize scarce/limited resources and delivery system difficulties.
   Corollary: When possible, interventions first consider/are aimed at changing institutions, policies, and settings (e.g., schools, welfare system, community settings), rather than individuals.
5. Congruent with/attentive to other agendas of settings/communities in which they are mounted; respect "hosts" and the ways other regularities may impact prevention initiative.
6. Timing of interventions is critical, with developmental appropriateness and continuity (e.g., strengths and vulnerabilities acquired at earlier ages effect possible impacts of later prevention efforts) considered in the design of preventive initiatives. Viewed as part of "developmental ladders" with consideration of adequacy of other "rungs" in deciding about necessary elements.
7. Dosage and fidelity levels receive careful consideration. Do not expect "one-shot" or short-term interventions (except during critical transitions) to have enduring effects. Continuity, booster sessions, comprehensiveness, and developmentally keyed follow-up are necessary. Initiatives must also be mounted as intended for fair test.
8. Theory and research based (as are their evaluations); are "intentional"; can articulate links between actions, aspects of developmental pathways to be changed, and outcomes to be achieved. They are experimental tests of hypotheses about causality.

the ways in which these principals may be manifested in actual practice. First, the characteristic of comprehensiveness is an overarching one that is further defined and addressed by each of the other features in Table 2. That is, comprehensive programming will reflect a multisystem–multilevel perspective; attend to the timing, dosage, and fidelity of the intervention; focus on natural settings and systems; and strive to be scientific and replicable. It must also be made clear that to simply instruct most professionals or members of a community to attempt to create a "comprehensive prevention strategy and system" (as for example, is being attempted by the U.S. Center for Substance Abuse Prevention's Community Partnership Program) may be so overwhelming that they will be left with little sense of where to start.

To facilitate this task what is required is an organizing heuristic or framework that is consistent with, and builds upon, the T–E perspective and that provides a systematic approach to breaking this larger task down into more manageable "bite-sized" ones. Here, the concept of a "developmental ladder' is one that is especially useful (Felner, Silverman, & Adix, 1991). This approach makes explicit that comprehensive prevention approaches must be both (1) *horizontally comprehensive*, i.e., comprehensive at particular life stages and critical risk periods, and (2) *vertically comprehensive*, reflecting a life-span perspective. The latter aspect builds on the understanding that the timing of preventive interventions is critical. A developmental ladder-based prevention system attempts to get each member of the target population through each life stage and developmental transition undamaged and, having been exposed to the requisite developmentally enhancing experiences, to be prepared to master the tasks of the next phase of his or her life.

A developmental ladder approach to developing a comprehensive prevention system for a community provides a highly specific and easily applied framework for thinking about what needs to be done to address the health and social problems and well-being of a community. Now, rather than asking, "What elements of a prevention system need to be in place for our entire community?" (clearly a question that will rapidly become unfocused given the diversity of needs at different ages and levels), those involved can ask, for example, "For families with children ages 0–3, 3–5, in elementary school, having an elderly parent, etc...., what conditions are particularly hazardous during "X" or "Y" developmental phase?" "What experiences are especially important to provide?," and "What resources are necessary?" A community can then examine whether, for each developmental phase, the requisite actions, conditions, and resources are in place.

A developmental ladder approach also addresses an additional key requirement of effective prevention efforts. Prevention programs have been shown to have the capacity to create enduring positive consequences and to reduce vulnerability to the development of later problems in the face of life's challenges (cf. Felner et al., 1991; Price et al., 1988). But, it is also the case that effective efforts at one life stage may be eroded if severe conditions of risk are confronted at latter stages or if necessary developmental experiences are lacking. Further, the effectiveness of programming later in life may be undermined by difficulties and vulnerabilities acquired previously. Illustratively, the research on the Perry Preschool Project (Schweinhart & Weikart, 1988), and Project Head Start (McKey, Condelli, Ganson, Barrett, McConkey, & Plantz, 1985) has demonstrated the potential enduring effects of preschool programming in obtaining a wide range of desired outcomes. These same data also reveal, however, that at least some of the gains may be lost if the preschool experience is surrounded or followed by schooling, familial, or community conditions that do not adequately allow the child to take full advantage of their newly acquired competencies.

Hence, there is a need for both comprehensive programming within life stages as well as for ongoing, complementary programming across each life stage, including "booster sessions," as discussed below. Inherent in the use of a developmental ladder strategy for prevention programming is just such integrated, ongoing preventive efforts. That such programming is required should not be taken as evidence that prevention programs at any one stage are not effective. To reach such a conclusion based on these data would be a little like saying that just because a person may develop problems latter in life, there are no positive benefits to having positive parent–child interactions during infancy. Rather, just as is the case for such naturally occurring positive developmental conditions, adequate prevention efforts at each life stage are necessary, but not always sufficient, conditions for obtaining the outcomes we seek.

Employing a developmental ladder perspective, we now turn to a consideration of representative prevention efforts that have demonstrated their efficacy and that might comprise critical elements of the "rungs" in a community's ladder (Table 3). Although we have organized these efforts by the age of the target cohort of youth, it should be understood that, as discussed above, T–E programs will, by definition, focus on both these individuals and at least one of their primary developmental system contexts. Thus, in the case of children and youth, this means that initiatives that target those at particular ages must implicitly, if not explicitly, also target, at minimum, primary caregivers (i.e., parents, teachers) in the relevant environments to meet the assumptions of a T–E approach to prevention.

Prenatal and Infant/Toddler Programs

Teenaged mothers, single mothers, and mothers suffering from severe economic hardships are all groups whose children more frequently experience pre- and post-natal complications, as well as maternal care patterns that place them at risk for a wide array of difficulties in later life. These infants also frequently require expensive medical procedures early in life. A particularly troubling feature of these patterns is the degree to which research has shown that, for relatively minimal expenditures of professional and economic resources, these enormous human and societal costs can be avoided. The enduring, positive impacts, on both infants and their parents, of comprehensive, multifaceted programming that changes the resource context of young mothers and infants from such high-risk populations have repeatedly been demonstrated. Common strategies are efforts to increase the levels of emotional and instrumental support available to young mothers, the accessibility and affordability of quality child care, early stimulation efforts to enrich the developmental contexts of the infant, and health care for the entire family.

The work of Olds (1988) provides a carefully evaluated example of one such strategy to safely get infants and families over the first rung of our ladder. This effort targeted a set of first-time mothers who fit into one or more of the risk groups noted above. The program strategies were carried out by pediatric nurses during pregnancy and the first two years of life. Three major activities were carried out with the mother (or both parents when possible): (1) parent education relating to nutrition and infant development; (2) efforts to increase the support provided to the mother by family and friends; and (3) linkage of the family to other formal health and human services. When compared to matched controls, women in the program improved their health habits and health care during pregnancy. Further, especially for teenaged mothers, there were significant increases in infants' birth weights and reductions in premature deliveries. Additionally, among women who had multiple (three) risk markers (poor, unmarried, and teenaged) there was a 75% reduction in the incidence of cases of child abuse and neglect. Across all groups the incidence of harsh care and discipline was lower for the program groups, and the mothers' attitudes toward their children was more positive. Given the impor-

TABLE 3. Illustrative Preventive and Enhancing Conditions and Interventions That Must Be Considered as Part of Comprehensive Community Strategies

Developmental "rung"/level	
Prenatal–2 years old	Prenatal care and well-baby health services; adequate nutrition; stable stimulating family environments; nurturing family/community/child care contexts; community/workplace policies that promote positive parent–child relationship formation (e.g., family leave policies)
3–5 years old	Quality preschool and child care programs that promote development of school readiness in cognitive, social, and emotional domains; stable, stimulating, nurturing caretaking environments; additional well-child health-care services
Elementary (grades K–5)	Developmentally, instructionally, and resource appropriate schools; quality child care/non-school hours programs and supervision; safe, nurturing, stable environment; health-enhancing nutrition and practices; experiences that promote social competence and values; safe neighborhoods and adequate contexts for play and positive peer interaction; media, school, and community policies that promote exposure to positive role models and reduce exposure to negative ones (ongoing throughout all developmental levels)
Middle school (grades 6–8) and high school (grades 9–12)	Schools and non-school settings structured for, and able to meet, developmental-, cultural-, and gender-diversity needs of early, middle, and late adolescents and that match their learning styles (relevant, hands-on, experiential); transitional risk reduction; appropriate non-school hours supervision; programming/recreational/vocational opportunities and experiences that promote social competencies, values, and aspirations; comprehensive health education; reduction of high-risk characteristics of major developmental environments; exposure to prosocial choices and role models; orientation and prep for workforce and post-secondary education
Young adult/ post-secondary	Educational/vocational experiences (e.g., lifelong learning approaches) that are required for a workforce with ever-increasing literacy and numeracy skills, and in which the jobs of the future may not yet be in place; self-sufficiency; school-to-workforce transitional programming and attention by public/private sector; workplace conditions that maximize adaptation and productivity of culturally and gender-diverse populations
Career development and family-raising years	Conditions that support young and developing families and that recognize range of needs of familes, e.g., quality and affordable child care; affordable housing finance policies; workplace policies that support families' education and reduce unnecessary work–family stresses; policies that promote economic and residential self-sufficiency; work environments that promote growth and adaptation of increasingly diverse populations; wellness programming in workplaces; public- and private-sector educational options for ongoing employment-skill development and redevelopment/career changes to match changing societal and personal circumstances; housing policies to ensure safe/affordable housing for families; health care; literacy and employment retraining efforts for those where workforce changes require new skill levels; policies that promote safety connectedness to community (e.g., gun control; community planning efforts that stabilize neighborhoods); programming that promotes adaptation to predictable and unpredictable family and life transitions; family recreational policies and programs in communities
Later mid-life	Retirement planning; health care; literacy enhancement and employment retraining and placement for those where workforce changes require new skill levels; safe community policies (e.g., gun control); programming that promotes adaptation to predictable and unpredictable family and life transitions; recreational skill/interest development program for fitness and wellness in later life; ongoing lifelong learning involvements; health care
Retirement	Policies and programming that promote continued involvement in, and feelings of contribution to, community and residental continuity; retirement transition programming and opportunities for interest/recreational expansion; health care; programming that promotes adaptation to predictable and unpredictable family and life transitions; educational programming (lifelong learning models) and opportunities that expand interests and allow for ongoing exploration of new interests; education of physicians and population to combat false negative expectations about loss of functions and abilities, and to reduce possibility of development of prescription substance abuse
Elderly	Health and social-service efforts and policies to promote residential stabilization and non-isolation from age-diverse communities (e.g., in home healthcare and homemaker support services); policies and programs that provide for maximum mobility in community and connectedness (e.g., volunteer programs; adequate and appropriate public transportation); community safety policies; ongoing lifelong educational programming and opportunities

tance of these conditions as risk factors in serious childhood and adolescent problems, the importance of this programming for the prevention of psychopathology is clear.

The Houston Parent–Child Development Center Program (H-PCDC) (Johnson, 1988) illustrates a preventive strategy with parents and infants that is complimentary to that represented by Olds' work, as it focuses a little further "up the ladder." The H-PCDC approach starts with the assumption that many adjustment problems in childhood arise from problematic interactions with important caregivers, especially parents. Starting at 12 months of age, children were enrolled in a program that combines in-home and daycare center elements during the child's second year of life. Much like Olds' program, a year of home visits was also provided, but in this program the visits were made by nonprofessionals. These visits sought to improve the mother's understanding of her child's development, especially of her impact on the child's development. Family workshops were also provided to increase the involvement of fathers and siblings in caring for the child.

During a second year in the program, mothers and children participated in center-based activities including (1) involving the child in cooperative play with peers, (2) additional child care and homemaking education for the mother, and (3) videotaped, structured mother–child situations that were used in feedback sessions with the mother to enhance her interactions with the child.

At the end of the program period, project children were found to have significantly higher I.Q. scores. Additional findings showed that project mothers provided more educationally stimulating home environments, used more praise, provided higher levels of affection, and were less critical and controlling—all patterns that have been previously shown to be related to better adaptive outcomes in children.

Longer-term evaluations were conducted when the children were 4–7 years of age and again 5 to 8 years after the program was completed. At the initial follow-up point, mothers reported greater behavior problems for control group males than project males. Further, at the second follow-up point, teachers who were unaware of which children had received the interventions also reported far more behavior problems in school by control children than those who were in the H-PCDC. Control children were also four times more likely to require special services than project children.

These results are especially interesting for prevention advocates and policy since the findings demonstrate that the program's effects are not only detectable 5 to 8 years after the program ended, but in a setting (the school) that is different from the one where the intervention took place (the home). Demonstration of the generalization of effects across settings is important if prevention is to claim broad-based effects on disorder. Also noteworthy is that there was an increase in the desired differences between the groups across the two follow-up points. Although differences were initially slight, control children developed far more problems by follow-up points than did project children. This pattern is similar to that reported by the Perry Preschool Project (Schweinhart & Weikart, 1988). Combined, these studies suggest that the targeting and reduction of relatively minor, early conditions of risk and vulnerabilities is effective in short-circuiting the evolution of more serious problems, including those that may have more prolonged incubation periods. These results are highly supportive of, and congruent with, those that would be predicted from the T–E view of developmental pathways to disorder, in which initially small transactional difficulties will, in a recursive fashion, grow larger and more severe if unchecked and repeated in other settings with which the child comes into contact during development.

A number of other programs have demonstrated the importance and potential long-term pay-off of preventive efforts that increase the psychological, physical, and material circumstances of infants and toddlers (cf. Committee on Economic Development, 1991). Cumulatively, these programs demonstrate the central importance of this first rung of the developmental ladder in providing a base for what follows.

Preschool Programs

The now-classic studies of High/Scope on the Perry Preschool program (Schweinhart & Weikart, 1988) are discussed above. Along with Head Start evaluations and a myriad of similar programs, these interventions have shown their potential for producing enduring gains in developmental outcomes—especially for children who are experiencing conditions that provide problematic levels of social and cognitive stimulation.

Illustratively, a 15-year follow-up evaluation of the children who participated in the Perry Preschool program (Schweinhart & Weikart, 1988) revealed that, when contrasted to the outcomes of a non-preschool comparison group, those who received the preschool programming had a broad array of more positive life outcomes, including being less likely to require special services while in school, having lower drop-out rates and higher rates of literacy, fewer arrests, less welfare dependency, and lower levels of unemployment. As noted above, an intriguing aspect of the findings was that their strength, and the degree to which the programming impacted relatively more severe life problems, appeared to increase over time. Further, consistent with the cost-efficacy arguments for prevention, the authors showed that for every dollar spent early on, the program returned from three to six dollars in long-term savings in costs associated with the higher levels of programming needed to address the greater difficulties in school and life found in the comparison sample.

School-aged Children and Adolescents

A wide array of preventive efforts have shown promise with school-aged children and adolescents. One major focus has been on the promotion of social competence. Most recent efforts of this type seek to enhance the development of cognitive, affective, and behavioral skills that will enable students to engage in successful transactions with their proximal developmental contexts and to master relevant developmental tasks (Caplan & Weissberg, 1989). Often, these programs are classroom-based and consist of curricula delivered by teachers or socially relevant outsiders, such as the police officers who deliver the Drug Abuse Resistance Education (D.A.R.E.) programs.

These curriculum-based efforts have yielded inconsistent results. Some have shown short-term effects on student behavioral and social adjustment (cf. Elias & Clabby, 1992; Shure & Spivack, 1988; Caplan & Weissberg, 1989). However, consistent with the need for a developmental ladder perspective, these results have often eroded when not followed by booster sessions or continuation of the programming in follow-up years. Many other efforts have failed to yield even initial effects or generalization (Furman, Giberson, White, Gavin, & Wehner, 1989). There appear to be at least two primary reasons for these disappointing findings. The efficacy of these efforts may be limited by the fidelity, dosage, and consistency with which program elements are implemented (Felner & Felner, 1989; Furman et al., 1989). In this vein, Furman et al. (1989) note that, "Regardless of whether a program is formally adopted [by a school system] it is not clear what proportion implement the program effectively or, for that matter, at all" (p. 356). Even among those schools and teachers that are committed to implementing such programs, other demands placed on them by the system may result in the implementation being at dosage levels far below those required to obtain changes in attitudes, behaviors, or skills (Connell, Turner, & Mason, 1985).

The concept of "level of dosage" applies to the numbers of sessions and exposures that a student may receive within a specified period. Consistent with a developmental approach, for adequate levels of dosage to be present, these exposures must take place over a sufficient age span. This will enhance the adequacy of dosage, as well as allow new competencies to be addressed that are required by developmental tasks that emerge at different ages. In this way, programming may be more sensitive to the readiness of children and youth to benefit from what is being taught. Caplan and Weissberg (1989) underscore the importance of such an approach, stating, "Recognition of the developmental tasks, changes, concerns, and pressures motivating behavior is essential if we are to create effective [social competence promotion] programs that facilitate current and future adaptive functioning" (p. 371). Extending this view to policy recommendations, the National Mental Health Association's Commission on Prevention of Mental-Emotional Disabilities has recommended that comprehensive social competence curricula be provided for students from preschool through high school (Long, 1986).

Transitions and milestones are the focus of a second major thrust of prevention efforts with children and adolescents. This work has focused on facilitating adaptation to normative and non-normative developmental and ecological transitions. Illustratively, Pedro-Carroll and Cowen (1985) focused on the non-normative transition of divorce in their The Children of Divorce Intervention Project (CDIP). The program reflects a selected strategy, as all children experiencing parental divorce are referred for services. The program takes place in a group format during the school day for children in grades four through six, and has three primary components: (1) an affective element that attends to the expression of divorce-related feelings; (2) a cognitive skill-building component that teaches skills for coping with divorce-related tasks; and (3) a segment designed to enhance self-esteem. Group leaders include trained paraprofessionals, teachers, school administrators, and school mental-health personnel.

Program evaluation has found participants improved more than untreated controls in terms of levels of anxiety, as well as teacher and parent ratings of adjustment. Replications have also shown that when compared with students from intact families, adjustment scores of participants approached those of the comparison group following receipt of the intervention (Pedro-Carroll, Cowen, Hightower, & Guare, 1986).

A second set of selected prevention efforts for this age group again uses the occurrence of a significant transition as the condition of risk on which to base targeting. These programs seek to enable children and adolescents to successfully negotiate the normative transitions between elementary, middle, and high schools. One of these interventions, The School Transition Environment project (STEP) was developed by Felner and his colleagues (Felner, Ginter, & Primavera, 1982; Felner & Adan, 1988; Felner, Brand, Adan, Mulhall, Flowers, Sartain, & DuBois, 1993). The project has as its primary focus alterating of the ecology of the school context, rather than attempting to change specific individuals directly.

STEP employs a multicomponent strategy to reduce the level of risks that confront students during these school transitions, especially when they are moving to schools that have multiple schools "feeding" into them. Program elements focus on reducing the flux and complexity of the school environment, reducing exposure to older students, and increasing the levels of peer and teacher support available.

These goals are accomplished in several straightforward ways. First, the project creates smaller social and learning environments in the larger school context by assigning entering students to "core" academic classes in groupings of approximately 60–110 students, so that all of those students who share core classes are drawn from the team. In this way, the number of other students that STEP children need to interact with during most of the day is significantly reduced.

To reduce the fear and confusion students may feel when attempting to adapt to an often overwhelming new school setting, core classes were scheduled in rooms that were in close physical proximity to one another. Finally, teachers' roles were restructured to make them the administrative-counseling link between the school, the student, and the student's family. Each team also had the same group of teachers for all of their core classes, who met together at least weekly to discuss students who may need assistance and to coordinate instructional approaches. All components are based on the T–E model of adaptation to life transitions that specifies that modification of key elements of the environment may facilitate the accomplishment of the adaptive tasks that accompany major transitions (Felner, 1984; Felner, Rowlison, & Terre, 1986).

Evaluation of the original program, as well as replications in a variety of different school types (e.g., middle schools, high schools; rural and urban settings), have been conducted. A five-year study of students in the original STEP trial showed an approximately 50% reduction in drop-out rates (from nearly 48% to less than 25%), compared to control students. Moreover, consistent with a view that there are non-specific early pathways to disorder, control students in a second evaluation trial showed significant negative shifts across a broad array of developmental outcomes, including self-concepts, behavioral and emotional difficulties, delinquent acts, and reported likelihood of illicit substance use. These declines were significantly greater than those shown by students in the STEP project, who generally avoided significant negative changes in adjustment in these domains, thus achieving critical goals of prevention.

Creating developmentally enhancing contexts, such as the changes in the resource contexts reflected in the infant and preschool programs discussed above and the changes in the overall ecology of a setting as reflected in STEP, is a strategy that has both great potential efficacy and is integral to a T–E model of prevention. As should be clear from our discussion, this is the "first" option of a T–E model; such models are models of choice over those that seek to change attributes of specific individuals. Unfortunately, they have often failed to be identified as falling under the rubric of prevention, at least by the mental health and human service community. Further, the most overlooked, but in many ways most promising, of these initiatives are those that seek to understand the ways in which elements of the school, community, peer, or home environment may be structured or reorganized to improve their match to the developmental needs and competencies of the populations that inhabit them.

To correct this overly narrow view of prevention, what must be recognized is that legitimate prevention efforts will include those changes in social and educational policies and programming that increase the developmental appropriateness and resources and reduce the conditions of risk in significant human contexts, even when the primary goals of these initiatives are improved mental health outcomes. School and welfare reform and transformation efforts; restructuring of work-sites to increase worker participation, satisfaction, and productivity; community development efforts to change opportunity structures, safety, sense of community, and resource patterns for families (Chavis & Wandersman, 1990; Felner, 1992; Garbarino, 1990; Perkins, Florin, Rich, Wandersman, & Chavis, 1990); family support programs (Weiss & Jacobs, 1988); and social and recreational "youth development programming" (Carnegie Council on Adolescent Development, 1992; Reppucci, 1987) are but a few of the domain of initiatives that seek to change the ecology of the peoples' lives and that have not, in the past, been adequately recognized for their potential as core strategies in preventive initiatives.

A major set of these initiatives for children and their families has been clustered under the label of "Schools of the Future" (Holtzman, 1992). These efforts use the school as a hub around which to build coordinated, comprehensive human service and educational efforts. The most ambitious of these efforts focus both on employing school settings as points of coordination and delivery for health and social service and programs and on the implementation of educational transformation and reform efforts that seek to increase the nature of participation by parents in the schools and their governance.

Preliminary evaluations of these initiatives have shown they may have enormous potential for increasing the success of children in school, as well as for decreasing related social, emotional, behavioral, and health problems. Taking diverse forms, such as Comer's Social Development Program (Comer, 1988; Haynes, Comer, Hamilton-Lee, 1988), and Zigler's School of the 21st Century (Zigler, 1989), a wide array of similar school–community efforts is undergoing continuing development. Although varying somewhat in their specifics, based on local conditions, resources, and focus, these programs share certain common points of emphasis. Typically, they include child-care and family-support services, integrating social service prevention and intervention delivery into "one-stop shopping." They also include efforts to enhance the development of target children from the prenatal period through adolescence. More specific elements include such activities as home visits and preschool programming, afterschool programs that provide child care and developmentally enhancing experiences, access to adequate preventive and illness-related health care for children and family members, and increased involvement of parents in social service and school governance (cf. Holtzman, 1992).

Summarizing the data on these efforts, Holtzman states

> [they] are cited for improving school climate, reducing dropouts, improving achievement levels, social behavior, and self-esteem of students; improving teacher morale; and increasing the involvement of parents and other community members in the educational enterprise. The results are sufficiently promising, especially for inner-city schools in low income neighborhoods, to justify a major effort devoted to a comprehensive experimental programming covering the full range of proven innovations for children from birth through adolescence (pp. 12–13).

The Schools of the Future initiatives discussed by Holtzman (1992) have primarily focused on students at the elementary level or below. At the same time, the Carnegie Corporation has undertaken a complementary national initiative in collaboration with a number of states to implement the recommendation of the *Turning Points* report, written by their Task Force on the Education of Young Adolescents (Carnegie Corporation, 1989). Their focus is on the comprehensive transformation of middle-grade schools, including the creation of learning teams and other elements of smaller learning environments and replacing such practices as "tracking" with others, such as cooperative learning and heterogeneous-ability learning groups, that reduce development risk and enhance developmental outcomes. Noteworthy is the link between these reforms and those taking place in the workplaces of the nation, where team and cooperative models are rapidly becoming the recommended norm. Other recommendations of this group for middle-grade school transformations include shifts in instructional practices toward interdisciplinary integration, greater decision-making powers by teachers, the use of community-advisory teams, teacher-based advisory programming, increased levels of parental involvement, the provision of comprehensive health care and health education, and increases in the community experiences of students through programs such as service learning. A critical goal of the overall transformation process is to match the characteristics of the school environment to the developmentally appropriate needs and abilities of students.

Data on these reforms are highly promising (Felner, Mulhall, Sartain, Standiford, Brand, & Kasak, 1992), showing patterns of improvement in achievement and socioemotional well-being for adolescents similar to those reported for the elementary-school efforts. Further, a noteworthy feature of these comprehensive school-reform efforts is that they create school-community contexts that are more supportive of, and congruent with, the goals of more traditional school-based prevention efforts, thus potentially increasing the efficacy of these programs. As anyone who has worked with schools knows, the degree to which there is time set aside during which teachers can engage in social development programming with youth, and the degree to which they perceive such activities as part of their role, will have a profound effect on whether they implement such efforts and the levels of fidelity with which they do so. Teacher advisory periods, such as those advocated by *Turning Points*, are ideal times for activities such as the delivery of curriculum-based prevention efforts. Additionally, the developmental philosophies of such schools help teachers understand the importance of attending to social development as a means of enhancing academic outcomes, increasing the probability that they may actually attend to teaching social skills or competencies. Further, the team/integrative curriculum approach in *Turning Points*-based middle schools provides a means by which strategies can be implemented to provide for students' applications of the competencies learned throughout the school day—a feature that has been identified as critical for obtaining generalization and maintenance (Caplan & Weissberg, 1989). In this way genuinely ecologically enmeshed, multilevel interventions can and will take place within a school setting.

There are numerous other preventive efforts that may be targeted to children and families that are more ecologically congruent with the existing regularities and systems of their lives than those of the earlier generations of such efforts. For families in poverty, and for economically disadvantaged neighborhoods and communities, the comprehensive prevention efforts that target changes throughout the context are not only advisable but necessary for almost any of the individual program efforts to be viable. Parents who are concerned about their children cannot and will not go to work or to obtain additional education if it means leaving their children without adequate adult supervision and support in high-risk neighborhoods. Indeed, it is important to understand that social programs and policies that require parents to go to work or pursue training without providing for high-quality child care are, in fact, asking parents to engage in what may well be chargeable neglect! These are precisely the kinds of problematic policies that may emerge without sufficient attention to the way in which what appear to be dysfunctional behaviors are, in fact, found to be adaptive ones when contextual regularities are considered. Such analyses are critical as we attempt to develop family policies that respect the interrelated needs and demands of all of the members and that will have far greater potential for efficacy. Indeed, given the changing nature of society, quality child care and afterschool programming that provides both supervision as well as social and educational development aspects may be one of the most powerful setting-level interventions that may be mounted, for all families, under the "flag" of prevention. Additional family-support programs, such as those that provide homeless families and/or those who are socially and educationally disadvantaged with coordinated and necessary stabilization, medical, human-service, and food resources, also fall into this category.

Space does not allow us to address the full range of T–E-based programs that may address the needs of families and adults. But the metaphor of a developmental ladder is one that is equally viable as we go up through later ages, with a careful analysis of the needs, risks, and opportunities for development and acquisition of new competencies associated with each age (e.g., school to work transition points, anticipable stresses during the work life of adults, barriers to living productively and with good health in older age) can well serve any community's efforts to develop systematic prevention efforts, especially when such analyses are informed by an understanding of the unique characteristics of the community context that may interact with the more general developmental-level conditions. For example, communities that are moving from rust-belt industries to high-tech economies have work-age adults who are facing substantially different challenges, risks, and requirements for new competencies in the workplace than do adults in communities where the economic base is more stable. An essential point here is that a T–E perspective on prevention will shift our focus to the enhancement of all of the developmental settings in a person's/family's life and their interrelationships when considering the necessary and sufficient elements of adequate prevention initiatives. These shifts will move us naturally away from narrow program-based prevention efforts toward more comprehensive and population-focused preventive strategies. It will also lead us to the recognition that if we did some of the "basics" of positive, proactive, wellness development (Cowen, this volume), e.g., good prenatal care, adequate child care and preschool programs, developmentally appropriate and adequate schooling, family-support resources, and the removal of policies that impede the positive development of families, we might not have to do some of the "fancy" programs of which human services are so fond.

Reforming Policy and Practice at the Federal, State, and Local Levels

In our quest to achieve more effective prevention programs, knowing what works and having an adequate framework to guide these efforts are, unfortunately, still not sufficient conditions to ensure that these more effective strategies will actually emerge. The understanding of what it takes for effective and well-conceived programming is generally not reflected in either the nature of state- and federal-funding initiatives, nor in the practices of field professionals. Prevention initiatives funded by federal and state agencies are often organized more by the accident of who funds them and/or by focusing on highly specific outcomes (e.g., teen births, substance abuse, conduct disorders, depression), than by a basis on the understandings discussed above. Illustratively, state and federal agencies currently fund separate initiatives to prevent teenage pregnancy, child abuse, substance abuse, school failure, youth suicide, school aggression, gang membership, illiteracy, pre- and perinatal complications, and welfare dependency, to name but a few of these fragmented and often uncoordinated efforts. Even among efforts that focus on a common single outcome (e.g., substance abuse) there may be multiple state and/or federal agencies involved, each of which has their own separate initiative. At best, these are typically only loosely coordinated. At worst, they may fight over turf and create needless and wastefully duplicative programs.

Such fragmentation is a very poor use of resources, typically leaving each initiative with just enough resources to not be effective. As we have seen, this organization is also the opposite of what we would do if our efforts were based on theory and research. A major priority of policymakers in many states, as well as of several federal initiatives (cf. Virginia Department of Mental Health, Mental Retardation, and Substance Abuse, 1988; the U.S. Center for Substance Abuse Prevention's Community Partnership Program) is to develop a more integrative approach, given the growing recognition of the interrelatedness of the programs of concern, the need to reduce fragmentation for the cost-efficient expenditure of resources, and the growing understanding that such disjointed services are neither effective nor appropriate. Comprehensive family-support programs (cf. Moynihan, 1986; Schorr, 1989; Weiss & Jacobs, 1988) and the Schools of the Future (Holtzman, 1992), with their emphasis on positive development and meeting the needs of whole families, are more effective policy metaphors than are the traditional categorical approaches.

Bringing about the required enduring shifts in how funding agencies and staff in educational settings and human-service agencies think about what they are doing and translating that to action will not be easy tasks. To ask those who have been working in these agencies and policy systems to change what they do may be difficult and may be met with resistance, even among those who are favorably inclined. Those working within existing systems will be limited in their ability to frame what they do by their personal and professional socialization experiences (Sarason, 1981). Instead of simply criticizing prevention professionals, researchers must offer these individuals new ways of "thinking about what they are thinking about." The T–E perspective offered above is one such step. Further, the prevention field in general, and prevention researchers in particular, must attend to the development of an infrastructure and technology transfer capacity that will allow for the effective dissemination to, and implementation of, what we have learned by those who live in our communities.

Much has been made in recent years of the need for those in local communities to be fully involved in generating the solutions to the social and health problems they face. This call should not be mistaken for a move to an abdication of professional involvement. Rather, much can be gained by all involved through focused, careful collaborations among policymakers, educational/social program professionals and, importantly, community members. In this vein, Rappaport (1977) cited the need to recast the role of the mental health professional to that of "community collaborator," rather than expert. In such collaborations, the definitions of problems and issues to be addressed, and of the resources required to address them, can and must be provided and shaped by the community members. Prevention professionals, providers, and policymakers can then serve as partners by identifying a range of strategies and community-change models that have been attempted, including their strengths or weaknesses. These groups must then work together to take those state-of-the-art efforts that are identified as most appropriate to the needs that have been defined and mold them to local community conditions through a dynamic ongoing process between providers and constituents.

A key step in accomplishing these goals is the establishment of settings such as the Center for Social and Community Development at Rutgers University (Chavis, 1992), or the Center for Prevention Research and Development, Institute of Government and Public Affairs, at the University of Illinois (Felner, 1992), whose explicit missions are to evolve and expand the land grant missions of universities. Now, instead of focusing solely on the traditional issues of agriculture, university-based settings must create formal partnerships with local communities, and social welfare and educational agencies at state, local, and federal levels, to solve the social problems that we confront.

In the preceding pages we have presented what we see as a framework that can guide the development of the next generation of prevention efforts and serve as a foundation on which to build a systematic knowledge base for a science of prevention. As prevention moves toward its next generation of efforts, the contributions of those who provide the shoulders on which we stand in gaining our current vision should not be underestimated or underappreciated. Given this perspective and their "boost," we hope that the perspective provided in this chapter further changes our ways to "think about what we are thinking about" in the continued evolution of a science of prevention, and moves us further from the bounds of the procrustean, individually focused bed in which it was born.

REFERENCES

Albee, G. W. (1959). *Mental health manpower trends.* New York: Basic Books.

Albee, G. W. (1982). Preventing psychopathology and promoting human potential. *American Psychologist, 32,* 150–161.

Albee, G. W. (1986). Toward a just society: Lessons from observations on the primary prevention of psychopathology. *American Psychologist, 41,* 891–898.

Barker, R. G. (1968). *Ecological psychology: Concepts and methods for studying the environment of human behavior.* Stanford, CA: Stanford University Press.

Bond, L. A., & Wagner, B. M. (Eds.). (1988). *Families in transition.* Beverly Hills, CA: Sage.

Britt, D. W. (1991). Constructing adaptability: Proactive and reactive coping changes in response to an environmental jolt and increased organizational strain. *Journal of Applied Social Psychology, 8,* 1–18.

Bronfenbrenner, U. (1979). *The ecology of human development: Experiments by nature and design.* Cambridge, MA: Harvard University Press.

Cantwell, D. P., & Baker, L. (1989). Stability and natural history of DSM-III childhood diagnoses. *Journal of the American Academy of Child and Adolescent Psychiatry, 28,* 691–700.

Caplan, M. Z., & Weissberg, R. P. (1989). Promoting social competence in early adolescence: Developmental considerations. In B. H. Schneider, G. Attili, J. Nadel, & R. P. Weissberg (Eds.), *Social competence in developmental perspective* (pp. 371–386). Boston: Kluwer Academic.

Carnegie Council on Adolescent Development. (1989). *Turning points: Preparing America for the 21st century.* New York: Carnegie Corporation.

Carnegie Council on Adolescent Development. (1992). *A matter of time: Risk and opportunity in the nonschool hours.* New York: Carnegie Corporation.

Center for Substance Abuse Prevention. (1991). *The future by design: Community prevention system framework for alcohol and other drug prevention.* Washington, D.C.: The Circle.

Chavis, D. M., & Wandsersman, A. (1990). Sense of community in the urban environment: A catalyst for participation and community development. *American Journal of Community Psychology, 18,* 55–82.

Comer, J. P. (1988). Educating poor minority children. *Scientific American, 259,* 42–48.

Committee for Economic Development. (1991). *The unfinished agenda: A new vision for child development and education.* New York: Committee for Economic Development.

Connell, D. B., Turner, R. R., & Mason, E. F. (1988). Summary of the findings of the school health education evaluation: Health from effectiveness, implementation, and costs. *Journal of School Health, 1988; 55,* 316–323.

Cowen, E. L. (1980). The wooing of primary prevention. *American Journal of Community Psychology, 8,* 258–284.

Cowen, E. L. (1983). Primary prevention in mental health: Past, present, and future. In R. D. Felner, L. A. Jason, J. N. Moritsugu, & S. S. Farber (Eds.), *Preventive psychology: Theory, research, and prevention* (pp. 11–25). New York: Pergamon.

Dryfoos, J. G. (1990). *Adolescents at risk: Prevalence and prevention.* New York: Oxford University Press.

Eccles, J. S., & Midgley, C. (1989). Stage/environment fit: Developmentally appropriate classrooms for early adolescents. In R. E. Ames & C. Ames (Eds.), *Research on motivation in education, Vol. 3* (pp. 139–186). New York: Academic Press.

Elias, M. J., & Clabby, J. F. (1992). *Building social problem-solving skills: Guidelines from a school-based programs.* San Francisco: Jossey-Bass.

Felner, R. D. (1984). Vulnerability in childhood: A preventive framework for understanding children's efforts to cope with life stress and transitions. In M. C. Roberts & L. Peterson (Eds.), *Prevention of problems in childhood: Psychological research and applications* (pp. 133–169). New York: Wiley-Interscience.

Felner, R. D. (Invited Address) (1992). *An ecological analysis for enhancing the developmental outcomes of children in poverty.* Fifth Annual Conference on Stress and Coping in Childhood and Adolescence, American Psychological Association (Committee on Children and Youth) and the University of Miami, Miami, FL.

Felner, R. D., & Adan, A. M. (1988). The school transitional environment project: An ecological intervention and evaluation. In R. H. Price, E. L. Cowen, R. P. Lorion, & J. Ramos-McKay (Eds.), *Fourteen ounces of prevention: A casebook for practitioners* (pp. 111–122). Washington, D.C.: American Psychological Association.

Felner, R. D., DuBois, D. L., & Adan, A. M. (1991). Community-based intervention and prevention: Conceptual underpinnings and progress toward a science of community intervention and evaluation. In C. E. Walker (Ed.), *Clinical psychology: Historical and research foundations* (pp. 459–510). New York: Plenum.

Felner, R. D., Farber, S. S., & Primavera, J. (1980). Children of divorce, stressful life events and transitions: A framework for preventive efforts. In R. H. Price, R. F. Ketterer, B. C. Bader, & J. Monahan (Eds.), *Prevention in mental health: Research, policy and practice* (pp. 81–108). Beverly Hills: Sage.

Felner, R. D., Farber, S. S., & Primavera, J. (1983). Transitions and stressful life events: A model for primary prevention. In R. D. Felner, L. A. Jason, J. N. Moritsugu, & S. S. Farber (Eds.), *Preventive psychology: Theory, research, and prevention* (pp. 191–215). New York: Pergamon.

Felner, R. D., & Felner, T. Y. (1989). Prevention programs in the educational context: A transactional-ecological framework for program models. In L. Bond & B. Compas (Eds.), *Primary prevention in the schools* (pp. 13–49). Beverly Hills, CA: Sage.

Felner, R. D., Ginter, M. A., & Primavera, J. (1982). Primary prevention during school transitions: Social support and environmental structure. *American Journal of Community Psychology, 10,* 277–290.

Felner, R. D., Jason, L. A., Farber, S. S., & Moritsugu, J. N. (1983). An overview of preventive psychology. In R. D. Felner, L. A. Jason, J. N. Moritsugu, & S. S. Farber (Eds.), *Preventive psychology: Theory, research, and practice* (pp. 3–10). New York: Pergamon.

Felner, R. D., & Lorion, R. P. (1985). Clinical child psychology and prevention: Toward a workable and satisfying marriage. *Proceedings: National Conference on Clinical Child Psychologists,* 41–95.

Felner, R. D., Mulhall, P., Sartain, B., Standiford, S., Brand, S., & Kasak, D. (1992). The evaluation of the impact of middle grades restructuring on school regularities, climate, and student outcomes. Presentation to Annual Meeting of the National Middle School Association, San Antonio, TX.

Felner, R. D., Rowlison, R. T., & Terre, L. (1986). Unraveling the Gordian Knot in life change events: A critical examination of crisis, stress, and transitional frameworks for prevention. In S. W. Auerbach & A. L. Stolberg (Eds.), *Children's life crisis events: Preventive intervention strategies* (pp. 39–63). New York: Hemisphere/ McGraw-Hill.

Felner, R. D., Silverman, M., & Adan, A. M. (1989). Primary prevention: Relevance of principles for the prevention of youth suicide. *Report of the Secretary's Task Force on Youth Suicide, Volume 3: Prevention and intervention in youth suicide* (pp. 23–30), DHHS Publication No. (ADM) 88-1623. Washington D.C.: U.S. Government Printing Office.

Felner, R. D., Silverman, M., & Adan, A. M. (1992). Risk assessment and prevention of youth suicide in educational contexts. In R. Maris, A. Berman, J. Maltsberger, & R. Yufit (Eds.). *Assessment and prediction of suicide* (pp. 420–447). New York: Guilford.

Felner, R. D., Silverman, M. M., & Adix, R. S. (1991). Prevention of substance abuse and related disorders in childhood and adolescence: A developmentally based, comprehensive ecological approach. *Family and Community Health: The Journal of Health Promotion and Maintenance, 14*(3), 1–11.

Furman, W., Goberson, R., White, A. S., Gravin, L. A., & Wehner, E. A. (1989). Enhancing peer relations in school systems. In B. H. Schneider, G. Attili, J. Nadel, & R. P. Weissberg (Eds.), *Social competence in developmental perspective* (pp. 355–377). Boston: Kluwer Academic.

Garbarino, J. (1990). The human ecology of early risk. In J. P. Shonkoff & S. J. Meisels (Eds.), *The handbook of early intervention* (pp. 78–96). New York: Cambridge University Press.

Gordon, R. S. (1983). An operational classification of disease prevention. *Public Health Reports, 98,* 107–109.

Hawkins, J. D., Catalano, R. F., & Miller, J. Y. (1992). Risk and protective factors for alcohol and other drug problems in adolescence and early adulthood: Implications for substance abuse prevention. *Psychological Bulletin, 112*(1), 64–105.

Haynes, N. M., Comer, J. P., & Hamilton-Lee, M. (1988). The school development program: A model for school improvement. *Journal of Negro Education, 57,* 11–21.

Healthy People 2000: National Health Promotion and Disease Prevention Objectives. DHHS Publication. Washington, D.C.: U.S. Government Printing Office, 1990.

Holtzman, W. H. (Ed.). (1992). *School of the future.* Austin, TX: American Psychological Association and Hogg Foundation.

Jencks, C., & Peterson, P. E. (1991). *The urban underclass.* Washington, D. C.: The Brookings Institution.

Jessor, R., & Jessor, S. L. (1977). *Problem behavior and psychosocial development: A longitudinal study of youth.* New York: Academic.

Johnson, D. L. (1988). Primary prevention of behavior problems in young children: The Houston parent–child development center. In R. H. Price, E. L. Cowen, R. P. Lorion, & J. Ramos-McKay (Eds.), *Fourteen ounces of prevention: A casebook for practitioners* (pp. 44–55). Washington, D. C.: American Psychological Association.

Joint Commission on Mental Illness and Health. (1961). *Action for mental health.* New York: Basic Books.

Kellam, S. G., & Brown, C. H. (1982). *Social, adaptational and psychological antecedents of adolescents psychopathology ten years later.* Baltimore, MD: Johns Hopkins University Press.

Kellam, S. G., Brown, C. H., Rubin, B. R., & Ensminger, M. E. (1983). Paths leading to teenage psychiatric symptoms and substance abuse: Developmental epidemiological studies in Woodlawn. In S. E. Guze, F. J. Earls, & J. E. Bartlett (Eds.), *Child psychopathology and development.* New York: Raven.

Kliztner, M. D. (1987). *Report to congress on the effectiveness of state, federal, and local drug prevention/education programs: Part 2. An assessment of the research on school-based assessment programs.* Vienna, VA: Center for Advanced Health Studies.

Lamb, M. (1992). Developmental issues in addressing poverty. Fifth Annual Conference on Stress and Coping in Childhood and Adolescence, American Psychological Association (Committee on Children and Youth) and the University of Miami, FL.

Lamb, H. R., & Zusman, J. (1979). Primary prevention in perspective. *American Journal of Psychiatry, 136,* 12–17.

Lewin, K. (1951). *Field theory in social science: Selected theoretical papers.* New York: Harper.
Long, B. B. (1986). The prevention of mental-emotional disabilities: A report from the national mental health association commission. *American Psychologist, 41,* 825–829.
Lorion, R. P. (1991). Targeting preventive interventions: Enhancing risk estimates through theory. *American Journal of Community Psychology, 19,* 859–866.
Lorion, R. P., Price, R. H., & Eaton, W. W. (1989). The prevention of child and adolescent disorders: From theory to research. In D. Schaffer, I. Phillips, N. B. Enzer, M. M. Silverman, & V. Anthony (Eds.), *Prevention of mental disorders, alcohol and other drug use in children and adolescents: OSAP Prevention Monograph-2* (pp. 55–96). DHHS Publication No. (ADM) 89-1646. Washington, D.C.: U.S. Government Printing Office.
McKey, R. H., Condelli, L., Gansen, H., Barrett, B. J., McConkey, C., & Plantz, M. C. (1985). *The impact of Head Start on children, families, and communities.* DHHS Publication No. (OHDS) 90-31193. Washington, D.C.: U.S. Government Printing Office.
Mednick, S. A. Griffith, J. J., & Mednick, B. R. (1981). Problems with traditional strategies in mental health research. In F. Schulsinger, S. A. Mednick, & J. Knop (Eds.), *Longitudinal research: Methods and uses in behavioral science* (pp. 3–15). Boston: Martinus Nijhoff.
Moynihan, D. P. (1986). *Family and nation.* Orlando, FL: Harcourt Brace Javonovich.
Olds, D. (1988). Prenatal/early infancy project. In R. H. Price, E. L. Cowen, R. P. Lorion, & J. Ramos-McKay (Eds.). *Fourteen ounces of prevention: A casebook for practitioners* (pp. 9–23). Washington, D. C.: American Psychological Association.
Pedro-Carroll, J. L., & Cowen, E. L. (1985). The children of divorce intervention project: An investigation of the efficacy of a school-based prevention program. *Journal of Consulting and Clinical Psychology, 53,* 603–611.
Pedro-Carroll, J. L., Cowen, E. L., Hightower, A. D., & Guare, J. C. (1986). Preventive intervention with latency-age children of divorce: A replication study. *American Journal of Community Psychology, 14,* 277–290.
Perkins, D. D., Florin, P., Rich, R. C., Wandsersman, A., & Chavis, D. M. (1990). Participation and the social and physical environment of residential blocks: crime and community context. *American Journal of Community Psychology, 18,* 83–116.
Pillow, D. R., Sandler, I. N., Braver, S. L., Wolchick, S. A., & Gersten, J. C. (1991). Theory based screening for prevention: Focusing on mediating processes in children divorce. *American Journal of Community Psychology, 19,* 809–837.
President's Commission on Mental Health. (1978). *Report to the President. Vol. 1.* Stock No. 040-000-0390-8. Washington, D.C.: U.S. Government Printing Office.
Price, R. H. (1980). Risky situations. In D. Magnusson (Ed.), *The situation: An interactional perspective.* Hillsdale, NJ: Erlbaum.
Price, R. H. (1983). The education of prevention psychologist. In R. D. Felner, L. A. Jason, J. N. Mortisugu, & S. S. Farber (Eds.), *Preventive psychology: Theory, research, and prevention* (pp. 290–296). New York: Pergamon.
Price, R. H., Cowen, E. L., Lorion, R. P., & Ramos-McKay, J. (Eds.). (1988). *Fourteen ounces of prevention: A casebook for practitioners.* Washington, D.C.: American Psychological Association.
Rappaport, J. (1977). *Community psychology: Values, research, and action.* New York: Holt, Rinehart, and Winston.
Rappaport, J. (1987). Terms of empowerment/exemplars of prevention: Toward a theory for community psychology. *American Journal of Community Psychology, 15,* 121–148.
Reppucci, N. D. (1987). Prevention and ecology: Teenaged pregnancy, child sexual abuse, and organized youth sports. *American Journal of Community Psychology, 15,* 1–22.
Richters, J., & Weintraub, S. (1990). Beyond diatheses: Toward an understanding of high risk environments. In J. Rolf, A. S. Masten, D. Cicchetti, K. H. Nuechterlein, & S. Weitraub (Eds.), *Risk and protective factors in the development of psychopathology* (pp. 67–96). Cambridge, UK: Cambridge University Press.
Ross, J. G., Saavedra, P. J., Shur, G. H., Winters, F., Scaramuzzo, E., & Felner, R. D. (1992). The effectiveness of an after-school program for primary grade latchkey students on precursors of substance abuse. *Journal of Community Psychology, Special Issue,* pp. 22–38.
Rutter, M. (1981). Stress, coping, and development: Some issues and some questions. In N. Gannezy & M. Rutter (Eds.), *Stress, coping, development in children.* New York: McGraw-Hill.
Rutter, M. (1989). Isle of Wight revisited: Twenty-five years of child psychiatric epidemiology. *Journal of Child and Adolescent Psychiatry, 28,* 633–653.
Sameroff, A. J., & Chandler, M. J. (1975). Reproductive risk and the continuum of caretaking casualty. In F. D. Haeres, M. Hetherington, S. Scarr-Salapatek, & G. Siegal (Eds.), *Review of Child Development Research, Vol. 4.* Chicago: University of Chicago Press.
Sameroff, A. J., & Fiese, B. H. (1989). Conceptual issues in prevention. In D. Schaffer, I. Phillips, N. B. Enzer, M. M. Silverman, & V. Anthony (Eds.), *Prevention of mental disorders alcohol and other drug use in children and adolescents: OSAP Prevention Monograph-2* (pp. 23–54). DHHS Publication No. (ADM) 89-1646. Washington, D.C.: U.S. Government Printing Office.

Sameroff, A. J., Seifer, R., Barocas, R., Zax, M., & Greenspan, S. (1987). I.Q. scores of 4-year-old children: Social-environmental risk factors. *Pediatrics, 79*(3), 343–350.

Sarason, S. B. (1981). *Psychology misdirected.* New York: Free Press.

Sarason, S. B. (1982). *The culture of the school and the problem of change.* 2nd ed. Boston: Allyn & Bacon.

Sarason, S. B., & Doris, J. (1979). *Educational handicap, public policy, and social history: A broadened perspective on mental retardation.* New York: Free Press.

Schorr, L. B. (1988). *Within our reach: Breaking the cycle of disadvantage.* New York: Doubleday.

Schweinhart, L. J., & Weikart, D. P. (1988). The High/Scope Perry Preschool Program. In R. H. Price, E. L. Cowen, R. P. Lorion, & J. Ramos-McKay (Eds.), *Fourteen ounces of prevention: A casebook for practitioners* (pp. 53–66). Washington, D.C.: American Psychological Association.

Seidman, E. (1983). Unexamined premises of social problem solving. In E. Seidman (Ed.), *Handbook of Social Intervention* (pp. 48–67). Beverly Hills: Sage.

Seidman, E. (1987). Toward a framework for primary prevention research. In J. A. Steinberg and M. M. Silverman (Eds.), *Preventing mental disorders: A research perspective* (pp. 2–19). DHHS Pub. No (ADM)87-1492. Washington, D.C.: U.S. Government Printing Office.

Seidman, E. (1988). Back to the future, community psychology: Unfolding a theory of social intervention. *American Journal of Community Psychology, 16*, 3–24.

Seidman, E. (1990). Pursuing the meaning and utility of social regularities for community psychology. In P. Tolan, C. Keys, F. Chertok, & L. Jason (Eds.), *Researching community psychology: Issues of theory and methods* (pp. 91–100). Washington, D.C.: American Psychological Association.

Seidman, E., & Rappaport, J. (Eds.). (1986). *Redefining social problems.* New York: Basic Books.

Shure, M. B., & Spivack, G. (1982). Interpersonal problem-solving in young children: A cognitive approach to prevention. *American Journal of Community Psychology, 10*, 341–356.

Silverman, M. M. (1989). Commentary: The integration of problem and prevention perspectives: Mental disorders associated with alcohol and drug use. In D. Schaffer, I. Phillips, N. B. Enzer, M. M. Silverman, & V. Anthony (Eds.), *Prevention of mental disorders alcohol and other drug use in children and adolescents: OSAP Prevention Monograph-2* (pp. 7–22). DHHS Publication No. (ADW) 89-1646. Washington, D.C.: U.S. Government Printing Office.

Sroufe, L. A., & Rutter, M. (1984). The domain of developmental psychopathology. *Child Development, 55*, 17–29.

Virginia Department of Mental Health, Mental Retardation, and Substance Abuse. (1988). *A comprehensive plan of prevention.* Richmond, VA.

Weiss, H. B., & Jacobs, F. H. (1988). Introduction: Family support and education programs, challenges and opportunities. In H. B. Weiss and F. H. Jacobs (Eds.), *Evaluating family programs.* New York: Aldine de Gruyter.

Wilson, W. J. (1987). *The truly disadvantaged: The inner-city, the underclass, & public policy.* Chicago: University of Chicago Press.

W. T. Grant Foundation. (1988). *The forgotten half: Non-college youth in America.* New York: W. T. Grant Foundation.

Zigler, E. F. (1989). Addressing the nation's child care crisis: The school of the 21st century. *American Journal of Orthopsychiatry, 59*, 485–491.

Zigler, E. F. (1990). Forward. In S. J. Meisels and J. P. Shonkoff (Eds.), *Handbook of early childhood intervention* (pp. ix–xiv). New York: Cambridge University Press.

CHAPTER 2

Empowerment Theory

Psychological, Organizational and Community Levels of Analysis

MARC A. ZIMMERMAN

Empowerment is both a value orientation for working in the community and a theoretical model for understanding the process and consequences of efforts to exert control and influence over decisions that affect one's life, organizational functioning, and the quality of community life (Perkins & Zimmerman, 1995; Rappaport, 1981; Zimmerman & Warschausky, 1998). A distinction between the values that underlie an empowerment approach to social change and empowerment theory is necessary. The value orientation of empowerment suggests goals, aims, and strategies for implementing change. Empowerment theory provides principles and a framework for organizing our knowledge. The development of empowerment theory also helps advance the construct beyond a passing fad and political manipulation.

A theory of empowerment suggests ways to measure the construct in different contexts, to study empowering processes, and to distinguish empowerment from other constructs, such as self-esteem, self-efficacy, or locus of control. One definition of empowerment is useful, but appears to be limited to the individual level of analysis:

> Empowerment may be seen as a process where individuals learn to see a closer correspondence between their goals and a sense of how to achieve them, and a relationship between their efforts and life outcomes (Mechanic, 1991).

Another definition explicitly incorporates person–environment interaction:

> Empowerment is an intentional, ongoing process centered in the local community, involving mutual respect, critical reflection, caring, and group participation, through which people lacking an equal share of valued resources gain greater access to and control over those resources (Cornell Empowerment Group, 1989).

A definition by Rappaport (1984) accounts for the fact that empowerment may occur at multiple levels of analysis: "Empowerment is viewed as a process: the mechanism by which

MARC A. ZIMMERMAN • Department of Health Behavior and Health Education, School of Public Health, University of Michigan, Ann Arbor, Michigan 48109.

Handbook of Community Psychology, edited by Julian Rappaport and Edward Seidman. Kluwer Academic/Plenum Publishers, New York, 2000.

people, organizations, and communities gain mastery over their lives," but does not provide details about the process across levels of analysis. These definitions suggest that empowerment is a process in which efforts to exert control are central. These conceptual definitions also suggest that participation with others to achieve goals, efforts to gain access to resources, and some critical understanding of the sociopolitical environment are basic components of the construct. Applying this general framework to an organizational level of analysis suggests that empowerment may include organizational processes and structures that enhance member participation and improve organizational effectiveness for goal achievement. At the community level of analysis, empowerment may refer to collective action to improve the quality of life in a community and to the connections among community organizations and agencies. Organizational and community empowerment, however, are not simply the aggregate of many empowered individuals.

This chapter begins with a brief discussion of the value orientation underlying an empowerment approach to social change. Next, I briefly describe empowerment as theory. Finally, I examine the construct of empowerment at the individual, organizational, and community levels of analysis. These sections include a discussion of the parameters of empowerment, a brief review of relevant research, and suggestions for future research at each level of analysis. The chapter emphasizes the individual level because most of the research to date has been devoted to this level of analysis, but this focus is not intended to suggest its relative importance.

EMPOWERMENT AS A VALUE ORIENTATION

Empowerment suggests a distinct approach for developing interventions and creating social change. It directs attention toward health, adaptation, competence, and natural helping systems. It includes the perspective that many social problems exist due to unequal distribution of, and access to, resources. Some individuals are best served by mutual help, helping others, or working for their rights, rather than having their needs fulfilled by a benevolent professional (Gallant, Cohen, & Wolff, 1985). An empowerment approach goes beyond ameliorating the negative aspects of a situation by searching for those that are positive. Thus, enhancing wellness instead of fixing problems (Cowen, Chapter 4, this volume), identifying strengths instead of cataloging risk factors, and searching for environmental influences instead of blaming victims characterizes an empowerment approach.

Empowerment calls for a distinct language for understanding lay efforts to cope with stress, adapt to change, and influence our communities. Rappaport (1985) describes how an empowerment-oriented language can help redefine our roles as professional helpers. He suggests that the traditional language used to describe the helping process unwittingly encourages dependence on professionals, creates the view that people are clients in need of help, and maintains the idea that help is unidirectional. The language of professionals limits the discovery of indigenous resources and reduces the likelihood of people helping each other. An empowerment approach replaces terms such as "client" and "expert" with "participant" and "collaborator."

An empowerment approach to intervention design, implementation, and evaluation redefines the professional's role relationship with the target population. The professional's role becomes one of collaborator and facilitator rather than expert and counselor. As collaborators, professionals learn about the participants through their cultures, their worldviews, and their life struggles. The professional works with participants instead of advocating for them. The professional's skills, interests, or plans are not imposed on the community; rather, professionals become a resource for a community. This role relationship suggests that what professionals do will depend on the particular place and people with whom they are working, rather than on the technologies that are predetermined to be applied in all situations. While interpersonal assessment and evaluation skills will be necessary, how, where, and with whom they are applied cannot be automatically assumed, as occurs in the role of a psychotherapist with clients in a clinic. Fawcett et al. (1994) describe eight case studies that exemplify innovative roles for professionals interested in promoting empowerment among those with whom they are working. They provide a framework of empowering strategies that focus on capacity-building for individuals and groups, and creating environments that support the development of empowerment.

Kelly (1971) describes several qualities of a community psychologist that are consistent with an empowerment approach. These include giving away the byline, tolerance for diversity, coping effectively with varied resources, and creating an eco-identity (i.e., identifying with the community). These qualities suggest a capability to learn about the context within which one is working, and to accept and acknowledge the values of that context. Kelly (1970) also identifies several strategies for training that would help prepare community psychologists for applying an empowerment approach, including field-assessment skills, integrating theory and practice, and identifying resources in the community.

An empowerment orientation also suggests that community participants have an active role in the change process, not only for implementing a project, but also in setting the agenda. The professional works hard to include members of a setting, neighborhood, or organization so they have a central role in the process. Participants can help identify measurement issues and help collect assessment and evaluation data. The evaluation process not only includes participants in its planning and implementation, but the results are also shared. Feeding back information to the community and helping to use it for policy decisions is a primary goal. An empowerment approach to evaluation focuses as much attention on how goals are achieved as on outcomes. This approach suggests that both quantitative and qualitative methods are necessary for evaluation (Lincoln & Guba, 1986). Kelly (1988) describes a process for prevention research that is consistent with an empowerment approach, and several investigators describe a participatory approach to research (Brown, 1983; Chesler, 1991; Israel, Schulz, Parker, & Becker, 1998; Pasmore & Friedlander, 1982; Peters & Robinson, 1984; Rappaport, 1990; Serrano-Garcia, 1984). Fetterman (1996) has also described empowerment evaluation as a process that not only involves participants, but also helps them develop skills for self-evaluation.

EMPOWERMENT AS THEORY

A theory of empowerment includes both processes and outcomes (Swift & Levine, 1987). The theory suggests that actions, activities, or structures may be empowering, and that the outcome of such processes result in a level of being empowered. Both empowerment processes and outcomes vary in their outward form because no single standard can fully capture its meaning for all people in all contexts (Rappaport, 1984; Zimmerman, 1995). The behaviors necessary for a 16-year-old mother to become empowered are different from the behaviors for a recently widowed middle-aged man. Similarly, what it means to be empowered for these two individuals is not the same. Thus, empowerment is context and population specific. It takes on different forms for different people in different contexts.

A distinction between empowering processes and outcomes is critical in order to clearly define empowerment theory. Empowering processes are ones in which attempts to gain control, obtain needed resources, and critically understand one's social environment are fundamental. The process is empowering if it helps people develop skills so they can become independent problem-solvers and decision-makers. Empowering processes will vary across levels of analysis. For example, empowering processes for individuals might include organizational or community involvement; empowering processes at the organizational level might include shared leadership and decision-making; and empowering processes at the community level might include accessible government, media, and other community resources.

Empowered outcomes refer to operationalization of empowerment so we can study the consequences of citizens' attempts to gain greater control in their community, or the effects of interventions designed to empower participants. Empowered outcomes also differ across levels of analysis. When we are concerned with individuals, outcomes might include situation-specific perceived control, skills, and proactive behaviors. When we are studying organizations, outcomes might include organizational networks, effective resource acquisition, and policy leverage. When we are concerned with community-level empowerment, outcomes might include evidence of pluralism, the existence of organizational coalitions, and accessible community resources.

A thorough development of empowerment theory requires exploration and description at multiple levels of analysis. Citizens who unite to stop a chemical company from dumping toxic waste near their children's school are trying to exert control in their environment. They might create an organization to address the problem and educate their community. The organization could join other similar organizations so they can increase their base of support. Their community could then unite to elect officials that represent their concerns and allow them more access to governmental decision-making. Mechanisms of empowerment include individual competencies and proactive behaviors, natural helping systems and organizational effectiveness, and community competence and access to resources.

Each level of analysis, although described separately, is inherently connected to the others. Individual, organization, and community empowerment are mutually interdependent and are both a cause and a consequence of each other. The extent to which elements at one level of analysis are empowered is directly related to the empowering potential of other levels of analysis. Similarly, empowering processes at one level of analysis contribute to empowered outcomes at other levels of analysis. Empowered persons are the basis for developing responsible and participatory organizations and communities; it is difficult to imagine an empowering community or organization devoid of empowered individuals. Efforts to understand empowering processes and outcomes are not complete unless multiple levels of analysis are studied and integrated. An examination of empowerment theory (i.e., empowering processes and outcomes) at the individual, organizational, and community levels of analysis follows.

PSYCHOLOGICAL EMPOWERMENT

Empowerment at the individual level of analysis may be referred to as psychological empowerment (Zimmerman, 1990a; Zimmerman & Rappaport, 1988). Psychological empowerment (PE) includes beliefs about one's competence, efforts to exert control, and an understanding of the socio-political environment. The specific actions one takes to achieve goals are not as important as simply being involved and attempting to exert control. Understanding one's socio-political environment—critical awareness—refers to the capability to analyze and understand one's social and political situation. This includes an ability to identify those with power, their resources, their connection to the issue of concern, and the factors that influence their decision-making. Sue and Zane (1980) describe this process as understanding causal agents. A critical awareness also includes knowing when to engage conflict and when to avoid it, and the ability to identify and cultivate resources needed to achieve desired goals (Kieffer, 1984).

One way individuals can develop these analytic skills is through participation in activities and organizations. They may model others or gain experience by organizing people, identifying resources, or developing strategies for social change. Berger and Neuhaus (1977) suggest that increased opportunities for people to become involved in community organizations (e.g., churches, neighborhood groups, service organizations) will help to decrease a sense of powerlessness, alienation, and withdrawal from community living. These organizations, which they call mediating structures (because they mediate between large impersonal organizations and individual lives), provide opportunities for learning new skills, developing a sense of community, building a sense of control and confidence, and improving community life.

Thus, an empowered person might be expected to exhibit a sense of personal control, a critical awareness of one's environment, and the behaviors necessary to exert control. These different dimensions of PE can be identified as intrapersonal, interactional, and behavioral components (Zimmerman, 1995). The intrapersonal component includes personality (e.g., locus of control), cognitive (e.g., self-efficacy), and motivational aspects of perceived control (Zimmerman & Rappaport, 1988). Perceived control may be specific to personal, interpersonal, or sociopolitical life domains (Paulhus, 1983). The interactional component of PE refers to how people use analytic skills (e.g., problem-solving) to influence their environment. The behavioral component of PE refers to taking action to exert control by participating in community organizations or activities.

Empowering processes at the individual level of analysis include experiences to exert control by participation in decision-making or problem-solving in one's immediate environment. This may be achieved through participation in community organizations or activities, being involved in work-site management teams, or learning new skills. Processes such as applying cognitive skills (e.g., decision-making), managing resources, or working with others on a common goal may all have empowering potential. Table 1 summarizes empowering processes and empowered outcomes for the individual, as well as the organizational and community levels of analysis.

TABLE 1. A Comparison of Empowering Processes and Empowered Outcomes across Levels of Analysis

Levels of analysis	Process ("empowering")	Outcome ("empowered")
Individual	Learning decision-making skills	Sense of control
	Managing resources	Critical awareness
	Working with others	Participatory behaviors
Organizational	Opportunities to participate in decision-making	Effectively compete for resources
	Shared responsibilities	Networking with other organizations
	Shared leadership	Policy influence
Community	Access to resources	Organizational coalitions
	Open government structure	Pluralistic leadership
	Tolerance for diversity	Residents' participatory skills

Research Related to Psychological Empowerment

Three areas of research—perceived control, citizen participation, and direct efforts to develop empowerment theory—are reviewed briefly below as they pertain to psychological empowerment.

Perceived Control

Perceived control is the belief that one can influence outcomes. The outcome can be achieving a goal or avoiding an undesirable situation. Individuals react differently to situations perceived as controllable versus those seen as uncontrollable (see Gatchel, 1980; Langer, 1983, for reviews). Investigators have found perceived control to reduce psychological stress (Fleming, Baum, & Weiss, 1987; Revicki & May, 1985; Vinokuv & Caplan, 1986) and predict positive health behaviors (Labs & Wurtele, 1986; Sallis, Haskell, Fortman, Vranizan, Taylor, & Soloman, 1986; Seeman & Seeman, 1983; Visher, 1986). Perceived control is also related to social action and political involvement (Gurin, Gurin, Lao, & Beattie, 1969; Lefcourt, 1976; Zimmerman, 1989). The research literature is saturated with distinct measures of perceived control that can be categorized in personality, cognitive, and motivational domains (Zimmerman, 1986). The integration of personality, cognitive, and motivational domains of perceived control provides a basis for studying the intrapersonal component of PE.

The personality domain—locus of control—refers to one's beliefs about the cause of success and failure in one's life, and represents a disposition that includes a generalized expectancy about the relationship between one's actions and outcomes (Lefcourt, 1976; Rotter, 1966). The cognitive domain—self-efficacy—refers to the judgments one makes concerning how well one can perform behaviors necessary to achieve desired goals (Bandura, 1977). Self-efficacy may help determine what activities people engage in, how much effort they will expend to achieve goals, and how long they persevere in the face of adversity (Bandura, 1982). A particularly relevant situation-specific aspect of self-efficacy for PE is political efficacy (Craig & Maggiotto, 1982; Zimmerman, 1989).

The motivational domain of perceived control refers to the notion that mastery of the environment satisfies an intrinsic need to influence the environment (De Charms, 1968; White, 1959). Several investigators have reported that motivational deficits are associated with a perceived lack of control (Alloy, 1982; Glass & Singer, 1972; Sherrod, Hage, Halpern, & Moore, 1977). PE, however, includes more than simply feelings of control; it also includes behaviors to exert control.

Citizen Participation

Participation in community organizations (e.g., neighborhood associations, mutual help groups, social change groups) is one way to exercise a sense of competence and control. Participants in a variety of community organizations have reported an increase in activism and involvement, greater perceived competence and control, and a decrease in alienation. This has been found for individuals involved in welfare rights organizations (Levens, 1968; Zurcher, 1970), nursing-home residents (Langer & Rodin, 1976), members of neighborhood associations (Carr, Dixon, & Ogles, 1976; Chavis & Wandersman, 1990; Florin & Wandersman, 1984), and union members (Denney, 1979).

Stone and Levine (1985) compared activists and nonactivists in the Love Canal environmental conflict—a crisis that affected a thousand families who lived next to an abandoned toxic chemical site. Stone and Levine (1985) collected interview data from 39 individuals during the early stages of the citizen movement, and again several months later. Twenty-four of the respondents were activists. They were compared with their uninvolved neighbors on perceptions of how the Love Canal crisis had affected them personally, and how it influenced their social lives. These researchers found that activists felt better about themselves and reported stronger feelings of political efficacy than non-activists. They also found that activists lost some friends, but were more likely to have developed new friendships. Although research describing naturally occurring events cannot include random selection of people to participation and non-participation groups and, therefore, cannot address the possibility that individuals who chose to participate may already feel more empowered than those who do not participate (i.e., self-selection bias), the longitudinal nature of Stone and Levine's research lends support for the notion that efforts to exert control may have empowering potential.

Fawcett and his colleagues (1980, 1984; Balcazar, Seekins, Fawcett, & Hopkins, 1990) have reported community interventions for increasing individual control over important aspects of their lives. Their work illustrates how human-service professionals can help design and implement what they call social technologies. They use principles of learning theory to train individuals to either solve community problems or enhance community resources. The training provides individuals with the skills and knowledge necessary to gain control in their lives. Fawcett, Seekins, Whang, Muiu, and Suarez de Balcazar (1984) have trained leaders to chair meetings effectively, educate neighbors about the impact of new roadways in their neighborhood, and help handicapped individuals enhance the enforcement of parking regulations and increase awareness of the disabled. Balcazar et al. (1990) describe the results of the training for disabled persons.

Development of Psychological Empowerment Theory

Two studies suggest that psychological empowerment is a combination of personal beliefs of control, involvement in activities to exert control, and a critical awareness of one's environment. The studies provide converging evidence using different research methods. Kieffer (1984) used a qualitative approach to describe the development of PE among community leaders. He conducted in-depth interviews with 15 individuals, including migrant workers, housewives, and miners who emerged as local leaders in grass-roots organizations. He reported that individuals felt more powerful as a result of their involvement, even if they did not actually gain more power. Kieffer (1984) concluded that empowerment encompasses the development of participatory competence that is composed of a positive sense of competence and self-concept, construction of an analytical understanding of the social and political environment, and cultivation of personal and collective resources for social action.

Zimmerman and Rappaport (1988) used a quantitative approach to examine the common variance among several measures of perceived control in student and community samples. They examined the relationship among 11 measures representing personality, cognitive, and motivational domains of perceived control, and participation. Participation was measured in three ways: (1) as an analogue of participation; (2) the level of participation in community organizations; and (3) the extent of involvement in community activities. The analogue measure used responses to hypothetical scenarios in which respondents were asked to indicate whether they would try to change the situations described. Level of involvement in community organizations was a composite of the number of months involved, the number of hours volunteered in a month, the number of leadership positions held, and attendance at organizational meetings for each organization in which respondents listed membership. Extent of involvement in community activities was measured by a 26-item activity checklist that included voting, signing a petition, boycotting a product, organizing people, and writing a letter to an editor. Groups of individuals defined by the participation measures were then compared on the 11 indicators of empowerment.

Results of a discriminant function analysis indicated that the combined variance of the 11 measures of perceived control formed one dimension that distinguished high-participation groups from low- or no-participation groups. Similar results were found for students and community samples across the participation measures. Group differences remained when age, socioeconomic status, sociability, and social desirability were controlled statistically. The dimension that distinguished groups was identified as one component of PE because it represented three domains of perceived control. The results support the notion that PE includes personal control, a sense of competence, a desire to exercise control, and participation. A study using similar measures of participation, comparable measures of perceived control, and a random sample of urban residents replicates these findings (Zimmerman, Israel, Schulz, & Checkoway, 1992).

These studies suggest that psychological empowerment includes intrapersonal, interactional, and behavioral components (Zimmerman, 1995). The intrapersonal component refers to perceived control or beliefs about competence to influence decisions that affect one's life. The interactional component refers to the capability to analyze and understand one's social and political environment (i.e., critical awareness). This includes an ability to understand causal agents (those with authoritative power), their connection to the issue of concern, and the factors that influence their decision-making. A critical awareness also includes knowing when to engage conflict and when to avoid it, and the ability to identify and cultivate resources needed to achieve desired goals. The behavioral component includes participation in collective action, involvement in voluntary or mutual help organizations, or solitary efforts to influence the sociopolitical environment. The specific actions one takes to achieve goals are not as important as attempting to exert control and being involved with others to do so. Empowered individuals have some combination of a sense of control, critical awareness of their sociopolitical environment, and involvement in their community. One component does not necessarily lead to another, nor are they hierarchically ordered. Rather, these components may be found in varying degrees in an individual. It is possible, for example, to participate in collective actions but have little critical awareness or sense of control. Similarly, a person may be astute about causal agents that affect one's life, but take no action to influence those agents. All three of the components would be expected to a large degree in the most highly empowered individuals, but some amount of any of them would suggest some level of PE.

Directions for Future Research

Although the perceived control literature, research on individual outcomes of participation, and comparative analyses of leaders and non-leaders or participants and non-participants are useful starting points, research on PE requires attention to the development of a theoretical framework that is particular to the construct. One research direction is to look at the interaction between perceived control and the development of personal resources. Zimmerman (1990a) has posited the idea of learned hopefulness, which addresses the positive psychological consequences of control experiences. The model, a counterpart of learned helplessness theory, focuses on the positive consequences of efforts to control outcomes. Learned hopefulness is a process by which individuals develop and use personal resources in an effort to exert control in their lives. The resources one develops may include specific skills (e.g., leadership, problem-solving), social support, or knowledge about causal agents. The final outcome in the learned hopefulness model, consistent with an empowerment value orientation, is PE, rather than the decrease in self-concept and motivation found in the learned helplessness literature.

A significant barrier for studying PE is the development of appropriate measurement devices. The development of a universal global measure of PE, however, may not be feasible or conceptually sound, given that the specific meaning of the construct is context- and population-specific. This suggests that measures of PE need to be developed for each specific population with which one is working. Similarly, measures of PE in one life domain may not be appropriate to other settings of an individual's life. Measurement development must include the research participants to help create measures and to test and refine them. The research may also require intense observation and involvement with a particular population in a particular context as a first step in the research process. In-depth study of the research setting and population would not only add to our understanding of PE, but would also add insight into the organizational and community settings in which it develops.

Zimmerman and Zahniser (1991) describe the development of a socio-political control scale, and suggest that it measures two aspects of the intrapersonal component of PE that may be particularly relevant for members of voluntary organizations or individuals involved in community organizing. Items from ten measures that represented personality, cognitive, and motivational domains of perceived control were empirically selected and factor-analyzed. A two-factor solution was replicated across two samples and validity analyses were consistent across three samples. The factors were identified as policy control and leadership confidence; however, the limits of self-report scales designed to measure the intrapersonal aspects of empowerment are perhaps more instructive for future research than the scale itself.

Self-report measures can provide us with a convenient tool for data collection, but it is important to keep in mind the limits of such measures. Research that simply labels individuals based on their response to self-report items may not be the best way to develop the construct of PE. Self-report scales tend to suggest a static level of competence, an idea that is antithetical to the concept of empowerment. PE is not a trait that some of us are born with and others are not, nor is it a normally distributed individual difference variable; rather, it is earned, developed, and ongoing (Zimmerman, 1990b). All people have the potential to empower themselves. Measures must be population- and situation-specific and must include relevant aspects of perceived control, knowledge of causal agents, and participation (Zimmerman, 1995). Future research could also begin to examine the relationship among the intrapersonal, interactional, and behavioral components of PE for different populations and settings.

ORGANIZATIONAL EMPOWERMENT

A distinction must be made between what the organization provides to members, and what the organization achieves in the community. Organizations that provide opportunities for people to gain control over their lives are empowering organizations. Organizations that successfully develop, influence policy decisions, or offer effective alternatives for service provision are empowered organizations. Although a distinction between empowering and empowered organizations is made, organizations may have both characteristics.

An empowering organization may have little impact on policy, but may provide members with opportunities to develop skills and a sense of control. Hobby clubs, for example, are typically not interested in political issues or community decision-making, but they do require leadership, resource management, and coordination of activities. They also provide settings in which people with similar interests share information and experiences and develop a sense of identity with others. Organizations with shared responsibilities, a supportive atmosphere, and social activities are expected to be more empowering than hierarchical organizations (Maton & Rappaport, 1984; Prestby, Wandersman, Florin, Rich, & Chavis, 1990). Several investigators suggest that formal organizational practices may play a central role in empowering members (Conger & Kanungo, 1988; Heil, 1991; Klein, this volume). Maton and Salem (1995) examined three community organizations to identify common empowering themes. They described four vital characteristics of an empowering organization: (1) a culture of growth and community building; (2) opportunities for members to take on meaningful and multiple roles; (3) a peer-based support system that helps members develop a social identity; and (4) shared leadership with commitment to both members and the organization. Gruber and Trickett (1987), however, point out that empowering organizational structures may also work to undermine the act of empowerment if members do not share real decision-making power.

Empowered organizations are those that successfully thrive among competitors, meet their goals, and develop in ways that enhance their effectiveness. Empowered organizations may or may not provide opportunities for members to develop a sense of empowerment, but they do become key brokers in the policy-decision process. Empowered organizations may extend their influence to wider geographical areas and more diverse audiences. They are also expected to effectively mobilize resources such as money, facilities, and members (Ferree & Miller, 1985; Jenkins, 1983; McCarthy & Zald, 1978). One may to efficiently compete for limited resources is to connect with other organizations to share information and resources, and to create a strong base of support. Table 1 presents characteristics of empowering and empowered organizations.

Research Related to Organizational Empowerment

Empowering Organizations

Research on the characteristics of an empowering organization can be found in studies of organizational structure. Organizations with participatory decision-making structures may enhance opportunities for members to develop a sense of PE. The voluminous literature on participative decision-making in organizations suggests that participation leads to greater job satisfaction and productivity (Miller & Monge, 1986). Jackson (1983), for example, used a Solomon-four group design in a hospital setting to evaluate an intervention designed to increase employee participation in decision-making. She found participation reduced role conflict and role ambiguity, and increased perceived control and job satisfaction. Bartunek and Keys (1982) found similar results for an intervention designed to increase teachers' roles in school decision-making. An organization that provides opportunities for member participation in decision-making could be considered an empowering organization.

Social climate may also be a factor in determining the empowering potential of community organizations. Dougherty (1988) studied the relationships among social climate, participation, and personal and political efficacy for members of a neighborhood association. She found high levels of task orientation increased members' perceived control over neighborhood and local government policy. McMillan et al. (1995) also found that organizations that were task-focused and included pluralistic decision-making structures were more empowering than less focused and inclusive settings. Maton (1988) examined the relationship between organizational characteristics and members' self-esteem, psychological well-being, and group appraisal among 144 members from three different self-help groups. He found members from groups with shared roles and responsibilities reported more well-being and self-esteem than members in groups where control was concentrated in a single leader. He also found that groups in which members perceived high levels of order and organization reported more benefits from group involvement than members in less organized settings.

Empowered Organizations

Riger (1984) describes several factors that may influence the survival of feminist-movement organizations. She examined ideology, goal orientation, and decision-making procedures for several women's organizations. She found that unresolved conflict between ideology and the decision-making process often led to the demise of the organization. For example, strict adherence to collective decision-making was not always the most effective way to solve organizational conflict, but other types of decision-making processes were not congruent with the organizations' ideology, so members did not use them. Riger (1984) recommends that understanding the development and resolution of ideological conflicts in politically oriented organizations may help to insure their survival and enhance their empowering potential. Conflict-management issues may help distinguish between empowered organizations and those with less impact on policy.

Another approach to studying empowered organizations is to investigate how they develop and influence social policy. Checkoway and his colleagues (1980, 1982) report the development of a health-care consumer advocacy group. They describe how the consumers gained control of a county health planning board and proceeded to insure that their health-care needs were met. They included an analysis of the factors that contributed to the groups' success: (a) planning step-by-step procedures for achieving goals; (b) choosing issues of a broad concern that were also specific enough to appeal to many people; (c) collecting data to support their point of view; and (d) holding public meetings to present their findings and rally support. They also found that the group created alliances with other organizations to help them achieve their goals.

Zimmerman, Reischl, Seidman, Rappaport, Toro, and Salem (1991) describe the expansion strategies used by a mutual help organization for individuals experiencing emotional difficulties. The organization grew from 12 groups and a $30,000 per year budget to 100 groups and a $500,000 per year budget in a little over five years. The organization mobilized resources from a variety of sources, delineated responsibility for obtaining different resources, and targeted particular providers for specific resources. The organization also used the strategy of creating underpopulated settings (Barker, 1960; Perkins, Burns, Perry, & Nielsen, 1988) as a way to encourage individual involvement. The organization would create a setting before the necessary personnel were available to maintain it. These strategies appeared to avoid overtaxing resource pools, reduce job ambiguity, and encourage member participation.

Snow, Zurcher, and Elkind-Olson (1980) examined the membership recruitment strategies of several community organizations. They examined case studies of emerging organizations and queried university students about their involvement and recruitment experiences. They found that organizations that were linked to other groups and tapped social networks outside the organization grew faster and developed larger memberships than more isolated groups. Organizations, like individuals, may have a better chance of becoming empowered if they are connected to other groups and exploit existing resources to foster development. Networking has been found to be related to organizational longevity and success for advocacy (Kelly, 1986) and citizen protest (Lindgren, 1987) groups.

Directions for Future Research

Future research on the empowering potential of organizations could examine the relationship between skills learned from involvement and organizational characteristics. These issues can be examined for different types of organizations (e.g., policy change, community service, problem amelioration) and different organizational structures (e.g., participatory decision-making, decentralized authority). The social climate of organizations could also be used to distinguish different types of settings. For example, social climate variables such as organization, cohesion, self-discovery, and task orientation may be especially relevant for empowerment in some organizations, but not others.

Research on empowered organizations can expand on resource mobilization theory and research. Studies that describe processes for identifying, obtaining, and managing resources may help distinguish empowered organizations from organizations less effective in the policy process. Comparative studies of organizations with different resource mobilization strategies can help us understand the factors that may influence organizational empowerment. Research could examine the type of organizations that connect with other organizations, and the effects of networking on organizational survival and goal achievement.

Another research direction could be to evaluate the effectiveness of community organizations. Crosby, Kelly, and Schaefer (1986) describe six criteria for evaluating the success of citizen participation. They suggest that effective participation includes: (1) pluralistic representation; (2) skill-training and shared information for decision-making; (3) equal input at all stages of the decision-making process; (4) long-term evaluation of costs; (5) adaptable methods so several different tasks and decisions can be worked on; and (6) being seriously considered in final decisions. These criteria can be applied to different types of organizations as a way to examine empowering processes and empowered outcomes.

COMMUNITY EMPOWERMENT

An empowered community is one that initiates efforts to improve the community, responds to threats to quality of life, and provides opportunities for citizen participation. Iscoe (1974) identifies a community in which its citizens have the skills, desire, and resources to engage in activities to improve community life as a competent community. Cottrell (1983) describes a competent community by the extent to which interdependent components of a community work together to effectively identify community needs, develop strategies to address the needs, and perform actions to meet those needs. Minkler (1990) suggests that shared leadership and its development are critical for developing competent communities.

The structure and relationships among community organizations and agencies also helps to define the extent to which a community is empowered. An empowered community is expected to comprise well-connected organizations (i.e., coalitions) that are both empowered and empowering. It also has settings for citizen involvement in activities such as neighborhood crime prevention, planning commissions, and health care. This requires several different types of voluntary organizations, resource accessibility for all members of the community, and equal opportunities for involvement.

An empowering community also includes accessible resources for all community residents. Resources include recreational facilities (e.g., parks, playing fields), protective services (e.g., police, fire), health and mental health care (e.g., emergency medical services), and general services (e.g., media, sanitation). Empowering communities, for example, are expected to have media resources available to residents. These might include accessible radio and television stations, as well as editorial pages open to multiple perspectives. A balanced presentation of the news helps to encourage critical discourse among residents, increases the chances that problem solutions would represent a variety of viewpoints, and suggests a tolerance for diversity. White (1981) provides a useful analysis of the power of the media and the importance of citizen involvement for influencing television programming (see also McAlister, this volume). Empowering processes in a community also include an open governmental system that takes citizen attitudes and concerns seriously, and includes strong leadership that seeks advice and help from community members. The town meetings popular in New England are a good example of a participatory governmental structure. Table 1 summarizes the characteristics of empowering and empowered communities.

Research Related to Community Empowerment

O'Sullivan, Waugh, and Espeland (1984) report a case study of a Native American community's successful efforts to stop a relocation effort. Community leaders wanted to build a dam that would flood their tribal homeland. The Fort McDowell Yavapai Indians, a community of only 350 people, fought business interests and federal government regulatory agencies to prevent the flooding. Their efforts included using community surveys to show the psychological impact of relocation, uniting with local environmental groups, and exploiting the media to stop plans to build the dam. This is an excellent example of community empowerment because it highlights media accessibility, coalitions among organizations, and the critical awareness among residents to successfully influence causal agents.

Maynard (1986) describes how a town in New Hampshire successfully persuaded the U.S. Department of Energy to change its plans for building a nuclear waste repository in their community. She describes how the community obtained information on nuclear waste, informed each other of the implications of living near the dump site, and organized to remove their community from a list of potential sites being considered. This is a good example of united community leadership, competent residents seeking information on the issues, and dissemination of information throughout the community for individuals to make their own choices about the proposed dump site.

Freudenberg and Golub (1987) describe the development of the NYC Coalition to End Lead Poisoning. The coalition included housing activists, health educators, physicians, social workers, and community organizers. The coalition was established after early lead poisoning prevention efforts failed to maintain vigilance on the issue. They used small group meetings, community organizing, coalition-building, and mass-media coverage to alert residents about the problem of lead poisoning, and to motivate the city to develop more preventive efforts. This case study provides an example of the processes involved in an empowering community. Minkler (1985) describes efforts to foster social support and social activism among low-income elderly. Other examples of community-empowerment processes and outcomes can be found for toxic waste issues (Levine, 1982), welfare and civil rights (Pivan & Cloward, 1977), arson prevention (Maciak, Moore, Leviton, & Guinan, 1998), community health and mental health services (Cravens, 1981), and neighborhood associations (Alinsky, 1971; Fish, 1973). These case studies emphasize the importance of organizational coalitions, media involvement, and pluralistic leadership.

Community network analysis may be a useful approach for describing empowered communities (Galaskiewicz, 1979; Morrissey, Tausig, & Lindsey, 1986). Galaskiewicz (1979) examined organizational networks in a community and identified monetary, informational, and supportive networks. The monetary network was bipolar with a private and public sector. The information networks were separated by activities, and included television and radio stations, newspapers, colleges, and organizations such as the Chamber of Commerce and United Way. The support networks were the least well-defined and included hospitals and social service agencies. He also studied the extent and density of the networks, and reported that the most central organizations were those with the most available resources.

Morrissey et al. (1986) studied mental health system networks in two communities. They interviewed agency directors about their organizational affiliation with other similar service organizations in the community and found little evidence for a formally coordinated system of services for the chronically mentally ill, but the agencies did play a role in connecting disjointed agency sectors. They also found that institutionally based and community-based services worked primarily independently of one another. Community network analysis suggests that organizational relationships may be useful for identifying factors that enhance or inhibit community involvement and understanding resource accessibility.

Directions for Future Research

The structure and content of community networks may help to identify the level of integration, shared problem-solving, and cooperation among organizations in a community. Organizational network analysis is particularly relevant for community empowerment because it can be used to describe the nature of resource exchange and the amount of integration among community organizations. Network analysis can also be useful for understanding the connections among causal agents and their relationships with resource distribution and accessibility.

Future research at the community level of analysis could also begin to identify environmental factors associated with empowerment. Some areas within a city may be more empowering than others because they have active neighborhood associations, access to government officials, and shared leadership. Environmental factors such as housing and common spaces may help influence the empowering potential or the level of empowerment within a given section of a city. It may be easier, for example, to organize residents living in high-density housing where accessible meeting places are available than in more dispersed housing conditions with limited public space. Perkins, Florin, Rich, Wandersman, and Chavis (1990) found that the physical environment of a neighborhood was related to residents' level of participation in a neighborhood association.

Research on community empowerment could also begin to examine how empowered individuals work together to create competent communities. This research might examine how leadership develops in the community and the organizations or settings in which it develops. The opportunities for getting involved and their accessibility to residents may be an important part of research on leadership development. Research on community empowerment might also examine the source and flow of different resources, and study how individuals unite to gain access to a greater share of community resources.

CRITICAL ANALYSIS

While empowerment theory is a fundamental concept in community psychology, it remains somewhat enigmatic. It is certainly not a panacea for solving community problems, conducting research, or understanding natural helping systems. In some instances, it may actually be used as an excuse to hold individuals responsible for their life situations, and provide a rationale for relieving institutional responsibility to take care of people and communities through structural interventions. It is a useful construct that is consistent with our values, helps redefine our roles as professionals and our community collaborators, and gives us a conceptual framework to understand community participation. Yet it is not a remedy for all problems and is not applicable in all contexts. Conversely, the difficulty in measuring empowerment has led some to dismiss its usefulness, but that does not diminish its validity as a vital concept for the field. Empowerment may be most useful as a heuristic for our work. One could argue that empowerment is only of interest to the extent that it results in some other outcome. Zimmerman et al. (1997) describe an intervention designed to prevent the spread of HIV/AIDS among Mexican males living on the border between the United States and Mexico. The intervention used an empowering process whereby participants were involved in developing, implementing, and evaluating the intervention. Participants soon took over leadership of the project by setting the agenda for topics covered, developing resources for the intervention, planning strategies to distribute condoms, providing assistance to people with HIV/AIDS, conducting community education campaigns, and forming partnerships with other organizations. The evaluation of the intervention included attitudes, knowledge, and behavior related to HIV/AIDS prevention, but did not assess individual empowerment outcomes (i.e., psychological empowerment). The results indicated that participants engaged in more preventive behaviors than did non-participants. This study suggests that empowering strategies may be beneficial regardless of the effects they may have on the level of empowerment achieved for participants (psychological).

Another issue raised about empowerment is that it is equivalent to power. The two constructs are fundamentally connected, but they are not the same (Zimmerman, 1995). Power that refers to authority is not analogous to empowerment. Several researchers have reported instances in which politically disenfranchised groups with no official authority struggled to influence those with governmentally mandated power and succeeded (e.g., Freudenberg & Golub, 1987; Minkler, 1985; O'Sullivan, Waugh & Espeland, 1984). They may not have gained any real authoritative power, but they did influence the decisions of those in power. Empowerment may be more closely linked to social power (Speer & Hughey, 1995), which refers to the application of resources to hinder or facilitate community decision-making. While this type of power is not authoritative power, it does involve the capability to reward (or punish) causal agents, influence public debate and policy, and shape community ideology and consciousness. Speer and Hughey (1995) suggest that community organizations provide the means by which disenfranchised individuals gain social power. Power is linked to empowerment because the theory includes issues regarding the struggle for power, power relationships, and efforts to exert control over, or influence on, community power structures, but they are distinct constructs.

Although empowerment theory has consistently included multiple levels of analysis, the preponderance of research has been on psychological empowerment. This may lead to the erroneous conclusion that empowerment is solely an individual-level construct. Efforts to understand organizational and community empowerment are clearly necessary to help move the theory beyond the individual bias of psychology. The theory may also unintentionally suggest that conceptions of control, participation, and community favor traditionally masculine and Western standards. This, too, may be an erroneous assumption because the particular definition or meaning of the concepts in empowerment theory depends on the population with whom one is working, and the context in the which the work is being done. Zimmerman (1995) points out that empowerment is an open-ended construct that may not be fully captured by a single operationalization uniformly applied because, by its very nature, it takes on different forms in distinct populations, contexts, and times. In the final analysis, empowerment theory is an effort to provide a conceptual framework for understanding processes and outcomes associated with the continuing struggle to make our lives, organizations, and communities closer to our ideal. The closer the correspondence between our goals, our sense of how to achieve them, and our efforts to succeed, the closer we are to being empowered.

SUMMARY AND CONCLUSIONS

Participation, control, and critical awareness are essential aspects of empowerment. At the individual level of analysis, these factors include a belief in one's ability to exert control (intrapersonal component), involvement in decision-making (behavioral component), and an understanding of causal agents (interactional component). At the organizational level of analysis, these factors refer to settings that provide individuals with opportunities to exert control and organizational effectiveness in service delivery and the policy process. At the community level of analysis, these factors refer to the contexts in which organizations and individuals interact to enhance community living, and insure that their communities address local needs and concerns.

Social change and policy developed from an empowerment perspective requires a redefinition of terms and methods. Professional help that limits itself to experts giving advice in an office or to intrapsychic adjustment to current social realities is antithetical to an empowerment approach. An empowerment approach is concerned with resources and formal settings for enhancing natural helping systems and creating opportunities for participatory decision-making. The focus is on enhancing strengths and promoting health, rather than fixing problems and addressing risk factors.

Empowerment theory connects individual well-being with the larger social and political environment, and suggests that people need opportunities to become active in community decision-making in order to improve their lives, organizations, and communities. Individual participants may develop a sense of empowerment even if wrong decisions are made because they may develop a greater understanding of the decision-making process, develop confidence to influence decisions that affect their lives, and work to make their concerns known. Organizations may be empowering even if policy change is not achieved because they provide settings in which individuals can attempt to take control of their own lives. Communities may enhance opportunities for residents to participate in the policy process even if some battles are lost. A community can be empowered because the citizens engage in activities that maintain or improve their collective quality of life.

Empowerment is a multilevel construct that requires us to think in terms of health promotion, self- and mutual-help, and multiple definitions of competence. Research on empowerment will add to our understanding of individual adaptation, organizational development, and community life. Empowerment is an individual-level construct when one is concerned with intrapersonal and behavioral variables, an organizational-level construct when one is concerned with resource mobilization and participatory opportunities, and a community-level construct when sociopolitical structure and social change are of concern. We can begin to learn about the contexts in which empowerment takes place and the processes by which empowerment develops if we study the settings that provide opportunities for natural helping systems to flourish and grow.

ACKNOWLEDGMENTS. I would like to thank James G. Kelly, Thomas A. Reischl, and the editors of this Handbook, Julian Rappaport and Ed Seidman, for their thoughtful comments on earlier drafts of this chapter. I would also like to extend special thanks to Deborah A. Salem, whose support and comments on earlier drafts made this chapter possible, and to Mary Jane Ormsby, for her assistance in formatting the manuscript.

REFERENCES

Alinsky, S. (1971). *Rules for radicals.* NY: Vintage.

Alloy, L. B. (1982). The role of perceptions and attributions for response-outcome noncontingency in learned helplessness: A commentary and discussion. *Journal of Personality, 50,* 443–479.

Balcazar, F. E., Seekins, T., Fawcett, S. B., & Hopkins, B. L. (1990). Empowering people with physical disabilities through advocacy skills training. *American Journal of Community Psychology, 18,* 281–296.

Bandura, A. (1977). Self-efficacy: Towards a unifying theory of behavior change. *Psychological Review, 84,* 191–215.

Bandura, A. (1982). Self-efficacy mechanism in human agency. *American Psychologist, 37,* 122–147.

Barker, R. G. (1960). Ecology and motivation. *Nebraska Symposium on Motivation, 8,* 1–44.

Bartunek, J., & Keys, C. (1982). Power equalization in schools through organizational development. *Journal of Applied Behavioral Science, 18,* 171–183.

Berger, P. J., & Neuhaus, R. J. (1977). *To empower people: The role of mediating structures in public policy.* Washington, D.C.: American Enterprise Institute for Public Policy Research.

Brown, L. D. (1983). Organizing participatory research: Interfaces for joint inquiry and organizational change. *Journal of Occupational Behavior, 4,* 9–19.

Carr, T. H., Dixon, M. C., & Ogles, R. M. (1976). Perceptions of community life which distinguish between participants and nonparticipants in a neighborhood self-help organization. *American Journal of Community Psychology, 4,* 357–366.

Chavis, D. M., & Wandersman, A. (1990). Sense of community in the urban environment: A catalyst for participation and community development. *American Journal of Community Psychology, 18,* 55–81.

Checkoway, B. (1982). The empire strikes back: More lessons for health care consumers. *Journal of Health Politics, Policy, and Law, 7,* 111–124.

Checkoway, B., & Doyle, M. (1980). Community organizing lessons for health care consumers. *Journal of Health Politics, Policy, and Law, 5,* 213–226.

Chesler, M. A. (1991). Participatory action research with self-help groups: An alternative paradigm for inquiry and action. *American Journal of Community Psychology, 19,* 757–768.

Conger, J. A., & Kanungo, R. N. (1988). The empowerment process: Integrating theory and practice. *Academy of Management Review, 13,* 471–481.

Cornell Empowerment Group. (1989). Empowerment and family support. *Networking Bulletin, 1,* 1–23.

Cottrell, L. S., Jr. (1983). The competent community. In R. Warren & L. Lyon (Eds.), *New perspectives on the American community* (pp. 398–432). Homewood, IL: Dorsey.

Craig, S. C., & Maggiotto, M. (1982). Measuring political efficacy. *Political Methodology, 8,* 85–109.

Cravens, R. B. (1981). Grassroots participation in community mental health. In W. Silverman (Ed.), *Community mental health.* New York: Praeger.

Crosby, N., Kelly, J. M., & Schaefer, P. (1986). Citizen panels: A new approach to citizen participation. *Public Administration Review, 46*, 170–178.

De Charms, R. (1968). *Personal causation.* New York: Academic.

Denney, W. M. (1979). Participant citizenship in a marginal group: Union membership of California farm workers. *American Journal of Political Science, 23*, 330–337.

Dougherty, D. (1988). *Participation in community organizations: Effects on political efficacy, personal efficacy, and self-esteem.* Doctoral Dissertation, Boston University, Boston, MA.

Fawcett, S. B., Mathews, R. M., & Fletcher, R. K. (1980). Some promising dimensions for behavioral community technology. *Journal of Applied Behavior Analysis, 13*, 505–518.

Fawcett, S. B., Seekins, T., Whang, P. L., Muiu, C., & Suarez de Balcazar, Y. (1984). Creating and using social technologies for community empowerment. *Prevention in Human Services, 3*, 145–171.

Fawcett, S. B., White, G. W., Balcazar, F. E., Suarez-Balcazar, Y., Mathews, R. M., Paine, A. L., Seekins, T., and Smith, J. F. (1994). A contextual-behavioral model of empowerment: Case studies involving people with physical disabilities. *American Journal of Community Psychology, 22*, 471–486.

Ferree, M. M., & Miller, F. D. (1985). Mobilization and meaning: Toward an integration of social psychological and resource perspectives on social movements. *Sociological Inquiry, 55*, 38–61.

Fetterman, D. M. (1996). Empowerment evaluation: An introduction to theory and practice. In D. M. Fetterman, S. J. Kaftarian, & A. Wandersman (Eds.), *Empowerment evaluation: Knowledge and tools for self-assessment and accountability* (pp. 3–46). Thousand Oaks, CA: Sage.

Fish, J. (1973). *Black power/white control: The struggle of the Woodlawn Organization in Chicago.* Princeton, NJ: Princeton University Press.

Fleming, I., Baum, A., & Weiss, L. (1987). Social density and perceived control as mediators of crowding stress in high density residential neighborhoods. *Journal of Personality and Social Psychology, 52*, 899–906.

Florin, P., & Wandersman, A. (1984). Cognitive social learning and participation in community development. *American Journal of Community Psychology, 12*, 689–708.

Freudenberg, N., & Golub, M. (1987). Health education, public policy, and disease prevention: A case history of the New York City Coalition to End Lead Poisoning. *Health Education Quarterly, 14*, 387–401.

Galaskiewicz, J. (1979). *Exchange networks and community politics.* Beverly Hills, CA: Sage.

Gallant, R. V., Cohen, C., & Wolff, T. (1985). Change of older persons' image, impact on public policy result from Highland Valley Empowerment Plan. *Perspective on Aging, 14*, 9–13.

Gatchel, R. (1980). Perceived control: A review and evaluation of therapeutic application. In A. Baum & J. Singer (Eds.), *Advances in environmental psychology* (pp. 1–22). Hillsdale, NJ: Erlbaum.

Glass, D. C., & Singer, J. E. (1972). *Urban stress: Experiments on noise and social stressors.* New York: Academic.

Gruber, J., & Trickett, E. J. (1987). Can we empower others? The paradox of empowerment in the governing of an alternative public school. *American Journal of Community Psychology, 15*, 353–371.

Gurin, P., Gurin, G., Lao, R. C., & Beattie, M. (1969). Internal-external locus of control in the motivational dynamics of negro youth. *Journal of Social Issues, 25*, 129–153.

Heil, W. B. (1991, August). *Re-reviewing participation in decision-making: Toward a multidimensional model.* Paper presented at the Ninety-Ninth Annual Convention of the American Psychological Association, San Francisco, CA.

Iscoe, I. (1974). Community psychology and the competent community. *American Psychologist, 29*, 607–613.

Israel, B. A., Schulz, A. J., Parker, E. A., & Becker, A. B. (1998). Review of community-based research: Assessing partnership approaches to improve public health. *Annual Review of Public Health, 19*, 173–202.

Jackson, S. E. (1983). Participation in decision-making as a strategy for reducing job-related strain. *Journal of Applied Psychology, 68*, 3–19.

Jenkins, J. C. (1983). Resource mobilization theory and the study of social movements. *Annual Review of Sociology, 9*, 527–553.

Kelly, J. G. (1970). Antidotes for arrogance: Training for community psychology. *American Psychologist, 25*, 524–531.

Kelly, J. G. (1971). Qualities for the community psychologist. *American Psychologist, 26*, 897–903.

Kelly, J. G. (1986). Context and process: An ecological view of the interdependence of practice and research. *American Journal of Community Psychology, 14*, 581–589.

Kelly, J. G. (1988). A guide to conducting prevention research in the community: First steps. *Prevention in Human Services, 6*, 1–174.

Kieffer, C. H. (1984). Citizen empowerment: A developmental perspective. *Prevention in Human Services, 3*, 9–36.

Labs, S. M., & Wurtele, S. K. (1986). Fetal health locus of control scale: Development and validation. *Journal of Consulting and Clinical Psychology, 54*, 814–819.

Langer, E. J. (1983). *The Psychology of Control.* Beverly Hills, CA: Sage.

Langer, E. J., & Rodin, J. (1976). The effects of choice and enhanced personal responsibility for the aged: A field experiment in an institutional setting. *Journal of Personality and Social Psychology, 34*, 191–198.

Lefcourt, H. (1976). *Locus of control: Current trends in theory and research.* Hillsdale, NJ: Erlbaum.

Levens, H. (1968). Organizational affiliation and powerlessness: A case study of the welfare poor. *Social Problems, 16*, 18–32.

Levine, A. G. (1982). *Love Canal: Science, politics, and people.* Lexington, MA: Lexington Books.

Lincoln, Y. S., & Guba, E. G. (1986). But is that rigorous?: Trustworthiness and authenticity in naturalistic evaluation. In D. D. Williams (Ed.), *Naturalistic evaluation: New directions for program evaluation* (pp. 73–84). San Francisco: Jossey-Bass.

Lindgren, H. E. (1987). The informal-intermittent organization: A vehicle for successful citizen protest. *Journal of Applied Behavioral Science, 23*, 397–412.

Maciak, B. J., Moore, M. T., Leviton, L. C., & Guinan, M. E. (1998). Preventing Halloween arson in an urban setting: A model for multisectoral planning and community participation. *Health Education & Behavior, 25*, 194–211.

Maton, K. I. (1988). Social support, organizational characteristics, psychological well-being, and group appraisal in three self-help group populations. *American Journal of Community Psychology, 16*, 53–78.

Maton, K. I., & Rappaport, J. (1984). Empowerment in a religious setting: A multivariate investigation. *Prevention in Human Services, 3*, 37–70.

Maton, K. I., & Salem, D. A. (1995). Organizational characteristics of empowering community settings: A multiple case study approach. *American Journal of Community Psychology, 23*, 631–656.

Maynard, J. (1986, May 11). The people of New Hampshire against the nuclear dump. *New York Times Magazine*, pp. 20–22, 24–25, 40.

McCarthy, J. D., & Zald, M. (1978). Resource mobilization and social movements: A partial theory. *American Journal of Sociology, 82*, 1212–1241.

McMillan, B., Florin, P., Stevenson, J., Kerman, B., & Mitchell, R. E. (1995). Empowerment praxis in community coalitions. *American Journal of Community Psychology, 23*, 699–727.

Mechanic, D. (1991, February). *Adolescents at risk: New directions.* Paper presented at the Seventh Annual Conference on Health Policy, Cornell University Medical College.

Miller, K. I., & Monge, P. R. (1986). Participation, satisfaction, and productivity: A meta-analytic review. *Academy of Management Journal, 29*, 727–753.

Minkler, M. (1985). Building supportive ties and sense of community among inner-city elderly: The tenderloin senior outreach project. *Health Education Quarterly, 12*, 303–314.

Minkler, M. (1990). Improving health through community organization. In K. Glanz, F. M. Lewis, & B. K. Rimer (Eds.), *Health behavior and health education: Theory, research, and practice* (pp. 257–287). San Francisco: Jossey-Bass.

Morrissey, J. P., Tausig, M., & Lindsey, M. L. (1986). Interorganizational networks in mental health systems: Assessing community support programs for the chronically mentally ill. In W. R. Scott & B. L. Black (Eds.), *The organization of mental health services* (pp. 197–230). Beverly Hills, CA: Sage.

O'Sullivan, M. J., Waugh, N., & Espeland, W. (1984). The Fort McDowell Yavapai: From pawns to powerbrokers. *Prevention in Human Services, 3*, 73–97.

Pasmore, W., & Friedlander, F. (1982). An action-research program for increasing employee involvement in problem solving. *Administrative Science Quarterly, 27*, 343–362.

Paulhus, D. (1983). Sphere-specific measures of perceived control. *Journal of Personality and Social Psychology, 44*, 1253–1265.

Perkins, D., Burns, T., Perry, J., & Nielsen, K. (1988). Behavior setting theory and community psychology: An analysis and critique. *Journal of Community Psychology, 16*, 355–371.

Perkins, D. D., Florin, P., Rich, R. C., Wandersman, A., & Chavis, D. M. (1990). Participation and the social and physical environment of a residential block: Crime and community context. *American Journal of Community Psychology, 18*, 55–82.

Perkins, D. D., & Zimmerman, M. A. (1995). Empowerment theory, research, and application. An introduction to a special issue. *American Journal of Community Psychology, 23*, 569–579.

Peters, M., & Robinson, V. (1984). The origins and status of action research. *Journal of Applied Behavioral Science, 20*, 113–124.

Pivan, F. F., & Cloward, R. A. (1977). *Poor people's movements: Why they succeed, how they fail.* New York: Vintage Books.

Prestby, J. E., Wandersman, A., Florin, P., Rich, R., & Chavis, D. M. (1990). Benefits, costs, incentive management, and participation in voluntary organizations: A means to understanding and promoting empowerment. *American Journal of Community Psychology, 18*, 117–149.

Rappaport, J. (1981) In praise of paradox: A social policy of empowerment over prevention. *American Journal of Community Psychology, 9,* 1–25.

Rappaport, J. (1984). Studies in empowerment: Introduction to the issue. *Prevention in Human Services, 3,* 1–7.

Rappaport, J. (1985). The power of empowerment language. *Social Policy, 16,* 15–21.

Rappaport, J. (1990). Research methods and the empowerment social agenda. In P. Tolan, C. Keys, F. Chertok, & L. Jason (Eds.), *Researching Community Psychology* (pp. 51–63). Washington, D.C.: American Psychological Association.

Revicki, D., & May, H. J. (1985). Occupation stress, social support, and depression. *Health Psychology, 4,* 899–906.

Riger, S. (1984). Vehicles for empowerment: The case of feminist movement organizations. *Prevention in Human Services, 3,* 99–118.

Rotter, J. B. (1966). Generalized experiences for internal versus external control of reinforcement. *Psychological Monographs, 80,* 1014–1053.

Sallis, J. F., Haskell, W. L., Fortman, S. P., Vranizan, K. M., Taylor, C. B., & Soloman, D. S. (1986). Predictors of adoption and maintenance of physical activity in a community sample. *Preventive Medicine, 15,* 331–341.

Seeman, M., & Seeman, T. (1983). Health behavior and personal autonomy: A longitudinal study of the sense of control in illness. *Journal of Health and Social Behavior, 24,* 144–160.

Serrano-Garcia, I. (1984). The illusion of empowerment: Community development within a colonial context. *Prevention in Human Services, 3,* 173–200.

Sherrod, D. R., Hage, J. N., Halpern, H. L., & Moore, B. S. (1977). Effects of personal causation and perceived control on responses to an adverse environment: The more the control the better. *Journal of Experimental Social Psychology, 13,* 14–27.

Snow, D. A., Zurcher, L. A., & Elkind-Olson, S. (1980). Social networks and social movements. *American Sociological Review, 45,* 787–801.

Speer, P. W., & Hughey, J. (1995). Community organizing: An ecological route to empowerment and power. *American Journal of Community Psychology, 23,* 729–748.

Stone, R. A., & Levine, A. G. (1985). Reactions to collective stress: Correlates of active citizen participation. *Prevention in Human Services, 4,* 153–177.

Sue, S., & Zane, N. (1980). Learned helplessness theory and community psychology. In M. S. Gibbs, J. R. Lachenmeyer, & J. Sigal (Eds.), *Community psychology: Theoretical and empirical approaches* (pp. 121–143). New York: Gardner.

Swift, C., & Levine, G. (1987). Empowerment an emerging mental health technology. *Journal of Primary Prevention, 8,* 71–94.

Vinokuv, A., & Caplan, R. D. (1986). Cognitive and affective components of life events: The relations and effects of well being. *American Journal of Community Psychology, 14,* 351–370.

Visher, S. C. (1986). The relationship of locus of control and contraception use in the adolescent population. *Journal of Adolescent Health Care, 7,* 183–187.

White, D. M. (1981). "Mediacracy": Mass media and psychopathology. In J.M. Joffe & G. W. Albee (Eds.), *Prevention through political action and social change.* Hanover, NH: University Press of New England.

White, R. W. (1959). Motivation reconsidered: The concept of competence. *Psychological Review, 66,* 297–333.

Zimmerman, M. A. (1986). *Citizen participation, perceived control, and psychological empowerment.* Unpublished doctoral dissertation, University of Illinois, Urbana-Champaign.

Zimmerman, M. A. (1989). The relationship between political efficacy and citizen participation: Construct validation studies. *Journal of Personality Assessment, 53,* 554–566.

Zimmerman, M. A. (1990a). Toward a theory of learned hopefulness: A structural model analysis of participation and empowerment. *Journal of Research in Personality, 24,* 71–86.

Zimmerman, M. A. (1990b). Taking aim on empowerment research: On the distinction between psychological and individual conceptions. *American Journal of Community Psychology, 18,* 169–177.

Zimmerman, M. A. (1995). Psychological empowerment: Issues and illustrations. *American Journal of Community Psychology, 23,* 581–600.

Zimmerman, M. A. Israel, B. I., Schulz, A., & Checkoway, B. (1992). Further explorations in empowerment theory: An empirical analysis of psychological empowerment. *American Journal of Community Psychology, 20,* 707–728.

Zimmerman, M. A., Ramirez-Valles, J., Suarez, E., de la Rosa, G., & Castro, M. A. (1997). An HIV/AIDS prevention project for Mexican homosexual men: An empowerment approach. *Health Education & Behavior, 24,* 177–190.

Zimmerman, M. A., Reischl, T. R., Rappaport, J., Seidman, E., Toro, P. A., & Salem, D. A. (1991). Expansion strategies of a mutual help organization. *American Journal of Community Psychology, 19,* 251–278.

Zimmerman, M. A., & Rappaport, J. (1988). Citizen participation, perceived control, and psychological empowerment. *American Journal of Community Psychology, 16,* 725–750.

Zimmerman, M. A., & Warschausky, S. (1998). Empowerment theory for rehabilitation research: Conceptual and methodological issues. *Rehabilitation Psychology, 43*(1), 3–16.

Zimmerman, M. A., & Zahniser, J. H. (1991). Refinements of sphere-specific measures of perceived control: Development of a sociopolitical control scale. *Journal of Community Psychology, 19*, 189–204.

Zurcher, L. A. (1970). The poverty board: Some consequences of "maximum feasible participation." *Journal of Social Issues, 26*, 85–107.

CHAPTER 3

Individualism, Collectivism, and Community Psychology

COLLIN VAN UCHELEN

INDIVIDUALISM, COLLECTIVISM, AND PSYCHOLOGICAL RESEARCH

A continuing challenge for researchers in community psychology is conceptualizing community phenomena at a collective level with appropriate theoretical constructs (Heller, 1989). However, the pervasiveness of an individualistic ideology in psychology makes it difficult to conceptualize psychological phenomena in terms of a collectivistic perspective. Individualism, and its conceptual counterpart, collectivism, are basic assumptive world views that vary within and across cultures. While both individualism and collectivism influence the nature and expression of psychological phenomena, psychological theory and practice generally assume an individualistic perspective. Awareness of the hidden bias of individualism is particularly important for those who wish to be sensitive to cultural diversity (Vega, 1992). In developing constructs that reflect a collectivistic perspective, the individualism embedded within our discipline must be identified and challenged.

In the following, I describe individualism and collectivism, and highlight the prominence of individualism in psychological research. I illustrate some ways to identify individualistic assumptions through a critical analysis of psychological conceptualizations of power and control. I discuss the implications of this critique for developing a more collectivistic perspective that highlights the shared and relational aspects of power and control. I then present some additional examples of community psychology research that provide collectivistic perspectives on psychological phenomena. Finally, I conclude by summarizing themes from these examples that may be useful to those interested in adding such perspectives to their own research.

COLLIN VAN UCHELEN • Cross Cultural Psychiatry Program, Department of Psychiatry, University of British Columbia, Vancouver, British Columbia, V6T 2A1, Canada.

Handbook of Community Psychology, edited by Julian Rappaport and Edward Seidman. Kluwer Academic / Plenum Publishers, New York, 2000.

Individualism and Collectivism

Individualism and collectivism represent contrasting sets of values, norms, assumptions, and ideologies that vary across cultures and are expressed in social behavior (Bellah, Madsen, Sullivan, Swidler, & Tipton, 1985; Triandis, 1989a, 1989b; Triandis, Bontempo, Villareal, Asai, & Lucca, 1988). Individualism is associated with independence, autonomy, agency, emotional detachment from others, and competition (Triandis, 1989a). Collectivism involves cooperation, emotional attachment to others, concern with others' opinions, and attention to family and relatives (Triandis, 1989a). Cultures as a whole can be characterized in terms of their individualism and collectivism (e.g., the United States is highly individualistic, while the People's Republic of China is more collectivistic).

Triandis (1989a) characterizes individualism and collectivism as follows:

> In individualist cultures most people's social behavior is largely determined by personal goals that overlap only slightly with the goals of collectives, such as the family, the work group, the tribe, political allies, coreligionists, fellow countrymen [sic], and the state. When a conflict arises between personal and group goals, it is considered acceptable for the individual to place personal goals ahead of collective goals. By contrast, in collectivist cultures social behavior is determined largely by goals shared with some collective, and if there is a conflict between personal and group goals, it is considered socially desirable to place collective goals ahead of personal goals (p. 42).

Individuals in a given culture vary in the extent to which they are individualistic or collectivistic with respect to given social settings. The more a person identifies with the collective, the more congruence between individual and collective aims. In highly collectivistic settings, the discrepancy between individual and collective aims may diminish entirely (Triandis, 1989a).

Individualism in Psychological Research

The differences between individualism and collectivism are readily apparent when comparing social phenomena in diverse cultures, and are well described in the field of cross-cultural psychology (see Triandis, 1995). An overview of the nature and correlates of individualism and collectivism may be of interest to community psychologists; however, here I address what I see as one of the primary implications of this research for our field. Essentially, that is the general tendency to represent psychological phenomena in terms of an individualistic perspective. To a large extent, this tendency reflects the individualistic cultural context within which psychology originated and operates (Pepitone, 1981). Consequently, many of the conceptual and methodological tools of our trade encode and reproduce the prevailing ideology of individualism of Western society (Fox, 1985; Hogan, 1975; Prilleltensky, 1989). This critique has been made about psychological research on achievement motivation (Spence, 1985), the self (Heelas & Lock, 1981; Lykes, 1985; Markus & Kitayama, 1991; Sampson, 1985), control (Furby, 1979; Weisz, Rothbaum, & Blackburn, 1984), self-efficacy and learned helplessness (Stam, 1987), empowerment (Riger, 1993; Surrey, 1991; van Uchelen, 1989), power (Miller, 1976, 1987), psychotherapy (Wallach & Wallach, 1983), development (Gilligan, 1982), and the notion of mental health (Sampson, 1977).

The ideology of individualism is embedded in basic assumptions about the nature of individual and social reality (Watt, 1989). For example, Sampson (1977, 1985, 1988) observes that, in much of psychology, the person is conceived of as a self-contained and autonomous individual. This view is prevalent in individualistic societies wherein the person is constructed in terms of rigid self/nonself boundaries that clearly delineate the individual from the surrounding social field (Heelas & Lock, 1981; Sampson, 1985, 1988). This is an *independent* view of the person (Markus & Kitayama, 1991), emphasizing individuation and autonomy. In this view, the boundaries of the individual are at the skin.

The independent view of the person, however, is not universal. Conceptions of the person vary both across and within cultures and settings (Geertz, 1975; Heelas & Lock, 1981; Lykes, 1985; Markus & Kitayama, 1991; Sampson, 1988; Shweder & Bourne, 1982; Zeigler, 1990). In contrast to the independent self, an *interdependent* view of the person is based on relatedness, social embeddedness, and interdependence. In this view, the boundaries of the self are permeable and fluid. One's identity is inextricably linked to, and constituted in terms of, one's relationships with others (e.g., family or collective), geographic settings (e.g., home or land), or transpersonal realms (spiritual force or ancestry). The interdependent conception of the person is applicable in collectivistic cultures in which the collective is seen as part of the self, and the self as part of the collective (Triandis, 1989a, 1989b). Within collective contexts, the self is often experienced in terms of the overlap between the individual and surrounding social context[1] (Markus & Kitayama, 1991; Triandis, 1989b; see also Miller, 1984).

Consequences of Individualistic Assumptions

Individualistic assumptions embedded in theory and methods have several consequences of importance to our discipline. The misapplication of individualistic concepts or measures to collectivistic phenomena can misrepresent or bias the way collective processes are understood, resulting in incomplete, inaccurate, and insensitive representations of the phenomena of interest. When phenomena operate in accord with individualism, we will be able to account for their variance with individualistic models (Spence, 1985). However, when the phenomena of interest are primarily collectivistic, individualistic theoretical models will be inadequate (Spence, 1985; Weisz, Rothbaum, & Blackburn, 1984).

For example, one way that individualism is incorporated in theory occurs in *cost-benefit* models that assume behavior or decision-making occurs in order to maximize benefit to the individual. As an alternative, some theorists are recognizing that people also behave in ways that prioritize the gain to the collective. Using dilemma games, Dawes, van de Kragt, and Orbell (1990) have shown that when individuals identify with a collective entity, they behave in ways that maximize gain to the entire collective. Similarly, Fiske (1992) describes a collectivistic model of *communal sharing* to understand behavior that maximizes the collective good. Utilizing theoretical models that incorporate collectivistic values will improve the fit of our theory to collectivistic community phenomena.

To the extent that our discipline is influenced by individualism, it hampers our ability to conceptualize phenomena in ways that articulate collectivistic perspectives. Given that community psychologists are often interested in phenomena that occur on a collective or community level, it is especially important to become aware of how individualistic assumptions are

[1]A third alternative is suggested by Lykes (1985), who introduces the notion of social individuality. She contends that the individualistic (independent) and collectivistic notions of self represent only two models of how the self is experienced. Social individuality refers to a synthesis of these two models, representing the self as an ensemble of social relations. Although Lykes (1985) draws a distinction between collectivist and social-individuality views of the self, both these views hold much in common when contrasted with the independent view of the self. For the purpose of this chapter, then, I will refer to both the collectivist and social-individuality concept of the self as an "interdependent" view of the self. This is consistent with the terminology used by Markus and Kitayama (1991), and simplifies the presentation at hand.

incorporated into theoretical models of collective phenomena. Such phenomena include responses to community threat (O'Sullivan, Waugh, & Espeland, 1984), participation in neighborhood organizations (Chavis & Wandersman, 1990), and involvement in self-help groups (Levine, 1988)..

Another consequence of individualistic assumptions in our theory and methods is that it can lead to culturally insensitive research. As a discipline, community psychology values cultural diversity (Rappaport, 1977; Vega, 1992). One way in which cultural differences are manifested is through individualism and collectivism (Triandis, 1989a). These terms define a primary dimension of cultural variation occurring both between and within cultures. Many collectivistic subcultures exist in the context of more individualistic dominant cultures (e.g., Asian, Latino, and Native American communities exist within the United States). Although community psychology emerged within the context of the highly individualistic culture of the United States, its values represent a challenge to be accepting of, and sensitive to, the diversity within society. Yet, given that many community researchers and activists are embedded within an individualistic society, it is likely that the ideology of individualism is incorporated into our work. The individualistic influence becomes problematic when measures or constructs misrepresent the nature of phenomena that occur in collectivistic settings, subcultures, or groups. Psychologists who work with such settings should pay particular attention to the consequences of their research with the collectivistic aspects of the phenomena of interest.

CHALLENGING INDIVIDUALISTIC ASSUMPTIONS

Recognizing the ways in which individualistic assumptions operate in our own discipline is quite difficult. As a cultural ideology, individualism is both elusive and influential (Watt, 1989). Examining its influence in our discipline is like asking those who know only one language to reveal the ways in which it constrains and shapes the nature of their experiences and their ability to communicate about them. To know this, it is useful to have the perspective afforded by knowing another language. In the same vein, community psychologists can learn the conceptual language of collectivism as a step toward recognizing and challenging individualism embedded in our own theory and methodology.

An illustration of evaluating the individualistic bias in psychological constructs is presented below. This example highlights a few of the individualistic assumptions contained in psychological concepts of power and control. In particular, I focus on how the discourse on control assumes an independent conception of the person, defines power and control in terms of dominance, and incorporates an individualistic view of control in the notion of mental health. This reveals the subtle ways that individualism enters into psychological theory, and lays the groundwork for a more collectivistic view of power and control.

Example 1: Individualism in Concepts of Power and Control

The relationship between powerlessness and human distress is a major concern of community psychology (Joffe & Albee, 1981). Similarly, the concept of *empowerment* has provided a focus for theory and research in the field (Kieffer, 1984; Lord & Hutchinson, 1993; Maton & Rappaport, 1984; Pretsby, Wandersman, Florin, Rich, & Chavis, 1990; Rappaport, 1981, 1984, 1987; Riger, 1993; Zimmerman, 1990; Zimmerman & Rappaport, 1988). Although empowerment is a multilevel phenomenon that spans the individual, group, and community levels of analysis, the construct still reflects individualistic ideology to the extent that it incorporates individualistic views of power and control (Chavis & Wandersman, 1990; Riger, 1993; van Uchelen, 1989).

Psychological conceptualizations of control may misrepresent the collective aspects of power because of individualism inherent in theory and methods. On the level of theory, individualism is reflected in independent definitions of the person (Sampson, 1988), the centrality of individual dominance in constructs of power and control (Eisler, 1987; Fine, 1989; Furby, 1979; Gergen, 1989; Miller, 1976), and individual agency as an ideal of psychological health (Gergen, 1989; Sampson, 1977, 1988; van Uchelen, 1989). On the level of methodology, power is operationalized in terms of individualistic measures of personal control over desired outcome (Chavis & Wandersman, 1990; Furby, 1979; Gurin, Gurin, & Morrison, 1978; Seeman, 1972, 1983; Stam, 1987). A critical examination of how power and control are conceptualized and measured must be undertaken if community psychologists are to understand a more collectivistic perspective of this topic.

Control and Conceptions of the Person

Within the Euro-American cultural context, the individual is seen as the unit from which action or agency emanates (de Charms, 1968). Internal control implies a locus of control internal to the person. In contrast, if the locus of control is believed to be external to the individual, control then presumably rests within a realm outside of (or external to) the person. The conception of the person is thus a key aspect in the meaning of control.

The underlying assumption of locus of control is that the individual is taken as the fundamental unit of reference or agent to which locus of control beliefs pertain (Sampson, 1988). To the extent that a person holds an independent view of self, the assumption of the self as an autonomous agent and source of control is not problematic. Given the prevalence of the independent view of self within individualistic cultures, it makes sense to conceptualize locus of control, in its most basic form, as either internal or external to the autonomous individual.

However, when the self is seen in interdependent terms, it is no longer accurate to view the autonomous individual as the unit to which the experience of power and control pertain. If the self is viewed (and experienced) as inextricably linked to, and constituted by, a network of relations embedded in the collective context, then conceptualizations of control may need to be revised to accommodate a more encompassing view of the person. The meaning of internal control would need to refer to something that both includes and goes beyond the individual as the point of reference. A collectivistic conceptualization of control would allow us to use an interdependent view of a person who experiences and realizes power in the context of relationships within the collective. The concept of locus of control (Rotter, 1966), as it is commonly used, is unable to accommodate this conceptual shift because it presumes an independent notion of the person.

A Feminist Critique of Power as Domination

Feminist theorists have revealed another individualistic assumption embedded in our concepts of power and control. Writing on the topic of power, Miller (1976, 1987) has noted that the traditional meaning of power and control assumes dominance as a defining feature.

She distinguishes between having power *for* oneself and exercising power *over* others. Miller suggests that the dominant conception of power is one that emphasizes "the ability to advance oneself, and, simultaneously, to control, limit, and if possible destroy the power of others" (1976, p. 116). This view combines a notion of self-power ("the capacity to implement") with that of dominion or dominance over others. Miller challenges the necessity of linking these two components. She opposes the understanding of power that assumes dominance as an essential characteristic—an understanding that she suggests reflects a patriarchal emphasis on interpersonal domination and subordination.

As an alternative, Miller (1976) calls for an understanding of power that gives primacy to self-power without dominance. She suggests that women often experience a sense of power in the context of relationships that enable one to develop one's own resources and capacities (see also Eisler, 1987; Fine, 1989; McClelland, 1975; Starhawk, 1987; Surrey, 1991). In this view, an individual's power is developed in the context of relationships that enhance the power of the self and of others.

A similar critique of power as dominance is advanced by hooks (1984), who maintains that a reconceptualization of power in terms of life-affirming and creative action to end domination provides an alternative definition of power based on the experiences of working-class women of color. She notes that this type of power occurs in feminist groups in the form of task rotation, consensus decision-making, and internal democracy. This alternative view of power is expressed through women's resistance to definitions of their reality advanced by those in traditional positions of authority. The critiques offered by Miller (1976, 1987) and hooks (1984) name patriarchy as an overarching condition that enlists individualism and domination as essential components of traditional definitions of power (see also Fine, 1989; Gergen, 1989; Janeway, 1980).

Control and the Western Ideal

Another individualistic assumption embedded in the discourse on psychological concepts of control is the ideal of internal control as a desirable characteristic for psychological health (Waterman, 1984). Sampson (1977, 1985, 1988) and Gergen (1989) critique Western psychology's image of the ideal person: An autonomous, self-contained individual with a high level of internal personal control. This ideal is reflected in the individualistic goals and approaches of contemporary clinical psychotherapy (Wallach & Wallach, 1983), and in the policy objectives of community mental health (Sampson, 1977).

In his 1977 paper, Sampson illustrates how the ideal of the self-contained individual is a defining feature of mental health. For example, a common measure of success in the treatment of those who are labelled as mentally ill is autonomous functioning and independent living. After discharge from psychiatric hospitalization, ex-patients often live collectively in residential halfway houses. The goal is to graduate from these group homes into independent living arrangements. This reflects an understanding of interdependent living as merely a transitional phase on the road to independent living as the final goal. However, the reality of independent living for these citizens is often experienced as a lonely, isolated, and alienated existence in single-room occupancy accommodations. Failure to maintain independence is viewed as a deterioration in functioning. The failure is located within the individual and in his or her inability to live independently, while the individualistic criterion of independence as a hallmark of mental health is rarely called into question.

As an alternative, Sampson (1988) and Gergen (1989) suggest an ideal of interdependence and social embeddedness. This alternative ideal is based on an ethic of caring (Gilligan, 1982; Noddings, 1984) and communion (Bakan, 1966; Wiggins, 1991), rather than domination and individualism. Gergen (1989) advocates relinquishing the ideal of autonomous individualism and individualistic conceptions of control, and proposes that theoreticians explore a new concept of control based on the ideal of interdependence.

Individualism in Measures of Control

The individualistic bias of measures of control (e.g., Rotter, 1966; Seeman, 1972) is manifested in the relationship between externality and collectivism. In collectivistic settings, identity is commonly experienced in terms of the interdependent view of the self. In these circumstances, the locus of control is in the collective or context of which the person is a part. However, the individual may not experience him or herself as powerless because control comes about through identifying with the collective. In this case, control is located both in the individual and the collective, although it is not framed in this way. With individualistic measures, the outcome is one in which collectivism correlates with external locus of control. This can lead to the erroneous conclusion that collectivists are more powerless than individualists. This conclusion pivots on an individualistic conception of control and power. The challenge is to rethink the conceptualization and measurement of power and control in a way that does not make collectivists appear powerless.

Incorporating Collectivistic Perspectives in Community Psychology Conceptualizing Control in the Collective Field

I have argued that individualistic concepts of power and control may not be congruent with the ways control is experienced when the self is constituted in relational terms. This points to the importance of tailoring theoretical constructs to the contexts for which they are used. I use the term "field control" (Sampson, 1988) to refer to a collectivist conceptualization of control. Field control refers to a conception of control that is based on an interdependent view of the person. The term calls attention to the context or field as an important element in one's experience of having control. Field refers to the locus or sphere of control that encompasses both the individual and the collectivity of which he or she is a part; control refers to actual and experienced competence, efficacy, capacity, and ability that exists within the collective field.

The defining feature of field control is sharing control and power within the collective. It is not control *over* other members of the collective, nor does it suggest that the individual is personally controlled by the collective. Rather, field control occurs when one has a voice in the collective without domination based on hierarchical authority. The concept of field control suggests a shift from an individualistic understanding of control based on an independent view of the self, to a collectivist view of control that is based on an interdependent view of the person embedded in the collective.

Researchers who study empowering processes and contexts can benefit from an examination of the theoretical and experiential dynamics of a more collectivistic view of power and control. To the extent that individualistic concepts and measures of control are used as empirical indicators of empowerment among collectivistic groups and settings, researchers may not only fail to see the collectivistic manifestation of control in these contexts (Chavis & Wandersman, 1990), but may also inadvertently conclude that collectivistic participants are powerless because of the implicit individualistic criteria incorporated in measures of power or control. Field control may be better suited to conceptualizing control in collectivistic settings because it incorporates an interdependent concept of the person embedded in the collective. Using a more collectivistic concept of power and control can contribute to a broader understanding of the nature of empowerment in collectivistic settings.

Example 2: Synergistic Community

Another example of research that challenges individualistic assumptions is seen in the work on synergistic community reported by Katz and colleagues (1984; Katz and Seth, 1987). Synergistic community is a state in which a community becomes highly cohesive and members freely contribute psychological resources to the collective. This creates an expanding or synergistic phenomenon in which members experience a connection with the energy of the entire community—a resource that is greater than the sum of its parts (Katz, 1984). In this state, the more one contributes his or her psychological resources to the community, the more resources are available to all community members.

The concept of synergistic community was used by Katz (1984) to understand traditional approaches to community healing among African !Kung and Fiji islanders. Katz observed this phenomenon among the !Kung in activities that involved the entire village in ritual singing and dancing aimed at community healing. These activities both expressed and reaffirmed community solidarity. Katz has also applied the idea of synergistic community to conceptualize collective phenomena occurring in self-help groups and in community responses to threat (Katz & Seth, 1987).

The concept of synergistic community challenges individualistic assumptions through employing an interdependent conception of the self. In synergistic communities, the individual is defined and experienced in an interdependent and contextualized manner. Members of a synergistic community have a sense of self-embedded-in-community (Katz & Seth, 1987). This inclusive view of the person invokes the power of the collective in the context of shared activity, resources, and identity. Katz observes that synergistic community is less likely to occur when community members invoke independent views of the person.

A second individualistic assumption identified in Katz's research is the scarcity paradigm of human resource availability. Within the scarcity paradigm, resources are seen as finite and limited (Katz, 1984). Even though valued resources may be psychological (e.g., support or information) rather than material, the scarcity paradigm fosters competition for access to them. Recasting psychological resources within a synergy paradigm, however, brings a new set of assumptions to the fore: collaboration, cooperation, and equality. In this view, the resources are seen as renewable, expanding, and accessible to all. For example, among the !Kung, Katz notes that the healing energy, *num*, created by participation in the community healing rituals is available to all members of the community.

Katz's use of non-individualistic concepts illuminates collectivistic properties in his subject matter. By adopting an interdependent conception of the person and a synergy paradigm of resource availability, Katz interprets his data in a way that focuses attention on its communal or collective features. Although a more individualistic theoretician may interpret Katz's material in a more individualistic manner, the collectivistic concepts employed by Katz are appropriate to the values of the communities that he studied. This work provides compelling ideas to articulate collectivistic aspects of community phenomena.

Example 3: Psychological Sense of Community

Research on the psychological sense of community introduces another challenge to individualistic assumptions. The relationship between individuals and the communities to which they belong has been a notable substantive focus of community psychology. Studies of the psychological sense of community (Sarason, 1974; McMillan & Chavis, 1986) represent the move from individualistic to collectivistic concepts and methodology in our field.

The psychological sense of community (PSC) can be conceptualized by focusing on an individual's experience in the context of the community of which he or she is a part. The work of McMillan and Chavis (1986) illustrates this view. They delineate four components of PSC: membership, influence, integration/fulfillment of needs, and shared emotional connection. This conceptualization draws attention to various aspects of the individual's experiences in the context of collective social fields. These experiences will vary within individuals, depending on the nature and tenure of their relationships with the communities to which they belong.

The conceptualization of psychological sense of community advanced by McMilland and Chavis (1986) is sensitive to context and illustrates an interactional perspective (Altman & Rogoff, 1987). Although this concept focuses on the individual experience of community, it explicitly acknowledges the importance of the community context. This perspective moves the researcher a step closer to a collective point of view through recognizing the linkage between an individual's experience and the group or collective.

Building on the individual level of analysis, research by Buckner (1988) illustrates a conceptualization of PSC at the collective or community level of analysis. Buckner (1988) proposes a construct called cohesion, which is a collective-level conceptualization of the individual-level concept of PSC. Cohesion is measured by aggregating PSC data for all the individuals in a given community. The aggregated value forms an index of community cohesion that quantifies the sense of community for the entire sample. Using this index, the researcher can compare various communities on their cohesion. In this manner, the concept of psychological sense of community is shifted from the individual to the collective level. This shift is achieved methodologically through aggregating data for the entire collective, and conceptually through re-expressing the original individual-level concept in appropriate collective-level terms.

Empirical and conceptual aggregation provides a useful methodological tool for advancing collective-level concepts. Although based on the individual level, Buckner's work provides an illustration of moving closer toward a collective level of analysis. Community researchers should consider using this approach with other concepts for which appropriate and meaningful aggregations can be made from the individual level to the collective level.

Example 4: Framing Research Questions

My final example of employing collectivistic perspectives focuses on how psychological phenomena is framed by the nature of our research questions. An example of this comes from my own work in collaboration with First Nations (Aboriginal) communities in Western Canada (Heiltsuk Wellness Project, 1994; van Uchelen, Davidson, Quressette, Brasfield, &

Demerais, 1997). This research focuses on indigenous views of health and wellness, and the strengths that exist in the lives of Aboriginal people and their communities.

One of the preliminary interview questions we developed for this research asked participants to speak about their own personal views of wellness. Transcripts of preliminary interviews revealed that participants often referred to other people's experiences and perspectives on wellness, rather than describing their own individual views. Their responses focused on the health of their family members and the health-promoting traditions of their community and Nation as a whole. When participants were asked about their individual strengths, they commonly identified collective-level strengths (e.g., sense of community, strong family ties, and shared cultural traditions).

Based on the collectivistic nature of the responses to the original individual-focus interview questions, we added revised questions that asked about wellness in general and the strengths of the community as a whole. This framed the phenomenon of interest in terms of the collective, rather than individual, level. In this way, the questions were asked in a manner appropriate to the collectivism of the cultural setting. This allowed the research team to learn that it is through relating the stories of others in their community that participants revealed their own views on wellness and strength.

The results of these studies highlight the importance of collectivistic phenomena such as the well-being of the collective (e.g., friends, family, clan, community) and collective strengths within the community. Our findings underscore the relational context within which wellness and strength have meaning. The prominence of community and connection is consistent with McCormick's (1997) identification of interdependence as a recurrent theme in accounts of healing in a sample of Canadian First Nations people. Both McCormick's and our own findings highlight the salience of collectivistic values in Aboriginal views of wellness and strength (see also Trimble, Manson, Dinges, & Medicine, 1984).

Asking research questions in a manner that focuses on individual experience is a way in which the phenomena of interest can become framed in individualistic terms. This may obscure important features of the phenomena under study. In collectivistic settings, it is especially important to phrase research questions in ways that allow participants to articulate collectivistic views. This highlights the need to tailor methods to be appropriate for the particular sample and phenomena being studied.

SUMMARY

I have described ways in which individualistic assumptions enter into the conceptual/theoretical discourse of psychological constructs. These include: (a) constructing the individual in terms of an independent view of the person that introduces artificial distinctions between the individual and the collective social field, (b) holding individual dominance and agency as essential components in definitions of power and control, and (c) viewing the agentic and self-contained individual as an ideal of mental health. Research on synergistic community questions the applicability of an individualistic scarcity paradigm to understand the allocation of psychological resources among collectivistic settings.

I provided a few illustrations of research that utilizes theoretical concepts or methods to yield more collectivistic understandings of social phenomena. Ways of incorporating concepts or methods that are more compatible with collectivistic phenomena include reconceptualizing power and control vis-à-vis an interdependent view of the self embedded in the collective social field. In addition, studies of community cohesion illustrate the utility of aggregating individual-level constructs to the community level of analysis. Finally, posing research questions that refer to the collective level may be useful for collectivistic groups that do not frame their own experiences in individualistic terms.

CONCLUSIONS

I have attempted to explicate ways in which individualistic assumptions are codified into psychological constructs. The extent to which these assumptions constrain and distort our understanding of the phenomena we study is an important matter to address in community psychology research and practice. One of the hallmarks of community psychology is an appreciation for diversity (Rappaport, 1977; Vega, 1992). Examining the assumptions of individualism underlying psychological concepts and measures is one way the investigator can begin to build sensitivity to diversity into the research process.

The critique I have made is not intended to challenge the value of individualism as an ideology *per se*. To the extent that community phenomena operate according to individualistic principles, individualistic research (both in theory and method) may go far in explaining the phenomena at hand. What is emphasized here, rather, is that the individualistic assumptions should not be the unexamined default version of reality that becomes encoded in our research.

Individualistic and collectivistic assumptions in our understanding of psychological phenomena render different constructions of social reality. Without scrutiny, the individualist position has been adopted, unwittingly, in our discipline. Individualistic assumptions can be identified and exposed in the process of conducting community research. Once identified, the researcher will be in a position to evaluate the appropriateness of the assumptions underlying the project at hand.

The researcher need not abandon all components of the individualist view in favor of adopting collectivist perspectives. Rather, the increased awareness that one's perspective rests on such assumptions can mitigate against the tendency for the ideology to remain hidden (Parker & Shotter, 1990). Exposing the ideology can, in turn, facilitate more sensitive (and sensible) theory and understanding. To this end, it is incumbent upon community researchers to begin to scrutinize theoretical constructs and methods for such implicit assumptions. The challenge is to be cognizant of both individualistic and collectivistic assumptions in order to recognize how they may shape the research of our field.

ACKNOWLEDGMENTS. I wish to thank Julian Rappaport for unfailingly encouraging me to develop and articulate my critique of individualism in our field, and M. Brinton Lykes for her part in stimulating discussions on this topic. I also wish to thank Sheila Woody and Loraine F. Lavallee for incisive feedback on earlier drafts of the manuscript, and Michelle Anderson for her support. Finally, I wish to acknowledge Hilistis Pauline Waterfall of the Heiltsuk Nation for encouraging me to look at the First Nations people in British Columbia as exemplars of a more collectivistic way of living.

REFERENCES

Altman, I., & Rogoff, B. (1987). World vies in psychology: Trait, interactional, organismic, and transactional perspectives. In D. Stokols & I. Altman (Eds.), *Handbook of environmental psychology* (pp. 7–40). New York: Wiley.

Bakan, D. (1966). *The duality of human existence.* Boston: Beacon.

Bellah, R. N., Madsen, R., Sullivan, W. M., Swidler, A., & Tipton, S. M. (1985). *Habits of the heart: individualism and commitment in American life.* New York: Harper and Row.

Buckner, J. C. (1988). The development of an instrument to measure neighborhood cohesion. *American Journal of Community Psychology, 16,* 771–791.

Chavis, D. M., & Wandersman, A. (1990). Sense of community in the urban environment: A catalyst for participation and community development. *American Journal of Community Psychology, 18,* 55–81.

Dawes, R. N., van de Kragt, A. J. C., and Orbell, J. M. (1990). Cooperation for the benefit of us—not me or my conscience. In J. J. Mansbridge (Ed.), *Beyond self interest* (pp. 97–110). Chicago: University of Chicago Press.

de Charms, R. (1968). *Personal causation.* New York: Academic.

Eisler, R. (1987). *The chalice and the blade: Our history, our future.* San Francisco: Harper.

Fine, M. (1989). Coping with rape: Critical perspectives on consciousness. In R. K. Unger (Ed.), *Representations: Constructions of gender* (pp. 186–200). Amityville, NY: Baywood.

Fiske, A. P. (1992). The four elementary forms of sociality: Framework for a unified theory of social relations. *Psychological Review, 99,* 689–723.

Fox, D. R. (1985). Psychology, ideology, utopia, and the commons. *American Psychologist, 40,* 48–58.

Furby, L. (1979). Individualistic bias in studies of locus of control. In A. Buss (Ed.), *Psychology in social context* (pp. 169–190). New York: Irvington.

Geertz, C. (1975). On the nature of anthropological understanding. *American Scientist, 63,* 47–53.

Gergen, M. M. (1989). Loss of control among the aging?: A critical reconstruction. In P. S. Fry (Ed.), *Psychological perspectives of helplessness and control in the elderly* (pp. 261–290). North-Holland: Elsevier Science.

Gilligan, C. (1982). *In a different voice: Psychological theory and women's development.* Cambridge, MA: Harvard University Press.

Gurin, P., Gurin, G., & Morrison, B. M. (1978). Personal and ideological aspects of internal and external control. *Social Psychology, 41*(4), 275–296.

Heiltsuk Wellness Project. (1994). *Heiltsuk wellness: A shared vision.* Waglisla, B. C.: Heiltsuk Tribal Council.

Heller, K. (1989). The return to community. *American Journal of Community Psychology, 17,* 1–15.

Heelas, P. L. F., & Lock, A. J. (Eds.). (1981). *Indigenous psychologies: The anthropology of the self.* London: Academic.

Hogan, J. (1975). Theoretical egocentrism and the problem of compliance. *American Psychologist, 30,* 533–540.

hooks, b. (1984). *Feminist theory: From margin to center.* Boston: South End Press.

Janeway, E. (1980). *Powers of the weak.* New York: Knopf.

Joffe, J. M., & Albee, G. W. (Eds.). (1981). *Prevention through political action and social change.* Hanover, NH: University Press of New England.

Katz, R. (1984). Empowerment and synergy: Expanding the community's healing resources. *Prevention in Human Services, 3,* 201–226.

Katz, R., & Seth, N. (1987). Synergy and healing: A perspective on Western health care. *Prevention in Human Services, 5,* 109–136.

Kieffer, C. (1984). Citizen empowerment: A developmental perspective. *Prevention in Human Services, 3,* 9–36.

Levine, M. (1988). An analysis of mutual assistance. *American Journal of Community Psychology, 16,* 167–183.

Lord, J., & Hutchinson, P. (1993). The process of empowerment: Implications for theory and practice. *Canadian Journal of Community Mental Health, 12,* 5–23.

Lykes, M. B. (1985). Gender and individualistic vs. collectivist bases for notions about the self. *Journal of Personality, 53,* 356–383.

Markus, H. R., & Kitayama, S. (1991). Culture and the self: Implications for cognition, emotion, and motivation. *Psychological Review, 98,* 224–253.

Maton, K. I., & Rappaport, J. (1984). Empowerment in a religious setting: A multivariate investigation. *Prevention in Human Services, 3,* 37–72.

McClelland, D. C. (1975). *Power: The inner experience.* New York: Irvington.

McCormick, R. M. (1997). Healing through interdependence: The role of connecting in First Nations healing practices. *Canadian Journal of Counselling, 31*(3), 172–184.

McMillan, D. W., & Chavis, D. M. (1986). Sense of community: A definition and theory. *Journal of Community Psychology, 14,* 6–23.

Miller, J. B. (1976). *Toward a new psychology of women.* Boston: Beacon.

Miller, J. B. (1984). The development of women's sense of self. *Work in Progress* no. 12. Wellesley, MA: Stone Center Working Papers Series.

Miller, J. B. (1987). Women and power. *Women and Therapy, 6,* 1–10.

Noddings, N. (1984). *Caring: A feminine approach to ethics and moral education.* Berkeley: University of California Press.

O'Sullivan, M. J., Waugh, N., & Espeland, W. (1984). The Fort McDowell Yavapai: From pawns to powerbrokers. In J. Rappaport, C. Swift, and R. Hess (Eds.), *Studies in empowerment: Steps toward understanding and action* (pp. 73–97). New York: Haworth.

Parker, I., & Shotter, J. (Eds.). (1990). *Deconstructing social psychology.* London: Routledge.

Pepitone, A. (1981). Lessons from the history of social psychology. *American Psychologist, 36,* 972–985.

Pretsby, J. E., Wandersman, A., Florin, P., Rich, R., & Chavis, D. M. (1990). Benefits, costs, incentive management, and participation in voluntary organizations: A means to understanding and promoting empowerment. *American Journal of Community Psychology, 18,* 117–149.

Prilleltensky, I. (1989). Psychology and the status quo. *American Psychologist, 44,* 795–802.

Rappaport, J. (1977). *Community psychology: Values, research, and action.* New York: Holt, Rinehart and Winston.

Rappaport, J. (1981). In praise of paradox: A social policy of empowerment over prevention. *American Journal of Community Psychology, 9,* 1–25.

Rappaport, J. (1984). Studies in empowerment: Introduction to the issue. *Prevention in Human Services, 3,* 1–7.

Rappaport, J. (1987). Terms of empowerment/exemplars of prevention: Toward a theory for community psychology. *American Journal of Community Psychology, 15,* 121–144.

Riger, S. (1993). What's wrong with empowerment. *American Journal of Community Psychology, 21*(3), 279–292.

Rotter, J. B. (1966). Generalized expectancies for internal versus external control of reinforcement. *Psychological Monographs, 80*(1, Whole No. 609).

Sampson, E. E. (1977). Psychology and the American ideal. *Journal of Personality and Social Psychology, 35,* 767–782.

Sampson, E. E. (1985). The decentralization of identity: Toward a revised concept of personal and social order. *American Psychologist, 40,* 1203–1211.

Sampson, E. E. (1988). The debate on individualism: Indigenous psychologies of the individual and their role in personal and societal functioning. *American Psychologist, 43,* 15–22.

Sarason, S. (1974). *The psychological sense of community.* San Francisco: Jossey-Bass.

Seeman, M. (1972). Alienation and engagement. In A. Campbell & P. E. Converse (Eds.), *The human meaning of social change* (pp. 467–527). New York: Russell Sage Foundation.

Seeman, M. (1983). Alienation motifs in contemporary theorizing: The hidden continuity of the classic themes. *Social Psychology Quarterly, 46,* 171–184.

Shweder, R. A., & Bourne, E. (1982). Does the concept of person vary cross-culturally? In A. J. Marsella & G. M. White (Eds.), *Cultural conceptions of mental health and therapy* (pp. 97–137). Boston: Reidel.

Spence, J. T. (1985). Achievement American style: The rewards and costs of individualism. *American Psychologist, 40,* 1285–1295.

Stam, H. J. (1987). The psychology of control: A textual critique. In H. J. Stam, T. B. Rogers, & K. J. Gergen (Eds.), *The analysis of psychological theory: Metapsychological perspectives* (pp. 131–156). Washington: Hemisphere.

Starhawk (1987). *Truth or dare: Encounters with power, authority, and mystery.* San Francisco: Harper.

Surrey, J. L. (1991). Relationship and empowerment. In J. V. Jordan, A. G. Kaplan, J. Baker Miller, I. P. Stiver, & J. L. Surrey (Eds.), *Women's growth in connection: Writings from the Stone Center* (pp. 162–180). New York: Guilford.

Triandis, H. C. (1995). *Individualism and collectivism.* Boulder, CO: Westview.

Triandis, H. C. (1989a). Cross-cultural studies of individualism and collectivism. In J. Berman (Ed.), *Nebraska symposium on motivation, 1989* (pp. 41–133). Lincoln: University of Nebraska Press.

Triandis, H. C. (1989b). The self and social behavior in differing cultural contexts. *Psychological Review, 96,* 506–520.

Triandis, H. C., Bontempo, R., Villareal, M., Asai, M., & Lucca, N. (1988). Individualism and collectivism: Cross-cultural perspectives on self-ingroup relationships. *Journal of Personality and Social Psychology, 54,* 323–338.

Trimble, J. E., Manson, S. M., Dinges, N. C., & Medicine, B. (1984). American Indian concepts of mental health: Reflections and directions. In P. B. Pedersen, N. Sartorius, & A. J. Marsella (Eds.), *Mental health services: The cross-cultural context* (pp. 199–221). Beverly Hills, CA: Sage.

van Uchelen, C. (1989). *Healing mechanisms of self help: Toward a non-individualistic conception of control.* Paper presented at the Second Biennial Conference on Community Research and Action, East Lansing, MI.

van Uchelen, C., Davidson, S. F., Quressette, S., Brasfield, C., & Demerais, L. (1997). What makes us strong: Urban Aboriginal perspectives on wellness and strength. *Canadian Journal of Community Mental Health, 16*(2), 37–50.

Vega, W. A. (1992). Theoretical and pragmatic implications of cultural diversity for community research. *American Journal of Community Psychology, 20,* 375–391.

Wallach, M. A., & Wallach, L. (1983). *Psychology's sanction for selfishness: The error of egoism in theory and therapy*. San Francisco: Freeman.

Waterman, A. S. (1984). *The psychology of individualism*. New York: Praeger.

Watt, J. (1989). *Individualism and educational theory*. Dordrecht, The Netherlands: Kluwer Academic.

Weisz, J. R., Rothbaum, F. M., & Blackburn, T. C. (1984). Standing out and standing in: The psychology of control in America and Japan. *American Psychologist, 39*, 955–969.

Wiggins, J. S. (1991). Agency and communion as conceptual coordinates for the understanding and measurement of interpersonal behavior. In D. Cicchetti & W. Grove (Eds.), *Thinking clearly about psychology: Essays in honor of Paul E. Meehl*. Minneapolis: University of Minnesota Press.

Zeigler, R. M. (1990). The inseparable self. Unpublished manuscript, University of Illinois at Urbana-Champaign.

Zimmerman, M. A. (1990). Taking aim on empowerment research: On the distinction between individual and psychological conceptions. *American Journal of Community Psychology, 18*, 169–177.

Zimmerman, M. A., & Rappaport, J. (1988). Citizen participation, perceived control, and psychological empowerment. *American Journal of Community Psychology, 16*, 725–750.

CHAPTER 4

Community Psychology and Routes to Psychological Wellness

Emory L. Cowen

The main purpose of this chapter is to develop and illustrate the concept of "routes to psychological wellness," which, I believe, has much orienting value in framing fruitful questions for psychologists and others to pose and fruitful activities for psychologists and others to undertake. I use the term to identify what Rappaport (1987) called the phenomena of interest, i.e., "the entire class of phenomena that we want our research to undertake, predict, explain or describe; that we want our applications and interventions to stimulate, facilitate or create; and our social policies to encourage" (p. 129).

Although the concept of routes to psychological wellness remains amply fuzzy, it is broader and more integrative than the phenomena of interest that have occupied the mental health fields and the emergent field of community psychology. At the same time there are domains of overlap between its issues and the focal issues of those two fields. The concept is sufficiently comprehensive to enfold other concepts, such as primary prevention, empowerment, competence, and heightened resilience (invulnerability) in children, that have themselves been advanced either as significant orienting concepts or, indeed, as the phenomena of interest for community psychology. It also vivifies a point made by Rappaport (1981) and underscored by others (Levine & Perkins, 1987; Sarason, 1987), i.e., that intrinsically complex human and social problems require multiple, divergent, and changing solutions.

Although the chapter's primary focus is neither on mental health nor community psychology, the concept of routes to psychological wellness can best be developed by considering briefly some of its historical antecedents in those fields. Mental health's unifying themes, starting with its vestigial precursors in primitive man and continuing to the present time, have been the quests to understand and repair things that go wrong psychologically (Zax & Cowen, 1976). Although the field has, to be sure, changed over time, those changes have primarily involved: (1) a broadening in the number and types of conditions considered to fall within its

Portions of this chapter were presented in an invited address to the First Biennial Conference on Community Research and Action, Columbia, South Carolina, May 21, 1987.

Emory L. Cowen • Center for Community Study, University of Rochester, Rochester, New York 14620.

Handbook of Community Psychology, edited by Julian Rappaport and Edward Seidman. Kluwer Academic / Plenum Publishers, New York, 2000.

realm—a point punctuated by the bulk of DSM III-R, (2) an evolution in the explanatory concepts used to comprehend diverse forms of psychological dysfunction, and (3) a growing sophistication in the methods used to contain or repair such dysfunction. Within mental health's own defining context, some of those changes have been seen as sufficiently sweeping as to be called revolutions (Hobbs, 1964; Zax & Cowen, 1976). I personally doubt that noteworthy revolutions have occurred, as the field's energies and resources, its transmitted wisdoms, and its training practices have centered unswervingly around a self-limiting search for fuller understandings of the vagaries of damaged psyches and better ways to fix them.

I do not mean to imply that mental health has been unconcerned with psychological wellness. Rather, the particular way it has construed issues of wellness, i.e., that psychological wellness is, or should be, a matter of concern when it breaks down—indeed, the more flagrant the breakdown the greater the reason for concern (Joint Commission on Mental Illness and Health, 1961; Goldstein, 1982)—is narrow and restrictive. That de facto definition of phenomena of interest, and the foci and activities that derive from it, has obscured a broader, potentially more useful proposition—that greater progress toward the ideal of psychological wellness can be achieved by building and enhancing steps than by the sum of society's most powerful and effective efforts to repair established deficits in wellness. Implicit in the concept of routes to psychological wellness is the conviction that wellness must be a matter of prime concern at all times, not just when it fails. Indeed, the occurrence of a genuine, as opposed to a pseudo mental health revolution may depend on that conceptual leap or redefinition of phenomena of interest.

Domains are susceptible to ferment and re-examination when their guiding concepts and practices fail to address satisfactorily a field's problems as defined (or redefined). Thus, the need to resolve refractory problems and/or to encompass new knowledge lead to paradigm shifts (Kuhn, 1970; Rappaport, 1977, 1987) that entail major refocusings of phenomena of interest and derivative activities. Growing dissatisfaction with the classically defined mental health field has long been apparent. Indeed, expressed in somewhat different words, such dissatisfaction has been a focal theme of three major national reports, spanning several decades, which have reviewed and made recommendations about the state of the field (Joint Commission on Mental Health of Children, 1969; Joint Commission on Mental Illness and Health, 1961; President's Commission on Mental Health, 1978).

Given that the concerns reflected in those reports, and related ones, have been considered in detail in many sources (e.g., Cowen, 1973, 1977, 1980, 1983; Levine & Perkins, 1987; Prevention Task Panel Report, 1978; Rappaport, 1977; Zax & Cowen, 1976), only a brief summary is provided here. (1) Mental health (repair) resources were insufficient to meet spontaneous demand for services, much less underlying need (Albee, 1959; Arnhoff, Rubenstein, & Speisman, 1969; Levine & Perkins, 1987; Zax & Cowen, 1976). (2) De facto allocations of mental health services, for overdetermined reasons, followed the rule that help was least available where it was most needed (Cowen, Gardner, & Zax, 1967; Lorion, 1973, 1974; Manson, 1982; Rappaport, 1977; Ryan, 1971; Sanua, 1966; Schofield, 1964). Such glaring distributional inequities led the President's Commission on Mental Health (1978) to highlight the unmet needs of the "unserved and underserved" throughout its final report. (3) Major mismatches between mental health's traditional service-delivery modes and the ways in which large segments of the population defined, perceived, and dealt with their problems, created conditions under which those groups saw traditional mental health services as inappropriate or irrelevant (Rappaport, 1977; Reiff, 1967; Reiff & Riessman, 1965; Ryan, 1971; Zax & Cowen, 1976). (4) Notwithstanding a dedicated effort by competent, committed mental health professionals, the serious problems that major mental disorders (e.g., schizophrenia) posed could not be solved (Cowen, 1982b; Goldstein, 1982; Zax & Cowen, 1976). (5) Mental health's most finely honed repair strategies (e.g., psychotherapy) had limited efficacy, less because of default in skills or effort, and more because the very conditions they were called on to remediate were rooted and change-resistant (Albee, 1982; Cowen, 1973; Levine & Perkins, 1987; Rappaport, 1977). Under such circumstances even the most sophisticated, costly and time-consuming repair efforts have a guarded prognosis.

Ensuing searches for viable alternatives have reflected different implicit views of the root causes of those unresolved problems. The first and simplest competing notion, without challenging mental health's past underlying assumptions, emphasized the need to augment the reach, improve the timing, and increase the efficacy of restorative services for the psychologically troubled. This was the thrust of the early community mental health movement, highlighted in the very first sentence of the Swampscott Conference report marking the birth of this new field: "Traditional approaches to the mental health problem are being challenged today by *new concepts of community service*" (emphasis added) (Anderson et al., 1966, p. 1). In the new regime, services, still primarily restorative, were to be located in community settings where people in need could find them sooner, more readily, at lower cost, and hopefully in more ecologically valid formats.

Moving one important step beyond, new community psychology thrusts began to question whether repairing dysfunction was the only or best approach to psychological wellness, and whether there might not be viable alternatives to mental health's passive–receptive mode of waiting for dysfunction to find its way into society's formal repair system. Harbingers of this broadened view also appeared in the Swampscott report when, for example, it envisioned appealing new, professional roles such as "change agents, social system analysts, consultants in community affairs and students generally of the whole man in relation to all his environments" (Anderson et al., 1966, p. 26). This later development, closer to community psychology's present core, turned attention to person–environment relationships, social policy and planning, justice and empowerment and, to some extent, programs to promote wellness (Levine & Perkins, 1987; Rappaport, 1977). In so doing, it tilted an axis away from mental health's classic repair loci—office, clinic, hospital, consulting room—to the community and its important settings (schools, churches, informal groups, etc.). A cautionary note however: the word "community" in community psychology refers to a locus and perhaps an instrumentality, not *ipso facto* to a specific way to redefine phenomena of interest or derivative assumptions and practices.

If one recasts the Procrustean question that has long guided the mental health fields, i.e., How can we best repair psychological malfunction? into the broader questions of: How does psychological wellness come about and how can it be promoted?, then (1) community institutions, settings, and processes become important study foci in their own right insofar as they relate to wellness; and (2) the community offers settings that are more relevant and functional than the consulting room to actions and interventions that can enhance the well-being of large numbers of people. For those reasons, the community and its key settings must be one significant action-arena in a comprehensive approach to routes to psychological wellness.

Several points implied in the preceding discussion bear highlighting. The first is that there is, or should be, some continuity in what has transpired in mental health for many centuries and the broadening developments of the past quarter century in community mental health and community psychology, including some of the latter's intriguing evolutionary buds. One key continuity element lies in the prime dependent variables, i.e., psychological wellness-related variables, on which these fields have focused. A noteworthy difference, however, is the shift in emphasis in viewing such variables—away from a heroic, if socially doomed, effort to undo established deficit, to the promotion of wellness in different life stages, settings, and circumstances. That shift is powered by several gnawing concerns: What if repairing deficits in wellness can, at best, account (for whatever reasons) for only a small fraction of the universe of instances relevant to psychological wellness? And what if it is easier, farther reaching, and more effective to facilitate wellness, whether through steps in person formation and/or education, or by modifying settings, practices, and social policies, than to struggle after the fact to remediate failings in wellness (Cowen, 1985).

Although community psychology has, to be sure, moved in those new directions, it has done so more in *ad hoc* than planful ways. The planful emergence of a field is catalyzed by a set of guiding concepts or views that some call "theory." Although theory can range in breadth, it has orienting value, whatever its scope. This is what Lewin had in mind when he observed that there is nothing as practical as a good theory. But theory does not develop in a vacuum; it is theory about something. As Rappaport (1987) suggested, theory coheres around phenomena of interest. Phenomena of interest reflect values. To the extent that people have different phenomena of interest in mind, or even if related phenomena of interest differ in breadth, planful inputs deriving from theory will differ, although they may be ascribed to a common generic banner. Presently, community psychology is indeed a common generic banner for which there are many referents. Too little, as Rappaport (1987) stressed, has been done to develop unifying theory and that gap has hampered the field's development.

Although one important goal of this chapter is to sketch further orienting theory, my position is strongly shaped by two limiting considerations. The type of theory I have in mind (1) does not start with the concept of community psychology, though community is important to it; and (2) is intended to reflect and embrace domains (i.e., dependent variables or outcomes) that have been central to the roots and phenomena of interest both of the classic mental health field and the community-psychology movement. To address meaningfully the problems that result from the restrictiveness of prior frameworks, however, requires redefinition of the phenomena of interest to the more comprehensive, proactive concept of routes to psychological wellness—how it comes about and the potentially diverse ways in which psychological and other knowledge can be developed and applied to enhance it.

To understand the full panorama of routes to psychological wellness will require ways of framing issues, knowledge bases, and methodologies that differ substantially from those that have guided the inquiry and activities of the mental health fields and community psychology (Cowen, 1982a, 1984b). On the other hand, relevant feeder-strands from both those fields, especially community psychology's more recent thrusts, can be meaningfully applied to the redefined phenomena of interest and profitably extended. In the final reckoning, however, the concept of routes to psychological wellness is proposed, unlike empowerment, not as a way to construe community psychology's phenomena of interest (Rappaport, 1987), but rather as an overarching phenomenon of interest in its own right. Within that enlarged frame, a key question for community psychology is: How can its present and future knowledge bases illuminate the broader topic of routes to psychological wellness? Kelly (1986) reflected a similar orientation when he described the purpose of community research as "understanding those social processes that promote the health and well-being of individuals and organizations" (p. 584).

PSYCHOLOGICAL WELLNESS: A CLOSER LOOK

Having proposed the concept of routes to psychological wellness as a unifying theme around which to coalesce future efforts, let me try to clarify my use of the term, if only in a preliminary and approximate way. One thing such usage points to is the domain's prime dependent variables or, in layman's terms, what we hope to see happen as a result of our inquiry and efforts.

Although I have, thus far, referred to psychological wellness as if it were an entity or state, in fact, I see it as a continuous rather than a binary concept. Moreover, it is a concept with significant developmental, cultural, situational, temporal, and, no doubt, value determinants. Precisely because of those realities, many essays have been written (e.g., Jahoda, 1958), and many more will be written, about the definition and manifestations of psychological wellness.

Enduringness and breadth are important aspects of the concept of psychological wellness I am proposing. Its basic temporal stability differs from (i.e., considerably transcends) the momentary satisfaction of seeing a good movie or watching one's favorite football team win the Super Bowl. It implicates important facets of a person's life and involves recuperability in the face of adversity. Even so, the term is used to describe a predominant condition, not a flawless or invariant state. I recognize that happenings ranging from hassles of daily living to, more importantly, the (often) unpredictable and uncontrollable occurrence of stressful life events and circumstances act to disrupt wellness.

I use the term broadly and accept, indeed urge, considerable latitude in how it is assessed and inferred. I do not at all mean to restrict it to specific indicators such as Rorschach records, teachers' ratings of school children's adjustment, or self-reports of anxiety or depression, which some have found to be unsatisfying, if not downright irritating (Bronfenbrenner, 1977; Rappaport, 1981). On the other hand, I believe that the concept implies: (1) the presence of "name, rank, and serial number" marker-outcomes, such as eating well, sleeping well, and working well—mindful perhaps of Freud's earthy notion of adaptation, i.e., Leben und Arbeiten; and (2) higher-order elements, such as a sense of control over one's fate, a feeling of purpose and belonging, and a basic satisfaction with oneself and one's existence—each of the latter backed by external validating signs.

Were I to be taken to court and sued over the i-dottings and t-crossings of that gross concept definition, I would not fight the case. It is simply a loose mark-up of a set of outcomes that help to place boundaries around the phenomena of interest. If outcome terms such as wellness, adaptation, or adjustment produce allergic reactions, widely used alternatives such as "life satisfaction" (Rappaport, 1987) or "gratifications in living," i.e., the obverse of problems in living (Rappaport, 1981), can be substituted.

Let me next advance several position statements, or perhaps, more accurately, assertions, that seem at this time to pertain importantly to the overarching concept of psychological wellness:

1. Psychological wellness, as I have suggested, is a more-or-less, rather than an either-or, condition. Using the term as an absolute is simply a shorthand of convenience. Appropriate goals for psychologists and others to pursue are to develop knowledge about the nature of wellness and routes to wellness, and to apply such knowledge in ways that strengthen wellness in many people. Kelly (1975) made much the same point: "If we as community psychologists are going to prevent distress, we must understand the variety of conditions, processes and events that produce conditions of healthiness" (p. 206).

2. The literal factors that define psychological wellness differ at different ages and under different environmental circumstances. Hence, specific routes to wellness may differ for different groups at different times.

3. Psychological wellness is not a "once-and-forever" condition (Werner & Smith, 1982). Just as early wellness can be undermined by later adversities, natural or engineered conditions, processes, and events, to use Kelly's (1975) terms, can enhance wellness.

4. It is easier and more promising to promote wellness from the start than to repair rooted defects in wellness.

5. Input strands to psychological wellness become more complex as one passes from early childhood to adulthood, both because of the greater number of systems in which a person interacts and the importance of those systems to wellness at later times. This point can be cast within Bronfenbrenner's (1977, 1979) ecological-system framework. Wellness for the infant, to the extent that it is even perceived as relevant, is defined largely by behavior within the family microsystem. For children, the school experience and the mesosystems that reflect interrelationships among school, family, and peer groups are of central importance to psychological wellness. Later, society's influence is less immediately obvious; exosystems and macrosystems underlying the formal and informal social structures that relate, for example, to justice, empowerment, and life opportunity, have greater and more direct impact on psychological wellness.

6. Psychological wellness has significant person-related (both dispositional and experiential), transactional, and environmental determinants. A comprehensive theory of wellness requires that each of these strands be seriously reflected, and their relevance at different time points and under different conditions be understood.

7. A person's psychological wellness, at all stages of development, is affected by multiple, cross-setting, interaction systems that significantly reflect "aspects of the environment beyond the immediate situation containing the subject" (Bronfenbrenner, 1977, p. 514). Indeed, even within delimited system (e.g., the family), wellness outcomes are shaped by transactional elements that transcend individuals (Cicchetti & Toth, 1987; Sameroff, 1977; Sameroff & Chandler, 1975; Werner, 1987), i.e., ways in which "specific characteristics of the child transact with the caretaker's mode of functioning" (Sameroff, 1977, p. 49).

8. Many factors either contribute to, or impede, psychological wellness. Some, but not all, of those factors are psychological. Examples of non-psychological factors include such "taken-for-granteds" as having a job, food to eat, and a decent place to live. Accordingly, a rich understanding of the roots of, and routes to, psychological wellness will require major inputs from other than mental health sources and collaboration among groups that have not frequently interacted in the past (Cowen, 1982a).

Sources of Impact on Psychological Wellness

To the extent that routes to psychological wellness is the shared phenomenon of interest, any variable that bears on such wellness is theoretically pertinent. Qualifying the verb "bears on" with the adverbs "significantly" and "enduringly" helps to prioritize domains on which to focus and to end-run a legion of potential wellness-related variables, such as the titanium paints, yoghurts, and unpolished rices spoofingly cited in Kessler and Albee (1975).

The following sources of influence have important and enduring effects in advancing or restricting people's psychological wellness: (1) the family context in which a child grows up and the nature of the child's formation and early experiences; (2) the effectiveness of the child's total educational experience, a good deal of which takes place in schools; (3) the nature and shaping impact of the significant social settings and systems in which a person interacts; (4) the extent to which the broad societal surround, i.e., its exosystems and macrosystems (Bronfenbrenner, 1977), as well as its specific mediating structures, including family, neighborhood, church, volunteer organizations (Rappaport, 1981), are just, empowering, and provide opportunities consonant with a person's abilities.

Sometimes nature's normal course leads spontaneously to early wellness. When that happens, we should click our heels and shout "Hallelujah!" Natural routes to wellness must be studied actively and systematically, and knowledge so gained applied to enhance wellness. Although there has been limited *ad hoc* study of this topic (e.g., Block & Block, 1980; Murphy & Moriarity, 1976; White, Kaban, & Attanuci, 1979), it is mute testimony to the mental health field and its *de facto* phenomena of interest that studies of dysfunction and its causes outnumber studies of wellness at least tenfold. That imbalance needs to be redressed. The orienting concept of routes to psychological wellness can help to further that goal.

Education, defined broadly or narrowly, formally or informally, is a potentially powerful route to psychological wellness. A person's educational experiences provide the knowledge and skill bases needed to master essential life tasks. They also significantly shape self views of competence and, from those, a sense of control of one's destiny. Education's potential for enhancing wellness is reflected in long-term findings from Project Head Start (Cowen, 1986; Levine & Perkins, 1987; Rickel, Dyhdalo, & Smith, 1984; Zigler & Valentine, 1979) and related educational programs for disadvantaged children, such as Perry Preschool Project (Berrueta-Clement, Schweinhart, Barnett, Epstein, Weikart, 1984; Berrueta-Clement, Schweinhart, Barnett, & Weikart, 1987).

Targeted to young, inner-city, relatively low IQ, high-risk children, the Perry program included both a saturated, enriched preschool component for children, and a parallel intensive, home-based educational program for parents. Participants and randomly assigned, matched no program controls have been followed for two decades. Wellness benefits to participants have been apparent throughout in terms of such bellwether criteria as superior academic performance; higher rates of high school graduation and post-secondary educational and vocational training; better employment and earnings records; and lower rates of teenage pregnancy, welfare assistance, delinquency, and crime. In interpreting those long-term findings, the authors view the educational experience itself as the key link in a chain of positive program outcomes, i.e., "... children at-risk of educational failure achieve enhanced success in early schooling; early success is linked to later success and to higher educational attainment at the end of secondary education. School success, in turn, is linked to reduced rates of misbehavior and delinquency" (Berrueta-Clement et al., 1987, p. 226).

Education's potential as a force for psychological wellness has not been sufficiently harnessed. Value-laden decisions about education's proper timing, content, and formats, sometimes made planfully sometimes by default (Sarason, 1971, 1983), can operate, in fact, either to advance or impeded wellness. That most people in modern society go through a formal educational system both challenges us, and provides opportunities, to develop ways of engineering educational experiences that not only meet the school's mandated objective of transmitting knowledge, but serve concurrently to advance psychological wellness.

Although natural and educational routes sometimes result in wellness, that is far from a universal outcome (Glidewell & Swallow, 1969). Indeed, institutions, settings, and processes built around the goals of managing, containing, and repairing deficits in psychological wellness or problems in living expressed in many forms, have become a hallmark of modern society. The costs associated with such problems, both to affected individuals and to society, are staggering (President's Commission on Mental Health, 1978). Hospitals, clinics, community mental health centers, and the practice of psychotherapy and related strategies of amelioration all reflect directly the magnitude of the problems created by breakdown in psychological wellness. Deficits in wellness also entail phenomenal cost to the welfare, delinquency, criminal justice, substance abuse, educational, and legal systems, among others. Such problems are widespread, not isolated, in modern society; their fallout is extensive (Levine & Perkins, 1987).

Consideration of factors that predispose deficits in wellness may hold a key to families of promising, though different, routes to wellness. Threats to, or failings in, wellness come about through malfunction at any of the source levels cited above. Specifically, (1) A child's givens and/or early development may fail to provide the necessary conditions (e.g., a secure relationship, care and concern, good physical health, support, or sound models) for psychological wellness. (2) A child's continuing formation, including the formal and informal educational processes to which he or she is exposed, may not provide the essential skills, competencies, and self views that mediate wellness; (3) Events or circumstances may occur that undermine psychological wellness. (4) Key social institutions may operate in ways that pose impediments to people's wellness. (5) People's lives may be overrun by injustice, lack of opportunity to use skills, exclusion, and disempowerment.

Although any of these elements and their interactions can seriously undermine wellness, they are likely to be salient at different times and to occur in relationship to different systems, institutions, and mediating structures. Whereas formation and skill acquisition are vital in the earlier years, deterrents to wellness that stem from disempowerment become more salient later on. Stressful life events and circumstances harbor wellness-detracting elements throughout the lifespan. One aspect of this array of deterrents stands out. Much more than classic (e.g., psychodynamic) notions of disturbance in wellness, they implicate community, institutions, and social forces. But not equally so! Collectively, they suggest that systematic furtherance of the goal of wellness calls for a multilevel, multimethod approach in which a focus on community determinants is one, but not the only, important element.

To the extent that deficit in wellness reflects the absence of early essential ingredients and/or the failure to acquire skills and competencies that significantly mediate wellness, then families, schools, and underlying processes of education are central areas on which to focus efforts to enhance wellness. To the extent that injustice and disempowerment deprive people of opportunity—indeed, of hope—then the institutions, policies, and practices that comprise a society's exosystems and macrosystems and, as such, are *de facto* providers of opportunity, justice, and empowerment, must be focal concerns. To the extent that profoundly stressful experiences pose jugular threats to psychological wellness, then the promotion of conditions and skills that can defuse such threats and strengthen both immediate wellness and future resilience should be prime goals. In summary, the problems created by malformation and failings in psychological wellness, as well as steps designed to enhance wellness, "pull" for a range of divergent, and at times, seemingly antagonistic, solutions.

EXEMPLAR CONCEPTS WITHIN A WELLNESS FRAMEWORK

Earlier, I suggested that my use of the concept of routes to psychological wellness was sufficiently broad to embrace diverse exemplar constructs that have themselves been used as orienting concepts, in whole or part, for community psychology. The next sections consider several such exemplars, including competence, empowerment, and heightened resilience (invulnerability) in children. Notwithstanding obvious and major surface differences among those concepts, they find a structural unity when the inclusive concept of routes to psychological wellness is used to define the phenomena of interest.

Competence

At an entirely personal level, I must confess that I have great respect for competence in others, be they automobile mechanics, TV-repair persons, jewelers, dentists, electricians or most certainly, commercial airline pilots and surgeons. Competence default in some of those instances is life-threatening; in others it creates major hassles in everyday living. Basically, competence means doing well and appropriately that which a person's abilities and life role suggest that he or she should be doing. The person, in other words, produces positive outcomes and avoids negative ones in mandated life spheres. Theorists, using the term "effectance motivation," have long stressed the motivational centrality of perceiving oneself as competent and effective in interactions with physical and social environments (Connell, 1988; Deci & Ryan, 1985; Harter, 1974, 1978; White, 1959, 1979). Seeing oneself as competent depends in some measure on whether one has acquired relevant competencies. Both self-efficacy (Bandura, 1979) and learned-helplessness (Abramson, Seligman, & Teasdale, 1978) theorists have emphasized the instrumental value of the sense of competence in controlling culturally and individually defined outcomes, and in giving people a sense of mastery over their own fate.

The concept of competence applies to all stages and walks of life; only the specific competencies of relevance change. When one discharges one's mandated tasks competently, it draws appreciation, respect, and positive regard from others and, by eliciting personal satisfaction, helps the person to form an image of self as effective and worthwhile (Deci & Ryan, 1985). Relevant competencies, as noted, differ at different points in the life cycle. Many relate to one's current life tasks, whether those have to do with school work for the 7-year-old or job performance for the 37-year-old. Others involve more generic interpersonal skills: communication skills, listening skills, interaction skills, social problem-solving skills, and appropriate assertiveness skills. There is much evidence to suggest that the presence of such skills relates to psychological wellness; their underdevelopment relates to problems in living (e.g., Spivack, Platt, & Shure, 1976).

Many important life skills and competencies are formed in childhood (Anderson & Messick, 1974), shaped more by educational experiences, both formal and informal, and modeling than by what we normally think of as empowering processes. Consistent with that view, Werner (1987) reported that competence in such basic educational skills as reading and writing was "a major ameliorative factor among resilient youth who coped well in spite of poverty and family distress" (p. 41). One step further, to build a small and perhaps useful bridge, I would suggest that acquiring relevant competencies may be the single most important pathway that children have to empowerment, at least to the aspect of empowerment defined phenomenologically as a sense of control over one's fate.

To the extent that acquiring relevant life and interpersonal competencies favors wellness outcomes, a comprehensive approach to wellness must pay heed both to natural pathways to competence and actions designed to strengthen adaptive competencies throughout the lifespan. Community psychology's faults in this sphere lie less in its failure to recognize this proposition and more in the narrowness of the models it has used to test it (Cowen, 1986; Cowen & Work, 1987), and the questionable ecological validity (Bronfenbrenner, 1977) of the criteria used to evaluate the efficacy of those models (Rappaport, 1981).

Empowerment

The term "empowerment," with good reason, has become increasingly visible and respected on the community psychology scene (Albee, 1982, 1986; Kessler & Albee, 1975; Levine & Perkins, 1987; Rappaport, 1981, 1984, 1987; Rappaport, Swift, & Hess, 1984; Swift, 1984; Swift & Levin, 1987). It speaks to phenomena of much interest both in their own right and to the broader topic of routes to psychological wellness. A stated goal for empowerment theorists is to promote policies and conditions, both at broad- and narrow-band levels, that "enhance possibilities for people to gain control over their own lives" (Rappaport, 1981, p. 15).

The concept arises out of wrenching, non-repressible realities: (1) that vast, and very different, segments of our population are disempowered; and (2) there are striking associations between such disempowerment and problems of living (Rappaport, 1977). Among the prominent disempowered groups cited in Swift and Levin's (1987) stimulating essay are ethnic minorities, the elderly, physically and emotionally disabled persons, children, women, and the homeless.

Although the concept of empowerment has broad appeal, it is not automatically self-defining. Indeed, several authors (Cowen, 1986; Swift & Levin, 1987) have highlighted a potentially important gross distinction between defining it objectively, i.e., as equal access to resources and opportunities, or phenomenologically, i.e., as a sense of control over one's fate. There is reason to question whether those two processes are the same, or even closely related, in terms of the operations that define them or the outcomes they might be expected to generate (Cowen, 1986; Gruber & Trickett, 1987).

To date, the still evolving, complex concept of empowerment has been used in molar, approximate ways. Even so, the implicit assumption has been made that the empowerment process will reduce problems and increase gratifications in living. As Rappaport (1981) put it: "... people are likely to benefit psychologically from more rather than less control over their lives and resources" (p. 19). Although logic and observation across many situations offer support for that view, it requires further empirical documentation that takes into account differing notions of empowerment and the differing contexts and groups to which those notions pertain (Cowen, 1986; Gruber & Trickett, 1987). What seems clearest at this point are the compelling associations between disempowerment, injustice, and lack of opportunity and problems of living. To the extent that disempowerment is a major deterrent to psychological wellness, and I am persuaded that it is, the development of conditions that enhance people's empowerment should be seen as another essential route to follow in the quest for psychological wellness.

The strongest development of the empowerment thesis to date is in Rappaport's (1987) argument that empowerment, as the gateway to what he earlier (1977) called "a more equitable, fair and just society," should be the overarching phenomenon of interest for community psychology. Without questioning the importance of empowerment, within a theory organized around the broader concept of routes to psychological wellness, it can only reflect one key set of such routes (Cowen, 1985, 1986; Kahn, 1986; Muñoz, 1986; Stokols, 1986). To sharpen the issue, I would suggest that empowerment without competence, just as competence without empowerment, limits psychological wellness and, conversely, that the presence of both can advance wellness by giving people a fuller sense of mastery over their environments and control over their fates. Perhaps that, in part, is what Swift and Levin (1987) had in mind when they proposed that for the disempowered to use resources effectively, they "must be both motivated and competent to do so" (p. 15). Those authors appropriately identified education and training as key pathways to competence enhancement.

The intent of the preceding argument is not at all to downgrade the potential importance of empowerment as a route to psychological wellness. Rather, it is to underscore a point made by Rappaport in the larger context of the need for divergent solutions to complex social problems, i.e., "Should empowerment become dominant as a way of thinking, I have no doubt that it too will force one-sided conclusions" (1981, p. 21).

Heightened Resilience in Children

In a framework built around routes to psychological wellness, there are other relevant worlds beyond the energizing concepts of competence and empowerment—worlds of support and compassion, of social ecology, of person–environment fits, among others. Let us turn attention to another of those worlds. Based both on my profound biases and my reading of an impressive body of research literature (Compas, 1987; Dohrenwend & Dohrenwend, 1981; Garmezy & Rutter, 1983; Honig, 1986a, 1986b; Johnson, 1986; Kornberg & Caplan, 1980), I would argue that important variations in psychological wellness can occur even under optimal conditions of competence and empowerment. Muñoz (1986) makes a similar point.

One reason is that all of us, at any time, are susceptible to unanticipable, uncontrollable assaults on wellness. One lives in the shadow of chronic violence or abuse; a close family member passes away; parents divorce; one loses his or her job; roots are torn up when one moves; unanticipable disaster (e.g., earthquake, fire, flood, tornado) destroys one's world; the terror of aggression and war is visited upon us. The negative effects of such experiences, individually and cumulatively, can be extensive for the competent as well as the less competent, for the empowered as well as the disempowered. Accordingly, a framework that features routes to psychological wellness must direct serious attention to events and circumstances that significantly impair such wellness. Although the latter typically cannot be prevented from occurring, how they are handled is a potent force that can favor or obstruct future wellness. Passivity or inaction in the face of such conditions, when there is knowledge showing that certain actions can prevent damage and/or promote wellness, betrays just as much of a value as planful effort to intervene to forestall predictable misfortune.

The issue at stake is not just one of circumscribed, unfortunate events. More deadly is a situation of chronic exposure to multiple profound stressors known to exact staggering psychological tolls and to predispose significant problems in living for many people who experience them. The last statement is both a summary of empirical fact (Garmezy & Rutter, 1983; Honig, 1986b) and a cue for introducing the concept of heightened resilience (invulnerability) in children (Anthony & Cohler, 1987; Cowen & Work, 1988; Garmezy, 1976, 1982, 1983, 1985; Garmezy, Masten, & Tellegen, 1984; Garmezy & Nuechterlein, 1972; Garmezy & Tellegen, 1984; Masten & Garmezy, 1985; Werner, 1987; Werner & Smith, 1982). That concept extends naturally what we know about stressful life events and circumstances and their harmful psychological effects.

Many children in modern society grow up in worlds of chronic, profound buffetings aptly labeled by Garmezy (1983) as "stressors of marked gravity." For the great majority, those grim realities have serious short- and long-term consequences. Some few, however, propelled by a special resilience that stems from sources not yet well understood, not only surmount the most profound life adversity, but show unusual adaptive skills and competence on the face of it. Werner (1987) described them colorfully as children who, notwithstanding heavy exposure to life-stressors, "worked well, played well, loved well and expected well" (p. 28).

These are the children of heightened resilience, i.e., "survivors," who come in nature's crucible to find adaptive ways of coping with stressors of marked gravity and, thus, to achieve a sense of mastery of their environments and control of their own destinies. How does that happen? What factors enable them to beat the heavy odds? And how can such information be harnessed both to forestall the dramatically harmful effects of chronic, profound stress and, more basically, to promote wellness?

Although children with this unusual resilience in the face of chronic and profound life stress are few in number, in a theory built around routes to psychological wellness, they are far more important than their limited numbers imply. Garmezy (1982) clearly recognized that point when he spoke of the significant "long-range benefits" that could accrue to society "were we to study the forces that move such children to survival and to adaptation" (p. xix). Although present theory and empirical findings point to the presence of a triad of stress protective factors in the histories of these special youngsters (Cowen & Work, 1987; Garmezy,

1983; Werner, 1987; Werner & Smith, 1982; Rutter, 1983), our knowledge of those factors, and more generally about pathways to resilience, is still very limited. That void too must be filled.

NEXT STEPS

Competence, empowerment, and heightened resilience! These phenotypically disparate concepts, perhaps paradoxically, find genotypic synchrony in a framework in which routes to psychological wellness is the overarching phenomenon of interest. Within such a proactive framework, each exemplifies the umbrella construct, but speaks to different routes and threats to wellness, timepoints in the life span, and circumstances. Although each offers promising early observational and/or empirical signposts, none can yet be seen as "money in the bank." A nagging voice of reality reminds us that it is easier to say that these qualities or processes should enhance wellness than to establish such linkages empirically. The latter is the stuff needed to nourish effective planning of long-term strategies to promote psychological wellness.

I am thus suggesting the need for active, multipronged efforts to identify the determinants of psychological wellness and, on that basis, to formulate policies and programs to enhance wellness. Within such a framework, one can imagine clusters of scholars and practitioners spearheading at least three, multilevel families of effort built around (1) the initial formation of wellness, including the microsystems, mesosystems, transactional processes, community forces, and policies that favor such development; (2) social policy and planning that takes cognizance of society's exosystems and macrosystems, including empowerment steps designed to enhance wellness both at the broad societal, and more delimited setting levels; and (3) antidotes to menacing life events and circumstances that pose jugular threats to wellness.

The intentional use of the phrase "clusters of scholars and practitioners," rather than "community psychologists" or even "psychologists," hints at several points that bear further comment. Although community psychologists surely have relevant inputs to make to the systematic study of routes to psychological wellness, they are not alone in that respect. As one case in point, I would argue that clear understandings of the early formation of wellness will require coordinated contributions, not only from community psychologists; but from educators; child-development specialists, particularly in social and emotional development; system analysts, and people in planning and policy-making roles for children, to mention several obvious input groups. In like manner, optimal development and application of empowerment notions within a routes to wellness framework calls for linkages among community psychologists; urban planners; political scientists; and representatives of the legal, criminal justice, and welfare systems, among others, as implied in a monograph on that topic (Rappaport et al., 1984).

Considerations such as these prompted me to suggest elsewhere (Cowen, 1982a, 1984b) the needs to (1) form new cross-disciplinary groupings to catalyze, and strengthen the ecological validity of, the study of wellness; and (2) modify community psychology training to broaden perspectives on the intrinsically complex strands of wellness and facilitate the new types of alliances needed to advance the development of wellness-enhancing programs. To achieve the latter goal may entail yet another type of alliance, i.e., between those with primary interests in the development and the application of knowledge (Price & Smith, 1985). Ultimate gain from a routes to wellness framework, measured as enhanced wellness at a population level, depends in some appreciable measure on the effectiveness of the latter alliance.

The three primary domains cited above illustrate, rather than exhaust, promising routes to pursue in seeking to advance psychological wellness. Each can be better prosecuted in community contexts and with a community mindset than on prior, self-limiting individually targeted, restorative battlegrounds.

Although I have thus far described the three domains largely as if they were circumscribed and self-contained, that is not, in fact, the case. Bronfenbrenner's (1977) penetrating analysis stressed the interdependence and joint impact of multiple settings on their "elements." The nub of his argument, pertinent to the main thesis of this chapter, is that an ecologically sound research approach must go "beyond the immediate setting containing the person to examine larger contexts, both formal and informal, that affect events within the immediate setting" (p. 527). One can perceive in that view useful potential bridges across the domains specified above, as, for example, the hypothesis that gain from skill- or competence-training programs for children may be greater, more enduring, and generalize further for youngsters who come from empowered, rather than disempowered, home settings. That possibility is consistent both with (1) Forehand, Walley, and Furey's (1984) suggestion that skill enhancement or distress-reducing programs are likely to work best in familial contexts characterized by "adequate health care, housing, employment and opportunity and status for parenthood" (p. 361), and (2) Levine and Perkins' (1987) interpretation that Head Start's success reflects the effective blending of essential competence building and social setting-change elements.

PRIMARY PREVENTION AND ROUTES TO WELLNESS

In proposing, indeed spotlighting, the concept of routes to psychological wellness as a fruitful matrix for defining a domain's prime phenomena of interest, I have thus far avoided using the term "primary prevention." It may be appropriate now to comment briefly on its place in the broader thesis being advanced. Within psychology's established framework, the concept of primary prevention has become steadily more visible and influential (APA Task Panel on Promotion and Prevention, 1987; Cowen, 1986; Felner, Jason, Moritsugu, & Farber, 1983; Roberts & Peterson, 1984), even though differences in views remain about its centrality and importance to that field (e.g., Cowen, 1985; Rappaport, 1981, 1987).

Central to the position being developed in this chapter is the conviction that there are many different potential routes to psychological wellness. Within that elasticized framework, the concept of primary prevention, like the concepts of competence, empowerment, and heightened resilience, is subordinate to (an exemplar of) the overarching concept of routes to psychological wellness. Otherwise put, although each of these exemplar concepts, and others, can contribute significantly to the ultimate goal of advancing wellness, each is insufficient by itself to cover the full range of potentially relevant instances. Sameroff (1977) made a similar point in a more specific context: "... if a child's characteristics are seen as an ongoing adaptation to a particular set of life circumstances, then we are offered a multiplicity of possibilities for changing those circumstances and thereby changing the prognosis for that child" (p. 61).

Earlier, I suggested that nature itself, including formal and informal educational processes, sometimes results in wellness. That, *per se*, is one important route, or set of routes, to wellness. More often, however, failures of nature leave residues of human and social misfortune. Metaphorically, primary prevention can be seen as a systematized effort to improve nature's "minor-league batting average" in the wellness ballpark. Languaged up, within a routes to wellness framework, primary prevention is an important exemplar or family of routes, consisting of intentional, conceptually and empirically grounded interventions to enhance psychological wellness from ground zero, and/or to defuse deterrents to wellness (Cowen, 1980, 1985; Levine & Perkins, 1987). It is the application of knowledge to promote wellness—something that can happen in many ways, on many turfs, at different times. Choices about specific areas will necessarily reflect people's interests, skills and values. All such work, however, is bound by its prospective relevance to the phenomena of interest, i.e., routes to psychological wellness. Prospective relevance is defined by the strength of the underlying generative knowledge bases on which primary prevention programs rest (Cowen, 1980, 1984a).

SUMMARY

I have used the broad concept of routes to psychological wellness to identify and bound a domain with a unified theme and set of challenges. Although psychological wellness is a desired goal at all stages of life, its manifestations and salient contributing strands vary substantially at different time points, under different circumstances, and for different groups.

Sometimes wellness comes about naturally. Such instances are to be cherished, understood, and harnessed. More often, however, limiting aspects of people, settings, policies, and environments impose *de facto* barriers to psychological wellness. Education offers one potentially important pathway to wellness. Another called primary prevention can be seen as a systematic network of efforts, based on a generative discernment of impediments to, and correlates of, wellness, to intervene in ways that improve nature's batting average and enhance wellness.

The more specific concepts of competence, empowerment, and heightened resilience, individually and interactively, are also subservient to the integrative concept routes to psychological wellness. Each speaks meaningfully to real, but different, aspects of a lifespan view of wellness that takes into account age-related, situation-related, and group-related determinants of, and impediments to, wellness. Thus, the three concepts are alike as important keys to a full and faithful quest for wellness, but different in the wellness issues they address, the time points and groups to which they apply, and their defining strategies and operations.

And what of community psychology? Within the proposed framework, community psychology is an important means, not an integral end—a means of addressing more meaningfully and richly some challenging questions about psychological wellness that were scarcely perceived, much less engaged, under the yoke of earlier, more restrictive, conceptual paradigms. A community orientation and ensuing set of activities, simply put, offers access to important strands of the wellness issue.

There are many potential routes to psychological wellness and many different ways in which it can be obstructed. The task at hand is to develop and evaluate strategies for advancing wellness and restricting its obstruction. No single "magic bullet" can offer such sweeping benefit. Phenotypically disparate concepts such as competence, empowerment, and heightened resilience, as well as other concepts not developed in this chapter, must be allies, not competitors, in such a quest. They share legitimacy as needed exemplars of a comprehensive, multipronged thrust to promote wellness. The diversity of that thrust is consistent with the biological axiom that genetic variation increases the likelihood of evolutionary success and, indeed, with the praise of paradox.

ADDENDUM: WELLNESS AND PREVENTION SCIENCE

This section describes some recent developments that pertain to wellness-related issues considered in this chapter. Primary prevention's emergence was significantly hampered by several major problems beyond the ample skepticism (Lamb, 1983; Marlowe & Weinberg, 1983) of professionals habituated to ways of traditional mental health. One very important problem was the lack of a solid research base showing the approach to be effective. Much progress has since been made in this area. Durlak & Wells (1997) ambitious meta-analysis, for example, established the overall efficacy of 177 primary prevention programs. In parallel, the influential Institute of Medicine Report (Mrazek & Haggerty, 1994), based on 209 studies, concluded that the field's undergirding research base had gotten much stronger.

Other examples that reflect this same research solidification process include (1) Durlak's 1995 book describing successful school-based prevention programs, and his 1997 volume documenting primary prevention's efficacy in averting behavior and emotional problems, poor physical health and injury, maltreatment, and learning problems, (b) Albee and Gullotta's 1997 volume describing, in-depth, 15 successful primary prevention projects, and (c) Weissberg and Greenberg's 1998 review providing extensive evidence of the efficacy of a number of major primary prevention programs. Collectively, these sources suggest that primary prevention has come of age (Cowen, 1997a) and is now a significant element in mental health's overall armamentarium.

A second early primary prevention concern, i.e., the absence of an agreed-upon definition (evidenced in non-overlapping—indeed often unrelated—usages of the term), has followed a more complex, polarized course. Although today's dominant view of primary prevention is much clearer than when the term first entered the popular mainstream, that sharpened definition has come at the expense of several hidden costs that bear further consideration.

Early efforts to define the term (Cowen, 1973; Prevention Task Panel, 1978) included two main prongs: (a) preventing serious psychological disorder and (b) building psychological health (Cowen, 1994, 1996, 1997a). Over time, however, the term's de facto usage by planners and funders came to rivet on the first objective and downplay the second (Cowen, 1999). Within that narrower framework, the notion of a "science of prevention" was envisioned, with a prime goal of preventing or moderating "major human dysfunctions" (Coie et al., 1993). Consistent with that view, Koretz (1991) identified as the special mandate for NIMH's newly established Preventive Intervention Research Centers (PIRCS) the "prevention of specific disorders and dysfunctions." Five fairly narrow steps were articulated by which this new science of prevention was to proceed (Mrazek & Haggerty, 1994; Muehrer, 1997): (1) identifying the serious disorder one sought to prevent; (2) reviewing existing knowledge about risk and protective factors relating to that disorder; (3) doing pilot studies on that base and evaluating their efficacy; (4) extending effective pilots to large-scale preventive trials; and (5) promoting community-wide applications of effective program models.

Although the risk-disorder prevention model makes good sense in its chosen sphere of operation, several factors limit its broader applicability. First, pathways between risk and disorder are often complex, reflecting the operation of two principles: (1) multicausality, i.e., a given disorder can come about as a result of many different risk factors, and (2) multifinality, a given factor can predispose a broad range of maladaptive outcomes (Cicchetti & Rogosch, 1996; Durlak, 1997). Hence, approaches built on presumed risk-disorder connections are susceptible to (a) overlooking people at risk for a given dysfunction, who reach that point as a result of factors other than those targeted by a program; (b) including people whose risk status predisposes them to adverse consequences other than those that a program seeks to address; and (c) identifying risk factors late enough in an unfolding process so that a program's helping potential is sharply limited. Consistent with the principal of multifinality, the case has been made, with increasing frequency, that building wellness from the start and maintaining it may protect people against the ravages of major psychological dysfunction as, or more effectively than, later targeted prevention programs built around identified risk for specific disorders (Cowen, 1994, 1999, 2000).

Awareness of intrinsic limitations of a primary prevention approach based on a risk detection-disorder prevention strategy increases the appeal of wellness-enhancement alternatives. At the core of the latter approach are the goals of building well from the start and striving to foster and maintain wellness thereafter. Cowen (1997b) argued that (a) the goals of disorder prevention and wellness enhancement are basically complementary, rather than competing or mutually exclusive; and (b) wellness enhancement is the broader notion—broad enough to encompass a risk-disease prevention approach within its scope.

One significant source of encouragement for further developing a wellness-enhancement framework was Durlak & Wells (1997) meta-analysis finding that wellness-oriented prevention programs were at least as effective as those oriented to problem reduction. Others have also called attention to the appeal and potential of a wellness-enhancement approach (Albee, 1996; Cicchetti, Rappaport, Sandler, & Weissberg, 2000; Durlak, 1997; Durlak & Wells, 1997; Elias, 1995; Masten & Coatsworth, 1998).

Although a wellness enhancement thrust is now clearly visible, because it is still young many of its important challenges remain to be resolved. These include identifying all major components of the approach and developing further evidence of their efficacy; intensifying program-development work on facets of the approach that can best be engaged now; and refining articulation of a comprehensive, lifespan approach to wellness, and identifying real-life complexities involved in pursuing it. Subsequent writings have sought to take these issues several logical steps beyond the points made here. Illustratively, Cowen (1994) identified a family of five important (albeit on the surface somewhat different) wellness-enhancement strategies: (1) promoting wholesome caregiver–child attachment relationships; (2) helping children to acquire early, stage-salient competencies; (3) engineering wellness-enhancing formative environments, as for example schools (Battistich et al., 1989, 1995; Dryfoos, 1994); (4) strengthening people's ability to cope with stress; and (5) enhancing people's sense of empowerment and having control of their fate.

Although these strategies may at first seem disparate, they share the common goal-oriented genotype of enhancing wellness. Each strives to advance this goal in relevant ways for particular groups, developmental stages, and life circumstances. For any of these strategies, wellness-enhancement steps can take different forms under different conditions. Thus, whereas empowerment steps for poor, minority, inner-city residents call for a social framework of justice and opportunity, for a 3- or 4-year-old, the sense of empowerment and control of one's fate may result from caregiver provision of autonomy support (Ryan, Deci, & Grolnick, 1995; Ryan & Stiller, 1991).

The early rooting of wellness seemed to be a sensible starting point for fleshing out a wellness-enhancement approach (Cowen, 1997c, 1997d) both because it is a relatively more accessible, controllable component within a broad wellness enhancement framework, and because it establishes a base (solid or porous) on which later wellness developments must rest. Accordingly, Cowen (1999) developed a ministructural model built around elements thought to favor the early rooting of wellness. The model's four main input strands included two relatively less modifiable ones ("givens" such as temperament, intelligence, and physical attractiveness, and acute and chronic stressors intrinsic to a child's life situation), and two other potentially more modifiable ones (the nature of the caregiver–child attachment relationship, and the extent to which the child acquires stage-salient competencies).

However useful that starter analysis, it is limited in several key respects. Although it identifies elements that favor early wellness, it does not consider determinants of those wellness-enhancing conditions (e.g., life-history pathways that subserve a sound, current parent–child relationship), and it deals only with how early wellness is formed, which, though an important piece in the wellness jigsaw puzzle, is but one aspect of it. Otherwise put, although early wellness is likely to facilitate later wellness, it hardly guarantees such an outcome.

These gaps stimulated a next step toward marking up a lifespan wellness-enhancement approach (Cowen, 1999) built on the base of Bronfenbrenner's (1977) proposed framework for research on human development (of which psychological wellness, of course, is one focal aspect). Bronfenbrenner identified four increasingly complex layers of influence on human development: (1) microsystems, i.e., key settings of influence that people inhabit (e.g., home, school, worksite); (2) mesosystems, i.e., networks of interrelated settings that affect individuals at any point in time; (3) exosystems, i.e., formal and informal social structures (e.g., communities, mass media) that shape the nature and operating ways of important settings; and (4) the macrosystem, i.e., a matrix of highly influential blueprints, sometimes visible in rules and laws, but often hidden, that powerfully shape the nature of a society's political, economic, legal, and educational systems. Bronfenbrenner's analysis highlights the great complexity and changing aspects of influence sources that shape wellness at any point in time, and over the course of a lifetime.

As one moves from microsystem- to macrosystem-wellness-enhancement steps, focal issues become more complex and diffuse; access lines and opportunities for control and constructive change, more difficult. Sources of knowledge and expertise needed to bring about such change become increasingly diverse. Hence, it is much easier to worship wellness enhancement than to make it happen. As Sarason (1998) pointed out, the latter is a tall order because macrosystems are incredibly complex and highly change-resistant. Even so, a much deeper knowledge of how, precisely, micro-, meso-, exo-, and macrosystems affect wellness is essential to the sound development of a psychology of wellness. And, as such knowledge is accreted, the need to develop technologies for its effective application (i.e., for constructive social change) will become even greater.

Systematic enhancement of psychological wellness differs in concept, method, and complexity from today's dominant notion of primary prevention in mental health. Over time, the importance of this distinction has become clearer. Wellness enhancement is an ideal that will not be realized quickly or easily. It is realistic today to see it as a beacon that can gainfully guide conceptual formulations and research in mental health in ways that may, over time, significantly enhance life satisfaction for many people.

REFERENCES

Abramson, L. Y., Seligman, M. E., & Teasdale, J. D. (1978). Learned helplessness in humans: Critique and reformulation. *Journal of Abnormal Psychology, 87*, 49–74.

Albee, G. W. (1959). *Mental health manpower trends.* New York: Basic Books.

Albee, G. W. (1982). Preventing psychopathology and promoting human potential. *American Psychologist, 37*, 1043–1050.

Albee, G. W. (1986). Lessons from observations on the primary prevention of psychopathology. *American Psychologist, 41*, 891–898.

Albee, G. W. (1996). Revolutions and counterrevolutions in prevention. *American Psychologist, 51*, 1130–1133.

Albee, G. W., & Gullotta, T. P. (1997). *Primary prevention works*. Thousand Oaks, CA: Sage.

Anderson, L. S., Cooper, S., Hassol, L., Klein, D. C., Rosenblum, G., Bennett, C. C. (1966). *Community psychology: A report of the Boston Conference on the Education of Psychologists for Community Mental Health*. Boston, MA: Boston University.

Anderson, S., & Messick, S. (1974). Social competence in young children. *Developmental Psychology, 10*, 282–293.

Anthony, E. J., & Cohler, B. J. (Eds.). (1987). *The invulnerable child*. New York: Guilford.

APA Task Panel on Promotion and Prevention (1987). Washington, D.C.: American Psychological Association.

Arnhoff, F. N., Rubenstein, E. A., & Speisman, J. C. (1969). *Manpower for mental health*. Chicago: Aldine.

Bandura, A. (1979). Self efficacy: Toward a unifying theory of behavioral change. *Psychological Review, 84*, 191–215.

Battistich, V., Schaps, E., Watson, M., & Solomon, D. S. (1995). Prevention effects of the Child Development Project: Early findings from an ongoing multisite demonstration trial. *Journal of Adolescent Research, 11*, 12–35.

Battistich, V., Solomon, D. S., Watson, M., Solomon, J., & Schaps, E. (1989). Effects of an elementary school program to enhance prosocial behavior and children's cognitive social problem solving skills and strategies. *Journal of Applied Developmental Psychology, 10*, 147–169.

Berrueta-Clement, J. R., Schweinhart, L. J., Barnett, M. W., Epstein, A. S., & Weikart, D. P. (1984). *Changed lives: The effects of the Perry Preschool program on youths through age 19*. Ypsilanti, MI: High/Scope Educational Research Foundation.

Berrueta-Clement, J. R., Schweinhart, L. J., Barnett, W. S., & Weikart, D. P. (1987). The effects of early educational intervention on crime and delinquency in adolescence. In J. O. Burchard & S. N. Burchard (Eds.), *Prevention of delinquent behavior* (pp. 220–240). Newbury Park, CA: Sage.

Block, J. H., & Block, J. (1980). The role of ego-control and ego resiliency in the organization of behavior. In W. A. Collins (Ed.), *Development of cognition, affect, and social relations. The Minnesota Symposia on Child Psychology, Vol. 13* (pp. 39–101). Hillsdale, NJ: Erlbaum.

Bronfenbrenner, U. (1977). Toward an experimental ecology of human development. *American Psychologist, 32*, 513–531.

Bronfenbrenner, U. (1979). *The ecology of human development: Experiments by nature and design*. Cambridge, MA: Harvard University Press.

Cicchetti, D., Rappaport, J., Sandler, I., & Weissberg, R. P. (2000). *The promotion of wellness in children and adolescents*. Thousands Oaks, CA: Sage.

Cicchetti, D., & Rogosch, F. A. (1996). Equifinality and multifinality in developmental psychopathology. *Development and Psychopathology, 8*, 597–600.

Cicchetti, C., & Toth, S. L. (1987). The application of a transactional risk model to intervention with multi-risk maltreating families. *Bulletin of the National Center for Clinical Infant Programs, 7*, 1–8.

Coie, J. D., Watt, N. F., West, S. G., Hawkins, J. D., Asarnow, J. R., Markman, H. J., Ramey, S. L., Shure, M. B., & Long, B. (1993). The science of prevention: A conceptual framework and some directions for a national research program. *American Psychologist, 48*, 1013–1022.

Compas, B. E. (1987). Coping with stress during childhood and adolescence. *Psychological Bulletin, 101*, 393–403.

Cowen, E. L. (1973). Social and community interventions. *Annual Review of Psychology, 24*, 423–472.

Cowen, E. L. (1977). Baby-steps toward primary prevention. *American Journal of Community Psychology, 5*, 1–22.

Cowen, E. L. (1980). The wooing of primary prevention. *American Journal of Community Psychology, 8*, 258–284.

Cowen, E. L. (1982a). The special number: A complete roadmap. In E. L. Cowen (Ed.), Research in primary prevention in mental health. *American Journal of Community Psychology, 10*, 239–250.

Cowen, E. L. (1982b). Choices and alternatives for primary prevention in mental health. In M. P. Goldstein (Ed.), *Preventive intervention in schizophrenia: Are we ready?* (pp. 178–191). Washington, DC: NIMH Primary Prevention Series, Government Printing Office.

Cowen, E. L. (1983). Primary prevention in mental health: Past, present and future. In R. D. Felner, L. Jason, J. Moritsugu, & S. S. Farber (Eds.), *Preventive psychology: Theory, research, and practice in community interventions* (pp. 11–25). New York: Pergamon Press.

Cowen, E. L. (1984a). A general structural model for primary prevention program development in mental health. *Personnel and Guidance Journal, 62*, 485–490.

Cowen, E. L. (1984b). Training for primary prevention in mental health. *American Journal of Community Psychology, 12*, 253–259.

Cowen, E. L. (1985). Person centered approaches to primary prevention in mental health: Situation focused and competence enhancement. *American Journal of Community Psychology, 13*, 87–98.

Cowen, E. L. (1986). Primary prevention in mental health: A decade of retrospect and a decade of prospect. In M.

Kessler & S. E. Goldston (Eds.), *A decade of progress in primary prevention* (pp. 3–42). Hanover, NH: University Press of New England.

Cowen, E. L. (1994). The enhancement of psychological wellness: Challenges and opportunities. *American Journal of Community Psychology, 22,* 149–179.

Cowen, E. L. (1996). The ontogenesis of primary prevention: Lengthy strides and stubbed toes. *American Journal of Community Psychology, 24,* 235–249.

Cowen, E. L. (1997a). The coming of age of primary prevention: Comments on Durlak and Wells' meta-analysis. *American Journal of Community Psychology, 25,* 153–167.

Cowen, E. L. (1997b). On the semantics and operations of primary prevention and wellness enhancement: Or, will the real primary prevention please stand up? *American Journal of Community Psychology, 25,* 245–255.

Cowen, E. L. (1997c). Psychological wellness in children. In H. Friedman (Ed.). *Encyclopedia of mental health* (pp. 689–698). San Diego, CA: Academic.

Cowen, E. L. (1997d). Schools and the enhancement of psychological wellness: Some opportunities and some limiting factors. In T. P. Gullotta, R. P. Weissberg, R. L. Hampton, B. A. Ryan, & G. R. Adams (Eds.). *Healthy children 2010: Establishing preventive services* (pp. 97–123). Thousand Oaks, CA: Sage.

Cowen, E. L. (1999). In sickness and in health: Primary prevention's vows revisited. In D. Cicchetti & S. L. Toth (Eds.), *Rochester Symposium on Developmental Psychopathology: Developmental approaches to prevention, Vol. 9* (pp. 1–24). Rochester, NY: University of Rochester Press.

Cowen, E. L. (2000). Psychological wellness: Some hopes for the future. In D. Cicchetti, J. Rappaport, I. Sandler, & R. P. Weissberg (Eds.), *The promotion of wellness in children and adolescents.* Thousand Oaks, CA: Sage.

Cowen, E. L., Gardner, E. A., & Zax, M. (Eds.). (1967). *Emergent approaches to mental health problems.* New York: Appleton-Century-Crofts.

Cowen, E. L., & Work, W. C. (1988). Resilient children, psychological wellness and primary prevention. *American Journal of Community Psychology, 16,* 597–607.

Deci, E. L., & Ryan, R. (1985). *Intrinsic motivation and self-determination in human behavior.* New York: Plenum.

Dohrenwend, B. P., & Dohrenwend, B. S. (1981). Socioenvironmental factors, stress and psychopathology. *American Journal of Community Psychology, 9,* 128–164.

Dryfoos, J. G. (1994). *Full-service schools: A revolution in health and social services for children, youth, and families.* San Francisco: Jossey-Bass.

Durlak, J. A. (1995). *School-based prevention programs for children and adolescents.* Thousand Oaks, CA: Sage.

Durlak, J. A. (1997). *Successful prevention programs for children and adolescents.* New York: Plenum.

Durlak, J. A., & Wells, A. M. (1997). Primary prevention programs for children and adolescents: A meta-analytic review. *American Journal of Community Psychology, 25,* 115–152.

Elias, M. J. (1995). Primary prevention as health and social competence promotion. *Journal of Primary Prevention, 16,* 5–24.

Felner, R. D., Jason, L. A., Moritsugu, J. N., & Farber, S. S. (Eds.). (1983). *Preventive psychology: Theory, research and practice.* New York: Pergamon.

Forehand, R. L., Walley, P. B., & Furey, W. M. (1984). Prevention in the home. In M. E. Roberts & L. Peterson (Eds.), *Prevention of problems of childhood: Psychological research and applications* (pp. 342–368). New York: Wiley.

Garmezy, N. (1976). *Vulnerable and invulnerable children: Theory, research and intervention.* Washington, D.C.: American Psychological Association.

Garmezy, N. (1982). Foreword. In E. E. Werner & R. S. Smith (Eds.), *Vulnerable but invincible: A study of resilient children* (pp. xiii–xix). New York: McGraw-Hill.

Garmezy, N. (1983). Stressors of childhood. In N. Garmezy & M. Rutter (Eds.), *Stress, coping, and development in children* (pp. 43–84). New York: McGraw-Hill.

Garmezy, N. (1985). Stress resistant children: The search for protective factors. In J. E. Stevenson (Ed.), *Recent research in developmental psychopathology. Journal of Child Psychology and Psychiatry, Book Supplement No. 4* (pp. 213–233). Oxford: Pergamon.

Garmezy, N., Masten, A. S., & Tellegen, A. (1984). Studies of stress-resistant children: A building block for developmental psychopathology. *Child Development, 55,* 97–111.

Garmezy, N., & Nuechterlein, K. (1972). Invulnerable children: The fact and fiction of competence and disadvantage. *American Journal of Orthopsychiatry, 42,* 328–329.

Garmezy, N., & Rutter, M. (Eds.). (1983). *Stress, coping, and development in children.* New York: McGraw-Hill.

Garmezy, N., & Tellegen, A. (1984). Studies of stress-resistant children: Methods, variables and preliminary findings. In F. Morrison, C. Ford, & D. Deating (Eds.), *Advances in applied psychology (Vol. 1)* (pp. 1–52). New York: Academic.

Glidewell, J. C., & Swallow, C. S. (1969). *The maladjustment in elementary schools: A report prepared for the Joint Commission on the Mental Health of Children.* Chicago: University of Chicago Press.

Goldstein, M. J. (1982). *Preventive intervention in schizophrenia: Are we ready?* Washington, D.C.: NIMH Primary Prevention Series, Government Printing Office.

Gruber, J., & Trickett, E. J. (1987). Can we empower others? The paradox of empowerment in the government of an alternative public school. *American Journal of Community Psychology, 15*, 353–371.

Harter, S. (1974). Pleasure derived by children from cognitive challenge and mastery. *Child Development, 45*, 661–669.

Harter, S. (1978). Effectance motivation reconsidered: Toward a developmental model. *Human Development, 21*, 34–64.

Hobbs, N. (1964). Mental health's third revolution. *American Journal of Orthopsychiatry, 34*, 822–833.

Honig, A. S. (1986a). Stress and coping in children (Part 1). *Young Children*, (May), 50–63.

Honig, A. S. (1986b). Stress and coping in children (Part 2): Interpersonal family relationships. *Young Children*, (July), 47–59.

Jahoda, M. (1958). *Current concepts of positive mental health.* New York: Basic Books.

Johnson, J. H. (1986). *Life events as stressors in childhood and adolescence.* Newbury Park, CA: Sage.

Joint Commission on Mental Health of Children (1969). *Crisis in child mental health: Challenge for the 1970's.* New York: Harper & Row.

Joint Commission on Mental Illness and Health (1961). *Action for mental health.* New York: Basic Books.

Kahn, R. L. (1986). Comments on Kelly. *American Journal of Community Psychology, 14*, 591–594.

Kelly, J. G. (1975). Community psychology: Some priorities for the immediate future. *Journal of Community Psychology, 3*, 205–209.

Kelly, J. G. (1986). Context and process: An ecological view of the interdependence of research and practice. *American Journal of Community Psychology, 14*, 581–589.

Kessler, M., & Albee, G. W. (1975). Primary prevention. *Annual Review of Psychology, 26*, 557–591.

Koretz, D. S. (1991). Prevention-centered science in mental health. *American Journal of Community Psychology, 19*, 453–458.

Kornberg, M. S., & Caplan, G. (1980). Risk factors and preventive intervention in child psychotherapy: A review. *Journal of Prevention, 1*, 71–133.

Kuhn, T. S. (1970). *The structure of scientific revolutions* (2nd ed.). Chicago: University of Chicago Press.

Lamb, H. R. (1983). The argument against primary prevention. In H. A. Marlowe & R. B. Weinberg (Eds.). *Primary prevention; Fact or fallacy* (pp. 17–28). Tampa: University of South Florida.

Levine, M., & Perkins, D. V. (1987). *Principles of community psychology. Perspectives and applications.* New York: Oxford University Press.

Lorion, R. P. (1973). Socioeconomic status and traditional approaches reconsidered. *Psychological Bulletin, 79*, 263–270.

Lorion, R. P. (1974). Patient and therapist variables in the treatment of low-income patients. *Psychological Bulletin, 81*, 344–354.

Manson, S. M. (Ed.). (1982). *New directions in prevention among Native American and Alaska native communities.* Portland, OR: Oregon Health Sciences University.

Marlowe, H. A., & Weinberg, H. B. (1983). *Primary prevention: Fact or fallacy.* Tampa: University of South Florida.

Masten, A. S., & Coatsworth, J. D. (1998). The development of competence in favorable and unfavorable environments: Lessons from research on successful children. *American Psychologist, 53*, 205–220.

Masten, A. S., & Garmezy, N. (1985). Risk, vulnerability and protective factors in developmental psychopathology. In B. B. Lahey & A. E. Kazdin (Eds.), *Advances in child clinical psychology (Vol. 8)* (pp. 1–52). New York: Plenum.

Mrazek, P. J., & Haggerty, R. J. (Eds.). (1994). *Reducing risks for mental disorders: Frontiers for preventive intervention.* Washington, D.C.: National Academy Press.

Muehrer, P. (1997). Introduction to Special Issue: Mental health prevention science in rural communities and contexts. *American Journal of Community Psychology, 25*, 421–424.

Muñoz, R. F. (1986). Current issues in prevention. In M. Kessler & S. E. Goldston (Eds.), *A decade of progress in primary prevention* (pp. 391–397). Hanover, NH: University Press of New England.

Murphy, L. B., & Moriarty, A. E. (1976). *Vulnerability, coping and growth: From infancy to adolescence.* New Haven: Yale University Press.

President's Commission on Mental Health (1978). *Report to the President* (Vol. 1). Washington, D.C.: U.S. Government Printing Office, Stock No. 040-000-00390-8.

Prevention Task Panel Report (1978). *Task Panel reports submitted to the President's Commission on Mental Health* (Vol. 4) (pp. 1822–1863). Washington, D.C.: U.S. Government Printing Office, Stock No. 040-000-00393-2.

Price, R. H., & Smith, S. S. (1985). *A guide to evaluating prevention programs in mental health.* Rockville, MD: National Institute of Mental Health.

Rappaport, J. (1977). *Community psychology: Values, research, and action.* New York: Holt, Rinehart & Winston.

Rappaport, J. (1981). In praise of paradox: A social policy of empowerment over prevention. *American Journal of Community Psychology, 9*, 1–25.

Rappaport, J. (1984). Studies in empowerment: Introduction to the issue. *Prevention in Human Services, 3*, 1–7.

Rappaport, J. (1987). Terms of empowerment/exemplars of prevention: Toward a theory of community psychology. *American Journal of Community Psychology, 15,* 121–148.

Rappaport, J., Swift, C., & Hess, R. (Eds.). (1984). Studies in empowerment: Steps toward understanding and action. *Prevention in Human Services, 3,* 1–230.

Reiff, R. (1967). Mental health manpower and institutional change. In E. L. Cowen, E. A. Gardner, & M. Zax (Eds.), *Emergent approaches to mental health problems* (pp. 74–88). New York: Appleton-Century-Crofts.

Reiff, R., & Riessman, F. (1965). The indigenous nonprofessional: A strategy of change in community action and community mental health programs. *Community Mental Health Journal, Monograph No. 1.*

Rickel, A. U., Dyhdalo, L. L., & Smith, R. L. (1984). Prevention with preschoolers. In M. C. Roberts & L. Peterson (Eds.), *Prevention of problems in childhood: Psychological research and applications* (pp. 74–102). New York: Wiley.

Roberts, M. C., & Peterson, L. (Eds.). (1984). *Prevention of problems in childhood: Psychological research and applications.* New York: Wiley.

Rutter, M. (1983). Stress, coping and development: Some issues and some questions. In N. Garmezy & M. Rutter (Eds.), *Stress, coping and development in children* (pp. 1–41). New York: McGraw-Hill.

Ryan, R. M., Deci, E. L., & Grolnick, W. S. (1995). Autonomy, relatedness and the self: Their relation to development and psychopathology. In D. Cicchetti & D. J. Cohen (Eds.), *Developmental psychopathology: Theory and methods, Vol. 1* (pp. 618–655). New York: Wiley.

Ryan, R. M., & Stiller, J. (1991). The social contexts of internalization: Parent and teacher influence on autonomy, motivation, and learning. In R. P. Pintrich, & M. L. Maehr (Eds.), *Advances in motivation and achievement: Goals and self-regulatory processes, Vol. 7* (pp. 115–149). Greenwich, CT: JAI Press.

Ryan, W. (1971). *Blaming the victim.* New York: Random House.

Sameroff, A. J. (1977). Concepts of humanity in primary prevention. In G. W. Albee & J. Joffe (Eds.), *Primary prevention of psychopathology, Vol. 1* (pp. 42–63). Hanover, NH: University Press of New England.

Sameroff, A. J., & Chandler, M. J. (1975). Reproductive risk and the continuum of caretaking casualty. In F. D. Horowitz, M. Hetherington, S. Scarr-Salapatek, & G. Siegel (Eds.), *Review of child development research* (pp. 187–244). Chicago: University of Chicago Press.

Sanua, V. D. (1966). Sociocultural aspects of psychotherapy and treatment: A review of the literature. In L. E. Abt & L. Bellak (Eds.), *Progress in clinical psychology, Vol. VIII.* New York: Grune & Stratton.

Sarason, S. B. (1971). *The culture of the school and the problem of change.* Boston: Allyn-Bacon.

Sarason, S. B. (1983). *Schooling in America: Scapegoat and salvation.* New York: The Free Press.

Sarason, S. B. (1987, May). *The barometers of community change.* Address given at APA division 27's First Biennial Conference on Community Research and Action, Columbia, SC.

Sarason, S. B. (1998). *Political leadership and educational failure.* San Francisco: Jossey-Bass.

Schofield, W. (1964). *Psychotherapy: The purchase of friendship.* Englewood-Cliffs, NJ: Prentice-Hall.

Spivack, G., Platt, J. J., & Shure, M. B. (1976). *The problem-solving approach to adjustment.* San Francisco: Jossey-Bass.

Stokols, D. (1986). The research psychologist as a social change agent. *American Journal of Community Psychology, 14,* 595–599.

Swift, C. (1984). Empowerment: An antidote for folly. *Prevention in Human Services, 3,* ix–xv.

Swift, C., & Levin, G. (1987). Empowerment: The greening of prevention. In M. Kessler, S. E. Goldston, & J. M. Joffe (Eds.), *The present and future of prevention: In honor of George Albee* (pp. 99–111). Newbury Park, CA: Sage.

Weissberg, R. P., & Greenberg, M. T. (1998). School and community competence-enhancement and prevention programs. In W. Damon, I. E. Siegel, & K. A. Renninger (Eds.), *Handbook of child psychology, 5th ed., Vol. 4: Child psychology in practice* (pp. 877–954). New York: Wiley.

Werner, E. E. (1987). Vulnerability and resiliency in children at risk for delinquency: A longitudinal study from birth to young adulthood. In J. D. Burchard & S. N. Burchard (Eds.), *Prevention of delinquent behavior* (pp. 16–43). Newbury Park, CA: Sage.

Werner, E. E., & Smith, R. S. (1982). *Vulnerable but invincible: A study of resilient children.* New York: McGraw-Hill.

White, B. L., Kaban, B. T., & Attanuci, J. S. (1979). *The origins of human competence: Final report of the Harvard Preschool Project.* Lexington, MA: D. C. Heath.

White, R. W. (1959). Motivation reconsidered: The concept of competence. *Psychological Review, 66,* 297–333.

White, R. W. (1979). Competence as an aspect of personal growth. In M. W. Kent & J. E. Rolf (Eds.), *Primary prevention of psychopathology, Vol. 3: Social competence in children* (pp. 5–22). Hanover, NH: University Press of New England.

Zax, M., & Cowen, E. L. (1976). *Abnormal psychology: Changing conceptions* (2nd ed.). New York: Holt, Rinehart and Winston.

Zigler, E., & Valentine, J. (Eds.). (1979). *Project Head Start: A legacy of the war on poverty.* New York: Free Press.

CHAPTER 5

Toward an Integration of Behaviorism and Community Psychology

*Dogs Bark at Those They Do Not Recognize**

G. ANNE BOGAT AND LEONARD A. JASON

The field of behavioral community psychology has emerged during the last 25 years as a subspecialty of community psychology and applied behavior analysis. It attempts to understand and change community problems through the application of behavioral theory and technology. The field has spawned several textbooks (e.g., Glenwick & Jason, 1980; Nietzel, Winett, MacDonald, & Davidson, 1977), a special issue of *Journal of Community Psychology* (Glenwick & Jason, 1984), and a compendium of articles originally appearing in the *Journal of Applied Behavior Analysis*, entitled *Behavior Analysis in the Community 1968–1986* (Society for the Experimental Analysis of Behavior, 1987). In addition, several recent chapters elaborate the contributions that behavioral researchers can make to community psychology (e.g., Burgoyne & Jason, 1991; Fawcett, 1990). These different sources present compelling theoretical and empirical data to demonstrate the utility and scope of such an approach; yet most contain one of two types of caveats. The first expresses regret that behavioral community psychology has yet to tackle large societal problems. Some authors (e.g., Fawcett, Mathews, & Fletcher, 1980) even suggest that there may be insurmountable obstacles to using behavioral technologies to promote far-reaching community change. The second is that, unfortunately, a synthesis of community approaches and behavioral technology has been delayed because of difficulties delineating turf, choosing problems best suited for a collaboration between the two approaches, and agreeing upon definitions of concepts (Glenwick & Jason, 1993).

These two caveats make quite different points as to the nature of integrating behaviorism

*This is a translation of a "fragment" from the pre-Socratic philosopher Heraclitus of Ephesus.

G. ANNE BOGAT • Department of Psychology, Michigan State University, East Lansing, Michigan 48824.
LEONARD A. JASON • Department of Psychology, De Paul University, Chicago, Illinois 60614.

Handbook of Community Psychology, edited by Julian Rappaport and Edward Seidman. Kluwer Academic / Plenum Publishers, New York, 2000.

with community psychology; however, the conclusion reached is the same: To date, although the behavioral perspective has been adopted by some community psychologists, it has not been wholeheartedly embraced by the dominant ecological model (Duffy & Wong, 1996; Jason & Bogat, 1983; Jason & Crawford, 1991; Jason & Glenwick, 1984). At this point in the history of community psychology, this state of affairs seems perplexing. This chapter will examine why, to date, there has been such minimal collaboration between the two fields, and how a more meaningful partnership might best be effected. Any discussion of the difficulties integrating these two approaches must necessarily consider three separate aspects of behaviorism: its philosophy concerning human behavior, the theories that result from this philosophy, and the technology used to test these theories.

PHILOSOPHICAL DIFFERENCES

One of the major determinants in the formation of community psychology was a basic discontent with the asocial nature of psychology. [See Sarason's (1981) penetrating analysis of clinical psychology's pertinacious pursuit of the "self-contained" individual.] Early behaviorists anticipated community psychologists by stressing the importance of the context of behavior. Kantor consistently admonished psychologists for ignoring the role of the environment. "Despite the fact that psychological events always consist of fields, psychologists persist in locating their data in or at the organism" (Kantor, 1958, p. 83). His interbehavioral psychology takes its name from his insistence on the importance of understanding individuals' behavior as "interbehavior" with the environment. Skinner's radical behaviorism also was concerned with the environment and its influence on behavior, although he conceded that "... the selective role of the environment in shaping and maintaining the behavior of the individual is only beginning to be recognized and studied" (1971, p. 25). Finally, the early rhetoric of the applied behaviorists embraced sociological theories concerned with the influence of culture and society on behavior. For instance, Ullmann and Krasner (1969), in their behavioral approach to abnormal behavior, focused quite strongly, at least in their introductory comments, on the importance of labeling theory.

Thus, the behaviorists, with their emphasis on studying environments and person–environment interactions, helped legitimize these pursuits within the academic community, and hence paved the way for community psychologists. Historically, then, the link between community psychology and behaviorism should have been a natural one; however, there are, as will be discussed below, philosophical differences that have hindered collaboration.

For some years, the field of clinical psychology debated the merits of integrating behavior therapy with more traditional, psychoanalytic therapies. Messer and Winokur (1980) suggested that, in part, the differences between these therapeutic approaches emanated from contrasting assumptions about viewpoints and visions of reality. Portions of their argument also highlight the philosophical differences in community psychology between behaviorism and the mainstream community-ecological model. First, behavioral and community psychology approaches tend to stress contrasting viewpoints on reality (taken from Rychlak, 1968). Behaviorists tend to develop ideas about the world based on their "vantage point as observer, regardless of the subject's viewpoint" (Messer & Winokur, 1980, p. 822). In contrast, community-ecological psychology approaches emphasize respect for cultural relativity; an emphasis on collaborative, rather than a merely professional, relationship with settings; implementing programs responsive to community needs; etc. All of these values uphold the importance of each person's competency, not just the professional's, in defining and solving problems.

Kelly and colleagues (1987, 1990, 1998; Kingry-Westergaard & Kelly, 1990) have provided detailed and insightful recommendations for collaborative relationships between social scientists and citizens. In one paper Kelly (1987) asks "Why worry about creating a collaborative relationship or creating social settings?" His answer is instructive:

> *I believe that the very process of creating social settings is a process which can be empowering and thereby preventive.* When the professional initiates a process where citizens actively co-design service delivery, citizens are validated for taking action that is synonymous with what is known about the practice of good mental health. They are identifying resources, receiving support while creating resources, and having the autonomy and free choice to use these resources for the development of their own needs and aspirations (p. 4; emphasis in the original)

In principle, behaviorists could easily support the above-stated viewpoint of community psychology. In practice, however, behaviorists often frame reality differently. Behavioral community psychologists, like community psychologists, seek to enhance those mediational factors that enable people to control their lives. However, behavioral community psychologists also believe that certain setting and consequence events, some of which people are not even aware, can and should be modified so that deleterious influences on human behavior are reduced. In other words, a person's recognition of the aversive consequences of a particular problem is not the sole reason for motivating a change. Behaviorists feel comfortable creating change by controlling reinforcers and contingencies.

This viewpoint is also manifested by the written descriptions of behavioral research. Willems (1974) suggested that the behaviorist's "skill and ingenuity in picking crucial behaviors and deciding upon category systems needs to be made more public and explicit and it needs to be subjected to study. It is, after all, diagnosis *par excellence*" (p. 20; emphasis in the original). This is only one piece of important information (from a community psychologist's perspective) that is missing. Behaviorists rarely chronicle how they came to define a behavior or an environment as a problem (were they independent observers, agents of the setting, agents of concerned citizens?) or how a particular intervention was decided upon (were persons other than the investigators involved in planning and implementing the intervention?). The absence of these types of person and setting descriptions cannot represent a total lack of interest in the collaborator's perspective (applied research cannot be conducted without some contact with persons in the setting), but it does indicate the behaviorist's tendency to formulate a problem and its solution from the observer's vantage point.

For example, in a series of truly innovative studies, Twardosz, Cataldo, and Risley (1974) examined the influence of an open environmental design in a child-care center. A community psychologist might describe this research as the creation of an alternative setting. As part of this narrative, the community psychologist would detail the process of collaboration between a group of university researchers and the staff of a daycare center that resulted in optimal learning and supervision environments for children. However, Twardosz et al. do not conceptualize their research as the creation of alternative settings. They do not mention how the collaboration was enacted or the difficulties establishing and monitoring environmental changes. The reader is provided only a thumbnail sketch of the setting; the major portion of the paper describes the interventions and documents changes in the children's behavior.

Returning to Messer and Winokur's argument, behavioral psychologists and traditional psychologists differ not only on their viewpoint of reality, but also on their basic *visions* of reality, of which there are four: the romantic,[1] the ironic, the tragic, and the comic.

[1]These four visions are based on Schafer's (1976) reworking of Frye's (1957) four mythic forms. According to Schafer (1976), the romantic vision is "a perilous, heroic, individualistic journey … which ends after crucial struggles with exaltation" (p. 31). We believe that neither behaviorism nor community psychology adheres to a romantic vision.

> The ironic vision ... is characterized chiefly as a readiness to seek out internal contradictions, ambiguities, and paradoxes.... The tragic vision emphasizes [that] ... conflict is endemic in life; it cannot be eliminated, but only confronted with the muted hope of partial mastery.... The comic vision is in many ways antithetical to the tragic: It emphasizes the familiar, controllable, and predictable aspects of situations and people. Conflict is viewed as centered in situations, and it can be eliminated by effective manipulative action or via the power of positive thinking (Messer & Winokur, 1980, p. 823).

Although both behaviorism and community psychology encompass some aspects of the ironic, the tragic, and the comic, behaviorists' predominant vision of reality most closely approximates the comic, whereas some combination of ironic and tragic visions is the regnant perspective of most community psychologists.

Perhaps community psychology's ironic vision is best exemplified by Rappaport's (1981) exhortation for community psychologists to pursue paradox. He suggested that all social problems are inherently paradoxical; they contain internal antinomies that cannot be resolved. Community psychologists need to search out these paradoxes and emphasize the aspect of the social problem that is being ignored. Paradoxes imply ambiguity. With a historical tradition specifically founded on an opposition to conceptualizations that result in ambiguous outcome criteria, behaviorists do not embrace the ironic vision.

The tragic vision in community psychology is closely tied to the ironic vision. Rappaport stated that the purpose of community psychology is not to find the one best solution to a social problem. "I do not believe that there are no solutions, only that given the nature of social problems there are no permanent solutions and no single 'this is the only answer possible' solutions, even at any moment in time" (Rappaport, 1981, p. 9). Because *all* social problems, by definition, are paradoxical, they require divergent types of solutions. Behaviorists believe there are specific, convergent solutions to target problems and that, in time, effective behavioral strategies will be discovered for currently insolvable problems. (Some writers qualify this by saying the social change will be at microlevels of society or "first-order" change.) This perspective is at the heart of behaviorists' comic vision.

The merit in this approach is obvious. Behaviorists can take exceedingly complicated problems and construe them in such a way as to create manageable and researchable topics. "What is chaos to others yields functional and critical dimensions of behavior to them [behaviorists]" (Willems, 1974, p. 20). But this propensity for ascertaining simple problems and solutions in the midst of complex social problems worries community psychologists. Sarason (1972) illustrated such reservations when he criticized Skinner's theory, not for being wrong, but for being incomplete.

These unstated differences in the viewpoint and visions of reality between behaviorism and mainstream community psychology underpin some community psychologists' skepticism concerning the applicability of behaviorism to major social problems. However, it is also possible that these differences can serve as an important adjunct to the dominant community-ecological model. Such integration could occur both at the theoretical and technological levels of research.

THEORETICAL ISSUES

When discussing philosophical differences between behaviorism and the dominant community model, we purposely blurred all distinctions between different behavioral theories. However, within the behavioral perspective, and thus within behavioral community psychology, there are two major paradigms: behavior analysis and behavior therapy. Behavior analysts (BAs) adhere to a more strictly operant approach, are more apt to collect time-series data, and are more closely identified with the work of B. F. Skinner. Behavior therapists (BTs) value cognitive events, use traditional, experimental designs as well as time-series designs, and are more closely linked with such early theorists as Wolpe, Lazarus, and Eysenck. Hence, the theoretical differences between these two approaches can be vast. BAs control and influence behavior by altering either the antecedents (the environment or setting) or the consequences (rewards or punishments) associated with them. They eschew the notion of hypothetical constructs; their theory is based on the understanding and manipulation of observable, quantifiable events. In contrast, BTS are willing to consider the theoretical importance of unobservable phenomena. They suggest that cognitive processes (e.g., feelings, beliefs) help to explain the individual's interaction with his or her environment, and are thus important to modify.

Either a BA or a BT approach can be used to conceptualize a particular community problem. For example, a BA approach at the organizational level has been effective in drastically reducing passive smoke in public settings (Jason & Liotta, 1982). This study was undertaken in two phases. In the first, "no smoking" signs were posted in one section of a school cafeteria. The signs, used as prompts or stimuli, moderately reduced the number of persons smoking in that area of the cafeteria. In the second phase of the study, the prompts were maintained and consequence controls were added. Those persons smoking in this section were told: "This is a non-smoking area, please don't smoke here." The addition of the consequence control resulted in a dramatic reduction in the number of persons smoking in that section. Following this demonstration project, the cafeteria's employees instituted the consequence controls. Significant reductions in smoking were maintained over a three-month follow-up period.

A BT framework can be used to combat the problem of smoking at a community level (Jason, McMahon, Salina, Hedeker, Stockton, Dunson, & Kimball, 1995; Jason, Salina, McMahon, Hedeker, & Stockton, 1997). Following a media intervention, 14 one-hour meetings were held for the subsequent six months at companies in the greater Chicago metropolitan area. Meetings were first scheduled relatively frequently, when abstainers needed the most support, and then gradually reduced. In addition, participants were able to earn money for quitting and remaining abstinent (Jason et al., 1995). At the 24-month follow-up, 38% of the participants who received support groups and incentives were abstinent, compared to 22% of those receiving support groups only (Jason et al., 1997).

Behavioral theory has been used to address many other community problems besides smoking (e.g., preventing child injury, Peterson & Mori, 1985; reducing speeding and accidents, Van Houten et al., 1985; decreasing residential energy consumption, Winett, Leckliter, Chinn, Stohl, & Love, 1985; increasing immunization of preschool children, Yokley & Glenwick, 1984; increasing safe sex behavior, Winett, 1993; increasing blood donations, Ferrari & Jason, 1990; and helping parents reduce their children's television watching, Jason & Hanaway, 1997). In fact, one of the most widely implemented primary-prevention programs helps to develop social problem-solving skills among children—an approach very much within the rubric of a cognitive behavioral paradigm (Weissberg & Greenberg, 1997).

Despite all the evidence that behavioral theories can be used to conceptualize social problems, two widely held misperceptions about behavioral theories may continue to impede constructive dialogue between those advocating a behavioral approach and those espousing the dominant community model: Behavioral theories are only relevant for individual-level interventions, and are too narrowly focused to offer solutions for large and multifaceted social problems.

The primary criticism directed against behavioral theory is that is can only describe individual behavior. It is true that, at present, most behavioral community interventions have been conceptualized at an individual level; however, this is not proof that the theory cannot accommodate higher-order change.

For example, many behavioral community psychologists have studied the problem of litter. The general tactic of this research is the institution of feedback and reinforcement techniques that encourage individuals to dispose of their trash properly (see Geller, Winett, & Everett, 1982). This literature has been faulted for being fairly insignificant, as well as for focusing at an individual, tertiary level of analysis (Glenwick & Jason, 1993). We believe that behavioral theory can be employed to reframe the issue of litter so that there will be general agreement as to its significance as a social problem, the level of analysis will be the community or society, and the level of intervention will be primary prevention. Arguments analogous to the one that follows could be applied to other social problems that behavioral theory might address.

In the early 1970s, when the first behavioral study on litter was published, few would have envisioned the scenario that occurred in 1986–1987, when a tugboat towing a garbage barge spent nine months looking for a state (six turned it down) or foreign country (three declined) in which to dump its 3000 tons of refuse. As the century draws to a close, waste management has become a problem of staggering magnitude, and behaviorists appear almost prescient in their early attention to this problem.

Mainstream community psychologists would agree that waste disposal is an important problem; however, they would not necessarily concur that theory and tertiary interventions focused on individual citizens can solve it. The behaviorists construed the solution as one of encouraging proper disposal rather than as one of (a) encouraging less extraneous packaging, (b) developing new, non-biodegradable, and dangerous by-products of packaging, or (c) manufacturing goods of superior quality that can be recycled and repaired. These solutions are clearly more difficult to research and influence; interventions for their implementation require primary prevention strategies to create more broad-based social changes.

The determination of whether a problem is important rests more with one's philosophical perspective than with some objective truth. For the behaviorist, who maintains a comic vision, a valid intervention emphasis is litter itself. This focus creates an unambiguous, "familiar, controllable, and predictable" problem amenable to behavioral theory and technology. For the community psychologist, who adheres to a tragic/ironic vision, litter and its disposal would be viewed as only one component of a multifaceted ecological system. In examining the entire system, the community psychologists might note that an intervention focused on points a–c in the previous paragraph might ultimately have a larger impact on waste disposal than would an individual-focused intervention. Further, the community psychologist would be concerned about the unintended effects of an individual-centered intervention; for example, would it thwart or prevent organizational and societal change because public sentiment comes to assume that the genesis of the problem is the individual, not society?

An integration of all three visions of reality creates a context in which the problem of litter, and the behavioral community psychology interventions directed toward it, have significance. Weick (1984), in detailing the importance of small wins when approaching social problems, suggests a way of integrating these visions. He provides examples of successful small endeavors (e.g., Alcoholics Anonymous, the evolution of gender neutrality in American language) as examples of changes that may be construed as minor, but when taken together, show results. His description of the politics of small wins evokes the comic viewpoint:

> [s]mall wins may sound hopelessly naive, since they rely heavily on resources such as hope, faith, prophecies, presumptions, optimism, and positive appraisals ... naive beliefs favor optimism. Many of the central action mechanisms for small wins ... gain their energy from the initial belief that people can make a difference.... We justify what we do, not by belief in its efficacy but by an acceptance of its necessity (pp. 47–48).

The behavioral community psychologist's concern with reinforcing the proper disposal of litter has a greater significance when considered within the framework of small wins.

> [a] small change is either a change in a relatively unimportant variable (people tend to agree on what is an important change) or a relatively unimportant change in an important variable.... Small wins often originate as solutions that single out and define as problems those specific, limited conditions for which they can serve as the complete remedy (Weick, 1984, p. 43).

Changing American culture to decrease the production of wasteful packaging and its sometimes toxic by-products, for example, is a tall order for the social science researcher. The scope of the problem is so large that its solution, whether implemented by the behavioral community psychologist or the mainstream community psychologist, could not be successfully conceptualized without the concerted efforts of many individual citizens. But litter is not a pressing problem for most citizens (or most social scientists); witness the reluctance of many states to institute returnable bottle laws. Even the citizen concerned about the problems of refuse often cannot envision what steps to take to help solve the problem.

Alinsky (1971) noted that most American citizens do not participate in the important decisions affecting their lives. He suggested that when the alienation is very severe, the community organizer needs to create conditions in which small victories can occur. Thus, in discussing why he was willing to work on small problems (such as making one apartment building more habitable), he said: "we organize to get rid of four-legged rats so we can get on to removing two-legged rats" (p. 68).

The research on proper litter disposal is a first step—in behavioral terms, a successive approximation—toward the ultimate goal. If such a project were properly implemented, it could mobilize community concern about the problem, create a small win, and bring the public's (and the research community's) attention to the problem. Bringing the citizenry's attention to the smaller problems of litter (e.g., aesthetics, pollution of rivers) is the first step toward tackling the larger, social problems that create such refuse. And then, to paraphrase Alinsky, although they start out fighting for hamburger, before you know it they want filet mignon.

Can behavioral theory be used to conceptualize a primary prevention research project that addresses the social problem of litter? Community principles posit that resources for change are frequently available; unfortunately, our inability to appreciate the universe of alternatives limits our interventions and, hence, our effectiveness (Sarason, 1971). The reluctance of most behaviorists to engage in higher-level interventions is based largely on the erroneous perception that they lack access to the necessary reinforcers to effect important or large-scale social change.

There are many strategies that might be implemented. We will discuss one, the boycott, which works on behavioral principles. To the extent that the policies implemented by a business generate money, they are reinforcing. The object of a boycott is to change the reinforcers: to let businesses know that if they continue with a certain policy, they will lose a substantial amount of money. Suppose our goal is to encourage packaging companies to produce more biodegradable and recyclable packaging—a preventive, non-individual-focused intervention for the problem of litter. There are many organizations, with substantial memberships, concerned about these types of problems (e.g., Greenpeace). As a social scientist, one might work with these organizations to implement a strategic boycott of certain businesses that use non-biodegradable and non-recyclable packaging. If a large business no longer found it profitable to use this type of packaging, they would begin to order an alternative product.

According to Alinsky (1971), boycotts are only effective if staged against some, but not all, of the problem businesses. Although in the past few years businesses have become more ecologically minded, non-biodegradable and non-recyclable packaging is still a problem. It is unrealistic to expect the average American to stop using all products that have this type of packaging. For a boycott to work, the citizens must have an alternative source to obtain the product. Environmental groups might be organized in several cities to boycott just one or two products. The membership of these groups would have to be willing to boycott if necessary, but the threat of a boycott might provide enough pressure to change the business policies. If the threat was insufficient, the boycott would be enacted.

Encouraging one or two large companies to use more ecologically sound packaging would not change the practices of all American businesses. However, if the boycott received sufficient media exposure, other businesses would become aware that they could also be targeted for a boycott, and ecological awareness among citizens as a whole would be increased. The boycott would be a "middle-size win" on the road to major social change.

A second criticism of behavioral theory is that it is too narrow to provide comprehensive answers for complex social problems. According to this viewpoint, social problems are believed to involve "mixed questions" that require expertise from many fields (Adler, 1965; Fawcett, 1990); therefore, behaviorism cannot possibly provide all the necessary theory. However, this criticism is not solely applicable to behavioral theory; community psychologists have long advocated multidisciplinary research approaches. Often, behavioral theories and techniques are sufficient to explain and invoke change in socially significant behaviors; however, in some circumstances, their power could be amplified if principles within other subareas (e.g., developmental, organizational, and community psychology) are coupled with behavioral theory.

For example, while behaviorists have demonstrated that social skills can be taught, the gains often do not endure. Strain (1985) has suggested this is because "the intervention techniques (e.g., reinforcement, modeling, coaching, group contingencies) most widely used to improve the peer social performance of young children have no conceptual or empirical link to the target behaviors ... [nor] to the natural processes of peer influence" (p. 194). Attention to developmental principles (e.g., observing the ways in which children naturally socialize and gain peer acceptance) will enable psychologists to teach relevant social skills that may endure in children's repertoires.

Attention to developmental research can also aid our efforts to help infants who experience prenatal and birth complications (Jason, 1992). For example, Sameroff (1987) reports that many early infant difficulties remedy themselves, *except* when the infant is born into a low socioeconomic family. In these situations, the child–environment transactions and the environment, rather than the individual, should be the focus of the psychologist's interventions (Jason & Glenwick, 1984).

Thus, behavioral theory can usefully be applied to conceptualizations at the individual, group, community, and societal levels. When integrated with other psychological theories, behaviorism can further enrich our understanding of particularly complex social problems. But the integration of behaviorism with community psychology need not take place just at the theoretical level. Behaviorism can provide community psychologists with a wealth of relevant technology for conducting and evaluating research.

TECHNOLOGICAL ISSUES

We use the term "behavioral technologies" to refer to those intervention techniques and experimental methods used by behaviorists. As stated earlier, the particular technologies employed will depend, in part, on whether the behaviorist adheres to a BA or a BT paradigm. Intervention techniques include modification of antecedent and consequent stimuli, self-instruction, role-playing, institution of environmental design changes, and modeling. When evaluating their interventions, behaviorists choose from a variety of experimental designs, including traditional control-group designs; reversal (or A-B-A-B) designs; multiple-baseline designs across time, individuals, settings, or situations; changing-criterion designs; and simultaneous treatment designs. (See Miltenberger, 1997, for excellent, brief descriptions of each of these.) At least one of the commonalities between the technological approaches of the BT and the BA paradigms is their emphasis on the measurement of objective, quantifiable outcomes (cf. Jason, 1991; Mahoney, Kazdin, & Lesswing, 1974).

Historically, community psychologists who were critics of behaviorism conceded that behavioral technologies had proven themselves in the "laboratory and highly financed, small demonstration projects" (Reppucci & Saunders, 1974, p. 658), or when applied to problems confronted by clinical psychology and community mental health (Rappaport, 1977). However, three general criticisms were advanced by these commentators to contend that behavioral technologies were probably not applicable to most applied settings or to the problems of community psychology. Some of these same biases hold sway today and may underpin community psychologist's reluctance to employ behavioral technologies.

First, behavioral techniques are viewed as not particularly powerful or generalizable. In the previous section, we noted that, for certain social problems, the generalizability of behavioral theory and technology can be greatly enhanced by paying closer attention to real-world (rather than researcher-generated) reinforcers. Power and generalizability might also be promoted through "contextually appropriate" technology; that is, effective, inexpensive, decentralized, flexible, sustainable, simple, and compatible behavioral interventions (Fawcett et al., 1980). For example, many of the early behavioral community-psychology demonstration projects established interventions that were simply not cost effective. Everett, Hayward, & Meyers (1974) evaluated a token reinforcement procedure to increase bus ridership on a college campus; the intervention did increase the number of bus riders (more people will ride the bus if you pay them to do so) but, financially, the college could not sustain such an intervention. The field has since moved from an interest in merely documenting effective, potent interventions to considerations of generalizability; thus, cost effectiveness has become one of many issues that behavioral community psychologists emphasize when developing and evaluating their interventions.

Furthermore, behaviorists, in their many reviews of the application of behavioral principles to community problems (e.g., Bogat & Jason, 1997; Glenwick & Jason, 1993; Jason & Bogat, 1983), find that these interventions can be effective in less structured environments. Behavioral interventions have included programs to promote social network development among elderly community residents (Bogat & Jason, 1983), to help students cope with the stress of transferring schools (Bogat, Jones, & Jason, 1980; Jason, Weine, Johnson, Warren-Sohlberg, Filippelli, Turner, & Lardon, 1992; Warren-Sohlberg, Jason, Weine, Lantz, & Reyes, 1998), to stop store vendors from illegally selling cigarettes to minors (Jason, Berk, Schnopp-Wyatt, & Talbot, in press; Jason, Billows, Schnopp-Wyatt, & King, 1996), to provide youngsters anticipating tonsillectomies relevant coping strategies (Peterson & Shigetomi, 1981), to increase the use of child safety seats for newborns (Alvarez & Jason, 1993), to enhance job interview skills for immigrants (Jung & Jason, 1998), and to promote health efforts in the media (Jason, 1998). The settings, and their inherent problems, are identical to those with which mainstream community psychologists must cope.

A second criticism is that behaviorists do not often consider who controls the reinforcers in their interventions. Interestingly, many behavioral technologies do not involve the control of reinforcers: For example, in Yokley and Glenwick's (1984) study to increase the immunization of preschool children, only one of their four experimental interventions employed a reinforcer: "(a) a mailed general prompt, (b) a mailed specific prompt, (c) a mailed specific prompt plus expanded clinic hours ..., and (d) a mailed specific prompt plus a monetary incentive" (p. 243). These conditions were compared to contact and no contact control groups. The results revealed that the greatest number of immunizations occurred in the specific prompt plus monetary incentive group, but gains nearly as significant were attained by the two specific prompt groups. Prompts, which occur prior to behavior, do not entail the use of reinforcers.

Of course, many behavioral community psychology interventions do employ reinforcers, and behaviorists are aware that their technology has sometimes been used to maintain the status quo, often with the implicit approval of the researcher. For instance, behavior modification procedures in the classroom have often been used to reinforce conformity (Winett & Winkler, 1972). Psychologists are rightly concerned with the kind of power that may be abused in these situations. However, for many non-behaviorists, this concern can quickly conjure up images of George Orwell's *1984* and the rigid control behaviorists might exert. As Heller and Monahan (1977) conclude: "current behavioral techniques are least effective when they are utilized simply as devices for automatic conditioning and are much more effective when they involve cooperation and active cognitive participation" (Heller & Marlatt, 1969, p. 243). A full consideration of the problem of power and its misuse in psychology or in behaviorism lies beyond the scope of this chapter. But it takes only a cursory knowledge of the history of psychology to recognize that abuses of power existed long before the advent of applied behavioral technologies. If, as the historian Lord Acton suggested, "Power tends to corrupt and absolute power corrupts absolutely," then it should be some measure of comfort to know that the most successful behavioral interventions rely on the cooperation of the participants.

The third broad criticism of behavioral community psychology is that it may be difficult, or even impossible, to implement. This criticism had its genesis in a 1974 article by Reppucci and Saunders, who listed seven difficulties encountered when implementing behavior modification in natural settings: the problem of institutional constraints, the problem of external pressure, the problem of language, the problem of two populations, the problem of limited resources, the problem of perceived inflexibility, and the problem of compromise. Reppucci and Saunders' concern was that because behavior modification programs failed to address these points explicitly, the reader might be left with the mistaken impression "that implementation of an effective behavior modification program is a straightforward, trouble-free affair" (p. 650).

We have argued in the previous section that this omission may, in large part, result from the behaviorists' viewpoint of reality. For example, Stokes and Fawcett (1977) consulted with the Sanitation Workers' Association of a city in order to change the ways citizens packaged their refuse. Their research barely mentions the questions of importance to Reppucci and Saunders: "Where should one seek to enter a setting? Where will the points of conflict arise? What will constitute a viable support system? What is a realistic time perspective for change?" (p. 660), and yet these concerns had to be addressed prior to the implementation of the research.

Although some writers have doubts about the utility of behavioral technologies in applied settings, there are some interventions in community psychology with behavioral underpinnings (e.g., as mentioned earlier, those programs that attempt to enhance problem-solving skills). Unfortunately, in these interventions and others, experimental designs advocated by the behaviorists are rarely employed. Because space precludes discussing the merits of all the possible approaches, we will limit our comments to the multiple baseline technique.

The multiple baseline technique is useful when the number of subjects is small, a reversal design would be unethical, or subjects cannot be assigned randomly to no-treatment control groups (Glenwick & Jason, 1984). Briefly, the technique involves charting one or more behaviors until they stabilize; this is the baseline phase. Then, the experimental manipulation is implemented and its effect on the behavior is charted. Data can be collected at the individual, group, community, or societal levels. The prominence of multiple baseline techniques in behavioral research reflects behaviorists' interest in the process of the intervention—the constant transaction between the individual and the environment. The collection of ongoing data, not merely pretest and posttest markers, provides the researcher, the change agent, and the participant with immediate feedback concerning the intervention. Thus, the intervention is, in effect, a totally flexible one that can be specially adapted for individual persons or settings. In the peer tutoring research of the second author, children's competencies in various academic subjects are charted daily. This enables the tutor to immediately ascertain whether the pupil is making adequate progress. If there are problems, the tutoring procedure is revised.

We have emphasized throughout this chapter that the behavioral viewpoint of reality results in a tendency to emphasize the researchers', rather than the participants', view of the world. However, some behavioral designs, especially multiple baseline, clearly allow for a type of data collection that is much more likely to consider the subject's point of view. The community psychologist, with stated values concerning true collaboration with settings, respect for cultural diversity, and implementing programs responsive to community needs, has attended most closely to these issues when *designing* projects, and less so when *evaluating* them. Program evaluations in mainstream community psychology have often focused on documenting overall, comprehensive change through control-group designs that rely on statistical techniques comparing mean scores. Such designs are obviously useful, but they may obscure real differences between project participants. Of particular interest are those subjects who do not benefit from, or may be harmed by, our interventions. Community psychologists have begun to explore other statistical procedures (e.g., causal modeling, subject clustering) that allow for a more complete understanding of their interventions; however, the search for alternatives should include behavioral techniques, which can help community psychologists evaluate the integrity of their interventions (Bogat & Jason, 1997).

CONCLUSION

This chapter has attempted to demonstrate the value of integrating aspects of behavioral philosophy, theory, and technology with mainstream community psychology. Of course, this position necessarily implies that the work of behavioral community psychologists can benefit from the integration of perspectives held by mainstream community psychologists (cf. Fawcett et al., 1980; Jason, 1991; Jason & Glenwick, 1984).

The practice of community psychology involves Herculean tasks, and behaviorism offers no panacea for these difficulties. But behaviorism does offer important ideas that, if successfully integrated with community psychology, could help customize our interventions, as well as provide avenues through which to begin working on major social problems using the small wins or successive approximations approach. We hope we have provided a starting point to begin conceptualizing this integration.

REFERENCES

Adler, M. J. (1965). *The conditions of philosophy.* New York: Atheneum.

Alinsky, S. (1971). *Rules for radicals.* New York: Random House.

Alvarez, J., & Jason, L. A. (1993). The effectiveness of legislation, education, and loaners for child safety in automobiles. *Journal of Community Psychology, 21,* 280–284.

Bogat, G. A., & Jason, L. A. (1983). An evaluation of two visiting programs for elderly community residents. *International Journal of Aging and Human Development, 17,* 267–280.

Bogat, G. A., & Jason, L. A. (1997). Interventions in the school and community. In R. T. Ammerman & M. Hersen (Eds.). *Handbook of prevention and treatment with children and adolescents: Intervention in the real world contest* (pp. 134–154). New York: Wiley.

Bogat, G. A., Jones, J. W., & Jason, L. A. (1980). School transitions: Preventive intervention following an elementary school closing. *Journal of Community Psychology, 8,* 343–352.

Burgoyne, N. S., & Jason, L. A. (1991). Incorporating the ecological paradigm into behavioral preventive interventions. In P. M. Martin (Ed.), *Handbook of behavior therapy and psychological science: An integrative approach* (pp. 457–472). New York: Pergamon.

Duffy, K. G., & Wong, K. Y. (1996). *Community psychology.* Boston: Allyn and Bacon.

Everett, P. B., Hayward, S. C., & Meyers, A. W. (1974). The effects of a token reinforcement procedure on bus ridership. *Journal of Applied Behavior Analysis, 7,* 1 –9.

Fawcett, S. B. (1990). Some emerging standards for community research and action: Aid from a behavioral perspective. In P. Tolan, C. Keys, F. Chertok, & L. A. Jason (Eds.), *Researching community psychology: Integrating theories and methodologies* (pp. 64–75). Washington, D.C.: APA.

Fawcett, S. B., Mathews, R. M., & Fletcher, R. K. (1980). Some promising dimensions for behavioral community technology. *Journal of Applied Behavior Analysis, 13,* 505–518.

Ferrari, J. R., & Jason, L. A. (1990). Incentives in blood-donor recruitment. *Evaluation and the Health Professions, 13,* 373-377.

Frye, N. (1957). *Anatomy of criticism.* New York: Atheneum.

Geller, E. S., Winett, R. A., & Everett, P. E. (1982). *Preserving the environment: New strategies for behavior change.* New York: Pergamon.

Glenwick, D. S., & Jason, L. A. (Eds.). (1980). *Behavioral community psychology: Progress and prospects.* New York: Praeger.

Glenwick, D. S., & Jason, L. A. (1984). Behavioral community psychology: An introduction to the special issue. *Journal of Community Psychology, 12,* 103–112.

Glenwick, D. S., & Jason, L. A. (1993). Behavioral approaches to prevention in the community: a historical and theoretical overview. In D. S. Glenwick & L. A. Jason (Eds.), *Promoting health and mental health in children, youth and families* (pp. 3–13). New York: Springer.

Greene, B. F., Winnett, R. A., van Houten, R. V., Geller, E. S., & Iwata, B. A. (1987). *Behavior analysis in the community 1968–1986 from the Journal of Applied Behavior Analyses.* Reprint Series, Vol. 2. Lawrence, KS: Society for the Experimental Analysis of Behavior.

Heller, K., & Marlatt, G. A. (1969). Verbal conditioning, behavior therapy, and behavior change: Some problems in extrapolation. In C. M. Franks (Ed.), *Behavior therapy: Appraisal and status* (pp. 569–588). New York: McGraw-Hill.

Heller, K., & Monahan, J. (1977). *Psychology and community change.* Homewood, IL: Dorsey.

Jason, L. A. (1991). Participating in social change: A fundamental value for our discipline. *American Journal of Community Psychology, 19,* 1–16.

Jason, L. A. (1992). Eco-transactional behavioral research. *The Journal of Primary Prevention, 13,* 37–72.

Jason, L. A. (1998). Tobacco, drug, and HIV preventive media interventions. *American Journal of Community Psychology, 26,* 145–187.

Jason, L. A., Berk, M., Schnopp-Wyatt, D. L., & Talbot, B. (1999). Effects of enforcement of youth access laws on smoking prevalence. *American Journal of Community Psychology, 27,* 143–160.

Jason, L. A., Billows, W., Schnopp-Wyatt, D., & King, C. (1996). Reducing the illegal sales of cigarettes to minors: Analysis of alternative enforcement schedules. *Journals of Applied Behavior Analysis, 29,* 333–344.

Jason, L. A., & Bogat, G. A. (1983). Preventive behavioral interventions. In Felner, R. D., Jason, L. A., Moritsugu, J. N., & Farber, S. S. (Eds.), *Preventive psychology: Theory, research and practice* (pp. 128–143). New York: Pergamon.

Jason, L. A., & Crawford, I. (1991). Toward a kinder, gentler, and more effective behavioral approach in solving community problems. *Journal of Applied Behavior Analysis, 24*, 649–651.

Jason, L. A., & Glenwick, D. S. (1984). Behavioral community psychology: A review of recent research and applications. In M. Hersen, R. M. Eisler, & P. M. Miller (Eds.), *Progress in behavior modification* (Vol. 18) (pp. 85–121). New York: Academic.

Jason, L. A., & Hanaway, E. K. (1997). *Remote control: A sensible approach to kids, TV, and the new electronic media.* Sarasota, FL: Professional Resource Press.

Jason, L. A., & Liotta, R. (1982). Reducing cigarette smoking in a university cafeteria. *Journal of Applied Behavior Analysis, 15*, 573–577.

Jason, L. A., McMahon, S. D., Salina, D., Hedeker, D., Stockton, M., Dunson, K., & Kimball, P. (1995). Assessing a smoking cessation intervention involving groups, incentives, and self-help manuals. *Behavior Therapy, 26*, 393–408.

Jason, L. A., Salina, D. D., McMahon, S. D., Hedeker, D., & Stockton, M. (1997). A worksite smoking intervention: A 2 year assessment of groups, incentives, and self-help. *Health Education Research, Theory and Practice, 12*, 129–138.

Jason, L. A., Weine, A. M., Johnson, J. H., Warren-Sohlberg, L., Filippelli, L. A., Turner, E. Y., & Lardon, C. (1992). *Helping transfer students: Strategies for educational and social readjustment.* San Francisco: Jossey-Bass.

Jung, R. S., & Jason, L. A. (1998). Job interview social skills training for Asian-American Immigrants. *Journal of Human Behavior in the Social Sciences, 14*, 11–25.

Kantor, J. R. (1958). *Interbehavioral psychology.* Bloomington, IN: Principia.

Kelly, J. G. (April, 1987). *Beyond prevention techniques: Generating social settings for a public's health.* Invited address at the Tenth Erich Lindemann Memorial Lecture, Harvard Medical School, Boston, MA.

Kelly, J. G. (1990). Changing contexts and the field of community psychology. *American Journal of Community Psychology, 18*, 769–792.

Kingry-Westergaard, C., & Kelly, J. G. (1990). A contextualist epistemology for ecological research. In P. Tolan, C. Keys, F. Chertok, & L. Jason (Eds.), *Researching community psychology. Issues of theory and methods* (pp. 23–31). Washington, D.C.: American Psychological Association.

Mahoney, M. J., Kazdin, A. E., & Lesswing, N. J. (1974). Behavior modification: Delusion or deliverance? In C. M. Franks & G. T. Wilson (Eds.), *Annual review of behavior therapy, theory and practice* (pp. 11–40). New York: Brunner/Mazel.

Messer, S. B., & Winokur, M. (1980). Some limits to the integration of psychoanalytic and behavior therapy. *American Psychologist, 35*, 818–827.

Miltenberger, R. (1997). *Behavior modification: Principles and procedures.* Pacific Grove, CA: Brooks/Cole.

Nietzel, M. T., Winett, R. A., MacDonald, M. L., & Davidson, W. S. (1977). *Behavioral approaches to community psychology.* New York: Pergamon.

Peterson, L., & Mori, L. (1985). Prevention of child injury: An overview of targets, methods, and tactics for psychologists. *Journal of Consulting and Clinical Psychology, 53*, 586–595.

Peterson, L., & Shigetomi, C. (1981). The use of coping techniques to minimize anxiety in hospitalized children. *Behavior Therapy, 8*, 464–467.

Rappaport, J. (1977). *Community psychology: Values, research, and action.* New York: Holt, Rinehart and Winston.

Rappaport, J. (1981). In praise of paradox: A social policy of empowerment over prevention. *American Journal of Community Psychology, 9*, 1–25.

Reppucci, N. D., & Saunders, J. T. (1974). Social psychology of behavior modification: Problems of implementation in natural settings. *American Psychologist, 29*, 649–660.

Rychlak, J. F. (1968). *A philosophy of science for personality theory.* Boston: Houghton Mifflin.

Sameroff, A. J. (1987). Transactional risk factors and prevention. In J. A. Steinberg & M. M. Silverman (Eds.), *Preventing mental disorders: A research perspective* (pp. 74–89). U.S. Department of Health and Human Services (Pub. No. 87-1492). Washington, D.C.: U.S. Government Printing Office.

Sarason, S. B. (1971). *The culture of the school and the problem of change.* Boston: Allyn and Bacon.

Sarason, S. B. (1972). *The creation of settings and the future societies.* San Francisco: Jossey-Bass.

Sarason, S. B. (1981). An asocial psychology and a misdirected clinical psychology. *American Psychologist, 36*, 837–836.

Shafer, R. (1976). *A new language for psychoanalysis.* New Haven, CT: Yale University Press.

Skinner, B. F. (1971). *Beyond freedom and dignity.* New York: Knopf.

Stokes, T. F., & Fawcett, S. B. (1977). Evaluating municipal policy: An analysis of a refuse packaging program. *Journal of Applied Behavior Analysis, 10,* 391–398.

Strain, P. S. (1985). Programmatic research on peers as intervention agents for socially isolate classmates. In B. H. Schneider, K. H. Rubin, & J. E. Ledingham (Eds.), *Children's peer relations: Issues in assessment and intervention* (pp. 193–205). New York: Springer-Verlag.

Tandon, S. D., Azelton, L. S., Kelly, J. G., & Strickland, D. A. (1998). Constructing a tree for community leadership: Contexts and processes in collaborative inquiry. Unpublished manuscript.

Twardosz, S., Cataldo, M. F., & Risley, T. R. (1974). Open environment design for infant and toddler day care. *Journal of Applied Behavior Analysis, 7,* 529–546.

Ullmann, L. P., & Krasner, L. (1969). *A psychological approach to abnormal behavior.* Englewood Cliffs, NJ: Prentice-Hall.

Van Houten, R., Rolider, A., Nau, P. A., Friedman, R., Becker, M., Cholodovsky, I., & Scherer, M. (1985). Large-scale reductions in speeding and accidents in Canada and Israel: A behavioral ecological perspective. *Journal of Applied Behavior Analysis, 18,* 87–93.

Warren-Sohlberg, L., Jason, L. A.,Weine, A. M., Lantz, G. D., & Reyes, O. (1998). Implementing and evaluating preventive programs for high-risk transfer students. *Journal of Educational and Psychological Consultation, 9,* 307–329.

Weick, K. E. (1984). Small wins: Redefining the scale of social problems. *American Psychologist, 39,* 40–49.

Weissberg, R. P., & Greenberg, M. T. (1997). School and community competence-enhancement and prevention programs. In W. Damon (Series Ed.), I. E. Sigel & K. A. Reinninger (Vol. Eds.), *Handbook of child psychology: Vol. 4, Child Psychology in practice* (5th edition). New York: Wiley.

Willems, E. P. (1974). Behavioral technology and behavioral ecology. *Journal of Applied Behavior Analysis, 7,* 151–165.

Winett, R. A. (1993). Media-based behavior change approaches for prevention. In D. S. Glenwick & L. A. Jason (Eds.), *Promoting health and mental health in children, youth, and families* (pp. 181–204). New York: Springer.

Winett, R. A., Leckliter, I. N., Chinn, D. E., Stahl, B., & Love, S. Q. (1985). Effects of television modeling on residential energy conservation. *Journal of Applied Behavior Analysis, 18,* 33–44.

Winett, R. A., & Winkler, R. C. (1972). Current behavior modification in the classroom: Be still, be quiet, be docile. *Journal of Applied Behavior Analysis, 5,* 499–504.

Yokley, J. M., & Glenwick, D. S. (1984). Increasing the immunization of preschool children: An evaluation of applied community interventions. *Journal of Applied Behavior Analysis, 17,* 313–325.

CHAPTER 6

Cognition in Social Context

Contributions to Community Psychology

PATRICK O'NEILL

Nobel prize winner Jacques Monod was fascinated by the impact of ideas on the fate of human groups. He believed that the power of an idea was independent of its truth. "The performance value of an idea," he said, "depends upon the change it brings to the behavior of the person or the group that adopts it." (1972, p. 166). Ideas, whether they be true or false, are agents and products of the evolutionary struggle for survival. "The human group upon which a given idea confers greater cohesiveness, greater ambition, and greater self-confidence thereby receives from it an added power to expand which will insure the promotion of the idea itself." If Monod is right, the study of ideas is indispensable for the adequate analysis of topics in community psychology. The way people think about a social problem may encourage them to confront it, and will affect the form and outcome of that confrontation.

Since the term "cognitive community psychology" was coined (O'Neill, 1981) the use of cognitive variables in community psychology research has been on the rise (a brief sampling: Chavis & Wandersman, 1990; Constantino & Nelson, 1995; Florin & Wandersman, 1984; Lavoie, Jacob, Hardy, & Martin, 1989; Lavoie, Vézina, Piché, & Boivin, 1995; Mitchell, Davidson, Chodakowski, & McVeigh, 1985; O'Neill, 1989; O'Neill & Hern, 1991; Pancer & Cameron, 1994; Rich, Edelstein, Hallman, & Wandersman, 1995; St. Lawrence, Eldridge, Reitman, Little, Shelby, & Brasfield, 1998; Van Uchelen, Davidson, Quressette, Brasfield, & Demerais, 1997; Vinokur & Caplan, 1986).

This chapter will review prototypical research that takes a cognitive approach to social and community psychology. I will begin by introducing three levels of analysis that will be used throughout the chapter. I will then review recent studies of stereotyping that may advance our understanding of intergroup conflict. Turning from stereotyping to social action, I will present three current lines of research, each of which reflects a different level of analysis. The chapter will conclude with some reflections on the problems and prospects involved in combining several levels of analysis to look at issues in our field.

A central theme of this book is that phenomena can be analyzed on different levels, and

---

PATRICK O'NEILL • Department of Psychology, Acadia University, Wolfville, Nova Scotia B0P 1X0, Canada.

Handbook of Community Psychology, edited by Julian Rappaport and Edward Seidman. Kluwer Academic / Plenum Publishers, New York, 2000.

that we must be clear in community psychology about the level on which we are working at any given moment. In this chapter I will refer to three levels of analysis: the individual, the interpersonal, and the community. At the *individual* level, phenomena are explained by a person's beliefs, motives, or feelings, without reference to interpersonal transactions or social context. At the *interpersonal* level, the focus is on the transaction between two or more people. At the *community* level, reference is made to group identification to explain social events.

A problem may take different shapes when approaches on different levels of analysis; consider, for example, child abuse. At the individual level, a researcher might focus on characteristics of parents who abuse their children (e.g., Rickel, 1989) or of children who are abused (victims often blame themselves; see O'Neill, 1998). At the interpersonal level one might target the family, looking at the dynamics of parent–child interactions or intrafamily transmission of abuse over generations (e.g., Braun, 1993). On the community level, Garbarino has studied a variety of important factors in the incidence of abuse, including lack of community identity and cohesion (Garbarino & Kostelny, 1992). One might also, at this level of analysis, look at the way abuse is defined among community groups (e.g., Campbell, 1999) or construed in historical context (e.g., Hacking, 1991, 1995), or one might use a gender-power analysis to explain the underlying motivation for abuse and its tolerance (e.g., Brickman, 1992). One may also employ systems theory to understand a community's response to cases of abuse (e.g., O'Neill & Hern, 1991).

None of these levels of analysis gives a picture of reality that is true while the other levels' versions are false. As Prilleltensky & Nelson (1997) point out, when one way of looking at a problem is in the foreground, the other ways tend to fade into the background. They argue, and few community psychologists would disagree, that mainstream psychology overemphasizes the individual level of analysis while neglecting community, social, and cultural explanations. They also note that community psychology has been more receptive than mainstream psychology to broader analyses. It may even be that the balance has been tipped, and community psychology has not incorporated all that it might from such areas as cognitive social psychology (O'Neill, 1981; O'Neill & Trickett, 1982).

Social cognition, loosely defined as the study of knowledge structures, decision-making, and information processing, might seem to represent an obvious individual-level approach to research. But, in fact, it cuts across all three levels. Consider the following explanations for social action: Activists tend to be those who believe in their power to affect change and that social conditions are often unjust (individual level); people escalate their demands when a person in authority makes small, grudging concessions (interpersonal level); collective action occurs when people identify with a group that they perceive as being unfairly treated (community level). Notice that social cognition plays a role in each of these propositions. At the individual level, beliefs are involved; at the interpersonal level, information is transmitted; at the community level, identification processes are invoked.

STEREOTYPING AND INTERGROUP RELATIONS

An ideal of community psychology is the promotion of tolerance. The community should value diversity of lifestyle, cultural and religious practices, sexual orientations, and other aspects of human variation. The model community would not, in Rappaport's (1977) words, rank order people on a single criterion; it would, instead, maximize the ability of all to live according to a standard of life selected by the persons themselves. A goal of many community interventions is to promote tolerance for diversity and an appreciation of the various adaptations people make to their environments (O'Neill & Trickett, 1982). The reduction of prejudice is a valid objective of community psychology.

The formation of negative stereotypes of other groups is associated with prejudice and discrimination (Oakes, Haslam, & Turner, 1994; O'Neill, 1981). This section will review current work on stereotyping, and will consider its implications for community psychology. The essence of the problem of negative ethnic stereotypes can be captured in the following brief example. A tourist from the United States drives through Quebec on vacation. The tourist is treated rudely by a French-speaking waitress. On the basis of this single encounter, the tourist decides that the French in Quebec are rude and dislike U.S. tourists. Later the tourist meets Quebeckers who do not fit the stereotype, but they are discounted as exceptions to the rule.

As illogical as this scenario seems, there is considerable research evidence to support it. People often generalize from extremely small samples (Tversky and Kahneman, 1971), and may even generalize on the basis of single cases (Hamil, Wilson, & Nisbett, 1980; Nisbett & Borgida, 1975; Zuckerman, Mann, & Bernieri, 1982). Once a belief is in place, though, it is hard to shake, even when the person is presented with counter-examples (Wilder, 1984), or is told that the information on which the belief was based was false (Anderson, Lepper, & Ross, 1980; Anderson, 1983).

What are the conditions that lead people to create stereotypes on the basis of small samples, then to cling to these stereotypes, even when they are discredited? In terms of formation, there is some evidence that people generalize without considering whether a sample case was randomly drawn from a larger group (Nisbett and Borgida, 1975). They may even generalize in the face of information that the sample case is *atypical* (Hamil, Wilson, & Nisbett, 1980), although there is contradictory evidence on this point (Zuckerman et al., 1982). They tend to generalize more when they view the target group as homogeneous. The perceived homogeneity of out-groups, compared to their own group, leads people to make more extreme judgments—good or bad—about out-group members than about members or their own group (Linville & Jones, 1980).

Turning to the perseverance of stereotypes, we find that a belief is more resistant to discomfirming evidence when the person has worked out a scenario that makes the belief seem plausible (Anderson et al., 1980). A tourist with a causal scenario about why the French in Quebec might have reason to be rude to English speakers will be more likely to cling to the belief that they *are* rude, even when faced with strong evidence to the contrary.

Weber and Crocker (1983) propose three competing models of what may happen when a person who believes a stereotype is confronted with disconfirming evidence. In the bookkeeping model, the stereotype is modified gradually, one example at a time. In the conversion model, the stereotype changes radically in response to sudden or salient instances. In the subtyping model, new stereotypic structures are developed to accommodate instances not easily assimilated by existing stereotypes. If the subtyping model is correct, for example, a tourist who expects rudeness from Quebeckers may, when confronted with a friendly merchant, develop a subtype: Merchants are friendly to get business. The initial stereotype stays in place, but becomes more complex.

In experiments to test these models, Weber and Crocker (1983) found that when disconfirming evidence is dispersed across many members of a group, the stereotype tends to change slowly, as a function of the number of disconfirming examples. When the disconfirming evidence is concentrated in a few members, however, subtypes are developed. Dramatically inconsistent individuals (such as the friendly merchant) are seen as unrepresentative of the group as a whole. The conversion model is probably most relevant to the development of a stereotype in the first place. We know that, as the conversion model predicts, people often generalize on the basis of a single vivid case. The bookkeeping and subtyping models are relevant to changing entrenched stereotypes. The three models, and the conditions under which they operate, offer one solution to the paradox that we stereotype quickly on the basis of inadequate evidence, then we cling to the belief, even when confronted with good evidence that it is false.

Other promising lines of research into stereotyping focus on salience and vividness. Salience is a function of differential attention. Novel stimuli are salient. The tourist who is snubbed by a Quebec waitress generalizes to Quebeckers rather than to waitresses. Why? Because the tourist has been served by many waitresses, but has never before encountered a French-speaking waitress in Quebec. Salience has been shown to play a role in formation of stereotypes (Forgas, 1983).

The vividness of information also seems to contribute to stereotyping. Vivid information is emotionally interesting, concrete, imagery-provoking, and proximate in a sensory, temporal, or spatial way (Nisbett & Ross, 1980). An interaction with a rude waitress is more emotional than an interaction with a friendly waitress; it has more impact when it happens to you, personally, than when you hear about it from someone else. Vividness, salience, and other cognitive variables influence what we remember. Moods also affect memory (Alvaro, McFarland, & Beuhler, 1998; McFarland & Beuhler, 1997).

The role of vividness and salience in belief formation, and the role of causal explanations in belief maintenance, have other applications relevant to community psychology. For example, they are implicated in the perceived correlation between social class and criminal behavior. Tittle (1982) examined various theories of crime that assume a correlation between social class and criminal behavior. He suggested that there is a lack of evidence for the criminality of the lower class, yet the belief remains strong despite its fragile empirical basis. Social scientists, for instance, devote a good deal of mental energy to devising theories to account for a correlation that may not exist. Tittle offered several explanations for the strength of this belief, including one based on a cognitive view of stereotyping. He noted that "there is a robust tendency for humans, even those with trained scientific minds, to form their judgments about phenomena on the basis of the most recent, the most dramatic, or the most personally relevant piece of information" (p. 354). Once a person decides that a relationship exists—between social class and criminal behavior, in this case—that belief is hard to shake, especially when the person has thought of a causal theory to explain the relationship. Thus, in Tittle's view, once we have thought of reasons why the lower class should be drawn to criminal behavior, our stereotype tends to withstand evidence that there is little or no relationship between class and crime.

In another community-based application of social cognition, Yates and Aronson (1983) used findings concerning the impact of vivid information to recommend ways in which the general public could be persuaded to conserve energy in residential buildings. The National Energy Conservation Act of 1978 led to a program in which major gas and electric utility companies in the United States offered customers a variety of conservation services. The companies were required to provide useful, reliable, and accurate information to customers in all socioeconomic subgroups. The information was to be provided by auditors trained to act as effective communicators. Yates and Aronson made a number of specific suggestions about how these communicators might convey information in ways that would be vivid and personally relevant.

Although there are many potentially interesting applications of research on belief formation and maintenance, stereotyping on the basis of group membership has still drawn the most attention from investigators.

Beyond the Individual Level of Analysis

Much of the research on stereotyping has an individual focus, but we ought not slight the importance of interpersonal and community levels of analysis when we consider prejudice and discrimination. Forgas (1983) warns against relying on individual cognition to understand stereotyping. People learn about one another through interaction, and our interactions are shaped by group identification.

The importance of considering various levels of analysis is demonstrated by the problem of so-called realistic group conflict. Sherif (1956) created artificial groups, pitted them against one another, and then looked for ways to resolve the resulting conflict. His work has been taken as a demonstration that actual competition underlies prejudice. But the community level of analysis, where group loyalties are real, not artificial, gives a somewhat different interpretation. Kinder and Sears (1981) studied voting behavior in two Los Angeles mayoral elections, each involving one white and one black candidate. Realistic group conflict, based on direct threats to whites' neighborhoods, jobs, children's schooling, or families' safety, had almost *no* effect on voting. Instead, voting by whites was influenced by what Kinder and Sears call "symbolic racism"—sociocultural prejudice related to long-standing group identification.

Some research programs include design features that highlight more than one level of analysis. For instance, Dubé combines the interpersonal and community levels. She looks at interactions between people with strong group identifications, such as the French and English in Quebec. She asks: Under what conditions can members of different groups become friends?; are these conditions different than those required for friendship between members of the same group? (Simard, 1981). By using real interactions, she has discovered aspects of intergroup relations that are hard to pinpoint in the laboratory. For instance, similarity was extremely important in cross-cultural friendships; friendship required that persons from two different groups be more similar to one another than would be necessary within a group. Language is an obvious barrier when two people are not fluent in each other's language, but Dubé's research showed that the barrier is still up even when the two potential friends are bilingual; participants thought it was extremely important that their mother tongue be used in conversation with the other person.

Up to this point, I have followed the usual social psychological approach of assuming that stereotypes are necessarily false, since they are simplifications, and that they are generally bad, since they are implicated in prejudice and discrimination. I want to move away from these conventions, because matters are not as simple as they seem.

First, are stereotypes necessarily false? Campbell's work on the basis of stereotypes (e.g., Campbell, 1967; LeVine & Campbell, 1972) was, for a time, a rare exception to the consensus that they are indeed false. Referring to cross-cultural studies, Campbell pointed out that the main components in negative stereotypes believed by one group about another were usually ways in which the groups really did differ. For example, a group that avoided alcohol was most likely to emphasize the drunkenness of one that did not. Campbell was concerned about the creation of cultural identities and the way stereotypes fed into those identities.

It has taken mainstream psychology some decades to follow Campbell's lead. The new turn is marked by a book of research published by the American Psychological Association, *Stereotype accuracy: Toward appreciating group differences.* The book opens with a frank discussion of the political difficulties in studying this topic: "The idea that stereotypes may have some degree of accuracy is apparently anathema to many social scientists and laypeople. Those who document accuracy run the risk of being seen as racists, sexists, or worse" (Lee, Jussim, & McCauley, 1995, p. xiii).

There is, in fact, a considerable body of evidence that stereotypes of one group by another do have a grain of truth. McCauley (1994) reported accurate judgment of real group differences in studies involving race, gender, and college major.

Are stereotypes always a bad thing? To be sure, they are, by definition, a simplification of complex material. Such simplification is not a good thing when judging a job candidate. But the same may not hold true at the community level, when the unit of analysis is the group rather than the individual member.

Stereotypes reflect ethnic and national traditions, not just ethnocentric prejudice. Groups are often proud of their ability to "laugh at themselves," especially when their own cherished traditions incorporate some aspect of the stereotype. Consider the following joke, which former French President Giscard d'Estaing used to tell when speaking at official functions in European capitals. In heaven, he said, the chefs are French, the police are English, the engineers are German, the administrators are Swiss, and the lovers are Italian. In hell, he continued, the chefs are English, the police are German, the engineers are Italian, the administrators are French, and the lovers are Swiss. His joke plays on both positive and negative aspects of traditional stereotypes drawn from ideas about national virtues and vices—ideas that must be generally accepted for the joke to work. As a personal aside, I tried this story out while enrolled in a language course in Tours, France, before a group of fellow students that included representatives of all the groups mentioned in the joke. Only one of the two Swiss claimed not to understand what was so amusing.

When we employ different levels of analysis in our work, we bring some of our underlying assumptions into question. In a sense, the mainstream attack on cultural stereotypes reflects the melting-pot view of the ideal society. Stereotypes contradict the polite fiction that people are really all the same. The main alternative to the melting pot is the ideal of society as a mosaic, made up of different ethnic groups who treasure their traditions, even while they cooperate with one another in democratic institutions.

There is ongoing debate about how far one can or should go in respecting group traditions in a liberal democracy; see, for instance, Geertz (1986) on diversity, Rorty (1991) on ethnocentrism, Taylor (1995) on the politics of recognition, and Fish (1997) on "boutique multiculturalism."

However this debate plays out, there is no doubt that our notions about the ideal society have shifted from the melting pot to some form of the mosaic. With that shift, we need to reexamine the mainstream view in psychology that stereotypes are necessarily pernicious. Taylor has explored this question in research in Canada, where the mosaic ideal has been in place longer than it has in the United States. He points out that in a multicultural society, members of ethnic groups are encouraged to retain their cultural diversity and preserve their heritage. Ethnic categories are positively valued. As Taylor (1981) says, in that context: "Stereotypes can be an important mechanism for recognizing, and expressing, ethnicity" (p. 163).

In considering the implications of the cognitive bases of stereotyping for intergroup relations, our target should not be the stereotyping process itself, which will almost certainly prove to be well-defended against our assaults. Instead, we should worry about the application of stereotypes to individuals in situations that matter to them as individuals. We should be concerned when stereotypes are used to promote one culture-bound perspective as being universally appropriate (LeVine & Campbell, 1972).

SOCIAL COGNITION AND SOCIAL CHANGE

We have seen that social cognition has implications for the ideal of a tolerant community, however far one is prepared to go down the road to multiculturalism. Social cognition also has much to offer another social ideal, that of the just community. In such a community, resources would be distributed equitably and citizens would be involved in the policy decisions that affect their lives. In advancing this ideal, community psychologists often find themselves helping groups that have been deprived of resources, or that have little access to decision-making, or both. Thus, empowerment has become a major theme in community psychology (Prilleltensky, 1994; Seidman & Rappaport, 1986) but, as with the melting pot versus multiculturalism, there is controversy in the field about the assumptions reflected in empowerment (see Carroll, 1994; Riger, 1993).

Social action is a vehicle for empowerment, and as such, it has a central place in research done by community psychologists (e.g., O'Neill, Duffy, Enman, Blackmer, Goodwin, & Campbell, 1988; Steiner & Mark, 1985). In this section, three research programs into social action will be described. It may be useful, before presenting this work, to consider classical theory about the conditions under which people will engage in social action. As Dubé & Guimond (1986) point out, it is usual for psychologists to take as their essential task "the identification of the conditions under which people feel frustrated, dissatisfied, or unjustly treated" (p. 201).

In the classical view, people demand social change when conditions are already improving. This has been termed the revolution of rising expectations. In his analysis of the origins of the French Revolution, de Tocqueville (1856/1955) noted that conditions had improved before the start of the revolution. He was one of the first scholars to draw from that fact a now-familiar conclusion: When an oppressive regime relaxes its pressure, its subjects will take up arms against it: "... the most perilous moment for a bad government is one when it seeks to mend its ways" (p. 177). There are other examples of escalating demands for change as conditions were improving: the Puritan revolution in England, the American Revolution, and the Russian Revolution.

Different levels of analysis give us different explanations for the fact that people demand social change in the context of improving social conditions. At the individual level, one concentrates on characteristics of the person and ignores the transaction between the deprived and the powerful. Thus, one may rely on an intrapsychic explanation of the sort used by Le Bon (1879). He was a conservative journalist who despised collective social action, considering it a function of crowd behavior in which people descend several rungs on the evolutionary ladder and are swept into impulsive, irrational actions. Reiff (1968) noted that such explanations are still used to account for social phenomena such as wars, strikes, riots, and political movements. He criticized so-called expert opinion that attributed urban riots to self-destructive or suicidal impulses, low self-esteem of black males raised in a matriarchal society, and a loss of conscience and self-imposed controls due to mass hysteria.

These intrapsychic explanations operate on an individual level of analysis. On the interpersonal level, the researcher focuses on transactions between two or more parties contending for scarce resources. Social cognition emphasizes the informational content of interactions. A move by either side provides the other with information about the nature of the relationship, the balance of power between the parties, and so on. Concessions may inform the disadvantaged about the motives, character, or strength of the person making those concessions. Social cognition also alerts us to the potential importance of the way participants view themselves and the world. Some beliefs may lead people to interpret information in a manner that leads to renewed demands for change.

Moving to the community level of analysis, one considers the sense of community (Sarason, 1974) that leads people to identify with particular groups. When historical examples of social change are explained on the individual or interpersonal levels, the analysis may omit the important fact that such collective action involves large groups of people interacting with one another. Tajfel (1978) encourages us to look for the effects on beliefs and behavior that come from people perceiving themselves to be members of a group, dealing with people who they perceive as members of other groups.

Research on Social Action

I turn now to three examples of research on social action. The first, at the interpersonal level, created a series of simulations of escalating demands for social change. The second, at the individual level, used psychometric methods to probe belief sets that facilitate participation in social action. The third, at the community level, related group identification and militancy.

Simkus (1986)[1] used laboratory simulations to explore the variables affecting the relationship between an improvement in conditions and an escalation of demands. She wanted to know what information is conveyed to the disadvantaged by the way in which the powerful respond to requests or demands. She speculated that the manner in which such requests or demands are dealt with tells the disadvantaged group a good deal about the balance of power between the parties and about the amount of conflict in the relationship.

Participants played the role of clerks who worked on tasks and received pay from managers. Clerks were told that the managers had discretion over what to pay them. Various manipulations were used to vary the clerks' perceptions of the manager's fairness. Clerks could send messages to the managers expressing satisfaction with the pay, requesting increases, or threatening strike action. The managers responded by giving large or small raises, refusing to give raises, threatening to fire the clerk, and so on.

Using the basic procedure, Simkus could make alterations in experimental conditions to test hypotheses about the effect of concessions on future demands. At several points in the simulation, participants were asked to complete questionnaires that assessed several dependent variables. The most important of these was whether the clerk would, at that moment, go on strike; neither the clerk nor the manager could earn any more points until the strike ended. Other dependent variables included perception of the manager's strength and the likelihood that she or he would back down if threatened, perception of conflict in the relationship, contentment, and aspiration level.

To summarize the most important of Simkus' many findings:

- Do those with power risk rebellion when they give in to a demand? Not necessarily. A large improvement in conditions of the relatively powerless actually decreased the probability of escalating demands. Small improvements, on the other hand, increased escalation. When the disadvantaged asked for change and were given large benefits, they become content and overestimated the friendliness of their relationship with the powerful.
- Small improvements indicated to the powerless that the person in power was not as strong as they had supposed.

[1]Shortly after completing her doctorate, Nora Simkus died while climbing Mount Kenya. She did not have an opportunity to distill her findings into a research paper. Readers are referred to her dissertation, available from *Dissertation Abstracts International.*

- The threat of escalating demands was greatest when small improvements seemed to be a direct response to action by the powerless, who perceived their relationship with the powerful as antagonistic.
- Finally, the perception of conflict was increased when small improvements came in a long series, doled out by the powerful with apparent reluctance.

In a related study, Martin, Brickman, & Murray (1984) used choice of legitimate or illegitimate forms of collective behavior as a dependent variable. Participants were more likely to consider extreme methods when they had frequent contact with one another, when their own participation was important for the success of the simulated business firm, and when they were given an example of others in the same position mobilizing for action.

Analogue studies always have ecological validity problems. We can never be sure that we have captured all of the important variables in a simulation. But laboratory control permits one to look at the moves and countermoves of people who relate to one another in power imbalance. Latané & Wolf (1981) pointed out the inadequacy of considering only one side of the equation in social change. Their alternative was to consider a social force field that includes the resources that each side can bring to bear in any attempt at influence.

The research by simkus (1986) and by Martin, Brickman, & Murray (1984) raises some intriguing possibilities for persons attempting to hold their power positions, as well as those who are trying to improve their lot. For those in power, the results suggest that escalating demands may be avoided if one makes significant improvement in conditions, and if benefits are given with an openhandedness that symbolizes power rather than weakness. The worst response to discontent is to make small improvements grudgingly, over a long period of time, when the discontented have the power to mobilize and have as an example others who have mobilized.

For the disadvantaged and those who would empower them, the lesson might be to emphasize the degree of conflict in the relationship. The experiments suggest that organizers should emphasize the potential power of their constituency and the lack of power of the adversary. Organizers should make it seem that each benefit granted by the powerful is actually a concession won through the active efforts of the people. These ideas drawn from simulations are consistent with the approach actually used by well-known organizers such as Saul Alinsky and Si Kahn. Alinsky (1971) emphasized conflict in the relationships between the powerful and the powerless by the use of terms such as "battle" and "war" to characterize social action. Kahn (1970) and Alinsky (1971) both claimed that the first actions by a new organization must be successful to give the people a sense of their own power.

Individual Differences and Social Action

The experimental results described help us to think about the information conveyed by transactions between those with and without power. But people have different ways of organizing information and drawing implications from it. We should consider the way information is interpreted by those who make demands. Fiske (1987) advocates the study of activists to "provide insight into how other citizens can make themselves heard" (p. 215). The following research project compared activists and nonactivists to see how they differ in the way they think about social conditions and their own power to bring about change.

It will be recalled that Simkus, in her simulations, created conditions that conveyed information about the power balance between clerk and manager, and the unfairness of the manager. But those in a disadvantaged position in society vary in their readiness to accept and interpret such information. They bring to each new encounter their present beliefs about the fairness of social arrangements and about their potential ability to have an impact on the political process.

Community psychologists have found that the perception that one has control over events is a factor in such diverse phenomena as ability to cope with stress (Vinokur & Caplan, 1986), response to the threat of rape (Riger, Gordon, & LeBailly, 1982), and women's willingness to insist on protected sex to avoid HIV infection (St. Lawrence, Eldridge, Reitman, Little, Shelby, &Brasfield, 1998).

A citizen's feeling a sense of personal power should predict his or her participation in social action. Stokols (1975) suggests that both the fact and the form of participation will be influenced by whether the citizen perceives that he or she has viable options for action. Weick (1984), in his small-wins theory, says that the massive scale on which social problems are often conceived gives the citizen a sense of powerlessness. Reformulating such problems on a smaller scale gives the citizen a sense of control. Florin & Wandersman (1984) found that expectancies about the success of grass-roots organizations predicted participation in community development.

Another cognitive variable that may predict willingness to engage in social action is the belief that social conditions are often unjust. Those who believe in the just-world hypothesis (Lerner & Miller, 1978) might blame the victim rather than recognize oppression. The distinction between person-blame and situation-blame has proven useful in community psychology theory (Ryan, 1971) and research (Mitchell et al., 1985). Blaming social conditions, rather than victims, is probably a component of the belief system of potential activists (O'Neill & Trickett, 1982).

My colleagues and I developed two short belief scales to study the importance of cognition in citizen participation in social action (O'Neill et al., 1988). The purpose of the scales was to investigate the hypothesis that citizen participation in social action is more likely when citizens believe that social conditions are unjust, and that they have the power to act effectively. Our model of the relationship between these beliefs and social action is shown in Table 1.

Existing tests of internality (Rotter, 1966) and belief in a just world (Rubin & Peplau, 1975) were modified, creating independent measures of belief in personal power and belief in possible injustice in society. Internal consistency and stability for the personal power (PP) and injustice (Ij) scales were established using conventional psychometric procedures. In addition, because there were French and English versions of both scales, it was possible to use an innovative test–retest method; bilingual participants were given the scales first in one language, then in the other (O'Neill & Thibeault, 1986).

TABLE 1. A Two-Dimensional Model Relating Belief Sets to Citizen Participation in Social Action

		Personal power	
		High	Low
Injustice	High	Social action	Oppression
	Low	Individual achievement	Fatalism

The personal power scale predicted results in an experiment relevant to the internal locus of control; the injustice scale predicted the outcome in an experiment that focused on victim blame. The scales were found to be independent of one another. Once the scales had been shown to be stable and independent, and to predict the outcomes of theoretically relevant experiments, they were given to activists and nonactivists.

The first comparison, done in the province of Nova Scotia, involved three groups that might be expected to fall into different quadrants of the model shown in Table 1 (O'Neill et al., 1988). We compared the board members of a transition house for battered women, university students, and single mothers on the waiting list for service from Big Brothers/Big Sisters. The transition-house board members were highly involved in social action, and were expected to have high scores on both the injustice and personal power scales. University students were thought to be more oriented toward achievement, and were predicted to have high scores on the PP scale, but low ones on the Ij scale. Most single mothers are in a powerless position in society, so their personal power scores were expected to be low. We used single mothers on the waiting list for service, because service from Big Brothers/Big Sisters have been shown to improve well-being and social adjustment (Campbell & O'Neill, 1985). Ij scores of single mothers were expected to be high, since they would have had many opportunities to see the just-world hypothesis disproved in their own lives.

The transition-house board had worked for several years to establish a shelter for battered women. This board had forcefully confronted various levels of government to get support for its project. The majority of board members, male as well as female, described themselves as feminists. Data were collected at the end of the second year of the board's efforts, when it seemed likely that the transition house would not receive the needed government support. By the end of the third year the group had, in fact, succeeded in establishing a transition house.

As expected, the transition-house board scored high on both scales. University students were high in personal power but low on the injustice scale (they tended to blame the victim). Single mothers were high on the injustice scale but low in perceived personal power. The results supported the hypothesis that activism is associated with a combination of a sense of injustice and a belief in one's personal power. The data were also consistent with the theory that activism requires these two cognitive sets, but, of course, that causal theory cannot be directly tested with a correlational design.

Data from other activist groups have supported the model. Chiasson (1986) noted that the results indicating that students tended to believe in a just world were samples based on university students in general. She predicted that students who were members of activist groups on the campus would have scores similar to non-student activists. Her prediction was confirmed.

The scales were given to a group of activists in Vancouver whose members were in more than 40 groups or causes, from the peace movement to single mother's action organizations. These activists, most of whom belonged to more than one group, had scores on both scales that put them in the activist quadrant. The pattern of results from the activist groups, students, and single mothers, is shown in Table 2.

Support for the model also came from subsequent work in Montreal in which we varied the social class of activists. At the extremes, groups included a working-class community group that organized when people learned that a toxic-waste dump was to be located in their neighborhood, and a group of businessmen who organized to save parkland from being developed by two universities.

Longitudinal research is needed to determine whether personal power and a sense of injustice are not only associated with activism, but actually facilitate it. It is possible,

TABLE 2. Mean Scores for Community Groups and University Students in a Model with Two-Belief Dimensions: Personal Power and Injustice

		Personal power scale						
		9	8	7	6	5	4	3
	9							
	8		+ Vancouver activists					
			+ transition house					
	7		+ student activists				+ single mothers	
Injustice scale	6							
			+ university students					
	5							
	4							
	3							

especially with regard to personal power, that being involved in social action increases one's belief in the ability to control events. But even in the absence of longitudinal data, there is some reason to doubt the alternative hypothesis. None of the activist groups (in Nova Scotia, Vancouver, or Montreal) had achieved significant successes at the time that the members filled out our scales. The highest mean score on the personal power scale was recorded by the neighborhood group fighting against the toxic waste dump in Montreal, although it probably had the bleakest outlook of any group. (More than 3,000 of the projected 10,000 truckloads of toxic waste were already in the dump before residents knew what was happening and formed their organization.) It seems reasonable to speculate that activists are drawn into the arena of action in part because they believe they can influence events, a belief presumably based on a particular history of control over reinforcement [consistent with the Rotter's (1954) social learning theory.]

The view that a belief in personal power encourages social action is consistent with Fiske's (1987) analysis of antinuclear activists. She states that these activists have a strong sense of political efficacy: "The antinuclear activist believes that nuclear war is preventable, not inevitable, and that citizens working together can influence government action to decrease the chance of a nuclear war" (p. 213). Her advice to psychologists who wish to motivate citizens to become activists was "First, find a way to give people a sense of political efficacy" (p. 215).

Group Identification and Social Change

On a community level of analysis, we find that collective action is undertaken by people who have a strong sense of identity with their group. For example, Gurin, Miller, & Gurin (1980) found that group identification among African-Americans was strongly related to discontent with the group's power position and with a collective orientation toward social change. Action is also more likely when the disadvantaged group has identified another specific group as having treated them unfairly.

This research group also investigated the situation in which those who identify strongly with one group perceive that *another* group is being treated unfairly. Tougas, Veilleux, & Dubé (1987) assessed the attitudes of men and women toward affirmative action designed to enhance the status of women in the workplace. They also measured whether participants believed that women were being treated unfairly. They found, not surprisingly, that the women were more militant the more they perceived that their group was being treated unfairly; again, the relationship between relative deprivation and militancy operated at the group, rather than at the personal, level. The more interesting finding concerned male participants. Their perception that women were being treated unfairly was associated with favorable attitudes toward affirmative action. This is a phenomenon that has hitherto been ignored in relative deprivation research: an advantaged group being favorable to programs that will diminish its own advantage, based on group members' perception that a disadvantaged group is being treated unfairly.

The community level of analysis also encourages us to include the situational context that makes social action more or less likely to succeed. Leiter and I did a series of simulations to look at whether strong group identification affects the ability of group members to work together (O'Neill & Leiter, 1986). We found that shared assumptions about the cause of a problem create a sense of identity among group members. But, while this cohesion gives the group a sense of mission, it also makes the group more inflexible and less responsive to possibilities that might arise that would permit the group to achieve its goals, perhaps in novel ways.

In this section, three current research programs concerning social action have been described. Taken together, these programs indicate that social cognition and individual differences are important considerations in the study of empowerment and social change. The programs were complementary, each operating at a different level of analysis. The next section will deal directly with levels of analysis.

LEVELS OF ANALYSIS

The main contribution of community psychology may, in the end, be its ability to integrate several levels of analysis to produce a comprehensive understanding of social phenomena. Explanations of problems, such as prejudice and social action, that neglect the setting or the person are inadequate (Rappaport, 1977). Community psychology has brought the person and the setting into the foreground simultaneously (Tracey, Sherry, & Keitel, 1986), and has focused on the interaction between the two (Florin & Wandersman, 1984; O'Neill & Trickett, 1982; Trickett, Kelly, & Todd, 1972).

In this chapter I have used the individual, interpersonal, and community levels; in other chapters, authors divide the space in different ways; by including an organizational level, for instance. Whatever levels we find helpful, we must be clear about how they work and how they yield explanations that give us new insights. Working on only one level has its dangers; but so, too, does moving carelessly from one level to another. Mills (1967) highlighted these issues in a classic paper in which he identified the macroscopic and molecular styles of social science research. His points are useful for community psychologists.

The macroscopic approach is that which emphasizes the broad sweep of a social problem, as in:

QUESTION: What brings on escalating demands for social change?
ANSWER: A recent improvement in social conditions.

The problem with this level of analysis is that it is not tied to controlled observation. When we are convinced, Mills suggests, it is because the answer seems to make sense, as does de Tocqueville's (1856/1955) analysis of the French Revolution. But the fact that an answer seems to make sense does not mean that it is right. Simkus (1986) pointed out that revolutions often come from a worsening, rather than a bettering, of conditions. What does seem to be true is that revolutions rarely follow long periods of unchanging conditions (Gurr, 1970). Even if the explanation were not an overstatement, we would still need to know how an improvement in social conditions translates into a multitude of individual decisions to do something.

Looking at the question and the answer entirely on the molecular level, however, is also unsatisfying:

QUESTION: What encourages people to join local social action groups?
ANSWER: A sense of injustice and a belief in their personal power, as indicated by high scores on the injustice and personal power scales.

Now the concepts are operational. But where are the broader social implications? We have neither explored nor explained the relationship between our social action groups and an upsurge of collective action. Social action groups flourish in some conditions and not in others, a fact that is left out when we give an answer that refers only to the beliefs of members.

We cannot solve the levels-of-analysis problem by posing the question on one level and answering it on another. Confusion of levels can lead to ludicrous simplifications, such as Le Bon's (1879) well-known dismissal of revolution as the mere madness of crowds. In the social change example, a mix-up of levels might lead us to see injustice and personal power scores of members of some social action groups to answer the question: What brings on escalating demands for social change in society? In Mills's (1967) terms, we have unduly stretched a variable. The beliefs of members of some social action groups have been inappropriately generalized to explain a broad social phenomenon.

Another sort of mix-up occurs if we refer to a recent improvement in social conditions to explain why people joined particular social action groups. Now we have falsely concretized a concept, treating an improvement in social condition as though it could be measured in the way we measured the beliefs of group members about injustice and personal power. Furthermore, we have not explained why some people join social action groups, while others stay home, no matter how favorable the conditions for action may be.

Levels of analysis, then, must be handled with some care. We should be sure that questions and answers are on the same level, while finding creative ways to shuttle between levels so that our explanations are as comprehensive as possible.

CONCLUSIONS AND FUTURE DIRECTIONS

This chapter has presented work on social cognition that seems especially relevant to the community field. The focus was on research conducted in the time since an earlier review outlined a cognitive approach to community psychology (O'Neill, 1981). Two general areas were explored in the chapter: stereotyping of one group by another, and cognitive approaches to understanding social action.

Recent work on stereotyping highlights the fact that people form beliefs on the basis of extremely weak evidence, then cling to those beliefs even when presented with strong evidence that they are false. Vividness and salience of information seem to be important in stereotype formation, while intuitive theories that "explain" perceived correlations are important in stereotype maintenance. The ubiquity of stereotyping makes it unlikely that the process itself can be modified, or at least modified enough to have an impact on real examples of prejudice among groups. At the same time, the shift in emphasis from a melting-pot ideal to a multicultural ideal forces us to examine our assumptions about the negativity of stereotypes *per se*. Future work on the role of stereotypes in intergroup hostility will have most relevance for community psychology when it examines and explains the basis for *negative* stereotypes.

Three research programs into cognitive aspects of social action were reviewed. The first employed a laboratory simulation to discover what information is conveyed by various transactions between the powerful and the disadvantaged. The second looked at the beliefs that are associated with activism—beliefs about social injustice and one's power to effect change. The third was concerned with group identification as a factor in social action. These lines of research each produced data that have intriguing possibilities that will, in turn, require further testing. It is necessary to discover whether transactions in a laboratory setting hold good for community groups, whether the beliefs of activists are actually causes of social action, and whether people who believe that a group is being unfairly treated would be willing to suffer a personal cost to help resolve the inequity.

The work reviewed in this chapter testifies to the fruitfulness of including social cognition in our attempts to understand and intervene in social conditions and community processes.

ACKNOWLEDGMENTS. I would like to thank Seanna O'Neill, Roger Bouthillier, Rachel Thibeault, Christine Richards, and Heather Sears, who were research assistants on work with the personal power and injustice scales reported in this paper. In particular, Seanna collected data from the sample of social activists in Vancouver, and Roger and Rachel worked on the Montreal phase of the project. I am also grateful to Janice Best for her helpful comments on a draft of this chapter, and to Heather Turner for her work with the text. Inquiries can be sent by e-mail to pat-oneill@acadiau.ca.

REFERENCES

Alinsky, S. (1971). *Rules for radicals*. New York: Random House.

Alvaro, C., McFarland, C., & Beuhler, R. (1998). *Self-focused attention and the relationship between moods and memory*. Paper presented at the annual convention of the American Psychological Association, San Francisco, August.

Anderson, C. A. (1983). Abstract and concrete data in the perseverance of social theories: When weak data lead to unshakable beliefs. *Journal of Experimental Social Psychology, 19*, 93–108.

Anderson, C. A., Lepper, M. R., & Ross, L. (1980). Perseveration of social theories: The role of explanation in the persistence of discredited information. *Journal of Personality and Social Psychology, 39*, 1037–1049.

Braun, B. G. (1993). Dissociative disorders: The next ten years. In B. G. Braun & J. B. Parks (Eds.), *Proceedings of the tenth international conference on multiple personality/dissociative states*. Chicago: Rush-Presbyterian–St. Luke's Medical Center.

Brickman, J. (1992). Female lives, feminist deaths: The relationship of the Montreal Massacre to dissociation, incest, and violence against women. *Canadian Psychology, 33*, 128–143.

Campbell, D. T. (1967). Stereotypes and the perception of group differences. *American Psychologist, 22*, 817–829.

Campbell, R. E. (1999). *Defining child abuse: An examination of parents' and child welfare agents' beliefs*. Doctoral dissertation, University of Guelph, Guelph, Canada.

Campbell, R. E., & O'Neill, P. (1985). Social support for single mothers: A study of Big Brothers/ Big Sisters. *Canadian Journal of Community Mental Health, 4*, 81–87.

Carroll, M. A. (1994). Empowerment theory: Philosophical and practical difficulties. *Canadian Psychology, 35*, 376–381.

Chavis, D. M., & Wandersman, A. (1990). Sense of community in the urban environment: A catalyst for participation and community development. *American Journal of Community Psychology, 18*, 55–81.

Chiasson, S. (1986). Women's Awareness Network Team Support: Its beginnings. Unpublished honor's thesis, Acadia University, Wolfville, Nova Scotia, Canada.

Constantino, V., & Nelson, G. (1995). Changing relationships between self-help groups and mental health professionals: Shifting ideology and power. *Canadian Journal of Community Mental Health, 14,* 55–70.

de Tocqueville, A. (1856/1955). *The old regime and the French revolution.* (S. Gilbert, trans.). Garden City, NY: Doubleday.

Dubé, L., & Guimond, S. (1986). Relative deprivation and social protest: The personal-group issue. In J. M. Olson, C. P. Herman, & M. P. Zanna (Eds.), *Relative deprivation and social comparison: The Ontario symposium. Vol. 4.* Hillsdale, NJ: Erlbaum.

Fish, S. (1997). boutique multiculturalism, or, why liberals are incapable of thinking about hate speech. *Critical Inquiry, 23,* 378–396.

Fiske, S. T. (1987). People's reactions to nuclear war. *American Psychologist, 42,* 207–217.

Florin, P. R., & Wandersman, A. (1984). Cognitive social learning and participation in community development. *American Journal of Community Psychology, 12,* 689–708.

Forgas, J. P. (1983). The effects of prototypicality and cultural salience on perceptions of people. *Journal of Research in Personality, 17,* 153–173.

Garbarino, J., & Kostelny, K. (1992). Child maltreatment as a community problem. *Child Abuse and Neglect, 16,* 455–464.

Geertz, C. (1986). The uses of diversity. *Michigan Quarterly Review, 25,* 105–123.

Guimond, S., & Dubé-Simard, L. (1983). The relative deprivation theory and the Quebec nationalist movement: The cognitive emotion distinction and the personal-group deprivation issue. *Journal of Personality and Social Psychology, 44,* 526–535.

Gurin, P., Miller, A. H., & Gurin, G. (1980). Stratum identification and consciousness. *Social Psychology Quarterly, 43,* 30–47.

Gurr, T. R. (1970). *Why men rebel.* Princeton, NJ: Princeton University Press.

Hacking, I. (1991). The making and molding of child abuse. *Clinical Inquiry, 17,* 253–288.

Hacking, I. (1995). *Rewriting the soul: Multiple personality and the sciences of memory.* Princeton, NJ: Princeton University Press.

Hamil, P., Wilson, T., & Nisbett, R. (1980). Insensitivity to sample bias: Generalizing from atypical cases. *Journal of Personality and Social Psychology, 39,* 579–589.

Kahn, S. (1970). *How people get power.* New York: McGraw-Hill.

Kinder, D. R., & Sears, D. O. (1981). Prejudice and politics: Symbolic racism versus racial threats to the good life. *Journal of Personality and Social Psychology, 40,* 414–431.

Latané, B., & Wolf, S. (1981). The social impact of majorities and minorities. *Psychological Review, 88,* 438–453.

Lavoie, F., Jacob, M., Hardy, J., and Martin, G. (1989). Police attitudes in assigning responsibility for wife abuse. *Journal of Family Violence, 4,* 369–388.

Lavoie, F., Vézina, L., Piché, C., and Boivin, M. (1995). Evaluation of a prevention program for violence in teen dating relationships. *Journal of Interpersonal Violence, 10,* 517–525.

Le Bon, G. (1879). *The crowd: A study of the popular mind.* London: T. F. Unwin.

Lee, Y.-T., Jussim, L. J., & McCauley, C. R. (1995). *Stereotype accuracy: Toward appreciating group differences.* Washington, D.C.: American Psychological Association.

Lerner, N. J.,& Miller, D. T. (1978). Just world research and the attribution process: Looking back and looking ahead. *Psychological Bulletin, 85,* 1030–1051.

LeVine, F. A., & Campbell, D. T. (1972). *Ethnocentrism, theories of conflict, ethnic attitudes and group behaviour.* Toronto: Wiley.

Linville, P. W., & Jones, F. F. (1980). Polarized appraisals of out-group members. *Journal of Personality and Social Psychology, 38,* 689–703.

Martin, J., Brickman, P., & Murray, A. (1984). Moral outrage and pragmatism: explanations for collective action. *Journal of Experimental Social Psychology, 20,* 484–496.

McCauley, C. R. (1994). Are stereotypes exaggerated? In Y.-T. Lee, L. J. Jussim, & C. R. McCauley (Eds.), *Stereotype accuracy: Toward appreciating group differences* (pp. 238–239). Washington, D.C.: American Psychological Association.

McFarland, C., & Beuhler, R. (1997). Negative affective states and the motivated retrieval of positive life events: The role of acknowledgment. *Journal of Personality and Social Psychology, 73,* 200–214.

Meissen, G. J., Mason, W. C., & Gleason, D. F. (1991). Understanding the attitudes and intentions of future professionals toward self-help. *American Journal of Community Psychology, 16,* 699–714.

Mills, C. W. (1967). Two styles of social science research. In I. L. Horowitz (Ed.), *Power, politics and people: The collected essays of C. Wright Mills* (pp. 553–567). New York: Oxford University Press.

Mitchell, C. N., Davidson, W. S., Chodakowski, J. A., & McVeigh, J. (1985). Intervention orientation: Quantification of "person-blame" versus "situation-blame" intervention philosophies. *American Journal of Community Psychology, 13*, 543–552.

Monod, J. (1972). *Chance and necessity.* (A. Wainhouse, trans.). New York: Vintage.

Nisbett, R. S., & Borgida, F. (1975). Attribution and the psychology of prediction. *Journal of Personality and Social Psychology, 32*, 932–943.

Nisbett, P., & Ross, L. (1980). *Human inference.* Englewood Cliffs, NJ: Prentice-Hall.

Oakes, P. J., Haslam, S. A., & Turner, J. C. (1994). *Stereotyping and social reality.* Cambridge, MA: Basil Blackwell.

O'Neill, P. (1981). Cognitive community psychology. *American Psychologist, 36*, 457–469.

O'Neill, P. (1989). Responsible to whom? Responsible for what? Some ethical issues in community intervention. *American Journal of Community Psychology, 17*, 323–341.

O'Neill, P. (1998). *Negotiating consent in psychotherapy.* New York: New York University Press.

O'Neill, P., Duffy, C., Enman, M., Blackmer, E., Goodwin, J., & Campbell, R. E. (1988). Cognition and citizen participation in social action. *Journal of Applied Social Psychology, 18*, 1067–1083.

O'Neill, P., & Hern, R. (1991). A systems approach to ethical problems. *Ethics & Behavior, 1*, 129–143.

O'Neill, P., & Leiter, M. P. (1986). Shared assumptions: A citizen action group simulation. *Canadian Journal of Behavioural Science, 18*, 115–125.

O'Neill, P., & Thibeault, R. (1986). Evaluation des prédispositions à l'action sociale. *La Revue Canadienne de Santé Mentale Communautaire, 5*, 49–62.

O'Neill, P., & Trickett, E. J. (1982). *Community consultation.* San Francisco: Jossey-Bass.

Pancer, S. M., & Cameron, G. (1994). Resident participation in the Better Beginnings, Better Futures prevention project: Part I—The impacts of involvement. *Canadian Journal of Community Mental Health, 13*, 195–211.

Prilleltensky, I. (1994). Empowerment in mainstream psychology: Legitimacy, obstacles, and possibilities. *Canadian Psychology, 35*, 358–373.

Prilleltensky, I., & Nelson, G. (1997). Community psychology: Reclaiming social justice. In D. Fox & I. Prilleltensky (Eds.), *Critical psychology: An introduction.* London: Sage.

Rappaport, J. (1977). *Community psychology: Values, research, and action.* New York: Holt, Rinehart and Winston.

Reiff, R. (1968). Social intervention and the problem of psychological analysis. *American Psychologist, 23*, 524–530.

Rich, R. C., Edelstein, M., Hallman, W. K., & Wandersman, A. H. (1995). Citizen participation and empowerment: The case of local environmental hazards. *American Journal of Community Psychology, 23*, 657–676.

Rickel, A. U. (1989). *Teen pregnancy and parenting.* New York: Hemisphere/Taylor & Francis.

Riger, S. (1993). What's wrong with empowerment? *American Journal of Community Psychology, 21*, 279–292.

Riger, S., Gordon, M. T., & LeBailly, N. K. (1982). Coping with urban crime: Women's use of precautionary behaviors. *American Journal of Community Psychology, 10*, 369–386.

Rorty, R. (1991). On ethnocentrism: A reply to Clifford Geertz. In R. Rorty, *Objectivity, relativism, and truth.* Cambridge: Cambridge University Press.

Rotter, J. B. (1954). *Social learning and clinical psychology.* Englewood Cliffs, NJ: Prentice-Hall.

Rotter, J. B. (1966). Generalized expectancies for internal versus external control of reinforcement. *Psychological Monographs, 80* (1, Whole No. 609).

Rubin, Z., & Peplau, A. (1975). Who believes in a just world? *Journal of Social Issues, 31*, 65–89.

Runciman, W. O. (1966). *Relative deprivation and social justice.* Berkeley: University of California Press.

Ryan, W. (1971). *Blaming the victim.* New York: Pantheon.

Sarason, S. B. (1974). *The psychological sense of community: prospects for a community psychology.* San Francisco: Jossey-Bass.

Seidman, E. S., & Rappaport, J. (1986). *Redefining social problems.* New York: Plenum.

Sherif, M. (1966). *In common predicament: Social psychology of intergroup conflict and cooperation.* Boston: Houghton Mifflin.

Simard, L. (1981). Intergroup communications. In Gardner, R. C., & Kalin, R. K. (Eds.), *A Canadian social psychology of ethnic relations.* Toronto: Methuen.

Simkus, N. (1986). *Effects of improvement size on contentment, aspiration level, perceived strength, perceived conflict, and instrumental action escalation.* Doctoral dissertation, University of Western Ontario, London, Ontario, Canada.

St. Lawrence, J. S., Eldridge, G. D., Reitman, D., Little, C. E., Shelby, M. C., & Brasfield, T. L. (1998). Factors influencing condom use among African-American women: Implications for risk reduction intervention. *American Journal of Community Psychology, 26*, 7–28.

Steiner, P. A., & Mark, M. M. (1985). The impact of a community action group: an illustration of the potential of time series analysis for the study of community groups. *American Journal of Community Psychology, 12*, 12–20.

Stokols, P. (1975). Toward a psychological theory of alienation. *Psychological Review, 82*, 26–44.

Tajfel, H. (1978). *Differentiation in social groups*. London: Academic.

Taylor, C. (1995). *Philosophical arguments*. Cambridge, MA: Harvard University Press.

Taylor, D. (1981). Stereotypes and intergroup relations. In Gardner, R. C., & Kalin, R. K. (Eds.), *A Canadian social psychology of ethnic relations*. Toronto: Methuen, 1981.

Tittle, C. R. (1982). Social class and criminal behavior: A critique of the theoretical foundation. *Social Forces, 62*, 334–358.

Tougas, F., Veilleux, F., & Dubé, L. (1987). Privation relative et programmes d'action positive. *Canadian Journal of Behavioural Science, 19*, 167–175.

Tracey, T. J., Sherry, P., & Keitel, M. (1986). Distress and help-seeking as a function of person-environment fit and self-efficacy: A causal model. *American Journal of Community Psychology, 14*, 657–676.

Trickett, E. J., Kelly, J. C., & Todd, D. N. (1972). The social environment of the high school: Guidelines for individual change and organizational redevelopment. In S. Golann & C. Eisendorfer (Eds.), *Handbook of community mental health*. New York: Appleton-Century-Crofts.

Tversky, A., & Kahneman, P. (1971). Belief in the law of small numbers. *Psychological Bulletin, 76*, 105–110.

Van Uchelen, C. P., Davidson, S. F., Quressette, S. V. A., Brasfield, C. R., & Demerais, L. H. (1997). What makes us strong: Urban Aboriginal perspectives on wellness and strength. *Canadian Journal of Community Mental Health, 16*, 37–50.

Vinokur, A., & Caplan, R. D. (1986). Cognitive and affective components of life events: Their relations and effects on well-being. *American Journal of Community Psychology, 14*, 351–370.

Walker, I., & Pettigrew, T. F. (1984). Relative deprivation theory: An overview and conceptual critique. *British Journal of Social Psychology, 23*, 301–310.

Weber, R., & Crocker, J. (1983). Cognitive processes in the revision of stereotypic beliefs. *Journal of Personality and Social Psychology, 45*, 961–977.

Weick, K. (1984). Small wins: Redefining the scale of social problems. *American Psychologist, 39*, 40–49.

Wilder, D. A. (1984). Intergroup contact: The typical member and the exception to the rule. *Journal of Experimental Social Psychology, 20*, 177–194.

Yates, S. N., & Aronson, F. (1983). A social psychological perspective on energy conservation in residential buildings. *American Psychologist, 38*, 435–444.

Zuckerman, M., Mann, K., & Bernieri, F. (1982). Determinants of consensus estimates: attribution, salience, and representativeness. *Journal of Personality and Social Psychology, 42*, 839–852.

CHAPTER 7

Understanding and Changing Social Systems

An Ecological View

JAMES G. KELLY, ANN MARIE RYAN, B. EILEEN ALTMAN, AND STEPHEN P. STELZNER

INTRODUCTION: THE ECOLOGICAL POINT OF VIEW

A preventive orientation affirms how social systems can be organized to have a positive impact on the development of those individuals who make it up. Here, the authors affirm that an ecological approach to social systems is useful to build a *community-based* community psychology, a psychology that is attentive to the promotion of competent individuals in responsive social systems.

The essence of the ecological perspective is to construct an understanding of the interrelationships of social structures and social processes of the groups, organizations, and communities in which we live and work. The concept of interdependence is the basic axiom of the ecological perspective (Kelly, 1966, 1968, 1979a, 1979b; Kelly & Hess, 1987; Kelly, Dassoff, Levin, Schreckengost, Stelzner & Altman, 1988; Muñoz, Snowden, & Kelly, 1979; Kingry-Westergaard & Kelly, 1990; Trickett, 1984, 1987, 1996). Designing change processes, creating new organizations and services, or reducing the noxious impacts of environmental and social factors, requires a working sense of not only the current interdependencies of people and structures, but the potential of creating, and facilitating new interdependencies.

The axiom of interdependence has been affirmed by R. A. Rappaport: "the ecosystem concept itself is a vital element in the construction, maintenance and reconstruction of the

JAMES G. KELLY • Department of Psychology, University of California, Davis, Davis, California 95616. ANN MARIE RYAN • Department of Psychology, Michigan State University, East Lansing, Michigan 48824. B. EILEEN ALTMAN • 1156 High Street, Santa Cruz, California 95064. STEPHEN P. STELZNER • Department of Psychology, College of St. Benedict, St. Joseph, Minnesota 56374.

Handbook of Community Psychology, edited by Julian Rappaport and Edward Seidman. Kluwer Academic / Plenum Publishers, New York, 2000.

webs of life upon which, by whatever name we call them, we are absolutely dependent" (Rappaport, p. 69, 1990).

This chapter has been prepared in the spirit of Rappaport's assertion. The authors have also drawn on the writings and research of Barker (1968, 1987); Bateson (1972, 1979); Bronfenbrenner (1979, 1986); Kahn (1968), Katz & Kahn (1978); Raush, Barry, Hertel, & Swain (1974); Raush (1977, 1979); Sarason (1972); Scott (1981); Stokols (1987, 1988); Trickett (1984, 1996); and Wicker (1987).

To create a resourceful social system requires that the initiator have a view of how people and social systems affect each other. The ecological perspective is proposed as a point of view that can elaborate structures and processes for both people and social systems.

Scott (1981) has summed up the concept of social system in the following statement:

> Organizations are first and foremost, systems of elements, each of which affects and is affected by the others. Goals are not the key to understanding the nature and functioning of organizations, no more than are the participants, the technology, or social structure. And no organization can be understood in isolation from the larger environment. We will miss the essence of organization if we insist on focusing on any single feature to the exclusion of all others (Scott, 1981, pp. 18–19).

The larger environment, within which an organization exists, also becomes a focus from an ecological perspective. As Scott expresses it:

> The interdependence of the organization and its environment receives primary attention in the open systems perspective. Rather than overlooking the environment ... the open systems model stresses the reciprocal ties that bind and interrelate the organization with those elements that surround and penetrate it. The environment is perceived to be the ultimate source of materials, energy, and information, all of which are vital to the continuation of the system (Scott, 1981, pp. 119–120).

Here the term "environment" refers to those factors, forces, and events that are outside the immediate social system. If the focus for prevention, for example, is an elementary school classroom, the classroom is considered to be the social system, and includes the various structures and events within it (Weinstein, 1991; Gump, 1987). The term environment refers to those parts of the school beyond the particular classroom and includes the surrounding community. Events, concerns, and themes in the larger community, as environmental factors, are considered to affect the classroom.

An ecological approach to social systems has at least two distinguishing features. First, it places the focus of analysis upon the transactions between persons *and* systems, and not only on the independent qualities of persons *or* systems. An ecological analysis focuses on the social system as a unified whole, as well as on the analysis of persons and their interrelationships within the system. An ecological analysis also attempts to understand the system's relationships with other systems (Aldridge, 1979; Aldwin & Stokols, 1988; Allen, Stelzner, & Wielkiewicz, 1998; Capra, 1996; Katz & Kahn, 1978; von Bertalanffy, 1968, 1975; Buckley, 1968; McKelvey, 1982; Miller, 1978; Sameroff, 1980; Scott, 1981).

Second, the *balance* of social structures and social processes, rather than either of these in isolation, is seen as the source of effective system functioning. *Structures* are those elements of a social system that provide the opportunities or settings in which a member of the system interacts with other participants in the system—a framework in which to interact; while *processes* are the actions in the system that allow structures to be created, changed, or simply acted upon—how persons relate within the structure. Each structure and each process is treated in terms of its relationship with all other social structures and social processes. In any social system, structures and processes are developed in response to constraints and opportunities that inevitably arise for persons within that system.

Structures may be policies, procedures, events and the settings for those events, or organizational elements and characteristics that provide access to meaningful resources within the social system. The structures within a social system indicate "what" makes up the characteristic elements of the system.

Processes are a series of social actions that make use of the structures of the system, and the interpersonal exchanges that take place within and between the various structures. The processes indicate "how" interactions take place within the social system. Processes consist of linked behavioral exchanges (Umbarger, 1983). The understanding of process has long been of interest to community psychologists (Kelly, 1979b; Klein, 1968), and a particular focus of consultation literature (cf., Kelly & Hess, 1987; Smith & Corse, 1986; Juras, Mackin, Curtis, & Foster-Fishman, 1997; Thomas, Gatz, & Luczak, 1997). Process is a major topic that organizational and clinical psychologists consider when working on organizational and personal change. The proponents of an ecological view observe how the various structures and various processes are, in fact, linked and woven together, affecting each other and creating a dynamic and unique expression of the particular system at a particular time (Capra, 1996).

In real life, social systems can be stifling. A common understanding of the term "social system" may suggest that a person's sense of self is subsumed under the needs of the system. Accordingly, meeting the needs of a person is seen as secondary to meeting the needs of the system. This common view of a social system means that an individual not only is subordinate to the system, but also that he or she is given few of the tools necessary to maintain a balance between satisfying personal needs and satisfying the needs of the particular social system.

An ecological perspective encourages the design of preventive interventions that promote the creation of social structures that better connect persons with the system in a positive manner, and encourage processes within that system that will allow persons to have a meaningful influence on the system itself. The goal of this type of intervention is to stimulate a social system so that individuals have opportunities to develop *personal* and *social resources*.

This chapter will elaborate a conceptual framework for putting the ecological perspective into practice. This will be done by first introducing eight concepts about the structures and process of social systems, which will be helpful in understanding how structures and processes interact. The latter part of the chapter will discuss concepts from two other perspectives, open-systems theory and developmental theory. This is done to illustrate connections between ecological concepts with which readers may be more familiar. It is hoped that this elaboration of the ecological perspective will enhance the work of community psychologists to generate lasting, growth-promoting, systemic changes.

EIGHT CONCEPTS ABOUT STRUCTURE AND PROCESS

In the following section, eight concepts are presented that provide an ecological framework for the analysis of social systems. They are divided into two main categories, four concepts defining structure and four concepts defining processes. These two concepts are considered basic and interdependent components of a social system. Together these eight concepts constitute an ecological approach to social systems, and represent the continued elaboration of an ecological perspective (Kelly, 1987; Kelly & Hess, 1987; Kelly et al., 1988; Kingry-Westergaard & Kelly, 1990; Trickett, 1987). The concepts are also presented as heuristic ideas to help design preventive interventions for social systems. Accompanying each of the eight concepts is an illustration of how an elementary school can be viewed as an ecological system.

Structure

The four defining concepts of structure are: *personal resource potentials*, *social system resources*, *social settings*, and *system boundaries*. Each concept is estimated to make a unique and essential contribution to the quality of life within the social system.

Personal resource potentials refer to the opportunity for people within a social system to offer particular qualities, skills, or information that help promote the social competence of other participants in the system (e.g., recognizing participants for accomplishments that might otherwise go unnoticed). The concept of personal resource potential as a structural variable refers to the potential of environmental pathways that can make it easy for the competencies of persons to be expressed. For example, there may be an individual within the system who has a knack for creating spontaneous occasions for celebration, or initiating friendships, or encouraging emotional release. It is necessary for the system to have in operation norms, values, and roles that can facilitate the expression of such behavior. In contrast, there may be norms, values, or roles that prevent this person from expressing these qualities. Personal resource potentials may be low in an organization lacking a history of expressing spontaneity, improvised occasions, or a commitment to informally recognize participants.

A basic notion of personal resource potential is that there does exist the potential for social ties to develop between and among participants in social systems, and that "resource opportunities" can be created as a result of those ties. The concept is similar to Granovetter's (1973) discussion of "weak ties" in personal social networks, or to the notion of personal communities articulated by Wellman, Carrington, and Hall (1988). The concept of personal resource potential is, however, not a reference to social networks often described in the social support literature (Gottleib, 1981; Naparstek, Biesel, & Spiro, 1982; Pilisuk & Parks, 1986; Maguire, 1983; Vaux, 1988). The term personal resources refers to an "open" social system in which participants are able to express useful personal qualities that have an impact on other participants in the system. Often these qualities will not be recognized as valuable, or may even appear to be slightly unconventional (Chaleff, 1995).

When personal resource potentials are present in a system, or when social norms to support the development of personal resources are present, other persons can seek out informal ties. A low level of personal resource potential may indicate that environmental constraints are restricting the development of personal resources. For example, work overload within a "closed" organization can limit the opportunities for participants of that organization to engage in the type of behaviors described above (e.g., traditions to support the maintenance of friendship). In the same way, environmental constraints can also limit the expression of social norms that promote the development of persons as resources (e.g., prohibiting conversation between assembly-line workers). Some persons who serve as resources often are not immediately recognized or acknowledged by others in the system. This can be a result of these persons occupying a lower social position, such as custodian or secretary.

In an elementary school, for example, the secretary may deal with a student's problem before it reaches crisis proportions. One diagnostic clue to whether a system is "open" is the extent to which persons serve as personal resources for each other, independent of their social position. The custodian may have established trust and rapport with students, but may not have access to certain information that could be useful in alleviating a problem, such as the availability of tutoring. Persons who serve as personal resources can have a larger impact when social system resources are made available to them. Ultimately, those who serve as personal resources contribute to the quality of life of the participants in a social system (Allen, Stelzner, & Wielkiewicz, 1998).

The personal resources for the elementary school are potentially all persons in the school who can be a part of any program designed to improve the functioning of the system. This includes school secretaries, the building engineer, custodians, school bus drivers, street-crossing guards, other children, and parents, as well as the principal and teachers. *All* participants and persons directly related to the system serving the children become possible resources for an intervention, independent of their social or economic position, their primary or secondary affiliation, or their explicit or implicit roles.

Social system resources are groups, procedures, or events that influence the development of social systems. Social system resources, like personal resources, are available to promote the social competence of individuals within the system. In this case, however, the resource might be a specific occasion (e.g., a student or an "apprentice" given the opportunity to put new skills into practice) or a sympathetic group of people (e.g., a corporate board that contributes informational, financial, or political resources to a school or community service organization). Social system resources not only include information, money, and influence, but also traditions, customs, and observances that facilitate feelings of integration and of being a part of a social system. It is telling of a social system whether persons can access resources beyond those of individuals. Social system resources can make it possible to enhance the development of persons within the system, as well as to activate social relationships with other social systems. Once again, it is critical that there are norms and values that encourage the creation of such occasions or relationships.

Social system resources might also include a state or municipal law that helps to achieve the aims of a particular organization, such as laws guaranteeing equal access to resources (e.g., education for the handicapped or school athletic programs for women). Social system resources might also be influential persons who can sanction the work of the group, such as local celebrities, politicians, or business leaders. Some social system resources, like personal resources, can be hidden or unacknowledged, such as anonymous benefactors to community organizations or precedent-setting laws or policies.

As with personal resources, there will be constraints within the system that prevent the development of social system resources, such as norms and values that are at odds with the pursuit of a particular resource (e.g., a social action group that does not trust the political process). Social system resources are sometimes expected to increase or decrease with changes in the accessibility of personal resources. For example, not having a person with the time for, or understanding of, lobbying, greatly decreases the opportunity for influencing the legislative process. The reverse is also true, of course, in that increases or decreases in social system resources may result in increases or decreases in personal resources. Finally, social system resources can reflect the system's values and norms regarding the use of current resources and the creation of new resources.

The way in which resources are defined and appreciated informs the community psychologist about just how much difficulty there is in perceiving and drawing upon the potential latent sources within a social system. *An ecological perspective assumes that there are many more resources within a social system than are perceived to be available.* The community psychologist, in using an ecological approach, focuses upon social system resources in order to determine how unidentified resources can be identified and tapped.

The social system resources of a specific elementary school are the commitments and the social norms that make it possible for all of the participants in the system to express support, to spontaneously create solutions for the management of the school, and so on. Resources that can be brought to bear on the problem can be inside or outside the elementary school. Such resources can be community volunteer organizations, such as Big Sisters or Big Brothers, community recreational programs, or specially trained teachers in subject areas not already offered in the school. The concept of social system resources also refers to surplus energy in the form of untapped commitment and affiliation on the part of the participants in the system, as well as other community resources that the school can employ to carry out its activities and to cope with external demands.

Social settings are specific places or sites, both informal and formal, that provide an opportunity for the creation of both personal and social system resources (Sarason, 1972). Social settings are expected to enhance a sense of identity and integration; they provide an opportunity for participants to share experiences, and to develop personal affiliations and a sense of community. Social settings are specific places in which significant social interaction occurs, such as the local high school athletic contest, the employee lounge, city council chambers, a local restaurant, the board room, the area around a photocopier, a park, and so on (Barker, 1968). Such places host social interactions or events that may develop new resources, or may maintain resources already established. Subsequently, each of these settings has the potential to be a place in which the individual may come into contact with potentially valuable personal and social system resources, which in turn may be useful to the individual and the entire social system.

Some social settings, like some personal and social system resources, are not expected to be well-known or acknowledged by participants (e.g., restrooms). Whether acknowledged or not, social settings are expected to affect the transmission of cultural values, social norms, and rules of conduct that govern the social system; they make it possible for persons to be interdependent with the larger social system. They represent concrete expressions of the system's way of life, and illustrate how structure and process within the system are balanced. It is within these social settings that participants in the social system learn how the structures and processes of the system come together.

In an elementary school, social settings denote those places within or outside the school that can become sites for creating a milieu for informal help and support. These can be places such as the school cafeteria, the playground, sports facilities, the teachers' lounge, the gymnasium, a local candy store, the secretaries' office, the neighborhood library, as well as hallways and classrooms (Newman, 1979). Social settings can also be occasions created by the participants to informally acknowledge each other, to celebrate holidays or birthdays, and to take time out to have fun after an arduous period of work. These can be locations where the competencies of all the participants in the system can be developed and where social support and guidance can be provided. A natural social setting can serve as an indigenous "intervention." A social setting provides the personal and social system resources for social support while the participants learn new skills. The social support generated can help a child or teacher in social settings become integrated within the system, so that they then can more easily create personal meaning for their roles within the social system.

Social settings are expected to be affected by the quality of system boundaries. *System boundaries* refer to the relationships between social systems (e.g., one organization and another; one neighborhood and another), and specifically refer to the formal and informal interaction and communication that exists between two or more systems. System boundaries represent the degree to which a particular system makes it easy or difficult for persons inside one social system to establish reciprocal relationships with persons outside the system.

Personal and social system resources are created and affected by the level of informational exchange between systems. Local school systems may multiply the resources available to the students within that system if there is open communication and accessibility between the schools and area businesses, government organizations, or senior-citizen centers. Stevenson, Florin, & Mitchell (1998) found, for example, that the extent of interorganizational linkages within 35 Rhode Island communities predicted the implementation of substance-abuse prevention programs. It is likely that both systems or communities in such an exchange gain resources (e.g., any one community organization receives experienced advice, while all the business, government, or community organizations become more informed).

System boundaries offer the opportunity for personal and social system resources to be shared or exchanged among social systems. The extent of perceived permeability of system boundaries makes it possible for socialization processes to be developed and for social norms to be established in order to initiate, develop, and maintain joint or collaborative efforts (Ashkenas, 1997; Kanter, 1996; Kahn, 1989; Davis, Kahn, & Zald, 1990; Ulrich, 1997). The extent of perceived permeability of system boundaries can sanction persons from different systems to appreciate alternative lifestyles and philosophies. System boundaries are ecological structures that can facilitate the development of values for diversity and social engagement between persons and systems. Tight impermeable system boundaries are expected to generate processes that are limiting, insulating, and restrictive of the development of persons and systems.

In an elementary school, system boundaries focus on the intensity and the extent of communication and personal relationships between the participants of the school and other social systems, such as other elementary schools, the adjacent junior high or high school, the neighborhood, the school board, and parent groups. How the participants of the school actually go about identifying resources in their own and other communities, and how they develop collaborative relationships with other community groups, can assist the school, as a system, in responding to unexpected changes or crises, such as the addition of a large number of children from another culture to the school, or the opportunity to absorb a new curriculum.

The quality and diversity of personal and social system resources, the functions of social settings, and the nature of system boundaries, as structures, can set limits on the capacity of a social system to develop its participants. These same structures also can provide opportunities for the participants to become interdependent with the system.

Process

As structure defines the *what* of the system, process defines the *how*—the specific actions or operations that represent how the unique character of the system is expressed. Processes are indices of how the values and social norms of the social system are expressed. They are also apt illustrations of how the system responds to entropy, as it moves toward the natural process of disorganization and decay. Negative entropy is initiated within social systems to reduce decay and generate resources, such as social settings and permeable system boundaries (von Bertalanffy, 1968, 1975; Glidewell, 1987; Katz & Kahn, 1978).

The four processes that are proposed to illustrate an ecological approach to systems are: reciprocity, networking, boundary spanning, and adaptation.

Reciprocity refers to the various ways in which the participants in a social system define and create give-and-take exchanges. For example, organizational members may see value in maintaining reciprocal interpersonal relationships with members of a "lower" organizational status, such as secretaries or custodians. These relationships may lead to modified or expanded roles for many members of the organization, and may open up the system to an expanded exchange of personal and environmental resources.

For example, in a school, teachers may develop informal relationships with secretaries and school clerks when discussing the teacher's concerns about specific children. The secretary's listening and sympathetic ear make it possible for the teacher to be responsive to the secretary's own concerns. This emerging reciprocity can stimulate a recognition among the teachers and secretaries that the personal resources of each other can become a larger resource for the whole school in understanding and responding to parents and children.

An important feature of such exchanges is whether the participants are aware of the expression of reciprocity or whether the participants develop give-and-take relationships without much self-conscious awareness. To a large extent, the existence of personal and social system resources will depend upon the participants of the system developing a norm of reciprocity. It may be necessary for the system to develop social settings in which the value of mutual exchange is promoted. For example, many organizations provide seminars or workshops that promote various forms of interpersonal communication, which can facilitate reciprocity.

What is important is whether members of the organization believe or expect that reciprocity is possible or forthcoming at some future time. The presence of actual reciprocal deeds between persons is not expected to be realized; it is the promise of reciprocity that is most defining for the individual and the system.

An analysis of how reciprocity is created and maintained is important in understanding social system functioning, including how the system provides resources to facilitate reciprocity. Reciprocity is an essential concept because it defines a special type of interdependence among participants in a social system. Reciprocal processes help to sustain the openness of the structures of systems. The skills learned in developing reciprocal relationships can enhance the networking ability of participants.

In an elementary school, reciprocity represents how the principal, teachers, children, and the various staff members go about exchanging information, wisdom, help, and emotional support. When teachers, parents, children, principal, secretaries, and custodial staff develop meaningful and satisfying exchanges, independent of their primary social roles, they are giving and receiving information in a more "open" manner. The various personal and social system resources, when interdependent, increase the chances of creating a sense of community as individuals carry out their various roles in the school.

Networking refers to the various actions that participants take to establish communication with other participants, both within their own social system and with persons from other systems. Networking focuses on the specific steps taken by participants in order to become acquainted and connected with other persons. Reciprocity involves a deep, intimate relationship in which there is a commitment to being helpful to each other. Networking primarily involves establishing contacts with others; these contacts over time may lead to relationships in which reciprocity is expressed.

The operation of networks can reveal how the social norms of a particular system are understood by participants in the system. Networks can suggest what behaviors are valued and how participants go about identifying valued resources. The actions that people take to share information and establish ties with new persons may be taken for granted. Yet, the networking process is important in the creation of resources because networking enables new resources to be identified—resources that were not previously known or acknowledged. For example, Paris (1998) found that networking served as a means of generating medical students' interest in geriatric medicine, enabling new resources to be brought to an area of medicine that needed renewed attention.

One positive consequence of networking is that those persons who actively engage in the process can appreciate how others function at the boundaries of systems, where additional resources can be identified and created. For example, Morrison, White, and Van Velsor (1987) found that women who broke through the "glass ceiling" and became top corporate executives actively engaged in networking. However, networks can also be limiting. For example, Drentea (1998) found that women who networked were more likely to take jobs with a greater ratio of women to men, whereas those who used other means of searching for jobs were more likely to take those with fewer women in them. That is, networking was gendered.

In the elementary school, networking refers to how teachers and students share information with each other and with other key personal resources in the school and the larger community. A value that is expressed in the concept of networking is that it is acceptable for a teacher, principal, or student not to be restricted to their primary role in the elementary school. What is valued instead is for parents, teachers, and students to seek out and share information, wisdom, and facts with others within the school, or with other schools in the neighborhood. Networking validates the concept that learning includes drawing upon personal and social system resources and extending communication to others not within the person's own immediate life space or daily interaction (Galbraith, 1997; Senge, 1997). Tjosvold (1997) found that productive networking by dentists required developing cooperative goals and sharing views open-mindedly. The ability to build cooperative goals and reduce competitive ones among the dentists required a shared purpose, interconnected roles, and sympathy. Likewise, the school principal can become informed about the operation of a local business; a teacher can become informed about how new employees in another school learn their roles; students can learn how children in another town go about the tasks of learning a special skill. Useful knowledge for the creation of personal and social system resources is created out of the process of networking.

Boundary spanning refers to participants in one social system establishing relationships and communications with participants in other systems in order to explicitly identify and exchange resources between systems. In particular, boundary spanning refers to the creation and acting out of roles within a system that make it possible for participants in one or more systems to create exchanges. Boundary spanning, in contrast to networking, involves the formal enactment of social norms to sanction and support a participant to exchange resources for the benefit of the system as a system.

For the exchange process to work, each particular system must sanction persons to carry out the exchange role (Aldrich, 1979, pp. 243–264; Scott, 1981, pp. 179–206). Boundary spanning roles may develop from perceived environmental constraints or dangers that can affect the resources of systems. For example, a threat to a human-service organization's funding may result in the creation of a liaison person between the organization and the funding sources. The creation of boundary spanning roles also may derive from perceived environmental opportunities. For example, participants in a local school system may develop a relationship with the local college or university, hoping to draw upon the expertise of faculty who can offer training, consultation, or general information useful to achieve the school's goals. Part of the boundary spanning, in this case, may involve a person from the school offering his or her own expertise to the college, i.e., as part-time instructor. The survival of a social system may depend upon how effectively participants in a system create resources with persons of other systems. The boundary spanning function illustrates how a social system can benefit from the exchange of resources while preserving the integrity of each of the collaborating systems.

In an elementary school, boundary spanning refers to the processes by which the teachers and students assume roles specifically to exchange information with teachers, students, and administrative staff in other schools or other systems. Boundary spanning represents a value and policy of the school as a system to identify resources beyond the school itself by encouraging teachers and students, as representatives, to develop collaborative exchanges with another school, or with community groups. Under the concept of boundary spanning, teachers and students assume roles wherein they develop collaborative alliances with other persons from other systems, and are acknowledged and valued in their own school for their collaborative work. This particular skill is quite important. The teacher or student who fulfills a boundary spanning role can then understand the ways in which the two systems work separately and together, and can make this knowledge available to the participants in their own system. Boundary spanning functions are particularly valuable at a time of crisis when systems need to create and use resources.

Adaptation refers to the processes that the participants in a social system generate to respond to the demands of their system, particularly those requirements imposed by external environments. These adaptations may develop as a result of reciprocity, networking, or boundary spanning. The processes of adaptation are expected to vary from social system to social system and from individual to individual.

It is implicit in the concept of adaptation that the process facilitates the development of competencies in individuals and resources of the social system. Adaptation refers to the multiple ways in which individuals, in responding to external demands, preserve their own unique qualities while also developing new qualities. Adaptation does not refer to passive adjustment or acquiescence; *adaptation refers to an active effort to influence the social structure and the processes of a system while responding to the demands activated by the external environmental system.*

For example, adaptation refers to the ways in which teachers, students, and all of the participants respond to the demands placed upon their system by external events. In the case of the elementary school, the steps that the faculty adopt to respond to a financial emergency or to a change in the ethnicity of the school population indicates how the school as a system alters its methods of teaching or administration to better utilize its resources or create new ones.

The concept of adaptation takes its meaning from the elaboration of the other seven concepts, and refers to the sum of the processes the system and participants carry out to change their structures in response to changing environmental conditions. A changing environmental condition makes it possible for the participants to enlarge their own options for development and change. The elementary school as an adaptive system can continue to sustain its own processes of self-definition while responding to unexpected demands from outside systems.

Summary

Each of these four structures and each of these four processes are proposed as ecological concepts for viewing social systems. When these eight concepts are considered, the efficacy of preventive interventions is expected to be enhanced. A preventive intervention is considered ecologically effective when that intervention stimulates efficient use of social structures, such as personal and social system resources, social settings, and permeable system boundaries. An effective preventive intervention stimulates efficient use of social processes, such as reciprocity, networking, boundary spanning, and adaptation.

These eight concepts are presented as generic ideas to enhance the local support and implementation of a preventive intervention, no matter what the specific topic of interest may be (e.g., teenage pregnancy, substance abuse, child abuse, school dropout rate, etc.). The structures and processes outlined above are heuristic ideas that make it possible for a community-based preventive intervention to anchor the proposed intervention.

The process of planning a preventive program involves a process of (1) creating personal and social system resources, and (2) arranging social settings that can serve as viable structures for the support of the prevention program. Social systems that include permeable boundaries can enable participants to activate processes that facilitate interdependence between the participants of the system and other systems. The ecological perspective also proposes that the processes of reciprocity, networking, and boundary spanning can contribute to the continued adaptation of the system.

When a community psychologist works with a social system, such as an elementary school, the focus is often on the assessment of individual children who are not responding to schooling. The difficulties of the individual child are often the primary concern. The preceding discussion has illustrated an alternative emphasis. The social system of the *entire* school, including relationships with other systems, becomes the major concern. The social system is construed as a contributor to the relative health of the participants and their relationships to each other and the system.

The preceding comments present the vocabulary of an ecological system. The following comments relate the ecological system to six operational concepts. These six concepts will be discussed in terms of how they facilitate the implementation of an ecological point of view.

When viewing the structure of a system, Katz and Kahn (1978) affirmed the potency of *values*, *norms*, and *roles* as central to define the way of life of the system. These three concepts will be discussed as they facilitate an understanding of the ecology of systems. When viewing the concepts of system processes, the concepts of *entry*, *socialization*, and *development* are also generic. These three processes will be discussed in terms of how they illuminate the evolution of systems.

VALUES NORMS, AND ROLES: MAINTAINING AND CHANGING STRUCTURES AND PROCESSES

Norms, roles, and values are often presented in the literature primarily as tools for describing systems, not for designing preventive interventions. When mentioned in the context of designing an intervention, discussion often focuses on an isolated concept or technique for changing roles or changing values, rather than examining how changing norms, roles, and values can affect change in the structure and processes of a system. This section illustrates the ways in which an assessment of values, norms, and roles can facilitate an understanding of the structures of social systems.

Katz and Kahn (1978) define values as the generalized ideological justifications for behavior, and norms as the general expectation of participants in a system or subsystem. Roles are defined as the specific forms of behavior associated with given positions. All three of these concepts have implications for the functioning of a social system and the individuals within the system. The design and implementation of community interventions can be enhanced by examining these three components and their interrelationships with the eight concepts presented above.

Values

In considering a system's values, the community psychologist can note the pervasiveness of specific values, the extent to which certain values have led to established patterns of social interaction, and the extent to which values block changes in goals and/or criticisms of practices. For example, in the literature, much attention has been paid to hiring and the extent to which people are selected by a system because of their congruence with its values (Cable & Judge, 1997; Kristof, 1996). The expression of values can influence how personal and social system resources are communicated and how social settings can become potential resources for the system. One way in which individuals within a social system can identify others as personal resources is through value congruency, i.e., those who hold the same or compatible beliefs about the goals of an organization may serve as personal resources for each other. Participants in systems vary in their awareness of commonly held values, and in the methods and processes by which discrepancies in values are addressed or managed. By looking at the value implications for both the system and the individual members, the community psychologist can approach the design of interventions from multiple levels.

Rappaport, Seidman, Toro, McFadden, Reischl, Roberts, Salem, Stein, and Zimmerman (1985) noted that the shared values of mental health practitioners led to an advocacy of deinstitutionalization for the mentally ill. Those same values regarding care of the chronically mentally ill have now led to a criticism of deinstitutionalization practices because of inadequate community care. The values that led to changes in the use of mental health system resources were not integrated with the networking and boundary spanning necessary to create social settings within the community for the mentally ill. However, values can also inhibit changes in structure and process. The belief that mental health professionals are the preferred helpers for the chronically ill has led the mental healthcare system to neglect developing structures and processes for self-help and other non-professional help. By neglecting self-help approaches to the mentally ill, very personal and social system resources that are necessary for the maintenance of the mentally ill person outside the hospital are often missed. Professional treatment and self-help treatment are interdependent, yet seldom joined.

Norms

Related to the concept of values is the concept of norms. Norms translate the concept of values into behavioral regulants that then create social regulation for the individuals. Katz and Kahn (1978) outline several functions for norms: (1) integrating people into the system; (2) furnishing a frame of reference that can facilitate adjusting to, and working within, the system; and (3) providing the moral and social justification for system activities. Interventions can be enhanced if they establish norms to incorporate these functions into a system. Norms can constrain or facilitate the definition, elaboration, and creation of personal and social system resources.

Norms provide the participants with the orienting framework for what behaviors are appropriate and acceptable (Deutsch & Gerard, 1955). For example, are there restrictions about how an individual becomes a resource for others in the system and about whether being a resource is acknowledged by others in the system? Is the expression of reciprocity helped by the shared expectation that it is appropriate for participants to be resources to each other? It is often uncertain whether expressions of goodwill and spontaneous acts of helping are individual expressions of reciprocity, or whether these expressions are influenced primarily by social norms. Rappaport et al. (1985) examined the extent to which a norm for networking affected the personal resources available to members of a group.

In the case of the organization GROW, reciprocity *is* a norm. A goal of GROW is that members become personal resources for one another outside of the organization. The organization presents itself as "a sharing and caring community." Thus, GROW creates norms for reciprocity via networking, and provides the opportunity for members to become resources to each other (Zimmerman et al., 1991). Researchers in this setting attended the organization's meetings, as well as other social functions, to fully understand GROW as a system and how the value of sharing and caring had an impact on the behavior of members.

Examining the extent to which behavior that has been labeled a norm by system members can facilitate an understanding of a system and its processes (Cialdini & Trost, 1998). For example, a norm regarding the use of resources may be followed by all system members. Although individuals in a social system may appear as if they are subscribing to a social norm, the behavioral consensus may not be the result of consensus in the belief, but may instead be due to convention, partial integration of some members into the system, or unequal power distribution within the system (Katz & Golomb, 1974). The GROW researchers (Stein, personal communication; Luke, Rappaport, & Seidman, 1991) focused on how GROW's norm for participation at meetings—the group method—was actually governing the behavior of the self-help groups. In evaluating norms, a community psychologist should consider whether the norm emphasizes generating proactive social influence or conformity, two contrasting bases for benefiting one's social status.

Norms can lead directly to the development of social structures within an organization. For example, the norm of reciprocity in turn can lead members to create different social settings. Social norms in one setting of the system can influence the activities in another setting. Biddle (1986) noted that although it is often assumed that the sharing of beliefs about norms results in better system integration, little research has been conducted to show under what conditions differences in beliefs about norms are functional (i.e., promote system development. Norms can emphasize the ongoing interdependence between structures and processes in social systems. For example, the presence of a social process for reciprocity can help establish a social norm for giving help. Individuals then have a predictable standard to guide their own behavior and to integrate that behavior within the social system. Qualities of personal relationships (e.g., personal resources) can, in turn, affect the workings of the system beyond the interactions of any pair of individuals. Reciprocal processes between individuals can generate other structures, such as informal feedback mechanisms, that help establish norms or values for giving help within the system. From an ecological perspective, it is useful to examine exactly how the availability of personal and social system resources can affect the awareness of social norms for such salient processes as reciprocity and networking.

Roles

The roles of the various individuals within the system should also be examined. The behavior of an individual is, in part, determined by others who have certain role expectations by which the individual's performance is evaluated. Role messages sent to community members differ in specificity and intensity. Parents, for example, may receive different messages from different sources regarding what their role should be in the local school setting, i.e., community leaders advocating parent involvement in decisions affecting their children, teachers suggesting that parents defer matters to the discretion of teachers, and a school board sending a weak or an insincere message to "get involved." Enacting the role of "parent" in the school system is thus affected by the messages sent by others in the system and how the parent perceives these messages. The ways in which these messages are sent, received, and acted upon can affect how parents adopt the roles of being personal resources or boundary spanners, or contribute to the socialization of other parents to the system.

A community psychologist working from an ecological perspective might ask about the roles of individuals and their interrelationships within a system. For example, to what extent is there agreement on role expectations? Biddle (1986) notes that role expectations can be norms or preferences or beliefs, each of which can be learned through different experiences. For example, the role expectations presented to GROW group members revolve around the norm of helping others and serving as a personal resource, and include expectations of sharing one's own experiences and coping strategies and guiding others (Stein, personal communication; Roberts et al., 1991). When planning an intervention, an examination of all three (norms, preferences, beliefs) of these modes of transmitting role expectations, and the ways in which they are transmitted in a particular system, can be helpful in learning more about how roles are influenced in that particular setting (King & King, 1990).

Glidewell (1987), in an experimental five-year community intervention program, illustrated how citizens, when trained, increased their effectiveness in focusing on school issues. What is compelling is that Glidewell illustrated the sequence of processes that the training initiated. These processes, in turn, helped to activate citizens themselves to become personal resources within the community. The training initiated a sequence that involved the following competencies: negotiating skills, which (one month later) influenced school board decisions which in turn were followed by changes in citizens' risk-taking, which in turn affected the self-esteem of the citizens and increased attendance at board meetings, which in turn affected their negotiating skills, which then began a new cycle. This training activated community resources and stimulated an engaged community for at least 24 months. In this case, the training affected the roles that citizens played in their community by activating a series of interdependent sequential processes that expanded their competencies to be personal resources to each other and social system resources in the community.

Further questions about roles include: What kinds/methods of role prescriptions in this specific social system evoke the most effective performance and the fewest undesirable side effects? How is reciprocity evidenced within an individual's role set? How does the taking of multiple roles by an individual, i.e., involvement in more than one subsystem, affect the enactment of each role? What are the boundary-spanning roles in a social system, how did they come about, and how does their enactment affect the resources of the system? Where does role conflict exist within the system and how does it affect both system and individual functioning?

The concerns expressed above about role functioning and role expectations can help illuminate the importance of the structures and processes in a social system. Social settings will remain undeveloped sources of support and integration for system participants preoccupied with role expectations that are in conflict or ambiguous. When participants devote their finite energies to clarifying role expectations and creating a workable structure that fulfills their own needs, system boundaries also remain closed to the opportunities that may develop as a result of boundary spanning. Kahn (1990) discusses how role characteristics can affect personal engagement and disengagement at work (or within the system) by influencing an individual's role conflict, ambiguity can be reduced or eliminated. However, participants in social systems can be expected to have more energy available to make use of, or help increase, the resourcefulness of the system by developing personal and system resources within the various social-setting and boundary-spanning opportunities. Reducing role ambiguity also allows participants to create social norms so that new participants can continue that resourcefulness.

How the participants in the system create norms for the elaboration of roles defines how many equally valid ways there are for interpreting, expressing, and acknowledging roles. Norms can facilitate or constrain the expression of resourceful behavior by an individual, groups of individuals, or the system as a whole.

Pfeffer (1981, 1982, 1985) noted that interventions that focus on a systemwide level, rather than on the individual level, implicitly incorporate the notion of roles and attempt to work with them. For example, a program to prevent teenage pregnancy, aimed at an individual level, would focus on changing the attitudes and behaviors of individual teens. An ecological perspective would look at the key persons with whom teenagers interact (peers, teachers, parents, employers), as possible resources to involve in the intervention. An examination of these key resources and their interrelationships pinpoint how personal resources can be created as "help" for the specific teenager. In addition, the examination of these role relationships can illuminate the ways in which social system resources and social settings can nurture and support the socialization of the individual teenager into various potential adaptive roles. In this case, those who are part of the specific teenager's role relationships can become personal resources who may help the teenager gain access to social system resources. An ecological perspective can direct the attention of community psychologists to include those social settings in which persons in the role set create social norms for reciprocity and networking that give that teenager a sense of support and integration.

STRUCTURES AND PROCESSES TO CREATE NEGATIVE ENTROPY

Besides considering the structure of the system in terms of the roles, norms, and values, the community psychologist can also examine how that structure is maintained and changed. Katz and Kahn (1978) note that all organizations move toward disorganization and death (entropy). In order to survive, organizations need to maintain negative entropy, that is, import more energy than is expended. This requires efficient utilization of personal and social system resources and social settings. In examining the structure of a system, the community psychologist must consider what social system processes exist to support negative entropy. For example, how does the system ensure continuing membership? How does the system obtain and ensure adequate resources? The maintenance of negative entropy depends upon the interdependence of the social structures and social processes. The operation of the various structures, such as personal and social system resources, contribute to the activation of various processes, such as networking and boundary spanning.

Due to an ongoing shortage of resources, one way GROW maintains negative entropy is through chronic "understaffing" of positions within the organization (Stein, 1988; Zimmerman et al., 1991; Luke et al., 1991). This concept of "understaffing" is derived from Barker's concept of "undermanning" (Barker, 1968; Schoggen, 1989). The concept is based upon empirical research that has found that if there are a relatively smaller number of people than roles to be performed, these fewer people will assume the needed roles. If there are more activities needed to be performed than persons to perform them, a social setting can emerge for those participants in the undermanned setting. The persons in the undermanned setting can develop skills and competencies, increasing their chances of being personal resources (Schoggen, 1989). Understaffing can provide a mechanism to express an organizational value—the competence of all members. Rather than simply filling positions, GROW advocates "understaffing" so that the organization can continue its commitment to its mission by attracting members' energy and excitement. By involving more of the individual members' energy, there is less opportunity for the individual to be located and restricted to the performance of one role, thereby reducing the loss of energy that can be channeled to the group.

A defining quality of a generative social system is the capacity for the system to reduce decaying processes of entropy. One criteria for evaluating the effectiveness of a preventive intervention is the extent to which an intervention can enhance the flexibility of roles, norms, and values, which in turn reduces entropy (Nicholson, 1984). Interventions for combating entropy can be conducted with a focus on roles, norms, or values. An example of combating entropy at the role level is given by Glidewell (1972) in his description of the helping triad in which input and output are balanced through the existence of separate persons performing roles.

Surplus energy or organizational slack is necessary for system growth. In addition to being useful in controlling the entropic process, organizational slack refers to the resources that the participants consciously have stored and saved to facilitate the adaptation and renewal of the system (Katz & Kahn, 1978). With organizational slack, a social system is able to move beyond combating entropy to generating system change (Katz & Khan, 1978). This is accomplished through the structures of the system by encouraging the utilization of roles, norms, and values to create surplus energy. Participants in systems can choose not only whether surplus energy will be utilized for growth or maintenance, but also how the growth will occur (e.g., adding members, training, adding coordination mechanisms). When structure and process are balanced, "slack" can be restored and protected.

A hallmark of an adaptive system is the capacity of the participants in its different subsystems to generate resources and create interdependence. Organizational slack can be used in an integrated system for the participants to establish values, norms, and roles for communication, interchange, involvement, and concerted activities among and between various subsystems. In this sense, it is expected that organizational slack can enhance the integration of the system (Schneider, 1990).

An excellent incorporation of the concept of entropy and systems thinking is provided in Wicker's (1987) discussion of behavior-setting theory. Settings are seen as self-regulating and their demise can be attributed to such factors as loss and non-replacement of resources; the faltering or breakdown of operating, maintenance, or adaptive circuits; failure to sense significant environmental changes; excessive stability; or unfavorable outside conditions. As Wicker points out, these sources are in many cases highly interdependent. Entropy usually occurs when there are either long-term deficiencies or when needed changes are not implemented in the setting. Wicker also provides examples of how the stability/flexibility of a setting needs to be maintained in order to insure survival. Social settings are often the sites or locations by which the processes of the system are activated. The concepts suggested by Wicker provide a framework for evaluating just how interventions can be designed to stimulate the operation of social settings, particularly the ways that settings can create opportunities, structures, and norms for the development of personal and social system resources.

The process for reducing entropy is one that involves a continuous to and fro from establishing stability to facilitating flexibility. Persons need to predict the behavior of others; they also need opportunities to change their social structures in order to increase the possibility of their needs being met and their aspirations being validated. How persons participate in creating values, norms, and roles to balance stability and flexibility defines the openness of the system. Community-based interventions can focus on creating stability in norms (e.g., instituting a regular decision-making process), roles (e.g., relegating certain functions to specific persons), and values (e.g., creating a sense of community and pride in a neighborhood group). An intervention can also create flexibility in norms (e.g., allowing exceptions to the norms), roles (e.g., having several skilled members of the organization skilled to be interchangeable in dealing with a particular type of problem), and values (e.g., increasing recognition of differences in cultural beliefs). *The process of designing a preventive intervention is a process of determining the balance between stable and flexible components of the system. Both are needed, but often at different points in the system's evolution.*

ESSENTIAL SYSTEM PROCESSES: ENTRY, SOCIALIZATION, DEVELOPMENT

Three processes essential to the long-term functioning of systems will be examined: (1) entry, (2) socialization, and (3) development. These three processes are ongoing activities of a system and can serve as focal points for preventive interventions. They provide a convenient rubric to elaborate the development of personal resources and social settings, and are considered generic processes that can affect how reciprocity, networking, boundary spanning, and adaptation are expressed. The processes of entry, socialization, and development have been discussed in the literature of various disciplines without being brought together (Brim & Wheeler, 1966; Clausen, 1968). This present discussion is an effort to integrate these generic concepts with the purpose of designing preventive interventions.

Entry

Entry refers to the processes by which an individual from one system enters a new system. In the family therapy literature, this process is called joining (Umbarger, 1983). The entry process provides consultants with diagnostic information about the system, the consultee, and the consultant's response to the system. The entry process affects how the consultant will work within the system (Smith & Corse, 1986). For example, if a consultant enters a system aloof and as an "expert," it may be difficult for the consultant to develop an in-depth understanding of the particular system if the system is wary of "experts." In addition to the importance of understanding the entry process for consultants or therapists to assess and help the system, an analysis of entry is also important in understanding how individuals within the system begin to become connected to each other via shared entry experiences (Glidewell, 1959; Mann, 1983; Smith & Corse, 1986; Keys, 1986).

Systems set up both formal and informal structures (Katz & Kahn, 1978) such as interviews, planned greetings and introductions, welcoming social occasions, rites of passage, and graduation, to facilitate entry. As long as these structures are congruent with both the host community and the needs of individuals in the community, the entry process for new participants can be accomplished. When there is a lack of congruence between individuals' needs and the larger community, innovative structures can be devised to facilitate entry. To be effective, these novel structures should draw on the existing environmental and personal resources in the community. Aronson, Stephan, Sikes, Blaney, and Snapp's (1978) jigsaw classroom is an example of a social structure devised to facilitate the entry of children of color into a white-dominated educational system. The children in these classrooms are encouraged to cooperate with each other in order to reach a common goal. This idea of cooperative or collaborative learning has been further examined by David and Roger Johnson in a wide variety of classroom situations, from elementary school to college (Johnson & Johnson, 1989; Johnson, Johnson, & Holubec, 1991; Johnson, Johnson, & Smith, 1991). They suggest that such a structure not only can facilitate learning, but allows the students to develop social skills necessary for success in a wide variety of social systems. These methods draw on the social setting of the classroom, the personal resources of students, and the social system resources of learning tasks to facilitate an adaptive new structure for entry, as well as to facilitate the development of new personal and social system resources.

As another example, suppose that a consultant to an elementary school discovers that the children who are not responding to schooling tend to be relatively new immigrants to the community. The school as a system may reflect the larger community's norm of mistrusting "outsiders." A closed boundary may exist between the new children and long-term residents. The "dysfunctional" children, who are dysfunctional in terms of responding to the norms of the "insiders," are then not able to "enter" the system of the school and as a result may perform poorly in an unwelcoming social setting. Using an ecological perspective, the community psychologist can assess the formal and informal structures and processes that exist to facilitate entry. In many schools it is likely that there are already existing social settings, such as playgrounds or cafeterias, that, with the help of identified personal and social system resources, can be adapted to reduce the boundary between the incoming minority children and the long-term residents. The kind of intervention suggested here for entry does not focus on the "presenting problem"—the dysfunctional child—but instead focuses upon how settings and resources can support and neutralize negative responses to newcomers. The community psychologist who views the school as a potentially open system can help members recognize their latent resources and create processes to mobilize these resources.

There are many unexplored issues related to entry. Miller and Jablin (1991) proposed a model of newcomer information-seeking that encourages those studying entry processes to consider both the what and the how of information-seeking as individuals join organizations. The following questions focus on how a systems approach can be applied to entry: (1) Do highly structured processes facilitate entry for some people but limit it for others? If so, could such an entry process be an inadvertent form of discrimination? (2) Do subsystems with little formalized entry procedures foster mistrust, anger, or premature structure-building if they are embedded within a larger system that has highly formalized entry procedures? (3) What kind of effective structures can be created to facilitate the entry process into the community for "displaced" groups in our society (e.g., deinstitutionalized mental patients, ex-convicts, immigrants)? (4) What kinds of entry structures are most adaptive at various phases in the evolution of systems? (5) Do different entry processes have a greater or lesser potential to generate personal and social system resources and to facilitate or impede such processes as reciprocity, networking, and boundary spanning?

Socialization

Accompanying the entry process is the process of socialization. It is defined as those processes by which people acquire the knowledge, skills, and dispositions that assist them in being contributing members of their society (Brim & Wheeler, 1966). The socialization process has been discussed in the developmental and organizational psychology literature. Katz and Kahn (1978) discuss socialization into organizations in terms of the acquisition of values, norms, and roles. In developmental psychology, socialization in childhood and early life is characterized by the acquisition of fundamental values and competencies, while socialization in adulthood involves the acquisition of various behaviors related to specific role contexts (Brim & Wheeler, 1966). Families, schools, and peers are the primary socialization mechanisms for children acquiring values, but for adults, socialization into various role contexts can often be quite haphazard. We are socialized by orientation programs, trial and error, identification with a group doing a similar task, and by informal communication and informal group affiliations.

Each social system is assumed to have unique ways of generating its socialization processes. These exist to ease the individual into the system by gradually diffusing the boundary between her or him and the larger system, and then recreating a new permeable boundary that includes the particular individual.

Such a change in system boundaries can then facilitate the individual's adaptation to the system and the system's adaptation to the individual. Schein (1990) noted that although the goal of socialization is to perpetuate the organization's culture, individuals respond differently to the same tactics, and thus both group and individual socialization methods should be considered. Further, Meyer, Irving, and Allen (1998) showed that people hold different work values, leading them to respond to the same experience during socialization in different ways. Ashford and Black (1996) found that individuals differed in the extent to which they would be proactive during socialization (e.g., seeking information rather than waiting to be provided with it).

New teachers in a school could be routinely and systematically introduced to each current teacher in an orientation that not only takes into account structure and process, but also considers the unique cultural norms and values there. In addition, new teachers can be shown where all the important social settings are for exchanging informal information with colleagues. Before the end of the new teacher's first day, each of the veteran teachers can make a point of stopping by to chat and fill the newcomer in on some of the "inside history" of the school. This seemingly innocuous and common-sense process can facilitate quick entry into the school and begin the teachers' socialization process within the course of a single day. New teachers become aware of the personal resources available to them and the social settings for drawing on those resources; they can begin to visualize their own contributions to their new environment.

An ecological framework is a conceptual resource for the community psychologist to assess the socialization process. Some signs that the socialization process is *not* being effectively accomplished are: (1) people leave the system within a short time; (2) people who have been in the system for a relatively long time do not network; (3) people experience a great deal of role ambiguity; (4) there is an absence of processes for orienting newcomers; and (5) there is an absence of links between organizational norms and roles and peoples' needs.

In a policy-reform organization described by Kelly, Ryan, Altman, and Stelzner (1987), there is little formal socialization for helping new members move into participative decision-making roles, a value that the organization particularly espouses. This lack of a socialization structure, along with the fact that this organization has a strong leader, leaves new members unsure of how to participate in the ongoing operation of the organization. Some people drop out of the organization because of the perceived lack of opportunities to contribute to a broader definition of the organization's direction. Because the organization still accomplishes a great deal of its forward-reaching goals, remaining members have not pushed for a change in the socialization process. Nonetheless, the organization seems at risk because it is losing valuable personal resources because of an inadequate socialization process.

Kelly et al. (1987) also described another policy-reform organization that does have a well-defined structure for socializing new participants. New members of the system read published literature about the organization and then meet with members of each of the organizational units. The explicit goal is to socialize new people by providing them with a historical perspective of the organization, thereby allowing new staff members to see their roles in perspective. Their relationship to the larger system becomes clearer and the boundaries between themselves and the larger system loosen. Such a socialization process helps new individuals to better understand how to use their personal resources by acquainting them with the social system resources and the social settings of the organization.

Research on socialization from an ecological perspective might address such questions as: (1) What kinds of socialization processes are adaptive for different persons and various kinds of systems? Do less formal (traditional) systems require more or less explicit socialization? (2) How do the developmental needs of members interact with the socialization needs of a complex system in order for members to emerge as personal resources? (3) How can the socialization process be structured to facilitate the interdependence of structures and processes within the organization? (4) How can socialization processes facilitate participants learning about networking and boundary spanning roles and, (5) What types of personal and social system resources can facilitate socialization?

Development

Development is defined in terms of the degree of organizational structure attained by a system. If a system increases in differentiation and hierarchic integration, the person-in-environment system is seen as a developing system (Kaplan, 1966). The concept of development presented here is derived from Wapner's (1987) review of an organismic–developmental systems perspective.

The most developmentally advanced system exists when the members of the system control their transactions with it. As a system increases in size and complexity, it is expected to have more trouble using the greater and more varied personal resources that are available to it. In this situation, fewer people tend to be invited to contribute their personal resources, and more people become isolated from access to social system resources (Glidewell, 1972). Wapner makes a distinction between systems that just become larger and more complex, and those that develop as supportive environments. When the developing system becomes more complex, it generates processes that provide social system resources for the development of personal resources.

The development process in social systems is often made difficult by the tendency of conventional, large, and complex systems to rely less on personal resources and more on formal roles to accomplish tasks. Nonetheless, many organizations have set up "open" structures that can facilitate the developmental process. Trist (1981) discusses several companies that have created industrial plants under a "new organizational paradigm" that enhances the developmental process. These plants are characterized by fewer levels, functions, and numbers of management personnel; less total workforce; payment for knowledge, not for what a person does at a particular time; individuals in progressively evolving work roles; supervisors who are either nonexistent or are facilitators, trainers, and planners; and information that is shared for the purpose of problem-solving. This kind of organizational structure is committed to developing personal resources, and therefore allows for greater commitment and innovation within the system (Vondracek, Lerner, & Schulenberg, 1986). Kanter (1983) describes a similar type of organizational structure in her discussion of companies that promote innovation.

An important diagnostic question for the community psychologist is how a social system appreciates the process of development. The commitment that a system expresses for the development of personal resources can affect both the stability and the long-term viability of the system. One way to assess a system's value for the development of personal resources is to see how the participants talk about it. If they describe themselves as being a "part of a family" or the environment as being "stimulating," the system may be encouraging the development of personal resources. This is the way employees describe Hallmark Cards, which is rated as one of the "100 Best Companies to Work for in America" (Levering, Moskowitz, & Katz, 1984). If on the other hand, system members see themselves as expendable and the system as cold and impersonal, the system is not expected to be fully developing its personal resources. If the consultant believes that the system is not adequately developing its personal resources, he or she might look for ways to restructure the system under the kind of organizational paradigm that Trist (1981) and Kanter (1983) describe.

While there is certainly a risk that systems may not be developing their personal resources, a complementary risk is for systems to rely solely on personal resources without providing adequate social system resources. Without the availability of social system resources, individuals experience "burnout" leaving the system without the personal resources that it previously developed. Cherniss (1980) describes aspects of the work setting that lead to quick burnout for new public-service professionals. These include little formal orientation for new members; a heavy workload; little intellectual stimulation, challenge, and variety; extensive client contact; little professional autonomy; little clarity or consistency of institutional goals; poor leadership and supervision; and high professional isolation. For example, Brown and O'Brien (1998) suggested that those consulting with shelter workers should recognize the need to teach coping strategies and develop support networks because of the high levels of burnout.

Some additional research questions about the process of development are: (1) How do some systems evolve to appreciate the development of personal resources? What kinds of systemwide interventions are useful to counteract lack of such appreciation? (2) How can systems effectively balance individual developmental needs with the developmental needs of the system? (3) How can non-traditional community organizations ensure that adequate social system resources are created to counteract the large drain on personal resources? (4) How can the development process be so designed so that social settings can be places or occasions to validate the concept of development as a shared value? (5) How can the structures and processes of the organization be enhanced so that the development process is adaptive?

THE RELATIONSHIP BETWEEN STRUCTURE AND PROCESS

Before concluding, we will offer some further comments about the relationship between structure and process. In the beginning of the chapter we mentioned that the ecological perspective affirms that the design of interventions focuses upon the interdependence of structures and process. As the preceding comments have illustrated, the various structures and processes are inextricably related. The question is whether the participant who is living in the system every day has a point of view that encourages reflection about how personal resources influence reciprocity, and how social settings impact upon such processes as boundary spanning. The ecological point of view helps to constantly focus on the organic connections between how social systems regulate and how the participants adapt to those regulations and codes for behavior. The relationship between structure and process is a pivotal axiom for the expression of an ecological point of view.

As anthropologists have noted (Vincent, 1986), the conceptual distinctions between system, structure, and process are often difficult to make in practice. Social structures and processes develop because of the activities that are necessary to manage a system. In order for the system to "work," there must be a balance between its structure and processes. If the structures that are set up to facilitate processes become too rigid, entropy ensues and the system becomes less adaptive to the environment and for the individuals within it.

Trist and Bamforth's (1951) classic study of coal mining illustrates the way that structures organized to maximize production can create debilitating conflicts between subsystems. By relying exclusively on creating *structures* for production without attending to the concomitant *processes* of production, the coal-mining industry became too segmented and, in effect, lowered its productivity. In addition, the conflicts between the rigidly bounded subsystems limited the human effectiveness of the industry.

There are numerous examples in the corporate world of systems that struggle under the constraints of too much structure, thereby reducing the chances for individual resources to contribute to the system, inhibiting the very processes for which the structures were originally developed (Kanter, 1983). Partly in response to the rigid structures that are experienced in many organizations, some community psychologists have questioned the validity of structures, particularly those that are hierarchical. Also, many community organizers and community-development professionals place a great value on reflecting and understanding egalitarian-horizontal decision-making processes. There is a danger, however, in not creating some clear structures to facilitate the processes for a system. For example, Freeman (1972) described the "tyranny of structurelessness" in self-directed women's groups that began as consciousness-raising groups, but then turned their energies to specific social change or service interests. These groups adopted the position that formal group structures perpetuated inequalities among members. This "structurelessness" was adaptive when the groups' purpose was the process of facilitating personal insight. However, when the groups' purpose became the accomplishment of an external task, the participants found that they devoted a tremendous amount of time and energy to their own internal processes, informal leaders were often resented and undercut, and they were less effective in accomplishing their goals. Social psychological research also provides an example of this phenomenon. In their now-classic study, Kelley and Thibaut (1969) demonstrated that leaderless groups tend to reproduce the status structure of the larger culture (in the United States, a hierarchical one) from which the participants are drawn. Thus, by not creating some *new* structures for carrying out the valued functions of a system, there is a danger that the very structure that is not desired is unwittingly recreated. In this situation, the participants have less control over the change process because they are operating "as if" a hierarchical structure does not exist when, in fact, a hierarchical structure is operating.

The evolution of alternative community organizations provides examples of systems that fail because of a lack of attention to structure in favor of process. Gruber and Trickett (1987) and Trickett (1991) described the failure of a policy council at an alternative public school. This particular alternative school failed primarily because inequalities in access to information existed and the ideology of egalitarianism in meetings perpetuated, rather than ameliorated, those inequalities. Thus, because individuals had differential access to social system resources, the system lost personal resources.

Moore, Soltman, Manar, Steinberg, and Fogel (1983) identified specific characteristics of ineffective child-advocacy efforts in the schools. At the top of their list is inadequate attention to group-management activities essential to building and maintaining an effective advocacy organization. Thus, just as there is a danger for systems to become entropic when their structures are too rigid to adapt their own processes to a changing environment, there is an equal danger for systems to disintegrate if process becomes the exclusive focus of the system members.

The balance and interplay between structure and process presents some difficult problems. Balancing the two in "real" systems is still rare. Community psychologists should be aware of their own biases toward structure *or* process. Individual preferences will doubtless affect the way one approaches, assesses, and intervenes in systems.

The ecological thinking that is suggested to affect workable, balanced systems is not easy, particularly since there is little research that conceptualizes systems without an orientation toward either a hierarchical or participatory mode. This search for balance raises more research questions: (1) As systems evolve over time, how can they balance their investment in structure with a responsiveness to process? (2) How can systems with undeveloped structures adapt to external demands? (3) Is there a tendency to create too much structure when a system is in crisis? (4) How can a system adapt to crises with minimal loss of personal resources? (5) What sort of social settings are there in communities and organizations that can create a good balance between structure and process? (6) How can an appropriate type of structure be determined to facilitate a particular process within a system?

CONCLUSIONS

This chapter presented ecological concepts for viewing social systems in the design of a preventive intervention. Emphasis was given to both the structures and the processes of social systems. The purpose is to suggest that, by including the social system as a critical resource in the work of community psychologists, the design and evaluation of preventive interventions and community services can be enriched. The meaning of the concepts of structure and process in social systems for the field of community psychology were elaborated by the presentation of eight concepts. These concepts guided the discussion and understanding of how systems impact individuals, and even more importantly, how systems can be helped to respond to the needs of the members of the system.

The field of community psychology offers a novel and compelling opportunity to conduct research and create services so that persons in social systems can create their own resources and settings to enhance their quality of life. An ecological perspective is directed to that purpose, and includes an explicit value framework to help clarify how a system can be a resource and not be stultifying.

The following quotation, by the late Joan Kelly, is an apt expression of the authors' point of view in preparing this chapter. This quotation is a compelling challenge for future work. The authors hope that the point of view presented here is one resource for meeting this challenge.

> Our social institutions allow us to express and share so little of our real human needs that we are forced to lock them up inside ourselves. We all bear witness to the results: the explosions and implosions of these pent-up feelings are the stuff of the private tragedies and public violence and the disorder of our everyday life. Let us acknowledge, then ... that the personal is political; that the test of a social system is its ability to translate the personal into the public and at the same time to make community a real part of one's daily, personal life through meaningful participation in the decisions that shape us all (Kelly, J., 1984, p. xvii).

ACKNOWLEDGMENTS. The following persons read earlier drafts of the chapter and gave the authors constructive feedback: Daniel Cervone, Nancy Dassoff, Paul Dolinko, Peter Graves,

Christopher Keys, Mary Kripner, Lynn Ostergren, Janice Schreckengost, Cathy Stein, Alan Wicker, and Marc Alan Zimmerman. The following persons read later revisions of the chapter and also offered helpful suggestions and commentaries: Seán Azelton, Rebecca Burzette, Cecile Lardon, and Lynne O. Mock. The authors thank each of them and the volume editors, Julian Rappaport and Ed Seidman, for their interest and contributions to this work.

REFERENCES

Aldridge, H. E. (1979). *Organizations and environments*. Englewood Cliffs, NJ: Prentice-Hall.

Aldwin, C., & Stokols, A. (1988). The effects of environmental change on individuals and groups: Some neglected issues in stress research. *Journal of Environmental Psychology, 8*, 57–75.

Allen, K. E., Stelzner, S. P., & Wielkiewicz, R. M. (1998). The ecology of leadership: Adapting to the challenges of a changing world. *The Journal of Leadership Studies, 5* (2), 62–82.

Aronson, E., Stephan, C., Sikes, J., Blaney, N., & Snapp, M. (1978). *The jigsaw classroom*. Beverly Hills: Sage.

Ashford, S. J., & Black, J. S. (1996). Proactivity during organizational entry: The role of desire for control. *Journal of Applied Psychology, 81*, 199–214.

Ashkenas, R. (1997). The organization's new clothes. In F. Hesselbein, M. Goldsmith, & R. Beckhard (Eds.), *The organization of the future* (pp. 99–108). San Francisco: Jossey-Bass.

Barker, R. G. (1968). *Ecological psychology*. Stanford: Stanford University Press.

Barker, R. G. (1987). Prospecting in environmental psychology: Oskaloosa revested. In D. Stokols & I. Altman (Eds.), *Handbook of environmental psychology* (pp. 1413–1432). New York: Wiley.

Bateson, G. (1972). *Steps to an ecology of mind*. New York: Ballantine.

Bateson, G. (1979). *Mind and nature*. New York: Dutton.

Bertalanffy, L. von (1968). *General system theory*. New York: George Braziller.

Bertalanffy, L. von (1975). *Perspectives on general system theory*. New York: George Braziller.

Biddle, B. J. (1986). Recent developments in role theory. In *Annual review of sociology* (pp. 67–92). Palo Alto, CA: Annual Reviews.

Brim, J., O. G., & Wheeler, S. (1966). *Socialization after childhood: Two essays*. New York: Wiley.

Bronfenbrenner, U. (1979). *The ecology of human development*. Cambridge, MA: Harvard University Press.

Bronfenbrenner, U. (1986). Ecology of the family as a context of human development. *American Psychologist, 32*, 513–531.

Brown, C., & O'Brien, K. M. (1998). Understanding stress and burnout in shelter workers. *Professional Psychology: Research and Practice, 29*, 383–385.

Buckley, W. (Ed.). (1968). *Modern systems research for the behavioral scientist*. Chicago: Aldine.

Cable, D. M., & Judge, T. A. (1997). Interviewers' perceptions of person-organization fit and organizational selection decisions. *Journal of Applied Psychology, 82*, 546–561.

Capra, F. (1996). *The web of life: A new scientific understanding of living systems*. New York: Anchor.

Chaleff, I. (1995). *The courageous follower: Standing up to and for our leaders*. San Francisco: Berrett-Koehler.

Cherniss, C. (1980). *Professional burnout in human service organizations*. New York: Praeger.

Cialdini, R., & Trost, M. (1998). Social influence: Social norms, conformity, and compliance. In D. Gilbert, S. Fiske, & G. Lindzey (Eds.), *The Handbook of Social Psychology* (pp. 151–192). New York: McGraw-Hill.

Clausen, J. A. (Ed.). (1968). *Socialization and society*. Boston: Little, Brown & Company.

Davis, G. F., Kahn, R. L., & Zald, M. N. (1990). Contracts, treaties, and joint ventures. In R. L. Kahn & M. M. Zald (Eds.), *Organizations and nation-states: New perspectives on conflict and cooperation* (pp. 19–54). San Francisco: Jossey-Bass.

Deutsch, M., & Gerard, H. B. (1955). A study of normative and informational social influences upon individual judgment. *Journal of Abnormal and Social Psychology, 51*, 629–636.

Drentea, P. (1998). Consequences of women's formal and informal job search methods for employment in female-dominated jobs. *Gender and Society, 12*, 321–338.

Freeman, J. (1972). The tyranny of structurelessness. In A. Koedt, E. Levine, & A. Rapone (Eds.), *Radical feminism*. New York: Quadrangle.

Galbraith, J. R. (1997). The reconfigurable organization. In F. Hesselbein, M. Goldsmith, & R. Beckhard (Eds.), *The organization of the future* (pp. 87–98). San Francisco: Jossey-Bass.

Glidewell, J. C. (1959). The entry problem in consultation. *The Journal of Social Issues, 15*(2), 51–59.

Glidewell, J. C. (1972). A social psychology of mental health. In C. Eisdorfer, & S. E. Golann (Eds.), *Handbook of community mental health.* New York: Appleton-Century-Crofts.

Glidewell, J. C. (1987). Induced change and stability in psychological and social systems. *American Journal of Community Psychology, 15,* 741–772.

Gottlieb, B. H. (Ed.). (1981). *Social networks and social support, (Vol. 4), Sage studies in community mental health.* Beverly Hills: Sage.

Granovetter, M. (1973). The strength of weak ties. *American Journal of Sociology, 78,* 1360–1380.

Gruber, J., & Trickett, E. J. (1987). Can we empower others? The paradox of empowerment in the governing of an alternative public school. *American Journal of Community Psychology, 15,* 353–371.

Gump, P. (1987). School and classroom environments. In D. Stokols & I. Altman (Eds.), *Handbook of environmental psychology* (pp. 691–732). New York: Wiley.

Johnson, D. W., & Johnson, R. T. (1989). *Cooperation and competition.* Edina, MN: Interaction Book Company.

Johnson, D. W., Johnson, R. T., & Holubec, E. J. (1991). *Cooperation in the classroom: Revised.* Edina, MN: Interaction Book Company.

Johnson, D. W., Johnson, R. T., & Smith, R. A. (1991). *Active learning: Cooperation in the college classroom: Revised.* Edina, MN: Interaction Book Company.

Juras, J. L., Mackin, J. R., Curtis, S. E., & Foster-Fishman, P. G. (1997). Key concepts of community psychology: Implications for consulting in educational and human service settings. *Journal of Educational and Psychological Consultation, 8,* 111–133.

Kahn, R. L. (1968). Implications of organizational research for community mental health. In J. W. Carter, Jr. (Ed.), *Research contributions from psychology to community mental health* (pp. 60–74). New York: Behavioral Publications.

Kahn, R. L. (1989). Nations as organizations: Organizational theory and international relations. *Journal of Social Issues, 45*(2), 181–194.

Kahn, W. A. (1990). Psychological conditions of personal engagement and disengagement at work. *Academy of Management Journal, 33,* 692–724.

Kanter, R. M. (1983). *The change masters: Innovation for productivity in the American corporation.* New York: Simon & Schuster.

Kanter, R. M. (1996). World class leaders: The power of partnering. In F. Hesselbein, M. Goldsmith, & R. Beckhard (Eds.), *The leader of the future* (pp. 39–98). San Francisco: Jossey-Bass.

Kaplan, B. (1966). The comparative developmental approach and its application to symbolization and language in psychopathology. In S. Arieti (Ed.), *American handbook of psychiatry, Vol. 3.* New York: Basic Books.

Katz, D., & Golomb, N. (1974). Integration, effectiveness and adaptation in social systems: A comparative analysis of kibbutzim communities. Part 1. *Administration and Society, 6,* 283–316. Part II, 1975, *6,* 389–422.

Katz, D., & Kahn, R. L. (1978). *The social psychology of organizations* (2nd ed.). New York: Wiley.

Kelly, H. H., & Thibaut, J. W. (1969). Group problem solving. In G. Lindzey (Ed.), *The handbook of social psychology, Vol. 4.* Reading, MA: Addison-Wesley.

Kelly, J. (1984). *Women, history, and theory.* Chicago: University of Chicago Press.

Kelly, J. G. (1966). Ecological constraints on mental health services. *American Psychologist, 21,* 535–539.

Kelly, J. G. (1968). Toward an ecological conception of preventive interventions. In J. W. Carter, Jr. (Ed.), *Research contributions from psychology to community mental health* (pp. 75–99). New York: Behavioral Publications.

Kelly, J. G. (Ed.). (1979a). *Adolescent boys in high school.* Hillsdale, NJ: Lawrence Erlbaum.

Kelly, J. G. (1979b). 'Tain't what you do, it's the way that you do it. *American Journal of Community Psychology, 7,* 244–261.

Kelly, J. G. (1994). Beyond prevention techniques: Generating social settings for a public's health. In D. Satin (Ed.), *Insights and innovations in community mental health* (pp. 125–146). New York: Guilford.

Kelly, J. G., & Hess, R. E. (Eds.). (1987). *The ecology of prevention: Illustrating mental health consultation.* New York: Haworth.

Kelly, J. G., Ryan, A. M., Altman, B. E., & Stelzner, S. P. (1987). *Preserving the efficacy of policy reform organizations: Reflections from two case studies.* Paper presented at the First Biennial Conference on Community Research and Action, Columbia, SC.

Kelly, J. G., Dassoff, N., Levin, I., Schreckengost, J., Stelzner, S., Altman, E. (1988). *A guide to conducting prevention research in the community: First steps.* New York: Haworth.

Keys, C. B. (1986). Organization development: An approach to mental health consultation. In F. V. Mannino, E. J. Trickett, M. F. Shore, M. G. Kidder, G. Levin (Eds.), *Handbook of mental health consultation* (pp. 81–112). Washington, D.C.: U.S. Government Printing Office.

King, A., & King, W. (1990). Role conflict and role ambiguity: A critical assessment of construct validity. *Psychological Bulletin, 107*(1), 48–64.

Kingry-Westergaard, C., & Kelly, J. G. (1990). A contextualist epistemology for ecological research. In P. Tolan, C. Keys, F. Chertok, & L. Jason (Eds.), *Researching community psychology: Issues of theory and methods* (pp. 24–31). Washington, D.C.: American Psychological Association.

Klein, D. C. (1968). *Community dynamics and mental health.* New York: Wiley.

Kristof, A. L. (1996). Person-organization fit: An integrative review of its conceptualizations, measurement, and implications. *Personal Psychology, 49,* 1–49.

Levering, R., Moskowitz, M., & Katz, M. (1984). *The 100 best companies to work for in America.* Reading, MA: Addison-Wesley.

Levin, G. *Handbook of Mental Health Consultation: Washington, D.C.* U.S. Government Printing Office, No. ADM 86-1446, 81-112.

Luke, D. A., Rappaport, J., & Seidman, E. (1991). Setting phenotypes in a mutual help organization: Expanding behavior setting theory. *American Journal of Community Psychology, 19,* 147–167.

Maguire, L. (1983). *Understanding social networks.* Beverly Hills: Sage.

Mann, P. A. (1983). Transition points in consultation: Entry, transfer, and termination. In S. Cooper, W. F. Hodges (Eds.), *The mental health consultation field.* New York: Human Sciences.

Mannino, F. V., Trickett, E. J., Shore, M., Shore, M. F., Kidder, M. G., & Levin, G. (Eds.). (1986). *Handbook of mental health consultation.* U.S. Department of Health and Human Services, Government Printing, Washington, D.C.

McKelvey, B. (1982). *Organizational systematics.* Berkeley: University of California Press.

Meyer, J. P., Irving, P. G., & Allen, N. J. (1998). Examination of the combined effects of work values and early work experiences on organizational commitment. *Journal of Organizational Behavior, 19,* 29–52.

Miller, J. G. (1978). *Living Systems.* New York: McGraw-Hill.

Miller, V. D., & Jablin, F. M. (1991). Information seeking during organizational entry: Influences, tactics, and a model of the process. *Academy of Management Review, 16*(1), 92–120.

Mitchell, R. E., & Trickett, E. J. (1992). An ecological metaphor for research and intervention in community psychology. In M. S. Gibbs, J. R. Lachenmeyer, & J. Sigal (Eds.), *Community psychology and mental health* (2nd Ed.) (pp. 13–28). NY: Gardner.

Moore, D. R., Soltman, S. W., Manar, U., Steinberg, L. S., & Fogel, D. S. (1983). *Standing up for children: Effective child advocacy in the schools.* (Available from Designs for Change, 200 S. State St., Suite 1900, Chicago, IL 60604).

Morrison, A. M., White, R. P., & Van Velsor, E. (1987). *Breaking the glass ceiling: Can women reach the top of America's largest corporations?* Reading, MA: Addison-Wesley.

Muñoz, R. F., Snowden, L. R., & Kelly, J. G. (1979). *Social and psychological research in community settings.* San Francisco: Jossey-Bass.

Naparstek, A. J., Biegel, D. E., & Spiro, H. R. (1982). *Neighborhood networks for humane mental health care.* New York: Plenum.

Newman, P. R. (1979). Persons and settings: A comparative analysis of the quality and range of social interaction in two high schools. In James G. Kelly (Ed.), *Adolescent boys in high school: A psychological study of coping and adaptation* (pp. 187–217). Hillsdale, NJ: Lawrence Erlbaum.

Nicholson, N. (1984). A theory of work role transitions. *Administrative Science Quarterly, 29,* 172–191.

Paris, B. E. (1998). The development of a medical student interest group in geriatrics. *Educational Gerontology, 24,* 199–205.

Pfeffer, J. (1981). *Power in organizations.* Boston: Pitman.

Pfeffer, J. (1982). *Organizations and organization theory.* Boston: Pitman.

Pfeffer, J. (1985). Organizations and organizational theory. In G. Lindzey & E. Aronson (Eds.), *Handbook of social psychology* (3rd ed.). New York: Random House.

Pilisuk, M., & Parks, S. H. (1986). *The healing web: Social networks and human survival.* Hanover, MA: University Press of New England.

Rappaport, J., Seidman, E., Toro, P. A., McFadden, L. S., Reischl, T. M., Roberts, L. J., Salen, D. A., Stein, C. H., & Zimmerman, M. A. (1985). Collaborative research with a mutual help organization. *Social Policy,* 12–24.

Rappaport, R. A. (1990). Ecosystems, populations and people. In E. F. Moran (Ed.), *The ecosystem approach in anthropology: From concept to practice* (pp. 41–72). Ann Arbor: The University of Michigan Press.

Raush, H. L. (1977). Paradox, level, and junctures in person–situation systems. In D. Magnuson & N. S. Endler (Eds.), *Personality at the crosswards: Current issues in interactional psychology* (pp. 287–305). New York: Wiley.

Raush, H. L. (1979). Epistemology, metaphysics, and person situation methodology. In L. R. Kahle (Ed.), *New directions for methodology: Person-situation interactions* (pp. 93–106). San Francisco: Jossey-Bass.

Raush, H. L., Barry, W. A., Hertel, R. K., & Swain, M. A. (1974). *Communication, conflict and marriage.* San Francisco: Jossey-Bass.

Roberts, L. J., Luke, D. A., Rappaport, J., Seidman, E., Toro, P. A., & Reischl, T. M. (1991). Charting uncharted terrain: A behavioral observation system for mutual help groups. *American Journal of Community Psychology, 119,* 715–737.

Sameroff, A. J. (1980). Developmental systems: Contexts and evolution. In P. Mussen (Ed.), *Handbook of child psychology, Vol. 1* (pp. 237–294). New York: Wiley.

Sarason, S. B. (1972). *The creation of settings and the future of societies.* San Francisco: Jossey-Bass.

Schein, E. H. (1990). Organizational culture. *American Psychologist, 45*(2), 109–119.

Schneider, B. (Ed.). (1990). *Organizational climate and culture.* San Francisco: Jossey-Bass.

Schoggen, P. (1989). *Behavior settings.* Stanford: Stanford University Press.

Scott, W. R. (1981). *Organizations.* Englewood Cliffs, NJ: Prentice Hall.

Senge, P. M. (1997). Leading learning organizations: The bold, the powerful, and the invisible. In F. Hesselbein, M. Goldsmith, & R. Beckhard (Eds.), *The organization of the future* (pp. 41–58). San Francisco: Jossey-Bass.

Smith, K. K., & Corse, S. J. (1986). The process of consultation: Critical issues. In F. V. Mannino, E. J. Trickett, M. F. Shore, M. G. Kidder, & G. Levin (Eds.), *Handbook of mental health consultation* (DHHS Publication No. ADM 86-1446). Washington, D.C.: U.S. Government Printing Office.

Stevenson, J., Florin, P., & Mitchell, R. (1998). *Predicting intermediate outcomes for prevention coalitions: A developmental perspective.* Paper presented at the American Psychological Association Annual Convention, San Francisco, CA.

Stokols, D. (1987). Conceptual strategies of environmental psychology. In D. Stokols and I. Altman (Eds.), *Handbook of environmental psychology, Vol. 1* (pp. 41–70). New York: Wiley.

Stokols, D. (1988). Transformational processes in people–environmental relations. In J. E. McGrath (Ed.), *The social psychology of time: New perspectives* (pp. 233–254). Newbury Park, CA: Sage.

Thomas, K. G., Gatz, M., & Luczak, S. E. (1997). A tale of two school districts: Lessons to be learned about the impact of relationship building and ecology on consultation. *Journal of Educational and Psychological Consultation, 8,* 297–320.

Tjosvold, D. (1997). Networking by professionals to manage change: Dentists' cooperation and competition to develop their business. *Journal of Organizational Behavior, 18,* 745–752.

Trickett, E. J. (1984). Toward a distinctive community psychology: An ecological metaphor for the conduct of community research and the nature of training. *American Journal of Community Psychology, 12,* 261–279.

Trickett, E. J. (1987). Community interventions and health psychology. An ecologically oriented perspective. In G. Stone (Ed.), *Health psychology: A discipline and a profession* (pp. 151–163). Chicago: University of Chicago Press.

Trickett, E. J. (1991). *Living an idea: Empowerment and the evolution of an alternative high school.* Brookline, MA: Brookline Books.

Trickett, E. J. (1996). A future for community psychology: The contexts of diversity of contexts. *American Journal of Community Psychology, 24*(2), 203–234.

Trist, E. L. (1981). The sociotechnical perspective: The evolution of sociotechnical systems as a conceptual framework and as an action research program. In A. H. Van de Ven & W. F. Joyce (Eds.), *Perspectives on organization design and behavior.* New York: Wiley.

Trist, E. L., & Bamforth, K. W. (1951). Some social and psychological consequences of the long-wall method of coal-getting. *Human Relations, 4,* 3–38.

Ulrich, D. (1997). Organizing around capabilities. In F. Hesselbein, M. Goldsmith, & R. Beckhard (Eds.), *Organizing around capabilities* (pp. 189–196). San Francisco: Jossey-Bass.

Umbarger, C. C. (1983). *Structural family therapy.* Orlando, FL: Grune & Stratton.

Vaux, A. (1988). *Social support: Theory, research, and intervention.* New York: Praeger.

Vincent, J. (1986). System and process, 1974–1985. *Annual Review of Anthropology, 15,* 99–119.

Vondracek, F. W., Lerner, R. M., & Schulenberg, J. E. (1986). *Career development: A life-span developmental approach.* Hillsdale, NJ: Erlbaum.

Wapner, S. (1987). A holistic, developmental, systems-oriented environmental psychology: Some beginnings. In D. Stokols & I. Altman (Eds.), *Handbook of environmental psychology, Vol. 2.* New York: Wiley.

Weinstein, C. S. (1991). The classroom as a social context for learning. *Annual Review of Psychology, 42,* 493–525.

Wellman, B., Carrington, P. J., & Hall, A. (1988). Networks as personal communities. In Wellman & Berkowitz (Eds.), *Social structures: A network approach* (pp. 130–184). New York: University of Cambridge Press.

Wicker, A. W. (1987). Behavior settings reconsidered: Temporal stages, resources, internal, dynamics, context. In D. Stokols & I. Altman (Eds.), *Handbook of environmental psychology* (pp. 613–654). New York: Wiley.

Zimmerman, M. A., Reischl, T. M., Seidman, E., Rappaport, J., Toro, P. A., & Salem, D. A. (1991). Expansion strategies of a mutual help organization. *American Journal of Community Psychology, 19,* 251–278.

PART II

PEOPLE IN CONTEXT

Empirically Grounded Constructs

Part I presented many of the key theoretical orienting assumptions and conceptual issues of concern to community psychologists. Its aim was to orient the reader to the community psychology story and to broadly map that part of the psychological universe with which community psychology discourse is concerned. Part II moves us from the large-scale theoretical and conceptual maps of Part I to some of the more focused area maps also used by many community psychologists. This section provides background empirical information that orients the community psychologist to key issues in public health and epidemiology, mental health and well-being, stress and social support, and neighborhood and organizational development.

The chapters in this section are particularly concerned with what is known about connections between individual psychological well-being and important social contexts. The contexts invoked here range from the private experience of stress to public engagement with neighborhood, work, and life. Each of these contexts is of concern to many other subfields within the psychological sciences, but here they are approached from the perspectives of community psychology—looking *both* to and beyond the individual, and through a lens that takes for granted the desire to prevent problems before they occur, to work as collaborators with the people of concern, and to seek a more equitable distribution of social and psychological resources. The chapters here should all be read with these aims in mind. The authors each refer to quite specific empirical literature, some presented in detail, some summarized, and some being the inferential basis for raising a set of new questions and research directions considered to be important for further development of the larger community psychology agenda.

The maps of Part II are designed to help the community psychologist locate a set of particular problem areas and associated empirical work that links the concerns of individual people to social and organizational contexts. While the particular contexts and empirical foundations are necessarily selective, they are historically among the most basic concerns of the field. Work reported here touches on the transitions from childhood to adult life, and points to problem areas where considerable empirical research has already been conducted. Indeed, the problem for the mapmaker is less one of locating empirical research and more one of focusing us on particular empirical foundations that point to those directions likely to be fruitful for future research and intervention with respect to the field's agenda for preventively oriented, empowering relationships between the research, service, and local communities.

The section opens with Zautra and Bachrach's introduction of key concepts from public health and psychiatric epidemiology as they apply to issues of both dysfunction and well-being. In their view, in order to evaluate and design better community interventions, information is needed about both well-being and distress, a combination that is often overlooked in traditional research with the identified mentally ill. All people, even the most distressed, experience positive aspects of life, while even the most well-functioning community residents also experience problems in living. These authors call attention to maps that detail both sides of this complicated reality. They point to both commonly used assessment procedures and designs for the conduct of epidemiological research. They draw on two research traditions: the application of public health methods to the study of mental disorders (detection of psychopathology), and social-indicator research designed to index the quality of life in particular geographical areas. Psychiatric epidemiology, complicated by the problem of defining disease, is supplemented here by considerations of wellness. With their emphasis on subjective well-being and wellness (see also Cowen in Part I) the community psychologist's concern with proactive, as well as reparative, functions is emphasized.

Sandler, Gensheimer, and Braver link developments in our understanding of stress with the community psychologist's concerns about intervention. At the individual level of analysis they draw on the work of a cognitively oriented basic psychology that emphasizes the appraisal of life experiences. However, they also make clear (in ways that are central to a community psychology viewpoint) that prevention of environmental stressors includes political action, and here the link between individual skills and the ability to cope with, change, and control life circumstances becomes apparent.

The stress research literature is reviewed with respect to three identifiable themes, each of which has implications for programs of action: stress as a study of transactional processes, measurement of the parameters of life experiences that are stressful, and locating sources of protection and resilience. These authors suggest interventions at multiple levels of analysis, including with individuals, settings, and systems. Interventions may range from enhancing the availability of environmental resources, to the teaching of skills, to the development of strategies for crisis intervention. Interestingly, Sandler and his colleagues seem to propose exactly the type of targeted intervention that Felner questions in Chapter 2, and it may be useful to look for points of both tension and agreement in these two different versions of prevention.

For many psychologists the word "stress" immediately conjures up images of "social support" (as a resource for stress reduction). Ignored for many years as the helping professions became increasingly preoccupied with individual (and especially individualistic) therapeutic approaches that deemphasized reliance on social ties, community psychologists were among the most active in reviving the notion that social support may be an important factor in mediating, moderating, or otherwise influencing the quality of one's life experiences. Social support might be understood as a genuine resource enhancing the material, psychological, and emotional well-being of individuals; and also perhaps as a linkpin set of processes that connect individuals (for better or worse) with collectivities such as family, friends, organizations, and communities. Barrera provides a broad review of the empirical literature in this important domain. He also makes it clear that conflicted support and negative consequences are a part of the picture.

For those interested in social policy (see Phillips, Chapter 17), some of this work may have implications beyond the interpersonal. Ways to think about how to interpret psychological data so that we can better connect social policy to individual experience are sorely needed, since most policymakers know very little about the impact of a social policy on individual lives, and most psychologists ignore the implications of their work for public policy. This is properly an important domain for the community psychologist. For example, following Barrera's analysis of the negative consequences of support, one might ask if there are important differences between institutionalized forms of support that convey negative messages of stigmatized status (subsidies based on economic need as defined by "poverty" or "disability"), as opposed to those that are associated with more universal entitlements defined by mutuality (such as Medicare or Social Security for those who have worked, or GI-Bill-type educational entitlements for those who have served their country). Some economists and sociologists have argued this point from logic and archival data (Wilson, 1987; Remnick, 1996), but little psychological information is available with respect to how such programs are actually perceived by the public and interpreted and experienced by the recipients themselves. This is but one example of issues addressed in the empirical literature of psychological and interpersonal processes that may be profitably applied to broader social issues, a variety of which are addressed throughout this volume.

Wandersman and Florin shift our attention from general considerations of social support to a specific social context—the neighborhood. They emphasize the personal benefits of citizen participation in the life of one's most local geographical community. They review what is known about the impact of participation with respect to personal, interpersonal, physical, and social outcomes. This chapter points us to a large empirical literature on the correlates of citizen participation with respect to individual, group, and organizational characteristics. It can also serve as a starting point for many of the issues of collaboration that are of more general interest to community psychologists. Wandersman and Florin suggest that much of what can be learned from empirical research on local neighborhood participation is applicable to issues of participation in other contexts. Some of these same issues, for example, are addressed through a different empirical literature reviewed by Klein, Ralls, and Douglas (in the context of work settings) in their Chapter.

Klein and her colleagues draw connections between empowerment theory and organizational theory (see also Shinn and Perkins, Part IV). Issues of worker participation and both satisfaction and effectiveness (productivity) are addressed. Empirical studies based on models of organizational power lead these authors to focus on increasing worker expertise. Similarities and differences between this viewpoint and the conceptions of empowerment suggested by both Zimmerman and van Uchelen in Part I point to the importance of understanding empowerment in terms of contextualized goals and values, and of asking exactly how it is to be defined in particular contexts by particular researchers.

This section provides a sample of the field's empirical foundations. The sort of empirical maps suitable for a handbook in a field as broad as community psychology can, at best, locate certain main roads to be followed and anticipate the variety of paths to be encountered. Those who pursue the main roads highlighted here will undoubtedly encounter both alternative pathways and uncharted courses as they set out on their own journey in conjunction with community residents and research participants.

REFERENCES

Remnick, D. (1996). Dr. Wilson's neighborhood. *The New Yorker*, April 29 & May 6, pp. 96–107.

Wilson, W. J. (1987). *The truly disadvantaged* (pp. 3–19, 109–164). Chicago: University of Chicago Press.

CHAPTER 8

Psychological Dysfunction and Well-Being

Public Health and Social Indicator Approaches

ALEX J. ZAUTRA AND KENNETH M. BACHRACH

The study of health and well-being of communities has its roots in two relatively recent research traditions: psychiatric epidemiology and social indicator research. Psychiatric epidemiology applies public health methods to the study of mental disorder, while social indicator research attempts to determine the quality of life in our neighborhoods, our cities, and in the county as a whole. The two approaches complement one another to provide measures and developing methodologies that show great promise in understanding mental health problems and in charting the prospects for psychological well-being within communities.

The epidemiological methods that characterize public health approaches have undergone profound development in recent years (Kelsey, Whittemore, & Evans, 1996). In its most elementary form, the method relies on counts of "cases" of discasc, and provides detailed analysis of the distribution of both mental health and substance abuse problems among groups and neighborhood areas through careful sampling of the community under study. The increasing sophistication in methods and the development of multifactor etiological models has led researchers to address questions of cause of disordered behavior through the identification of the optimal set of predisposing risk factors and "triggers," in rather than searching for a single underlying causal agent. There is also mounting evidence that the course, as well as onset, of severe cases of mental illness are influenced by the presence of social and physical environmental constraints. Some of these developments in identification of psychosocial risk factors associated with psychiatric conditions, most notably, the study of stressful life events and the potential salubrious effects of social networks, are discussed in Barrera and Sandler's chapters (this volume). This chapter will focus on recent gains in methods of identifying psychological problems, including new measures of "caseness" and their applicability to understanding a

---

ALEX J. ZAUTRA • Department of Psychology, Arizona State University, Tempe, Arizona 85287. KENNETH M. BACHRACH • Tarzana Treatment Center, Tarzana, California 91356.

Handbook of Community Psychology, edited by Julian Rappaport and Edward Seidman. Kluwer Academic / Plenum Publishers, New York, 2000.

community's mental health. We include a discussion of social indicator research because the focus on disease states that characterizes psychiatric inquiries into the community is unduly restrictive. Attainment of quality of life is an equally compelling goal for communities and individuals as the more delimited objective of the eradication of disease, and is no more elusive. Research evidence shows newer measures of subjective well-being are not full of caprice, as once was feared, although they certainly are influenced by contextual variables at least as much as measures of mental distress and disorder. We shall expand on these points.

The chapter is organized to first provide a brief review of the current state of our knowledge from psychiatric epidemiology, and in going so we note some of the major methodological problems that confront that research effort. We then turn to a discussion of a subset of social indicators referred to as measures of subjective well-being, and review the promise those measures hold for enriching our knowledge base within community psychology.

PSYCHIATRIC EPIDEMIOLOGY

Basic Concepts

Kleinbaum, Kupper, and Morgenstern (1982) have identified four major goals of epidemiology:

1. To describe the health status of populations.
2. To examine the etiology of disease by identifying causative factors.
3. To predict disease occurrence and its distribution in the population.
4. To control the distribution or spread of disease by preventing new cases and eradicating existing cases.

The concern for the welfare of populations, and the emphasis placed on preventive methods, has made this approach among the most widely adopted perspectives among researchers within community psychology.

The most common measures of health and illness relied on in epidemiology are estimates of *point prevalence*, the number of cases of disorder existing within the community at a given point in time, and *incidence*, the number of new cases over a designated time period. *Relative risk* for contracting a disease is another common indicator; relative risk is a comparison of the probabilities of becoming ill between groups that differ in some important characteristic. *Odds ratios*, in particular, have been used to communicate levels of risk within a readily understood conceptual framework; the odds of having a disease is the probability of contracting a disease over a specified time period divided by the probability of not contracting the disease. The relative odds of contracting lung cancer, for example, between smokers and non-smokers is about 10 to 1.

The application of these public health methods to the study of mental health problems is the focus of psychiatric epidemiology. Psychiatric disorders define a special set of disease entities within epidemiology; they pose complex problems in case identification and differentiation. Most mental health problems (with the possible exception of manic–depressive disorder and some forms of dementia) lack specific biochemical markers associated with disordered behavior. The distinction between "sick" and "well" is not always clear-cut in functional terms either. The establishment of a set of operational rules to guide the classification of mental disorders (Spitzer, Endicott, & Robins, 1978) has made psychiatric diagnosis among clinicians more reliable. Even in those circumstances, however, only manifestations of the disorder are in evidence—manifestations that may arise from a multitude of underlying conditions and may be treated by a number of different methods. Nevertheless, the operational definitions of caseness have greatly improved the reliability of judgments among studies of mental disorder among researchers who have adopted these common definitions.

Of great significance to public health is the heterogeneity in long-term prognosis among those who develop mental disorders. Harding, Zubin, and Strauss (1987) reviewed studies of chronicity in schizophrenia and found evidence of full recovery among 20–34% of those initially labeled chronically ill. Evidence of such variability in recovery has led to an increasing number of investigations into the course of the disorder. Special attention has been given to the prediction and prevention of relapse through studies of the patients' families (Falloon, 1988; Vaugh & Leff, 1976), as well as the care and treatment provided by mental health care providers. Early detection of disordered behavior of children has been associated with poor outcomes in some studies (Gersten, Langner, Eisenberg, & Simcha-Fagan, 1975), due perhaps to labeling of the person and the social stigma attached to that label (Horwitz, 1982; Scheff, 1974). Others (Gove, 1980) have argued that when effective treatments are available, early detection should result in beneficial results. It is estimated that one-third of the homeless suffer from some major mental disorder (Levine & Rog, 1990). The treatment of these people and their impact on the communities in which they live has become a major public health issue in recent years due to the growing numbers and visibility of these indigent and often disturbed people.

The counterpoint to these studies of the poor is a recent report from Vaillant and Schnurr (1988) who followed an initially healthy group of 188 college freshman for 45 years. He found that a quarter of them eventually warranted a DSM-III diagnosis during the follow-up years; nearly half evidenced significant psychiatric impairment at some point, but most recovered. Risk for severe psychological disturbance appears high even for the healthiest groups; this state is not irreversible provided the person has adequate resources with which to cope with his or her difficulties.

Epidemiological investigations in general, and especially those that pursue etiological evidence concerning mental disorders, cannot isolate a single cause of the disease. Instead, these studies rely on the careful examination of risk factors that may increase the odds of the person developing a disorder, but which by themselves are neither necessary nor sufficient causes of the disorder. Such factors are studied to see if they covary with the disease state, precede the occurrence of the disease in time, and survive critical tests of spuriousness through the examination of other potential explanatory mechanisms.

Research Designs

The most common study design in psychiatric epidemiology is a *cross-sectional field survey* of a representative sample of a community population. Such a design can accomplish much in the way of describing the population and providing clues to possible risk factors through an examination of the covariates of disordered states. *Cohort studies* examine groups of people over time who differ in one or more risk factors to determine if there are differences in incidence rates due to initial differences in the risk factors under study. This design is optimal for the testing of causal hypotheses, but is rarely accomplished in psychiatric epidemiology, as it is necessary to track very large cohorts in order to detect differences in incidence for disorders that have low base rates. A useful compromise is the *retrospective case-control design*, where the history of known cases are examined to identify features that distinguish them from similar controls. Three problems plague this design. First, it is very difficult to distinguish antecedent events from consequences, *post hoc*. Recall may be differentially affected by the presence of a disorder, for example. Second, often the researcher himself cannot avoid searching for significance in the data set, increasing the probability of chance findings. Third, it is impossible to match cases and controls perfectly, which allows for the possibility that other (unmeasured) differences between cases and controls are responsible for both the disorder and the identified antecedent risk factor. The success of this design depends, therefore, on the development and testing of a limited set of *a priori* hypotheses concerning etiology, in the veridicality of historical information gathered, and the adequacy of sampling methods for identifying and testing carefully matched controls.

Defining a Case

The most nagging issue in the psychiatric epidemiologic literature has been defining caseness. The issue of caseness centers around three questions: (1) What is the unique subset of affects, cognitions, and behaviors associated with a specific psychiatric disorder; (2) How much symptomatology needs to be reported or observed to warrant the classification of psychologically impaired?, and (3) How long should the symptoms persist in order to judge them to be associated with an underlying pathological state of the person and not due to a transitory reaction to a stressful life circumstance? When there is no agreement as to how these questions should be answered, the consequence is the prevalence rates of mental disorders range widely—from less than 1% to over 60% in studies conducted around the world (Dohrenwend & Dohrenwend, 1969; Schwab & Schwab, 1978). These large variations in rates raised questions regarding both the reliability of measurement and the validity of the criterion employed to define mental disorders.

The problem of reliability has been dealt with by using structured and standardized interview schedules to decrease error variance due to administration and interviewer differences. Also, multiple "expert" raters have been employed to enhance and check reliability. The issue of validity is much stickier because there is no single agreed upon "gold standard" for judging mental disorder. Most researchers have little trouble differentiating severely disturbed individuals from those who show no sighs of psychopathology. The problem occurs towards the middle of the mental health continuum, where there are no clear-cut distinctions between normal and abnormal behavior.

Most of the early studies, from the 1950s until the mid-1970s, had two common characteristics: (1) mental disorder was defined on a continuum, and (2) specific diagnoses were rarely made. In place of a differential diagnosis, level of impairment in functioning was assessed as a common denominator of illness severity. In recent years the zeitgeist has changed, resulting in a move away from global ratings of psychological distress/impairment to an attempt to identify prevalence rates of specific disorders. There has been a concerted effort to reestablish medicine within psychiatry including the use of specific psychiatric labels. The reasons for this are many, including political and economic pressures to demonstrate the scientific basis of psychiatry (Klerman, 1986). The publication of the 1980 *Diagnostic and Statistical Manual of Mental Disorders* (DSM) (American Psychiatric Association, 1980) provided more objective criteria for making diagnoses, which allowed for reliable classification of cases and non-cases by diagnosticians. This was a significant methodological advance for investigations of mental disorders as specific disease entities because it provided a standard set of criteria for research, permitting comparison of findings across studies. Whether the classification of disordered behavior into highly differentiated diagnostic entities is really more than convenient fiction is still a subject of much debate (for example, Mirowsky & Ross, 1989). We shall provide some examples of these difficulties as we review current efforts.

Measuring Psychological Distress: Instrument Development

The type of research instruments employed in psychiatric epidemiologic studies have varied depending on the needs of the investigators. In general, however, there has been a move away from the reliance on clinicians and human decision-making to define caseness and toward the use of trained administrators and computerized scoring. From the MidTown Manhattan study came the Langner 22-item screening inventory (Langner, 1962), one of the most widely used "first generation" measures of psychiatric condition. The measure provided scores on global impairment in functioning (for more recent advances in this approach see National Institute of Mental Health, 1985). Since that time a "second generation" of inventories have been developed that have numerous symptom dimensions, such as somatization, depression, and psychoticism. Another refinement is their inclusion of intensity measures, which allows the respondent to report his or her subjective level of symptomatic distress. The questions on these newer inventories tend to be more specific and allow for less interpretation on the part of the respondent. The SCL-90-R (revised) (Derogatis, 1977) represents one of these second-generation screening inventories. One of its most attractive features is that it was developed on psychiatric outpatients and focuses on measuring neurotic symptomatology. The nine symptom dimensions of the SCL-90-R are somatization, obsessive–compulsive, interpersonal sensitivity, depression, anxiety, hostility, phobic anxiety, paranoid ideation, and psychoticism. Each of the 90 items can be rated on a five-point scale ranging from "not at all" to "extremely."

Questions have been raised by researchers as to whether these screening inventories actually measure distinct forms of psychological upset. Dohrenwend and his colleagues (1980) have argued that most screening inventories assess *demoralization*, a non-specific form of distress (see Frank, 1973). Dohrenwend et al. (1980) contend that demoralization is the psychological equivalent to temperature in assessing one's physical condition. An elevated score tells you something is wrong, but not what it is.

THE EPIDEMIOLOGIC CATCHMENT AREA PROGRAM

Development of the Diagnostic Interview Schedule

This dissatisfaction with general impairment measures, and the desire to advance knowledge of rates of specific mental health problems using present psychiatric nomenclature led to the development of a new and comprehensive research instrument: The NIMH Diagnostic Interview Schedule (DIS). This set of measures was developed by Robins, Helzer, Croughan, and Ratcliff (1981) to collect data for a large multicommunity survey project entitled the Epidemiologic Catchment Area (ECA) program. The ECA program was an outgrowth of questions and recommendations made by the 1978 Report of the President's Commission on Mental Health (Regier, Myers, Kramer, Robins, Blazer, Hough, Eaton, & Locke, 1985). The primary objective of the ECA program was to obtain prevalence rates of specific mental disorders, rather than prevalence rates of global impairment (Eaton, Regier, Locke, & Tanke, 1981).

Four respected instruments developed during the 1970s were considered for incorporation into the DIS: The Present State Examination (PSE) (Wing, Cooper, & Sartorius, 1974), the Psychiatric Epidemiological Research Interview (PERI) (Dohrenwend et al., 1980), the Schedule for Affective Disorders and Schizophrenia (SADS) (Spitzer & Endicott, 1977), and the Renard Diagnostic Interview (RDI) (Helzer, Robins, & Crougham, 1978). The DIS needed to employ DSM-III criteria, make psychiatric diagnoses in the absence of key informants or medical records, and be reliably administered by trained lay interviewers in a reasonable length of time. Only the RDI met all of these criteria, so it was developed to meet the needs of the ECA program. The DIS was designed to make lifetime diagnoses using the Feighner criteria (Feighner, Robins, Guze, Woodruff, Winokur, & Muñoz, 1972), and make distinctions between current and past diagnoses. The Folstein-McHugh Mini Mental State Examination (Folstein, Folstein, & McHugh, 1975) was used to assess cognitive impairment.

The ECA Communities

The five sites selected for the ECA program included New Haven, Connecticut (Yale University); Baltimore, Maryland (Johns Hopkins University); St. Louis, Missouri (Washington University); five contiguous counties in the Piedmont area of North Carolina (Duke University); and Los Angeles, California (University of California at Los Angeles). Multiple sites were employed to assess special populations of interest (black, Hispanic, aged, rural, and urban) and to assess the replicability of findings across sites. At each site approximately 3000 community residents over age 18 were interviewed, along with 500 residents of institutions. Detailed information about the sampling and methodology has been described by Eaton and Kessler (1985).

ECA Estimates of Magnitude of Mental Health Problems

Roughly one in five persons in the previous six months or one in three persons during their lifetime experienced psychological problems significant enough to warrant a diagnosis of a DIS/DSM-III disorder or severe cognitive impairment. Rates were surprisingly consistent across sites, with the exception of a high rate of phobias in Baltimore. If phobias are excluded, 6-month and lifetime prevalence rates averaged 15% and 25%, respectively (Burnam, Hough, Karno, Escoban, & Telles, 1987; Karno et al., 1987).

These rates are quite similar to the well-known Stirling County and Midtown Manhattan studies conducted during the 1950s. The Midtown Manhattan study's estimated point prevalence impairment rate was 23%, while the Stirling County's lifetime impairment rate was 31.1% (28.7% mild, 2.3% moderate, and 0.1%, severe). In the Stirling County study, 57% of the sample were estimated to be psychiatric cases sometime during their life, but only 24% of the sample were judged to be both significantly impaired and psychiatric cases.

The leading lifetime diagnoses in the ECA sample were alcohol abuse or dependence (15%), phobias (12% with Baltimore site excluded), drug abuse or dependence (6.5%), major depressive episode (6%), dysthymia (3.5%), and antisocial personality (3%). The percentages in parentheses are gross estimates based on averages across ECA sites (Karno et al., 1987; Robins et al., 1984). The leading 6-month diagnoses were phobias (8% with Baltimore site excluded), alcohol abuse or dependence (5%), major depressive episode (3%), and drug abuse or dependence (2%). Dysthymia could not be estimated for 6-month prevalence rates since time of symptom onset was unknown.

Demographic Correlates of Lifetime Disorders

Gender

Men had substantially high rates for substance (particularly alcohol) abuse/dependence and antisocial personality, while women had higher rates for phobia and major depressive episode. Trends were found suggesting that women have higher rates than men for dysthymia and panic disorder. Few sex differences were found among the young—those in the 18 to 24 age group (Robins et al., 1984).

Age

People less than 45 years of age had rates of mental disorder two times higher than persons 45 years of age and older. Substance abuse/dependence and antisocial personality were found to be primarily young person's disorders, while cognitive impairment was most prevalent in those 65 years of age and older (Robins et al., 1984).

Ethnicity

Ethnic differences were only found at the Los Angeles site, where a large number of Mexican-Americans (n = 1243) were compared with non-Hispanic whites. Non-Hispanic whites had higher rates of drug abuse/dependence and major depressive episode than Mexican–Americans. Certain age and sex differences were found by ethnic group. Drug abuse/dependence was uncommon among Mexican–American women of any age and for men and women over 40 years of age of either ethnic group. Mexican–American males abused alcohol 5½ times more frequently than drugs, whereas non-Hispanic whites abused drugs and alcohol in nearly equal proportions. However, recent data suggest an increase in use of drugs among Mexican–American males. Substantial higher prevalence rates among native-born Mexican-Americans in comparison to immigrants have also been found, which suggests that exposure to American majority culture may lead to higher substance abuse (Burnam et al., 1987).

Education

College graduates had fewer psychiatric disorders than those with less education, but differences for specific disorders rarely were found across all sites. The only consistent finding across sites was for cognitive impairment, suggesting that the rate of decline in intellectual abilities leading to dementia is slower for those of greater educational attainment.

Urbanization

Overall rates of psychiatric disorder were found to be higher in inner-city areas (Robins et al., 1984). This finding is consistent with Faris and Dunham's (1939) early work based on hospital admission rates. Rates of substance use disorders, antisocial personality, and cognitive impairment were found also to be higher in urban, rather than rural, areas. Only panic disorder was more prevalent in rural/small town areas, according to Robins et al. (1984).

Utilization of Health and Mental Health Services

The practical utility of determining rates of mental disorder is in the estimation of service needs of the community. To what extent do those identified as ill actually seek services when such are available to them? As part of the ECA project, service-use rates were computed across different purposes of the visit and two types of provider groups: mental health specialty sector and general medical services.

On the average, 6–7% of the sample reported a mental health care visit to a provider during the 6 months preceding the DIS interview. Although more than twice as many persons with disorders saw a mental health service professional in the previous 6 months in comparison to those without disorders, 80% of persons with a recent DIS/DSM-III disorder did not see any provider for mental health reasons, while one-third of all mental health visits were for persons with no disorder (Shapiro, Skinner, Kessler, Von Korff, German, Tischler, Leaf, Benham, Cohler, & Regier, 1984). Clearly, diagnosis of mental disorder from the DIS interview is neither necessary nor sufficient cause for a person to seek mental health services.

Persons with a recent disorder utilized health care services more than persons with a past disorder or no lifetime history of a disorder. Nearly 70% of persons with a recent DIS/DSM-III disorder made either a health and/or mental health visit during the previous 6 months, averaging 4 to 5 visits per person. In contrast, utilization rates for the entire sample were roughly 10% lower, with visits averaging 2.5 to 2.8 per person across sites. Los Angeles had lower overall rates due to the consistent underutilization of services by Mexican-Americans with and without recent disorders (Hough, Landsverk, Karno, Burnam, Timbers, Escobar, & Regier, 1987).

Roughly one-third of persons with a recent disorder were untreated from any professional provider, nearly 60% utilized only the general medical care sector, while approximately 10% sought out the specialty mental health care sector. Women were more likely to seek help for mental health problems than men, but men who made a mental health visit were more likely to use the specialty sector. Mental health service use was particularly low for substance use disorders and cognitive impairment (Shapiro et al., 1984).

Methodological Limitations

The ECA program has provided the most comprehensive look at mental health problems and mental health service utilization in the United States of any study to date. Yet questions remain regarding both the validity and reliability of the findings. The interview relies heavily on self-reports; problems of recall, particularly for "lifetime" rates, are likely to bias results. For example, older adults had lower lifetime rates of most major mental disorders than younger samples, and it seems unlikely that differences in mortality rates among those with mental disorders can explain those findings fully. It seems plausible, however, that the elderly, being further in age from time when they were most likely to have experienced a major mental disorder (ages 18–36), remembered those occasions less readily. Underreporting of deviant affective symptoms and behaviors, such as heavy alcohol consumption, is also likely, and interviewer effects may be especially pronounced in this area (see Bradburn, 1983, for a review).

Anthony, Folstein, Romanoski, Von Korff, Nestadt, Chahal, Merchant, Brown, Shapiro, Kramer, and Gruenberg (1985) raised a number of questions as to how well the DIS compares with diagnoses reached by psychiatrists. They compared diagnoses made based on data collected with the DIS instrument with lay interviewers with those made by a psychiatrist who interviewed the same persons. Most of the interviews were performed within 90 days of the DIS interview. A total of 810 persons were interviewed using both methods: two-thirds had a DIS diagnosis and one-third were from a random sample of those with no DIS diagnosis. Significant differences in prevalence estimates were found in six of the eight disorders investigated; only manic–depressive episodes and schizophrenia had similar rates when comparing interview assessments. Compared with DIS-driven estimates, psychiatrists rated nearly twice as many participants as having alcohol-related disorders within the past month (6.9% compared with 3.9%), and one-half the number of major depressive episodes (1.1% in the past month compared with 2.3%). Level of agreement on individual cases was modest at best; less than half of those given diagnoses by the psychiatrists were given the same diagnosis by the DIS. Robins (1985) has pointed out that those with the most serious disorders were generally identified by both methods, and that low base rates for some disorders make high levels of agreement difficult to achieve.

There is still much debate on the utility of the DIS survey for use in identification of prevalence of specific mental disorders given findings such as those of Anthony et al. (1985). The rates of mental disorder overall appear to agree readily with past estimates, but the reliability of specific case assignments has yet to be persuasively demonstrated for the DIS interview. Much work needs to be done to identify the core disorders underlying the manifestations of clinical syndromes such as anxiety and depression. Boyd et al. (1984) found that having one DSM-III disorder increases the odds of having two or three coexisting disorders substantially. Such a finding suggests there might be much less differentiation in types of psychopathology at the core of many displays of symptomatology.

ANALYSIS OF COMMUNITY ECOLOGIES

A major limitation of the current approaches has been a concentration on individual attributes, both to define pathological states and to identify factors that place a person at greater risk for mental disorder. Missing in these accounts is an analysis of the distributions of disordered behavior at the level of community or neighborhood. Such approaches, often referred to as ecological or social-area analyses (Bell, 1966), provide a means of formally addressing the contribution of social and systems-level contexts on disordered behavior.

The different rates of phobic disorder across ECA sites are a "story foretold" of community differences that cannot be explained with reference to individual differences in subjects or assessment methods across sites. Over 23% of the Baltimore community was identified as having a phobic disorder at sometime in their lives; this rate was 2.5 times that of other areas. The dynamic interplay between individuals and the contexts within which they live, work, and seek psychiatric care may play an important role in determining these differences in rates of mental disorder.

Just as with studies of the individual, there are many potential sources of variability in rates of disorder in community life. The most straightforward approach to identifying ecological/systems variables at the community level is to rely on the development of neighborhood typologies based on sociodemographic characteristics aggregated across residents of the area, and rates of important social influences such as in and out migration, home ownership turnover, unemployment, and income variability (National Institute of Mental Health, 1975). Bloom (1975), for example, performed a cluster analysis of census tracts in Pueblo, Colorado, and found the census neighborhoods formed natural groupings. One such grouping, labeled the social disequilibrium cluster, was characterized by a high proportion of divorced, recent movers, and renter-occupied housing. This cluster had the highest rates of psychiatric admission.

The key characteristics that make social areas such as neighborhoods supportive of human adaptation are not likely to be contained solely in demographic profiles. Garbarino and Sherman (1980) compared survey results from two neighborhoods that had similar demographic profiles, yet differed in their rates of child maltreatment. The families in neighborhoods at higher risk for child abuse tended to see their neighborhoods as less supportive and reported more life stress than families from low-risk neighborhoods (see also Garbarino, Eckenrode, & Barry, 1997).

A key issue is how community characteristics interact with those of the person residing there to affect mental health outcomes. Robinson (1950) was among the first to point out that aggregate statistics can be highly misleading when used to interpret causes underlying individual behavior. For instance, the persons found exhibiting the disordered behavior in the Pueblo census tracts may not have had those characteristics that typify their neighborhood. Braucht (1979) was able to collect data on individual as well as neighborhood characteristics; he compared the sociodemographic characteristics of persons exhibiting suicidal behavior with the average background characteristics of the census tracts where they lived. He found that suicidal behavior rates were higher for those persons who did not fit the demographic profile of their neighborhoods.

How would incongruence affect disordered behavior? There are a number of possible mechanisms. Poor fit of the person's needs with environmental resources is thought to strain adjustment capacities, increasing vulnerability to disorder. The disorientation of psychiatrically impaired persons could increase the probability of their selecting unsuitable environments in which to live. Third, people different from their neighbors may stand out, and therefore may attract attention more readily. Minority races and ethnicities that are subject to prejudicial treatment may face additional hostilities from those in the majority within their neighborhoods.

The influence of neighborhood and community may also emerge as more than a linear function of its attributes. Spatial diffusion analyses (e.g., Haggett, Cliff, & Frey, 1971; Cliff, 1982) might detect evidence of behavioral contagion; maladaptive behavior patterns such as substance abuse may indeed spread quickly among those living adjacent physically and in similar life circumstances. Clearly, norms for social and disordered behavior can emerge from community groups in ways that are not fully understood at present. Research hypotheses regarding how to study these interactions between person and community to predict vulnerability and/or resistance to psychopathology within the community are still relatively unsophisticated. Such problems are likely to engage the interests of the community psychologists interested in public health problems in the years to come. This is a major limitation of the work of those attempting to account for the many manifestations of disordered behavior without examining the community contexts within which those behaviors are observed.

One Last Limitation of the Epidemiological Approach

A fundamental problem with epidemiological approaches is that they only study mental disorders and their variants. Because of this, their view of the person is limited to those measures associated with states of illness. They have no conceptual apparatus with which to characterize well-being and positive mental health, except as the converse of mental illness.

Yet it is a truism that mental health means more than the absence of mental disorder. Auden (1975) captured the essence of this limitation in "The Unknown Citizen," which he begins by describing what is known of one person's life in the following,

> He was found by the Bureau of Statistics to be
> One against whom there was no official complaint.

The last lines read:

> Was he free, was he happy? The question is absurd.
> Had anything been wrong, we should certainly have heard.

An accounting of well-being, personal happiness, and perceptions of quality of life are needed to more fully understand the person, his or her normal motivations, and aspirations for a better life. Such an approach has been the subject of intensive study and debate among social scientists. Within sociology, it is known as the study of indicators of quality of life. We turn now to a discussion of social indicator research.

SOCIAL INDICATOR RESEARCH

Basic Concepts

In order to understand the measurement of subjective well-being, it is useful to review the purposes of such assessments. Those purposes are very different from the public health concerns that prompted the development of indicators of mental disorder. Social indicators were developed to evaluate progress toward societal goals at the level of community, state, and nation. Bauer (1966) defined this approach as "The association and bringing together of those facts which are calculated to illustrate the conditions and prospects of society." Indeed, the prevalence of mental disorder in communities found through epidemiologic research would be an important social statistic with which to judge the quality of life in a given locale, but it would not be the only important statistic. Progress toward equitable distribution of goods and services, education, and the public's ratings of progress toward their own aspirations would also be considered to be important, perhaps more so, than the communities' control of abnormal or disordered behavior.

The origins of social indicators in the United States have been traced to provisions in the U.S. Constitution for a periodic population census. The interest among social scientists developed most rapidly in the late 1950s through the work of Bauer and his colleagues as a means of charting social progress by means other than economic indicators. Initial efforts relied solely on "objective" indicators—aggregate social statistics such as divorce rates or percent of population completing high school monitored over time as indicators of improvement or decline in a community's quality of life (see Gilmartin, Rossi, Lutomski, & Reed, 1979, for an annotated review).

Subjective indicators of well-being, such as measures of life satisfaction and perceived quality of life, were developed later to complement objective indicators. They were to provide a comprehensive assessment of the goodness, or quality of life, from the perspective of the citizen. The need for such measures was apparent from the outset. Campbell and Converse (1972) used the analogy of a ship steered toward a destination appraised "objectively" on its progress by estimates of speed and closeness to correct course. They asked rhetorically if one did not also need to know if the ship's destination was desirable to its passengers.

Unlike mental disorder, subjective well-being is more closely tied to ongoing life circumstances. The ebb and flow of life events, cognitions about those events, and vividness of memory for those events all play an important part in regulation of affective states. Stable dispositions to experience positive affects and retain high self-efficacy expectations also influence subjective well-being. Such effects of ongoing circumstances and personality differences are likely to be more pronounced for subjective well-being than estimates of mental disorder.

Developments in Measuring Subjective Well-Being

One of the earliest systematic attempts to measure subjective states was the nationwide studies of Cantril (1965), who explored citizen aspirations and level of fulfillment. He did so with "ladder" ratings; respondents were presented with an image of a ladder on a card, where the top of the ladder would be labeled a judgment such as "the best possible life," and the bottom, "the worst possible life." The respondent was asked to place himself or herself on the rung that represented the level he or she had reached. These ratings are self-anchored, unlike most of the scales currently in use; they do not depend on the assumption of communality in meaning of affect-laden terms (such as "very happy"). The average U.S. citizen places himself or herself slightly more than halfway up the ladder.

By and large, these methods have given way to Likert-type rating scales, having a range of five to seven response options that are assumed to represent a continuum of equally spaced intervals. These scales of life satisfaction have demonstrated superior psychometric properties; they show high internal consistency and moderate test-retest reliabilities. Two such scales are the Andrews and Withey (1976) Perceived Quality of Life Scale and the Campbell, Converse, and Rodgers (1976) Inventory of Life Satisfaction. Of the two, the Andrews and Withey (1976) measure has been subject to the most psychometric work. One of the single most useful items is the global measure of perceived life quality, "How do you feel about your life as a whole?" Respondents are given a seven-point scale with the options: delighted, pleased, mostly satisfied, mixed, mostly dissatisfied, unhappy, terrible. The average score for U.S. citizens based on national surveys falls between mostly satisfied and pleased.

These measures were written to cluster around life domains such as work, family life, health, income, leisure time, and neighborhood. Satisfaction within each domain is expected to affect (and be affected by) global ratings of quality of life, and also to measure specific concerns of the respondent. Those domains more central to the person, such as marriage, social life, and work contribute significantly more to overall well-being than those more peripheral aspects, such as ratings of satisfaction with local government. Nevertheless, measures of the less central aspects have been shown to be both reliable and stable indicators of specific domain satisfaction (Headey, Holmstrom, & Wearing, 1984). Some scales attempt to assess psychological domains like positive and negative affect (Bradburn, 1969) and other inferred states such as vitality (Neugarten, Havighurst, & Tobin, 1961).

Andrews and McKennell (1980) proposed that each measure of well-being may be decomposed into more basic cognitive and affective components. Reports of happiness, for example, are thought to assess mainly positive affects, reports of anxiety and sadness mostly negative affects, and reports of satisfaction derive from cognitions about affective states, as well as from the experience of both positive- and negative-feeling states. The cognitive algebra underlying these summary evaluations has not yet been examined.

A key finding in measurement of well-being is that positive states are not the inverse of negative states. Herzberg, Mausner, and Snyderman (1959), in investigations of working life, and Bradburn (1969), through national surveys of reports of happiness, were the first to present convincing data on this subject. Using very different methods, they showed that under some measurement conditions, positive and negative states define separate and independent affective domains. Research efforts over the past several years have led to the development of new and more psychometrically sound measures of positive and negative affect (Watson, Clark, & Tellegen, 1988).

There are two senses in which these states are evaluated as distinct: (1) the degree to which they are intercorrelated and (2) the degree with which they display distinct patterns of association with other variables. Both issues have important implications for evaluating the importance of including such measures in studies of mental health and well-being of community residents.

The research evidence reveals that the degree of (inverse) correlation between positive and negative states depends on a number of factors, including the length of the time interval (past day or past week; Diener, Horowitz, & Emmons, 1985), and the degree to which the measures ask for comparative judgments, such as "how much of the time" versus direct recall of experience. Reports of positive experiences are usually uncorrelated or positively correlated with number of negative events (Zautra & Reich, 1983). On the other hand, Veit and Ware (1983) report a correlation of −.72 between two dimensions of mental health, well-being and distress, when using a scale that asks for judgments of the amount of time the affect in question was experienced. Abbey and Andrews (1985) correlated depression and anxiety subscales from a measure of psychiatric distress with global ratings of well-being and found that well-being was correlated −.69 with depression and −.54 with anxiety. The level of correlation may also be age-dependent, with older samples showing less discrimination in reporting of affects (Zautra, Guarnaccia, & Reich, 1988). Current debates include claims that independence between affects is an erroneous consequence of correlated measurement error (Green, Goldman, & Salovey, 1993). Zautra, Potter, and Reich (1997) have presented a model that suggests that uncertainty underlining stressful events may promote a simpler affect structure, one in which positive and negative affects are more highly correlated, albeit inversely.

There is less ambiguity over the second question about positive and negative affects; they *do* appear to be associated with different life conditions. Zautra and Reich (1983) reviewed a number of studies to show that positive events tended to correlate only with increased well-being, whereas negative events primarily increased distress. Zautra, Guarnaccia, and Dohrenwend (1986) found their measure of small desirable events occurring in the past month was significantly associated with positive affect (r = .30) and was uncorrelated with negative affect. Small undesirable events occurring in the past month showed moderate correlations with negative affective states (r = .32). Bradburn (1969) demonstrated different demographic correlates of positive and negative affect. In his studies, negative affects were associated with divorced status and poverty, while positive affects tended to be associated with achievements such as advanced education, occupational status, and social participation. In a study of three samples of rheumatoid arthritis patients, Zautra et al. (1995) found that pain was associated with negative affect but not positive affect, while activity limitation was associated primarily with lower positive affect. Costa and McCrae (1980) investigated personality correlates of well-being and found that neuroticism tended to be associated with greater negative affect but not less positive affect; extraversion was associated only with positive affect. It is apparent from studies like these that the well-being of communities cannot be assessed with measures that identify differences in psychopathology exclusively. People differ in the degree of positive affects as well, something that can be missed in overconcern with the illness aspects of public health.

The Role of Cognition in Subjective Well-Being

A person's ratings of subjective well-being are affected greatly by the social and temporal comparisons they make. Dermer, Cohen, Jacobson, and Anderson (1979) had subjects review historical material that emphasized either positive or negative past events. Subjects who reviewed negative past events rated their present satisfaction significantly higher than those presented with past events that were positive. Michalos (1985) has proposed a "gap" model to explain such effects. He found that the perceived difference (or gap) between what one has and what others have, and what one had in the past compared with what one has present, can account for as much as 50% of the variance in subjective well-being ratings.

Self-efficacy expectations (Bandura, 1977) and the degree with which the person maintains a sense of personal mastery have been shown to play a substantial role in reports of subjective well-being as well as psychological upset (Abbey & Andrews, 1985). Some measures have been designed to assess this dimension directly, such as Pearlin and Schooler's (1978) personal mastery scale. Antonovsky (1979) has developed a measure of sense of coherence that taps the degree of purposeful engagement in work and community life. Kobasa (1982) has developed a tool to assess "hardiness" that is designed to assess perceptions of personal control, commitment to goals, and a willingness to interpret stressful events as challenges rather than threats. An assessment based on Jahoda's (1958) concepts of positive mental health has been offered by Ryff and Singer (1998); the inventory assesses the person's capacity for self-acceptance, positive relations with others, autonomy, environmental mastery, purpose in life, and personal growth. She has demonstrated that some of the scales chart new domains of well-being, unrelated to traditional measures of life satisfaction and positive affect. Although unproven as yet, these new measures represent exciting new ways of conceptualizing well-being that goes far beyond past efforts in providing means of identifying optimal functioning.

Demographic Differences in Well-Being

Among the most surprising initial findings in this research area was the relative lack of strong demographic correlates of well-being in nationwide surveys (Andrews & Withey, 1976). Perceptual measures were expected to conform to patterns of objective statistics such that people with less education and lower incomes would report consistently lower psychological well-being. While most studies find a relationship between income and education on the one hand, and well-being on the other, the size of the relationship is small, accounting generally for less than 5% of the variance (Campbell, Converse, & Rodgers, 1976, pp. 368).

Part of the explanation for such weak effects is that the use of a simple bivariate statistic is not sufficient to explain the complex affective and cognitive processes that are at work in judgments of well-being. Bradburn (1969) found that income was more strongly related to negative affect than positive affect, and was especially predictive of well-being at the lower end of the income continuum. Diener (1984) found that those who were very wealthy (net worth over 10 million dollars) were different from middle-class controls most on positive affective states. Thus the effects of income appear different at different levels; it also appears that there is a broad band in the income levels for whom money has no influence on happiness.

Marital status is perhaps the strongest demographic correlate of well-being, with divorce status most responsible for the effects observed (Haring-Hidore, Stock, Okun, & Witter, 1985; Zautra & Beier, 1978). There have been gender differences observed as well. Childrearing, in particular, lowers life satisfaction more for women than men, and marriage leads generally to greater rather than less well-being for men, but is more equivocal in its effects on women.

With the exception of the disabled elderly, age brings slightly greater well-being (Warr & Payne, 1982), but there are also fewer positive affective experiences according to Bradburn (1969). These losses are accompanied by less negative affect as well (Zautra, Kochanowicz, & Goodhart, 1984) and, it appears, a more subdued set of expectations for the future. It may be shifts in cognitions about life's events that are most responsible for the tendency of the older to be more satisfied—through a reduction in their personal requirements for happiness. However, attitudinal and cultural differences between cohorts at different ages might also explain differences between age groups (Kozma, DiFazio, & Stones, 1992). The consistent, yet small, effects on well-being due to social and demographic differences are due to other complexities as well. Unlike social status variables, such as education, where the measure is a cumulative index of status, like satisfactions and subjective well-being may likely be much more influenced by current events than the sum of past experiences. No one has yet attempted to identify the decay in influence of important events on perceptions of well-being and quality of life over time, but it is likely to be substantial given what has been uncovered to date. Schwartz and Clore (1986) investigated whether memories for past events would effect current levels of well-being. They instructed subjects to recall pleasant or unpleasant events; the degree to which the instructions requested the subject to construct a vivid image of the event greatly enhanced the effects of recall of past events on present state. More recent, as well as more crucial, events are most likely to produce vivid memory traces.

The Effects of Everyday Life Events on Subjective Well-Being

The manipulation of everyday experiences has also been shown to influence subjective estimates of well-being. Csikszentmihalyi (1975) tested whether the disruption of everyday desirable experiences would have adverse consequences. He asked a group of college students to "act in a normal way, doing all things you have to do, but do not do anything that is 'play' or 'non-instrumental.'" The experimental period lasted for 48 hours. After that time respondents reported increased physical symptoms including more tiredness, less relaxation, more headaches, and overall poorer physical health. Deprivation of very simple daily pleasures apparently had a significant detrimental affect on subjective appraisals of health status. Reich and Zautra (1983) induced college students to engage in more pleasurable activities than was usual during a two-week period. Analysis of pre versus post scores with a comparison group of controls revealed increases in perceived quality of life for those who engaged in more pleasurable events. In addition, those subjects reporting more stressful life events at the time of the experiment showed reduced psychological distress after engaging in pleasurable events.

Limitations of Subjective Assessments

The central issue among researchers in this field is whether to admit self-evaluations of affect *per se* as evidence of mental health. Jahoda (1958), in proposing criteria for positive mental health, steered away from reports of happiness because she thought such measures allowed for self-deception as well as the desire to provide socially desirable responses. Her search culminated with a list of attributes that were measurable as personality features.

Although no one is in a better position to judge subjective well-being than the person, social scientists remain understandably uneasy when the last word on the existence and level of the attribute is vested in a (likely fallible) respondent.

The issue is a thorny one for social scientists. Subjective estimates of well-being are internally consistent, fairly stable over time, and tend to change in patterns consistent with objective conditions, such as changes in life events. In addition, confirmatory factor analyses have revealed that the underlying structure of self-reports of life satisfaction and perceived quality of life are stable across groups, suggesting that components of well-being add up in similar ways even among those from vastly different backgrounds. The predictability of such states from observations of others are as good as that found in other measures of inferred states. Peer ratings of another person's happiness have been correlated with subject's ratings yielding modest, but consistently significant, correlations (Kammann, Smith, & McQueen, 1984). Apparently, observers rely on their own levels of well-being to anchor their ratings of others, leading to lower consensus between self and other.

Even with high agreement among raters, there is no assurance that what one person means by "very satisfied" will conform closely to the affective state that another person would reference with the same words. On the other hand, this basic assumption is supported by data from a number of cross-cultural studies of affect and emotion. There is mounting evidence of universal communalities in the interpretation of emotional displays (Ekman, 1982; Ekman & Davidson, 1994), and that peoples of vastly different cultural backgrounds have common structures of connotative language they use to communicate affects (Mehrabian, 1972; Osgood, 1965).

SUMMARY AND IMPLICATIONS

We have presented two conceptual frameworks with which to assess mental health problems in the community. One emphasizes the detection of psychopathology through the use of epidemiological methods; the other seeks to assess levels of subjective well-being through reliance on citizen reports of their own mental states. In our view any comprehensive assessment of mental health would be incomplete without attention to both realms of human experience. Such balanced appraisals yield different pictures of physical and mental health than those that would arise from only one perspective. Understanding of how a person evaluates his or her own life requires knowledge beyond the diagnosis of psychopathology or its absence. Without information on abnormal patterns of behavior, the investigator may be lulled into complacency, overlooking severe emotional and cognitive disturbance in the community that requires more intense observation and care than the typical quality of life intervention. Together, both sets of measures serve as useful criteria with which to evaluate the success of our efforts to improve quality and diminish distress within the community.

Well-being estimates are especially useful to identify psychosocial problems among those groups able to report on their own mental health and motivated to provide an accurate accounting. The study of normal variations in psychological distress and positive affective states is an important part of the psychology of communities, and would be all but ignored in an overmedicalization of mental health outcomes through the sole reliance on the identification of abnormal or just distressed states. Even those with the most severe mental disorders can be trusted to provide fairly reliable estimates of changes in their own quality of life. Programs designed to enhance the citizenship of the chronically mentally ill, for example, ought to observe an increase in the life satisfactions of their clients. Without improvements in well-being, one may well question whether any gains have been made from the intervention, beyond changes for the better in the minds of the interveners.

The detection of mental disorders has an important part to play in the identification of needs and development of psychological services. Communities differ in the extent and distribution of mental disorders, and estimates of need are greatly improved by such data. The application of increasingly sophisticated research designs is beginning to permit the testing of the etiological significance of psychosocial factors in the onset and course of psychiatric disorders. Such evidence is already leading to empirically grounded preventive and rehabilitative programs designed to stem the tide of psychiatric impairment within the community.

Models of risk for psychiatric illness and community need would benefit from incorporating positive resistance resources. Recent efforts to identify positive social supports that buffer a person from stressful life events reviewed in the chapter by Barrera in this volume show considerable promise. Recently, Dohrenwend (1987) reported significant differences between cases of major mental disorder and community controls on the number of recent positive social role experiences, after controlling for demographic and other social characteristics between groups. Those without mental disorder reported fewer positive events preceding their episode of illness. Such findings suggest that positive events may have substantial benefits, preventing setting off the trigger for those vulnerable to episodes of severe mental disorder.

The reaction of the person and his or her social network to psychiatric symptoms is of considerable importance in the long-term effects of acute emotional disturbance, and differences in well-being may play a decisive role in those reactions. In two studies that attempted to predict service utilization rates among neighborhoods served by community mental health centers, the differences in rates of service use by census tracts were predicted by survey estimates of the quality of life in those areas, independent of the community's demographic profiles and differences in survey estimates of psychiatric impairment (Zautra & Simons, 1978; Goodstein, Zautra, & Goodhart, 1982). Neighborhoods with greater subjective well-being relied less on clinical services. We interpret such findings as evidence of the benefits of a positive emotional climate within neighborhoods, reducing the need to resort to professional helping services.

Models of mental health and illness are likely to continue to evolve in coming decades as community psychologists and other social scientists work toward better definitions of disordered behavior and how to best define optimal functioning. In our view, attempts to do so will increasingly acknowledge the necessity of integrating positive states with evidence of psychopathology. Recent advances made in psychiatric epidemiology must reach an accommodation with the knowledge base found in studies of the normal problems of people attempting to pursue a satisfying life in their communities in order for us to see new breakthroughs in our conceptions of the public's mental health.

REFERENCES

Abbey, A., & Andrews, F. M. (1985). Modeling the psychological determinants of life quality. *Social Indicators Research, 16*, 1–34.

American Psychiatric Association, Committee on Nomenclature and Statistics. (1980). *Diagnostic and statistical manual of mental disorders* (3rd ed.). Washington, D.C.: American Psychiatric Association.

Andrews, F. M., & McKennell, A. C. (1980). Measures of self-reported well-being: their affective, cognitive and other components. *Social Indicators Research, 8*, 127–155.

Andrews, F. M., & Withey, S. B. (1976). *Social Indicators of well-being*. New York: Plenum.

Anthony, J. C., Folstein, M., Romanoski, A. J., Von Korff, M. R., Nestadt, G. R., Chahal, R., Merchant, A., Brown,

C. H., Shapiro, S., Kramer, M., & Gruenber, E. M. (1985). Comparison of the Lay Diagnostic Interview Schedule and a standardized psychiatric diagnosis. *Archives of General Psychiatry, 42*, 667–675.

Antonovsky, A. (1979). *Health, stress and coping: New perspectives on mental and physical well-being*. San Francisco: Jossey-Bass.

Auden, W. H. (1975). *Collected shorter poems: 1927–1957* (pp. 146–147). New York: Vintage.

Bandura, A. (1977). Self-efficacy: Toward a unifying theory of behavioral change. *Psychological Review, 84*, 191–215.

Bauer, R. A. (1966). Detection and anticipation of impact: The nature of the task. In R. A. Bauer (Ed.), *Social indicators* (pp. 1–67). Cambridge, MA: M.I.T. Press.

Bell, W. (1966). The utility of the Shevsky typology for the design of urban sub-area field studies. In G. Theodorson (Ed.), *Studies in human ecology*. Evanston, IL: Row, Peterson.

Bloom, B. (1975). *Changing patterns of psychiatric care*. New York: Human Sciences Press.

Boyd, J. H., Burke, J. D., Jr., Gruenberg, E., Holzer, C. E., Rae, D. S., George, L. K., Karno, M., Stoltzman, R., McEvoy, L., & Nestadt, G. (1984). Exclusion criteria of DSM-III: a study of co-occurrences of hierarchy-free syndromes. *Archives of General Psychiatry, 41*, 983–989.

Bradburn, N. M. (1969). *The structure of psychological well being*. Chicago: Aldine.

Bradburn, N. M. (1983). Response effects. In R. H. Rossi, J. D. Wright, & A. B. Anderson (Eds.), *Handbook of survey research* (pp. 289–328). New York: Academic.

Braucht, G. N. (1979). Interactional analysis of suicidal behavior. *Journal of Consulting and Clinical Psychology, 47*, 653–669.

Brickman, P., & Campbell, D. T. (1971). Hedonic relativism and planning the good society. In M. H. Appley (Ed.), *Adaptation level theory*. New York: Academic.

Burnam, M. A., Hough, R. L., Karno, M., Escoban, J. I., & Telles, C. A. (1987). Acculturation and lifetime prevalence of psychiatric disorders among Mexican–Americans living in Los Angeles. *Journal of Health and Social Behavior, 28*, 89–102.

Campbell, A., & Converse, P. (1972). Social change and human change. In A. Campbell & P. Converse (Eds.), *The human meaning of social change*. New York: Sage.

Campbell, A., Converse, P. E., & Rodgers, W. L. (1976). *The quality of American life*. New York: Sage.

Cantril, H. (1965). *The pattern of human concerns*. New Brunswick, NJ: Rutgers University Press.

Cliff, A. (1982). *Spatial diffusion. An historical geography of epidemics in an island community*. New York: Cambridge University Press.

Cohen, S., & Hoberman, H. M. (1982). Positive events and life events as buffers of life change stress. *Journal of Applied Social Psychology, 13*, 99–125.

Costa, P. T., Jr., & McCrae, R. R. (1980). Influences of extraversion and neuroticism on subjective well-being: happy and unhappy people. *Journal of Personality and Social Psychology, 38*, 668–678.

Crandall, R. (1976). Validation of self-report measures using ratings by others. *Sociological Methods and Research, 4*, 380–400.

Csikszentmihalyi, M. (1975). *Beyond boredom and anxiety*. San Francisco: Jossey-Bass.

Dermer, M., Cohen, S. J., Jacobson, E., & Anderson, E. A. (1979). Evaluative judgments of aspects of life as a function of vicarious exposure to hedonic extremes. *Journal of Personality and Social Psychology, 37*, 247–260.

Derogatis, L. R. (1977. *The SCL-90-R manual: Scoring, administration, and procedures for the SCL-90-Revised*. Baltimore: Johns Hopkins University School of Medicine, Clinical Psychometrics Unit.

Diener, E. (1984). Subjective well-being. *Psychological Bulletin, 95*, 542–575.

Diener, E., Horowitz, J., & Emmons, R. A. (1985). Happiness of the very wealthy. *Social Indicators Research, 16*, 263–274.

Dohrenwend, B. P. (1987) (Chair). Untangling psychosocial factors for psychopathology. Symposium held at American Psychological Association Meetings, New York, August.

Dohrenwend, B. P., & Dohrenwend, B. S. (1969). *Social status and psychological disorder: A causal inquiry*. New York: Wiley.

Dohrenwend, P., Shrout, P. E., Egri, G., & Mendelson (1980). Nonspecific psychological distress and other dimensions of psychopathology. *Archives of General Psychiatry, 37*, 1229–1236.

Eaton, W. W., & Kessler, L. G. (1985). Epidemiologic field methods in psychiatry: The NIMH epidemiologic catchment area program. Orlando, FL: Academic.

Eaton, W. W., Regier, D. A., Locke, B. Z., & Tanke, C. A. (1981). The epidemiologic catchment area program of the National Institute of Mental Health. *Public Health Reports, 96*, 319–325.

Ekman, P. (1982). *Emotion in the human face* (2nd ed.). Cambridge: Cambridge University Press.

Ekman, P., & Davidson, R. J. (Eds.). (1994). *The nature of emotion: Fundamental questions*. New York: Oxford University Press.

Falloon, I. R. (1988). Expressed emotion: current status. *Psychological Medicine, 18*, 269–274.

Faris, R. E. L., & Dunham, H. W. (1939). Mental disorders in urban areas. Chicago: University of Chicago Press.

Feighner, J. P., Robins, E., Guze, S. B., Woodruff, R. A., Jr., Winokur, G., & Muñoz, R. (1972). Diagnostic criteria for use in psychiatric research. *Archives of General Psychiatry, 26*, 57–63.

Folstein, M. F., Folstein, S. E., & McHugh, P. R. (1975). "Mini- mental state.": A practical method for grading the cognitive state of patients for the clinician. *Journal of Psychiatric Research, 12*, 189–198.

Frank, J. D. (1973). *Persuasion and Healing*. Baltimore: Johns Hopkins University Press.

Garbarino, J., Eckenrode, J., & Barry, F. D. (1997). *Understanding abusive families: an ecological approach to theory and practice*. San Francisco: Jossey-Bass.

Garbarino, J., & Sherman, D. (1980). High risk neighborhoods and high risk families: The human ecology of child maltreatment. *Child Development, 51*, 188–198.

Gersten, J. C., Langner, T. S., Eisenberg, J. G., & Simcha-Fagan, O. (1975). Spontaneous recovery and incidence of psychological disorder in urban children. *Psychiatry Digest, 1*, 35–43.

Gilmartin, J., Rossi, R. J., Lutomski, L. S., & Reed, D. F. B. (1979). *Social indicators: An annotated bibliography of current literature*. New York: Garland.

Goodstein, J., Zautra, A. J., & Goodhart, D. (1982). A test of the utility of social indicators for behavioral health service planning. *Social Indicators Research, 10*, 273–295.

Gove, W. R. (1980). Labeling and mental illness: A critique. In W. R. Gove (Ed.), *The labeling of deviance: evaluating a perspective* (pp. 35–81). New York: Halsted.

Green, D. P., Goldman, S. L., & Salovey, P. (1993). Measurement error masks bipolarity in affect ratings. *Journal of Personality and Social Psychology, 64*, 1029–1041.

Haggett, P., Cliff, A., & Frey, A. *Locational analysis in human geography (2nd edition)*. New York: Wiley.

Harding, C. M., Zubin, J., & Strauss, J. S. (1987). Chronicity in schizophrenia: Fact, partial fact or artifact? *Hospital and Community Psychiatry, 38*, 477–486.

Haring-Hidore, M., Stock, W. A., Okun, M. A., & Witter, R. A. (1985). Marital status and subjective well-being: A research synthesis. *Journal of Marriage and the Family, 47*, 947–953.

Headey, B., Holmstrom, E., & Wearing, A. (1984). Well-being and ill-being: Different dimensions? *Social Indicators Research, 14*, 115–139.

Helzer, J., Robins, L. N., & Croughan, J. (1978). *Renard diagnostic interview*. St. Louis: Washington University.

Herzberg, F., Mausner, B., & Snyderman, B. (1959). *The motivation to work*. New York: Wiley.

Hogan, R. (1983). A socio analytic theory of personality. In M. Page (Ed.), Nebraska Symposium on Motivation (pp. 55–89). Lincoln: University of Nebraska Press.

Horwitz, A. V. (1982). The social control of mental illness. New York: Academic.

Hough, R. L., Landsverk, J. A., Karno, M., Burnam, M. A., Timbers, D. M., Escobar, J. I., & Regier, D. A. (1987). Utilization of health and mental health services by Los Angeles Mexican Americans and non-Hispanic Whites. *Archives of General Psychiatry, 44*, 702–712.

Jahoda, M. (1958). *Current concepts of positive mental health*. New York: Basic Books.

Kammann, R., Smith, R., & McQueen, M. (1984). Low accuracy in judgments of other's happiness. Unpublished manuscript, University of Otago, Dunedin, New Zealand.

Karno, M., Hough, R. L., Timbers, D. M., Escobar, J. I., Burnam, M. A., Santana, F., & Burke, J. B. (1987). Lifetime prevalence of specific psychiatric disorders among Mexican Americans and nonhispanic Whites. *Archives of General Psychiatry, 44*, 695–701.

Kelsey, J. L., Whittemore, A. S., & Evans, A. S. (Eds.). (1996). *Methods in Observational Epidemiology*. New York: Oxford University Press.

Kleinbaum, D. G., Kupper, L. L., & Morgenstern, H. (1982). *Epidemiologic Research: Principals and Qualitative Methods* (pp. 20–22). New York: Van Nostrand Reinhold.

Klerman, G. L. (1986). Scientific and public policy perspectives on the NIMH Epidemiologic Catchment Area (ECA) program. In J. Barrett & R. M. Rose (Eds.), *Mental disorders in the community: findings from psychiatric epidemiology* (pp. 20–28). New York: Guilford.

Kobasa, S. C. (1982). The hardy personality: Toward a social psychology of stress and health. In G. S. Sanders and J. Suls (Eds.), *Social Psychology of Health and Illness* (pp. 341–352). Hillsdale, NJ: Erlbaum.

Kozma, A., DiFazio, R., & Stones, M. J. (1992). Long term and short-term affective states in happiness: age and sex comparisons. *Social Indicators Research, 27*, 293–301.

Langner, T. S. (1962). A twenty-two item screening score of psychiatric symptoms indicating impairment. *Journal of Health and Human Behavior, 3*, 269–276.

Levine, I. S., & Rog, D. J. (1990). Mental health services for homeless persons: Federal initiatives and current service trends. *American Psychologist, 45*, 963–968.

Mehrabian, A. (1972). *Non-verbal communication*. Chicago: Aldine-Atherton.

Michalos, A. C. (1985). Multiple discrepancies theory (MDT). *Social Indicators Research, 16*, 347–413.

Mirowsky, J., & Ross, C. E. (1989). Psychiatric diagnosis as reified measurement. *Journal of Health and Social Behavior, 30*, 11–25.

National Institute of Mental Health. (1975). *A typological approach to doing social area analysis*. DHEW Publication No. (ADM) 76-262, Superintendent of Documents, U.S. Government Printing Office, Washington, D.C. 20402.

National Institute of Mental Health—Series DN No. 5 (1985). Measuring social functioning in mental health studies: Concepts and instruments. Kane, R. A., Kane, R. L., & Arnold, S. DNNS Publ. No. (ADM) 85-1384. Washington, D.C.: Supt. of Docs., U.S. Printing Office.

Neugarten, B. L., Havighurst, R. J., & Tobin, S. S. (1961). The measurement of life satisfaction. *Journal of Gerontology, 16*, 134–143.

Osgood, C. (1965). Cross-cultural compatibility in attitude measurement via multi-lingual semantic differentials. In I. Steiner & S. Fishbein (Eds.), *Current studies in social psychology* (pp. 195–202). New York: Holt, Rinehart & Winston.

Pearlin, L. J., & Schooler, C. (1978). The structure of coping. *Journal of Health and Social Behavior, 19*, 2–21.

Regier, D. A., Myers, J. K., Kramer, M., Robins, L. N., Blazer, D. G., Hough, R. L., Eaton, W. W., & Locke, B. Z. (1985). Historical context, major objectives, and study design. *Archives of General Psychiatry, 41*, 934–941. Orlando, FL: Academic.

Robins, L. N. (1985). Epidemiology: reflections on testing the validity of psychiatric interviews. *Archives of General Psychiatry, 42*, 918–924.

Robins, L. N., Helzer, J. E., Croughan, J., & Ratcliff, K. S. (1981). National Institute of Mental Health Diagnostic Interview Schedule: Its history, characteristics, and validity. *Archives of General Psychiatry, 38*, 381–389.

Robins, L. N., Helzer, J. E., Weissman, M. M., Orvaschel, H., Gruenberg, E., Burke, J. D., Jr., & Regier, D. A. (1984). Lifetime prevalence of specific psychiatric disorders in three sites. *Archives of General Psychiatry, 41*, 949–958.

Robins, L. N., Regier, D. A., & Freedman, D. X. (1990). *Psychiatric disorders in America: The Epidemiological Catchment Area Study*. New York: Free Press.

Robinson, W. S. (1950). Ecological correlations and the behavior of individuals. *American Sociological Review, 15*, 351–357.

Ryff, C., & Singer, B. (1998). The contours of positive human health. *Psychological Inquiry, 9*, 1–28.

Scheff, T. J. (1974). The labeling theory of mental illness. *American Sociological Review, 39*, 444–452.

Schwab, J. J., & Schwab, M. E. (1978). *Socio-cultural roots of mental illness*. New York: Plenum.

Schwartz, N., & Clore, G. (1983). Mood, misattribution and judgments of well-being: Informative and directive functions of affective states. *Journal of Personality and Social Psychology, 45*, 513–523.

Shapiro, S., Skinner, E. A., Kessler, L. G., Von Korff, M., German, P. S., Tischler, G. L., Leaf, P. J., Benham, L., Cohler, L., & Regier, D. A. (1984). Utilization of health and mental health services: Three epidemiological catchment area sites. *Archives of General Psychiatry, 41*, 971–978.

Spitzer, R. L., & Endicott, J. (1977). *Schedule for affective disorders and schizophrenia*. New York: New York State Psychiatric Institute.

Spitzer, R. L., Endicott, J., & Robins, E. (1978). Research diagnostic criteria. *Archives of General Psychiatry, 35*, 773–782.

Srole, L., Langner, T. S., Michael, S. T., Opler, M. K., & Rennie, T. A. C. (1962). *Mental health in the metropolis: The Midtown Manhattan Study. Vol. I.* New York: McGraw-Hill.

Vaillant, G. E., & Schnurr, P. (1988). What is a case? *Archives of General Psychiatry, 45*, 313–319.

Vaugh, C., & Leff, J. (1976). The influence of family and social factors on the course of psychiatric illness: A comparison of schizophrenics and depressed neurotic patients. *British Journal of Psychiatry, 129*, 125–137.

Veit, C. T., & Ware, J. E., Jr. (1983). The structure of psychological distress and well-being in general populations. *Journal of Consulting and Clinical Psychology, 51*, 730–742.

Warr, P., & Payne, R. (1982). Experience of strain and pleasure among British adults. *Social Science and Medicine, 16*, 1691–1697.

Watson, D., Clark, L. A., & Tellegen, A. (1988). Development and validation of brief measures of positive and negative affect: the PANAS scales. *Journal of Personality and Social Psychology, 54*, 1063–1070.

Wing, J. K., Cooper, J. E., & Sartorius, N. (1974). *Measurement and classification of psychiatric symptoms*. London: Cambridge University Press.

Zautra, A., & Beier, E. (1978). Life crisis and psychological adjustment. *American Journal of Community Psychology, 6*, 125–135.

Zautra, A. J., Burleson, M. H., Smith, C. A., Blalock, S. J., Wallston, K. F., DeVellis, R. F., DeVellis, B. M., & Smith, T. W. (1995). Arthritis and perceptions of quality of life: an examination of positive and negative affect in rheumatoid arthritis patients. *Health Psychology, 14*, 399–408.

Zautra, A. J., Guarnaccia, C. A., & Dohrenwend, B. P. (1988). Measuring small life events. *American Journal of Community Psychology, 14*, 629–655.

Zautra, A. J., Kochanowicz, N., & Goodhart, D. (1983). Surveying the quality of life in the community. In R. Bell, M. Sundel, J. Aponte, S. Murrell, & E. Lin (Eds.), *Assessing health and human service needs* (pp. 191–209). New York: Human Sciences Press.

Zautra, A. J., Potter, P. T., & Reich, J. W. (1997). The independence of affects is context-dependent: An integrative model of the relationship between positive and negative affect. In K. W. Schaie & M. P. Lawton (Eds.), *Annual review of gerontology and geriatrics: Vol. 17. Focus on adult development* (pp. 75–103). New York: Springer.

Zautra, A. J., & Reich, J. W. (1983). Life events and perceptions of life quality: Developments in a two-factor approach. *Journal of Community Psychology, 11*, 121–132.

Zautra, A., & Simons, L. S. (1978). An assessment of a community's mental health needs. *American Journal of Community Psychology, 6*, 351–362.

CHAPTER 9

Stress

Theory, Research, and Action

IRWIN N. SANDLER, SANFORD BRAVER,
AND LEAH GENSHEIMER

Few theoretical perspectives have had as continuous a place in the history of community psychology as stress theory. There has, however, been considerable change in stress research over the past decade, which has added greater complexity to our understanding of the processes by which stress impacts on well-being. Concomitantly, our models of the change process have evolved over the past several decades to include multiple levels of conceptualizing interventions in social problems and assessing their effects. This chapter will take advantage of advances in both the stress theory and intervention domain by discussing the intervention implications of recent developments in our understanding of stress processes.

STRESS THEORY IN THE HISTORY OF COMMUNITY PSYCHOLOGY

The important place of stress theory in the history of community psychology can be seen in the seminal papers of Dohrenwend (1978) and Felner, Farber, and Primavera (1980) among others (Bloom, 1979; Caplan, 1964; Hobfoll, 1998; Sandler, 1979; Sandler, Wolchik, MacKinnon, Ayers, & Roosa, 1997). These papers are similar to the present chapter in that they described the implications of a stress theoretical framework for the action of community psychology. Dohrenwend (1978) described the activities of community psychology as having the common theme of counteracting the processes by which stress leads to psychopathology. According to this model, stressors occur either because of psychological characteristics of people or because of environmental factors over which the person has little control. The effects of these stressors may be to increase psychopathology, to increase psychological growth, or to

IRWIN N. SANDLER AND SANFORD BRAVER • Department of Psychology, Arizona State University, Tempe, Arizona 85287. LEAH GENSHEIMER • Department of Psychology, University of Missouri–Kansas City, Kansas City, Missouri 64110.

Handbook of Community Psychology, edited by Julian Rappaport and Edward Seidman. Kluwer Academic / Plenum Publishers, New York, 2000.

lead to no permanent change in the individual. Which of these outcomes occurs is a function of characteristics of the individual (e.g., coping abilities) or characteristics of the situation (e.g., social support, economic conditions). Dohrenwend (1978) described how the interventions of community psychology affect each step in the stress process. The occurrence of stressors can be prevented either by political action to change environmental conditions or by social-skill-building interventions that teach people to avoid stressful situations. Once stressors have occurred, their negative effects can be reduced by teaching individuals skills to cope with these stressors or by enhancing the availability of sources of material resources. Finally, crisis intervention helps to resolve the immediate situation induced by the stressful event and prevent the development of longer term psychopathology.

Felner, Rowlison, and Terre (1986) utilized a derivative of a stress model to develop action implications for community psychology with their concept of "transitional events." They conceptualized transitional events as including more than stress *per se* and as being distinct from related concepts of stressful life events or crisis events. Transitional events are those events that mark an extensive change in an individual's life and demand significant adaptation. The concept is concerned with adaptation to change, rather than simply with coping with negative affect. A transitional event consists of a series of smaller changes, each of which create their own adaptive tasks. It may be a positive event that requires adaptation (e.g., promotion or marriage) or it may be a negative event (e.g., demotion or divorce). This perspective is equally interested in promoting the positive outcomes as it is in preventing the negative outcomes of stress events. Interventions into transitional events may be individual-focused in helping to build the skills to effectively adapt to the demands of these events. For example, teaching recently unemployed workers effective job-searching skills may help them improve their economic status and their mental health (Caplan, Vinokur, Price, & van Ryn, 1989). Alternatively, they may focus on restructuring the environment to reduce the difficulty of the adaptive tasks confronting individuals in the situation. Widow-to-widow programs, for example, create settings of mutual support that help widows with the tasks of adapting to the death of a spouse (Silverman, 1989).

While these approaches have been important in linking stress and transition theory to models of action for community psychology, the past decade has witnessed important new developments both in research on stress processes and in the development of models of action for community psychology. The goal of this chapter is to review major themes and recent findings in stress research, and to illustrate how they may be important in developing interventions. We will discuss the implications for each theme for the development of intervention programs. The chapter will apply Seidman's (1988) theory of action to develop an action research agenda for children of divorce, illustrating the link between stress theory and intervention.

THEMES IN THE CONCEPTUALIZATION OF STRESS

Stress is best thought of as a general rubric for a set of variables and processes, rather than as a psychological variable with specified hypothetico-deductive properties (Lazarus & Folkman, 1984; McGrath, 1970). The scientific utility of the term then is to refer to a family of research studies on related problems and processes, rather than to investigate a well-specified theoretical system. Our discussion of the conceptualization of stress will identify three important themes in this family of stress-research studies: stress as the study of transactional processes, conceptualization and measurement of stress, and individual and social environmental resources that affect adaptation to stress. Our thesis throughout this discussion is that each theme has important implications for action programs.

Stress as the Study of Transactional Processes

The study of stress is the study of relations between individuals and their environments as they influence each other over time. The implications of this formulation are quite different from earlier response-based or stimulus-based models of stress.

For example, a response-based model of stress might define stress by a particular response pattern, such as physiological arousal, negative affective state, or perceived psychological stress (Cohen, Karmack, & Mermelstein, 1983; Derogatis, 1982). According to McGrath (1970), such individual-based conceptions are intrinsically limited, however, in that they fail to address the issues of what leads to the stress response. They do not account for the fact that the various stress responses do not necessarily strongly relate to one another, and they may include as stressful stimuli many events that bring about similar responses, but which we would not ordinarily want to include as stressful (e.g., passion, exercise, surprise). As an environmental variable, stress would be defined in terms of specified properties of the situation. This approach does not account for individual differences in response to those situations in which some people may be challenged or invigorated but that may precipitate distress or depression in others.

A person–environment relational model provides a more adequate fit to the problems of interest in stress research. McGrath (1970) defined stress as a *perceived* imbalance between demands and response capabilities when the consequences of failing to meet these demands are perceived as important by the individual. This definition is similar to Lazarus and Folkman's (1984) later formulation that "psychological stress is a particular relationship between the person and the environment that is appraised by the person as taxing or exceeding his or her resources and endangering his or her well-being" (p. 19). Thus stress research is concerned with individual variables, such as values and skills, environmental variables (e.g., change, loss), and the perceived relation between the two that may result in outcomes such as negative affect and negative changes in physical or mental health.

Stress research is not simply concerned with these as separate variables, but also with the process by which they affect each other over time. Lazarus and Folkman (1984) refer to this as a transactional conception of stress. The transactional model views the person and the environment as being in a reciprocal bidirectional relationship. While the environment may cause change in the person, the person is also an active agent that can cause change in the environment. In a transactional model, the critical variables cannot be neatly categorized as either person or environment, but may be intrinsically relational in nature. For example, the variable of appraised environmental threat involves both a perceiver and an environmental stimulus. A transactional model is also dynamic in that it is concerned with processes that change over time as the person responds to environmental threat, and as the environment is changed as a result of the person's response.

Implications for Action

The conceptualization of stress as a transactional process has several implications for intervention development and evaluation. First, it suggests multiple variables as potential targets for intervention. By targeting individual variables, such as coping skills, we may impact on how a person is able to adjust to environmental stressors. For example, teaching emotion-focused coping skills to children living with an alcoholic parent may help to minimize the negative impact of this uncontrollable stressor on the child. Targeting environmental variables also may reduce the stressor's negative impact, or it may prevent the stressor from occurring at all. For example, Felner and Adan (1989) restructured the school environment uncertainty and increased social support for students in transition.

Second, since the model is reciprocal and bidirectional in nature, evaluation designs must assess anticipated outcomes across multiple variables. An intervention that targets individual variables holds potential for impacting environmental variables and vice versa. Change may reverberate throughout the system. Improving adaptational outcomes to a stressful situation may strengthen the person's coping ability and help him or her create less stressful future situations. For example, adaptive coping with an interpersonal loss may increase the person's belief in his or her ability to cope effectively (i.e., individual variable change), and lead him or her to make more adaptive choices in the future, decreasing the stressfulness of future environmental situations or reducing their occurrence (Sandler, Tein, Mehta, Wolchik, & Ayers, in press). Therefore, decreased occurrence of controllable stress events may be an outcome of a successful intervention, as may be changes in individual beliefs and/or skill level.

Third, the dynamic nature of the model suggests that processes may change over time. Researchers therefore need to design evaluations that are longitudinal in nature and that assess both proximal and distal effects in order to adequately evaluate the efficacy of intervention efforts and understand their full impact.

Conceptualization and Measurement of Stress

This section will discuss three issues in the assessment of stress. First we will discuss conceptual issues of what properties of events or transactions are stressful. Much of the research on the assessment of stress has involved testing different conceptual models of the properties that make an event stressful, the most prominent models being change and undesirability. Second we will address methodological issues in the assessment of life stress. The most significant of these issues is disentangling the potential contamination between the assessment of life stress and the effects of life stress on the individual. Third is the social ecology of the stress experience. Here the focus is on how, where, and when people experience stress in their lives. Included are variables such as whether stress is acute or chronic; whether it consists of single large experiences or smaller everyday experiences; and how the experience of stress related to people's normal course of social.

Conceptualization of the Stressful Quality of Events

The basic theoretical issue of which quality-of-life experiences are stressful can be seen to inform decisions on assessment. There is a long-standing debate in the life-stress-events literature on whether it is change or undesirability that is the central stress property of events. The initial work on life events (Holmes & Masuda, 1974; Holmes & Rahe, 1967) was based on the concept that change was a property of the event and the critical determinant of its stressfulness. The concept of stress as change is based on a homeostatic model in that change disrupts the steady state so that the person needs to readjust to bring about a new homeostatic balance. The more readjustment is required, the more the individual's resources may be exhausted so that they will be vulnerable to illness.

If change is the central stressful property, then it follows logically that whether change was perceived as positive or negative would make little difference on the stressful impact of the event. This change model was quickly challenged by an undesirability model, which stated that only events that were perceived as undesirable were stressful (Gersten, Langner, Eisenberg, & Orzeck, 1974; Vinokur & Selzer, 1975), while desirable changes were not. Theoretically an undesirable change might be stressful because it threatens an individual's physical or emotional well-being (Thoits, 1983), while this would not be true of desirable changes.

A great deal of research was generated to address the issue of whether stress results from change *per se* or from undesirable conditions (Turner & Wheaton, 1995). Zautra and Reich (1983) reviewed 17 studies that assessed the relationship of desirable and undesirable events with psychological distress. They reported that undesirable events essentially accounted for the relations between life events and psychological distress, while there was little evidence for a positive relationship between positive events and distress. While positive events do not directly relate to higher levels of distress, they are important and have been the subject of study in their own right. For example, several studies have reported that positive events buffer or reduce the effects of negative events on psychological distress (Cohen & Hoberman, 1983; Reich & Zautra, 1981). Positive events have also been consistently found to relate to positive psychological states, such as life satisfaction and positive affect (Reich & Zautra, 1988).

While change and desirability are the two dimensions of stressful experience that have received the most attention, various other dimensions have also been investigated, including loss, entrance, controllability, conflict, perceived long-term threat, and danger (Thoits, 1983; Sandler & Guenther, 1985; Paykel, 1978; Redfield & Stone, 1979). Sandler and Ramsay (1982) conducted an analysis of the dimensions of life events for children based on the similarity of their impact. They used factor analysis of perceived similarity judgements of events to identify independent event dimensions (e.g., loss, entrance, family troubles, physical harm). They found that two of these dimensions, family troubles and entrances, accounted for the relationship between events and symptomatology for a sample of inner-city children. They argued that rather than there being a single property of events that leads to stress, that there may be multiple stress-inducing event properties. As we will see later, this theme of the multidimensional nature of stress has received increasing conceptual attention (e.g., Swindle, Heller, & Lakey, 1988).

Lazarus (1991) has proposed that the subjective appraisal of the significance of the event for the person's goals and commitments are a critical determinant of their stressful impact. Folkman, Lazarus, Gruen, and DeLongis (1986) referred to these appraisals as the individual's perceived "stake" in the situation, and assessed six different stakes in a study of married couples. Sandler, Ayers, Suter, Schultz, and Twohey (in press) proposed that satisfaction of basic needs of physical safety, control, self-worth, and social relatedness described some of the common stakes that are threatened in stressful situations.

Methodological Issues in the Assessment of Life Stress

The most important methodological issue in the assessment of life stress involves obtaining valid reports that capture the theoretically important aspects of stress while avoiding contamination with measures of psychological symptomatology. The issue involves some very real dilemmas for the stress researcher for which there is no ideal solution; there is only a trade-off between problems. For example, some experiences that are clearly stressful, such as a decrease in school grades, increased arguments with parents, and beginning drug use, can also be seen as the consequence of stress. Relating these "stressors" to measures of conduct disorder will obtain correlations that may tell us more about the reliability of assessing conduct disorder problems than about the association between stress and symptomatology. Several critiques of life-event methodology point out that much of the association between stress and illness can be accounted for by confounded measurement of the stress and illness variables. For example, Dohrenwend and Shrout (1985) propose that one measure of life stress, the Hassles Scale (Kanner, Coyne, Schaefer, & Lazarus, 1981), is contaminated with psychological symptomatology because many of the items on the scale resemble symptoms. A second type of confounding may occur in assessing the individual's stressful response to the event. For example, several scales assess life stress as the respondent's report of the extent to which recent events have had a negative or stressful impact on them (Sarason, Johnson, & Siegel, 1978). It may be that distress ratings may be affected by respondents' psychological symptomatology at the time they complete the scale, thus inflating the relation between stress and symptomatology (Brown & Harris, 1978). Dohrenwend and Shrout (1985) argue that the Hassles Scale is subject to this problem because it asks respondents to report on events that made them feel hassled at least to a "somewhat severe" degree. They found that a single second-order factor accounted for the relation between the eight hassle dimensions, and that this factor also accounted for the relation between hassles and the measure of psychological symptomatology. They argue that this factor, which they label subjective upsetness, is shared between the Hassles Scale and the symptomatology measure, and thus is a source of confounding between the two.

The dilemma of stress researchers is that removing these sources of confounding between measures of stressful environmental occurrences and psychological symptomatology may artificially distort the transactional nature of the stress process that is being studied. Lazarus, DeLongis, Folkman, and Gruen (1985) state that

> some of the confounding ... reflects the fusion of variables in nature rather than being merely the result of measurement errors of researchers. If we try to delete the overlap in variables of genuine importance, we will be distorting nature to fit a simpler, mythical metatheory of separate antecedent and consequent variables (p. 778).

They propose that the transactional approach to stress requires that individual appraisals of the environmental events be assessed, for it is this relationship between events and persons that is significant. Several alternative solutions have been utilized by stress researchers. Dohrenwend and Shrout (1985) propose that both the events and peoples' responses should be assessed, but that they should be assessed separately. One method of assessing the stressor independently of the person's response has been to have objective raters, fully informed of the context within which the stressor occurred, judge how stressful it would be for the typical person in that situation (Brown & Harris, 1978; Wethington, Brown, & Kessler, 1995). A second approach has been to assess stress with as much fidelity to theory as possible, while using prospective longitudinal designs or multiple raters of psychological symptoms to check that any observed relationship does not simply reflect confounding between predictor (stress) and criterion (psychological symptom) variables.

Ecology of Stressful Experience

The issue here concerns how stressful experiences are embedded in people's lives: When and where do they occur? How long do they last? How frequent are they? How do they relate to the overall patterns of person–environment relations that structure and give meaning to people's lives? Several alternative dimensions can be employed to describe the ecology of life stress, including their size, frequency, and chronicity.

There has been considerable interest in contrasting stressors that differ in size, that is large versus small events. Originally the study of stressful events focused on events that were seen as major disruptions that threatened people's health and well-being. The study of the impact of major events has taken several different forms. Some researchers have studied the effects of single major experiences such as bereavement (Parkes, 1972), divorce (Bloom, Asher, & White, 1978), combat (Grinker & Spiegel, 1945), serious physical illness (Janis, 1958; Taylor, 1983), or unemployment (Catalano & Dooley, 1983; Kessler, Turner, & House, 1987). The assumption is that these experiences have important consequences in and of themselves, and the research objective is to identify these consequences and understand the processes by which they occur. For example, Bloom et al. (1978) reported that the problems of the divorced include elevated rates of psychopathology, motor vehicle accidents, physical health problems, and alcoholism. From an ecological point of view these events could be described as time-limited, they have a specifiable time of onset and cessation, although their effects may last for a long period. These events occur relatively infrequently and are not a part of people's everyday lives. For example, Tausig (1982) reported that the mean frequency of occurrence of 118 life events in a representative sample of adults over the prior 6 months was less than 5%.

Another approach to studying major stressors has been to study the cumulative impact of all those that occur within a defined recent time period. This approach is exemplified by such life-events scales as the Social Readjustment Rating Scale (Holmes & Rahe, 1967) and the Peri Life Events Scale (Dohrenwend et al., 1978). Such scales are often considered measures of major life events in that they include most of the single major events thought to have an important impact on people (e.g., death of a spouse, divorce). From an ecological point of view these events occur in a variety of settings (e.g., home, workplace), are time-limited, and may be either developmentally normative changes or unrelated to developmental processes. While each of these events is a relatively rare occurrence, cumulatively it is normative for several of these events to occur over the course of a year [e.g., Tausig (1982) reported that a mean of 4.4 events occurred during a 6-month period for a random sample of adults]. Very little has been written about how these events relate to the normal course of interactions in people's lives. For example, some events may be normal developmental occurrences (e.g., retirement, marriage), while others may occur in a near random manner over time (e.g., close friend seriously ill). It is also interesting to note that the events that are included on life-events scales are essentially events of convenience, in that there has been little systematic work to develop a representative list of major events. Dohrenwend et al. (1978), who have done the most extensive work to develop a representative list of events for residents in New York City, suggest that there may be different events that are important for samples in different geographic areas (e.g., rural vs. urban) or at different times, so that developing a universally applicable set of events may not be feasible.

In contrast to these major events, there has been considerable interest in small events. Kanner et al. (1981) proposed that the small events that characterize everyday life may have proximal effects that cumulatively have important impacts on people's health and well-being. They divided small events into negative hassles and positive uplifts, and found that hassles were more strongly related to psychological symptomatology than were major negative events. Other measures of small events have been developed by different authors (Lewinsohn & Amenson, 1978; Lewinsohn & Graf, 1973; Stone & Neale, 1984; Zautra, Guarnaccia, & Dohrenwend, 1986). The common elements of these small-event measures are that they occur more frequently than large events, and that they include events that occur across physical settings of home, workplace, school, and community. These scales are heterogeneous in many other ways. For example, the small-event scale of Zautra et al. (1986) specifies that small events are changes in people's everyday living patterns, while Stone and Neale (1984) include events that are part of ongoing daily activities, but that are not necessarily changes.

A related concept to that of small events is that of "tailor-made" events that assess the specific experiences that follow from major life events. The theoretical foundation for assessing these events is in the Felner et al. (1986) concept that much of the impact of major stressors, such as divorce, is that they cause the occurrence of multiple smaller events, each of which make adaptive demands on the individual. These tailor-made events are distinct from small events in that they are tied to the major event and represent the cascading stressful transactions that follow from it. Tailor-made life-event scales have been developed to assess the stress of major events such as parental divorce (Sandler, Wolchik, Braver, & Fogas, 1986) and parental alcoholism (Roosa, Sandler, Beals, & Short, 1988).

Another important ecological distinction between stressors is the dimension of chronicity versus acuteness. A chronic stressor is one that continues for a long period of time as part of the ongoing conditions of people's lives. Living in poverty, having a cold, rejecting a relationship with a parent or marital partner, and having a boring job, are all examples of chronic stressful conditions. Acute stressors are often thought of as changes that have a specifiable time of onset and duration, such as losing a job or a negative change occurring in a relationship with a significant other. For example, Brown and Harris (1978) assessed major ongoing difficulties as unpleasant problems (e.g., poor housing) that had gone on for at least 2 years and did not involve health problems. They found that these ongoing difficulties were related to the development of depression, independent of the effects of severe events. Gersten, Langner, Eisenberg, and Simcha-Fagan (1977) assessed ongoing stressful processes as social and familial variables that continue over a prolonged period of time (e.g., mental illness of a parent; cold, distant relationship with a parent). In a two-wave prospective longitudinal study of children and adolescents, they found that life-event changes did not add to the prediction of symptomatology after accounting for the effects of ongoing stressful processes. The effects of life-stress changes and ongoing stressful processes are not independent, of course, and we will shortly discuss several possible models of how they jointly affect the development of adjustment problems.

Another, more theoretically derived approach to conceptualizing chronic stress utilizes the concept of role strain (Pearlin, 1982, 1983). Pearlin proposes that social roles can be used to describe people's involvements in the major institutions of society: work, school, family, and so forth. Thus people are socialized to invest a great deal of importance in these roles so that role problems are significant sources of stress. Pearlin (1983) describes role strain as "the hardships, challenges, and conflicts or problems that people come to experience as they engage over time in normal social roles" (p. 8). He describes six different types of role strain. Role strain can be derived from the relationship between people and the tasks of the role; for example, noxious or dangerous work tasks may be sources of strain in the work role. Another source of role strain is interpersonal conflicts encountered with various role partners. For example, Pearlin describes role strains between marital partners as involving lack of perceived reciprocity, lack of recognition of worth, and failure to have the routine expectations of marriage fulfilled. Role conflict between incompatible facets of roles that people simultaneously play is another source of strain. For example, employed women may experience conflict between their working roles and their family roles. Pearlin describes being bound to an unwanted social role (role captivity) as a fourth type of role strain. Here the strain derives from the fact that the role is unwanted, but involves an obligation that the person cannot easily give up. For example, women who are homemakers but who would like to be employed outside the home experience role strain that leads to elevated levels of depression (Pearlin, 1975). Nonscheduled role transitions are another form of role strain that leads to stress. Pearlin describes these as "shifts in roles and statuses, particularly those involving loss, that are not tied to life-cycle movement" (p. 22). Pearlin proposes that the most stressful of these role transitions occur when they bring about changes in existing role relations. For example, aging parents or restructured family responsibilities following a parental divorce require stressful changes in the mutual responsibilities, tasks, and exchanges between role partners.

Mediating and Moderating Models of Stress

Ecological differences between stressful experiences can be looked at from a causal, as well as a descriptive, perspective. That is, the different types of stress may affect each other in complex ways to lead to the development of psychological and physical health problems. This may occur by a mediational model or a moderating model (Baron & Kenny, 1986).

In a mediational model, major stressful events lead to the development of psychological and physical health problems by increasing the occurrence of smaller negative events, or by worsening role strains or other negative ongoing life conditions. For example, Felner et al. (1986) propose in the concept of transactional ecological events that major events cause the occurrence of multiple smaller stressful events; the failure to cope with these events leads to psychological adjustment problems.

Pearlin, Lieberman, Menaghen and Mullan (1981) proposed that major life events have much of their effect on psychological symptomatology by creating role strains. Illustratively, in a prospective longitudinal study of adults in Chicago, they found that the effects of job disruption on depression was, in part, mediated by the creation of economic strains in the household. These economic strains include difficulty in acquiring the necessities (e.g., food, clothing, housing), as well as some of the desirable amenities (e.g., recreation, vacations), of life. They further found evidence that the effect of economic strain on depression was mediated by its effect of decreasing the person's sense of self-esteem and mastery.

An alternative version of a mediational model posits that chronic stressful conditions exert their effects by leading to increased major life events. Liem and Liem (1981), for example, point to a series of studies that indicate that lower social class status leads to psychological maladjustment through its effect of increasing the occurrence of stressful life events. This causal chain is consistent with evidence for an increased occurrence of major life stressors in the lower social class and from epidemiological studies on stress, social class, and psychological symptomatology (Dohrenwend, 1973).

It is interesting to consider the mutually causative processes by which negative chronic conditions and discrete events may operate to maintain people in a state of chronic exposure to stressful environments. For example, following divorce, the income of the women decreases by 30%, on average. Women may also experience role strain related to task overload and increased conflict with their children as they attempt to adapt to their new situation. Poor adaptation to the post-divorce situation may lead to a condition of chronic stress from unsatisfactory economic, family, and work conditions. In turn, these unsatisfactory ongoing conditions may make the person vulnerable to the occurrence of a future negative event. For example, unsuccessful attempts to deal with chronic strains may include poor decisions (e.g., bad marriage, inappropriate jobs) that over time lead to future negative events (e.g., divorce, job loss).

A second potential interrelation between ecologically different stress variables is that one stress variable may moderate or change the effect of another. For example, a stressful ongoing condition may create a context that exacerbates the stressful impact of discrete life stressors. For example, the context of economic poverty may lead a person to appraise events (e.g., illnesses, moving, accidents) more negatively because the person realistically perceives that he or she does not have the needed resources to cope with the event. Liem and Liem (1981) reviewed several studies that investigated whether the chronic stressful conditions associated with lower social class status exacerbated the stressful effects of discrete life events. One approach to testing this effect is to test for statistical interactions, whereby the impact of stressful events on psychological distress is greater for lower than for higher social class samples. Evidence for this effect has been obtained in several studies (e.g., Dohrenwend, 1973; Kessler, 1979). Brown and Harris (1978) discuss the complex interrelations between chronic stressful conditions (which they term major difficulties) and severe events in leading to depression. They propose that chronic major difficulties are part of the context that may enter into the person's judgement of whether an event poses a long-term threat. For example, a woman who is poor and also unsure of her relationship to her spouse may evaluate the event of becoming pregnant as having negative implications for her long-term well-being. Alternatively, a major event may lead a person to become more aware of the negative implications of his or her chronic negative condition. For example, a person who is unhappy and lonely because of the lack of an intimate relationship may become depressed at the marriage of a close friend or sibling.

Implications for Action

The issue that has the most significant implication for action involves the relationship between the ecologically different forms of stress. The important intervention issue is how to interrupt the cycle whereby stressful events lead to ongoing negative conditions and vice versa. For example, following the major event of divorce, interventions may be designed to assist the ex-spouses to establish stable and satisfying economic, social, and family roles (Bloom et al., 1982). Similarly, following parental divorce or parental death, interventions may be designed to facilitate the establishment of effective family relations and to prevent the occurrence of ineffective family functioning (Sandler, Gersten, Reynolds, Kallgren & Ramirez, 1988; Sandler et al., 1992; Wolchik et al., 1993). Such examples represent intervening at the individual and setting levels, but the cycle may also be interrupted at the policy level. For instance, chronic economic burdens associated with unemployment may be prevented through legislative actions such as unemployment insurance, maintenance of health care benefits, 60-day notification of plant shut-down, and job retraining programs. The short-term (proximal) outcomes of these interventions might be less stressful ongoing environmental conditions, while the long-term (distal) outcomes might be improved psychological well-being of the individuals.

Our knowledge of specific stressful events that follow major life events should be used in planning the design of interventions. Additional study would allow us to identify specific coping demands associated with such stressors, further contributing to intervention content ideas. For example, studies have shown that the major life event of divorce is associated with financial, social, parenting, and personal growth stressors (Weiss, 1975). Interventions teaching people how to cope with such stressors should contribute to their post-divorce adjustment.

Another variable that has intervention implications is positive life events. Their potential role in promoting positive well-being and buffering the effects of negative events suggests incorporating strategies to increase their occurrence in our interventions. For example, a positive divorce intervention may include teaching parents the importance of ways in which they might spend some "special time" with their children, doing activities of particular interest to them (Wolchik et al., 1993; Wolchik, West, Sandler, et al., in press).

Individual and Social Environmental Sources of Protection against the Negative Effects of Stress

There is general agreement that the effects of environmental stressors vary as a function of social environmental and personal resources available to the individual (Dohrenwend, 1978). While an in depth review of research on the functioning of these resources is beyond the scope of this chapter we will discuss the major variables which have been studied as social environmental and individual protective resources.

Social Support as a Social Environmental Source of Stress Protection

While social support generally encompasses the stress protection provided by an individual's social contacts, more fine-grained distinctions have been developed to distinguish between different ways of conceptualizing these social resources (Barrera, 1986). Barrera (1986) distinguishes between the concepts of social embeddedness, enacted support, and perceived social support. Social embeddedness refers to the characteristics of the individual's social network. Assessment of the social network is concerned with how to describe these ties, independent of the content of the exchanges that occur between network members (Wellman, 1981). Commonly used network measures in the social-support literature include the number of members of the network who provide some support, the number of different kinds of support provided by members (multiplexity), the degree of interrelations between members (density), and the different kinds of relations between the members and the individual (e.g., friends, family). Enacted support refers to the actual helping behaviors that are exchanged. Barrera and Ainley (1983) have described six different kinds of helping transactions based on a review of the support literature: advice and information, emotional support, physical assistance, recreation, and positive feedback. Perceived support refers to the individual's evaluation of the quality of support provided by the social network, that is, the degree to which it is seen as available and helpful. While these are each generally referred to as measures of social support, they should be seen as dynamically related, rather than as different measures of the same thing (i.e., social support). For example Wolchik, Beals, and Sandler (1989) developed a model in which more support received from the social network was indirectly related to lower symptomatology through its effect of increasing satisfaction with social support.

Research has enumerated several alternative models of how social support may be a protective resource for people in stressful situations (Barrera, 1986, 1988; Cohen & Wills, 1985; Wheaton, 1985). Sandler, Miller, Short, and Wolchik (1989) describe three of these models as *preventive*, *moderating*, and *counteracting* effects of support. In the preventive model, support prevents the occurrence of the stressful situation. For example, Brown, Harris, and BiFulco (1986) found that a strong and supportive family structure prevented children from being placed outside the home after the death of a parent, and this in turn was related to lower vulnerability to depression in adulthood.

In the moderating (or buffering) effect, support may reduce the negative impact of stressful events. This may occur by support (e.g., advice, emotional support) facilitating effective coping or changing the appraisal of the stressor to be less threatening (Thoits, 1986). Cohen and Wills (1985) conclude a major review of the stress-buffering literature with the finding that buffering effects are consistently found in studies that assess confidant relationships, in which the presence of support boosts self-esteem, and from measures of the perceived availability of support.

In the counteracting effect, support may have the direct effect of reducing distress, thus counteracting the distress-increasing effect of stress. This may occur because close social ties fulfill a basic human need; the absence of such ties leads to distress (Barrera, 1986; Cohen & Wills, 1985). Evidence of direct negative relations between support and psychological distress is abundant in empirical studies that use both cross-sectional and prospective longitudinal designs (Barrera, 1986; Cohen & Wills, 1985).

The preventive, moderating, and counteracting effects of support are not mutually exclusive. For example, in an effective help-seeking model, stress leads to obtaining more support and support moderates the negative effects of stress (Wheaton, 1985). This successful use of support may strengthen the social ties in the network, further counteracting the effects of the stressor. Finally, there may be a match between the demands of the stressful situation and the aid that can be provided by social support. If financial or material resources are needed, advice or emotional support may not provide effective assistance and would not be successful in moderating the effects of that stressor (Cohen & McKay, 1982).

Personal Resources as a Source of Stress Protection

The importance of personal dispositions as sources of resilience to the effects of life stress has received considerable recognition (Kobasa, Maddi, & Kahn, 1982; Cohen & Edwards, 1989; Antonovsky, 1979; Kim, Sandler, & Tein, 1997).

The belief that some personality characteristics make people relatively resistant to the negative effects of stress is consistent with considerable experiential evidence of people in highly stressful situations, such as being a victim of cancer or experiencing the death of a spouse (e.g., Antonovsky, 1979; Parkes, 1972; Taylor, 1983). Empirical support for a generally stress-resistant personality has been minimal, however, despite several encouraging leads (Cohen & Edwards, 1989). Cohen and Edwards (1989) reviewed research that investigated a wide range of different personality characteristics as sources of stress resistance. These characteristics included hardiness, social skills, social interest, anomie, locus of control, Type-A behavior pattern, coping styles, sensation seeking, self-esteem, private self-consciousness, as well as composite indices of personal assets. Overall, they report that, with some exceptions (i.e., locus of control), there is little consistent convincing evidence for a stress-buffering effect of personality variables. Illustratively, the variable that has received the most attention as a stress buffer is psychological hardiness (Kobasa, 1979). Hardiness is a composite variable including measures of locus of control, alienation, and psychological security. Kobasa described hardiness as consisting of a sense of control, commitment, and challenge in meeting life's stresses. While several studies found a stress-buffering role for hardiness, others did not, and the one study that attempted to disentangle the separate effects of the different component scales that make up hardiness found a buffering effect for only the alienation-from-self scale (Ganellen & Blaney, 1984). Despite the lack of consistent evidence for a buffering effect of personality, there is sufficient suggestive evidence to encourage further research along these lines. For example, it may be that personality variables provide protection for some specific stressful situations but not for others.

The view that personality may provide a more situation-specific influence on people's responses to stress rather than being a general stress-protective resource has been proposed by Swindle, Heller, and Lakey (1988). According to this model, different personality dimensions are relevant to determining responses to different classes of stress situations. A situation is perceived as stressful when it is appraised to be similar to prior situations that involved threat or danger. Situation-specific beliefs, expectations, and response tendencies for this kind of stress situation determine the individual's coping responses. For example, a person encountering a physical illness will construe it in the light of previous experiences with illnesses and will respond in accord with their beliefs about the effectiveness of coping with physical illness. According to this approach, rather than there being general personal characteristics that engender resistance to stress, different response tendencies enable effective coping in different situations. For example, faith may be helpful in a prisoner-of-war situation, direct action may be helpful in coping with business stressors, and help-seeking may be most effective when a symptom of physical illness is detected (Swindle et al., 1988).

This approach posits that stress resistance be conceptualized according to different types of stressors, rather than as a personality dimension relevant across all stress situations. This is essentially an interactionist model in which an event is stressful because it is construed as being a member of a class of events that have involved danger in the past, and in which situationally relevant personal dispositions such as values, beliefs, and expectancies influence the coping responses to the situations. Lazarus and Folkman (1984), in a similar vein, propose that the appraisal of events as stressful is, in part, a function of the individual's commitments and beliefs.

More fundamentally, however, Lazarus and Folkman (1984) propose that stress research focus on the process by which people cope with the demands of stressful events, rather than on the stable personal dispositions of the individual. They point out that personality dispositions are not good predictors of coping responses and that coping processes are probably more important determinants of the outcomes of stress experiences (Cohen & Lazarus, 1973). Lazarus and Folkman (1984) define coping as "constantly changing cognitive and behavioral efforts to manage specific external and/or internal demands that are appraised as taxing or exceeding the resources of the person" (p. 141). Three key features of this definition are that it is process-oriented and contextual, and it makes no presuppositions about what is "good" or "bad" coping. It is concerned with what people actually think and do, and how this changes over the course of the encounter (process-oriented), rather than with stable personal traits. It is shaped both by personal and situational variables (context-oriented). It does not consider certain strategies as inherently more desirable, but studies how outcomes may vary as a function of the match between situational demands and coping responses.

Three variables are central to the study of the coping process: appraisal, coping, and outcomes. Appraisals concern people's evaluations of the relevance of an environmental event for their well-being (primary appraisal) and of their prospects for dealing with the event (secondary appraisal). Primary appraisals can evaluate an event as being irrelevant (not significant for their well-being), benign (preserving or enhancing well-being), or stressful. Stress appraisals in turn are subdivided into harm/loss, threat, and challenge. Harm/loss involves an evaluation that some damage has already occurred to the person's physical well-being, social ties, or self-esteem. Threat involves the prospect of future harm or loss. Challenge appraisals recognize the demands of the event but focus on the potential gains to be achieved rather than the losses.

Secondary appraisals address the issue of what can be done to manage the threat to well-being or to maximize gains from the encounter. The individual considers the demands in relation to their coping options, the likelihood or success of these coping options, and his or her ability to apply these coping options effectively. The individual may ask how well his or her physical, psychological, social, or material resources enable him or her to handle the demands of the stressful situation. Secondary appraisals often involve perceptions of control over the likely outcomes of the situation. Folkman (1984) has pointed out that control appraisals are multifaceted. They may involve the perception of ability to reduce or avoid the harmful situation or to maintain emotional well-being in the new situation.

Coping refers to what is done in attempting to manage the demands of the situation. Two major functions of coping are to change the stressful person–environment relations (problem-focused coping) and to regulate the emotions (emotion-focused coping). These two functions are interdependent in that coping efforts are often directed towards accomplishing both functions, and success in accomplishing one affects success in accomplishing the other. For example, managing the level of arousal allows the individual to more effectively plan problem-solving strategies, and effective problem-solving may lower the level of negative arousal. People may employ multiple strategies to accomplish these functions. Folkman and Lazarus (1980) developed the "ways of coping" scale to assess the strategies people use to cope in identified stressful situations. Factor analysis of this scale and other related scales have identified several meaningful dimensions. For example Folkman, Lazarus, Dunkel-Schetter, DeLongis, and Gruen (1986) identified eight meaningful dimensions: confrontive coping, distancing, self-control, seeking social support, accepting responsibility, escape–avoidance, planful problem-solving, and positive reappraisal. Which strategies are used is determined by the personal and environmental resources available to the person, which determine the secondary appraisal of what the person can do to cope. These resources include individual skills, belief systems, available social networks, and material resources. Several studies report that if the person appraises that he or she can change the situation, he or she is more likely to use coping strategies that are likely to accomplish that goal (e.g., problem-solving); appraisals that one cannot change the situation are related to the use of more emotion-focused strategies (e.g., escape-avoidance) (Folkman & Lazarus, 1980; Folkman et al., 1986). Although some coping strategies have been found to relate to more satisfactory outcomes in empirical studies (Stone, Helder, & Schneider, 1988; Folkman et al., 1986), Lazarus and Folkman (1984) emphasize that the effectiveness of these strategies must be viewed in relation to situational demands. For example, denial may be helpful in alleviating distress in situations that cannot be changed, but may be maladaptive in situations where problem-focused strategies could be effective.

Implications for Action

Several models of action are suggested by the discussion of personal and social resources. First, since effective coping, personal, and social resources may be situation-specific, interventions for different stressors should be based on intensive study of targeted stressful situations. Future research to guide intervention planning should focus on such questions as: What are the stressors that follow a specific life event? What are the coping demands of these stressors? What modes of coping are more or less effective? What social resources are helpful? Knowledge of specific coping demands associated with different stressors should suggest potentially helpful intervention content that will teach specific skills, rather than more generic ones that may not be useful for a particular stressor. For example, more controllable stressors (e.g., geographic relocation, school transition) could be dealt with using problem-focused coping strategies, whereas less controllable situations (e.g., living with an alcoholic parent) could be more effectively handled by using emotion-focused coping strategies.

Second, the protective potential of social support suggests interventions that create supportive settings and reinforce effective coping. Programs could be designed to facilitate social networks that include experts on specific stressors (e.g., self-help groups such as Alanon), prevent the loss of support (e.g., Felner's [1982] school transition project), and/or teach coping skills, such as problem-solving, that may be generally helpful (e.g., component of Pedro-Carroll's Children of Divorce Project; Pedro-Carroll & Cowen [1987]).

A third area of intervention involves attempts to alter relevant individual dispositions, such as people's values, beliefs, and expectations—variables found to influence coping responses to a given situation. Interventions targeting communities could be designed to impact on values and beliefs that promote more positive well-being among community members. Although such interventions are, perhaps, more difficult to implement and systematically evaluate, they do hold potential for impacting on large numbers of people and reducing stress at a societal level. We have seen some examples of these changes throughout history, and we can speculate on the value of some more structured efforts. For example, the social stigma carried with divorce 20–30 years ago no longer exists, a consequence of both the high frequency of divorce in today's society and our acceptance of and expectation for women to work outside the home and be independent. The change in our culture's beliefs and expectations has reduced societal stress previously associated with divorce. Similarly, the stressor of being stigmatized as racially/ethnically different has been, and can further be, reduced by promoting positive beliefs about the value of individual differences among community residents (cultural/community values) and promoting a sense of prideful conditions of one's heritage (e.g., recall the "Black is Beautiful" campaign). Such efforts hold the potential to minimize or reduce societal environmental stressors and/or increase individuals' abilities to cope with the potential stress of being different.

CONCEPTUALIZING INTERVENTIONS FOR STRESS SITUATIONS

How does the existing research on stress inform the development of models of intervention in stress processes? To provide structure for our discussion of interventions, we will use the conceptual framework for primary prevention interventions developed by Seidman (1987). Our illustrations will be drawn from the intervention and theoretical literature concerning the adaptation of children of divorce. For each of Seidman's three levels of intervention we will provide illustrations of actual programs that intervene in divorce processes. We will discuss how theoretical issues concerning stress processes and empirical findings on the adaptation of children to the stress of parental divorce might further inform such interventions.

Seidman's framework proposes three levels for the locus of intervention: the population (or group), the setting, and the mesosystem. In this scheme, population reflects an aggregate of individuals who have some characteristics in common that puts them at risk for maladaptation. The individuals do not have any particular relationship or shared interest/goal, but they do share a common stress experience, such as parental divorce. The objectives of population-level interventions are to improve the coping skills of individuals in the populations. "Setting" is distinguished from "population" by the relationship that exists among its members. Setting is defined by three criteria: relationship between two or more individuals, sustained over time, and having a shared goal. Examples include family, peer group, and workplace. The objectives of interventions aimed at this level are to alter the relationships that exist *within* the setting for the long-term outcome of averting problems and promoting positive well-being. For instance, parenting programs would represent an intervention aimed at the family setting, since the objectives are to affect parent–child interactions. The third level, "mesosystem," refers to the relationships and connections *between* systems or settings. The objectives of intervention efforts at this level are to change existing relationships or to create new ones that impact on adaptation to stress. Interfaced within this model is the construct of "social regularities," that is, "patterns of social relations, connections, or linkages," (Seidman, 1988, p. 9). Social regularities refer to the settings or systems's rules of operation—the *status quo*. For example, regularities for children of divorce might refer to family members' patterns of interaction between the mother's and father's households.

Seidman conceptualizes both proximal and distal outcomes across each level. Proximal outcomes refer to the immediate effects on the level targeted for intervention. Distal outcomes reflect long-term effects and may occur at levels other than the one directly targeted for intervention. For group-level interventions, improved coping skills of individuals exposed to those stressors and improved adjustment are the proximal outcomes; the distal outcomes are maintenance of these individual-level improvements. For setting-level interventions, the proximal outcomes are improved functioning of the setting improvements and reduced maladjustment of the individual child. For mesolevel interventions, the proximal outcomes are improved interactions between settings; the distal outcomes are improved functioning of the settings and of the individual children within them.

Group Level Interventions for Children of Divorce

The objective of a group-level intervention for children of divorce is to facilitate adaptive coping with divorce-related stressors. The most successful example of a coping-enhancement program for children of divorce is Pedro-Carroll's Children of Divorce Intervention Program (CODIP) (Pedro-Carroll & Cowen, 1985, 1987; Pedro-Carroll & Alpert-Gillis, 1987; Pedro-Carroll, Cowen, Hightower, & Guare, 1986). This school-based program has been implemented in over 30 schools within the Rochester, New York, area (Pedro-Carroll & Alpert-Gillis, 1987). The CODIP involves a small group format and applies educational and cognitive-behavioral intervention strategies to teach children coping skills specific to the divorce situation. The intervention attempts to provide participants with support, build his or her competence in effective coping skills, teach anger control, enhance the child's self-esteem, and increase his or her understanding of divorce-related concepts and clarify misconceptions about divorce. The original program designed for children in grades four through six has been expanded and modified to fit the needs of children of different developmental stages and cultural backgrounds (Sterling, 1986; Alpert-Gillis, 1987).

Since 1982, a series of evaluations of this program have been conducted using true and quasi-experimental designs. Overall, these studies find some positive short-term program effects on children's adjustment, including gains on teacher's ratings of classroom adjustment; parents' ratings of school performance, peer relations, and feelings toward divorce; group leaders' reports of children's competence and problems; and the children's self-report of anxiety (Pedro-Carroll & Cowen, 1985; Pedro-Carroll et al., 1986). Long-term program effects on children's adjustment, however, have not yet been assessed, nor have mediational analyses been done to investigate the processes responsible for program effects.

While this program provides an encouraging example of the potential benefits of group-level interventions for children of divorce, it is useful to consider how the general stress literature and research on the stress of parental divorce may inform further development of such interventions. Two particularly important issues concern how stress research may inform the content of intervention strategies and the selection of participants in the program.

Two questions are particularly relevant to the content of interventions: (1) What are the stressors that affect children of divorce? and, (2) What cognitive, behavioral, or affective responses to these stressors lead to better mental health outcomes? From a transactional perspective, the stress of divorce can be disaggregated to consist of multiple, smaller stressors that follow and are set in motion by the divorce. "The Divorce Events Schedule for Children" (DESC) is a tailor-made life-event schedule specifically developed to assess these events (Sandler, Wolchik, Braver, & Fogas, 1986). The scale contains 62 items that often occur and are seen as being impactful following a parental divorce. Events for the scale were empirically generated from 100 key informants knowledgeable about the experiences of children following parental divorce (i.e., divorced parents and their children, psychologists, family practice lawyers). One interesting use of tailor-made life-events scales is to disaggregate the major stressors to identify their most stressful components. Wolchik, Sandler, Braver, and Fogas (1986) found that there was general consensus between parents', children's, and mental health professionals' ratings of the relative stressfulness of the events on the DESC, with the most stressful events involving interparental conflict, derogation of the parents, and blaming of the child for the divorce. Thus, these would seem to be the events for which children of divorce need the most coping assistance and might be the special focus of coping-enhancement programs.

Sandler, Tein, and West (1994) conducted cross-sectional and short-term prospective longitudinal studies of coping and psychological adjustment in preadolescent children of divorce. They assessed coping using a four-dimensional model, consisting of active coping, avoidant coping, distraction, and support-seeking. In the cross-sectional analysis, they found that avoidant coping was related to higher symptoms, while active coping buffered the effects of stress on children's conduct problems. In the prospective longitudinal analysis, active coping at time 1 had a significant negative relationship with depression at time 2, controlling for the effects of depression at time 1. Sheets, Sandler, and West (1996) studied children's negative appraisals for divorce-related stressful events. They defined negative appraisals as children's thoughts about the negative consequences of the stressors they experienced following their parents divorce. They found that negative appraisals related to higher symptoms in children (over and above reports of the occurrence of the events) using both cross-sectional and prospective longitudinal analyses. Sandler, Tein, Mehta, Wolchik, and Ayers (in press) studied children's perceptions of efficacy in dealing with the stressors that occurred following divorce. They found in both the cross-sectional and prospective longitudinal designs that perceived coping efficacy mediated the relations between coping efforts and children's internalizing problems. Active coping was related to increased perceptions of coping efficacy, which relate to decreased internalizing symptoms. Avoidant coping, however, relates to lower perceived coping efficacy, which mediates the positive relation between avoidant coping and internalizing symptoms. These findings have implications for the design of coping-enhancement programs for children of divorce. Such programs might increase active coping and perceived coping efficacy, and may decrease avoidant coping and negative appraisals of divorce stressors. If these variables are *causally* related to symptoms, changing them should lead to a decrease in symptoms. In fact, the activities of the Pedro-Carroll and Cowen (1985) program seem appropriate to improving coping and decreasing negative appraisals. However, their program evaluation design did not assess the program effects on these potentially mediating variables. Future research testing processes that mediate the effects of the program could greatly enhance our understanding of how the program exerts its effects and could also provide an experimental test of the causal relations between the mediating variables (e.g., coping) and psychological symptoms in children of divorce.

A second important issue for population-level interventions concerns defining the population to participate in the program. Although children of divorce are at risk for increased behavioral and emotional problems (Emery, Hetherington, & DiLalla, 1984), the effects of divorce on children are quite variable (Amato & Keith, 1991). For example, in a study of a nationally representative sample of American households, Zill (1978, 1983) found that 14% of the children from divorced families were reported by their parents as being in need of psychological help. While this is twice the rate of perceived need for help in non-divorce families, approximately 86% of the children of divorce were not seen as needing help. This finding has several important implications for the selection of participants for interventions for children of divorce. It may be that all children whose parents divorce do not need to participate in an intervention, and that resources could be more efficiently used by targeting those who are most at risk with a more intensive effort, rather than providing a less intensive intervention for a larger number of children. According to the transactional model, those most at risk should be children who have experienced more stressful environmental conditions following the divorce. For example, Pillow, Braver, Sandler, and Wolchik (1988) found that adjustment problems of children of divorce were related to the occurrence of more divorce-related stressful events, a worse relationship between the child and their custodial parent, and the occurrence of fewer stable positive events. Targeting a subgroup of more problematic divorces also has the advantage of increasing the statistical power of experimental tests of the intervention program to detect the effects of the intervention (Heller, Price, & Sher, 1980; Pillow et al., 1988). Heller et al. (1981) have shown that, given a constant effect size, the sample size needed to detect a significant difference between the intervention and control group decreases dramatically with an increase in the proportion of the population experiencing the problem of interest. Thus, the power of an experimental field trial of an intervention to detect significant effects could be increased by selecting a subpopulation of children of divorce who have a higher base rate of the problems to be impacted.

While population-level interventions may effectively change individual coping processes, they do not affect those variables that have most consistently been related to children's post-divorce adjustment—the social systems within which children live. Intervention at a higher level is needed to affect such changes.

Setting-Level Interventions for Children of Divorce

Setting-level interventions attempt to indirectly impact on the adjustment levels of the individual through altering relationships that exist within settings and are believed to mediate the impact of the stressor. Several interventions have been developed to impact on these setting-level variables, such as parenting programs designed to improve parent–child relationships (Stolberg & Garrison, 1985; Wolchik et al., 1993) and divorce mediation, designed to help parents reach divorce-related decisions (e.g., child-custody arrangements) in a less conflictual manner (Emery & Wyer, 1987).

Wolchik et al. (1993) developed a program to improve social–environmental factors that affect children's mental health following divorce. Based on the empirical literature, they identified five putative mediators of children's post-divorce adjustment: (1) quality of the custodial parent–child relationship; (2) contact with the noncustodial parent; (3) negative divorce-related events, including interparental conflict; (4) contact with and support from nonparental adults; and (5) discipline strategies. They hypothesized that improving these putative mediators would lead to a decrease in children's mental health problems. The program was designed to work with the residential mother, as someone who was in a position to influence each of these putative mediators. The program involved 10 weekly group sessions and two individual sessions. The intervention techniques were explicitly designed to change each of the putative mediating variables. For example, four skills were taught to improve the quality of the mother–child relationship: (1) increasing positive family activities, (2) increasing parent–child quality time, (3) providing positive attention for desirable behavior, and (4) improving mothers' listening skills. Parents were supported in using these skills to change their interactions with their children. The program was evaluated using a design in which families were randomly assigned to either the experimental or a wait-list comparison group. The program was found to improve the quality of the mother–child relationship, decrease the occurrence of negative divorce-related events, and improve the mothers' use of effective discipline strategies. The program also improved parent reports of mental health problems for children who initially had a higher level of problems. Analyses also showed that improvement in the quality of the mother–child relationship partially mediated the effects of the program on children's mental health.

These results provide encouraging support for the potential efficacy of working with the custodial mother to improve some social–environmental mediators of children's post-divorce adjustment. Nevertheless, the program did not affect other important aspects of the post-divorce environment. For example, the program did not affect the level of interparental conflict, the relationship between the child and the non-custodial father, or the economic well-being of the child following the divorce. In order to design programs to improve these factors, it may be necessary to conceptualize the problem at what Seidman terms the mesosystem level of analysis.

Mesosystem-Level Interventions for Children of Divorce

Mesolevel interventions are directed at altering the basic structural arrangements that exist between settings. It is anticipated that proximal changes at a mesolevel will have a subsequent distal impact on the settings in which children live, and subsequently on their adaptation. For illustrative purposes, we will discuss Wisconsin's Child Support Assurance System (CSAS), which includes mandatory wage garnishment of the noncustodial parent, an attempt to restructure the financial exchange between the post-divorce family settings of the father and mother.

Divorce is often an economic strain on the family, frequently producing downward economic mobility for the parties involved (Emery et al., 1984). Particularly hard hit are households of the divorced custodial mother. As much as a 30% drop in household income following divorce has been cited (Braver, Gonzales, Wolchik, & Sandler, 1989; Emery et al., 1984). As previously mentioned, reduced income of the custodial parent is likely to contribute further to the stress in the divorced household, either as a result of difficulties in acquiring the necessities of life or as a result of reductions in desirable amenities. Further, unless provisions are made, chronic economic strain may exacerbate the stressful impact of the discrete life stressor (Liem & Liem, 1981). For example, the economic strain experienced by the custodial parent may lead to his or her having a poorer post-divorce adjustment, which has been found to be significantly related to children's divorce adjustment (Kurdek & Berg, 1983).

The CSAS is a comprehensive reform package designed to address the numerous problems associated with our traditional private child-custody support payment system of the noncustodial parent, and those associated with our public support system of Aid to Families with Dependent Children and welfare (Garfinkel, 1988). As summarized by Garfinkel (1988, p. 13), within this plan all parents living apart from their children are obligated, under law, to share their income with their children. The amount is specified by an administrative standard primarily based upon the number of children the parent is obligated to support. Where possible, the obligation is collected through automatic payroll withholdings of the noncustodial parent, in a fashion similar to withholdings of social security and income taxes. Children are entitled to benefits equal to the child support paid by the noncustodial parent or the administratively assured minimum benefit, whichever is higher. If the noncustodial parent pays less than the assured amount, the difference is paid by the state. Further, in order to decrease dependence on the welfare system and make employment a more attractive option for low-income custodial parents, compensations for work expenses such as child care are incorporated within the package (Garfinkel, 1988). The plan is intended to correct many of the inadequacies of the current private child-support practices (e.g., reduce the rate of nonpayment, allow for changes in noncustodial parent's earning and cost of living), ensure the economic security of children regardless of the income levels of their parents, and reduce dependency of single mothers on the welfare system (Garfinkel, 1988).

Implementation of the plan began in 1983 and an evaluation has been completed of the program's effectiveness in increasing collection of child support and adherence to published income standards. The evaluation involved the comparison of child-support collection effectiveness and adherence to published income standards in the 10 piloted counties that used automatic income assignments, with these same 10 counties before they adopted the plan, and with a matched set of 10 other control counties that did not adopt the automatic income assignments. Unfortunately, the evaluation of the mandatory withholding of child-support aspect of the program indicates a somewhat disappointing level of improvement. Garfinkel and Klawitter (1992) report that whereas the compliance percentage (percentage of dollars paid to what was owed) increased 7% (from 55% before the program was instituted to 62% afterward) in the pilot counties, it increased 4% (from 55% to 59%) in the control counties. Thus only a 3% compliance increase is attributable to the program. This result is replicated in other studies. Pearson, Thoennes, and Anhalt (1993) report that wage-withholding in Colorado increases compliance only 7% (from 53% to 60%) and Gordon et al.'s (1991) report to the Office of Child Support Enforcement indicates that immediate withholding of child support produced a statistically non-significant impact on child-support compliance.

Why have such programs had less than satisfactory results? One possibility is the manner in which such policies are implemented by the enforcement bureaucracy. Policies that require heavy bureaucratic requirements take time to "work out the kinks" and function effectively. Garfinkle and Klawitter (1992) report some suggestive evidence that the Wisconsin program began operating slightly more effectively as the bureaucracy matured. On the other hand, some bureaucracies may never function well at all. On the other hand, some bureaucracies may never function well at all. Thus, 9 years after their inception of the program, Garfinkle and Klawitter (1992) reluctantly conclude that "routine income withholding will increase child support payment by [only] a modest amount ... it is no panacea" (p. 248).

A second possible reason for the poor results of these programs is that determinedly unwilling noncustodial parents can find ways to remain non-compliant even within a wage-withholding system. They may "dodge" the enforcement apparatus by such strategies as leaving the vicinity, changing jobs frequently, or commencing self-employment. The mandatory withholding policy ignores the motivation of the noncustodial parent and assumes that child-support payments can be increased by forcing payment. It assumes an adversarial relationship between the parents in which one's gain is the other's loss. However, if the motivation of the noncustodial parent is considered, alternative formulations of the problem are possible that may lead to more effective solutions.

Braver et al. (1993) recently reported the results of a 3-year longitudinal study of the predictors of child-support compliance. The study used a sizable, regionally representative sample, and was one of the first to systematically query noncustodial parents directly, as well as the surveying custodial parents and children. The results indicate that noncustodial parents *voluntarily* pay child support at very high levels (84–96% compliance) when they perceive that they have shared control of the post-divorce upbringing of the child and have input into the details of the divorce settlement. In contrast, by far the most important motivation for noncompliance appears to be the psychological reactance (Brehm, 1965) engendered by the loss of control over their own and their child's fate. When they feel disenfranchised and without the usual rights of parenthood, they "become in effect 'parents without children' ... [and] withdraw ... from the [usual] obligations of parenthood [as well]" (p. 20).

Viewed from this perspective, it is easy to see why the coercive approach of mandatory wage withholding, as well as other coercive approaches (c.f. Office of Child Support Enforcement, 1990; Pearson, Thoennes, & Tjaden, 1989) have experienced disappointing results: they have undoubtedly increased the perceived loss of control of the noncustodial parent, leading to even more reactance and resistance to payment. This perspective suggests alternative mesosystem-level interventions based on a reformulation of the problem.

The alternate formulation of the problem is how to construct a system that promotes a "cooperative parenting orientation" among both parents, allowing both to perceive high levels of control. It is important to note that Bay and Braver (1990) found that perceived control was not a "zero-sum game" in which what one parent gains in control, the other loses. Rather, the perceived level of control of the two parents was significantly *positively* correlated. In turn, these covaried with the degree of post-divorce conflict between the parents. If there was a high level of conflict, *neither* parent perceived that they had control, whereas both perceived high control when the conflict was well-managed.

How might a mesosystem-level intervention that promotes a cooperative parenting orientation and mutually high perceived control be designed? Our current "standard" domestic relations (family law) system, which promotes and contributes to adversarial and mutually coercive relationships between the parents, moves us in virtually the exact opposite from the desired direction. However, several more hopeful programs are rapidly being developed. Mediation as an alternative to litigation is being adopted in most jurisdictions (Myers et al., 1988; Pearson & Thoennes, 1989). By its nature, mediation attempts to mutually empower both parents, and provides an avenue for the parents to cooperate in settling of disputes. Joint legal (as opposed to residential) custody arrangements, which are presumptive in many states, promote the desirable sense that both parents retain for life their "parenthood" over their children. Many courts are also developing "divorce education" programs, in which all divorcing parents are compelled by the court to attend 2- to 4-hour sessions led by mental health personnel exhorting them to cooperative relationships (Kramer & Washo, 1993; Danner, 1991).

A mesosystem-level intervention that promotes a cooperative parenting orientation and mutually high perceived control should thus have multiple salutary effects on the child's well-being. First, it should reduce interparental conflict, one of the most influential factors relating to the child's adjustment (Emery, 1982; Amato & Keith, 1991). Since conflict with the ex-spouse is one of the most impactful stressors for the custodial parent (Tschann, Johnston, & Wallerstein, 1989; Hetherington, Cox, & Cox, 1976), contributing to his or her diminished parenting capability (Nelson, 1989; Jacobson, 1983), an indirect benefit to the child might also result. Second, such an intervention should increase the child's contact with the noncustodial parent. Braver et al. (1993) found that noncustodial parents who perceived substantial shared control visited from 7–11 times per month, a finding replicated by Kruk (1992). Numerous studies (Guidibaldi, Cleminshaw, Perry, & McLoughlin, 1983; Hess & Camara, 1979) have found that ample contact with the noncustodial parent increases child adjustment, especially where interparental conflict is minimized. Finally, if the intervention promotes the noncustodial parent's perceived control over the child's upbringing, child-support payments should increase.

CONCLUSIONS

This chapter reviewed major developments in theory and research on stress processes and discussed implications of such advances for the development of interventions—interventions consistent with models of action in community psychology. Three themes from the stress literature were identified as particularly important for the design of interventions: the transactional nature of stress processes, the ecology of stressful experiences, and social and personal resources that influence adaptation. Seidman's (1988) conceptualization of prevention programs was applied to the literature on children's adjustment to parental divorce to illustrate the connection between stress theory and intervention.

Our current knowledge of stress processes clearly indicates that we need to broaden our conceptualization of stressful situations. No longer can we think of stress solely in terms of single life events and/or individual effects. It is important that we use our existing knowledge base of stress theory and empirical findings to guide the development of our interventions. We have seen that stress is a complex interactive process involving multiple personal and environmental variables that affect each other over time. Consequently, stress processes must be analyzed from multiple levels, including the individual, setting, and mesolevels.

Such a comprehensive analysis will allow prevention researchers to articulate the anticipated chain of reactions or interactions among variables over time and across levels. This will indicate potential targets of intervention at each level in the stress process. Such planning should offer innovative ideas for the development of higher-level interventions (e.g., policies, settings), and should be useful in guiding the design of future evaluation efforts by indicating what proximal and distal outcomes are anticipated and, subsequently, need to be assessed. Overall, future action models for stress prevention must entail going beyond the study of individual effects of a single stressor, and move toward the study of stress processes across levels of analyses.

Acknowledgments. Support was provided by NIMH Grant #P50-MH39246 for the Arizona State University Preventive Intervention Research Center and T32-MH18387 for support training in prevention research.

REFERENCES

Alpert-Gillis, L. J. (1987). *Children of Divorce Intervention Program: Implementation of a program for young urban children.* Doctoral dissertation, University of Rochester, Rochester, NY.

Amato, P. R., & Keith, B. (1991). Parental divorce and the well- being of children: A meta-analysis. *Psychological Bulletin, 110*, 26–46.

Antonovsky, A. (1979). *Health, stress and coping*. San Francisco: Jossey-Bass.

Baron, R. M., & Kenny, D. A. (1986). The moderator-mediator variable distinction in social psychological research: Conceptual, strategic, and statistical considerations. *Journal of Personality and Social Psychology, 51*, 1173–1182.

Barrera, M. (1988). Models of social support and life stress: Beyond the buffering hypothesis. In L. H. Cohen (Ed.), *Life events and psychological functioning. Theoretical and methodological issues* (pp. 211–236). Beverly Hills, CA: Sage.

Barrera, M., Jr., & Aimley, S. (1983). Structure of social support: A conceptual and empirical analysis. *Journal of Community Psychology, 11*, 133–143.

Barrera, M. J. (1986). Distinctions between social support concepts, measures and models. *American Journal of Community Psychology, 14*, 413–445.

Bay, R. C., & Braver, S. L. (1990). Perceived control of the divorce settlement process and interparental conflict. *Family Relations, 39*, 382–387.

Bloom, B. (1979). Prevention of mental disorders: Recent advances in theory and practice. *Community Mental Health Journal, 15*, 179–191.

Bloom, B. L., Asher, S. L., & White, S. W. (1978). Marital disruption as a stressor: A review and analysis. *Psychological Bulletin, 85*, 867–894.

Bloom, B. L., Hodges, W. F., & Caldwell, R. A. (1982). A preventive program for the newly separated: Initial evaluation. *American Journal of Community Psychology, 10*, 251–264.

Braver, S. L., Gonzalez, D., Wolchik, S. A., & Sandler, I. N. (1985). Economics hardship and psychological distress in custodial mothers. *Journal of Divorce, 24*, 19–34.

Braver, S. L., Wolchik, S. A., Sandler, I. N., Sheets, V. L., Fogas, B., & Bay, R. C. (1993). A longitudinal study of noncustodial parents: Parents without children. *Journal of Family Psychology, 7*, 9–23.

Brehm, J. (1965). *A theory of psychological reactance*. New York: Academic.

Brothman, E., & Weisz, J. R. (1988). How to feel better when it feels bad: Children's perspectives on coping with everyday stress. *Developmental Psychology, 24*, 247–253.

Brown, G. W., & Harris, T. (1978). *Social origins of depression*. New York: Free Press.

Brown, G. W., Harris, T. O., & BiFulco, A. (1986). Long-term effects of early loss of parent. In M. Rutter, C. E. Izard, & P. B. Read (Eds.), *Depression in young people: Developmental and clinical perspectives* (pp. 251–284). New York: Guilford.

Caplan, G. (1964). *Principles of preventive psychology*. New York: Basic Books.

Caplan, R. D., Vinokur, A. D., Price, R. H., & van Ryn, M. (1989). Job seeking, reemployment and mental health: A randomized field experiment in coping with job loss. *Journal of Applied Psychology, 74*, 759–769.

Catalano, R., & Dooley, D. (1983). Health effects of economic instability: A test of economic stress hypothesis. *Journal of Health and Social Behavior, 24*, 46–60.

Cohen, S., & Edwards, J. R. (1989). Personality characteristics as moderators of the relationship between stress and disorders. In R. W. J. Neufeld (Ed.), *Advances in the investigation of psychological stress* (pp. 235–283). New York: Wiley.

Cohen, S., & Hoberman, H. (1983). Positive events and social supports as buffers of life change stress. *Journal of Applied Social Psychology, 13*, 99–125.

Cohen, S., Karmack, T., & Mermelstein, R. (1983). A global measure of perceived stress. *Journal of Health and Social Behavior, 24*, 385–396.

Cohen, S., & Lazarus, R. S. (1973). Active coping processes, coping dispositions, and recovery from surgery. *Psychosomatic Medicine, 35*, 375–389.

Cohen, S., & McKay, G. (1983). Social support, stress, and the buffering hypothesis: A theoretical analysis. In A. Barun, J. E. Singer, & S. F. Taylor (Eds.), *Handbook of psychology and health, Vol. 4* (pp. 253–267). Hillsdale, NJ: Lawrence Erlbaum.

Cohen, S., & Wills, T. (1985). Stress, social support, and the buffering hypothesis. *Psychological Bulletin, 98*, 310–357.

Danner, A. H. (1991). A court mandated parent divorce class. *The Advocate*, 17.

Derogatis, L. R. (1982). Self-report measures of stress. In L. Goldberg & S. Brezaite (Eds.), *Handbook of stress. Theoretical and clinical aspects* (pp. 270–294). New York: Free Press.

Dohrenwend, B. S. (1973). Social status and stressful life events. *Journal of Personality and Social Psychology, 28*, 225–235.

Dohrenwend, B. S. (1978). Social stress and community psychology. *American Journal of Community Psychology, 6*, 1–14.

Dohrenwend, B. S., Krasnoff, L., Ajkenasy, A. R., & Dohrenwend, B. P. (1978). Exemplification of a method for scaling life event: the PERI life events scale. *Journal of Health and Social Behavior, 19*, 205–229.

Dohrenwend, B. S, & Shrout, P. E. (1985). Hassles in the conceptualization and measurement of life stress variables. *American Psychologist, 40,* 780–785.

Emery, R. E. (1982). Interparental conflict and the children of discord and divorce. *Psychological Bulletin, 92,* 310–330.

Emery, R. E., Hetherington, E. M., & DiLalla, L. F. (1984). Divorce, children, and social policy. In H. W. Stevenson & A. E. Siegel (Eds.), *Child development research and social policy, Vol. 1* (pp. 189–266). Chicago: University of Chicago Press.

Emery, R. E., & Wyer, M. M. (1987). Child custody mediation and litigation: An experimental evaluation of the experience of parents. *Journal of Consulting and Clinical Psychology, 55,* 179–186.

Emery, R. E., & Wyer, M. M. (1987). Divorce mediation. *American Psychologist, 42,* 472–480.

Felner, R. D., & Adan, A. M. (1989). The school transitional environment project: An ecological intervention and evaluation. In R. H. Price, E. L. Cowen, R. P. Lorion, & J. Ramos-McKay (Eds.), *Fourteen ounces of prevention: A casebook for practitioners* (pp. 111–123). Washington, D.C.: American Psychological Association.

Felner, R. D., Farber, S. S., & Primavera, J. (1980). Children of divorce, stressful life events and transitions: A framework for preventive efforts. In R. H. Price, B. C. Ketterer, & J. Monahan (Eds.), *Prevention in community mental health: Research policy and practice, Vol. 1* (pp. 81–108). Beverly Hills, CA: Sage.

Felner, R. D., Rowlinson, R. T., & Terre, L. (1986). Unraveling the Gordian knot in life change inquiry. A critical examination of crisis, stress and transitional frameworks of procition. In S. M. Auerbusch & A. L. Stolberg (Eds.), *Crisis intervention with children* (pp. 39–63). Washington: Hemisphere.

Fogas, B. S. (1986). *Parenting behavior as a moderator for children after divorce.* Unpublished masters thesis, Arizona State University.

Folkman, S. (1984). Personal control and stress and coping processes: A theoretical analysis. *Journal of Personality and Social Psychology, 46,* 839–852.

Folkman, S., & Lazarus, R. S. (1980). An analysis of coping in a middle-aged community sample. *Journal of Health and Social Behavior, 21,* 219–239.

Folkman, S., Lazarus, R. S., Dunkel-Schetter, DeLongis, A., & Gruen, R. J. (1986). Dynamics of a stressful encounter: Cognitive appraisal, coping and encounter outcomes. *Journal of Personality and Social Psychology, 50,* 992–1003.

Ganellen, R. J., & Blaney, P. H. (1984). Hardiness and social support as moderators of the effects of life stress. *Journal of Personality and Social Psychology, 42,* 145–155.

Garfinkel, I. (1988). The evolution of child support. *Focus.* University of Wisconsin—Madison Institute for Research on Poverty. *11*(1), 11–16.

Garfinkel, I. (1992). *Assuring child support: An extension of social security.* New York: Russell Sage.

Garfinkel, I., & Klawitter, M. M. (1992). The effect of routine income withholding on child support collections. In I. Garfinkel, S. McLanahan, & P. K. Robins (Eds.), *Child support assurance: Design issues, expected impacts and political barriers as seen from Wisconsin* (pp. 229–253). Washington, D.C.: The Urban Institute Press.

Gersten, J. C., Langner, T. S., Eisenberg, J. G., & Orzeck, L. (1974). Child behavior and life events: Undesirable change or change per se. In B. S. Dohrenwend & B. P. Dohrenwend (Eds.), *Stressful life events: Their nature and effects* (pp. 159–171). New York: Wiley.

Gersten, J. C., Langner, T. S., Eisenberg, J. G., & Simcher-Fagan, O. (1977). An evaluation of the etiological role of stressful life-change events in psychological disorder. *Journal of Health and Social Behavior, 18,* 65–83.

Gordon, A. R., et al. (1991). *Income withholding, medical support and services to non-AFDC cases after the Child Support Enforcement Amendments of 1984.* Report of Office of Child Support Enforcement. Mathematical Policy Research Inc., Princeton, N.J.

Grinker, R. R., & Speigel, J. P. (1945). *Men under stress.* New York: McGraw-Hill.

Guidibaldi, J., Cleminshaw, H. K., Perry, J. D., & McLoughlin, C. S. (1983). The impact of parental divorce on children: Report of the nationwide NASP study. *School Psychology Review, 12,* 300–323.

Heller, K., Price, R. H., & Sher, K. J. (1980). Research and evaluation in primary prevention: Issues and guidelines. In R. H. Price, F. Ketterer, B. C. Bader, & J. Monahan (Eds.), *Prevention in mental health: Research, policy, and practice, Vol. 1* (pp. 285–313). Beverly Hills, CA: Sage.

Hess, R., & Camara K. (1979). Post-divorce family relationships as mediating factors in the consequences of divorce for children. *Journal of Social Issues, 35,* 79–96.

Hetherington, E. M., Cox, M., & Cox, R. (1976). The aftermath of divorce. In J. H. Stevens & M. Mathews (Eds.), *Mother/child father/child relationships* (pp. 149–176). Washington, D.C.: National Association for the Education of Young Children.

Hobfoll, S. E. (1998). *Stress, culture, and community: The psychology and philosophy of stress.* New York: Plenum.

Holmes, T. H., & Masuda, M. (1974). Life change and illness susceptibility. In B. S. Dohrenwend & B. P. Dohrenwend (Eds.), *Stressful life events: Their nature and effects* (pp. 45–73). New York: Wiley.

Holmes, T. H., & Rahe, R. H. (1967). The social readjustment rating scale. *Journal of Psychosomatic Research, 11,* 213–218.

Institute for Research on Poverty (April, 1985). *Preliminary report on the effects of the Wisconsin Child Support Reform Demonstration.* University of Wisconsin, Madison.

Jacobson, G. F. (1983). *The multiple crises of marital separation and divorce.* New York: Grune & Stratton.

Janis, I. L. (1958). *Psychological Stress: Psychoanalytic and behavioral studies of surgical patients.* New York: Wiley.

Kanner, A. D., Coyne, J. C., Schaefer, C., & Lazarus, R. S. (1981). Comparison of two modes of stress measurement: Daily hassles and uplifts versus major life events. *Journal of Behavioral Medicine, 4,* 1–39.

Kessler, R. (1979). Stress, social status and psychological distress. *Journal of Health and Social Behavior, 20,* 259–272.

Kessler, R., Turner, J. B., & House, J. S. (1987). Unemployment and health in a community sample. *Journal of Health and Social Behavior, 28,* 51–59.

Kim, L. S., Sandler, I. N., & Tein, J. Y. (1997). Locus of control as a stress moderator and mediator in children of divorce. *Journal of Abnormal Child Psychology, 25,* 145–155.

Kobasa, S. C. (1979). Stressful life events, personality and health: An inquiry into hardiness. *Journal of Personality and Social Psychology, 37,* 1–11.

Kobasa, S. C., Maddi, S. R., & Kahn, J. (1982). Hardiness and health: A prospective study. *Journal of Personality and Social Psychology, 42,* 168–177.

Kramer, L., & Washo, C. A. (1993). Evaluation of a court-mandated prevention program for divorcing parents: The Children First Program. *Family Relations, 42,* 179–186.

Kruk, E. (1992). Psychological and structural factors contributing to the disengagement of noncustodial fathers after divorce. *Family and Conciliation Courts Review, 30,* 81–101.

Kurdek, L. A., & Berg, B. (1983). Correlates of children's adjustment to their parents divorce. In L. A. Kurdek (Ed.), *Children and divorce, new directions for child development* (pp. 47–60). San Francisco: Jossey-Bass.

Lazarus, R. S. (1991). *Emotion and adaptation.* New York: Oxford University Press.

Lazarus, R. S., DeLongis, A., Folkman, S., & Gruen, R. (1985). Stress and adaptational outcomes: The problem of confounded measures. *American Psychologist, 40,* 770–779.

Lazarus, R. S., & Folkman, S. (1984). *Stress, appraisal and coping.* New York: Springer.

Lewinsohn, P. M., & Amenson, C. S. (1978). Some relations between pleasant and unpleasant mood related events and depression. *Journal of Abnormal Psychology, 87,* 644–654.

Lewinsohn, P. M., & Graf, M. (1973). Pleasant activities and depression. *Journal of Consulting and Clinical Psychology, 41,* 261–268.

Liem, R., & Liem, J. H. (1981). Relations among social class, life events and mental illness: A comment on findings and methods. In B. S. Dohrenwend & B. P. Dohrenwend (Eds.), *Stressful life events and their contexts* (pp. 234–256). New Brunswick, NJ: Rutgers University Press.

McGrath, J. E. (1970). A conceptual formulation for research on stress. In J. E. McGrath (Ed.), *Social and psychological factors in stress* (pp. 10–21). New York: Holt, Rinehart and Winston.

Myers, S., Gallas, B., Hanson, R., & Keilitz, S. (1988). Divorce mediation in the States: Institutionalization, use and assessment. *State Court Journal, 12,* 17–25.

Nelson, G. (1989). Life strains, coping, and emotional well-being: A longitudinal study of recently separated and married women. *American Journal of Community Psychology, 17,* 459–482.

Office of Child Support Enforcement. (1990). *Child Support Enforcement,* Fifteenth Annual Report to Congress, for the Period Ending September 30, 1990. Washington, D.C.

Parkes, C. M. (1972). *Bereavement.* New York: International Universities Press.

Paykel, R. S. (1978). Contribution of life events to causation of psychiatric illness. *Psychological Medicine, 8,* 245–253.

Pearlin, L. I. (1975). Status inequality and stress in marriage. *American Sociological Review, 40,* 344–357.

Pearlin, L. I. (1982). The social contexts of stress. In L. Golberger & S. Breznitz (Eds.), *Handbook of stress* (pp. 367–379). New York: Free Press.

Pearlin, L. I. (1983). Role strains and personal stress. In H. B. Kaplan (Ed.), *Psychological stress* (pp. 3–32). New York: Academic.

Pearlin, L. I., Lieberman, M. A., Menaghen, E. G., & Mullan, J. T. (1981). The stress process. *Journal of Health and Social Behavior, 22,* 337–356.

Pearson, J., Thoennes, N., & Anhalt, J. (1992). Child support in the United States: The experience in Colorado. *Family and Conciliation Courts Review, 31,* 226–243.

Pearson, J., & Thoennes, N. (1989). Reflections on a decade of divorce mediation research. In K. Kressel, D. Pruitt, & Associates (Eds.), *Mediation research: The process and effectiveness of third-party intervention* (pp. 17–35). San Francisco: Jossey-Bass.

Pearson, J., Thoennes, N., & Tjaden, P. (1989). Legislating adequacy: The impact of child support guidelines. *Law and Society Review, 23*, 569–590.

Pedro-Carroll, J., & Alpert-Gillis, L. (1987). *The Children of Divorce Intervention Program's Developmental and Cultural Considerations.* Paper presented at the 95th Annual Convention of the APA.

Pedro-Carroll, J., & Cowen, E. L. (1985). The Children of Divorce Intervention Program: An investigation of the efficacy of a school-based prevention program. *Journal of Consulting and Clinical Psychology, 53*, 603–611.

Pedro-Carroll, J., Cowen, E. L., Hightower, A. D., & Guare, J. C. (1986). Preventive intervention with latency-aged children of divorce: A replication study. *American Journal of Community Psychology, 14*, 277–290.

Pedro-Carroll, J. L., & Cowen, E. L. (1987). The Children of Divorce Intervention Program: Implementation and evaluation of a time limited group approach. In J. E. Vincent (Ed.), *Advances in family intervention, assessment and theory, Vol. 4*, Greenwich, CT: SAI.

Pillow, D., Braver, S., Sandler, I., & Wolchik, S. (1988). *Theory based screening of subjects for a prevention program for divorced parents.* Paper presented at the American Psychological Association Convention, San Francisco, CA.

Redfield, J., & Stone, A. (1979). Individual viewpoints of stressful life events. *Journal of Consulting and Clinical Psychology, 47*, 147–154.

Reich, J. W., & Zautra, A. (1981). Life events and personal causation: Some relationships with satisfaction and distress. *Journal of Personality and Social Psychology, 41*, 1001–1012.

Reich, J. W., & Zautra, A. J. (1988). Direct and stress-moderating effects of positive life experiences. In L. H. Cohen (Ed.), *Life events and psychological functioning. Theoretical and methodological issues* (pp. 149–180). Beverly Hills, CA: Sage.

Roosa, M. W., Sandler, I. N., Beals, J., & Short, J. L. (1988). Risk status of adolescent children of problem-drinking parents. *American Journal of Community Psychology, 16*, 225–239.

Sandler, I., Ayers, T., Suter, J., Schultz, A., & Twohey, J. (in press). Adversities, strengths, and public policy. In. B. Leadbetter, K. Maton, C. Schellenbach, & A. Solarz (Eds.), *Strengths basaed public policies.* Washington, D.C.: American Psychological Association.

Sandler, I., Gersten, J. C., Reynolds, K., Kallgren, C. A., & Ramirez, R. (1988). Using theory and data to plan support interventions: Design of a program for bereaved children. In B. H. Gottlieb (Ed.), *Marshaling social support formats, processes and effects* (pp. 53–83). Beverly Hills, CA: Sage.

Sandler, I., Miller, P., Short, J., & Wolchik, S. (1989). Social support as a protective factor for children in stress. In D. Belle (Ed.), *Children's social networks and social supports* (pp. 277–308). New York: Wiley.

Sandler, I. N. (1979). Life stress and community psychology. In I. G. Sarason & C. D. Spielberger (Eds.), *Stress and anxiety, Vol. 6* (pp. 213–232). New York: Wiley.

Sandler, I. N., & Guenther, R. T. (1985). Assessment of life stress events. In P. Karoly (Ed.), *Measurement strategies in health psychology* (pp. 555–600). New York: Wiley.

Sandler, I. N., & Ramsay, T. B. (1982). Dimensional analysis of children's stressful life events. *American Journal of Community Psychology, 8*, 285–302.

Sandler, I. N., Tein, J.-Y., Mehta, P., Wolchik, S., & Ayers, T. (in press). Coping efficacy as a mediator of the effects of coping on psychological symptoms for preadolescent children of divorce. *Child Development.*

Sandler, I. N., Tein, J.-Y., & West, S. G. (1994). Coping, stress and psychological symptoms of children of divorce: A cross-sectional and longitudinal study. *Child Development, 65*, 1744–1763.

Sandler, I. N., West, S. G., Baca L., Pillow, D. R., Gersten, J. C., Rogosch, F., Virdin, L., Beals, J., Reynolds, K. D., Kallgren, C., Tein, J.-Y., Kriege, G., Cole, E., & Ramirez, R. (1992). Linking empirically based theory and evaluation: The Family Bereavement Program. *American Journal of Community Psychology, 20*, 491–521.

Sandler, I. N., Wolchik, S. A., Braver, S. L., & Fogas, B. S. (1986). Significant events of children of divorce: Toward the assessment of risky situations. In S. M. Auerbach & A. L. Stolberg (Eds.), *Crisis intervention with children and families* (pp. 65–81). New York: Hemisphere.

Sandler, I. N., Wolchik, S. A., MacKinnon, D., Ayers, T., & Roosa, M. W. (1997). Developing linkages between theory and intervention in stress and coping processes. In S. A. Wolchik & I. N. Sandler (Eds.), *Handbook of children's coping: Linking theory and intervention* (pp. 3–41). New York: Plenum.

Sarason, I. G., Johnson, J. G., & Siegel, J. M. (1978). Assessing the impact of life changes: Development of the Life Experience Survey. *Journal of Consulting and Clinical Psychology, 46*, 932–946.

Seidman, E. (1987). Toward a framework for primary prevention research. In J. A. Steinber & M. M. Silverman (Eds.), *Preventing mental disorders: A research perspective* (pp. 2–19). Washington, D.C.: US Government Printing Office.

Seidman, E. (1988). Back to the future, community psychology: Unfolding a theory of social intervention. *American Journal of Community Psychology, 16*, 3–24.

Sheets, V., Sandler, I. N., & West, S. G. (1996). Negative appraisals of stressful events by preadolescent children of divorce. *Child Development, 67*, 2166–2182.

Silverman, P. R. (1989). Widow-to-Widow: A mutual help program the widowed. In R. H. Price, E. L. Cowen, R. P. Lorion, & J. Ramos-McKay (Eds.), *Fourteen ounces of prevention: A casebook for practitioners* (pp. 175–187). Washington, D.C.: American Psychological Association.

Sterling, S. E. (1986). *A school-based intervention program for early latency-aged children of divorce.* Unpublished doctoral dissertation, University of Rochester, Rochester, NY.

Stolberg, A. L., & Garrison, K. M. (1985). Evaluating a primary prevention program for children of divorce: The Divorce Adjustment project. *American Journal of Community Psychology, 13,* 111–124.

Stone, A. A., Helder, L., & Schneider, M. S. (1988). Coping with stressful events: Coping dimensions and issues. In L. H. Cohen (Ed.), *Life events and psychological functioning* (pp. 182–211). Beverly Hills, CA: Sage.

Stone, A. A., & Neale, J. M. (1984). New measure of daily coping: Development and preliminary results. *Journal of Personality and Social Psychology, 46,* 892–906.

Swindle, R. W., Heller, K., & Lakey, B. (1988). A conceptual reorientation to the study of personality and stressful life events. In L. H. Cohen (Ed.), *Life events and psychological functioning. Theoretical and methodological issues* (pp. 237–268). Beverly Hills, CA: Sage.

Tausig, M. (1982). Measuring life events. *Journal of Health and Social Behavior, 23,* 52–64.

Taylor, S. E. (1983). Adjustment to threatening events: A theory of cognitive adaptation. *American Psychologist, 38,* 1161–1173.

Thoits, P. A. (1983). Dimensions of life events that influence psychological distress: A evaluation and synthesis of the literature. In H. G. Kaplan (Ed.), *Psychosocial stress: Trends in theory and research* (pp. 33–103). New York: Academic.

Thoits, P. A. (1986). Social support as coping assistance. *Journal of Counseling and Clinical Psychology, 54,* 416–423.

*Tschann, J. M., Johnston, J. R., & Wallerstein, J. S. (1989). Resources, stressors, and attachment as predictors of adjustment after divorce: A longitudinal study. *Journal of Marriage and the Family, 51,* 1033–1046.

Turner, R. J., & Wheaton, B. (1995). Checklist measurement of stressful life events. In S. Cohen, R. C. Kessler, & L. U. Gordon (Eds.), *Measuring stress: A guide for health and social scientists* (pp. 29–59). New York: Oxford University Press.

Vinokur, A., & Selzer, M. L. (1975). Desirable versus undesirable life events: Their relationship to stress and mental distress. *Journal of Consulting and Clinical Psychology, 32,* 329–337.

Weiss, R. S. (1975). *Marital separation.* New York: Basic Books.

Wellman, B. (1981). Applying network analysis to the study of social support. In B. H. Gottlieb (Ed.), *Social networks and social support* (pp. 171–201). Beverly Hills, CA: Sage.

Wethington, E., Brown, G. W., & Kessler, R. C. (1995). Interview measurement of stressful life events. In S. Cohen, R. C. Kessler, & L. U. Gordon (Eds.), *Measuring stress: A guide for health and social scientists* (pp. 59–80). New York: Oxford University Press.

Wheaten, B. (1985). Models for the stress-buffering functions of coping resources. *Journal of Health and Social Behavior, 26,* 352–364.

Wolchik, S. A., Beals, J., & Sandler, I. N. (1989). Mapping children's social support networks: Conceptual and methodological issues. In D. Belle (Ed.), *Children's social networks and social support* (pp. 191–221). New York: Wiley.

Wolchik, S. A., Sandler, I. N., Braver, S. L., & Fogas, B. S. (1986). Events of parental divorce: Stressfulness ratings by children, parents and clinicians. *American Journal of Community Psychology, 14,* 59–74.

Wolchik, S. A., West, S. G., Sandler, I. N., Tein, J.-Y., Coatsworth, D., Lengua, L., Weiss, L., Anderson, E. R., Greene, S. M., & Griffin, W. A. (in press). The New Beginnings Program for divorced families: An experimental evaluation of theory-based single-component and dual-component programs. *Journal of Consulting and Clinical Psychology.*

Wolchik, S. A., West, S. G., Westover, S., Sandler, I. N., Martin, A., Lustig, J., Tein, J.-Y., & Fisher, J. (1993). The Children of Divorce Intervention Project: Outcome evaluation of an empirically based parenting program. *American Journal of Community Psychology, 21,* 293–331.

Zautra, A., Guarnaccia, C., & Dohrenwend, B. P. (1986). Measuring small life events. *American Journal of Community Psychology, 14,* 629–655.

Zautra, A., & Reich, J. (1983). Life events and perceptions of life quality: Developments in a two-factor approach. *Journal of Community Psychology, 11,* 121–132.

Zill, N. (1978). *Divorce, marital happiness and the mental health of children: Findings from the national survey of children.* Paper presented at the NIMH Workshop on Divorce and Children, Bethesda, MD, February.

Zill, N. (1983). *Happy, healthy and insecure.* New York: Doubleday Anchor.

CHAPTER 10

Social Support Research in Community Psychology

MANUEL BARRERA JR.

Social support is a central concept in community psychology. It is a concept that attempts to capture helping transactions that occur between people who share the same households, schools, neighborhoods, workplaces, organizations, and other community settings. From our own experiences, we are all aware of the benefits that can occur, both tangible and intangible, when neighbors help neighbors in both everyday tasks and emergencies. We are aware that in response to disasters, entire communities can become mobilized in rendering help to family, friends, neighbors, and complete strangers. Intuitively, we understand how the degree of caring expressed between community members can contribute to our psychological sense of community and the perceived safety of the places in which we live. In some of the most challenging moments of our lives, when we are faced with profound loss, serious threats to health, or personal adversity, we often seek out others for information, reassurance, advice, or concrete aid. Because our experience of social support is common and at times dramatic, it is easy to comprehend that as social scientists we became fascinated with trying to measure these natural resources, understanding their relation to adapting to adversity, and harnessing their power in planned interventions.

The concept of social support is connected to many of the other fundamental concepts in community psychology, such as the ecology of natural resources, psychological sense of community, prevention, adaptation to life stress, well-being, and even empowerment (Barrera & Perlow, in press; Bogat, Sullivan, & Grober, 1993; Cowen, 1994). From our social ecology perspective, informal helpers are viewed as natural resources that exist in communities. Gerald and Ruth Caplan and their colleagues were among the first to recognize the potential applications of natural support systems and mutual help in prevention and community mental health (Caplan, 1972; Caplan, 1976). Albee (1982) gave a prominent role to social support in his analyses that linked prevention to the epidemiology of psychopathology. Cowen (1994) described several pathways by which individuals achieve psychological well-being, which included attachment and competencies that are developed through social ties. Empowerment

---

MANUEL BARRERA JR. • Department of Psychology, Arizona State University, Tempe, Arizona 85287.

Handbook of Community Psychology, edited by Julian Rappaport and Edward Seidman. Kluwer Academic/Plenum Publishers, New York, 2000.

is defined as the process of gaining influence over events and outcomes of importance, a definition that incorporates both individuals' perceptions of personal control as well as behaviors to exercise control (Rappaport, 1987; Zimmerman, 1995). Perkins and Zimmerman (1995) saw empowerment as "a construct that links individual strengths and competencies, natural helping systems, and proactive behaviors to social policy and social change" (p. 569). It is difficult to identify a community psychology concept that is not related in some way to social support and social networks.

The once frenzied pace of social support research has slowed somewhat, but a deep literature has been built over the past 20 years. In their *Annual Review of Psychology* chapter on community and social interventions, Gesten and Jason (1987) commented that the literature on social support was the largest of any they reviewed. Subsequent *Annual Review* chapters concerned with social factors and psychopathology (Coyne & Downey, 1991), social interventions (Heller, 1990), and sociology (House, Umberson, & Landis, 1988), also featured social support. Still other reviewers noted that hundreds of articles dealing with social support were identified in *Psychological Abstracts* each year since "Social support networks" appeared as an index term (Shumaker & Brownell, 1984; Vaux, 1985). My own PsychLIT search of articles that contained the words "social support" in the title or abstract showed a rapid increase from 1978 (25 annual citations) to 1984 (555 annual citations) that then leveled off somewhat but there were still 707 citations in 1996 (Barrera, 1997). Only a fraction of this research could be considered community psychology literature, but these numbers reflect the tremendous interest in this concept throughout the subareas of psychology.

What has community psychology research taught us about social support? This chapter does not provide an exhaustive answer to this question, but it is intended to present some highlights. It is organized around six topics that have been focal points of research and have significance for community psychology: measurement, the empirical structure of support, the determinants of support, models of support's beneficial effects, negative influences of social interaction, and interventions. In addition to being a review of these topics, the chapter is intended to fit the spirit of a handbook by serving as a historical guide to key issues for those who are familiar with social support research, as well as those who are interested newcomers.

The terms "social network" and "social support" have appeared together prominently in the literature, such as in the title of Gottlieb's (1981) influential book *Social Networks and Social Support*. They are two generic and partially overlapping concepts. "Social network" is both a metaphor that conveys the idea that individuals or social units (such as community agencies) are linked to each other by various relationships, and an analytic strategy for investigating the properties of social systems (Wellman, 1981). Social network analysis has come to epitomize a "structural" approach to social support assessment because it emphasizes quantifiable methods of describing composition of the network and the pattern of linkages between network members. Characteristics such as network size, density, multiplexity, and reciprocity are some of the common quantifiable indicators used in network analysis (d'Abbs, 1982; Mitchell & Trickett, 1980). The concept of social network is much broader than that of social support. "Social support" is only one of many provisions that can define a linkage between network members. Linkages or relationships could be defined by political influence, communication of a contagious disease, business transactions, or any number of other types of exchange.

Social support is not confined to the study of social networks. This is apparent in many of the prominent measurement strategies, particularly those that assess perceived social support (e.g., Cohen, Mermelstein, Kamarck, & Hoberman, 1985; Procidano & Heller, 1983). With these strategies the goal is to evaluate individuals' appraisals of the availability or quality of support. There appears to be a growing trend to study the cognitive appraisal aspects of social support, rather than structural properties that are addressed in social network analysis (Lieberman, 1986), a trend that Coyne and DeLongis (1986) labeled the "cognitization" of social support. These measurement approaches are not intended to arrive at a number of supportive acquaintances or to quantify other structural characteristics. Thus, social network analysis complements other methods of conceptualizing and measuring social support.

In this chapter, the terms social support and social network are not used synonymously. To keep the focus on social support, only those social network analyses that are closely tied to this concept are relevant for review and discussion. However, this is not a radical restriction for the community psychology literature, which has almost always employed social network analysis as a method for studying social support.

Almost all social support research has treated the individual as the unit of analysis (Felton & Shinn, 1992). Although social network analysis lends itself to research strategies that use the network as the unit of analysis, most network analyses identify "ego-centric" or personal networks because they are based on the self-reports of one key informant, i.e., the actual research participant. Criterion measures in social support research frequently assess concepts such as psychological symptoms, physical health, life satisfaction, stress, and other concepts that also are evaluated with the individual as the unit of analysis. Research on the environmental determinants of social support structure and function (e.g., Oxley, Barrera, & Sadalla, 1981; Oxley & Barrera, 1984) might call for levels of analysis larger than the individual. For example, if we were interested in the influence of setting size and organizational structure on social support, communities, schools, work settings, religious congregations, or social groups could serve as units of analysis. Because research on these topics rarely appears in the literature, this review is limited to levels of analysis that almost always feature the individual.

There are other constraints to the chapter's scope that reflect options selected by the author. Because social support research emanates from several subfields within psychology (such as health, social, developmental, and clinical), and crosses many disciplinary boundaries (such as anthropology, sociology, and public health), difficult decisions were made to identify social support research that was most relevant to community psychology. There is growing literature on the relationships between personality variables and social support (e.g., Kobasa & Puccetti, 1983; Sarason, Shearin, Pierce, & Sarason, 1987), and the use of partners in clinical interventions (e.g., Mermelstein, Cohen, Lichtenstein, Baer, & Kamarck, 1986) that was not included in this review. Although there are critical conceptual issues that have been discussed in the literature, they were not featured so as to keep the spotlight on empirical findings. Readers are referred elsewhere for a discussion of conceptual issues, such as the definition of social support (Broadhead et al., 1983; Shumaker & Brownell, 1984; Vaux, 1988) and its distinctions from life stress (Barrera, 1986; Gore, 1981; Monroe, Bromet, Connell, & Steiner, 1986; Shinn, Lehmann, & Wong, 1984; Thoits, 1982).

SOCIAL SUPPORT ASSESSMENT

Development of Social Support Measures

One of the first challenges for social support research was the translation of intuitions and observations about natural helping transactions into the empirical development of social support measures. This has been a pivotal area of research for community psychologists because it has produced measurement tools that have made it possible to study substantive questions concerning theory and the application of social support principles. In addition, it has centered attention on issues of defining social support and clarified distinctions between its differing conceptualizations.

Researchers who are in need of social support/social network measures now have a number of options. There are many social support scales and social network measures that have adequate reliability and validity for many applications to community psychology research. The availability of options requires careful choices, however. Social support has been described as a meta-concept (Vaux, 1985) that encompasses several distinct concepts that are not highly related (Barrera, 1986). Concepts such as the frequency of help, number of supportive others, appraisals of support availability, and satisfaction with received support are just some that have been addressed in systematic scale-development efforts. It is clear that investigators must exercise judgment in selecting measures that fit the particular concepts of support that are specified in their research questions, rather than assuming that these measures are interchangeable.

Several excellent reviews surveyed this literature and provided careful analyses of individual measures (d'Abbs, 1982; Heitzman & Kaplan, 1988; House & Kahn, 1985; Sarason, Sarason, & Pierce, 1990; Tardy, 1985; Wolchik, Sandler, & Braver, 1987; Wood, 1984). Each analysis has a special orientation and scope. Wood's (1984) review is notable in that considerable attention was given to network measures. Seven measures of perceived social support, five measures for identifying network members, and several miscellaneous scales were featured. It included an orientation to network terminology such as density, clusters, boundary density, and multiplexity. Researchers who are unfamiliar with these terms will find her chapter valuable, as well as a small book by d'Abbs (1982) that is difficult to find, but contains impressive scholarship.

A review by Tardy (1985) included a discussion that delineated five characteristics of social support: direction (is support given or received?), disposition (availability or enactment of support), description/evaluation, content (or functions of support), and network. This author then selected seven specific measures that were clearly tied to the concept of social support and had at least some promising data regarding reliability and validity. These measures were the Arizona Social Support Interview Schedule (ASSIS; Barrera, 1981), the Inventory of Socially Supportive Behaviors (ISSB; Barrera, Sandler, & Ramsay, 1981), Perceived Social Support from Family and Friends (PSS-Fa, PSS-Fr; Procidano & Heller, 1983), the Social Relationship Scale (McFarlane, Neale, Norman, Roy, & Streiner, 1981), the Social Support Network Interview (Jones & Fisher, 1978), the Social Support Questionnaire (Sarason, Levine, Basham, & Sarason, 1983), and Social Support Vignettes (Turner, 1981). Tables contained in this article compared and contrasted the measures on the basis of characteristics such as direction, disposition, and content. In addition, the author summarized studies of each scale's psychometric properties.

Two reviews placed special emphasis on health outcomes (Heitzman & Kaplan, 1988; House & Kahn, 1985). Heitzman and Kaplan (1988) examined 19 separate methods for assessing some aspect of social support. Relative to other reviews, these authors were comprehensive in considering a range of formal social support measures and thorough in describing reliability and validity data. They concluded that several measures could be recommended on the basis of at least some supportive data. In addition to improving construct validity, the authors recognized the value of assessing the relationship between social support measures in order to discern areas of similarity and differences.

Wolchik et al. (1987) and Cauce, Reid, Landesman, & Gonzales (1990) provided reviews that focused on social support measures used in assessing children and adolescents. These authors found that the properties of only a few social support measures were evaluated with samples of children. Wolchik et al. (1987) noted that when psychometric properties were assessed, internal consistency reliabilities usually were adequate. On the other hand, stability (test–retest analyses) over intervals of 1–3 months were low. They found it difficult to interpret this lack of stability because interpersonal relationships of children can be expected to change over intervals of several months, particularly those children who experience upheavals such as parental divorce or separation. They argued that the more relevant psychometric question is *accuracy* of reporting, which might be assessed as stability of assessment over very brief intervals, such as a day or two.

Similar to reviewers of research with adults, Wolchik et al. (1987) identified the need for establishing the construct validity of social support measures used with children. In previous studies these social support measures have not always manifested strong relationships to measures of psychological distress or entered into interaction effects that are consistent with traditional models of buffering effects.

Social support research with children and adolescents has underscored the importance of distinguishing between subcomponents of the social support providers, particularly between parents and peers (Barrera & Garrison-Jones, 1992; Cauce & Srebnik, 1990; Wills, 1990; Wolchik, Beals, & Sandler, 1989). Wills (1990) pointed out that analyzing the effects of social support for adolescents is complicated because they belong to a number of networks, each capable of exerting a specific influence. Sensitivity to the social contexts of support (Hirsch, Engel-Levy, DuBois, & Hardesty, 1990) might lead us to make separate predictions about the influence of parents, siblings, school peers, or peers in formal organizations. In the literature on adolescent substance use (Wills & Vaughan, 1989) and depression (Barrera & Garrison-Jones, 1992), there are examples of studies in which parental support is positively related to good outcomes, while per support shows the opposite relationship (also see Barrera & Li, 1996). Drawing distinctions between types of providers will have special significance in future social support research with children as well as adults.

There have been a few developments that have not been discussed in published reviews. The psychometric properties of the Social Support Questionnaire (Sarason et al., 1983), perhaps the most widely used social support measure, received additional research (Sarason et al., 1987), including the development of a brief version (Sarason, Sarason, Shearin, & Pierce, 1987) and extensive comparisons with other social support instruments: (1) Social Network List (Stokes, 1983), (2) ISSB, (3) Family Environment Scale (Moos, Insel, & Humphrey, 1974), (4) ISEL (Cohen et al., 1985), (5) Perceived Social Support (Procidano & Heller, 1983), and (6) Inventory Schedule for Social Interaction (Henderson, Byrne, & Duncan-Jones, 1981). Studies conducted with university students showed that SSQ subscales of number (of support providers) and satisfaction (with support) were at least somewhat related to these other social support measures. However, the SSQ showed the strongest correlations with perceived social support scales, such as the ISEL and Perceived Social Support scale. These validation studies also reported extensive information on the relationship between the SSQ and individual difference variables such as social competence, depression, loneliness, and social anxiety.

Vaux developed measures of several different social support concepts, including social support appraisals (Vaux, Phillips, Holly, Thompson, Williams, & Stewart, 1986), perceived availability of supportive behavior (Vaux, Riedel, & Stewart, 1987), and network orientation (Vaux, Burda, & Stewart, 1986). Unfortunately, research describing these scales appeared in print after several major reviews had been completed.

Although Brown and colleagues made seminal contributions to the social support literature (e.g., Brown, Bhrolchain, & Harris, 1975), their approach for assessing social support is not well-known or often used by other researchers. The Self-Evaluation and Social Support (SESS) schedule is a semistructured interview that assesses both self-esteem and social support, particularly social support from intimates such as spouses and romantic partners. Its relative lack of use is almost certainly because it requires a large amount of time to administer (3–5 hours) and extensive training for both administration and scoring (Brown, Andrews, Harris, Adler, & Bridge, 1986; O'Connor & Brown, 1984). However, similar to his better-known interview methods for assessing life-stress events, the SESS appears to transform the richness of qualitative data (from an "ethnographic tradition") on confidant support and negative transactions into quantitative ratings. Despite the open-ended nature of questions and breadth of interview material that is rated, high inter-rater reliabilities were reported for a variety of scores that can be derived from the SESS (O'Connor & Brown, 1984). There are significant practical barriers to the use of the SESS, but it is a significant social support measure, particularly for epidemiological research on depression.

Conclusions

For each of the major domains of social support (social embeddedness, perceived social support, and enacted support), there are measures that have research to support at least some psychometric properties, most commonly internal consistency reliability. Almost every reviewer noted that measures usually lacked validity, especially construct validity. Careful evaluations of construct validity will encourage investigators to encounter questions that are central to the concept of construct validity. For example, what is "the theoretical network that surrounds the concept ... to generate theoretical predictions which, in turn, lead directly to empirical tests involving measures of the concept"? (Carmines & Zeller, 1979, p. 23). The significance of this question goes well beyond the pragmatic considerations of scale development. In construct validity, failures to confirm predictions can be interpreted as either a shortcoming of the scale or a shortcoming of the theory. In the past, construct validity for social support scales has meant that they were expected to show direct relationships to measures of illness or psychological distress, or to enter into interactions with stress measures that were consistent with the stress-buffering effect. As we draw distinctions between various social support concepts and expand the range of viable models of support effects (Barrera, 1986), validating all social support measures by demonstrating their direct effects on illness/distress criteria will be regarded as inappropriate or unnecessarily restrictive.

Although social support measures and social network analyses have been applied to a wide range of samples and problems, there are limitations to the range of samples that have been used in studies that were designed explicitly to evaluate the psychometric properties of measures. With only a few exceptions (Henderson et al., 1981; Jones & Fischer, 1978) university students serve as participants in these studies, particularly in the initial scale-development phases of various measures (Barrera et al., 1981; Cohen et al., 1985; Procidano & Heller, 1984; Sarason et al., 1983, 1987; Slavin & Compas, 1989; Vaux et al., 1986, 1987). The use of a readily available, inexpensive, and large pool of subjects is defensible for preliminary work, but it is disappointing when scale development is not extended to community samples for additional validation research.

Compared to the availability of social support scales for adults, measures suitable for use with children and adolescents are less well-developed (Belle, 1989). Extensions of research to children, particularly young children, will enrich the measurement literature because it will prompt investigators to consider assessment methods other than self-report. This will encourage the reconsideration of questions concerning the correspondence between phenomenological and externally observable measures of social support.

EMPIRICAL STRUCTURE OF SOCIAL SUPPORT

Theoretical Importance of Support Structure

There are numerous conceptual analyses of social support dimensions and rational taxonomies of social support functions (Barrera & Ainlay, 1983; Caplan, 1976; Cutrona & Russell, 1990; Gottlieb, 1978; Hirsch, 1980; House, 1981; Kaplan, Cassel, & Gore, 1977; Tolsdorf, 1976; Weiss, 1969). More recently, researchers have conducted empirical analyses to identify factors or clusters of social support elements. The value of these empirical approaches is in understanding questions concerning the structure of social support. Are there meaningful subtypes of social support that can be used to identify specific support functions or to capture dimensions underlying helping transactions? Answers to this question can then be used to address other questions that move beyond analyses of global-support indicators. Do different types of helpers provide different subtypes of support? Do dimensions or subtypes of support interact with specific categories of stress or show distinct relationships to measures of psychological distress? This last question in particular has special significance for one of the few theoretical perspectives to emerge in the social support literature.

The proposition that social support buffering effects are primarily observed when specific types of supportive provisions match specific needs was asserted by Cohen and McKay (1984) and by Cutrona in her development of "optimal matching" theory (Cutrona, 1990; Cutrona & Russell, 1990). This perspective is built on the critical assumption that social support can be disaggregated into conceptually and empirically distinct components. As a result, studies concerned with the structure of social support have provided an essential research base for tests of this theory.

Social Support Functions

Structure obviously is influenced by the content of the social support elements that are analyzed. One measure of supportive functions, the Inventory of Socially Supportive Behaviors (ISSB; Barrera et al., 1981), has been subjected to several factor, cluster, and confirmatory factor analyses by independent researchers (Barrera & Ainlay, 1983; Caldwell & Reinhart, 1988; Finch, Barrera, Okun, Bryant, Pool, & Snow-Turek, 1997; McCormick, Siegert, & Walkey, 1987; Newcomb, 1990; Stokes & Wilson, 1984). Although these studies employed different analytic procedures, there is substantial congruence between the observed structures.

In the first of these factor analyses, four factors were interpreted: directive guidance (advice), nondirective support (emotional support), positive social interaction, and tangible assistance (material aid and physical assistance) (Barrera & Ainlay, 1983). These factors resembled components that have been identified with some consistency in conceptual analyses of social support functions. This structure was replicated with an independent sample using confirmatory factor analysis (Finch et al., 1997). Other studies have found variations of this four-factor solution, sometimes simplified to just the three factors: emotional support, guidance, and tangible aid (Caldwell & Reinhart, 1988; McCormick et al., 1987; Tetzloff & Barrera, 1987).

For the most part, the analyses of social support structure described in the preceding studies all focused on the frequency of supportive acts and found factors that were structured around support types or functions. Other researchers have started with a broader view of identifying support dimensions. For example, Caldwell and Bloom (1982) proposed the following characteristics: (1) source of support, (2) network size, (3) geographic accessibility, (4) frequency of contact, (5) type of support, and (6) perceived adequacy. Hirsch and Rapkin (1986) investigated what they termed *network domains*: interactions with respect to work and general identities, positive and negative interactions, and key network members. These studies and others (e.g., Vaux et al., 1987) illustrate how a broader concept of social support can be factored into meaningful subcomponents.

Conclusions

Many critiques of social support research include pleas for researchers to conduct fine-grained analyses of specific subtypes of support. Indeed, there is evidence that meaningful structures can emerge. However, it is also true that there is a strong general factor of support that underlies several social support scales (Barrera & Ainlay, 1983; Caldwell & Reinhart, 1988; McCormick et al., 1987; Newcomb, 1990; Stokes & Wilson, 1984). One implication of this is that scoring schemes that ignore factor scores by unit weighting items will result in correlated subscales. Some researchers have allowed for correlated factors (Caldwell & Reinhart, 1988; Stokes & Wilson, 1984). This represents an appropriate reading of the nature of social support, particularly enacted support. For example, it is meaningful that directive guidance and emotional support (that includes nondirective elements) would be related to each other. In professional helping transactions, as well as naturally occurring supportive relationships, the active listening and reassurance that characterizes emotional support is often combined with advice and information of directive guidance. Although it would be convenient if support subtypes that are conceptually distinct would also be empirically orthogonal, this is seldom the case (Cohen et al., 1985; Newcomb, 1990; Tetzloff & Barrera, 1987). This certainly is not unique to measures of enacted support. Analyses of a well-known measure of perceived support, the ISEL, also show strong correlations between support subtypes (Brookings & Bolton, 1988).

Perhaps because there is a strong general dimension of support underlying its factor structure, it is rare to encounter examples of analyses in which subscales show distinct relations to subtypes of psychological distress or other outcomes (Caldwell & Reichert, 1988; Finch et al., 1997). Despite the appeal of the support specificity hypothesis and the theory of optimal matching (Cutrona & Russell, 1990), it is difficult to find support dimensions that are truly uncorrelated with each other in practical applications.

What is driving the factor structure of support scales? Why should items that reflect the frequency of support receipt emerge as dimensions that reflect the nature of the helping transaction? One possibility is that the factor structures are indicative of the need states of the individuals who receive support, which would be the case when support providers are sensitive to the needs of the focal aid recipient. Another possibility is that the structures indicate the helping styles of the supportive individuals, that is, the kinds of aid that they are likely to provide, somewhat independent of the needs of the aid recipient. Studies of support structure can contribute to our understanding of these issues and need not be viewed only as data-reduction efforts.

Structural analyses suggest that source of support and the valence of social interactions (support or rejection) are also meaningful dimensions for organizing social exchanges (Caldwell & Bloom, 1982; Hirsch & Rapkin, 1986; Pagel, Erdly, & Becker, 1987; Wolchik et al., 1989). Much more research is needed to establish the generalizability of these results. The few studies that found source of support to be a meaningful aspect of social support structure reinforce the distinctions that some researchers have drawn between family members and friends (Procidano & Heller, 1984), coworkers and supervisors (Dignam, Barrera, & West, 1986), and coworkers and family (LaRocco, House, & French, 1980; Kobasa & Puccetti, 1983). There is also a growing literature on the effects of positive and negative social exchanges that could be informed by this basic research. This topic is discussed further later in the chapter.

LINKAGES BETWEEN SOCIAL SUPPORT CONSTRUCTS

As discussed earlier, several writers have drawn distinctions between social support concepts, such as enacted support, social embeddedness, perceived availability, and support satisfaction (Barrera, 1981; Vaux, 1985). Failures to treat these as separate constructs not only limit our understanding of social support processes in models of psychological adaptation and well-being, but also obscure possible causal relationships between social support constructs (Barrera, 1988).

Because great emphasis was placed on social support's relation to psychological and health outcomes, there was a lack of research on factors that influenced the provision and perception of social support (Hobfoll, 1990; House et al., 1988). This was one of the conclusions of an international conference on social support conducted in Germany (Veiel & Baumann, 1992) and the subject of a special issue of the *Journal of Social and Personal Relationships* (Hobfoll, 1990). There is now a core of recent studies that has identified some of the factors that influence support receipt, perceived availability, and satisfaction with support.

Heller and Swindle (1983) proposed a model of social support and coping that began with ecological influences on the formation and maintenance of social connections (networks). The presence of social networks (along with the contributions of stress and personal characteristics) had a causal relationship to perceived social support. This cognitive appraisal of social support was then linked to reaction patterns such as support-seeking and other coping behaviors. Heller and Swindle are more elaborate than this cursory summary. For example, their model also shows the influence of personal characteristics such as social skills on the formation and maintenance of social networks.

Predictors of Obtained Support

Consistent with Heller and Swindle's hypothesis, Cutrona (1986a) found that a scale of perceived social support predicted the receipt of helping behaviors on days when stressful events were experienced. On days when no stressful event occurred, perceived social support was not related to subsequent helping behaviors. In general, more helping behaviors were experienced on those days when at least one stress event was reported. This finding was consistent with the results of other studies that found a positive relationships between stress and the receipt of socially supportive exchanges (Barrera et al., 1981; Dunkel-Schetter, Folkman, & Lazarus, 1987; Sandler & Barrera, 1984).

A somewhat different model was hypothesized and tested by Vaux and Wood (1987). In this model, the presence of social support resources (such as network indices) were found to influence the likelihood that supportive behaviors were enacted, and this, in turn, led to the perceived quality of social support (Vaux & Wood, 1987). This same study suggested that the beneficial effects of support resources and behaviors on psychological distress were mediated by the perceived quality of social support. This is consistent with other research that found psychological distress to be most highly correlated with appraisals of support adequacy and not structural or behavioral measures of social support (Barrera, 1986).

A study by Vinokur, Schul, and Caplan (1987) examined some determinants of an individual's perceptions of obtained support. Data were gathered from nearly 500 men and their "significant others," primarily wives and girlfriends. There were three separate assessment periods that extended over 12 months. Results from structural-equation modeling showed that perceptions of obtained support were substantially related to significant others' reports of the support they provided. This is a comforting finding to those who would like to believe that perceptions of obtained support have some basis in the social interactions that are reported by others. Results also showed that poor mental health and a generalized negative outlook (viewed as a relatively stable personality-like disposition) had smaller, but significant, influences on perceptions of obtained support.

In one of the few studies to examine environmental correlates of social support, Oxley and others tested the effects of setting size on social support (Oxley et al., 1981). Community size showed a direct and negative relationship to the average multiplexity of non-kin network relationships, a measure that captured the diversity of supportive ties. Community size also was negatively related to social network size, but this relationship was mediated by the segmentalization of social relationships and social participation.

Predictors of Perceived Availability and Satisfaction with Support

Intuitively, the receipt of social support should increase individuals' perceptions of social support availability. Indeed, there is some evidence of a positive relation between these two constructs. Research with new mothers and elderly subjects reported relationships between structural characteristics of networks and measures of perceived social support (Cutrona, 1986b). Although the results for the two samples differed somewhat, there was some suggestion that the number of supporters and frequency of contact with them was correlated with perceived support. Marital status for the elderly proved to be an important determinant of perceived support.

Newcomb (1990) identified a latent factor model for indicators taken from Sarason et al.'s (1983) Social Support Questionnaire and Barrera et al.'s (1981) ISSB. A latent factor labeled "perceived available support" was derived from the number of perceived available supporters and satisfaction with perceived available supports as determined from the SSQ. Four factors from the ISSB (emotional support, tangible assistance, cognitive information, and directive guidance) were indicators of the latent construct labeled "received social support." The correlation between these constructs was .32 in the modified latent factor model. Other studies have reported even stronger associations when the ISEL was the measure of perceived availability of social support (Cohen, McGowan, Fooskas, & Rose, 1984; Cohen & Hoberman, 1983).

Despite these demonstrations of a moderate relation between received support and perceived availability, the most thorough review of this literature concluded that there was only a weak association between the two constructs (Dunkel-Schetter & Bennett, 1990). In fact, when perceived availability of support is quantified by perceived network size, there is little relationship between received and perceived support (Barrera, 1981; Sandler & Barrera, 1984). In retrospect, it is understandable how the frequency of receiving supportive exchanges would be unrelated to the *number* of perceived supporters (network size), but moderately related to measures of perceived availability that captured types of support (ISEL) or satisfaction with support (such as Newcomb's use of SSQ-Satisfaction).

Because measures of support satisfaction have shown moderate to strong relationships to indices of psychological distress, there has been interest in identifying the correlates of support satisfaction (Hobfoll, Nadler, & Lieberman, 1986). In a study of numerous structural characteristics of social networks, only the presence of confidants had a direct relationship to support satisfaction (Stokes, 1983). Evidence of curvilinear relationships with support satisfaction was found for two network variables, i.e., network size and confidants. Satisfaction was greatest for midrange values of network size and lowest for extremely small and large networks. For the confidant measure, satisfaction ratings were positively related to the number of confidants up to moderate values, then leveled off as the number of confidants increased.

Although received support has not shown direct relations to measures of support satisfaction, Barrera and Baca (1990) hypothesized that support receipt would be related to satisfaction for those who had a positive orientation toward help receipt and low conflict in their networks. This hypothesis was tested with a sample of mental health clinic outpatients. Although received support did not show the predicted interactions with conflict and network orientation, frequency of received support, network orientation, and network conflict were all significantly related to satisfaction with obtained support (Barrera & Baca, 1990). As previously noted, Vaux and Wood (1987) also found that received support was correlated with support appraisals.

Conclusions

What factors influence the structure and functioning of social support? What had been a totally neglected area of research received serious attention for at least two reasons. First, as confidence increased that social support had beneficial effects, researchers moved on to investigate its antecedents. House et al. (1988), for example, concluded that the evidence for social support's health effects was as strong as the evidence that linked smoking to cancer. The authors asserted, however, that much more attention was needed to clarify the factors that shape social support structure and process, apart from social support's effects on distress and health. Second, greater interest in social support interventions demanded that we learn more about factors that could be manipulated to increase the availability and effectiveness of social support (Heller, Price, & Hogg, 1990).

Reviewers of the social support literature have observed that qualitative measures of social support, such as satisfaction and perceived availability, show stronger correlations with psychological adjustment than structural measures of support (Barrera, 1986; Cohen & Wills, 1985; Cutrona, 1986b). This observation gave rise to the obvious question: What are the determinants of perceived support? This question has enormous implications for the development of social support interventions. Does increasing the size of one's social network or frequency of interaction with network members increase the likelihood that support will be more satisfying or perceived to be more available? The tentative answer to these questions is yes, but the magnitude of relationship between quantitative and qualitative indices of support is not large (e.g., Cutrona, 1986b; Newcomb, 1990; Dunkel-Schetter & Bennett, 1990) and not always linear (e.g., Stokes, 1983).

With few exceptions (e.g., Oxley et al., 1981), there is almost no research on properties of communities or neighborhoods that might serve as determinants of support enactment or quality of supportive exchanges. The lack of research in this area is in sharp contrast to the literature on personality correlates of social support, such as locus of control (Lefcourt, Martin, & Saleh, 1984; Sandler & Lakey, 1982), hardiness (Blaney & Ganellen, 1990; Kobasa & Puccetti, 1983), and network orientation (Colletta, 1987); and intrapersonal characteristics such as sex, ethnicity, and age (Vaux, 1985). Identifying environmental determinants of supportive ties and exchanges is a critical research area for a community psychology of social support.

THE RELATIONSHIP OF SOCIAL SUPPORT TO PSYCHOLOGICAL DISTRESS AND WELL-BEING

Much of the initial interest in social support was stimulated by attempts to understand moderators of life stress (Cassel, 1976; Dean & Lin, 1977; Rabkin & Struening, 1976). Indeed, the most extensively studied model of social support depicts it as a moderator or "buffer" of stress (Cohen & Wills, 1985). Despite the dominance of this model, there are many other viable models for investigating and understanding social support influences (Barrera, 1986, 1988; Lin, 1986). The following discussion begins with a review of the stress buffer model and then proceeds to other models.

The Stress Buffer Model

Numerous reviews of social support have included at least some discussion of social support buffering effects (Barrera, 1988; Broadhead et al., 1983; Cohen & McKay, 1984; Cohen & Wills, 1985; Dean & Lin, 1977; Gottlieb, 1983; Heller & Swindle, 1983; Kaplan et al., 1977; Kessler & McLeod, 1985; Kessler, Price, & Wortman, 1985; Leavy, 1983; Lin, 1986; Mitchell, Billings, & Moos, 1982; Schradle & Dougher, 1985; Thoits, 1982; Wallston, Alagna, DeVellis, & DeVellis, 1983). Stress buffering is synonymous with expressions such as "stress moderating" or "stress conditioning," which reflect two equivalent effects: (1) the relation of support with outcomes (such as health or distress) is stronger under conditions of high stress than low stress (e.g., Cassel, 1976), and (2) the relation of stress with outcomes is stronger under conditions of low support than high support (e.g., Wilcox, 1981b).

Reviewers noted evidence congruent with buffer effects, but acknowledged that many studies failed to find evidence of buffering. These analyses revealed a variety of complexities in testing and interpreting these effects. Because stress-buffering effects are essentially interactions, they are usually tested with low statistical power relative to direct (main) effects. Interactions are also sensitive to the observed ranges of stress that constrain those studies relying on specialized high-stress samples, such as divorced parents or pregnant adolescents (Barrera, 1988). Lin (1986) and Wheaton (1985) observed that there are really several different patterns of findings that can be described as buffering effects, and there are different opinions in the statistical procedures that are used to test the buffer model (Cleary & Kessler, 1982; Finney, Mitchell, Cronkite, & Moos, 1984). In light of these complexities, it is not surprising that some studies do not detect these interactions and that reviewers do not always agree on those studies that have demonstrated social support's stress buffering (see Barrera, 1988).

Some attention has turned to the question of which factors determine when stress buffering is observed and when it is not. Two explanations have been offered. In the most extensive review of stress buffering, Cohen and Wills (1985) differentiated between structural (i.e., those assessing social integration) and functional measures (i.e., those evaluating the supportive functions that are provided by social relationships). They concluded that functional measures of support were likely to show stress buffering, whereas structural measures were likely to show main effects. However, the conclusion from my own review and analysis was that support for the stress buffer model was not remarkably different when functional measures were compared to structural measures (Barrera, 1988).

Another explanation is that buffering occurs when there is a match between the coping requirements that arise out of stressful conditions and the resources that are provided by socially supportive relationships (Cohen & Hoberman, 1983; Wilcox & Vernberg, 1985). Cutrona (1990) detailed the critical features of this perspective, which she labeled the "theory of optimal matching," and reviewed literature to examine the support for this theory (see also Cutrona & Russell, 1990). If such matching between resources and needs is required before buffering can be observed, some previous attempts to detect stress buffering might have been unsuccessful because they assessed support and stress globally, rather than examining the congruence between specific stressors and resources.

One analysis of optimal matching identified several assumptions that should be met in order to test this theory (Tetzloff & Barrera, 1987). First, support must be subdivided into meaningful subcategories. Second, these subcategories must be relatively uncorrelated with each other. Obviously, high correlations between subcategories of support would preclude the meaningful test of their specific effects. There are similar assumptions for subcategories of stress. Furthermore, corresponding stress and social support measures should not be highly correlated with each other if they are to be entered into interaction terms that can be unambiguously interpreted. There is assumed to be some conceptual correspondence between the subcategories of support and stress. Finally, strong tests of optimal matching require at least two distinct support types and two distinct stress types, so that conditions of matching can be contrasted with non-matches. Despite the appeal of this perspective, this complex set of assumptions needs to be met before the theory can be tested optimally. That it has been addressed directly in only a few studies and that these have provided only limited support is understandable. For example, a study of mothers who recently had separated from their husbands met each of these assumptions only after deliberate scaling manipulations for both stress and support measures (Tetzloff & Barrera, 1987). However, the study did not offer strong support for the benefits of matching. Instead, there were a number of direct effects for social support subcategories, even after accounting for stress variables.

Because few studies provide direct tests of stress-support matching, Cutrona and Russell (1990) reinterpreted studies that had examined interactions between at least some specific components of stress and social support. They reviewed studies that each included: (1) multiple components of support or one clearly identifiable component, (2) a sample of individuals who had all experienced the same stress event or analyses for subgroups who had experienced the same stressors, and (3) analyses that examined the relation between at least one component of support, one component of stress, and an outcome (health or psychological distress). Even though explicit comparisons between matches and mismatches within a given study could not be done in most cases, the reviewers interpreted the pattern of relationships across 42 studies that met criteria for inclusion. The authors made specific hypotheses about the stress dimensions that would match the provisions of supportive relations. For example, uncontrollable events were thought to require emotion-focused support, in contrast to controllable events, which would require support that fostered problem-focused coping. The "domain" or content of the stress event (e.g., financial strain, parenthood, bereavement) also was thought to determine the need for specific types of support.

Cutrona and Russell (1990) estimated that two-thirds of the stress events were consistent with their predictions from the theoretical model. However, their summary conclusion was that "for some events, certain kinds of social support can help achieve optimal adjustment, but that for other events, a broad range of social support components are required for recovery" (p. 359). Identifying which stressful conditions create a broad set of support needs and which create more specific needs will sharpen future tests of this theory. Although the practice of testing interactions between global stress and support scales has been sharply criticized, there is evidence that at least some stress events create the need for diverse kinds of support, and that there is a unidimensional core of support that runs through many social support scales, even those that show meaningful first-order factor structures (Newcomb, 1990).

To summarize, social support has moderated the relationship between stress and psychological disorder in many studies, but reviewers have expressed concern that observation of this effect is not reliable. Neither the distinction between functional and structural measures of support, nor the theory of optimal matching, has accounted adequately for the variability of stress buffering effects. The theory of optimal matching, however, deserves further testing, particularly in studies that directly compare the effects of stress-support matches and mismatches. Methodological features of some studies also have not provided for strong tests of stress-support interaction effects. These features include specialized samples that do not include a sufficient range of stress conditions, samples that lack adequate size to detect modest interaction effects, measures that have low reliability and/or validity, and assessment intervals that are not adequate to capture the processes leading to stress moderation.

Direct Effects of Support on Distress

Stress-buffering effects of social support became the dominant research topic, despite thoughtful discussions that proposed multiple pathways for social support's influence on psychological distress (Dean & Lin, 1977; Gore, 1981; Gottlieb, 1983; House, 1981; LaRocco et al., 1980). The only other model to receive serious consideration hypothesizes direct effects of social support on psychological distress, an effect that is thought to be independent of life stress. A number of early studies were presented as tests of whether social support exerted direct or buffering effects, as though these were the only plausible models of social support's influence (Aneshensel & Stone, 1982; Bell, LeRoy, & Stephenson, 1982; Cohen, Teresi, & Holmes, 1986; Fleming, Baum, Gisriel, & Gatchel, 1982; Thoits, 1982; Williams, Ware, & Donald, 1981).

Direct effects of social support on distress and illness were found in several studies that did not find evidence of stress buffering (Aneshensel & Stone, 1982; Bell et al., 1982; Costello, 1982; Lin, 1986; Tetzloff & Barrera, 1987; Williams et al., 1981). The early research that reported direct effects included some of the most methodologically sound studies, which used measures with good psychometric properties, large and carefully drawn samples, and prospective or panel designs (e.g., House et al., 1988; Newcomb & Bentler, 1988; Williams et al., 1981).

House and his colleagues, prolific reviewers of the social support literature, concluded that the evidence regarding the health benefits of social support were convincing and strongly suggestive of a causal effect (House et al., 1988). Much of their enthusiasm came from an analysis of large-scale, prospective studies of communities that assessed mortality and other health outcomes over time intervals of as long as 13 years. For example, the Alameda County study found that adults who lacked social support had a relative risk for death of 2.0 compared to those with high support. In the Tecumseh study, the relative risk was 2.0–3.0 for men and 1.5–2.0 for women. Findings from these studies are impressive because effects for rather crude measures of social relationships are found after accounting for baseline levels of physical health, physical activity, smoking, alcohol use, socioeconomic status, and other possible explanations of social support's prospective effect on health and mortality.

From their review of these prospective studies, House et al. (1988) suggested that the evidence for social support's health effects is as strong as the evidence linking smoking with cancer. They also concluded that: (1) the effects of social support on mortality were non-specific, that is, not restricted to any particular cause of death; (2) the relation of support to mortality was primarily due to extreme cases of social isolation; and (3) the effects were stronger for men than women.

The "direct effects model" sets itself apart from models that require the specification of stress, but its name does not convey the many mediators that are thought to transmit the effects of support to the outcomes of health and psychological distress. Among these mediators are enhanced self-esteem, maintenance of a healthy life style, immune-system functioning, and perceived stress (see Cohen, 1988; Uchino, Cacioppo, & Kiecolt-Glaser, 1996). There is growing research that identifies the mediators of social support's "direct" effect on health and psychological distress.

Stress Deteriorates Social Support

A negative relationship between the occurrence of stressful life events and social support, particularly measures of perceived social support, was observed in a few studies (see Barrera, 1988). A possible mechanism underlying this relationship is one in which stress deteriorates supportive relationships. This mechanism was most extensively studied in the Albany Area Health Survey (Dean & Ensel, 1982; Lin & Dean, 1984; Lin, Dean, & Ensel, 1986; Lin & Ensel, 1984). Because this study incorporated a panel design, it was possible to evaluate the influence of stress on social support prospectively. The results were consistent with more than one model of stress and social support, but there was evidence that stress was an antecedent condition that led to the decrease in social support. Deteriorated support, in turn, led to an increase in depressive symptoms.

There are a number of ways stressful events could contribute to the diminution of social support. For example, an individual who experiences traumatic events could encounter shunning or social avoidance by members of his or her social network. Network members who are normally supportive might avoid the victim of trauma because of the anticipated difficulty in knowing what to do or say (Wortman & Lehman, 1985). Social losses that result from events, such as residential relocation, divorce, and death of spouse could change the structure of social relationships (Leslie & Grady, 1985; Wilcox, 1981a). With divorce, for instance, in-laws and friends who were primarily connected through the spouse may fall out of one's social support network. Life stress could lead to the decreased use of social support if the stress mobilizes intrapersonal coping efforts that are used instead of interpersonal resources. Following an upheaval, some individuals might choose to withdraw from social interactions in order to solve problems without the added strain of social comparisons to others who are unaffected by the life stress. Also, events that result in physical disabilities might decrease mobility and the social contacts that help maintain supportive relationships (Schulz, Tompkins, & Rau, 1990). Unemployment for blue-collar workers could reduce social support by cutting into expenditures for leisure-time activities, eliminating contacts with co-workers, and straining marital relationships that are otherwise prime sources of support (Atkinson, Liem, & Liem, 1986). Thus, there are multiple mechanisms whereby stress could lead to a decrease in the availability, perceived adequacy, or utilization of social support.

Clarifying these mechanisms would be a valuable objective for future research. What are the nature of the events that are likely to lead to support deterioration? What are the characteristics of individuals and their networks who are vulnerable to support deterioration? A model for future research was provided by Kaniasty and Norris (1995) concerning the mobilization and deterioration of social support following natural disasters. They show that whether disaster stress leads to the mobilization or deterioration of support depends on the nature of support that is being assessed (received or perceived support), the providers of support (kin or kith), personal characteristics of the support recipients (e.g., race, gender), and the amount of time that has past since the disaster. They found evidence that a high level of helping activity immediately following a disaster (enacted support) led to a long-term depletion of supportive resources and perceptions of support. Longitudinal assessments of Kentucky flood victims showed declines in perceptions of support and in social embeddedness due to disruption of social events, religious activities, shopping, visiting, and participation in recreation. This research demonstrated how the Support Mobilization and Support Deterioration models are not incompatible when researchers draw distinctions between the different conceptualizations and measures of social support.

Insulation or Stress Prevention Model

Several models of social support seem to begin with the assumption that life stress is an antecedent to the mobilization of social support. A very different perspective views social support as a factor that prevents stressful events from occurring (Gore, 1981; Gottlieb, 1983; House, 1981; LaRocco et al., 1980). Two processes can be proposed as underlying stress prevention. First, the insulation of socially supportive relationships can shield individuals from experiencing the occurrence of stress events. For example, supportive ties cannot shield an individual from the death of a spouse, but they can assume some of the legal and financial responsibilities to protect the bereaved individual from some additional stress events. A second process consists of cognitive appraisals that influence the perception of the magnitude or salience of stress. Specifically, the perceived availability or adequacy of support modifies the cognitively appraised threat value of the stress event. The failure to receive an academic scholarship might be devastating for the student with no options for financial support and little reassurance from others about intellectual abilities. In contrast, this same event might be appraised as disappointing, but not tragic, for the student who perceives the certainty of reaffirmation of worth and financial supplies through social network resources.

Lin (1986) found evidence that social support prevented the occurrence of negative life events in an epidemiological, longitudinal study. A latent social support construct that included indicators such as community, network, confidant, and instrumental support predicted decreases in the frequency of undesirable life events one year later. Cross-sectional research focusing on perceived stress provided a very different illustration of stress prevention. A study of correctional officers hypothesized that supportive transactions between coworkers and supervisors would prevent job stress (i.e., role ambiguity) and thereby decrease burnout (Dignam et al., 1986). Causal modeling was consistent with these predictions.

Relative to other models, the stress prevention model has received little attention. Future studies of this model will need to determine if current concepts and measures adequately capture the kind of supportive exchanges that would prevent the occurrence of stress events or prevent them from being seen as threatening. Because many measures of support are built around notions of aid provision to individuals who are troubled or appraisals of aid that was received in response to experienced events, they are probably inappropriate for assessing support that could prevent stress. Just like the *prevention* of physical illness requires different behaviors than that needed for the *treatment* of illness, so too might the prevention of stress require different types of support than those provided after stress occurs.

DOES SOCIAL SUPPORT HAVE NEGATIVE CONSEQUENCES FOR RECIPIENTS?

The term *social support* connotes something that is helpful, positive, and desirable. To complement this focus on the positive, some researchers have attended to the negative aspects of social exchange (Coyne et al., 1988; Rook, 1984). In this context, they have discussed the stressful nature of social support, negative buffering effects, and negative reactions to help. Indeed, there is an extensive social psychological literature on recipients' reactions to aid, particularly negative reactions that stem from constraints on freedom, indebtedness, and loss of self-esteem (Fisher, Nadler, & Whitcher-Alagna, 1982).

Shumaker and Brownell (1984) presented a conceptual scheme that is useful for identifying different ways in which negative aspects of social interactions are relevant to the topic of social support. In this scheme, there are separate dimensions representing the donor's perceptions of aid and the recipient's perceptions; each of these dimensions has a positive and a negative pole. These authors noted that donor and recipient perceptions of aid are distinct from the effects of aid, and that there could be differences in the short- and long-term effects of aid. By considering the situations that involve the negative elements of these dimensions, we can identify several conditions that involve the negative perceptions or effects of aid.

Certain of these conditions are of particular interest. A fairly common situation occurs when acts perceived (intended) by the aid donor as positive are perceived by the recipient as negative. This would include situations such as when a donor's attempts to comfort or cheer a bereaved individual are perceived as insensitive or annoying, thus leading to short-term and possibly long-term negative effects on the recipient. A closely related situation is when helpers become so overinvolved and overprotective that the aid recipient feels restricted and smothered (Coyne et al., 1988). A somewhat separate condition would include aid that is not perceived by the recipient as positive, but that ultimately results in positive consequences. Parental directives such as "eat your vegetables," "do your homework," or "don't smoke cigarettes" are illustrative of this situation.

Acts initially perceived as positive by both the donor and the recipient can be negative in consequences determined by some external standard. Commiserating about poor working conditions with a coworker might be perceived as supportive by both helper and helpee, yet this emotion-focused non-change-oriented process might accentuate work stress rather than mitigate its effects. Another variation of this is when network members support each other in deviant acts such as addictive behaviors (Wills, 1990).

The most apparent negative interactions involve exchanges that would not be described as social support from either the donor or recipient perspective. Nevertheless, these interactions are relevant to the study of social support in that their effects on well-being can be contrasted with those of positive transactions and relationships (Rook, 1984). Purely negative social interactions also can be of interest when their sources are individuals who are key social support providers (Barrera, 1981). What is the effect of social support when it is provided by people who are perceived by the recipients as sources of conflict and interpersonal problems? In fact, the term "conflicted" support was used to identify social network members who had both positive and negative ties to an individual (Barrera, 1981; Sandler & Barrera, 1984).

Most of the studies that are concerned with negative aspects of social exchange involve one of three concepts: (1) help-seeking or help-receipt that is positively related to measures of psychological distress, (2) interpersonal conflict or problems, and (3) the negative buffering effect.

Positive Relationship of Distress to Measure of Help-Seeking and Help-Receipt

Many studies have found that some measures of social support are positively related to psychological distress or physical illness. In these studies, support measures have assessed concepts such as the frequency of help-receipt (Barrera, 1981; Cohen & Hoberman, 1983), frequency of discussing problems (Carveth & Gottlieb, 1979), and help-seeking (Coyne, Aldwin, & Lazarus, 1981; Fiore, Becker, & Coppel, 1983; Warheit, Vega, Shimizu, & Meinhardt, 1982). This research illustrates the possibility that the act of help-seeking or the help received had a deleterious effect on the recipients of support. However, it is at least as plausible that this relationship represents a "support mobilization" effect (Barrera, 1986). In this case, psychological distress causes individuals to seek out help, or support network members to contribute aid when they are made aware of the focal person's distress.

Dunkel-Schetter (1984) studied 79 cancer patients, 47 who were thought to have a good prognosis and 32 judged to have a poor prognosis. Different relationships between social support and well-being were found for the two groups. For patients with a good prognosis, social support was positively related to self-esteem and positive affect. Social support was not related to these outcomes for poor-prognosis patients.

On measures of physical health, social support was *positively* related to problems in functioning and symptoms for poor-prognosis patients only. Rather than concluding that social support had a negative effects on physical health. Dunkel-Schetter favored the interpretation that patients' deteriorating physical conditions *elicited* support or influenced patients' perceptions of family cohesiveness and other support resources.

In an article entitled "Does Help Help?," Lieberman and Mullan (1978) reported a longitudinal study of adults who experienced at least one of seven major life events over a 4–5 year interval. The study sought to determine if professional or informal help from one's social support network resulted in greater adjustment compared to those who did not seek help for these stressful events. Overall, the study did not provide strong support for the effectiveness of seeking help for major life events. Even after including statistical controls for age, sex, education, and race of the help recipient, a number of analyses suggested that those who obtained assistance from professionals and informal helpers were worse off than those who did not receive aid.

Lieberman and Mullan examined a number of correlates of help-seeking that might have accounted for its apparent deleterious effects. Help-seekers experienced life events as more troublesome than subjects who did not seek help. Controlling for the perceived aversiveness of events substantially reduced the number of analyses that showed help-seekers to be worse than non-help-seekers. Other variables, such as access to help, presence of coping skills, and the timing of stressful events, failed to account for participants' changes in adaptive functioning over the course of the study. In summary, there was not strong evidence that help was harmful when statistical controls were considered, but the results did not support the effectiveness of help in adjusting to these major life events.

Direct Effects of Conflict

Some research has investigated a concept Barrera (1981) labeled "conflicted support." This term was restricted to the number of social network members who were sources of both positive social support as well as negative transactions. In a study of pregnant teenagers, conflicted network size was significantly and positively related to anxiety and depression symptoms, whereas unconflicted network size was negatively (but not significantly) related to these same criteria (Barrera, 1981). Only unconflicted network size entered into a significant interaction with life stress in a manner that was consistent with a stress-buffering model. A second study of conflicted support was conducted with 45 university students (Sandler & Barrera, 1984). Similar to the previous study, conflicted network size was positively and significantly correlated with psychological distress, but unconflicted support was negatively (but not significantly) related to these same distress measures.

It is important to remember that individuals who comprised the conflicted network also were providers of positive social support. Yet conflicted network size did not contribute to the positive stress-buffering effects, and even potentiated the negative effects of life stress for the college-student sample. These findings suggest that decreasing the interpersonal conflict in social support networks might be as important as increasing the availability of individuals who provide positive social exchanges.

Rook (1984) compared the ability of several indices of positive and negative social relationships to predict the psychological well-being of elderly women. Her results generally supported the hypothesis that negative social contacts are stronger correlates of well-being than positive social contacts. The number of supportive functions fulfilled by subjects' networks was unrelated to well-being, but a parallel measure of the number of problems emanating from their network was significantly correlated with well-being. Similarly, the number of supportive individuals was unrelated to well-being, but the number of problematic others was inversely related to this outcome. Rook noted that questionnaire items concerning problematic social ties were more likely to contain affect-laden terms than were the positive support items. Restricting analyses to support items that conveyed closeness and comfort, two positive affect states, improved the correlation with well-being measures. There is potential conceptual overlap between psychological distress/well-being and the assessment of problematic social ties.

A study of caregivers who had spouses with Alzheimer's disease included the assessment of how upsetting their interactions were with members of their social networks (Fiore et al., 1983). Network members also were rated on the helpfulness of their contacts. Caregivers' depressive symptoms were not correlated with the perceived helpfulness of their interactions, but were significantly related to perceived upset. A 10-month follow-up to this study (Pagel et al., 1987) largely replicated these results. Perceived upset was related to depression at follow-up, but perceived helpfulness was not. Furthermore, perceived upset was negatively correlated with network satisfaction, but helpfulness was not a significant predictor of network satisfaction.

Negative Stress-Buffering Effects

Negative stress buffering occurs when the relationship between stress and measures of distress are stronger under conditions of high social support than low social support. Two studies illustrated negative stress buffering. In one study, a measure of enacted social support (the ISSB) showed these effects with anxiety, one of several outcome measures (Sandler & Barrera, 1984). This effect was not replicated in a second study reported in the same article. A separate social support scale, a network measure of conflicted support, potentiated the effects of stress. A significant interaction between conflicted support and stress revealed that stress was highly related to psychological distress for individuals with large conflicted networks. Those with small conflicted networks showed a nonsignificant correlation between stress and distress.

An epidemiological study of depression in rural counties of Tennessee, Oklahoma, and Ohio illustrated the complex results that can emerge when interactions between stress, social support, personal resources, and subject characteristics are considered simultaneously (Husaini, Neff, Newbrough, & Moore, 1982). The results cannot be summarized concisely because separate analyses were conducted for each of the eight social support indicators. Some of them measured qualitative dimensions of support appraisal (marital satisfaction, spouse satisfaction, spouse as confidant), some measured frequency of help-seeking (how often friends and relatives are called for help), and others assessed social embeddedness (number of close relatives, number of nearby friends, church attendance). As predicted by those who advocate drawing distinctions between these social support concepts (Barrera, 1986; Cohen & Wills, 1985; Vaux et al., 1986), the pattern of results varied with the social support measures that were included. For measures of perceived adequacy of support (marital satisfaction and spouse as confidant), the interactions of stress and support, and the triple interactions of stress, support, and personal competency, conformed to the predicted results. Stress was relatively unrelated to depression when social and personal resources were high. For support measures reflecting help-seeking and social embeddedness, findings emerged that were opposite to those predicted. For example, the relationship of stress and depression was stronger for those who were help-seekers than for those who were not. Similarly, there was a triple-interaction-like trend involving personal competence, support, and stress. For those low in social competence, the relationship between stress and depression was actually higher for those who sought the help of friends, had relatives nearby, and who attended church, than for those who did not have these social support resources.

Riley and Eckenrode (1986) found that for individuals who lacked personal resources, such as education and financial resources, social support was related to more negative affect. Like the social support measure in Husaini et al. (1982). Riley and Eckenrode's measure captured mobilized support. The direction of effects is uncertain, but similar to other studies, it is possible that those individuals who appear to be in need of support because they experience negative affect are those who are most likely to receive social support.

Conclusions

Concern with the negative aspects of social interaction and the potential harmful effects of aid has been a healthy development in social support research. The discovery of the deterioration effect in psychotherapy research added to the cynicism of some critics, but it also highlighted the importance of developing intervention methods and evaluating their effectiveness. Similarly, sensitivity to the potential negative influence of naturally occurring social support should stimulate research efforts directed at understanding these effects, and could inform the development of interventions that attempt to access social support resources.

Naturally, there is a danger of misinterpreting the research findings that have thus far been produced. It would be particularly unfortunate to confuse the harmful effects of network conflict, upset, and troubles with the deleterious influence of aid that is perceived by donors and recipients as positive support. At present there is much more evidence that network conflict contributes to psychological distress than there is on the negative effects of help.

When social support was found to be directly related to distress or was implicated in negative buffering effects, it was often operationalized as enacted support or mobilized helping behaviors. As described in this chapter and elsewhere (Barrera, 1986, 1988) there are alternatives to the explanation that support causes distress. These alternative models hypothesize pathways by which distress, even after controlling for the experience of stress events, can result in support-seeking or unsolicited aid provision. An underresearched topic concerns the role of social support networks in the initiation and maintenance of deviance or unhealthy behavior. For example, how might peer networks of adolescents promote substance abuse (Wills, 1990) or risky sexual behaviors? How might social support networks maintain problem drinking in their members? These questions have special relevance for social support because they involve social exchanges that might be perceived by donors and recipients as positive and satisfying, yet they ultimately contribute to undesirable consequences.

Social Support Interventions

In many areas of psychology there is an almost natural progression of research from cross-sectional field-based studies, through demonstrations of longitudinal research, and ultimately to interventions. To a large extent, this pattern fits the progression of research in the social support literature. Although the use of support groups and partners in therapy regimens pre-date serious research on social support, other interventions have been inspired by studies of social support (Gottlieb, 1988a). The development of support interventions is key for several reasons. First, it takes research on social support from the realm of correlations and observed relations between naturally occurring phenomena to the realm of manipulating supportive transactions in experimental research. Despite the persuasive findings from longitudinal research, manipulations of social support that result in improved functioning would fortify the empirical basis for social support's effectiveness. Second, the well-known action research adage that our understanding of psychological processes is elevated by attempting to change them, has true significance for social support research. At a time when social support is often conceptualized as a personality characteristic or cognitive factor, it is valuable to explore how different components of social support are altered and which factors influence perceptions of social support. Third, manipulating social support requires a technology for bringing about changes in either existing social systems or for adding new ones. There is a great need for practical solutions to delivering interventions, particularly in efforts to alleviate chronic problems or to provide services to those unlikely to receive traditional forms of professional care (Gottlieb, 1988a).

One starting point for systematic research on the creation and testing of social support interventions are typologies that organize what we already know and guide future efforts to formulate social support interventions. Gottlieb (1988b) identified five levels of support interventions: individual, dyadic, group, social system, and community. He also consolidated them into three basic support interventions: (1) support of a partner, (2) network-centered interventions, and (3) support groups (Gottlieb, 1988a). Support of a partner actually included two different strategies—using an existing support provider (such as a spouse) or adding a new partner. Partners who are spouses or members of existing networks have been used as adjuncts to interventions for a variety of disorders, particularly behavior excesses such as smoking and overeating (Cohen, Lichtenstein, Mermelstein, Kingsolver, Baer, & Kamarck, 1988). Similarly, there are well-known community-based interventions such as Big Brother–Big Sister organizations and Silverman's (1988) Widow-to-Widow program that make use of new, non-family supporters who receive some training to perform their roles.

Network-centered interventions include steps to mobilize existing supporters or improve the quality of support obtained from one's network. Mobilizing a network to support a caregiver who is attending a chronically ill spouse would be an example of a network intervention. These treatment or consultation programs are directed at the natural social support system rather than newly created networks. Support groups, on the other hand, are artificially created social units that compensate for the lack of natural supporters or constitute a peer group with special sensitivities and resources for supporting a member.

Vaux's (1988) description of social support interventions overlapped somewhat with that of Gottlieb. From Vaux's perspective, clinical interventions such as network therapy, family therapy, and couples therapy might be regarded as social support interventions because the extended family, nuclear family, and marital relationship are primary sources of social support. Similar to Gottlieb, he also discussed companionship therapy (linking a support recipient with a specific helper such as a Big Brother or peer advisor) and mutual aid groups. Vaux reviewed indirect social support interventions such as (1) consultation to support groups for improving their provision of social support; (2) enhancing support resources in the community, such as training cadres of community helpers (e.g., the Community Helpers Project, D'Augelli, Valiance, Danish, Young, & Gerdes, 1981); or (3) improving the helping skills of professionals who find themselves in support-donor roles, but who are not professional counselors (e.g., hairdressers, bartenders, classroom teachers).

Discussions of these typologies and other literature reviews point out the large gap between community psychology research on social support and social support interventions (Barrera & Prelow, in press; Bogat et al., 1993; Gottlieb, 1988a, 1988b; Heller et al., 1991). Almost all of the research on social support has been based on field-based, naturalistic studies, rather than evaluations of interventions. Field studies focus on existing social networks comprised of spouses, nuclear families, and close friends, whereas many intervention strategies attempt to add a new partner or a group consisting of individuals who were unknown to each other prior to the intervention. Also, understanding the supportive behaviors that contribute to beneficial outcomes would allow for a direct translation into intervention activities, but most often support is studied as "perception" or "satisfaction," which cannot be readily converted to targets for change (Gottlieb, 1988b).

Many of these gaps and their implications for social support intervention research were discussed by Heller et al. (1991) and eight researchers who were invited to comment on the paper's provocative findings. Heller et al. created an intervention that paired elderly women with telephone partners in an attempt to alleviate poor morale, loneliness, and depression. Despite numerous sensitivities to the substance of the intervention, the women's needs, and methodological issues, the intervention was not successful in increasing perceived support from friendships or improving participants' well-being. Among the various reactions to this study was the frequent recognition that we know little about methods for facilitating the development of intimacy between new acquaintanceships or incorporating new social support providers into the natural social support systems of individuals (Barrera, 1991).

Are social support interventions successful? In addition to Heller et al.'s (1991) failure to find a positive intervention effect, research on the effects of partners taking part in smoking cessation regimens shows significant failures (Cohen et al., 1988). However, some reviews of social support interventions have identified successful interventions that incorporated at least some components of social support (Barrera & Prelow, in press; Bogat et al., 1993). For example, Hobfoll and Stephens (1990) conceptualized the intervention methods used for treating soldiers within a social support paradigm. Soldiers who were treated near the front lines during active warfare were kept within the military community (rather than moved to more civilian settings), and were returned to the support of their units (Solomon & Benbenishty, 1986). These soldiers had about half the rate of posttraumatic stress disorder as soldiers who were not returned to their military units. In the most comprehensive review of social support interventions, Gottlieb (1988a) identified many other interventions that showed promising effects, even though some were limited by nonexperimental research designs.

For social support interventions directed at children, research programs by Olds and Felner are most prominent. With true experimental trials and many years of follow-up data, Olds and his colleagues have demonstrated the long-term effectiveness of an intervention in which visiting nurses provided young mothers with companionship, instruction in child care, and guidance in using community support services (Olds, 1988). Compared to controls, nurse-visited mothers had higher birthweight babies, and fewer preterm deliveries, injuries, ingestions, and emergency room visits (Olds, Henderson, & Kitzman, 1994).

Felner et al.'s (1982, 1993) School Transitional Environment Project (STEP) stands out as the best example of changing the social support in an environment to promote the wellness of adolescents. Transitions from middle school to high school can be marked by adverse changes in school achievement and behavior problems that are attributed to the "flux" of the social setting—a new school combined with a structure of constantly changing peer groups as students move from class to class throughout the school day. The initial STEP intervention was designed to ease the school transition by enhancing the homeroom teacher's role and clustering project students into the same classes. Homeroom teachers accepted responsibility for administrative and counseling function, thereby becoming the prime link between project students, their families, and the school. Rather than constantly changing classmates, project students took their four primary academic subjects with the other project students. Results showed that by the end of the school year, project students reported more teacher support, better grades, better self-concept, and less absenteeism than the control students. The 5-year follow-up evaluation of this initial intervention showed that STEP students experienced half the amount of school drop-outs and less absenteeism compared to students in the control condition (Felner et al., 1993).

Some of the studies that are showcased as support interventions actually contain many more elements than just manipulations of social support. As a result, the effectiveness of these interventions cannot be attributed unambiguously to changes in social support. It also is notable that many of the effective interventions that are cited involve professionals or professional settings (Olds, 1988; Sosa, Kennell, Klaus, Robertson, & Urrutia, 1980), rather than more natural supporters and environments. Because of the need to control the manipulations of social support and understand participants' involvement with the intervention, it is understandable that researchers might choose to work with highly trained intervention agents and relatively small, homogeneous populations. Although the combination of support with other treatment methods leads to interpretation problems, Heller (1990) argued that it is unlikely that support could stand alone as the sole intervention for most problems of living.

The National Institute of Mental Health brought together an interdisciplinary group of social support researchers who drafted guidelines for the development and evaluation of social support interventions (Gottlieb, 1988a). From the 12 specific recommendations that emerged from the conference, three basic principles have special prominence: (1) researchers should have a sense from theory and data as to why the manipulation of social support should make a difference in the outcome of interest, (2) they should have replicable methods for manipulating social support components, and (3) they should have a valid strategy for evaluating the effectiveness of the intervention. These principles should guide the planing and empirical test of future social support interventions. Exemplars of these principles are in the literature (e.g., Sandler, Gersten, Reynolds, Kallgren, & Ramirez, 1988).

Conclusions

What has social support research contributed to community psychology? More than 20 years of lively research has produced numerous measures of several distinct social support concepts, some understanding of their structural components, an appreciation for differences between support concepts, research data on social support's relationships to psychological distress and health for individuals experiencing a variety of stress/transition events, some awareness of the negative elements of social exchanges, and the emergence of interventions that are intended to harness salutary features of supportive relationships. By far the biggest contribution has been made to our understanding of the role of social support as a naturally occurring resource that can be brought to bear on the adaptation of community residents. Applications to quality of life, empowerment, psychological sense of community, or even prevention have been secondary to the central attention received by models of adaptation to stress.

What are the emerging topics in social support research? If we did not restrict our view to just the community psychology literature, we would find growing interest in microlevel analyses of supportive transactions, laboratory-based analogs of helping, interactions with personality variables, intrapersonal mediators (such as self-esteem) of support-distress relationships, and conceptualizations of social support as a perception, appraisal, or subjective experience of individuals. Lieberman (1986) and House et al. (1988) commented that the psychologizing of the social support construct has severed it from its sociological roots. According to Lieberman (1986), the psychologizing of social support has led to "a conceptual morass" that has compromised its knowledge base and its ability to inform public policy.

Even social support research published in community psychology journals has treated the individual as the primary unit of analysis. Treating the person as the unit of analysis has been consonant with social support research's dominant focus on stress, distress, physical health, and other consequences afflicting individuals. It is rare to find research on social support that addresses the interactions between environments and individuals, seeks to identify environmental determinants, or works with units of analysis other than the individual.

This review has not fully addressed the issues inherent in developing interventions based on manipulations of social support. Some have questioned whether sufficient knowledge has accrued to justify the implementation of social support interventions and have expressed cautious optimism about the prospects of developing such interventions in the near future (Brownell & Shumaker, 1985; Heller et al., 1990; Kiesler, 1985; Lieberman, 1986; Rook & Dooley, 1985). Also, it is arguable that methods touted as social support interventions, such as self-help groups, actually incorporate elements of naturally occurring supportive transactions (Lieberman, 1986). Other examples of "social support interventions" make heavy use of professionals such as teachers or nurses (see Barrera & Prelow, in press; Gottlieb, 1988a). The development of social-support-based interventions should go forward, despite our incomplete understanding of how social support promotes adaptation or well-being. We can remind ourselves of notable advances in medicine that have occurred serendipitously, and the number of effective interventions that are used although we are unable to fully unravel the secret to their efficacy. By postponing the development of social support interventions until we have more answers, we might be postponing opportunities to gain some insights into the important questions.

We should all expect a flurry of research on computer-based technology to be used in interventions of all types, particularly for chronic illness and substance use disorders, some of the same problems addressed by support groups (Salem, Bogat, & Reid, 1997). Many of these interventions will include social support components (e.g., chat rooms) that will allow participants to connect with each other and with professional caregivers in cyberspace, giving them 24-hour access to advice and information (Glasgow, Barrera, McKay, & Boles, 1998).

In addition to intervention research, community psychology ought to be concerned with community change, planned or unplanned, that disrupts naturally occurring social support. Even if we discover that our efforts to effectively change natural support systems or create artificial systems are unsuccessful, we could still be influential in preventing the erosion of valuable community resources such as social networks. For example, we know relatively little about the impact of residential relocation that is often imposed to accommodate highway construction, airport expansion, and the redevelopment of urban centers. We could also deepen our understanding of how social policies affect the development and utilization of social ties. These are some of the questions that could be addressed by the next generation of community psychology research on social support.

REFERENCES

Albee, G. W. (1982). Preventing psychopathology and promoting human potential *American Psychologist*, *37*, 1043–1050.

Aneshensel, C. S., & Stone, J. D. (1982). Stress and depression: A test of the buffering model of social support. *Archives of General Psychiatry*, *39*, 1393–1396.

Atkinson, T., Liem, R., & Liem, J. H. (1986). The social costs of unemployment: Implications for social support. *Journal of Health and Social Behavior*, *27*, 317–331.

Barrera, M., Jr. (1981). Social support in the adjustment of pregnant adolescents: Assessment issues. In B. H. Gottlieb (Ed.), *Social networks and social support* (pp. 69–96). Beverly Hills, CA: Sage.

Barrera, M., Jr. (1986). Distinctions between social support concepts, measures, and models. *American Journal of Community Psychology*, *14*, 413–445.

Barrera, M., Jr. (1988). Models of social support and life stress: beyond the buffering hypothesis. In L. H. Cohen (Ed.), *Life events and psychological functioning. Theoretical and methodological issues* (pp. 211–236). Newbury Park, CA: Sage.

Barrera, M., Jr. (1991). Social support interventions and the third law of ecology. *American Journal of Community Psychology*, *19*, 133–138.

Barrera, M., Jr. (1997). *Appraising the action validity of social support research: Implications for community interventions and public policy.* Presidential address to the Society for Community Research and Action (Div. 27), annual meeting of the American Psychological Association, Chicago.

Barrera, M., Jr., & Ainlay, S. (1983). The structure of social support: A conceptual and empirical analysis. *Journal of Community Psychology, 11,* 133–143.

Barrera, M., Jr., & Baca, L. M. (1990). Recipient reactions to social support: Contributions of enacted support, conflicted support and network orientation. *Journal of Social and Personal Relationships, 7,* 541–551.

Barrera, M., Jr., & Garrison-Jones, C. V. (1992). Family and peer social support as specific correlates of adolescent depressive symptoms. *Journal of Abnormal Child Psychology, 20,* 1–16.

Barrera, M., Jr., & Li, S. A. (1996). The relation of family support to adolescents' psychological distress and problem behaviors. In G. R. Pierce, I. Sarason, & B. Sarason (Eds.), *The handbook of social support and family relationships* (pp. 313–343). New York: Plenum.

Barrera, M., Jr., & Prelow, H. (in press). Interventions to promote social support in children and adolescents. In D. Cicchetti, J. Rappaport, I. Sandler, & R. Weissberg (Eds.), *The promotion of wellness in children and adolescents.* Beverly Hills, CA: Sage.

Barrera, M., Jr., Sandler, I. N., & Ramsay, T. B. (1981). Preliminary development of a scale of social support: Studies on college students. *American Journal of Community Psychology, 9,* 435–447.

Bell, R. A., LeRoy, J. B., & Stephenson, J. J. (1982). Evaluating the mediating effects on social support upon life events and depressive symptoms. *Journal of Community Psychology, 10,* 325–340.

Belle, D. (Ed.). (1989). *Children's social networks and social supports.* New York: Wiley.

Blaney, P. H., & Ganellen, R. J. (1990). Hardiness and social support. In B. R. Sarason, I. G. Sarason, & G. R. Pierce (Eds.), *Social support: An interactional view* (pp. 297–318). New York: Wiley.

Bogat, G. A., Sullivan, L. A., & Grober, J. (1993). Applications of social support to preventive interventions. In D. S. Glenwick & L. A. Jason (Eds.), *Promoting health and mental health in children, youth, and families* (pp. 205–232). New York: Springer.

Broadhead, W. E., Kaplan, B. H., James, S. A., Wagner, E. H., Schoenbach, V. J., Crimson, R., Heyden, S., Tibblin, G., & Gehlbach, S. H. (1983). The epidemiologic evidence for a relationship between social support and health. *American Journal of Epidemiology, 117,* 521–537.

Brookings, S. B., & Bolton, B. (1988). Confirmatory factor analysis of the Interpersonal Support Evaluation List. *American Journal of Community Psychology, 16,* 137–147.

Brown, G. W., Andrews, B., Harris, T., Adler, Z., & Bridge, L. (1986). Social support, self-esteem and depression. *Psychological Medicine, 16,* 813–831.

Brown, G. W., Bhrolchain, M. N., & Harris, T. (1975). Social class and psychiatric disturbance among women in an urban population. *Sociology, 9,* 225–254.

Brownell, A., & Shumaker, S. A. (1985). Where do we go from here? The policy implications of social support. *Journal of Social Issues, 41,* 111–121.

Caldwell, R. A., & Bloom, B. L. (1982). Social support: Its structure and impact on marital disruption. *American Journal of Community Psychology, 10,* 647–667.

Caldwell, R. A., & Reinhart, M. A. (1988). The relationship of personality to individual differences in the use of type and source of social support. *Journal of Social and Clinical Psychology, 6,* 140–146.

Caplan, G. (1976). The family as support system. In G. Caplan & M. Killilea (Eds.), *Support systems and mutual help: Multidisciplinary explorations* (pp. 19–36). New York: Grune & Stratton.

Caplan, R. (1972). *Helping the helpers to help.* New York: Seabury.

Carmines, E. G., & Zeller, R. A. (1979). *Reliability and validity assessment.* Beverly Hills, CA: Sage.

Carveth, W. B., & Gottlieb, B. H. (1979). The measurement of social support and its relation to stress. *Canadian Journal of Behavioral Science, 11,* 179–187.

Cassel, J. (1976). The contribution of the social environment to host resistance. *American Journal of Epidemiology, 104,* 107–123.

Cauce, A. M., Reid, M., Landesman, S., & Gonzales, N. (1990). Social support in young children: Measurement, structure, and behavioral impact. In B. R. Sarason, I. G. Sarason, & G. R. Pierce (Eds.), *Social support: An interactional view* (pp. 64–94). New York: Wiley.

Cauce, A. M., & Srebnik, D. S. (1990). Peer networks and social support: A focus for preventive efforts with youths. In L. A. Bond & B. Compas (Eds.), *Primary prevention in the schools* (pp. 235–254). Newbury Park, CA: Sage.

Cleary, P. D., & Kessler, R. C. (1982). The estimation and interpretation of modifier effects. *Journal of Health and Social Behavior, 23,* 159–169.

Cohen, C. I., Teresi, J., & Holmes, D. (1986). Assessment of stress-buffering effects of social networks on psychological symptoms in an inner-city elderly population. *American Journal of Community Psychology, 14,* 75–91.

Cohen, L. H., McGowan, J., Fooskas, S., & Rose, S. (1984). Positive life events and social support and the relationship between life stress and psychological disorder. *American Journal of Community Psychology, 12,* 564–587.

Cohen, S. (1988). Psychosocial models of the role of social support in the etiology of physical disease. *Health Psychology, 7*, 269–297.

Cohen, S., & Hoberman, H. (1983). Positive events and social supports as buffers of life change stress. *Journal of Applied Social Psychology, 13*, 99–125.

Cohen, S., Lichtenstein, E., Mermelstein, R., Kingsolver, K., Baer, J. S., & Kamarck, T. W. (1988). Social support interventions for smoking cessation. In B. H. Gottlieb (Ed.), *Marshaling social support: Formats, processes, and effects* (pp. 211–240). Newbury Park, CA: Sage.

Cohen, S., & McKay, G. (1984). Social support, stress, and the buffering hypothesis: A theoretical analysis. In A. Baum, S. E. Taylor, & J. E. Singer (Eds.), *Handbook of psychology and health, Vol. 4: Social psychological aspects of health* (pp. 253–267). Hillsdale, N.J.: Lawrence Erlbaum.

Cohen, S., Mermelstein, R., Kamarck, T., & Hoberman, H. M. (1985). Measuring the functional components of social support. In I. G. Sarason & B. R. Sarason (Eds.), *Social support: Theory, research, and applications* (pp. 73–94). Dordrecht, The Netherlands: Martinus Nijhoff.

Cohen, S., & Wills, T. A. (1985). Stress, social support, and the buffering hypothesis. *Psychological Bulletin, 98*, 310–357.

Colletta, N. S. (1987). Correlates of young mother's network orientations. *Journal of Community Psychology, 15*, 149–160.

Costello, C. G. (1982). Social factors associated with depression: A retrospective community study. *Psychological Medicine, 12*, 329–339.

Cowen, E. L. (1994). The enhancement of psychological wellness: Challenges and opportunities. *American Journal of Community Psychology, 22*, 149–179.

Coyne, J. C., Aldwin, C., & Lazarus, R. S. (1981). Depression and coping in stressful episodes. *Journal of Abnormal Psychology, 90*, 439–447.

Coyne, J. C., & DeLongis, A. (1986). Going beyond social support: The role of social relationships in adaptation. *Journal of Consulting and Clinical Psychology, 54*, 454–460.

Coyne, J. C., & Downey, G. (1991). Social factors and psychopathology: Stress, social support, and coping processes. *Annual Review of Psychology, 42*, 401–425.

Coyne, J. C., Wortman, C. B., & Lehman, D. R. (1988). The other side of support: Emotional overinvolvement and miscarried helping. In B. Gottlieb (Ed.), *Marshaling social support: Formats, processes, and effects* (pp. 305–330). Newbury Park, CA: Sage.

Cutrona, C. E. (1986a). Behavioral manifestations of social support: A microanalytic investigation. *Journal of Personality and Social Psychology, 51*, 201–208.

Cutrona, C. E. (1986b). Objective determinants of perceived social support. *Journal of Personality and Social Psychology, 50*, 349–355.

Cutrona, C. E. (1990). Stress and social support: In search of optimal matching. *Journal of Social and Clinical Psychology, 9*, 3–14.

Cutrona, C. E., & Russell, D. W. (1990). Type of social support and specific stress: Toward a theory of optimal matching. In B. R. Sarason, I. G. Sarason, & G. R. Pierce (Eds.), *Social support: An interactional view* (pp. 319–366). New York: Wiley.

d'Abbs, P. (1982). *Social support networks: A critical review of models and findings*. Melbourne, Australia: Institute of Family Studies.

D'Augelli, A. R., Valiance, T. R., Danish, S. J., Young, C. E., & Gerdes, J. L. (1981). The community helpers project: A description of a prevention strategy for rural communities. *Journal of Prevention, 1*, 209–224.

Dean, A., & Ensel, W. M. (1982). Modelling social support, life events, competence, and depression in the context of age and sex. *Journal of Community Psychology, 10*, 392–408.

Dean, A., & Lin, N. (1977). The stress-buffering role of social support: Problems and prospects for systematic investigation. *Journal of Nervous and Mental Disease, 165*, 403–417.

Dignam, J. T., Barrera, M., Jr., & West, S. G. (1986). Occupational stress, social support, and burnout among correctional officers. *American Journal of Community Psychology, 14*, 177–193.

Dunkel-Schetter, C. (1984). Social support and cancer: Findings based on patient interviews and their implications. *Journal of Social Issues, 40*, 77–98.

Dunkel-Schetter, C., & Bennett, T. L. (1990). Differentiating the cognitive and behavioral aspects of social support. In B. R. Sarason, I. G. Sarason, & G. R. Pierce (Eds.), *Social support: An interactional view* (pp. 267–296). New York: Wiley.

Dunkel-Schetter, C., Folkman, S., & Lazarus, R. S. (1987). Correlates of social support receipt. *Journal of Personality and Social Psychology, 53*, 71–80.

Felner, R. D., Ginter, M., & Primavera, J. (1982). Primary prevention during school transition: Social support and environmental structure. *American Journal of Community Psychology, 10*, 277–290.

Felner, R. D., Brand, S., Adan, A. M., Mulhall, P. F., Flowers, N., Sartain, B., & DuBois, D. L. (1993). Restructuring the ecology of the school as an approach to prevention during school transitions: Longitudinal follow-ups and extensions of the school transitional environment project (STEP). *Prevention in Human Services, 10*, 103–136.

Felton, B. J., & Shinn, M. (1992). Social integration and social support: Moving "social support" beyond the individual level. *Journal of Community Psychology, 20*, 103–115.

Finch, J. F., Barrera, M., Jr., Okun, M. A., Bryant, W. H. M., Pool, G. J., & Snow-Turek, A. L. (1997). Factor structure of received social support: Dimensionality and the prediction of depression and life satisfaction. *Journal of Social and Clinical Psychology, 16*, 323–342.

Finney, J. W., Mitchell, R. E., Cronkite, R. C., & Moos, R. H. (1984). Methodological issues in estimating main and interactive effects: Examples from coping/social support and stress field. *Journal of Health and Social Behavior, 25*, 85–98.

Fiore, J., Becker, J., & Coppel, D. B. (1983). Social network interactions: A buffer or a stress? *American Journal of Community Psychology, 11*, 423–439.

Fisher, J. D., Nadler, A., & Whitcher-Alagna, S. (1982). Recipient reactions to aid. *Psychological Bulletin, 91*, 27–54.

Fleming, R., Baum, A., Gisriel, M. M., & Gatchel, R. J. (1982). Mediating influences of social support on stress at Three Mile Island. *Journal of Human Stress, 8*, 14–22.

Gesten, E. L., & Jason, L. A. (1987). Social and community interventions. *Annual Review of Psychology, 38*, 427–460.

Glasgow, R. E., Barrera, M., Jr., McKay, H. G., & Boles, S. M. (1998). *Social support, health behaviors, and quality of life among participants in an internet-based diabetes support program: A multi-dimensional investigation.* Paper presented at the annual meeting of the American Diabetes Association.

Gore, S. (1981). Stress-buffering functions of social supports: An appraisal and clarification of research models. In B. S. Dohrenwend & B. P. Dohrenwend (Eds.), *Stressful life events and their contexts* (pp. 202–222). New York: Prodist.

Gottlieb, B. H. (1978). The development and application of a classification scheme of informed helping behaviours. *Canadian Journal of Behavioural Science, 10*, 105–115.

Gottlieb, B. H. (1981). *Social networks and social support.* Beverly Hills, CA: Sage.

Gottlieb, B. H. (1983). *Social support strategies: Guidelines for mental health practice.* Beverly Hills, CA: Sage.

Gottlieb, B. H. (1988a). Marshaling social support: The state of the art in research and practice. In B. H. Gottlieb (Ed.), *Marshaling social support: Formats, processes, and effects* (pp. 11–51). Newbury Park, CA: Sage.

Gottlieb, B. H. (1988b). Support interventions: A typology and agenda for research. In S. W. Duck (Ed.), *Handbook of personal relationships* (pp. 519–541). New York: Wiley.

Heitzmann, C. A., & Kaplan, R. M. (1988). Assessment of methods for measuring social support. *Health Psychology, 7*, 75–109.

Heller, K. (1990). Social and community intervention. *Annual Review of Psychology, 41*, 141–168.

Heller, K., Price, R. H., & Hogg, J. R. (1990). The role of social support in community and clinical interventions. In B. R. Sarason, I. G. Sarason, & G. R. Pierce (Eds.), *Social support: An interactional view* (pp. 482–507). New York: Wiley.

Heller, K., & Swindle, R. W. (1983). Social networks, perceived social support, and coping with stress. In R. D. Felner, L. A. Jason, J. N. Moritsugu, & S. S. Farber (Eds.), *Preventive psychology: Theory, research and practice* (pp. 87–103). New York: Pergamon.

Henderson, S., Byrne, D. G., & Duncan-Jones, P. (1981). *Neurosis and the social environment.* Sydney, Australia: Academic.

Hirsch, B. J. (1980). Natural support systems and coping with major life changes. *American Journal of Community Psychology, 8*, 159–172.

Hirsch, B. J., Engel-Levy, A., DuBois, D. L., & Hardesty, P. H. (1990). The role of social environments in social support. In B. R. Sarason, I. G. Sarason, & G. R. Pierce (Eds.), *Social support: An interactional view* (pp. 367–393). New York: Wiley.

Hirsch, B. J., & Rapkin, B. D. (1986). Social networks and adult social identities: Profiles and correlates of support and rejection. *American Journal of Community Psychology, 14*, 395–412.

Hobfoll, S. E. (1990). Introduction: The importance of predicting, activating and facilitating social support. *Journal of Personality and Social Psychology, 7*, 435–436.

Hobfoll, S. E., Nadler, A., & Lieberman, J. (1986). Satisfaction with social support during crisis: Intimacy and self-esteem as critical determinants. *Journal of Personality and Social Psychology, 51*, 296–304.

Hobfoll, S. E., & Stephens, M. A. P. (1990). Social support during extreme stress: Consequences and intervention. In B. R. Sarason, I. G. Sarason, & G. R. Pierce (Eds.), *Social support: An interactional view* (pp. 454–481). New York: Wiley.

House, J. S. (1981). *Work stress and social support.* Reading, MA: Addison-Wesley.

House, J. S., & Kahn, R. L. (1985). Measures and concepts of social support. In S. Cohen & S. L. Syme (Eds.), *Social support and health* (pp. 83–108). Orlando, FL: Academic.

House, J. S., Umberson, D., & Landis, K. R. (1988). Structures and processes of social support. *Annual Review of Sociology, 14,* 293–318.

Husaini, B. A., Neff, J. A., Newbrough, J. R., & Moore, M. C. (1982). The stress-buffering role of social support and personal competence among the rural married. *Journal of Community Psychology, 10,* 409–426.

Jones, L., & Fischer, C. S. (1978). A procedure for surveying personal networks. *Sociological Methods and Research, 7,* 131–148.

Kaniasty, K., & Norris, F. H. (1995). Mobilization and deterioration of social support following natural disasters. *Current Directions in Psychological Science, 4,* 94–98.

Kaplan, B. H., Cassel, J. C., & Gore, S. (1977). Social support and health. *Medical Care, 15,* 47–58.

Kessler, R. C., & McLeod, J. D. (1985). Social support and mental health in community samples. In S. Cohen & S. L. Syme (Eds.), *Social support and health* (pp. 219–240). Orlando, FL: Academic.

Kessler, R. C., Price, R. H., & Wortman, C. B. (1985). Social factors in psychopathology: Stress, social support, and coping processes. *Annual Review of Psychology, 36,* 531–572.

Kiesler, C. A. (1985). Policy implications of research on social support and health. In S. Cohen & S. L. Syme (Eds.), *Social support and health* (pp. 347–364). Orlando, FL: Academic.

Kobasa, S. C., & Puccetti, M. C. (1983). Personality and social resources in stress resistance. *Journal of Personality and Social Psychology, 45,* 839–850.

LaRocco, J. M., House, J. S., & French, J. R. P., Jr. (1980). Social support, occupational stress, and health. *Journal of Health and Social Behavior, 21,* 202–218.

Leavy, R. L. (1983). Social support and psychological disorder: A review. *Journal of Community Psychology, 11,* 3–21.

Lefcourt, H. M., Martin, R. A., & Saleh, W. D. (1984). Locus of control and social support: Interactive moderators of stress. *Journal of Personality and Social Psychology, 47,* 378–389.

Leslie, L. A., & Grady, K. (1985). Changes in mothers' social networks and social support following divorce. *Journal of Marriage and the Family, 47,* 663–673.

Lieberman, M. A. (1986). Social supports—the consequences of psychologizing: A commentary. *Journal of Consulting and Clinical Psychology, 54,* 461–465.

Lieberman, M. A., & Mullan, J. T. (1978). Does help help? *American Journal of Community Psychology, 6,* 499–517.

Lin, N. (1986). Modeling the effects of social support. In N. Lin, A. Dean, & W. Ensel (Eds.), *Social support, life events, and depression* (pp. 173–209). Orlando, FL: Academic.

Lin, N., & Dean, A. (1984). Social support and depression: A panel study. *Social Psychiatry, 19,* 83–91.

Lin, N., Dean, A., & Ensel, W. M. (1986). *Social support, life events, and depression.* Orlando, FL: Academic.

Lin, N., & Ensel, W. M. (1984). Depression-mobility and its social etiology: The role of life events and social support. *Journal of Health and Social Behavior, 25,* 176–188.

McCormick, I. A., Siegert, R. J., & Walkey, F. H. (1987). Dimensions of social support: A factorial confirmation. *American Journal of Community Psychology, 15,* 73–77.

Mermelstein, R., Cohen, S., Lichtenstein, E., Baer, J. S., & Kamarck, T. (1986). Social support and smoking cessation and maintenance. *Journal of Consulting and Clinical Psychology, 54,* 447–453.

Mitchell, R. E., Billings, A. G., & Moos, R. H. (1982). Social support and well-being: Implications for prevention programs. *Journal of Primary Prevention, 3,* 77–98.

Mitchell, R. E., & Trickett, E. J. (1980). An analysis of the effects and determinants of social networks. *Community Mental Health Journal, 16,* 27–44.

Monroe, S. M., Bromet, E. J., Connell, M. M., & Steiner, S. C. (1986). Social support, life events, and depressive symptoms: A one-year prospective study. *Journal of Consulting and Clinical Psychology, 54,* 424–431.

Moos, R. H., Insel, P. M., & Humphrey, B. (1974). *Family, work, and group environment scales: Combined preliminary manual.* Palo Alto, CA: Consulting Psychologist Press.

Newcomb, M. D. (1990). What structural equation modeling can tell us about social support. In B. R. Sarason, I. G. Sarason, & G. R. Pierce (Eds.), *Social support: An interactional perspective* (pp. 26–63). New York: Wiley.

Newcomb, M. D., & Bentler, P. M. (1988). Impact of adolescent drug use and social support on problems of young adults: A longitudinal study. *Journal of Abnormal Psychology, 97,* 64–75.

O'Connor, P., & Brown, G. W. (1984). Supportive relationships: Fact or fancy? *Journal of Social and Personal Relationships, 1,* 159–175.

Olds, D. L. (1988). The prenatal/early infancy project. In R. H. Price, E. L. Cowen, R. P. Lorion, & J. Ramos-McKay (Eds.), *Fourteen ounces of prevention: A casebook for practitioners* (pp. 9–23). Washington, D.C.: American Psychiatric Association.

Olds, D. L., Henderson, C. R., & Kitzman, H. (1994). Does prenatal and infancy nurse home visitation have enduring effects on qualities of parental caregiving and child health at 25 to 50 months of life? *Pediatrics, 93,* 89–98.

Oxley, D., & Barrera, M., Jr. (1984). Undermanning theory and the workplace: Implications of setting size for job satisfaction and social support. *Environment and Behavior, 16,* 211–234.

Oxley, D., Barrera, M., Jr., & Sadalla, E. K. (1981). Relationships among community size, mediators, and social support variables: A path analytic approach. *American Journal of Community Psychology, 9*, 637–651.

Pagel, M. D., Erdly, W. W., & Becker, J. (1987). Social networks: We get by with (and in spite of) a little help from our friends. *Journal of Personality and Social Psychology, 53*, 793–804.

Perkins, D. D., & Zimmerman, M. A. (1995). Empowerment theory, research, and application. *American Journal of Community Psychology, 23*, 569–579.

Procidano, M. E., & Heller, K. (1983). Measures of perceived social support from friends and from family: Three validation studies. *American Journal of Community Psychology, 11*, 1–24.

Rabkin, J. G., & Struening, E. (1976). Life events, stress, and illness. *Science, 194*, 1013–1020.

Rappaport, J. (1987). Terms of empowerment/exemplars of prevention: Toward a theory for community psychology. *American Journal of Community Psychology, 15*, 121–148.

Riley, D., & Eckenrode, J. (1986). Social ties: Subgroup differences in costs and benefits. *Journal of Personality and Social Psychology, 51*, 770–778.

Rook, K. S. (1984). The negative side of social interactions: Impact on psychological well-being. *Journal of Personality and Social Psychology, 46*, 1097–1108.

Rook, K. S., & Dooley, D. (1985). Applying social support research: Theoretical problems and future directions. *Journal of Social Issues, 41*, 5–28.

Salem, D. A., Bogat, G. A., & Reid, C. (1997). Mutual help goes on-line. *Journal of Community Psychology, 25*, 189–207.

Sandler, I. N., & Barrera, M., Jr. (1984). Toward a multimethod approach to assessing the effects of social support. *American Journal of Community Psychology, 12*, 37–52.

Sandler, I. N., Gersten, J. C., Reynolds, K., Kallgren, C. A., & Ramirez, R. (1988). Using theory and data to plan support interventions: Design of a program for bereaved children. In B. H. Gottlieb (Ed.), *Marshaling social support: Formats, processes, and effects* (pp. 53–83). Newbury Park, CA: Sage.

Sandler, I. N., & Lakey, B. (1982). Locus of control as a stress moderator: The role of control perceptions and social support. *American Journal of Community Psychology, 10*, 65–80.

Sarason, B. R., Sarason, I. G., & Pierce, G. R. (1990). Traditional views of social support and their impact on assessment. In B. R. Sarason, I. G. Sarason, & G. R. Pierce (Eds.), *Social support: An interactional perspective* (pp. 9–25). New York: Wiley.

Sarason, B. R., Shearin, E. N., Pierce, G. R., & Sarason, I. G. (1987). Interrelationships of social support measures: Theoretical and practical implications. *Journal of Personality and Social Psychology, 52*, 813–832.

Sarason, I. G., Levine, H. M., Basham, R. B., & Sarason, B. R. (1983). Assessing social support: The social support questionnaire. *Journal of Personality and Social Psychology, 44*, 127–139.

Sarason, I. B., Sarason, B. R., & Pierce, G. R. (1990). Social support: The search for theory. *Journal of Social and Clinical Psychology, 9*, 133–147.

Sarason, I. G., Sarason, B. R., Shearin, E. N., & Pierce, G. R. (1987). The short form of the Social Support Questionnaire and its theoretical implications. *Journal of Social and Personal Relationships, 4*, 497–510.

Schradle, S. B., & Dougher, M. J. (1985). Social support as a mediator of stress: Theoretical and empirical issues. *Clinical Psychology Review, 5*, 641–661.

Schulz, R., Tompkins, C. A., & Rau, M. T. (1988). A longitudinal study of the psychosocial impact of stroke on primary support persons. *Psychology and Aging, 3*, 131–141.

Shinn, M., Lehmann, S., & Wong, N. W. (1984). Social interaction and social support. *Journal of Social Issues, 40*, 55–76.

Shumaker, S. A., & Brownell, A. (1984). Toward a theory of social support: Closing conceptual gaps. *Journal of Social Issues*, 11–36.

Silverman, P. R. (1988). Widow-to-widow: A mutual help program for the widowed. In R. H. Price, E. L. Cowen, R. P. Lorion, & J. Ramos-McKay (Eds.), *Fourteen ounces of prevention: A casebook for practitioners* (pp. 175–186). Washington, D.C.: American Psychological Association.

Slavin, L. A., & Compas, B. E. (1989). The problem of confounding social support and depressive symptoms: A brief report on a college sample. *American Journal of Community Psychology, 17*, 57–66.

Solomon, Z., & Benbenishty, R. (1986). The role of proximity, immediacy and expectancy in frontline treatment of combat stress reaction among Israelis in the Lebanon war. *American Journal of Psychiatry, 143*, 613–617.

Sosa, R., Kennell, J., Klaus, M., Robertson, S., & Urrutia, J. (1980). The effect of a supportive companion on perinatal problems, length of labor, and mother–infant interaction. *New England Journal of Medicine, 303*, 597–600.

Stokes, J. P. (1983). Predicting satisfaction with social support from social network structure. *American Journal of Community Psychology, 11*, 141–152.

Stokes, J. P., & Wilson, D. (1984). The inventory of socially supportive behaviors: Dimensionality, prediction, and gender differences. *American Journal of Community Psychology, 12*, 53–70.

Tardy, C. H. (1985). Social support measurement. *American Journal of Community Psychology, 13*, 187–202.

Tetzloff, C. E., & Barrera, M., Jr. (1987). Divorcing mothers and social support: Testing the specificity of buffering effects. *American Journal of Community Psychology, 15*, 419–434.

Thoits, P. A. (1982). Conceptual, methodological, and theoretical problems in studying social support as a buffer against life stress. *Journal of Health and Social Behavior, 23*, 145–159.

Tolsdorf, C. (1976). Social networks, support, and coping: An exploratory study. *Family Process, 15*, 407–417.

Turner, R. J. (1981). Experienced social support as a contingency in emotional well-being. *Journal of Health and Social Behavior, 22*, 357–367.

Uchino, B. N., Cacioppo, J. T., & Kiecolt-Glaser, J. K. (1996). The relationship between social support and physiological processes: A review with emphasis on underlying mechanisms and implications for health. *Psychological Bulletin, 119*, 488–531.

Vaux, A. (1985). Variations in social support associated with gender, ethnicity, and age. *Journal of Social Issues, 41*, 89–110.

Vaux, A. (1988). *Social support: Theory, research, and intervention.* New York: Praeger.

Vaux, A., Burda, P., & Stewart, D. (1986). Orientation toward utilizing support resources. *Journal of Community Psychology, 14*, 159–170.

Vaux, A., Phillips, J., Holly, L., Thompson, B., Williams, D., & Stewart, D. (1986). The Social Support Appraisals (SS-A) scale: Studies of reliability and validity. *American Journal of Community Psychology, 14*, 195–218.

Vaux, A., Riedel, S., & Stewart, D. (1987). Modes of social support: The social support behaviors (SS-B) scale. *American Journal of Community Psychology, 15*, 209–237.

Vaux, A., & Wood, J. (1987). Social support resources, behavior, and appraisals: A path analysis. *Social Behavior and Personality, 15*, 107–111.

Veiel, H. O., & Baumann, U. (1992). *The meaning and measurement of social support.* New York: Hemisphere.

Vinokur, A., Schul, Y., & Caplan, R. D. (1987). Determinants of perceived social support: Interpersonal transactions, personal outlook, and transient affective states. *Journal of Personality and Social Psychology, 53*, 1137–1145.

Wallston, B. S., Alagna, S. W., DeVellis, B. M., & DeVellis, R. F. (1983). Social support and physical health. *Health Psychology, 2*, 367–391.

Warheit, G., Vega, W., Shimizu, D., & Meinhardt, K. (1982). Interpersonal coping networks and mental health problems among four race-ethnic groups. *Journal of Community Psychology, 10*, 312–324.

Weiss, R. S. (1969). The fund of sociability. *TransAction, 6*, 36–43.

Wellman, B. (1981). Applying network analysis to the study of social support. In B. H. Gottlieb (Ed.), *Social networks and social support* (pp. 171–200). Beverly Hills, CA: Sage.

Wheaton, B. (1985). Models for the stress-buffering functions of coping resources. *Journal of Health and Social Behavior, 26*, 352–364.

Wilcox, B. L. (1981a). Social support in adjusting to marital disruption: A network analysis. In B. H. Gottlieb (Ed.), *Social networks and social support* (pp. 97–115). Beverly Hills, CA: Sage.

Wilcox, B. L. (1981b). Social support, life stress, and psychological adjustment: A test of the buffering hypothesis. *American Journal of Community Psychology, 9*, 371–386.

Wilcox, B. L., & Vernberg, E. M. (1985). Conceptual and theoretical dilemmas facing social support. In I. G. Sarason & B. R. Sarason (Eds.), *Social support: Theory, research, and applications* (pp. 3–20). Dordrecht, The Netherlands: Martinus Nijhoff.

Williams, A., Ware, J. E., Jr., & Donald, C. A. (1981). A model of mental health, life events, and social supports applicable to general populations. *Journal of Health and Social Behavior, 22*, 324–336.

Wills, T. A. (1990). Multiple networks and substance use. *Journal of Social and Clinical Psychology, 9*, 78–90.

Wills, T. A., & Vaughan, R. (1989). Social support and substance use in early adolescence. *Journal of Behavioral Medicine, 12*, 321–339.

Wolchik, S. A., Beals, J., & Sandler, I. N. (1989). Mapping children's social support networks: Conceptual and methodological issues. In D. Belle (Ed.), *Children's social networks and social support* (pp. 191–220). New York: Wiley.

Wolchik, S. A., Sandler, I. N., & Braver, S. L. (1987). Social support: Its assessment and relation to children's adjustment. In N. Eisenberg (Ed.), *Contemporary topics in developmental psychology* (pp. 319–349). New York: Wiley.

Wood, Y. R. (1984). Social support and social networks: Nature and measurement. In P. McReynolds & G. J. Chelune (Eds.), *Advances in psychological assessment, Vol. 4* (pp. 312–353). San Francisco: Jossey-Bass.

Wortman, C. B., & Lehman, D. R. (1985). Reactions to victims of life crisis: Support attempts that fail. In I. G. Sarason & B. R. Sarason (Eds.), *Social support: Theory, research and applications* (pp. 463–489). Dordrecht, The Netherlands: Martinus Nijhoff.

Zimmerman, M. A. (1995). Psychological empowerment: Issues and illustrations. *American Journal of Community Psychology, 23*, 581–599.

CHAPTER 11

Citizen Participation and Community Organizations

ABRAHAM WANDERSMAN AND PAUL FLORIN

The noted black educator Benjamin Mays said: "nobody is wise enough, nobody is good enough, and nobody cares enough about you, for you to turn over to them your future or your destiny." Citizen participation creates the potential for schools, neighborhoods, and other institutions, environments, and services responsive to individuals and families. Citizen participation is defined as "a process in which individuals take part in decision making in the institutions, programs, and environments that affect them" (Heller, Price, Reinharz, Riger, & Wandersman, 1984, p. 339; see Churchman, 1987, for definitions of participation in different disciplines).

Advocates of citizen participation propose that multiple benefits result from citizen participation, including:

1. Participation improves the quality of the environment, program, or plan because the people who are involved in implementation or usage have special knowledge that contributes to quality.
2. Participation increases feelings of control over the environment and helps individuals develop a program, plan, or environment that better fits with their needs and values.
3. Participation increases feelings of helpfulness and responsibility and decreases feelings of alienation and anonymity (see Wandersman, 1979a).

Churchman (1987) suggests additional goals of participation, including furthering democratic values, building support for government or for planning, and raising political consciousness (see Berry, Portney, Bablitch, & Mahoney, 1984; Kweit & Kweit, 1981).

THE SCOPE OF PARTICIPATION

Citizen participation plays an important role in many different settings in our society including:

ABRAHAM WANDERSMAN • Department of Psychology, University of South Carolina, Columbia, South Carolina 29208. PAUL FLORIN • Department of Psychology, University of Rhode Island, Kingston, Rhode Island 02881.

Handbook of Community Psychology, edited by Julian Rappaport and Edward Seidman. Kluwer Academic / Plenum Publishers, New York, 2000.

- *Work settings*: An informal review of the psychological literature on participation suggests that the largest amount of participatory research is performed in the area of work. Japanese business success has increased U.S. interest in quality circles and other forms of participative management (Klein, this volume; Lawler, 1987).
- *Health care programs and environments*: Citizen participation in decision-making in health care can occur at different levels—doctor–patient (Katz, 1984), hospital (Carpman, Grant, & Simmons, 1986), and regional (Duhl, 1986).
- *Neighborhood planning and rehabilitation*: In the last two decades, neighborhood improvement and renewal has received considerable attention and funding in many countries (Checkoway, 1985; Susskind & Elliott, 1983). Resident participation has played an important role in many revitalization programs (see Churchman, 1987, for an extensive review).
- *Human service agencies* (e.g., social work agencies, prisons, police departments, and mental health centers): The importance of line staff participation in policy and program development is discussed in Toch and Grant (1982) and Frank, Cosey, Angevine, and Cardone (1985). The importance of client participation is illustrated by choice and control opportunities for elderly living in sheltered care environments (Moos & Lemke, 1984). (Interestingly, both Moos and Lemke and Frank et al. found interactive effects depending upon the resources and abilities of the individuals, indicating that participation is not preferred by everybody.)
- *Political participation*: Political participation involves participation in government and includes voting, working for a political party, and supporting or opposing a particular issue. It is the type of citizen participation often referred to by political scientists and government officials. Involvement in political participation is often seen as disappointingly low; for example, 49% of voting age Americans voted in the 1996 presidential election, while an even smaller percentage voted in state and local elections.

CENTRAL ISSUES IN CITIZEN PARTICIPATION

While the above areas provide a glimmer of the vast interest in citizen participation, we know that it is not an easy panacea for problems. It is a complex issue, often difficult to successfully accomplish. While there are hundreds of empirical studies in the area of participation (many of them in sociology, political science, and social work), they have left us with several basic issues that can be stated as questions:

1. What are the characteristics of people who participate? Why do they participate? Who are the people who do not participate? Why not?
2. What are the characteristics of organizations or environments that facilitate or inhibit effective participation? What are the characteristics of organizations that are effective and survive vs. those that die out?
3. What are the effects of different forms of participation? What are the benefits and costs to the individual who participates? How does participation affect the program or community in which it occurs?

Wandersman and his colleagues have developed frameworks to help clarify the important concepts in citizen participation in several content areas: planning environments (Wandersman, 1979b), community organizations (Wandersman, 1981), community mental health centers (Wandersman, Kimbrell, Wadsworth, Livingston, Myers, & Braithwaite, 1982), research

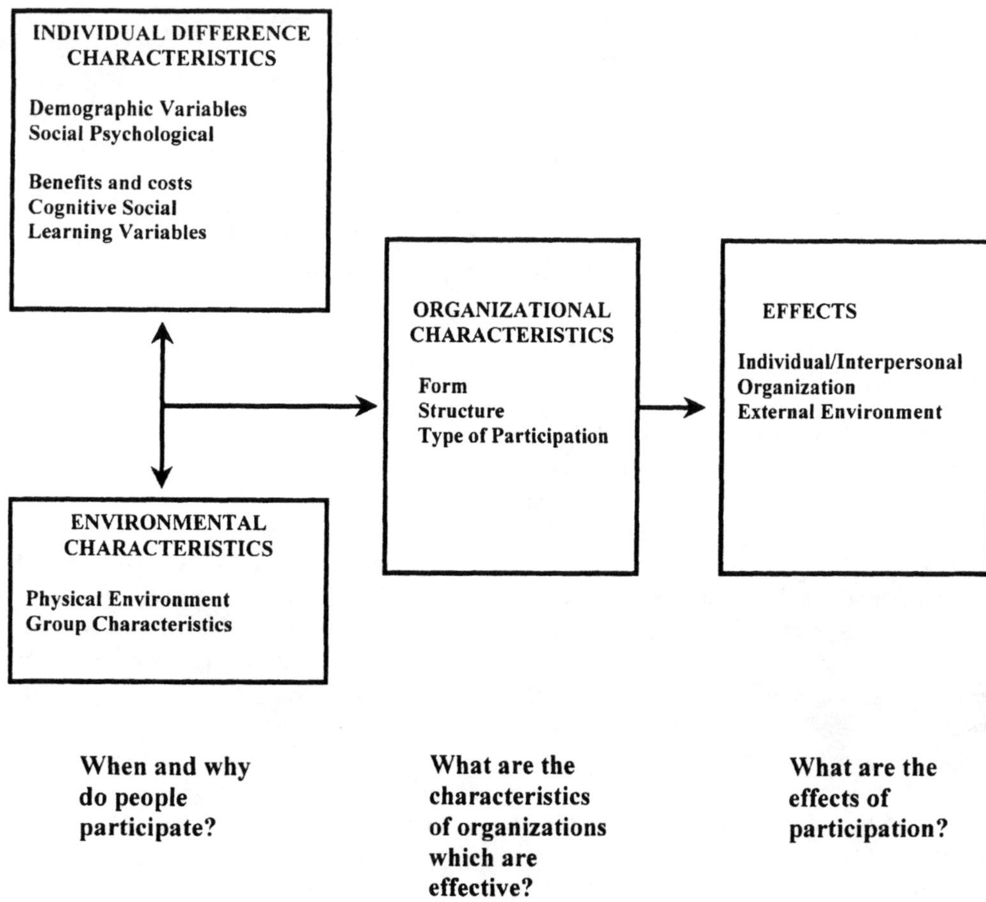

Figure 1. A framework of participation.

(Wandersman, Chavis, & Stucky, 1983), and community organizations formed in response to toxic hazards (Edelstein & Wandersman, 1987). In all of these areas, the frameworks describe the antecedents of participation, the process of participation, and the effects of participation. In Figure 1, we provide a general framework of citizen participation that relates the three sets of questions/issues to conceptual variables.

In this chapter, we will discuss the empirical literature on the three major issues of citizen participation. In order to make our literature review manageable, we have focused on the literature of citizen participation in neighborhood/community organizations (an area of particular relevance to community psychologists). However, we believe the issues and variables are relevant to all of the areas of citizen participation described in the scope of citizen participation. Many of the studies of citizen participation in neighborhood/community organizations were published in the 1970s and 1980s. This chapter is based upon a literature review conducted in 1992. In 1998, we updated the review by conducting a Psychlit and Medline search using the key words "citizen participation" and "participation in community organizations." We found few new studies in the updated review and none that challenged our belief that the issues and variables discussed below are relevant to all areas of citizen participation.

WHO PARTICIPATES, WHO DOES NOT PARTICIPATE, AND WHY?

A major puzzle in the citizen participation literature is "If participation is such a good thing, why don't more people participate?" Despite the desirable outcomes proposed as consequences of participation, relatively few people participate in government-initiated efforts or grass-roots groups (e.g., Cook & ISA Associates, 1993; Verba & Nie, 1972; Warren, 1963). The literature pertinent to individual characteristics and participation can be divided into demographic research and into social psychological research.

Demographic Variables

Many studies have related background demographic characteristics such as gender, age, marital status, education, and occupational status to voluntary action participation (cf. Smith, 1975). Demographic variables have been used in political science, sociology, and psychological studies to predict participation (Sundeen, 1988; Verba, Schlozman, Brady, & Nie, 1993). The relationship of socioeconomic characteristics and race to participation seem particularly important in the context of the residential environment. Piven (1968) identified several characteristics of the urban lower class that make participation less likely. These characteristics include being overwhelmed with concrete daily needs, having little belief in the ability to affect one's own world, and having fewer leadership skills. The work of a number of investigators suggests that middle-class people are more likely to participate than lower-class people, presumably because these social positions provide resources such as time and access to transportation (Alford & Scoble, 1968; Hyman & Wright, 1971; Milbrath, 1965; Smith, 1985; Sundeen, 1988). Controlling for socioeconomic status, blacks are more likely to participate in voluntary associations than whites (Orum, 1966; Williams, Babchuk, & Johnson, 1973; Florin, Jones, & Wandersman, 1986).

While demographic variables such as race and socioeconomic class have been related to participation, they have limited explanatory and predictive power. Research indicates that social background loses much of its direct explanatory power in predicting participation when intervening attitudes, personality, and situational variables are controlled statistically (Smith, 1975). It is possible that people who avoid participation in the larger society because of their own perceived inefficacy will respond with enthusiasm to an arena of concrete local concerns, such as activities that affect their own block or neighborhood. Therefore, general demographic characteristics, such as socioeconomic status or race, may be less relevant to participation in community organizations than characteristics such as specific relations to the community, or even marital status (Milbrath, 1965). Indeed, measures of investment in the locale, such as homeownership and length of residence, have been related to participation (Ahlbrandt & Cunningham, 1979; Babchuk & Thompson, 1962; Cohen, 1976; Litwak, 1961).

Generally, studies relating demographic variables to participation have focused on only one or two demographic variables. Two studies that have correlated several demographic variables with measures of participation found that they accounted for relatively little variance (Edwards & White, 1980; Vassar, 1978). Vassar (1978) investigated the relationship of gender, age, marital status, race, and socioeconomic status with block club membership and community projects membership and found 5% and 9% of variance accounted for, respectively. Edwards and White (1980) considered 11 demographic variables (age, sex, education, marital status, nuclear family size, community size, years lived in neighborhood, subjective assessment of health, yearly family income, education of the head of household, occupation of the head of the household) as predictors of various types of participation. The 11 variables accounted for only 8% of the variance in predicting participation in voluntary associations.

In a cross-cultural study of participation in block and neighborhood organizations in the United States and Israel, Wandersman, Florin, Friedmann, and Meier (1987) found that rootedness in the community was related to participation. Living in an area longer, intending to stay longer, and having more children can be seen as embedding an individual within a community, increasing both the opportunities and incentives to participate. Occupation, education, and race/ethnic status were not related to participation. This finding contrasts with much of the social science literature that has suggested the importance of education, occupation, and race for participation. For example, Williams and Ortega (1986) investigated the relationship of nine demographic variables with membership in five different types of voluntary organizations and found that only two variables (education and race) were related to all the types of organizations. The difference between the two studies may be due to the importance of the residential environment to working-class populations and the immediacy of the block/neighborhood organization. The similarity of the results in the United States and Israel on this issue indicates that these findings deserve attention and have important implications for expectations about who will and who will not participate.

Social Psychological Characteristics

In comparison to the many studies that have investigated demographic correlates of participation, very few have examined the relationship between participation and personality characteristics and attitudes (cf. Emmons, 1979; Parkum & Parkum, 1980; Smith, 1975; Tomeh, 1974). Some studies have explored the relationship between psychological characteristics of the individual and participation in voluntary organizations. An individual's participation in the community is associated with greater verbal and relational capabilities (Bronfenbrenner, 1960; Gough, 1952). Locus of control (a person's feeling of control over what happens) has been related to political activity (Gurin, Gurin, Lao, & Beattie, 1969) and to activity in the women's movement (Sanger & Alker, 1972).

Psychological empowerment (Zimmerman, 1990) and political efficacy (Hirlinger, 1992) have been associated with participatory behavior in several settings. Membership in a neighborhood organization has been shown to be related to favorable attitudes toward the neighborhood (Carr, Dixon, & Ogles, 1976). Chavis and Wandersman (1990) demonstrated in a longitudinal study that a sense of community could serve as a catalyst for participation in block associations, and Checkoway (1991) found that more active members and leaders in neighborhood associations rated community problems as more severe.

In the cross-cultural study by Wandersman et al. (1987) cited earlier, the striking aspect of the results from the social psychological set of variables was the overall consistency in the two different cultures. The results showed that 14 out of 16 social psychological variables were parallel across the samples, being either significant in both or nonsignificant in both. This suggests that the perceptions, attitudes, and beliefs leading to participation are the same and, by implication, the psychological processes that influence an individual's decision to become active are similar across the two cultures.

Group-Level Predictors

Research using block-aggregated survey and field-assessment data offers encouraging evidence that participation is related to malleable characteristics of community environments (Perkins, Florin, Rich, Wandersman, & Chavis, 1990). Noting that participation is unevenly distributed at the community level, Perkins et al. (1990) proposed an ecological framework for understanding the social and physical as well as the permanent and transient context of citizen participation in block associations. Block demographics and crime-related problems, perceptions, and fears, which were also part of their model, were largely unrelated to participation. However, they found that a combination of "catalysts" in the physical environment (such as poorly maintained properties) and "enablers" in the social environment (such as block satisfaction and neighboring behavior) were positively associated with collective participation.

The causal direction of this conclusion must be verified. But Perkins et al. (1990) argue that neighborhoods with little or no quality-of-life problems have nothing to organize about, and that neighbors who do not know, like, or interact with each other will not organize. However, when residents perceive physical deficiencies and when there is sufficient group social cohesion, they may organize and participate to rectify those problems. One implication of these community-focused, community-level correlates of participation is that conceptualizations of psychological empowerment might benefit from a more explicitly communitarian, or collectivist, orientation. "This would have the conceptual benefit of distinguishing empowerment from self efficacy and internal locus of control. It might also have the practical benefit of focusing interventions on collective action, which is likely to be more effective than individual action in solving collective problems" (Perkins et al., 1990, p. 108).

Why Do People Participate?

Based on her extensive review of the literature, Widmer (1984) concludes that many of the studies on why citizens participate actually focus on the characteristics of who participates. These studies have little to say about the motives of participants and the benefits they receive. "We need to know more about why people join organizations and what encourages them to devote time and energy to those organization's aims" (Gittell, 1980, p. 263).

Costs and Benefits

One approach to the issue of why people participate is represented by political economy theory (e.g., Moe, 1980; Olson, 1965; Rich, 1980). The theory suggests that a social exchange takes place in organizations in which participants will invest their energy only if they expect to receive some benefits (see Prestby, 1984, and Widmer, 1984, for a detailed review of costs, benefits, and incentives in voluntary organizations). Clark and Wilson's (1961) material, solidary, and purposive incentive typology has been widely cited. Material incentives are tangible rewards that can be translated into monetary value, such as wages, reduced taxes, and increased property values. Solidary incentives are derived from social interactions and include socializing, status, and group identification. Purposive incentives are derived from the suprapersonal goals of the organization and include bettering the community, doing one's duty, and feeling a sense of responsibility. The empirical literature on incentives in voluntary organizations is sparse. Knoke and Wood (1981) investigated incentives in voluntary organizations based on Clark and Wilson's typology. Most studies investigating incentives have looked only at leaders (e.g., Rich, 1980). Few studies have looked empirically at the costs involved in participation (e.g., time, money). While Oliver (1984) did explore the issue of costs of participation, she used indirect measures and did not directly ask respondents about the costs they experienced.

Wandersman et al. (1987) investigated the benefits and costs of participation in their cross-cultural study. They found two benefit factors (helping others and personal gains) and two cost factors (opportunity costs and organizational frustration). The absolute ratings suggested that both members and nonmembers agree that the greatest benefits are in making a contribution and helping others, rather than in self-interest or personal gains. In regard to costs, nonmembers perceived more costs than did members. The results suggest that nonmembers do not participate because they think it is costly. Possible reasons for the discrepancy between members and nonmembers is that nonmembers have an inaccurate perception of the costs or that their perception of members is based on those who are highly visible (i.e., leaders) who actually do work harder and bear more costs (see Friedmann, Florin, Wandersman, & Meier, 1988).

In the Block Booster Project, Prestby, Wandersman, Florin, Rich, and Chavis (1990), developed individual-level benefit and cost items as well as organization-level measures of incentive and cost-management strategies based on social exchange and political economy theory and voluntary organization research. These variables were applied to the examination of 29 block associations. Consistent with the finding of Wandersman et al. (1987), they found two benefit factors, consisting of personal and social/communal benefits, and two cost factors, consisting of personal and social/organizational costs. With respect to benefits and participation, Prestby et al. (1990) found that the most active participants reported receiving significantly more social/communal and personal benefits than less active participants, with personal benefits best distinguishing the most active participants. They propose that personal benefits, such as learning new skills, are likely to be exclusive to the high-level participants because they are contingent on participation. Regarding costs and participation, Prestby et al. found that the least active participants reported experiencing significantly more social/organizational costs than the active participants. In sum, social exchange and political economy theory were supported.

A review by Chinman and Wandersman (1999) summarizes the literature on costs and benefits and incentive/cost management. It also discusses costs and benefits in the context of different types of organizations, as well as their factor structures.

Taken as a whole, the social psychological and cost/benefit results lend empirical support to Henig's (1982) three-step model of mobilization wherein an individual perceives a condition, evaluates it as important to his or her well-being, and calculates that something can be done about it. This points to the importance of understanding more fully the processes through which an individual engages in a decision to participate in a particular organization.

Cognitive Social Learning Variables

Many psychologists agree that there is a complex interaction between the characteristics of the person and the environment that produces and sustains behavior. For this reason, an individual is likely to participate in only a few of the many organizations available. The organization(s) chosen are selected on the basis of the individual's own characteristics (e.g., needs, values, and personality) and the characteristics of the organization (e.g., purposes, efficacy, location).

The few studies that have organized multiple variables into conceptual frameworks have demonstrated the promise of a "process" approach to understanding and predicting participation. For example, Kaufman and Poulin (1994) organized seven variables thought relevant to participation within three constructs: participation accessibility, the desire to participate, and knowledge about participation. They were able to explain approximately 30% of the variance of participation in community prevention activities.

Mischel (1973, 1977) suggested five cognitive social learning variables as potentially useful in conceptualizing how the qualities of the person influence the impact of situations and how each person generates distinct patterns of behavior in interaction with the conditions of his or her life. Florin and Wandersman (1984) operationalized the cognitive social learning variables to predict participation in community settings. The five cognitive social learning variables are now called skills, view of the situation, expectations, values, and personal standards (Wandersman, Florin, Chavis, Rich, & Prestby, 1985). The set of cognitive social learning variables was compared with a larger set of traditional demographic and personality trait variables for ability to discriminate members from nonmembers, and they accounted for more of the variance in participation. Florin, Friedmann, Wandersman, and Meier (1989) replicated the results in a cross-cultural study of neighborhood participation in Israel.

Using structural equation modeling with these five cognitive social learning variables, Whitworth (1993) found that they accounted for nearly 50% of participation in neighborhood organizations, while Kerman (1996) found that they accounted for nearly 45% of behavioral intentions to participate in a community coalition.

The cognitive social learning variables are more likely to contribute to the practice of citizen participation because demographic and personality variables offer few practical suggestions for interventions to increase participation. A community organizer has little hope of changing age, personality, or status from renter to homeowner, while expectancies or skills are more amenable to change. This research is an example of the cognitive community psychology advocated by O'Neill (1981).

ORGANIZATIONAL CHARACTERISTICS AND PARTICIPATION

In this section, we review how organizational-level variables relate to the involvement and participation of members. We use a type of ecological analysis in examining individual behavior of the context of a setting (Moos, 1984; Trickett, Kelly, & Vincent, 1985). The approach is also an example of organizational analysis applied to community psychology phenomena (Keys & Frank, 1987). Finally, to the degree that neighborhood community development represents an empowerment process, these questions reflect a multilevel analysis of an empowerment context (Rappaport, 1987).

There are relatively few systematic studies of neighborhood community-development organizations. This is especially true when examining the organizational variables that facilitate members' involvement. There are multiple case studies that relate neighborhood characteristics to participation (Ahlbrandt & Cunningham, 1979; Crensen, 1983), that examine the role of community organizations in neighborhood mobilization (Henig, 1982), or that analyze the potential of different kinds of neighborhood groups to bring about social change (Lamb, 1975). Characteristics of leaders (Lamb, 1975) and specific strategies employed by community organizations (Henig, 1982) have also been examined for their association with mobilizing participation. But studies relating member involvement to organizational-level variables (i.e., characteristics of the internal structure, operations, and social climate of the community organization) are especially thin. Some literature does exist, including Knoke and Wood (1981) and Checkoway and Zimmerman (1992), who examined data from 90 neighborhood organizations and found that quality participation was related more to internal organizational adequacy than to the external strategy of the organization. The knowledge gap has significant practical implications. A major (perhaps the major) resource of small-scale voluntary associations, like block and neighborhood associations, is the members' participation. Members' time and energy must be mobilized into active involvement and performance of tasks. An organization that has many nominal members on paper, but cannot find anyone to do work, can hardly count itself as generating lots of participation. Knowledge of organizational variables that impact member involvement can be used to intervene to build capacity in such organizations (Chavis, Florin, Wandersman, & Rich, 1986; Florin, Chavis, Wandersman, & Rich, 1992).

The variables we examine here are those we commonly think of as describing characteristics of an organization. How many officers and committees does the organization have? Is it run loosely or with specific guidelines? Are decisions made at the top or with the involvement of many members? How much attention is given to ongoing communication among members? Do members feel as though the organization is cohesive or has "team spirit?"

The variables potentially associated with general organizational functioning and organizational maintenance present a wide array of choices. There is no tight theory of organizational functioning and maintenance in voluntary organizations that postulates a small and manageable number of variables (Smith, 1985). Here and in the next section (on organizational viability), we examine literature on selected variables from a framework developed for the Block Booster Project (Chavis et al., 1987; Florin et al., 1992). We review evidence on how the structure, decision-making style, and social climate of the voluntary organizations are related to members' involvement, satisfaction, and commitment.

Structural characteristics have been associated with member involvement. Structure refers to the way an association organizes its human resources for goal-directed activities, i.e., it is the way the members of an organization are arranged into relatively fixed relationships that largely define patterns of interaction, coordination, and task-oriented behavior (Steers, 1977). Structure includes such aspects as the levels of control, the number of formal officer roles for members to take part in within the organization, specialization (the degree to which activities are divided into specialized committees within the organization), and formalization (the degree to which rules and procedures are written and precisely defined).

Smith (1966) observed that members of voluntary associations prefer formal over informal groups, and this general finding also appears to apply to the members of neighborhood community-development associations. Milburn and Barbarin (1987) categorized 18 neighborhood associations into four groups according to the degree of structure present (highly structured, structured, unstructured, and highly unstructured). She found that the degree of structure present in the organization was strongly related to the degree of involvement in the organization among members. In a study of organizational viability of block associations, Prestby and Wandersman (1985) found that members in structured organizations were more involved and spent more time working for the organization outside of meetings.

How might more structure lead to greater member involvement? Members often join such an organization because they support it as a purposeful group and expect it to be task-oriented (Wandersman, Jakubs, & Giamartino, 1981; Pate, McPherson, & Silloway, 1987). More structure in an organization reduces ambiguities by delineating clear roles, task responsibilities, and operating procedures. This means a greater variety of options are open to engage or "hook" the members' energies and interests. A member can choose his or her level of involvement (e.g., officer, committee chair, committee member, general member) and area of involvement (e.g., to what committee to devote effort). McClure and DePiano (1983) found that role clarity was related to involvement in school advisory council participation. The clarity provided by more formalized procedures also allows for an orderly and predictable organization. Also, as Milburn and Barbarin (1987) observe, the clear role and task responsibilities allow the member to better manage time, committing only to those activities or tasks chosen, and needing, therefore, to be less vigilant of open-ended, free-wheeling commitments. Finally, to the degree that more structure relates to more success in accomplishing tasks and achieving success (Prestby & Wandersman, 1985), member involvement is reinforced and amplified.

Organizations conduct their business in particular ways. Most significant is the degree to which these organizations involve members in decision-making and how this relates to member commitment and involvement. Members in neighborhood community-development organizations may respond to more structure with greater involvement, but this does not imply that they simply want to be told what to do by leaders or that they do not want to have a say in the decision-making of the organization. Knoke and Wood (1981) found that increased participation in decision-making was related to members' commitment, time spent, and task performance. Prestby and Wandersman (1985) found members spent more time volunteering in block associations that used a democratic decision-making process as opposed to a mixed democratic/autocratic process or a solely autocratic one.

Social climate is a way of assessing the collective "personality" of an organization. The members' perceptions of organizational characteristics, such as relationships between members, leader support and control, and structural characteristics can be used to describe and contrast different organizational settings. Organizational researchers (e.g., Schneider, 1975) believe that the study of organizations should include participants' perceptions because they can make a great difference in organizational behaviors. Important social climate effects in several different kinds of settings have been documented (Moos, 1987). Earlier work has suggested that social climate is related to the activity level of block and neighborhood organizations (Yates, 1973). As with other organizational variables in neighborhood community development, research relating social climate variables to member commitment and involvement is virtually nonexistent. One study systematically examined social climate in such organizations (Giamartino & Wandersman, 1983). In the following, we briefly review the results from this study and then discuss a reanalysis of the same data, using a levels of analysis statistical method that sheds additional light on organizational climate influences in these organizations.

Giamartino and Wandersman (1983) used the Group Environment Scale to examine the relationship of 10 social climate dimensions to members' satisfaction, enjoyment, and time involvement. Using aggregate data from 172 members of 17 block associations (from the Neighborhood Participation Project), they found that the average level of satisfaction and enjoyment was significantly related to three social climate dimensions. Members were more satisfied and enjoyed their involvement more in associations that were perceived to have: (1) higher levels of "team spirit" and comraderie among members (cohesiveness), (2) higher degrees of structure and formalization of activities (order and organization), and (3) leaders who actively directed the group and enforced rules (leader control). Importantly, no significant relationships were found between any of the social climate dimensions and the average activity level of members in the organization (time spent on organizational activities in the previous 2 months). The message to the research community and practitioners working with small-scale voluntary community groups was that there was no empirical knowledge for taking action to increase the participatory activity of members through targeting particular climate dimensions. This could be a disheartening conclusion for leaders whose primary resource is the activity level of members. The data from the Giamartino and Wandersman study was later reanalyzed using a data analysis method unavailable to them at the time of their work (Florin, Giamartino, Kenny, & Wandersman, 1990). The data analysis method (Kenny & LeVoie, 1985) adjusts group-level correlations for the presence of individual effects. That is, when researchers aggregate climate scores within groups and then use the group as a unit of analysis, it is not known how much of the observed relationships were caused by an actual group interaction process that affects the member's response, and how much by the mere sum of (presumably preexisting) individual effects. The statistical program LEVEL (Kenny & Stigler, 1983) adjusts correlations at one level for the effects of the other. The adjusted group-level correlation shows how group interaction creates differences between groups beyond the sum of individual effects. It is more "pure group" than the usual group level, which simply aggregates individual member's scores. Adjusted group-level correlations revealed four sizeable correlations that were masked by the unadjusted group correlations. None of the GES subscales was related to time involvement at the individual level. Therefore, for a particular individual, personal perception of climate dimensions was unrelated to the amount of time they devoted to the organization. However, the adjusted group-level correlations suggest that group interaction itself has an effect such that the average time involvement of members is higher in groups that produce a climate that is (1) higher in cohesion, (2) lower in tolerance for independent action that is uncoordinated with the group, (3) higher in encouragement for sharing personal feelings and information, and (4) higher in tolerance for negative feelings or disagreements. The results have theoretical and practical implications. Researchers can construct models of the relationships among the relevant climate dimensions, hypothesized group processes, and an important behavioral outcome. Practitioners can be told about four different climate dimensions to target in their attempts to try to increase the average participation of members. There are important implications for reexamining group-level effects in social and community research, and for developing more sophisticated and articulated models of the relationship among social climate dimensions (Florin et al., 1990).

Organizational Characteristics and Organizational Viability

Small-scale community-development associations are vulnerable to rapid decline or failure because they rely on the energy and expertise of people who are volunteering their time, which they are free to withdraw at any time. Formation of such organizations may be relatively easy in comparison to maintaining the association after initial enthusiasm and excitement has faded (Miller, Malia, & Tsembersis, 1979). Therefore, it is important to investigate what factors help these associations survive and grow. There have been few systematic studies of organizational effectiveness and viability in voluntary organizations. Studies of neighborhood community development organizations are fewer still. There is literature that either surveys large numbers of such organizations and describes typical patterns and variations in operations, or describes individual organizations as examples worthy of emulation (National Commission on Neighborhoods, 1979). This type of work did not attempt to systematically measure organizational effectiveness. Organizational effectiveness was examined in larger, more sophisticated neighborhood community-development organizations with substantial funding and staff resources (Perlman, 1978). An example is Myers' (1984) comprehensive and systematic study that related factors from six internal and external organizational categories to an objective measure of effectiveness. The 99 neighborhood development organizations studied, however, had average annual budgets of around $250,000 and paid professional staffs. These organizations, like other community-development corporations (Pierce & Steinbach, 1987) or local social-service nonprofit organizations (Milofsky, 1987), are bureaucratized, with complex administrative structures and centralized decision-making to manage their considerable resources. They maintain their commitment to locale-based development and service, and can have enormous impacts on the entire neighborhood, which the less formal organizations cannot produce (Pierce & Steinbach, 1987). However, these are not the kind of neighborhood community-development organizations on which we are focusing. In the less formal organizations, the primary resource is the energy and involvement of members. These members have face-to-face contact and more decision-making participatory control. Therefore, the process and experience of participation in these less formal organizations is qualitatively different from resident involvement in the larger organizations (where participation is usually less direct and "hands on"). The very process of participation in the smaller and less formalized organizations produces its own effects related to the social fabric among residents and member attitudes and beliefs, including a sense of empowerment (see next section). These are the personal-level impacts that are lost when neighborhood organizations fail to survive. Indeed, failure of informal organizations to survive may decrease the expectations for the success of collective action, so that residents may not participate in the future. Retreat into the isolation of apathy and anomie is also possible. This more psychological and process approach to participation and organizational viability contrasts with a sanguine approach to organizational decline by those who hold a market-based economic analogy to community conditions (Milofsky, 1987). In the following we examine studies related to organizational viability in the less formal neighborhood community-development organizations.

There are several possible ways to think about organizational viability or effectiveness (Steers, 1977), and researchers have disagreed about the best way to measure viability (Smith, 1966). Agreement does exist on the common-sense notion that a primary indicator of viability in any organization is its ability to continue to exist or maintain itself. Organizations that cease to function are obviously less effective and viable. Cessation of functioning is a frequent occurrence in neighborhood community-development associations. Yates (1973) found that more than 50% of the block associations he studied became inactive after they had performed initial simple tasks. In the Neighborhood Participation Project, of the 17 active block associations studied, only 8 were found to be functioning one year later (Prestby & Wandersman, 1985; Wandersman et al., 1985). The Block Booster Project was also witness to the fragility of block associations. Thirty-two active block associations were selected for participation in the study in November 1984. By the study's end in May 1986, 12 of these 32 (37.5%) were no longer functioning.

Prestby and Wandersman (1985) examined several categories of variables related to differences between block associations that maintained operations and those that fell into inactivity and ceased operations. Several of these relate to the results of the previous section on organizational characteristics related to participation. Block associations that accomplished their goals and maintained their operations: (1) mobilized more of their internal resources (member commitment and satisfaction); (2) had more experienced, involved and visible leaders; (3) were more likely to involve their members directly in decision-making; (4) had social climates with higher levels of cohesiveness, structure, task focus, leader support, and leader control; (5) engaged in more fund-raising and recruitment activities; and (6) engaged in a greater number and wider variety of activities, thus providing a variety of participation options for residents.

In the Block Booster Project (Florin et al., 1992), data from a variety of sources was gathered on 28 active block associations from February 1985 to May 1985. By May 1986, eight of these block associations had lapsed into inactivity and ceased operations. "Inactivity" was operationalized as having had no meetings or activities during the preceding 6 months. The data gathered 12–15 months earlier was used to distinguish characteristics of those blocks that maintained operations from those who ceased functioning.

1. Block associations that maintained operations mobilized a greater proportion of the residents on their blocks into becoming members and mobilized a greater percentage of nominal members into being active members. The ability to mobilize resources and not actual block size accounted for larger numbers of members in those associations that maintained operations.
2. Associations that maintained operations engaged in more activities that offered a range of participation opportunities. All of the associations that remained active sponsored five or more different activities, while only half of those associations that eventually ceased operations did so.
3. Structural characteristics were associated with maintenance. Block associations that survived had a greater number of officers, twice as many committees (specialization), and were more likely to operate with rules and procedures written and precisely defined (formalization).
4. Organizations perform functions that focus their activities both quantitatively and qualitatively. Block associations that remained active.
   a. used a greater number of methods (e.g., newsletters, personal contact, telephone calls) to communicate with members.
   b. used more personalized outreach strategies to recruit new members (e.g., direct personal contact rather than reliance on word-of-mouth or general announcements).
   c. took a more proactive stance in the recruitment and preparation of new leaders (e.g., recruited potential leaders in preparation for future openings and assigned leadership responsibilities like chairing a committee to members who were not currently officers but were likely to be).
   d. used consensus and formalized (vote) decision-making procedures more often and attempted to delegate responsibilities for activities to a greater proportion of the membership (decentralization).
5. Block associations establish ties or linkages with sources of external resources. These ties often help maintain organizational viability (Knoke & Wood, 1981). Sixty-seven percent of the associations that maintained operations received helpfrom six or more external organizations, while only 17% of those associations that maintained operations received help from six or more external organizations.
6. Prestby et al. (1990) found that block associations that remained active and viable provided more membership incentive efforts and more membership cost-reduction efforts at a higher frequency than block associations that later became inactive or defunct. These results support social exchange and political economy theory, and suggest that incentive and cost-management efforts at the organizational level can positively influence organizational maintenance.

The ages of the block associations emphasized that maintenance is not something done once and then forgotten. The ages of block associations that became inactive averaged 6.9 years; some had been in existence for as long as 15 years. Maintenance takes an ongoing effort, no matter what the age of the block association.

Research results from the Block Booster Project identified specific structures and functions that distinguish which groups will remain active. Technical assistance training and materials were organized simply and concisely into four domains based on the findings: (1) structure of the organization, (2) activities related to mobilization of member resources, (3) promotion of decentralization and leadership development, and (4) identifying and accessing external resources. Checklists in each of these domains indicate the presence of "risk factors" associated with the organization's "health." The checklist can be cross-referenced to sections of a workbook/reference manual where recommendations for organizational change are found. Such a prototypical system for the provision of technical assistance was assessed as part of the Block Booster Project (Florin et al., 1992).

EFFECTS OF CITIZEN PARTICIPATION

Community development has been defined as the creation of improved physical, social, and economic conditions through an emphasis on the voluntary cooperation and self-help of residents (Rothman, 1970). Here citizen participation refers to citizen action (Langton, 1978), where citizens initiate and control activities designed to gain some influence over conditions affecting their lives. Citizen action in community development has been growing, and estimates of the numbers of neighborhood community-development organizations range from 8,000 to 60,000 nationally (Boyte, 1980; Langton, 1978). Where such organizations exist, participation rates generally range from 10–20% of the residents (Ahlbrandt, 1984; Podolefsky & DuBow, 1980; Skogan & Maxfield, 1980). This also represents only a portion of those who, in various surveys, report a willingness to do volunteer work for neighborhood improvement. Clearly, neighborhood community development is an area involving many people and much activity. Some see it as representing a social movement that has the potential to address many social problems at the local level, strengthen urban life, and expand democracy through the inclusion of formerly disenfranchised and disempowered groups (Boyte, 1980; Hallman, 1984; Perlman, 1979; Williams, 1985).

Community development captures the public's attention because of its emphasis on the traditional American values of participation and self-reliance. Its optimistic and humanistic views on the possibilities of achieving consensus and cooperation are further reasons why community development is a popular concept (Blakely, 1980; Heller et al., 1984). It also has appeal because its goals are sufficiently ambiguous, allowing for many hopes and desires to be seen as potential outcomes (Voth, 1979).

Some see neighborhood community development as a means of altering basic power relations between a community group and differing bureaucratic structures. Improving the physical conditions of the residential environment or altering social conditions, such as vandalism or crime, may also be the focus of a community group (Currie, 1982; Silberman, 1978). Some groups may strive to increase supportive, neighborly behaviors, while others focus on the individual in such areas as increasing citizenship skills and decreasing alienation (Currie, 1982; Howard, 1984; Silberman, 1978). Thus, proponents of community development have suggested many potential benefits of citizen participation in community-development efforts. Reports of successful efforts and case studies have supplied some concrete illustrations of several of these benefits. However, systematic research examining the effects of such participation on individuals, on their relationships with their neighbors, and ultimately on their environment is limited. In order to facilitate the evaluation of the effects of participation in neighborhood community development, we examine effects in three domains: (1) impacts on physical and social conditions, (2) impacts on interpersonal relationships, and (3) impacts on the participating individuals.

As mentioned above, much of the literature consists of case studies of particular neighborhood-development achievements. Collections of such case studies have been compiled to represent the range of potential impacts and provide examples of specific programs that might be adopted by others (Berkowitz, 1984; Hallman, 1984; Williams, 1985). Only a few multiple case studies have been conducted that examined multiple organizations using a systematic conceptual and measurement framework (Mayer, 1984; Crensen, 1983). The use of sophisticated quasi-experimental designs is rare.

In the following sections, we summarize results from studies that have examined the impact of neighborhood community-development organizations. We highlight the results of two projects that contribute to the literature by comparing blocks with and without small-scale community-development organizations (e.g., block associations) for multiple impacts. Because of the limited nature of the literature in some areas, supplemental material from outside the neighborhood community-development arena is included.

Impacts on Physical and Social Conditions

The majority of neighborhood community-development efforts usually have primary goals that focus on concrete conditions affecting neighborhood residents. Dissatisfaction with neighborhood conditions, such as poor housing, vacant buildings, litter and garbage, cluttered empty lots, inadequate municipal services, vandalism, and crime are factors that lead to the formation of neighborhood groups. Neighborhood development advocates recognize that because the neighborhood is an open system, large-scale forces, such as general demographic trends, industrial out-migration, suburban housing development, and general economic downturns affect metropolitan areas, and thus neighborhood conditions (Ahlbrandt & Cunningham, 1979; Downs, 1981; Schoenberg & Rosenbaum, 1980). Bartelt, Elesh, Goldstein, Leon, and Yancey (1987) present a detailed analysis of the powerful political economy forces of the city on neighborhood life. But neighborhood development advocates argue that neighborhood residents should work where they can hope to have an immediate impact. By creating such impacts, citizens may buffer or resist some of the negative effects of the larger external forces (Ahlbrandt & Cunningham, 1979; Checkoway, 1985).

Many neighborhood-development organizations are formed as a response to the threat or reality of physical deterioration. In a study of 153 neighborhood groups in the Chicago area, it was found that most of the groups were formed to address the physical conditions of their neighborhoods (Lavrakas, Normoyle, Skogan, Herz, Salem, & Lewis, 1980). These conditions can be directly affected by the self-help and mutual aid efforts of neighborhood residents. There are many case examples in the literature of how neighborhood organizations have successfully changed local physical conditions (e.g., Alterman & Frankel, 1985; Cassidy, 1980; Draisen, 1983; Godschalk & Zeisel, 1983; Harris, 1984; National Commission on Neighborhoods, 1979; Rohe & Gates, 1981, 1982; Schoeneberg & Rosenbaum, 1980; Wooley, 1985). These impacts range from relatively simple clean-up and beautification programs, to home-repair maintenance and improvement programs, to more ambitious building projects. The scope and impact of these programs are often determined by the degree to which a self-help/mutual aid neighborhood community-development effort evolves and expands into a more formalized neighborhood or community-development corporation (Hallman, 1984; Pierce & Steinbach, 1987). These larger and more structured organizations can have enormous positive impacts on neighborhood development. Some of these organizations have annual budgets in the millions of dollars, hundreds of employees, and operate extensive and sophisticated economic and social development projects (Pierce & Steinbach, 1987). Such formalization and bureaucratization, however, moves an organization away from the reliance on the voluntary efforts of residents as primary resource and away from more direct residential control of operations characteristic of the neighborhood self-help/mutual aid efforts that are our focus here.

Physical conditions on the block are important because they relate to neighborhood satisfaction, neighborhood confidence, and desire to move. Ahlbrandt and Cunningham (1979) and Zehner (1972) found that satisfaction with levels of upkeep in the microneighborhood explained 30% of the variance in overall satisfaction. Mitler et al. (1980) found satisfaction with neighborhood physical qualities and attractiveness accounted for over 40% of overall satisfaction. Ahlbrandt and Cunningham (1979) found that of those residents who planned to move within two years, 50% rated the neighborhood as a poor or fair place to live, as compared with 24% of those who did not plan to move. Physical conditions thus can affect satisfaction with, and confidence in, the block and neighborhood. In the Neighborhood Participation Project (Wandersman, Unger, & Florin, 1991), blocks with block associations were compared with similar blocks without block associations. A rating instrument was used by observers to assess the physical environment of the block in four areas: house, yard, semipublic, and public. Longitudinal results showed that blocks with block associations received significantly higher ratings of the physical environment in all four categories. Moreover, surveys of block residents showed that perceptions of the severity of problems there went down where there were block associations, while overall satisfaction increased. These results indicate that block associations organized for community-development purposes can have positive effects on the physical environment, and that changes in physical conditions are reflected in the perceptions of residents. Decreased confidence fanned by signs of physical deterioration can lead to fear that financial investments in property are endangered, leading to even less investment and promoting a downward spiral (Goetze, 1979). Physical improvements can thus have a stabilizing effect through increasing satisfaction and promoting confidence. Residents of blocks with block associations were more likely to invest in home improvements, demonstrating a confidence in making financial investments in their homes that is found less frequently among residents on blocks without associations. Similar results were found in the Block Booster Project (Chavis, Florin, Rich, & Wandersman, 1987) which gathered information from close to 1,000 residents on 47 blocks. Members of block associations were more satisfied with their blocks, planned to stay there longer, and homeowners demonstrated their greater confidence and commitment by a higher frequency of investment in home improvements.

Signs of physical decline are also related to the second major concern that prompts the formation of neighborhood groups—fear and concern about crime. Lewis and Maxfield (1980) demonstrated that physical deterioration, abandonment, and dilapidation contributed to fear of crime. Craik and Appleyard (1980) also found a relationship between signs of physical decline and feelings of insecurity. Halting physical deterioration and promoting physical improvements may be one avenue by which neighborhood development organizations may impact upon crime and fear of crime. Neighborhood development organizations can also address crime prevention directly. Organizations may be specifically formed to address this issue, e.g., crime-watch programs (Schneider & Schneider, 1978; Washnis, 1976). However, it is more typical that crime-prevention programs are sponsored by an existing neighborhood organization created for other purposes (Lavrakas et al., 1980). There are several studies that indicate that community crime-prevention programs do reduce crime rates (Latessa & Allen, 1980; Washnis, 1976; Whisenand, 1977). The effects of crime-prevention programs on fear of crime is less clear-cut. Some studies found that fear of crime was reduced (Chavis et al., 1987; Skogan & Maxfield, 1980; Washnis, 1976), while others found that it increased (Lavrakas & Herz, 1979). Still other studies found no relationship between participation and fear (Maxfield, 1977; Podoelfsky & DuBow, 1980; Rohe & Greenberg, 1982). Such discrepant findings indicate a complex relationship, with the need to study types of programs, severity of local crime, neighborhood make-up, and other situational factors as mediating variables.

Neighborhood community development can address social services provided to local residents. The actual mechanisms used to improve social-service delivery have varied greatly. Some neighborhood organizations organize and deliver their own social services provided entirely by volunteers. For example, neighborhood organizations have provided daycare and babysitting cooperatives, or designed and delivered programs for youth (e.g., summer employment programs) and the aged (e.g., senior escort services and home visits) (Boyte, 1980; Hallman, 1984). Neighborhood organizations may also influence various arrangements made by their city to decentralize and/or coordinate municipal services at the neighborhood level. The actual structural arrangements may range from task force, to multiservice centers, to neighborhood councils. Yin and Yates (1974) reviewed 215 case studies of decentralization and concluded that service delivery improved in 72% of the cases. Moreover, they found that such improvement of services happened most often in those decentralization programs in which residents had the most direct governing control over the service provided. A city may also form a partnership with a neighborhood organization where the city contracts with the organization to deliver services. When the partnership involves the neighborhood organization as a full and legitimate partner in goal formation, planning, and implementation, then genuine coproduction of services exists (Spiegel, 1987).

Impacts on Interpersonal Relationships

The spatial proximity of neighbors makes them particularly handy sources of aid (Unger & Wandersman, 1985). Neighbors do more than provide the loan of a cup of sugar; they are important sources of information and referral to needed services, such as childcare. Neighboring fosters a sense of identification with the area, develops a sense of community, and buffers feelings of isolation. Neighbors also serve as important sources for support for individuals by providing emotional and material aid. Warren (1981) found neighbors to be important components of helping networks, with 56% of respondents reporting they were helped by a neighbor during a life crisis the preceding year.

Impacts on interpersonal relationships include changes in socializing and mutual assistance among residents. This may be viewed as a secondary goal of community development or as the means to an end (e.g., promoting neighboring to increase mutual assistance toward the goal of reducing crime). But such impacts are seldom a primary goal of the organization.

Many studies have found a relationship between participation in formal community organizations and informal interactions among residents (Devereaux, 1960; Fellin & Litwak, 1963). Ahlbrandt and Cunningham (1979) and Hunter (1974) found that residents with more friends in their neighborhood and closer ties with their neighbors were more likely to be members of local community groups. These studies, however, do not indicate a direction of causality. Whether informal interaction was an impetus for, or the result of, participation was unclear. Other studies provide evidence that certain kinds of social ties with a neighborhood, specifically dense social networks (i.e., many of one's friends also know each other), can inhibit participation within a neighborhood organization (Crensen, 1978; Grannovetter, 1973, 1974, 1982).

A few studies have found an increase in neighboring as an effect of participation (Latessa & Allen, 1980). Using longitudinal data, Unger and Wandersman (1983) demonstrated that participation significantly increased the degree of neighboring. Neighboring was assessed prior to and after block associations were formed. Residents who became members of the block association showed a significant increase in neighboring, while the neighboring of those who did not participate stayed the same. Preliminary analyses of cross-sectional data from the Block Booster Project support the Unger and Wandersman finding. Neighboring was assessed on blocks with and without block associations. The neighboring of participants in block associations was significantly higher than that of nonparticipants, which was approximately the same as residents of blocks without associations. This suggests that block associations do increase neighboring among residents, but only for those who participate. There appear to be only minor spillover effects to nonparticipants.

Impacts on the Individual

Individual impacts, such as changes in attitudes, beliefs, and skills, accrue during the process of participation in neighborhood community development. These impacts, however, are often latent goals of neighborhood organizations. While these impacts play a role in both the theory and advocacy of participation in neighborhood community development, they are seldom directly articulated as a primary goal of the organization. Organizers and/or indigenous leaders may have the goal of "empowering" organizational members such that their skills are increased or their sense of political efficacy advanced; however, the actions of members are directed toward getting improved city services or reducing crime. Participants are usually asked to direct their attention and actions outward onto external conditions; seldom are they specifically asked to act in the service of creating change within themselves. These impacts are important, but they are not usually articulated as organizational goals.

Participation can result in changed attitudes and beliefs about various aspects of the environment, including attitudes towards one's neighbors, municipal services, or government in general. For example, some studies indicate that participation will increase individual satisfaction with one's neighborhood, and also will help to develop more positive attitudes toward other community members (Cunningham, 1979; Litwak, 1961). Ahlbrandt (1984) found statistically significant correlations between participation in neighborhood organizations and the belief that neighbors are interested in neighborhood problems. Cole (1974), studying 26 neighborhood programs in six midwestern localities, found that participation increased trust and confidence in the government in general. In the Block Booster Project (Chavis et al., 1987), members of block associations held significantly more positive attitudes toward their block and their neighbors than did nonmembers on the same blocks or residents of blocks without associations. Members were significantly more likely to think their block compared favorably with other blocks, to feel that conditions have improved and will continue to improve on their block, to express a higher sense of community with others on the block, and to plan on staying there longer. The cross-sectional nature of the data does not allow us to rule out the possibility that such associations may be the cause, rather than effect, of participation. However, the fact that nonmembers on blocks with associations were very similar to residents on blocks without associations suggests that participation can generate such differences in attitudes and beliefs. In the Neighborhood Participation Project, longitudinal analysis compared blocks with and without block associations over a one-year time interval. Positive ratings of the block went up on blocks with organizations and down on blocks without organizations. Furthermore, residents' perceptions of the severity of block problems decreased over the time interval on blocks with organizations and increased on blocks without organizations (Wandersman, Unger, & Florin, 1991). Using the same longitudinal data, Chavis and Wandersman (1990) found that participation increased individual's sense of community.

Participation in community-development activities can also lead to changes in individual's feelings about the self, such as personal efficacy (Bandura, 1986) in dealing with conditions affecting one's residential environment. These feelings might be related to the perception that community members can help themselves or can more effectively negotiate with those who control municipal services. Advocates have long promoted participation as increasing confidence and efficacy, while reducing alienation and powerlessness (cf. Churchman, 1987; Wandersman, 1979b). Studies of general participation in community organizations and studies of specific participation programs have found that participants have stronger feelings of personal and political efficacy than nonparticipants (Cole, 1974, 1981; Levens, 1968; Verba & Nie, 1972). Zimmerman and Rappaport (1988), using data collected from participants in a variety of community organizations, found greater participation to be related to higher scores on several measures reflecting the desire for, and actual experience of, personal and political efficacy. In the Block Booster Project, members of block associations were significantly more likely than nonmembers to demonstrate expectations of collective efficacy, such as thinking that residents can solve block problems by working together and expecting that residents would intervene on the block to maintain social control. The similarity between nonmembers and a comparison group of residents from blocks without associations suggests the role of participation in generating feelings of collective efficacy. In addition to attitudinal differences, members of block associations were significantly more likely than nonmembers to engage in collective (as opposed to individual) anticrime measures.

McMillan, Florin, Stevenson, Kerman, and Mitchell (1995) found that demographic variables were not related to psychological empowerment, but individuals who spent more time and played more roles in local community task forces (i.e., participated more) tended to be those who reported higher levels of psychological empowerment. McMillan et al. (1995) also found that community coalitions that generated higher levels of participation and empowerment among their members were more successful in influencing the policies and resource allocation of key community decision-makers (e.g., town council chairs, police chiefs, superintendents of schools) one year later.

In sum, empirical studies of participation thus suggest a strong association between participation and feelings about the self, but the cross-sectional nature of the data in most studies does not allow us to rule out the possibility that such associations may be the cause, rather than the effect, of participation. Most likely these variables both influence the decision to participate and are then themselves amplified in the participatory process in a reciprocal spiral of causality.

CONCLUSIONS

Community psychology has viewed the concept of empowerment as a central phenomenon of interest (Rappaport, 1987). Rappaport suggests that "empowerment is a process, a mechanism by which people, organizations, and communities gain mastery over their affairs" (p. 122). Community development deals essentially and directly with this process. Moreover, its particular mechanism (voluntary cooperation and self-help/mutual aid in locale-based organizations) involves another major and long-standing phenomenon of interest to community psychologists—a psychological sense of community (Sarason, 1974). The relationship between participation and sense of community is beginning to be articulated (Chavis & Newbrough, 1986; Chavis & Wandersman, 1990; Maton & Rappaport, 1984), but it is clear that successful community development involves both in reciprocal spirals of causality.

Empowerment concepts involve both an individual (psychological) dimension and a collective (political) dimension. Again, community development addresses both. Participants in community development develop skills and beliefs integral to empowerment (Kieffer, 1984). Skill development leads to individual competency-building and leadership development. The National Commission on Neighborhoods (1979) identified a crucial contribution of neighborhood community-development programs as "the growth and development of literally thousands of new neighborhood leaders, accepting new responsibilities in their neighborhoods and for their neighborhoods' improvement." We have seen that participation is associated with psychological manifestations of empowerment, such as perceived personal competence, political efficacy, expectations of successful group problem-solving, and a greater sense of civic duty. Neighborhood community development also impacts upon the actual power wielded by groups of neighborhood volunteers; this is important because "success, for empowerment activities, necessitates change ... in successful interventions members ... will achieve greater control over their lives" (Swift & Levin, 1987, p. 90). This form of collective empowerment extends beyond the sense of accomplishment and mastery inherent in self-help/mutual aid activities and speaks to these organizations obtaining increased mastery over their affairs by altering the distribution of power and decision-making authority within the community (Bachelor & Jones, 1981; Mamalis, 1983; May, 1973; Perlman, 1983). The relationships between neighborhood community-development organizations and the power wielded by municipal government can take many forms, from decentralization, to contracting for municipal and/or human services and partnerships in economic development, to integral roles in municipal planning and governance (Ahlbrandt, 1984; Hallman, 1984).

Neighborhood community-development organizations are potential empowerment mechanisms at the individual, organizational, and community levels. They represent very appropriate settings for the understanding and promotion of individual and collective empowerment. In a special section of the *American Journal of Community Psychology* on "citizen participation, voluntary community organizations and community development: insights for empowerment through research," Wandersman and Florin (1990) and their colleagues explore linkages between the concepts of citizen participation and empowerment through research and applications.

There are important roles open to community psychologists in relation to organizations that have citizen participation as a key component, such as neighborhood community-development organizations (Swift & Levin, 1987). One important role may be to combine research and action to increase the capacity of these organizations to function effectively (Florin et al., 1992). In this way, community psychology can contribute to a community-development movement that embodies many of the values of community psychology.

REFERENCES

Ahlbrandt, R. S., Jr. (1984). *Neighborhoods, people, and community.* New York: Plenum.

Ahlbrandt, R. S., & Cunningham, J. V. (1979). *A new public policy for neighborhood preservation.* New York: Praeger.

Alford, R. R., & Scoble, H. M. (1986). Community leadership: Education and political behavior. *American Sociological Review, 33,* 259–272.

Alterman, R., & Frenkel, A. (1985). Implementation of project outputs: Services provided and their beneficiaries. In R. Alterman, N. Carmon, & M. Hill (Eds.), *Comprehensive evaluation of Israel's Project Renewal,* Vol. 3. Haifa: Technion-Israel Institute of Technology, Samuel Neaman Institute for Advanced Studies In Science and Technology.

Babchuk, N., & Thompson, R. (1962). The voluntary association of Negroes. *American Sociological Review, 27.*

Bachelor, L., & Jones, B. (1981). Managed participation: Detroit's neighborhood opportunity fund. *Journal of Applied and Behavioral Science, 17*, 518–536.

Bandura, A. (1986). *Social foundations of thought and action.* Englewood Cliffs, NJ: Prentice-Hall.

Bartelt, D., Elesh, D., Goldstein, I., Leon, G., & Yancey, W. (1987). Islands in the stream: Neighborhoods and the political economy of the city. In I. Altman & A. Wandersman (Eds.), Neighborhood and community environments (pp. 163–190). New York: Plenum.

Berkowitz, B. (1984). *Community dreams.* San Luis Obispo, CA: Impact.

Berry, J. M., Portney, K. E., Bablitch, M., & Mahoney, R. (1984). Public involvement in administration: The structural determinants of effective citizen participation. *Journal of Voluntary Action Research, 13*, 7–23.

Blakely, E. J. (1980). Building theory for CD practice. In J. A. Christenson & J. W. Robinson, Jr. (Eds.), *Community development in America.* Ames: Iowa State University Press.

Boyte, H. C. (1980). *The backyard revolution: Understanding the new citizen movement.* Philadelphia: Temple University Press.

Bronfenbrenner, U. (1960). Personality and participation: The case of the vanishing variables. *Journal of Social Issues, 16*, 54–63.

Carr, T., Dixon, M., & Ogles, R. (1976). Perceptions of community life which distinguish between participants and nonparticipants in a neighborhood self-help organization. *American Journal of Community Psychology, 4*, 357–366.

Cassidy, R. (1980). *Livable cities.* New York: Hold, Rinehart and Winston.

Chavis, D. M., Florin, P., Rich, R., & Wandersman, A. (1987). *The role of block associations in crime control and community development: The Block Booster Project.* Final Report to the Ford Foundation. New York: Citizens Committee for New York City.

Chavis, D. M., Florin, P., Wandersman, A., & Rich, R. C. (1986). *Organization development for grassroots community development organizations.* Paper presented at the annual conference of the American Psychological Association.

Chavis, D. M., & Newbrough, J. R. (1986). The meaning of "community" in community psychology. *Journal of Community Psychology, 14*, 335–340.

Chavis, D. M., & Wandersman, A. (1990). Sense of community in the urban environment: A catalyst for participation and community development. *American Journal of Community Psychology, 18*, 55–81.

Checkoway, B. (1985). Neighborhood planning organizations: Perspectives and choices. *Journal of Applied Behavioral Science, 32*, 471–486.

Checkoway, B. (1991). Neighborhood needs and organizational resources: New lessons from Detroit. *Nonprofit and Voluntary Sector Quarterly, 20*, 173–189.

Checkoway, B., & Zimmerman, M. A. (1992). Correlations of participation in neighborhood organizations. *Administration in Social Work, 16*, 3–4, 45–46.

Chinman, M. J., & Wandersman, A. (1999). The benefits and costs of volunteering in community organizations. *Nonprofit and Voluntary Sector Quarterly, 28*, 46–64.

Churchman, A. (1987). Can resident participation in neighborhood rehabilitation programs succeed? Israel's Project Renewal through a comparative perspective. In I. Altman & A. Wandersman (Eds.), *Neighborhood and community environments* (pp. 113–162). New York: Plenum.

Clark, P. B., & Wilson, J. Q. (1961). Incentive systems: A theory of organizations. *Administrative Science Quarterly, 6*, 129–166.

Cohen, S. (1976). Factors influencing citizen participation and nonparticipation in a community design project. Masters thesis, Cornell University, Ithaca, NY.

Cole, R. L. (1974). *Citizen participation and the urban policy process.* Lexington, MA: D.C. Heath.

Cole, R. L. (1981). Participation in community service organizations. *Journal of Community Action, 1*, 53–60.

Craik, K. H., & Appleyard, D. (1980). Streets of San Francisco: Brunswick's lens model applied to urban inference and assessment. *Journal of Social Issues, 36.*

Crensen, M. A. (1978). Social networks and political processes in urban neighborhoods. *American Journal of Political Science, 22*, 578–594.

Crensen, M. A. (1983). *Neighborhood politics.* Cambridge: Harvard University Press.

Cunningham, J. V. (1979). *Evaluating citizen participation: A neighborhood organizer's view.* Washington: Civic Action Institute.

Currie, (1982). *Fighting crime.* Working Papers.

Devereaux, E. C., Jr. (1960). Community participation and leadership. *Journal of Social Issues, 16*, 29–45.

Downs, A. (1981). *Neighborhoods and urban development.* Washington, D.C.: Brookings Institution.

Draisen, M. (1983). Fostering effective citizen participation: Lessons from three urban renewal neighborhood in the Hague. In L. Susskind & M. Elliott (Eds.), *Paternalism, conflict and coproduction.* New York: Plenum.

Duhl, L. J. (1986). *Health planning and social change.* New York: Human Sciences Press.

Edelstein, M., & Wandersman, A. (1987). Community dynamics in coping with toxic contaminants. In I. Altman & A. Wandersman (Eds.), *Neighborhood and community environments* (pp. 69–112). New York: Plenum.

Edwards, J. M., & White, R. P. (1980). Predictors of social participation: Apparent or real? *Journal of Voluntary Action Research, 9*, 60–73.

Emmons, D. (1979). *Neighborhood activities and community organizations: A critical review of the literature.* Evanston, IL: Northwestern University, Center for Urban Affairs.

Fellin, P., & Litwak, E. (1963). Neighborhood cohesion under conditions of mobility. *American Sociological Review, 28*, 364–376.

Florin, P., Chavis, D., Wandersman, A., & Rich, R. (1992). A systems approach to understanding and enhancing grassroots organizations. The Block Booster Project. In R. Levine & H. Fitzgerald (Eds.), *Analysis of dynamic psychological systems* (Vol. II, pp. 215–243). New York: Plenum.

Florin, P., Friedmann, R., Wandersman, A., & Meier, R. (1989). *Cognitive social learning variables and behavior: Cross cultural similarities in person x situation behavior.* Unpublished manuscript.

Florin, P., Giamartino, G., Kenny, D., & Wandersman, A. (1990). Uncovering climate and group influence by separating individual and group effects. *Journal of Applied Social Psychology, 20*, 881–900.

Florin, P., Jones, E., & Wandersman, A. (1986). Black participation in voluntary organizations. *Voluntary Action Research*, 65–86.

Florin, P., & Wandersman, A. (1984). Cognitive social learning and participation in community development. *American Journal of Community Psychology, 12*, 689–708.

Frank, S., Cosey, D., Angevine, J., & Cardone, L. (1985). Decision making and job satisfaction among youth workers in community-based agencies. *American Journal of Community Psychology, 13*, 269–287.

Friedmann, R., Florin, P., Wandersman, A., & Meier, R. (1988). Local action on behalf of local collectives in the United States and Israel: How different are leaders from members in voluntary associations. *Journal of Voluntary Action Research, 17*, 36–54.

Giamartino, G., & Wandersman, A. (1983). Organizational climate correlates of viable urban block organizations. *American Journal of Community Psychology, 11*, 529–541.

Gittell, M. (1980). *Limits of citizen participation: The decline of community organizations.* Beverly Hills, CA: Sage.

Godschalk, D., & Zeisel, J. (1983). Coproducing urban renewal in the Netherlands. In L. Susskind, M. Elliott, et al. (Eds.), *Paternalism, conflict, and coproduction.* New York: Plenum.

Goetze, R. (1979). *Understanding neighborhood change: The role of expectations in urban revitalization.* Cambridge, MA: Ballinger.

Gough, H. G. (1952). Predicting social participation. *Journal of Social Psychology, 35*, 227–233.

Granovetter, M. S. (1973). The strength of weak ties. *American Journal of Sociology, 78*, 1360–1380.

Granovetter, M. S. (1974). Granovetter replies to Gans. *American Journal of Sociology, 80*, 527–529.

Granovetter, M. S. (1982). The strength of weak ties: A network theory revisited. In P. V. Marsden & N. Lin (Eds.), *Social structure and network analysis.* Beverly Hills, CA: Sage.

Gurin, P., Gurin, G., Lao, R., & Beattie, M. (1969). Internal-external control in the motivational dynamics of Negro youth. *Journal of Social Issues, 25*, 29–54.

Hallman, H. W. (1984). *Neighborhoods: Their place in urban life.* Beverly Hills, CA: Sage.

Harris, I. M. (1984). The citizens coalition in Milwaukee. *Social Policy, 15*, 9–16.

Heller, K., Price, R., Reinharz, S., Riger, S., & Wandersman, A. (1984). *Psychology and community change: Challenges of the future.* Homewood, IL: Dorsey.

Henig, J. (1982). *Neighborhood mobilization: Redevelopment and response.* New Brunswick, NJ: Rutgers University Press.

Hirlinger, M. W. (1992). Citizen-initiated contacting of local government officials: A multivariate explanation. *Journal of Politics, 54*, 552–563.

Hunter, A. (1974). *Symbolic communities.* Chicago: University of Chicago Press.

Hyman, H., & Wright, C. (1971). Trends in voluntary association membership of American adults: Replication based on secondary analysis of national sample surveys. *American Sociological Review, 36*, 191–206.

Katz, J. (1984). *The silent world of doctor and patient.* New York: The Free Press.

Kaufman, S., & Poulin, J. (1994). Citizen participation in prevention activities: A path model. *Journal of Community Psychology, 22*, 359–374.

Kenny, D. A., & LaVoie, L. (1985). Separating individual and group effects. *Journal of Personality and Social Psychology, 48*, 339–348.

Kenny, D. A., & Stigler, J. (1983). PROGRAM LEVEL: A FORTRAN program for group-individual analysis. *Behavior Research Methods and Instrumentation, 606.*

Kerman, B. D. (1996). *Towards an integrated model of participation in community based alcohol and other drug problem prevention coalitions.* Unpublished doctoral dissertation. Kingston: The University of Rhode Island.

Keys, C. B., & Frank, S. (1987). Community psychology and the study of organizations: A reciprocal relationship. *American Journal of Community Psychology, 15*, 239–251.

Kieffer, C. H. (1984). Citizen empowerment: A developmental perspective. In J. Rappaport & R. Hess (Eds.), *Studies in empowerment*. New York: Haworth.

Knoke, D., & Wood, J. R. (1981). *Organized for action: Commitment in voluntary associations*. New Brunswick, NJ: Rutgers University Press.

Kweit, M., & Kweit, R. (1981). *Implementing citizen participation in a bureaucratic society*. New York: Praeger.

Lamb, C. (1975). *User design*. Presented at the EDRA 6 Conference, Lawrence, KS.

Langton, S. (Ed.). (1978). *Citizen participation in America*. Lexington, MA: Heath.

Latessa, E. J., & Allen, H. F. (1980). Using citizens to prevent crime: An example of deterrence and community involvement. *Journal of Police Science and Administration, 8*, 69–74.

Lavrakas, P. J., & Herz, E. J. (1979). *An investigation of citizen participation in crime prevention meetings and other anti-crime activities* (working paper CP-20F). Evanston, IL: Northwestern University, Center for Urban Affairs.

Lavrakas, P. J., Normoyle, J., Skogan, W. G., Herz, E. J., Salem, G., & Lewis, D. (1980). *Factors related to citizen involvement in personal, household, and neighborhood anti-crime measures* (Executive Summary) Washington, D.C.: U.S. Department of Justice.

Lawler, E. E. (1987). *High-involvement management*. San Francisco: Jossey-Bass.

Levens, H. (1968). Organizational affiliation and powerlessness: A case study of the welfare poor. *Social Problems, 16*, 18–32.

Lewis, D. A., & Maxfield, M. G. (1980). Fear in the neighborhoods: An investigation of impact of crime. *Journal of Research in Crime and Delinquency, 17*, 160–189.

Litwak, E. (1961). Voluntary associations and neighborhood cohesion. *American Sociological Review, 26*, 258–271.

Mamalis, M. (1983). Housing "the co-op" way. *Architectural Psychology Newsletter, 13*, 22–25.

Maton, K. I., & Rappaport, J. (1984). Empowerment in a religious setting: A multivariate investigation. In J. Rappaport & R. Hess (Eds.), *Studies in empowerment*. New York: Haworth.

Maxfield, M. G. (1977). *Reactions to fear: Indirect costs and adaptive behavior*. Evanston, IL: Northwestern University Press.

May, J. (1973). Two model cities: Negotiations in Oakland. In G. Frederickson (Ed.), *Neighborhood control in the 1970s* (pp. 217–246). New York: Chandler.

Mayer, N. S. (1984). *Neighborhood organizations and community development: Making revitalization work*. Washington, D.C.: Urban Institute Press.

McClure, L., & Depiano, L. (1983). School advisory council participation and effectiveness. *American Journal of Community Psychology, 11*, 687–704.

McMillan, B., Florin, P., Stevenson, J., Kerman, B., & Mitchell, R. E. (1995). Empowerment praxis in community coalitions. *American Journal of Community Psychology, 23*, 699–727.

Milbrath, L. W. (1965). *Political participation: How and why do people get involved in politics?* Chicago: Rand McNally.

Milburn, N. G., & Barbarin, O. A. (1987). *Functional and structural aspects of neighborhood associations: Their effects on citizen participation*. Unpublished manuscript.

Miller, F. D., Malia, G., & Tsembersis, S. (1979, September). *Community activism and the maintenance of urban neighborhoods*. Paper presented to the 87th annual meeting of the American Psychological Association, New York.

Milofsky, C. (1987). Neighborhood-based organizations: A market analogy. In W. W. Powell (Ed.), *The nonprofit sector: A research handbook*. New Haven, CT: Yale University Press.

Mischel, W. (1973). Toward a cognitive social learning reconceptualization of personality. *Psychological Review, 80*, 252–283.

Mischel, W. (1977). The interaction of person and situation. In D. Magnusson & N. S. Endler (Eds.), *Personality at the crossroads: Current issues in interactional psychology* (pp. 333–352). Hillsdale, NJ: Erlbaum.

Moe, T. M. (1980). *The organization of interests: Incentives and the internal dynamics of political interest groups*. Chicago: The University of Chicago Press.

Moos, R. (1979). *Evaluating educational environments: Procedures, methods, findings and policy implications*. San Francisco: Jossey-Bass.

Moos, R. (1984). Context and coping: Toward a unifying conceptual framework. *American Journal of Community Psychology, 12*, 5–25.

Moos, R. (1987). Learning environments in context: Links between school, work, and family settings. In B. J. Fraser (Ed.), *The study of learning environments*. Perth, Western Australia, Curtin University of Technology.

National Commission on Neighborhoods (1979). *Neighborhoods: People building neighborhoods*. Washington, D.C.: Government Printing Office.

Oliver, P. (1984). If you don't do it, nobody else will: Active and token contributors to local collective action. *American Sociological Review, 49*, 601–610.

Olson, M. (1965). *The logic of collective action.* Cambridge, MA: Harvard University Press.

O'Neill, P. (1981). Cognitive community psychology. *American Psychologist, 36*, 457–469.

Orum, A. M. (1966). A reappraisal of the social and political participation of the Negroes. *American Journal of Sociology, 72*, 32–46.

Parkum, K., & Parkum, V. (1980). Citizen participation in community planning and decision making. In D. H. Smith (Ed.), *Participation in social and political activities.* San Francisco: Jossey-Bass.

Pate, A., McPherson, M., & Silloway, G. (1987). *The Minneapolis community crime prevention experiment: Draft evaluation report.* Washington, D.C.: Police Foundation.

Perkins, D. D., Brown, B. B., & Taylor, R. B. (1996). The ecology of empowerment: Predicting participation in community organizations. *Journal of Social Issues, 52*, 85–110.

Perkins, D. D., Florin, P., Rich, R. C., Wandersman, A., & Chavis, D. M. (1990). Participation and the social and physical environment of residential blocks: Crime and community context. *American Journal of Community Psychology, 18*, 83–115.

Perlman, J. (1979). Grassroots empowerment and government response. *Social Policy, 10*, 16–21.

Perlman, J. (1983). Citizen action and participation in Madrid. In L. Susskind & M. Elliott (Eds.), *Paternalism, conflict and coproduction* (pp. 207–238). New York: Plenum.

Perlman, J. E. (1978). Grassroots participation from neighborhood to nation. In S. Langton (Ed.), *Citizen participation in America.* Lexington, MA: Lexington Books.

Pierce, N. R., & Steinbach, C. F. (1987). *Corrective capitalism: The rise of America's community development corporations.* New York: Ford Foundation.

Piven, F. (1968). Participation of residents in neighborhood community-action programs. In H. B. Spiegel (Ed.), *Citizen participation in urban development*, Vol. 1. Washington, D.C.: NTL Institute.

Podolefsky, A., & DuBow, F. (1980). *The reactions to crime papers: Vol. II: Strategies for community crime prevention.* Evanston, IL: Northwestern University, Center for Urban Affairs.

Prestby, J. E. (1984). *Leaders and members in voluntary organizations.* Working paper, Department of Psychology, University of South Carolina.

Prestby, J. E., Wandersman, A., Florin, P., Rich, R., & Chavis, D. M. (1990). Benefits, costs, incentive management and participation in voluntary organizations: A means to understanding and promoting empowerment. *American Journal of Community Psychology, 18*, 117–149.

Prestby, J. E., & Wandersman, A. (1985). An empirical exploration of framework of organizational viability: Maintaining block organizations. *The Journal of Applied Behavioral Science, 21*, 287–305.

Rappaport, J. (1987). Terms of empowerment/exemplars of prevention: Toward a theory for community psychology. *American Journal of Community Psychology, 15*, 121–148.

Rich, R. C. (1980). The dynamics of leadership in neighborhood organizations. *Social Science Quarterly, 60*, 570–587.

Rohe, W., & Gates, L. (1981). Neighborhood planning: Promise and product. *The Urban and Social Change Review, 14*, 26–32.

Rohe, W., & Gates, L. (1982). Neighborhood planning and citizen influence. Paper presented at the Urban Affairs Association meeting. Philadelphia, PA.

Rohe, W., & Greenberg, S. (1982). *Participation in community crime prevention programs.* Chapel Hill, NC: University of North Carolina, Department of City and Regional Planning.

Rothman, J. (1970). Three models of community organization practice. In F. M. Cox, J. L. Erlich, J. Rothman, & J. E. Tropman (Eds.), *Strategies of community organization.* Itasca, IL: F. E. Peacock.

Sanger, P., & Alker, H. (1972). Dimensions of internal-external locus of control and the women's liberation movement. *Journal of Social Issues, 28*, 115–129.

Sarason, S. (1974). *The psychological sense of community: Prospects for a community psychology.* San Francisco: Jossey-Bass.

Schneider, B. (1975). Organizational climates: An essay. *Personnel Psychology, 28*, 447–479.

Schneider, A. L., & Schneider, P. R. (1978). *Private and public-minded citizen responses to a neighborhood-based crime prevention strategy.* Eugene, OR: Institute for Policy Analysis.

Schoenberg, S., & Rosenbaum, P. L. (1980). *Neighborhoods that work: Sources of viability in the inner city.* New Brunswick, NJ: Rutgers University Press.

Silberman, C. E. (1978). *Criminal violence, criminal justice.* New York: Random House.

Skogan, W. G., & Maxfield, M. (1981). *Coping with crime: Individual and neighborhood reactions.* Beverly Hills, CA: Sage.

Skogan, W. G., & Maxfield, M. G. (1980). *The reactions to crime papers. Volume I. Coping with crime: Victimization, fear and reactions to crime in three American cities.* Evanston, IL: Northwestern University, Center for Urban Affairs.

Smith, D. H. (1966). A psychological model of individual participation in formal voluntary organizations: Applications to some Chilean data. *American Journal of Sociology, 72,* 249–266.

Smith, D. H. (1975). Voluntary action and voluntary groups. In A. Inkeles, J. Coleman, & N. Smelser (Eds.), *Annual Review of Sociology,* Vol. 1. Palo Alto, CA: Annual Reviews.

Smith, D. H. (1985). Volunteerism: Attracting volunteers and staffing shrinking programs. In G. Tobin (Ed.), *Social planning and human service delivery in the voluntary sector.* Westport, CT: Greenwood.

Spiegel, H. (1987). Coproduction in the context of neighborhood development. *Journal of Voluntary Action Research.*

Steers, R. M. (1977). *Organizational effectiveness: A behavioral view.* Santa Monica, CA: Goodyear.

Sundeen, R. A. (1988). Explaining participation in coproduction: A study of volunteers. *Social Science Quarterly, 69,* 547–568.

Susskind, L., & Elliott, M. (1983). Paternalism, conflict and coproduction. In L. Susskind & M. Elliott (Eds.), *Paternalism, conflict and coproduction* (pp. 3–34). New York: Plenum.

Swift, C., & Levin, G. (1987). Empowerment: An emerging mental health technology. *Journal of Primary Prevention, 8,* 71–94.

Toch, H., & Grant, J. D. (1982). *Reforming human services: Change through participation.* Beverly Hills, CA: Sage.

Tomeh, A. K. (1974). Formal voluntary organizations: Participation correlates and interrelationships. *Sociological Inquiry, 43,* 89–122.

Unger, D., & Wandersman, A. (1983). Neighboring and its role in block organizations: An exploratory report. *American Journal of Community Psychology, 11,* 291–300.

Unger, D., & Wandersman, A. (1985). The importance of neighbors: The social cognitive, and effective components of neighboring. *American Journal of Community Psychology, 13,* 139–169.

Vassar, S. (1978). *Community participation in a metropolitan area: An analysis of the characteristics of participants.* Ph.D. dissertation, University of Illinois at Chicago.

Verba, S., & Nie, N. H. (1972). *Participation in America.* New York: Harper & Row.

Verba, S., Schlozman, K. L., Brady, H., & Nie, N. H. (1993). Citizen activity: Who participates? What do they say? *American Political Science Review, 87,* 303–315.

Voth, D. E. (1979). Problems in the evaluation of community development efforts. In E. J. Blakely (Ed.), *Community development research: Concepts, issues, and strategies.* New York: Human Sciences Press.

Wandersman, A. (1979a). User participation: A study of types of participation, effects, mediators and individual differences. *Environment and Behavior, 11,* 185–208.

Wandersman, A. (1979b). User participation in planning environments: A conceptual framework. *Environment and Behavior, 11,* 465–482.

Wandersman, A. (1981). A framework of participation in community organizations. *Journal of Applied Behavioral Science, 17,* 27–58.

Wandersman, A., & Florin, P. (Eds.). (1990). Citizen participation, voluntary community organizations and community development: Insights for empowerment through research. *American Journal of Community Psychology, 18.*

Wandersman, A., Chavis, D., & Stucky, P. (1983). Involving citizens in research. In R. Kidd & M. Saks (Eds.), *Advances in applied social psychology,* Vol. 2. Hillsdale, NJ: Erlbaum.

Wandersman, A., Florin, P., Chavis, D., Rich, R., & Prestby, J. (1985). Getting together and getting things done. *Psychology Today, 19,* 64–71.

Wandersman, A., Florin, P., Friedmann, R., & Meier, R. (1987). Who participates, who does not, and why? An analysis of voluntary neighborhood organizations in the United States and Israel. *Sociological Forum, 2,* 534–555.

Wandersman, A., Jakubs, J., & Giamartino, G. (1981). Participation in block organizations. *Journal of Community Action, 1,* 40–47.

Wandersman, A., Kimbrell, D., Wadsworth, J. C., Livingston, G., Myers, D., & Braithwaite, H. (1982). Assessing citizen participation in a community mental health center. In A. Jeger & R. Slotnick (Eds.), *Community mental health: A behavioral–ecological perspective* (pp. 373–388). New York: Plenum.

Wandersman, A., Unger, D., & Florin, P. (1991). The effects of block associations. Unpublished manuscript.

Warren, D. I. (1981). *Helping networks: How people cope with problems in the urban community.* Notre Dame, IN: University of Notre Dame Press.

Warren, R. (1963). *The community in America.* Chicago: Rand McNally.

Washnis, G. T. (1976). *Citizen involvement in crime prevention.* Lexington, MA: Heath.

Whisenand, P. M. (1977). *Crime prevention.* New York: Harper and Row.

Whitworth, D. (1993). *A structural equation model of a set of operationalized cognitive social learning variables and citizen participation in community organizations.* Ph.D. dissertation. The University of Rhode Island, Kingston.

Widmer, C. (1984). *An incentive model of citizen participation applied to a study of human service agency boards of directors.* Ph.D. dissertation, Cornell University, Ithaca, NY.

Williams, J., Babchuk, N., & Johnson, D. (1973). Voluntary associations and minority status: A comparative analysis of Anglos, Blacks, and Mexican Americans. *American Sociological Review, 38,* 637–646.

Williams, J., & Ortega, S. (1986). The multidimensionality of joining. *Journal of Voluntary Action Research, 15,* 35–44.

Williams, M. C. (1985). *Neighborhood organizations: Seeds of a new urban life.* Westport, CT: Greenwood.

Wooley, T. (1985). *Community architecture: An assessment of the case for user participation in design.* In S. Klein, R. Wener, & S. Lehman (Eds.), *EDRA 16/1985.* Washington, D.C.: EDRA.

Yates, D. (1973). *Neighborhood democracy.* Lexington, MA: Heath.

Yin, R. K., & Yates, D. (1974). *Street-level governments: Assessing decentralization and urban services.* Santa Monica, CA: Rand.

Zehner, R. B. (1972). Neighborhood and community satisfaction: A report on new towns and less planned suburbs. In J. F. Wohlwill & D. H. Carson (Eds.), *Environment and the social sciences: Perspectives and applications.* Washington, D.C.: American Psychological Association.

Zimmerman, M. (1990). Toward a theory of learned hopefulness: A structural model analysis of participation and empowerment. *Journal of Research in Personality, 24,* 71–86.

Zimmerman, M. A., & Rappaport, J. (1988). Citizen participation, personal control and psychological empowerment. *American Journal of Community Psychology, 16,* 725–750.

CHAPTER 12

Power and Participation in the Workplace

Implications for Empowerment Theory, Research, and Practice

KATHERINE J. KLEIN, R. SCOTT RALLS, VIRGINIA SMITH-MAJOR, AND CHRISTINA DOUGLAS

In the 1980s and 1990s, empowerment emerged as a central focus of research and a practical goal among community psychologists. Rappaport brought prominence to the term with his 1981 article on the subject, where he defined empowerment as the process of enhancing "the possibilities for people to control their own lives" (p. 15). Several authors have built on Rappaport's initial conceptualization in an effort to clarify the meaning of the term. Emphasizing the implications of empowerment for human service delivery models, Swift (1984) described empowerment as the antithesis of "the paternalistic model that has dominated human service delivery during this century" (p. xi). Empowerment, she argued, "insists on the primacy of the target population's participation in any intervention affecting its welfare" (p. xiv). Others have described empowerment as a corollary of citizen participation. Kieffer (1984), for example, described empowerment as "the transition from sense of self as helpless victim to acceptance of self as assertive and efficacious citizen" (p. 37). More recently, Perkins and Zimmerman (1995) proposed that "participation with others to achieve goals, efforts to gain access to resources, and some critical understandings of the sociopolitical environment are basic components of the construct" (p. 571). Elaborating further, Perkins and Zimmerman (1995) suggested that at the organizational level of analysis, "empowerment includes organizational processes and structures that enhance member participation and

KATHERINE J. KLEIN • Department of Psychology, University of Maryland, College Park, Maryland 20742. R. SCOTT RALLS • Vice President, Economic and Workforce Development, The North Carolina Community College System, Raleigh, North Carolina 27603. VIRGINIA SMITH-MAJOR • Department of Psychology, University of Maryland at College Park, College Park, Maryland 20742. CHRISTINA DOUGLAS • Center for Creative Leadership, Greensboro, North Carolina 27438.

Handbook of Community Psychology, edited by Julian Rappaport and Edward Seidman. Kluwer Academic / Plenum Publishers, New York, 2000.

improve goal achievement for the organization" (p. 571). Implicit in all these definitions of empowerment is the assumption that an individual's active participation in decision-making within the major organizations that substantively influence his or her daily life will engender both an increase in the individual's sense of personal power and effectiveness, and an increase in the organizations' abilities to meet the individual's needs.

The concept of empowerment within community psychology in many ways parallels the concept of worker participation in organizational psychology. As with empowerment, definitions of worker participation abound. Wagner described participation as "a process in which influence is shared among individuals who are otherwise hierarchical unequals" (p. 312). Miller and Pritchard (1992) suggested that worker participation refers to "systematic efforts to involve employees in problem-solving processes intended to improve efficiency and morale ... [including] employee involvement or participation programs such as quality circles, self-managing work teams, and problem-solving task forces" (p. 414). Lawler, Mohrman, and Ledford (1992) emphasized that employee involvement encompasses four mutually reinforcing processes: sharing information with employees, increasing employees' knowledge, rewarding employee performance, and redistributing power. Underlying these diverse definitions, however, is a common assumption within organizational research and theory, an assumption mirroring that of the empowerment literature—namely, that worker participation may engender an increase in both employee satisfaction and organizational effectiveness.

Although the community and organizational psychology assumptions are not identical, they are similar. Each emphasizes positive effects of participation in the workplace or other central organizations on both individual- and organizational-level outcomes. Both assumptions are value-based and controversial (Dachler & Wilpert, 1978; Riger, 1993). A key difference, however, is in the extent to which each assumption has been examined in theory, research, and practice. Although empowerment theory and research have burgeoned in recent years, participation has been studied by organizational psychologists for decades. Accordingly, in this chapter, we look to the workplace for possible lessons in empowerment. For the growing number of community psychologists interested in the workplace, our discussion of worker participation may prove useful in its own right. For others, the implications for empowerment in non-work, community settings may be most useful.

Below, we review four bodies of literature.[1] We begin by discussing theoretical models of organizational power because we believe that the concept of power, although often ignored within the worker-participation literature, is fundamental to that of worker participation and empowerment. In essence, power is the end point, the goal, while worker participation is a possible means to that end. We then review theoretical models of worker participation. Next, we provide a summary of empirical research on participation in the workplace. Finally, we describe examples of worker participation in practice, specifically, quality circles and total quality management. We conclude by highlighting key themes emerging from our review.

[1]We have not reviewed the small, but growing, organizational literature on empowerment *per se* because, in this literature, the term empowerment is used to refer to "a process whereby an individual's belief in his or her self-efficacy is enhanced" (Conger & Kanungo, 1988, p. 474) or to an individual's "intrinsic task motivation ... [based on his or her] sense of impact, competence, meaningfulness, and choice" (Thomas & Velthouse, 19909, p. 666). In contrast, we use the term "empowerment" to refer to a process whereby an individual's influence in workplace decision-making is enhanced. While programs to increase employee influence in organizational decision-making may enhance individual self-efficacy and/or intrinsic task motivation, this is rarely, if ever, the goal of such programs. Moreover, enhancing employee influence in organizational decision-making is but one of many possible strategies to enhance self-efficacy and intrinsic task motivation. Finally, we share Riger's (1993) concern that "psychology's emphasis on the cognitive processes of the individual leads us to study individuals' sense of empowerment rather than actual increases in power, thereby making the political personal."

THEORETICAL MODELS OF ORGANIZATIONAL POWER

The concept of power is fundamental to that of empowerment. Power is the ability to influence, to control, "to get things done the way one wants them to be done" (Salancik & Pfeffer, 1977, p. 417). Many organizational theorists have written extensively on the topic. Below, we review three prominent, even classic, theoretical models of organizational power.

Types of Power

The first model is French and Raven's (1960) analysis of the sources of individual power in the workplace. According to this model, power is best conceptualized not as a unidimensional phenomenon, but as a multifaceted one. Power derives from five different sources, each of which serves to define a different kind of power.

The first type of power is *legitimate* power. Legitimate power is based solely on the individual's position in the organizational hierarchy. One obeys legitimate power because one's superior has the right or authority to guide and influence others. The second type of power is *reward* power, which is based on the subordinate's expectation that he or she will receive praise, recognition, or pay for compliance. The third type of power is *coercive* power. The flip side of reward power, coercive power is based upon fear. One obeys coercive power in an effort to avoid punishment, whether the punishment is a reprimand, a failure to praise, or physical abuse. The fourth type of power is *expert* power. Expert power derives from special skill, expertise, or knowledge. One obeys expert power because the expert knows better, so the expert's directive is likely to be sound and helpful. Finally, the last type of power is *referent* power, which is based upon individual personality, attractiveness, or charm.

French and Raven use this schema to distinguish between sources of power available to an individual as a function of his or her organizational position, and sources of power available to the individual as a function of his or her personal characteristics. Legitimate power is positional; it derives solely from the individual's position in the organization. In contrast, reward and coercive power each have a positional and a personal component. That is, leaders may have the authority to dispense organizational rewards and punishment but, in addition, they may accrue further power because their subordinates desire to win their praise and avoid their punishment for personal reasons, divorced from organizational or positional considerations. Finally, expert and referent power derive from personal characteristics alone; the organization cannot confer such power.

This distinction between positional and personal sources of power elucidates the limits of nonmanagerial power. By virtue of their organizational status, the majority of nonmanagerial employees typically lack significant legitimate, reward, and coercive power. Their only sources of power are their expertise and their personal (referent) appeal.

Locus of Power

The second model is Salancik and Pfeffer's (1977) strategic-contingency analysis of organizational power. According to this model, power "accrues to organizational subunits (individuals, departments) that cope with critical organizational problems" (p. 417). That is, power accrues to people who have the ability to help the unit or organization thrive: "Power derives from a social situation in which one person has a capacity to do something and another person does not, but wants it done" (p. 420).

Salancik and Pfeffer's model has three important implications for the study of power. First, the model suggests that power is conferred upon an individual by others. Others define the critical contingencies faced by the organization, the critical skills necessary to cope with these contingencies, and the critical person (or people) who has these skills. One cannot simply declare oneself emperor; others must bow to one's throne.

Second, the model asserts that power is necessarily shared within complex organizations. That is, no single individual has the ability to tackle all organizational contingencies. Accordingly, Salancik and Pfeffer comment that power is shared in most organizations "out of necessity more than out of concern for principles of organizational development or participatory democracy" (p. 420).

Finally, the model suggests that organizations that do not recognize critical challenges and "assign" power accordingly will ultimately fail. Salancik and Pfeffer suggest that many organizations fall into this trap; they fail to recognize changing contingencies and thus do not make necessary changes in the distribution of organizational power. The failure to make these changes typically reflects the institutionalization of power in certain positions or departments. That is, those in power resist others' attempts to alter the power structure of the organization. This tension between organizational needs and individuals' self-serving tendencies explains why organizations often fail to anticipate changing circumstances, but instead respond to critical contingencies only after the fact.

The Amount of Power

The third model is Tannenbaum's expanding pie model of organizational power. The model is based on Tannenbaum and colleagues' cross-national study of 50 organizations in five countries (Tannenbaum, Kavcic, Rosner, Vianello, & Wiesner, 1974). In this study, the researchers asked employees at every level of each organization to rate how much power they had in the organization, how much power they should have, how much power others had, and how much power others should have.

Two key patterns of results emerged. First, a hierarchy of organizational power was apparent in every organization. In every organization, managers had more power (over more issues) than did rank-and-file organizational members. Second, the sum total of power in some organizations was higher than the sum total in others. That is, the total amount of power in organizations varied such that organizational members in some companies universally possessed less power than organizational members in other companies.

Tannenbaum (Tannenbaum et al., 1974; Tannenbaum, 1968) concluded that organizational power is not a zero-sum game. Rank-and-file members could, he argued, gain increased power with no ensuing loss in managers' and supervisors' power. This argument is compelling, although perhaps controversial, for it suggests that managers and supervisors need not fear worker-participation programs; subordinates' gain in power is not necessarily managers' loss.

Discussion

Four lessons for empowerment emerge, we believe, from the discussion of organizational power.

1. *Personal power is critical for the empowerment of non-managerial employees and, by extension, for the empowerment of other relatively powerless or disenfranchised group, organization, or societal members.* This proposition stems from French and Raven's distinction between personal and positional sources of employee power. Nonmanagerial employees can acquire and exercise personal power in the workplace; only rarely can they acquire or exercise positional power. Further, nonmanagerial employees are more likely to be awarded positional power if their preexisting personal power justifies the formal designation of position power. Finally, the acquisition of personal power is less dependent upon the cooperation and acquiescence of top managers than the acquisition of positional power; one's coworkers and immediate supervisors may recognize and "grant" one personal power, even if top managers do not.

   Expertise and personal charm are both personal sources of power, French and Raven suggest. Expertise, however, may be more readily acquired (e.g., through training, or even private, informal learning) than personal charm, and is likely to be a more effective and credible source of organizational power. Thus, expertise may prove an important instrument of empowerment.
2. *The exercise of expert power will typically yield more positive outcomes for the organization than the exercise of purely organizational forms of power. Thus, to the extent that empowerment efforts increase expertise, the organizational outcomes of those efforts should be positive.* This proposition stems from the combination of French and Raven's model and Salancik and Pfeffer's model. Together, they suggest that the exercise of expert power is likely to be adaptive for the organization, while the exercise of purely organizational or positional forms of power may well be detrimental to the organization. Expert power may be harnessed to effectively meet organizational contingencies. If, however, organizational power is institutionalized in a person or position, rather than allocated on the basis of individual expertise, the exercise of such power may well serve more to preserve and enhance the existing power hierarchy of the organization than to preserve and enhance the future of the organization itself. Accordingly, empowerment efforts based on the cultivation of expertise are likely to yield more positive organizational outcomes than empowerment efforts based on the simple acquisition of positional power.
3. *The holders of organizational power will not readily or willingly forfeit their power. Powerful organizational members may resist and attempt to subvert empowerment efforts.* Salancik and Pfeffer's model highlights managers' resistance to forfeiting their positional power. This tendency accounts for many organizations' failure to adapt successfully in response to changing organizational contingencies. It explains, as well, the difficulty of mounting successful empowerment efforts in a variety of groups and organizations. A less obvious point, however, is that the formerly unempowered may fall prey to this tendency as well. Having gained personal and/or positional power, the formerly unempowered may resist the further empowerment of any less powerful members of the organization.
4. *The environmental context of the organization will influence the extent of employee empowerment in the organization, as well as managers' receptiveness to such efforts.* Salancik and Pfeffer's model suggests that power sharing is likely to be based on organizational contingencies rather than on the larger benevolence of managers. That is, when faced with contingencies they cannot easily resolve on their own, managers are most likely to encourage and accept power sharing. For empowerment advocates,

> the key is to identify which organization contingencies may be effectively addressed by the unempowered. In this way, advocates may be more certain that their efforts to empower workers will be accepted by those already in power.

In sum, the power literature highlights the importance of expertise in the employee empowerment process. Employee expertise in addressing central organizational contingencies may well hold the key to realizing the individual and organizational benefits of empowerment. Nevertheless, efforts to increase employee expertise and power may be resisted by those who fear their own expertise, and power may be reduced as a result. We will return to these themes in our concluding comments. We turn now to an examination of the dynamics of power-sharing—participation—in the workplace.

THEORETICAL MODELS OF WORKER PARTICIPATION

The relationship of power to participation is that of result to process; employees achieve and exercise power in part by participating in organizational decision-making. Curiously, however, the literature on organizational power and on participation are quite distinct. Here, we briefly summarize the theoretical literature of worker participation, focusing on three key issues: (1) the values and assumptions of participation advocates, (2) the dimensions of participation, and (3) the hypothesized outcomes and mediating processes of participation. We conclude by noting some of the implications of this literature for research, theory, and practice in organizational and community psychology.

Values and Assumptions of Participation Advocates

Several authors (e.g., Dachler & Wilpert, 1978; Locke & Schweiger, 1979) have noted that worker participation is a value-laden topic. Worker participation is often advocated on moral, rather than empirical, grounds. However, the morals, or values, upon which advocates base their assertions vary from one group to another. To codify the array, Dachler and Wilpert (1978) described four basic value positions supporting worker participation: democratic theory, socialist theory, human growth and development theory, and productivity and efficiency theory. Not only do members of these four "camps" have different values, they also have different assumptions about the potential effects of participative practices within the workplace.

Democratic theorists advocate worker participation as an extension of political democratic values. If a society is truly democratic, they argue, citizens are allowed to exercise their individual rights not only in the voting booth, but also in the workplace. These theorists assume that worker participation will yield certain benefits for private organizations, but in addition, workplace democracy will help strengthen the foundations of national democracy. *Socialist theorists* advocate worker participation as the first step towards overcoming the specialization, powerlessness, alienation, and apathy of producers (workers) who, they argue, suffer from the separation of labor and capital. According to this view, worker participation will ultimately lead to the abolition of wage-labor relationships and the creation of a humanistic, egalitarian, proletarian society. *Human growth and development theorists* suggest that worker participation allows workers to fulfill their basic needs for self-actualization, responsibility, and self-esteem. In this view, worker participation is designed to overcome the debilitating psychological effects of traditional autocratic bureaucracies. Finally, *productivity and efficiency theorists* argue that worker participation is a means to overcome worker dissatisfaction, thereby reducing the costs of absenteeism, turnover, poor-quality work, and sabotage. More recent theorists within this "camp" (e.g., Scully, Kirkpatrick, & Locke, 1995) have argued that, whether employees are satisfied or not, participation is likely to increase organizational productivity and efficiency to the extent that employees with relevant knowledge and expertise are given the opportunity to influence organizational decision-making. In general, productivity and efficiency theorists are not interested in fundamentally altering the distribution of organizational power, but only in improving organizational performance by increasing morale and/or allowing employees to exercise their knowledge and expertise. U.S. advocates of worker participation typically fall into either this camp or the human development and growth camp.

Participation Dimensions

Several analysts (e.g., Cotton, Vollrath, Froggatt, Lengnick-Hall, & Jennings, 1988) have cautioned that the concept of "worker participation" encompasses a tremendous variety of participatory practices. Unfortunately, when organizational theorists write about worker participation, they are not always clear about exactly which forms of participation they are considering. In an effort to codify the array of practices, Klein, Smith-Major, and Ralls (1999) outlined eight dimensions along which participation programs and policies may vary.

First, worker participation may occur at different *levels of analysis* within an organization (Klein, Dansereau, & Hall, 1994). Worker participation may be an organization-level phenomenon, practiced across all units, managers, and employees of an organization. Alternatively, worker participation may be a unit-level phenomenon, such that some units may engage in high levels of participation, while other units may practice very little worker participation. Finally, worker participation may be a dyadic-level phenomenon, varying between supervisor–subordinate dyads. In other words, a supervisor may allow one or more of his or her subordinates to participate extensively in important decisions, while allowing other subordinates little opportunity to participate.

Second, worker participation may be *direct or representative*. When worker participation is direct, employees have the opportunity to personally influence decision-making. For example, they may offer suggestions for improvements in their work or attend quality circle meetings. When worker participation is representative, employees influence decision-making through their elected or appointed employee representatives, for example, fellow employees who sit on the company board of directors.

Third, participation may vary in the *amount of influence* it affords employees. Employees might have very broad decision-making responsibilities, or they might only be allowed to offer suggestions to their supervisors, who ultimately retain all authority to make decisions.

Fourth, worker-participation programs differ according to the *range of issues* over which workers have influence. Issues may vary from the trivial (e.g., deciding on the theme of a company party), to those of moderate importance and impact (e.g., determining how to perform certain job tasks), to those of much more importance and impact (e.g., influencing the company's decision on whether to merge with another business).

Fifth, worker participation may be either an organizational *intervention or the status quo*. When worker participation is an intervention, it represents a new program or practice, implemented by management to increase worker participation. In contrast, worker participation may not be a new intervention, but instead may represent the *status quo* within the organization, unit, or supervisor–subordinate dyad. When worker participation is an intervention, it is likely to be in the form of a formal program, like total quality circles or self-directed work teams. When participation is the *status quo*, it may either be an existing program or policy, long in place, or simply an informal cultural value or norm.

Sixth, worker participation may be *mandatory or voluntary*. Some formal programs like work teams require that employees participate. But there are many forms of participation that are voluntary, as when employees elect to offer suggestions to their supervisors.

Seventh, worker participation may be either an *ongoing or occasional* practice. If participation is ongoing, as in a self-directed work team, it is something that occurs everyday, and thus is an inextricable part of worklife. If participation is only occasional, such as a quality circle that only meets once a week, it may be less central to the organization.

And finally, worker participation may be a *unidimensional, isolated workplace practice* or it may be embedded within a *multidimensional constellation of complementary workplace practices*. When worker participation is an isolated program or practice, it is incongruent with other human resource and management practices. For example, workers may be organized into teams, and yet be rewarded on the basis of individual performance. In other cases, however, a particular program or practice is simply one among many congruent human resource and management practices, as when work teams are supported by group-incentive systems, team skills training, etc.

These eight dimensions may combine in different ways to form a variety of different types of worker participation (Klein et al., 1999). For example, an electrical engineer may have considerable autonomy in his or her job, deciding how to perform most tasks, which tasks have highest priority, and so forth. This engineer enjoys a form of participation that is individual-level, direct, moderate in influence over a range of job-related issues, the *status quo*, mandatory to the extent that he or she is expected to work in this manner, ongoing, and likely embedded in a context of related practices (e.g., appropriate skills training). Another example of worker participation is that which characterizes worker councils or worker representation on company boards or committees. This type of participation is organization-level, representative, of moderate influence over company-level issues, an intervention, mandated by management, occasional, and unidimensional.

Hypothesized Outcomes and Mediating Processes of Participation

Organizational theorists have offered several different models to explain the potential effects of worker participation. Often, the values and assumptions of the theorists are evident in the outcomes and mediating processes of interest in their models. So, for example, productivity and efficiency theorists offer models to explain participation's effects on organizational performance, while human growth and development theorists focus on how worker participation increases employee satisfaction. In fact, as most American organizational theorists fall within these two camps, most models focus on these two outcome variables—satisfaction and performance. Unfortunately, regardless of the theorist or model, few researchers adequately consider the variety of dimensions of worker participation, leading to some inevitable confusion about the outcomes and mediating processes of participation. Below, we briefly review some major models of worker participation, followed by an evaluation of the current state of theory about worker participation.

Need Satisfaction Models

One of the most common explanations of the hypothesized benefits of worker participation is that participation helps fulfill employees' high-order needs, such as independence, self-expression, and equality, and thereby leads to increased morale and, ultimately, to increased productivity (Miller & Monge, 1986). McGregor (1960), for example, wrote that:

> Participation ... offers substantial opportunities for ego satisfaction for the subordinate and thus can affect motivation toward organizational objectives.... The subordinate can discover the satisfaction that comes from tackling problems and finding successful solutions for them.... Beyond this there is a greater sense of independence and of achieving some control over one's destiny. Finally, there are the satisfactions that come by way of recognition from peers and superiors for having made a worth-while contribution to the solution of an organizational problem (pp. 130–131).

Members of the human growth and development tradition, including followers of the "human relations school of management" like McGregor, tend to advocate need-satisfaction models of worker participation.

Although the arguments of need-satisfaction models may be intuitively appealing, there are many reasons to question their validity. First, need theories such as Maslow's need hierarchy have come under considerable attack in recent decades (e.g., Pfeffer, 1982; Salancik & Pfeffer, 1977, 1978). Second, empirical research has demonstrated only a weak positive relationship between individual job satisfaction and performance (Ostroff, 1992), that is, even if attainment of high-order needs leads to job satisfaction, it may not necessarily lead to increased performance. Third, need-satisfaction models assume that workers will be satisfied if their suggestions are accepted and implemented by management, but research indicates that management often resists employee suggestions, finding them too expensive, impractical, and/or threatening (Klein, 1984; Lawler & Mohrman, 1991).

Finally, need-satisfaction models may not be relevant to all types of worker participation. For instance, need-satisfaction models appear most applicable to direct, rather than representative, worker participation, and individual-level, rather than unit- or organizational-level, participation. Expressing one's opinion through a representative's vote on a company board of directors is likely to be less "ego-gratifying" than personally voicing opinions to one's supervisor. And any improvements in individual morale and performance that result from need satisfaction would not necessarily translate to the unit or organizational level. Individual-level phenomena often do not "aggregate up" to higher levels of analysis (Goodman, Lerch, & Mukhopadkhay, 1994; Schneider & Klein, 1994).

Cognitive Models

Cognitive models focus on the potential effects of worker participation on unit and organizational performance, and thus tend to share the values and assumptions of theorists within the productivity and efficiency camp. In fact, in their purest form, cognitive models do not suggest a relationship between participation and satisfaction. Cognitive models "propose that workers typically have more complete knowledge of their work than management; hence if workers participate in decision making, decisions will be made with better pools of information" (Miller & Monge, 1986, p. 730). Followers of the cognitive school (e.g., Scully et al., 1995) thus suggest that participation will yield increased performance to the extent that it allows either: (1) managers to make more informed decisions than they would make in the absence of employee input, or (2) employees to make decisions themselves regarding issues over which they have critical, pertinent information. According to these models, the guiding principle of organizational decision-making should be "the rule of requisite knowledge: Assuming commitment to the values and vision of the firm, whoever has (or has the capacity to readily get) the requisite knowledge relevant to a given decision is either consulted or allowed to make the decision" (Locke, Alavi, & Wagner, 1997).

Cognitive models may not be equally relevant to all types of worker participation. For instance, they suggest a strong relationship between participation and unit- and organization-level, but not individual-level, performance. That is, the models focus on how individual participation enables organizations and units to make better decisions. In addition, cognitive models describe a form of participation that involves the upward transfer of knowledge—the communication of information from subordinates to managers—rather than the transfer of knowledge downward, a process better captured by the next model of participation's effects.

Commitment Models

Commitment models of the effects of worker participation suggest that worker participation increases employee support for organizational decisions. That is, employees are hypothesized to be more committed to decisions that they helped to make than to decisions in which they had no input. Accordingly, worker participation is hypothesized to increase employee commitment to a course of action and reduce employee resistance to change, and may thereby improve performance. Advocates of commitment models of the effects of worker participation tend to espouse the values of productivity and efficiency theorists.

Commitment models typically take one of two forms. Some commitment models emphasize that participative decision-making allows employees to shape a proposed new organizational program or action to their liking. Thus, for example, Kotter and Schlesinger (1979) posited that: "If the initiators involve the potential resistors in some aspect of the design and implementation of the change, they can often forestall resistance. With a participative change effort, the initiators listen to the people the change involves and use their advice" (p. 109).

Other commitment models draw on social psychological theories of cognitive dissonance (e.g., Festinger, 1957), commitment (e.g., Kiesler, 1971), self-perception (e.g., Bem, 1972), and rationalization (e.g., Aronson, 1983) to suggest that individuals become committed to a course of action as a result of their prior behaviors: "The degree of commitment derives from the extent to which a person's behaviors are binding. Four characteristics of behavioral acts make them binding and hence determine the extent of commitment: explicitness, revocability, volition, and publicity" (Salancik, 1983, p. 202). Thus, when individuals participate in decision-making and voice their support for a particular option freely, publicly, and explicitly, they are likely to become, subsequently, quite committed to that course of action.

Commitment models suggest, in sum, that worker participation provides a mechanism for overcoming resistance to change. Commitment models thus imply that participation may indirectly influence individual-, group-, or organizational-level performance (depending on the level of analysis of the participation program). That is, an individual's active, explicit, and public participation in making decisions increases his or her commitment to a course of action and may thereby improve performance, assuming, of course, that the chosen course of action is, in fact, efficacious. Commitment models do not suggest a clear or obvious link between participation and work satisfaction. Further, commitment models seem more applicable to direct employee participation than to indirect, representative forms of participation. Finally, the more influence employees are granted through their organization's participative decision-making practices, the more relevant commitment models become. Employees are, of course, more likely to be committed to decisions that they have shaped fundamentally than to decisions to which they only granted a nod of approval.

Contingency Models

Contingency models of the effects of worker participation focus on possible moderators of the relationships among participation, satisfaction, and performance. Thus, for example, "growth need strength" (Hackman & Oldham, 1975) may moderate the effects of participation on satisfaction and performance; need-satisfaction models may only apply to individuals who have stronger growth needs. Cognitive models (e.g., Locke et al., 1997) are often categorized as contingency models because they suggest that employee knowledge moderates the effects of worker participation on performance; participation is most effective if workers possess relevant knowledge and expertise. Vroom and Yetton's (1973) normative theory of leadership is, in fact, a contingency theory of worker participation, highlighting the fit between worker involvement in decision-making and the kind of decision to be made. If, for example, time was of the essence, Vroom and Yetton argued, then worker participation was probably inappropriate. If, on the other hand, management lacked adequate information to make the decision alone and employee acceptance of the decision was critical for implementation, workers should be involved in decision-making.

Organizational theorists (e.g., Burns & Stalker, 1961; Hage, 1980; Perrow, 1970) have long stressed the relationship between worker participation and organizational technology and environment. In essence, these authors argue that worker participation (or, more precisely, decentralization) is most appropriate for organizations that use nonroutine, rather than routine, technologies and work procedures. In such companies, the organizational structure cannot be highly bureaucratic and rigid because the nature of the work is variable and unpredictable. Worker expertise and input are necessary to effectively manage unexpected crises; managers lack the necessary information and resources to handle these crises alone. In a similar vein, these authors suggest that worker participation is most appropriate for organizations whose environments are characterized by uncertainty and rapid change. Again, the input of expert nonmanagers is necessary for the organization to respond effectively to quickly changing environmental demands.

Several recent commentators (e.g., Lawler & Mohrman, 1991; Pill & MacDuffie, 1996) have suggested another contingency model of participation. These scholars argue that participative practices are likely to have little effect on organizational performance in the absence of other supportive organizational policies and practices. The benefits of participation, they suggest, are contingent upon an organization's use of congruent management practices, such as goal-setting, group incentives, gain-sharing, and training. Implicitly or explicitly, authors of this new contingency school of participation effects note the many organizational forces that may counter the benefits of participation. These forces include managerial resistance to increases in employee influence; pay systems that reward individual, rather than group, contributions; and organizational pressures to produce a product quickly and efficiently, which may cause the slower process of participative decision-making, however beneficial it might prove, to be something of a frustration (Lawler & Mohrman, 1991).

Psychological-Contract Theory

Need satisfaction, cognitive, commitment, and contingency models dominate the theoretical and empirical literature on the benefits of worker participation. Although less well-known, psychological-contract theory offers another intriguing and rich perspective on worker participation—one that appears simultaneously familiar and novel. The psychological contract "is individual beliefs, shaped by the organization, regarding terms of an exchange agreement between individuals and their organization" (Rousseau, 1995, p. 9). The psychological contract specifies, often only tacitly, what an employee believes he or she owes his or her organization (e.g., punctuality, loyalty, performance up to standards), and what the employee believes the organization owes him or her in return (e.g., pay, benefits, opportunities for career development and promotions, respect, support). A "normative contract" emerges when a group of employees shares a common psychological contract. Normative contracts arise as a result of employees' shared organizational experiences and shared discussions (Rousseau, 1995).

The terms of psychological contracts may vary widely, of course. Some contracts are "transactional"—short-term, formal, written, closed-ended, narrow in scope, and financial (Rousseau, 1995). A temporary or "contract" worker may form such a contract with an organization. At the other end of the continuum are "relational contracts." The terms of such contracts are long-term, informal, open-ended, unwritten, broad in scope, and both financial and emotional. Over time, a long-term employee may forge such a contract with his or her organization, expecting that in exchange for his or her labor, long hours, loyalty, dedication, and creativity, he or she will receive praise, encouragement, support, recognition, stimulating assignments, opportunities for travel and advancement, pay raises, and bonuses.

How might psychological contract theory apply to the practice of worker participation? When an employee participates in organizational decision-making, he or she is giving the organization his or her ideas and creativity. The employee is investing—psychologically, cognitively, even emotionally—in the organization's future, particularly if his or her participation is direct and ongoing. The employee's participation in decision-making may thus render his or her psychological contract less transactional and more relational; the terms of the contract have changed. And what might the employee expect from his or her organization in return for his or her investment? To the extent that the employee perceives his or her participation to be an *extra* contribution to the organization, above and beyond the basic requirements of his or her job, the employee may expect *extra* benefits from the organization above and beyond the basic benefits of the job. Certainly, an employee would expect that his or her ideas would be taken seriously and carefully evaluated by supervisors and managers. But, the employee might well expect more, perhaps new authority, respect, and recognition, perhaps compensation for any financial benefits the organization receives as a result of implementing the employee's ideas, or, probably, both.

If an organization implements, as a new intervention, a group-level, mandatory, direct form of worker participation, employee's participation in decision-making is likely to become a part of the normative psychological contract, that is, shared by affected employees. Thus, employees as a group are likely to expect benefits in return for their suggestions. If employees' expectations are violated, that is, if the organization violates the normative expectation, employees might retaliate or exit. Surely, their enthusiasm for worker participation would wither, as might employee trust in management initiatives.

Unlike the established theories of the consequences of worker participation, reviewed above, the application of the psychological contract to worker participation does not suggest that worker participation necessarily leads to either increased satisfaction or performance. While the psychological contract "theory of worker participation" articulated here is clearly rudimentary, it suggests that employees may not perceive the opportunity to participate in organizational decision-making as a gift from management, but just the opposite. That is, employees may perceive their participation as their gift to management, to be compensated in respect, recognition, authority, and/or bonuses by management.

Discussion

The theoretical literature on worker participation hints at the complexity of studying and developing participation programs. The literature emphasizes the importance of attending to the values and assumptions that may drive the implementation of a participation program. It stresses the many different forms that a program may take. It attempts to describe and explain the possible outcomes of participation, as well as under what conditions those outcomes are most likely to occur. In an effort to summarize this literature, we highlight four implications of worker-participation theory, including possible lessons for empowerment beyond the workplace.

1. *For many, participation is a passion and a belief. This passion may potentially divert and obscure objective discussion of participation.* Both Dachler and Wilpert (1978) and Locke and Schweiger (1979) describe the value-laden passion with which many theorists endorse participation. Although this passion for participation is inspiring, if we are to engage in an open inquiry into the benefits of participation, we must make explicit the values and related assumptions that underlie and drive different participation models. Otherwise, the purposes and benefits of participation may be assumed rather than examined; drawbacks of, and alternatives to, participation may not be discussed. Ultimately, this may preclude both the careful planning required for the effective implementation of participation schemes and the precise analysis required for effective participation research. The passion for empowerment outside the workplace may have comparable effects. The challenge for workplace participation and community-empowerment enthusiasts is to harness the passion for participation and empowerment to good effect—to sound research and practice.
2. *The many dimensions of participation warrant greater attention within theories of participation.* Many participation theories devote little or no attention to the eight dimensions of worker participation as described above. As a result, these theories lack some of the specificity needed to guide participation research and theory. Thus, for example, researchers wishing to test the theoretical models outlined above may be uncertain which forms of participation to examine, and at which levels of analysis. Similarly, practitioners may, as we note below, be uncertain about which form of participation is most likely to fulfill both organizational and employee objectives.
3. *Not all workers view participation as a beneficial addition to their daily work. Not all organizations want or need participation.* While participation may be empowering and rewarding for some employees, for others it may be an extra chore on their list of job requirements. Participation theorists (Locke & Schweiger, 1978; Vroom & Yetton, 1973) have pointed to individual worker characteristics that may moderate the effects of participation. In a similar vein, other participation theorists highlight the importance of organizational characteristics (e.g., uncertainty, complexity, time pressures) in moderating the desirability of participation and its probable effects. Both individual and organizational characteristics may similarly moderate the effects of empowerment efforts outside the workplace.
4. *The development and evaluation of participation efforts pose a complex challenge for*

participation practitioners and researchers. The participation literature highlights the complexities and intricacies of participation. Should a participation program be voluntary or mandated, direct or indirect, job- or organization-focused? What are the consequences of these choices? How do these choices reflect the values underlying the participation effort? Which individual and organizational contingencies influence the success of participation? The answers to these questions are now largely unknown, despite years of participation research. This is unfortunate, for these questions are ones that empowerment advocates face whenever they design empowerment efforts, whether they be inside or outside the workplace. In the next section, we review what we do know, the current state of empirical research on worker participation.

EMPIRICAL RESEARCH ON WORKER PARTICIPATION

Participation research spans at least five decades, beginning with Coch and French's (1948) landmark study and continuing to the present (e.g., Scully et al., 1995). For the last twenty years, however, empirical research has been dominated not by original, primary research, but by major, comprehensive reviews and meta-analyses.

In 1979, Locke and Schweiger published the first major review of participation research. They reviewed over 50 studies of the relationship among participation, satisfaction, and productivity, and then coded each study's results as "participation superior," "participation inferior," or "no difference or contextual." Locke and Schweiger concluded that participative management practices typically do not lead to greater productivity than more directive management approaches, but do lead to higher employee satisfaction.

In an effort to provide a more precise assessment of the participation literature, Miller and Monge (1986) used meta-analysis (based on Hunter, Schmidt, & Jackson, 1982) to estimate the exact relationship among participation and both satisfaction and productivity. The meta-analysis strategy allows researchers to average study results, after weighting them for sample size and controlling, where appropriate, for measurement error and range restriction. Miller and Monge (1986) examined 47 studies and found a stronger weighted mean correlation between participation and satisfaction (.34) than between participation and productivity (.15). They also found several moderators of these relationships. The context of the study moderated the participation–satisfaction relationship, while both the type of decision to be made and the research setting moderated the relationship between participation and productivity.

Wagner and Gooding (1987a, 1987b) conducted a meta-analysis of 70 worker-participation studies to determine the influence of research design and situational moderators on the observed relationship between participation and several outcomes, including task performance and satisfaction. Wagner and Gooding's analysis highlighted the impact of percept–percept research design[2] on participation results. Wagner and Gooding (1987a) concluded that the correlation between worker participation and task performance was significantly larger in percept–percept studies (.45) than in multisource studies (.11). Similarly, the correlation between participation and satisfaction was larger in percept–percept studies (.42) than in multi-

[2]Percept–percept studies obtain independent and dependent variable data (e.g., data on participation and performance) from the same respondents, using the same questionnaire, at the same time. In contrast, multisource studies use at least one objective measure or assigned condition, different respondents for data on participation and outcome variables, and/or a longitudinal break between the collection of data on both participation and outcome variables from the same respondents.

source studies. In addition, after controlling for the effect of percept–percept bias, Wagner and Gooding (1987a) found that situational moderators like group size, task interdependence, task complexity, and performance standards had little effect on participation outcomes.

Cotton, Vollrath, Froggatt, Lengwick-Hall, and Jennings (1988) argued that the effects of participation reflect the form of the participation program—its formality, duration, focus, and so on. Accordingly, they sorted 91 studies into six groups as a function of the type of participation assessed in each study: (1) participation in work decisions (participation that is formal, direct, long-term, and with considerable influence over work-related issues); (2) consultative participation (essentially the same as the first category, except that workers have less influence in decision-making; (3) short-term studies of participation (participation of limited duration, ranging from a single laboratory session to training sessions of several days); (4) informal participation (no formal participation program, study participants report their perceived level of participation or influence in company decision-making); (5) employee ownership (formal, indirect participation as a function of ownership); and (6) representative participation (participation that is formal and indirect, with low to moderate influence over a variety of issues).

Using a traditional literature review (not meta-analysis), Cotton et al. (1988) found that the most positive effects occurred within three clusters: participation in work decisions, informal participation, and employee-ownership clusters. In each of these clusters, at least two-thirds of the studies reported that participation had a positive effect on satisfaction or performance. Summarizing their results, Cotton et al. concluded that participation is most effective in increasing employee satisfaction and performance when employees have a substantial amount of influence in decision-making and when the participation program is direct, permanent, focused on work-related issues, and of substantial duration.

More recently, Wagner (1994) conducted a meta-analysis of the studies that Cotton et al. (1988) had reviewed narratively. Wagner grouped the studies into Cotton et al.'s original six categories, but also specified whether a study used a percept–percept or multisource research design. He determined that percept–percept bias "seemed able to explain a primary finding of Cotton and his colleagues, namely, that information participation exerts significant influence on satisfaction" (p. 317). He also found that the effects of the six different forms of participation did not differ significantly. Finally, Wagner concluded that worker participation has a very small, but statistically significant, relationship to satisfaction and performance; across his multiple studies and reviews, the participation–satisfaction multisource correlation ranged from .15 to .25, while the participation–performance multisource correlation ranged from .08 to .16.

Discussion

The existing empirical literature has demonstrated that worker participation does, in fact, typically have a modest, positive effect on satisfaction and performance (Wagner, 1994), although the relative strength of the correlation among participation, satisfaction, and performance may reflect researchers' reliance on percept–percept designs (Wagner & Gooding, 1987a, 1987b). The literature also suggests that the effects of participation may vary as a function of the research setting (e.g., field or lab; Miller & Monge, 1986) and the nature of the participation (e.g., direct or indirect; Cotton et al., 1988).

Unfortunately, the empirical literature on worker participation is limited in several important respects. Accordingly, we offer one omnibus lesson regarding participation research:

The time is right for a return to original, theory-driven research on the effects of participation. Recent reviews and meta-analyses of participation have contributed a great deal to our understanding of the effects of worker participation. Yet many questions regarding the dynamics and effects of worker participation remain unanswered. The existence of multiple lengthy reviews of the literature may create the impression that organizational scholars have a thorough and multifaceted understanding of participation and its consequences. This simply isn't true. Thus, for example, we know very little about the consequence of different dimensions and forms of participation for individual satisfaction, individual performance, organizational performance, and the longevity of the participation program. We know very little about the individual characteristics (e.g., subordinate expertise, supervisor management style) and organizational characteristics (e.g., technology, industry, culture) that may mediate or moderate the effects of participation. We know very little about the multilevel dynamics and effects of participation. Indeed, the appropriate level of analysis for studying participation remains uncertain, and should be explored in both theory and research. We know very little about the antecedents of participation: Under what circumstances and for what reasons are organizations most likely to implement worker participation? Finally, we know very little about the negative consequences of participation. Proparticipation values may have made researchers myopic. What are the benefits and the costs of participation for individual employees, their supervisors, and the organization as a whole?

In sum, a lengthy and challenging agenda awaits researchers interested in the nature, dynamics, and consequences of worker participation. Some may find our critique of the existing literature discouraging. We do not mean to disparage past research, however, but only to suggest exciting opportunities for new research on workplace participation and, by extension, nonworkplace empowerment as well.

We turn now to an examination of participation programs that are relatively common in American businesses today. Studies of these programs shed further light on the dynamics of participation and suggest additional topics for future participation and empowerment research.

PARTICIPATION IN PRACTICE

In this section, we explore the practice of participation in the workplace. We focus primarily on quality circles (QCs), but also consider total quality management (TQM). Quality circles are groups of employees who meet regularly to solve work-related problems. Generally composed of 6–12 employees from the same work area, quality circles recommend solutions to management regarding productivity and quality problems. With regard to the dimensions of participative decision-making described earlier, quality circles are generally formal, voluntary, direct, occasional, and of limited influence over shop floor- and department-level issues. Quality circles gained tremendous popularity in the 1980s and early 1990s. Thus, for example, in the early 1990s, approximately 80% of Fortune 1000 companies were estimated to use quality circles to some extent (Lawler et al., 1992; Lawler, 1992; Milbank, 1992).

Later in the 1990s, total quality management (TQM) surpassed quality circles as the quality intervention of choice in American business. In a review of TQM theory, research, and practice, Hackman and Wageman (1995) reported that U.S. organizations typically employ the following five practices in the name of TQM: (1) short-term problem-solving teams with the overall objective of simplifying and streamlining work practices; (2) training in interpersonal skills, quality improvement processes, team-building, statistical analysis, supplier qualification training, and/or benchmarking; (3) top-down implementation, with each level of the organizational hierarchy carrying the TQM message to the next lower level; (4) closer relationships with suppliers in an effort to enhance the quality of component parts; and (5) data collection and reporting regarding customer demands and satisfaction. Together, the elements of TQM are designed to lead to "continuous improvement," that is, to

> ever better, less variable quality of the product or service itself; ever quicker, less variable response—from design and development through sales channels, offices, and plants, all the way to the final user; ever greater flexibility—in adjusting to customers' shifting volume and "mix" requirements; [and] ever lower cost—through quality improvement and non-value-adding (NVA) rework and waste elimination (Schonberger, 1992, p. 18).

Worker participation, in the form of short-term problem-solving teams, represents only one element of the multifaceted practice of TQM. Worker participation within the context of TQM is similar to worker participation in the form of quality circles (e.g., direct, formal, of limited influence). However, the total-quality movement, far more than the quality-circle movement, emphasizes the importance of buttressing worker involvement with an array of complementary management practices, including training, benchmarking, and measurement of customer service.

Research on Quality Circles and Total Quality Management

Despite the popularity of QCs and TQM programs, there is little high-quality research available on these topics. Far more common are anecdotal case studies of the consequences of the implementation of QCs and/or TQM in single companies (Ferris & Wagner, 1985; Hackman & Wageman, 1995). Writing over a decade ago, Steel and Shane (1986) described QC evaluation research as "at best, seriously flawed and, at worst, potentially misleading" (p. 451). More recently, Hackman and Wageman (1995) suggested that a full-fledged evaluation of a TQM program should include a rigorous assessment of: (1) the extent to which the organization has indeed implemented a multifaceted TQM program; (2) the effects of the TQM program on intermediate, process criteria (e.g., employee effort and knowledge); and (3) the effects of the TQM program on the ultimate, bottom-line goals of the program (e.g., productivity). Hackman and Wageman found no studies meeting these criteria. They concluded that while the results of studies of TQM have been strongly positive:

> [The results] are almost all based on case reports. In part, this problem exists because TQM has captured more attention from practitioners than from researchers: Many assessments of TQM are descriptions written by a member of the focal organization.... It is ironic that the designs and methodologies used in research on TQM fall far short of the standards of research design, measurement, and analysis that would be required or organization members studying their own work processes under TQM (Hackman & Wageman, 1995, p. 325).

Despite the general methodological inadequacies of QC and TQM research, a few QC studies may be instructive. Griffin (1988) compared 73 employees participating in quality circles with an individually matched group of nonparticipants drawn from a different (non-QC) plant in the same organization. Griffin found that the QC members' job satisfaction, organizational commitment, performance, and intentions to remain at the job improved gradually in the first 18 months and then decreased back to their initial levels. Griffin's findings reinforce Lawler and Mohrman's (1985) observations that most American quality circles follow a relatively short developmental cycle, marked by eventual disinterest on the part of managers and workers. Thus, quality circles, like many previously popular organizational interventions (e.g., management by objectives and T-groups), may fall into a familiar cycle of adoption, disappointment, and discontinuation (Wood, Hull, & Azumi, 1983).

Recent research also raises some questions about the effectiveness of total quality management programs. A 1991 survey of more than 300 electronics companies found that 73% of the companies reported having total quality programs, but the majority of these companies failed to make significant improvements in quality (Schaffer & Thomson, 1992). A 1992 Gallup survey of employees in companies with total quality programs found that a majority of respondents felt that their companies placed greater emphasis on the importance of quality, but only a third felt that their companies were doing anything effective to improve quality (American Society for Quality Control, 1990; Hyde, 1991).

Barriers to the Success of Participation in Practice

Although some organizations find their QC and TQM programs highly beneficial, many organizations find that their QC, TQM, and other high-involvement programs do not engender the expected gains in organizational performance and/or employee morale. Below, we explore some possible reasons.

Employee Frustration

QC and TQM programs typically allow employees to make suggestions, not final decisions. Thus, most QC and TQM programs increase employee power to a limited extent. Levitan and Johnson (1983) commented that "QCs and other participative arrangements are merely the same old attempts to increase workers' commitment to company goals without requiring managers to accept the burdens and risks of full participation" (p. 8). A 1992 Gallop survey of employees in companies with total quality programs found that while approximately two-thirds of the employees surveyed said they had been asked and were expected to participate in making organizational decisions, less than 15% said they had been given the power to make those decisions (American Society for Quality Control, 1990). When managers are unresponsive to employee suggestions, employees' commitment to the participative process may wane.

Many organizations implement worker participation in an attempt to change worker attitudes, rather than to make improvements in quality and productivity (Hayes, Wheelwright, & Clark, 1988; Hyde, 1991). Indeed, one survey found that the top reason given by American managers for implementing quality circles was to increase worker satisfaction, while the top reason given by Japanese managers was to improve product quality (Cole & Byosiere, 1986). Ultimately, this approach may backfire. Dean (1985) found that the main reason employees gave for participating in quality circles was the opportunity to participate in problem-solving, while the top reason for not wanting to participate was the belief that quality circles would have no effect. Dean (1985) concluded: "QC members have little motivation for going through the motions—they want results" (p. 326).

Managerial Resistance

Managerial concerns regarding QC, TQM, and related worker-involvement programs take, not surprisingly, a different form. Managers express concern that QC participants, having experienced a new level of influence in company decision-making, will desire still greater influence (Lawler & Mohrman, 1985). Indeed, Meyer and Stott (1985) found that employees participating in quality circles had difficulty limiting their focus to departmental, rather than organizational, issues, even though their mandate was to consider departmental concerns alone.

Middle managers often fear that the QC process will erode their authority over their employees and reduce, or render obsolete, their own role in the organizational hierarchy. Klein (1984) found that while most middle managers believed QC-type programs were beneficial to employees (72%) and to the organization (60%), relatively few (31%) believed QC-type programs were beneficial to middle managers. Middle managers may also resent top management's mandate that middle managers implement QC programs (Kanter, 1983). Meyer and Stott (1984) noted that supervisors often expressed annoyance that they were expected to involve their subordinates in decision-making, although they themselves lacked such influence with their own bosses.

Limited Employee Training

If QCs are to be successful, managers must provide employees with access to the expertise and information that employees need in order to make effective contributions and produce effective change (Ledford, Lawler, & Mohrman, 1988). Training is crucial to the success of most quality efforts, as many of the most significant cost-saving benefits are a direct result of the technical and problem-solving skills developed by employees (Wood et al., 1983). Unfortunately, less than 7% of the money spent on training in the U.S. goes to the frontline workers who participate in quality circles (Lawler, 1992). Further, the focus of the employee training that does exist may be misplaced. Although the use of scientific methods to solve quality problems is one of the hallmarks of TQM theory (e.g., Deming, 1986; Juran, 1974), American businesses devote more time and effort to interpersonal skills training than to training in scientific methods (Hackman & Wageman, 1995).

Failure to Support Worker Participation with Complementary Innovations in Other Human Resource Practices

In establishing quality circles and total quality management programs, many organizations appear to be hopping on the latest management bandwagon. In such cases, the quality program may be ill-suited to the practices and culture of the organization. Under these circumstances, the QC or TQM program is unlikely to be accepted and supported by organizational members. Indeed, no organizational intervention is likely to be effective unless it targets, or is already compatible with, multiple facets of the larger organization—its training, selection, socialization, job design, and reward systems, for example (Lawler, 1992; Schneider & Gunnarson, 1991; Schneider & Klein, 1994). Contemplating the future of TQM, Hackman and Wageman (1995) lamented: "The problem is that what many organizations are actually implementing is a pale or highly distorted version of what [the founders of TQM] laid out ... It is the difficult-to-implement portions of the program that are being finessed or ignored and the rhetoric that is being retained" (p. 338).

Discussion

The available literature provides a mixed, if incomplete, picture of the benefits and drawbacks of worker participation in practice. Below, we discuss three of the lessons suggested by the literature.

1. *Quality circle and total quality management programs do not provide organizations with a quick fix. Worker-participation programs require management commitment to sharing information, expertise, and power.* Many organizations adopt quality circles and TQM in the hope that these programs will boost productivity and morale. In some organizations, these programs do so. However, in others, a variety of problems plague QC and TQM programs. These problems include unrealistic employee expectations, employee disappointment and resentment, supervisor resistance, and uncertain long-term benefits for the company. To prevent or overcome these problems, organizations must have strong managerial support for participation, careful planning, supervisor and employee training, and ongoing evaluation.

2. *The failure of a quality program may highlight employees' limited influence in organizational decision-making, rendering labor–management relations worse than before.* Many employees enter quality interventions skeptical that management will give them real influence in the organization. If management withdraws its support for the intervention, employee skepticism may be reinforced. Further, supervisors and employees may resent the time and effort that they put into the unsuccessful program. Future attempts to gain employee input in the future may meet with resistance and cynicism. Surely organization efforts outside the workplace may face the same problems. If they fail, they too may heighten, rather than diminish, individual skepticism and hopelessness.

3. *Workplace quality and participation interventions cannot work alone; they are most effective when supported by a congruent organizational culture, strategy, and organizational environment.* Worker participation that is outside of, or parallel to, the real business and management of the organization is rarely effective (Lawler, 1992). Making participation central to the organizational culture, however, may prove a significant management undertaking. It may involve changing the reward structure to promote learning and participation, flattening management hierarchies, and educating employees about the inner financial workings of the company (Lawler, 1992). Training employees is critical. So, too, is commitment from top management (Lawler, 1992). Because the creation and maintenance of real avenues of worker participation may be time-consuming, expensive, and risky, extensive worker participation is not for every organization. Rather, worker participation may be most effective and appropriate in organizations best suited to realize the benefits of increased employee input, commitment and creativity, that is, organizations characterized by non-routine, complex tasks and an unpredictable business environment (Bowen & Lawler, 1992). Here, too, the lessons may apply to nonworkplace empowerment efforts; they too are most likely to be effective if they are but one element of a coordinated, multifaceted program to empower the unempowered.

CONCLUSIONS

Four important themes emerge from our review of the literature regarding organizational power and participation. First, the very phenomenon of worker participation is complex and multifaceted. Its complexity and variety have been overlooked in much of the theoretical and research literature, but should instead be embraced. Theoretical and empirical analysis of the many dimensions of participation will render a deeper, more textured, and ultimately more practical understanding of participation. Participation outside the workplace—empowerment—is no different. It too may take many forms and should be conceptualized and studied in all its complexity.

Second, the benefits of participation rest in large part upon employee expertise. The more expert employees are, the more their ideas will benefit the organization. The more expert employees are, the more their participation will be welcomed by organizational managers. The more expert employees are, the more they will seek opportunities to participate and gain satisfaction from participation. The selection, education, and training of skilled employees thus emerge as a potentially powerful empowerment strategy. To empower may be to cultivate expertise, not simply to allow input.

Counterbalancing the optimism of the second theme is the darker realism of the third: Managerial resistance to employee participation is to be expected. An increase in employee power may well threaten managerial rank and authority. Outside of the workplace, decision-makers may also resist the involvement and input of unempowered individuals. Thus, effective empowerment strategies may necessitate efforts both to increase the expertise and input of the unempowered and to address and assuage decision-makers' fears of participation. Unfortunately, existing theory and research shed little light on effective strategies for addressing and assuaging existing decision-makers' concerns and fears regarding participation and empowerment.

Fourth, employee participation is most likely to yield organizational benefits when employees are expert and when their organization's tasks are complex and rapidly changing. Under these circumstances, organizations are relatively likely to benefit from the organizational creativity and flexibility that participation may yield. This principle may hold for community organizations as well. When community organizations face complex, rapidly changing demands, they may welcome the input of formerly unempowered, but expert, individuals.

REFERENCES

American Society for Quality Control. (1990). *Quality: Everyone's job, many vacancies.* Milwaukee, WI: American Society for Quality Control.

Aronson, E. (1983). The rationalizing animal. In B. M. Staw (Ed.), *Psychological foundations of organizational behavior*, 2nd ed. (pp. 307–313). Glenview, IL: Scott, Foresman.

Bem, D. J. (1972). Self-perception theory. In L. Berkowitz (Ed.), *Advances in experimental social psychology, Vol.6* (pp. 1–62). New York: Academic.

Bowen, D. E., & Lawler, E. E., III. (1992). The empowerment of service workers: What, why, how, and when. *Sloan Management Review, 33*, 31–39.

Burns, T., & Stalker, G. M. (1961). *The management of innovation.* London: Tavistock.

Coch, L., & French, J. R. P., Jr. (1948). Overcoming resistance to change. *Human Relations, 1*, 512–532.

Cole, R. E., & Byosiere, P. (1986). Managerial objectives for introducing quality circles: A U.S.-Japan comparison. *Quality Progress, March*, 25–30.

Conger, J. A., & Kanungo, R. N. (1988). The empowerment process: Integrating theory and practice. *Academy of Management Review, 13*, 471–482.

Cotton, J. L., Vollrath, D. A, Froggatt, K. L., Lengnick-Hall, M. K., & Jennings, K. R. (1988). Employee participation: Diverse forms and different outcomes. *Academy of Management Review, 13*, 8–22.

Dachler, H. P., & Wilpert, B. (1978). Conceptual dimensions and boundaries of participation in organizations. *Administrative Science Quarterly, 23*, 1–39.

Dean, J. W. (1985). The decision to participation in quality circles. *Journal of Applied Behavioral Sciences, 21*, 317–327.

Deming, W. E. (1986). *Out of crisis.* Cambridge, MA: MIT Center for Advanced Engineering Study.

Ferris, G. R., & Wagner, J. A. (1985). Quality circles in the United States: A conceptual reevaluation. *Journal of Applied Behavior Sciences, 21*, 155–167.

Festinger, L. (1957). *A theory of cognitive dissonance.* Stanford, CA: Stanford University Press.

French, J., & Raven, B. (1960). The bases of social power. In D. Cartwright & A. Zanier (Eds.), *Group dynamics: Research and theory* (pp. 607–623). New York: Row, Peterson.

Goodman, P. S., Lerch, F. J., & Mukhopadhyay, T. (1994). Individual and organizational productivity: Linkages and processes. In D. H. Harris (Ed.), *Organizational linkages: Understanding the productivity paradox* (pp. 54–80). Washington, D.C.: National Academy Press.

Griffin, R. W. (1988). Consequences of quality circles in an industrial setting: A longitudinal assessment. *Academy of Management Journal, 31*, 338–358.

Hackman, J. R., & Oldham, G. R. (1975). Development of the Job Diagnostic Survey. *Journal of Applied Psychology, 60*, 159–170.

Hackman, J. R., & Wageman, R. (1995). Total quality management: Empirical, conceptual, and practical issues. *Administrative Science Quarterly, 40*, 309–342.

Hage, J. (1980). *Theories of organizations: Form, process, and transformation.* New York: Wiley.

Hayes, R. H., Wheelwright, S. C., & Clark, K. B. (1988). *Dynamic manufacturing.* New York: Free Press.

Hunter, J. E., Schmidt, F. L., & Jackson, G. B. (1982). *Meta-analysis: Culminating research findings across studies.* Beverly Hills, CA: Sage.

Hyde, A. C. (1991). Rescuing quality measurement from TQM. *The Bureaucrat. Winter 1990–91*, 16–20.

Juran, J. M. (1974). *The quality control handbook*, 3rd ed. New York: McGraw-Hill.

Kanter, R. M. (1983). *The change master.* New York: Simon and Schuster.

Katz, D. N., & Kahn, R. L. (1966). *The social psychology of organizations.* New York: Wiley.

Kieffer, C. (1984). Citizen empowerment: A developmental perspective. *Prevention in Human Services, 3*, 9–36.

Kiesler, C. A. (1971). *The psychology of commitment: Experiments linking behavior to belief.* New York: Academic.

Klein, J. A. (1984). Why supervisors resist employee involvement. *Harvard Business Review, 5*, 87–95.

Klein, K. J., Dansereau, F., & Hall, R. J. (1994). Levels issues in theory development, data collection, and analysis. *Academy of Management Review, 19*, 195–229.

Klein, K. J., Smith-Major, V. L., & Ralls, R. S. (1999). Worker participation: Current promise, future prospects. In A. Kraut & A. Koran (Eds.), *Evolving practices in human resource management: Responses to a changing world of work.* San Francisco: Jossey-Bass.

Kotter, J. P., & Schlesinger, L. A. (1979). Choosing strategies for change. *Harvard Business Review, 57*, 106–114.

Lawler, E. E. (1992). *The ultimate advantage: Creating the high-involvement organization.* San Francisco: Jossey-Bass.

Lawler, E. E., & Mohrman, S. A. (1985). Quality circles after the fad. *Public Welfare, Spring*, 37–45.

Lawler, E. E., & Mohrman, S. A. (1991). Quality circles: After the honeymoon, In B. M. Staw (Ed.), *Psychological dimensions of organizational behavior* (pp. 523–533). New York: McMillan.

Lawler, E. E., Mohrman, G. E., & Ledford, G. E. (1992). *Employee involvement and total quality management.* San Francisco: Jossey-Bass.

Ledford, G. E., Lawler, E. E., & Mohrman, S. A. (1988). The quality circle and its variations. In J. P. Campbell (Ed.), *Productivity in organizations* (pp. 255–294). San Francisco: Jossey-Bass.

Levitan, S. A, & Johnson, C. M. (1983). Labor and management: The illusion of cooperation. *Harvard Business Review, 61*, 8–16.

Locke, E. A., Alav, M., & Wagner, J. A., III. (1997). Participation in decision making: An information exchange perspective. In G. R. Ferris (Ed.), *Research in personnel and human resources management: Vol. 15* (pp. 293–331). Greenwich, CT: JAI Press.

Locke, E. A., & Schweiger, D. M. (1979). Participation in decision making: One more look. In B. M. Staw (Ed.), *Research in organizational behavior, Vol. 1* (pp. 265–339). Greenwich, CT: JAI Press.

McGregor, D. (1960). *The human side of enterprise.* New York: McGraw-Hill.

Meyer, G. M., & Stott, R. G. (1985). Quality circles: panacea or Pandora's box? *Organizational Dynamics, Spring*, 34–50.

Milbank, D. (1992). Unions' woes suggest how the labor force in the U.S. is shifting. *Wall Street Journal*, May 5, 1992.

Miller, K. I., & Monge, P. R. (1986). Participation, satisfaction, and productivity: A meta-analytical review. *Academy of Management Journal, 29*, 727–753.

Miller, K. I., & Pritchard, F. N. (1992). Factors associated with workers' inclination to participate in an employee involvement program. *Group and Organization Management, 17*, 414–430.

Ostroff, C. (1992). The relationship between satisfaction, attitudes and performance: An organizational level analysis. *Journal of Applied Psychology, 77*, 963–974.

Perkins, D. D., & Zimmerman, M. A. (1995). Empowerment theory, research, and application. *American Journal of Community Psychology, 23*, 569–579.

Perrow, C. (1970). *Organizational analysis: A sociological view.* Belmont, CA: Wadsworth.

Pfeffer, J. (1982). *Organizations and organization theory.* Cambridge, MA: Ballinger.

Pill, F. K., & MacDuffie, J. P. (1996). The adoption of high-involvement work practices. *Industrial Relations, 35*, 423–455.

Rappaport, J. (1981). In praise of paradox: A social policy of empowerment over prevention. *American Journal of Community Psychology, 9*, 1–25.

Riger, S. (1993). What's wrong with empowerment? *American Journal of Community Psychology, 21*, 279–292.

Rousseau, D. M. (1995). *Psychological contracts in organizations: Understanding written and unwritten agreements.* Thousand Oaks, CA: Sage.

Salancik, G. R. (1983). Commitment and the control of organizational behavior and belief. In B. M. Staw (Ed.), *Psychological foundations of organizational behavior*, 2nd ed (pp. 202–206). Glenview, IL: Scott, Foresman.

Salancik, G. R., & Pfeffer, J. (1977). Who gets power—and how they hold onto it: A strategic-contingency model of power. In J. Hackman, E. Lawler, & L. Porter (Eds.), *Perspectives on Behavior in Organizations* (pp. 417–429). New York: McGraw-Hill.

Salancik, G. R., & Pfeffer, J. (1978). A social information processing approach to job attitudes and task design. *Administrative Science Quarterly, 23*, 224–254.

Schaffer, R. H., & Thomson, H. A. (1992). Successful change programs begin with results. *Harvard Business Review, 70*, 80–89.

Schneider, B., & Gunnarson, S. (1991). Organizational climate and culture: The psychology of the workplace. In J. W. Jones, B. D. Steffy, & D. W. Bray (Eds.), *Applying psychology in business* (pp. 542–551). Lexington, MA: Lexington Books.

Schneider, B., & Klein, K. J. (1994). What is enough? A systems perspective on individual-organizational performance linkages. In D. H. Harris (Ed.), *Organizational linkages: Understanding the productivity paradox* (pp. 81–104). Washington, D.C.; National Academy Press.

Schonberger, R. J. (1992). Total quality management cuts a broad swath—through manufacturing and beyond. *Organizational Dynamics, 29*, 16–28.

Scully, J. A., Kirkpatrick, S. A., & Locke, E. A. (1995). Locus of knowledge as a determinant of the effects of participation on performance, affect, and perceptions. *Organizational Behavior and Human Decision Processes, 61*, 276–288.

Steel, R. P., & Shane, G. S. (1986). Evaluation research on quality circles: Technical and analytical implications. *Human Relations, 39*, 449–468.

Swift, C. (1984). Empowerment: An antidote for folly. In J. Rappaport, C. Swift, & R. Hess (Eds.), *Studies in empowerment: Steps toward understanding and action.* New York: Haworth.

Tannenbaum, A. S. (1968). *Control in organizations.* New York: McGraw-Hill.

Tannenbaum, A. S., Kavcic, B., Rosner, M., Vianello, M., & Wiesner, G. (1974). *Hierarchy in organizations: An international comparison.* San Francisco: Jossey-Bass.

Thomas, K. W., & Velthouse, B. A. (1990). Cognitive elements of empowerment: An "interpretive" model of intrinsic task motivation. *Academy of Management Review, 15*, 666–681.

Vroom, V. H. (1960). *Some personality determinants of the effects of participation.* Englewood Cliffs, NJ: Prentice-Hall.

Vroom, V. H., & Yetton, P. W. (1973). *Leadership and decision-making.* Pittsburgh, PA: University of Pittsburgh Press.

Wagner, J. A., III. (1994). Participation's effects on performance and satisfaction: A reconsideration of research evidence. *Academy of Management Review, 19*, 312–330.

Wagner, J. A., III, & Gooding, R. Z. (1987a). Shared influence and organizational behavior: A meta-analysis of situational variables expected to moderate participation-outcome relationships. *Academy of Management Journal, 30*, 524–541.

Wagner, J. A., III, & Gooding, R. Z. (1987b). Effects of societal trends on participation research. *Administrative Science Quarterly, 32*, 241–262.

Wood, R., Hull, F., & Azumi, K. (1983). Evaluating quality circles: The American application. *California Management Review, 26*, 37–52.

PART III

INTERVENTION STRATEGIES AND TACTICS

Part III emphasizes the kinds of roles and activities that flow from a community psychology worldview: consultant as partner, organizer as collaborator, creator and friend of alternative settings, concerned about, and willing to make use of, the media, and working to influence public policy and the dissemination of knowledge. These activities are the heart and soul of the field—the place where ideals turn to action, theory turns to works, and concepts become reality to be tested. We work with a wide range of constituencies and at multiple levels of analysis, from individuals to systems, but in most cases our aim is to work with and through others, rather than to provide direct services. We can often help to document the good work of other people, and thereby will both learn from it and help preserve it.

The roles played by human services professionals and their clientele tend to be defined by the implicit rules of social institutions in which they encounter each other (see Part IV). The mental health professional and the identified mental patient are bounded in an arrangement of mutual responsibilities and obligations. Teachers and their students, the consumers of public education and its producers, and the citizens who are provided with social welfare services are locked in their role relationships as much as are prisoners and guards, lawyers and clients, merchants and consumers. As community psychologists, we try to step outside the constraints of our presumed role relationships. Rather than selling our services as a commodity (even while looking for ways to earn a living, and to obtain grants, contracts, and jobs), we try to find ways to give services away, a surprisingly difficult task in a culture of faith in experts, with a symbiotic relationship among entrepreneurs and consumers. Even many former mental patients who have rejected professional control in favor of self and mutual help ironically refer to themselves as mental health "consumers." Community psychologists prefer to encourage a process rather than a product, an experience in participatory democracy as a means that is consistent with our ends. Such activity is not easily framed as the purchasable product of licensed and accredited experts, and hence the field has resisted such movements to define our roles and responsibilities.

Armed with concepts and frameworks (Part I), an awareness of social scientific empirical foundations (Part II), tempered by a desire to comprehend the social contexts (Part IV) in which we find ourselves (even when they differ from what we expected), the community psychologist enters the world of action—sometimes purposefully without specific predesigned program. The position taken is that it is undesirable to take action before one knows a great deal about the specific local setting and history and has developed a meaningful collaborative relationship with the people who are part of it. This is not the way expertise is typically sold, and for community psychologists there is a conscious tension between our own legitimation as experts and our desire to work with and for others, while learning from the people with whom we work.

The kind of expertise we offer is open to finding the ways to work with, rather than on, people, including those who are outside the mainstream of power and influence; yet this requires us to form alliances at both the grass-roots and the established centers of power. Only some of how to negotiate this can be known beforehand; it is as much craft as science. Everyday is an adventure in the unpredictable. If we are not to become disoriented, we require a very clear sense of our role relationship (as collaborators, and coworkers) with the people we encounter. Holding our conceptual and empirical maps before us, now in the world of social action, can be like trying to find our way home as a fog settles over us. We need vehicles with good headlights to contain and focus our work. These chapters provide such vehicles. They can serve as a means to move ourselves toward actions that are consistent with our concepts. The strategies and tactics presented here orient us to roles that remind us not only of where we want to go, but also of why we are out there in the first place. The ends do not justify the means, and what we seek is for our strategies and tactics (our ways of conducting our business) to reflect our goals and values.

We are guided by our goals, values, and assumptions about others, as well as by our understanding of the proper role relationship between ourselves and the people with whom we work. We are thrust, by both interest and necessity, toward an engagement with the world—its concrete organizations and implicit institutions, its assumptions, ideologies, and power struggles, its perspectives and ideologies. We do not wait for people to find us so as to adapt themselves to the culture of our office. We instead seek out the people of concern in the settings where they are actually engaged in their everyday lives. We risk being both audacious and intrusive as we become the visitors, the "other," who must learn the rules of engagement and the culture of everyday life in the varied settings where we try to do our work. We seek to build community strengths, prevent problems in living, empower others, collaborate for social change, and disseminate knowledge that fosters progressive values and social policies that are enabling, rather than demeaning. In some ways the community psychologist in action is operating to counter certain cultural assumptions about the relationship between experts as helpers and citizens as recipients of assistance. We are inclined to believe in the power of every person, and in our own capacity to share what we learn in ways that communicate such faith.

In the first chapter of this section, Trickett, Barone, and Watts provide a basic framework for thinking about consultation, a role that has historically served many community psychologists as a kind of transition activity from clinical work in their office to community mental health programs in other settings and with other professionals. Ultimately, the role of consultant has helped community psychologists to carve out a variety of new relationships in new settings, including work as activists in collaboration with grass-roots people and organizations beyond those narrowly defined as "mental health."

Trickett, Barone, and Watts take the implications of an ecological metaphor and apply them to the domain of consultation, which they see as having two goals: the development of indigenous resources in the host environment, and setting or community development through a process of "radiating effects." Their approach is emergent from the theoretical perspective associated with James G. Kelly and his colleagues. Reading this chapter, in conjunction with the conceptual paper by Kelly, Ryan, Altman and Stelzner in Part I, provides a particularly useful orientation to combining theory and action while keeping a critical eye on role relationships, as noted above.

Consultation is viewed as on ongoing process of learning, for the consultant as well as the client. The consultant is alert to unintended as well as intentional consequences of an intervention. Mechanisms to monitor, reevaluate, and change strategies and goals over time are crucial, and theory is a guide, but the consultant must learn to develop keen observation skills. Sometimes working in a group or using others as "consultants to the consultant" may make sense in this sort of work, which is often formative over time, rather than completely preplanned. Awareness of the power of social context is an important idea that alerts us to matters such as levels of trust, power, and community support for any intervention. Local ecology, including human diversity (both the clients' and the consultants'); system boundaries; and community influence, all affect the activity of the consultant. These authors remind us that personal status (race, class, and gender), as well as worldview, are central to the relationship. By use of specific examples they illustrate a more general approach to consultation issues including entry, reconnaissance, and assessment in local settings (see also the chapters by Linney and by Stewart in Part V).

Bill Berkowitz argues that community organizing, while more craft than science, should be a major theme of action and study for the field of community psychology. He begins such an analysis of the conditions that make for successful organizing. Berkowitz sees this work as intentional and relational. The organizer (a person or a group) tries to bring community residents together for joint action to improve the local quality of life in an enduring way. His focus is on geographical communities (neighborhoods) and in locality development, although community organizing may include social planning to create organizational structures, as well as social action to oppose external power. While the activity itself may be craftlike, the community psychologist can systematically describe the conditions that are conducive to successful organizing. We can learn from observation of, and work with, successful organizers; we can try to understand how settings, issues, and communication interact with leadership to influence outcomes. Such work requires a multiplicity of research methods (see Part V).

In this field of scholarship we may make good use of biographical observation and analysis of local organizers, as well as methods for dissemination of information in forms useful to the public (see also McAlister, this section, for suggestions with respect to media influence from an entirely different scholarly perspective). Perhaps somewhat disarmingly, and in a fashion rarely seen in the traditions of academic writing, Berkowitz suggests that those who want to encourage public life should themselves engage in it, a position that has shifted between background and foreground for community psychologists at different historical moments.

The creation of alternative settings (defined here by Cherniss and Deegan to include relatively permanent structures or groups created for a specific purpose, organizational settings, and small, circumscribed communities) is a topic that places us at the intersection between practical reality and ideal visions. One needs both vision and an astute sense of the possible. A fine line exists between creating a new setting and changing an existing one. The link between ideas and their implementation in concrete activity is, as a practical matter, at the center of community psychology. Understood as the creation of alternative settings, it rests on a history of utopian visions, as well as on sociological research on social movements, communes, and voluntary organizations. Cherniss and Deegan offer both theoretical analysis and practical advice. They point out that "alternative" does not refer only to new settings, and that a setting can be alternative in structure, goals, ideology, or technology. Their guidelines for intervention, many of which build on the writing of Sarason, ask us to attend to political realities such as sources of opposition, the role of leadership, anticipation of transitions, realistic time frames, budgets, conflicts, and factions. Read together with the preceding chapters on consultation and community organization, this chapter frames intervention strategies and tactics in yet another way, which forces us to attend to the nature of our role relationships to the people of concern.

The fourth chapter in this section, by McAlister, reminds us of the practical, technical skills and information available to psychologists who want to make use of the media. Starting from the observation that the mass media has "agenda-setting" effects, he suggests that community psychologists make conscious use of media resources for interventions that require attitudinal and behavioral change (social modeling). Much of this chapter serves to remind community psychologists of our access to a detailed knowledge base of social and behavioral techniques for the creation of individual change. But this knowledge base can be used for work consistent with the role relationships that the preceding three chapters discuss. The community psychologist as collaborator and consultant, as community organizer and supporter of alternative settings, can bring to his or her constituents access to a social and behavioral technology that can assist in effective use of mass media as a tool for generating new agendas for change and social support.

The chapter by Phillips shifts our attention to the role of the community psychologist in social policy, and to consideration of multiple levels of analysis and intervention. She begins with a discussion of the uneasy relationship between advocacy and psychology, and provides the reader with a perspective that both encourages and serves as a guide to a variety of considerations that will confront those who enter the world of work with government policymakers. However, she also points out that such work is often "bottom-up" as well as "top-down." Phillips reminds us that there are many potential connections between public policy considerations and community psychology, including our attention to multiple levels of analysis, value assumptions, issues of empowerment, and a willingness to address contemporary issues with both stories and statistics. She draws attention to dissemination of information (see also Mayer & Davidson in the following chapter).

How does our research become readable and accessible to policymakers, and how can our activity as psychologists be consistent with the desire to be useful participants in the creation and implementation of public policy? Phillips makes a strong case, and provides a variety of concrete examples, for the role of community psychology in developing strategies and tactics to engage in such work. Out of her specific examples a great deal of advice emerges that is applicable to work in policy, regardless of the specific substantive issues addressed.

Understanding (and enabling) the dissemination of innovations is an activity closely linked to engagement in the policy process. But, "actual on the ground" work at dissemination is also directly linked to implementation of programmatic change. Contrary to the notion that good research will naturally lead to the adoption of effective innovation, we often find that decision-making is not simply data driven. Dissemination is itself an intervention. It requires the skills of consultant, organizer, media consultant, and innovator in a multilevel effort that brings together many of the issues of the previous chapters concerned with strategies and tactics.

Mayer and Davidson view innovation as social change. They draw on the work of Fairweather and others at Michigan State University as they discuss dissemination tasks over time: adoption, implementation, and institutionalization. They review research on both adopters of innovation and on the nature of the innovations. But as they put it: "From the perspective of the community psychologist, adoption is only a prelude to implementation." Most importantly, their analysis is a useful one for evaluation of interventions. It highlights research questions of this form: When (and how) do changes become routine in an organization? Using this way of thinking, research on intervention outcomes can be linked with research on dissemination of successful programs. One is led to ask, Are programs successful if they demonstrate that they can be useful, but are never adopted after the demonstration? When is a program adopted? How much "fidelity" to the original is required? Dissemination of innovation becomes a domain of practice and research in the best traditions of community psychology's emphasis on action-oriented field research.

CHAPTER 13

Contextual Influences in Mental Health Consultation

Toward an Ecological Perspective on Radiating Change

EDISON J. TRICKETT, CHARLES BARONE, AND RODERICK WATTS

The origins of mental health consultation as a distinctive profession date back to the 1890s when Lightner Witmer's Philadelphia clinic began involving teachers and family members in the intervention processes of children and adolescents (see Levine & Levine, 1970). Throughout the following 60 years, consultation had a somewhat checkered history in terms of emphasis, and did not evolve a coherent conceptual framework until the writing of Caplan (1959, 1970). However, over the past quarter of a century, consultation has become an integral part of the mental health professions. Consultants report working in a wide range of settings around a variety of problems. Different models of consultation are evolving, research is becoming more sophisticated, and the ethical responsibility of the consultant is receiving increased attention (Dougherty, 1995; Grady, Gibson, & Trickett, 1981; Levin, Trickett, & Hess, 1990; Mannino, Trickett, Shore, Kidder, & Levin, 1986; Trickett, 1993).

This resurgence of interest in consultation was shaped by the social concerns of the 1960s, and reflected two issues of enduring importance to community psychology: (1) increasing local resources by providing indirect, rather than direct, service to clients, and (2) making a systemic difference. Two fundamental assumptions guided these emphases and goals. One was that many individuals other than mental health professionals could serve as potent resources for the psychological development of individuals. The second assumption was that

EDISON J. TRICKETT • Department of Psychology, University of Maryland, College Park, Maryland 20742. CHARLES BARONE • 3003 Van Ness Street, N.W., #W1129, Washington, D.C. 20008. RODERICK WATTS • Department of Psychology, De Paul University, Chicago, Illinois 60614.

Handbook of Community Psychology, edited by Julian Rappaport and Edward Seidman. Kluwer Academic / Plenum Publishers, New York, 2000.

consultation could be structured in such a way that its impact would radiate into the social system, thus creating systemic change.

The assumption that many individuals not in formal mental health roles can have a positive mental health impact has been amply vindicated over time. Not only did this assumption help sustain the paraprofessional movement (see Pearl & Riessman, 1965), but the domain of mental health consultation has broadened over the past 25 years. Consultants now work in an array of public and private settings, and with a diverse population of consultees, including citizens, teachers, bartenders, and lawyers involved in divorce mediation (see Dougherty, 1995; Kidder, Tinker, Mannino, & Trickett, 1986). For numerous reasons and in a variety of ways, indigenous individuals are defined as resources in the consultation process (Crocker, 1996).

The assumption that consultation could serve to radiate change in social settings has proved far more complex and difficult to document. In principle, change could be radiated through two distinct, though potentially related, processes: (1) increasing the effective behavior of individual consultees across settings and over time, and (2) demonstrating the systemic impact of the consultation over time. With respect to the first, consultation could be said to radiate change if the consultee generalized learning around a specific problem or issue to future situations. With respect to the second, the consultation would have been seen as radiating change if, as a consequence, new organizational policies were implemented, new structures and/or processes created, or future organizational issues were more effectively anticipated and handled. Empirical evidence is scant and, at best, mixed on the radiating potential of mental health consultation (see Dougherty, 1995; Schmuck & Miles, 1971; Mannino & Shore, 1975). However, the goal of consultation as a means for creating systemic impact remains a central legacy for community psychology. The purpose of the present chapter is to present a community psychology paradigm explicitly focused on this goal.

COMMUNITY PSYCHOLOGY AND MENTAL HEALTH CONSULTATION: RATIONALE FOR AN ECOLOGICAL PERSPECTIVE

As mental health consultation has evolved in the varying mental health professions, it has ben constrained by the norms, traditions, and paradigms of those professions (Kelly, 1986). While these perspectives have indeed broadened the role definitions and professional activities of psychologists, psychiatrists, psychiatric nurses, and social workers, they have not tended to focus on the opportunities for systemic impact inherent in the consultation role. Community psychology, whose "official" origins coincided with the renewed interest in consultation and whose political roots are similar, can contribute to the field by providing a distinctive framework for highlighting the two goals already mentioned: (1) the importance of viewing consultation as an opportunity to identify, nurture, and develop indigenous resources in the host environment, and (2) the importance of constructing consultation to increase its systemic impact. Both speak to the importance of attending to the "community" of community psychology.

While different perspectives within community psychology are of relevance to creating systemic impact through consultation, the focus of the present chapter is the ecological metaphor first articulated by Kelly, and on which he and his colleagues later elaborated (Kelly, 1968, 1971, 1979, 1986; Mills & Kelly, 1972; Trickett, Kelly & Todd, 1972; Trickett, Kelly, & Vincent, 1985; Trickett, 1984, 1986; Trickett & Birman, 1989; Trickett & Mitchell, 1992). The overarching thesis is that mental health consultation informed by community psychology begins with an appreciation of the ecology of communities and/or settings where the consultation occurs. In short, if consultation is to serve the goal of systemic impact, it must be grounded in an understanding of what the system is like. The ecological metaphor provides one such roadmap.

In addition to providing a heuristic for understanding the social context of the consultation, the ecological metaphor also involves assumptions about the general goals of consultation and about individuals. With respect to goals, emphasis is placed on conserving and increasing the indigenous resources for current and future problem-solving and community development. Thus, strengthening the local setting or community becomes the framework within which information is gathered and interventions are developed. Further, on an individual level, the sociocultural embeddedness of individuals receives explicit attention in how the consultation is conceptualized and implemented. One important aspect of this perspective is an emphasis on the positive value of cultural diversity (Trickett, Watts, & Birman, 1994). This emphasis affirms that social resources and opportunities are not randomly distributed across race, class, ethnicity, and gender, and that one's place in the social order—both as consultant and consultee—shapes one's perception of the issues in the consultation. Thus consultants, in particular, need to attend to how their sociocultural background has shaped their values and consultation goals. The ecological metaphor is thus intended to focus on the nature of social settings, the contextual embeddedness of individuals, and the goal of resource development in the service of system impact.

OVERVIEW OF THE CHAPTER

The remainder of the chapter is organized as follows. First, a brief overview of the ecological perspective on the goals and processes of mental health consultation is provided. Emphasis is placed on the implications of the perspective for the assessment of social settings and individual behavior. The basic premise is that ecologically based mental health consultation must, of necessity, be primarily concerned with how the social context affects the goals and processes of the consultation. Thus, the first part of the chapter presents the overall ecological perspective and provides a hypothetical example of how differing ecologies present mental health consultants with different kinds of challenges and opportunities to be useful.

The second part of the chapter presents examples from existing consultation literature of how the ecological environment surrounding the particular consultation affects various aspects of the consultative role, consultative processes, and the fate of interventions. Three different levels of the ecological environment (Bronfenbrenner, 1979) will be used for illustrative purposes. First is the influence that larger community norms, processes, and structures can have on consultation in a local setting. Here, case reports involving consultation in urban and rural areas will be described. Next is the impact of the ecology of the particular setting hosting the consultation on the consultation itself. The organizational structure, ideology, and organizational climate represent different kinds of influences here. Finally, a perspective on individuals emphasizing cultural diversity and, more generally, the sociocultural embeddedness of individuals, is presented. Here, issues of race, gender, and cultural differences between consultant and members of the host environment are highlighted as aspects of the ecology surrounding the consultation.

These three different aspects of the ecological environment all impact on the way the consultation is conceived and executed. Further, they represent some of the kinds of factors that influence the ability of the consultation to create systemic impact. They correspond roughly to the kinds of linkages postulated by O'Neill and Trickett (1983) to be useful in understanding mental health consultation more broadly; linkages of the host organization to the broader community, linkage among component parts of the host organization itself, and linkages between the consultant and various individuals and groups in the host organization.

An Ecological Metaphor for Mental Health Consultation

The development of an ecological approach to mental health consultation is more fully presented elsewhere and can only be outlined here (see Kelly, 1986; Trickett et al., 1985; O'Neill & Trickett, 1983; Trickett, 1986; Trickett & Birman, 1989). Rather than serving as a specific theory, the ecological approach described herein is best seen as a metaphor, a heuristic that alerts the consultant to look for certain kinds of data while developing, implementing, and evaluating consultative interventions. It is guided by the spirit of the positive development of the setting or community where the consultation occurs. Hence, its explicit and ultimate goal is linked to systemic impact.

No monolithic conception of the community is intended. Indeed, there may be circumstances in which the goal for one group in the community or setting may not be viewed as in the interest of the community as a whole. Still, within the ecological metaphor, the image of community development remains foremost as a way of organizing one's commitments, making strategic decisions, and assessing impact. Thus, understanding the local ecology becomes *the* critical diagnostic task for the consultant, since it surrounds any particular issue of concern to the locale.

The processes underlying an ecological approach to consultation flow from the goal of community development through enhancing local resources. The superordinate goal is to develop a collaborative and empowering relationship with the host environment, under the assumption that local empowerment facilitates the potential for community development and reinforces the notion of community control for choice and decision-making. Several more specific process goals are suggested by this general stance.

First is the task of structuring the consultation around an assessment of the indigenous resources in the setting and creating "the conditions for members to identify and acknowledge these natural resources" (Kelly, 1986, p. 6). This implies the importance of "getting to know the setting" as well as "getting to know the problem" around which consultation was requested. Thus, active and sustained inquiry across various groups in the setting promotes an understanding of how individuals and social structures may be resources for the intervention.

Second is the importance of developing processes to monitor both the intended and unanticipated consequences of the intervention. This is based on the belief that interventions designed to create systemic impact will also yield unanticipated consequences. While these consequences may be either desirable or undesirable, knowledge of how the intervention is radiating is a critical component of the intervention. The consultant who cares about systemic impact expresses that commitment through creating feedback mechanisms for assessing its multiple effects.

A third process emphasizes the evolutionary nature of the consultant's role. Here, priority is placed on developing ongoing collaborative processes for defining and redefining consultative strategies and goals over time. This implies that as the relationship between consultant and setting evolves and the setting becomes more comprehensible to the consultant, both the process and goals of the consultation may be revised. This may be in response to new knowledge about the setting, the recent availability of resources relevant to the defined problem, or the surfacing of latent dynamics that threaten to undermine the work. Processes might include regularized meetings with key system personnel or the creation of an internal review board to assess the implications of information developed by the intervention for future work.

The kinds of processes described above are intended to (1) serve as the goal of consultation as a collaborative and empowering activity, and (2) enhance the opportunities for the consultant to understand the local ecology of the consultation. Commitment to the development of such processes suggests that ecologically based mental health consultation requires, in the words of Kelly (1986), "a flexible, improvisational process" (p. 30). Responsibility to the local setting means a willingness to revise a favored technology to fit local circumstances or, indeed, to discard it entirely. It suggests the possibility that the specific role of the consultant may shift over time, or that differing roles may be adopted for differing segments of the community.

The intended result of these processes and consultative style is to develop an intervention that is integrated into the host environment in a way that becomes a resource for the setting. Processes for accountability and opportunity for sustained interaction between consultant and setting increase the potential for collaboration, mutual influence, trust, and knowledge about what the setting is like. Knowledge about the setting, in turn, provides the consultant with information that can increase the available intervention options. Flexibility of consultative style allows the consultant to take advantage of events as they unfold, to see and make connections among resources in the environment, and to resist the understandable temptation to impose a favored technology where it may be neither welcome nor useful. The superordinate goal of these processes, then, reflects the dual concern with empowering processes and community development goals.

ECOLOGICAL CONCEPTS FOR ASSESSING SOCIAL SETTINGS

Underlying the ecological approach to mental health consultation is the fundamental importance of the social context and the individual's embeddedness within it. Thus, the generative knowledge base for an ecological approach involves the development of perspectives on how social systems and communities may be characterized and how the reciprocal relationship between individuals and social settings can be understood and modified. Approaching this task requires the articulation of concepts about both settings and individuals that can guide research and intervention. Considerable substantive work has accumulated over the past 20 years in ecological/environmental psychology as well as interactional approaches to personality, and a review of the different paradigms underlying that work is beyond the scope of this chapter (e.g., see Magnussen & Endler, 1977; Moos, 1974, 1975, 1979; Barker, 1968; Stokols & Altman, 1987).

The ecological approach underlying the present chapter rests on the elaboration of four ecological processes, drawn by analogy from field biology, which serve as a heuristic for the mental health consultant in the assessment of both social settings and individual behavior. These processes—adaptation, cycling of resources, interdependence, and succession—taken together, help concretize the ecological mindset. Let us briefly describe them and their implications for the assessment of social settings and individuals.

The Adaptation Principle

At the level of the setting or community, the adaptation principle is perhaps the broadest, focusing on the overall nature of the social context and its adaptive requirements for individuals. In Sarason's (1972) terms, every setting has its own culture, its own distinctive way of being. This culture, through its norms, values, opportunity structures, processes, and aspirations, represents the social context within which individuals must cope. Like individuals, settings differ. They develop their own distinctive traditions and ways of celebrating; they embody different kinds of formal and informal means of making decisions and exercising power; they emphasize different goals for the future; and they evolve various ways of assessing and testing outsiders such as consultants. All these, and many other, setting differences contribute to their distinctive cultures that, in turn, influence the adaptive demands facing individuals. The general task for the ecologically oriented consultant is to "tune in" to how the particular setting functions and what combination of influences *in that particular setting* provide the most useful framework for designing and carrying out the intervention. Here, it is assumed that the same manifest problem may result from different sets of influences in contrasting settings. For example, in one school, problems of classroom management may be related to the leadership style of the principal, while in another it may involve conflicting norms and expectations between teachers and parents about appropriate behavior. Thus, the search is for an understanding of the particular ecology that surrounds and defines the consultative problem.

At the level of the individual, the adaptation principle contextualizes individual behavior and sensitizes the consultant to the potential ways that an individual's place in the larger social order influences the individual's perception of, and reaction to, the setting, the consultant, and the intervention. Here, such broader cultural factors as race, gender, social class, and religion all provide contextual markers for the consultant. The contextualization of individuals also reminds the consultant that individuals are constantly adapting to multiple contexts that may require different adaptive styles. Thus, information about the larger life sphere of individuals becomes salient in understanding individual behavior in any particular setting.

A further implication of the adaptation principle involves how the consultative intervention is assessed. If, for example, one component of the intervention involves change in the behavior of individuals or groups, the adaptation principle suggests the importance of assessing individual outcomes across settings in order to assess the generalizability of behavior across differing ecologies. This not only increases knowledge about how adaptive behavior may be linked to varying social contexts, it also increases the chances of spotting the unintended consequences of well-intentioned efforts.

The Cycling of Resources Principle

The cycling of resources principle represents another filter for the consultant to look through. Here the emphasis is on searching out, activating, or creating the potential and ongoing resources relevant to the problem-solving tasks at hand. Elsewhere (Kelly, 1980; Trickett et al., 1985), people, settings, and events have been nominated as different kinds of resources in the social context. A resource perspective suggests such questions as: What persons in the setting have the energy, talent, and commitment to work on the identified problem? What settings exist or need to be created in the larger organization to bring people together or provide a needed service? What event might be designed (see Vincent, 1987) to galvanize relevant community action? Resources may be easily identifiable or more latent and difficult to spot; they may be related to either formal or informal roles; they may exist in the setting or need to be imported from the outside on a temporary basis to build local resources.

The cycling of resources principle focuses most generally on how various aspects of the social setting can contribute to the improvement of the current situation. Applied to the individual level of analysis, the principle highlights the search for the strength and competencies that individuals bring to the setting. Emphasis is placed on finding those persons with energy, relevant knowledge, and a sensitivity to how the local culture works to become involved in shaping and implementing the intervention. The ecological assertion is that the dominant culture of the setting promotes the visibility of some individual skills and resources, while suppressing others. Thus, in addition to discovering those individuals whose talents are already appreciated in the setting, it is particularly important to search out more marginal members whose strengths are not currently being recognized or valued.

From the perspective of the cycling of resources principle, then, the consultant is alerted to (1) conceptualize the organization or community in terms of its resources of people, settings, and events; (2) assess local norms to understand how they highlight certain kinds of resources and inhibit others; and (3) get to know individuals in the setting in ways that extend beyond obvious job-related skills and role requirements. Because the development of resources in terms of both social structures and individuals remains the central intervention goal, the resource perspective is a critical one for the consultant.

The Interdependence Principle

The interdependence principle focuses on one critical aspect of the larger setting; namely, the way in which component parts of the setting are interconnected. Generally, this principle highlights the systemic nature of organizations and communities and promotes the image of a whole composed of interrelated parts. The connections between different parts of the system may be loose (i.e., change in one aspect of the system may have minimal impact on other aspects) or tight (i.e., change may have pronounced ripple effects in related parts of the setting). Thus, interventions will vary in the scope of their systemic impact. But the mindset for the ecologically oriented consultant is to look for the connections in order to understand the kinds of intended and unintended consequences that interventions inevitably produce.

There are many different ways to map out the kinds of interdependencies relevant to the issues of concern. For example, for schools facing a changing clientele, one issue suggested by the interdependence principle may be the fit between the current curriculum and the skills and aspirations of the changing student body. For an individual moving up the ladder of administrative responsibility it may be the new strain between role demands and his or her connections to individuals who were formerly peers. Interventions intended to have systemic impact must be responsive to such interconnections. Thus, they include such questions as: Who may be affected inadvertently by this intervention? How can I find this out? What can I do about it?

The interdependence principle mandates the same search for connections on the individual level as well. Here, the consultant probes the question of person–environment fit as a way of understanding individual behavior in any particular setting. The individual is seen as a person who is constantly negotiating multiple settings whose norms, roles, and expectations for the individual may vary considerably. For example, a student's school behavior may be more affected by how the student's neighborhood peers define appropriate ways of acting than by school norms about expected behavior (see Trickett, 1984). Thus, to understand school behavior it would be necessary to understand neighborhood norms and their salience for the individual. Such interdependence would, of course, assume heightened importance when the individual comes from a cultural background that differs in norms, values, and preferred coping styles from the dominant culture of the setting involved in the consultation (Trickett & Birman, 1990). Thus, on the individual level of analysis, the interdependence principle directs attention to the multiple contexts individuals must negotiate and the ways in which behavior in any one of those contexts may be connected to the larger ecology of the individual.

The Succession Principle

The succession principle represents the historical/temporal dimension of the setting involved in the consultation. As Kelly (1979) observes, settings go through cycles—of optimism and pessimism over their situation, of quiescence and turbulence, of expansion and retrenchment. They also develop, over time, traditions, ways of doing business, and, most generally, a culture. Both long-standing patterns and more transient cycles affect the nature of the consultative problems and the preferred interventions.

Here, the consultative stance focuses on the evolution of the setting with more particular reference to the history of those issues around which consultation is sought. Such information not only helps clarify how a particular situation became defined as a problem, but how that process reflects organizational history in addition to individual concerns. As such, it embeds individual behavior in organizational history. Attention to organizational history also aids the consultant in developing interventions that are sufficiently congruent with the culture of the setting to be acceptable.

The succession principle does not focus solely on the past, however. It pushes the consultant to seek out the larger vision that will guide the setting into the future. Awareness of these longer-range goals and hopes can, in like manner, inform interventions that serve future goals while simultaneously being responsive to setting history.

On the individual level of analysis, the succession principle focuses on the individual's transaction with the broader culture over time. Here, the emphasis is on those sociocultural influences that have affected the socialization of the individual and that shape his or her hopes, aspirations, and, most generally, world view. Family, community, and cultural contexts of enduring significance are seen as a framework for understanding and interpreting the significance of individual behavior and for assessing individual responses to any proposed intervention. Contextualizing individual history in such a way alerts the consultant to issues of cultural pluralism and social class as being central in, rather than peripheral to, assessing the impact of interventions on individuals. It further pushes community psychology in general to develop constructs and paradigms of intervention that attempt to blend or revise intervention technologies to reflect sociocultural circumstances.

ECOLOGY AND MENTAL HEALTH CONSULTATION: A HYPOTHETICAL EXAMPLE

We have briefly outlined the contours of an ecological perspective on mental health consultation consistent with the origins and commitments of community psychology. At its core is the emphasis on understanding the ecological context hosting the consultation. This context both constrains intervention options and is the ultimate object of intervention. The important implication, however, is that different environments present consultants with different types of challenges as they pursue their goal of systemic impact. Kelly (1974) presents a useful hypothetical example of how three important environmental variables may affect the options facing the consultant. These variables are (1) the level of *trust* accorded the consultant, (2) the level of *power* the setting allows the consultant to exercise, and (3) the level of community *support* for the intervention. Each of these variables depends on the transactions between the consultant and the particular ecology of the setting hosting the consultation.

In describing the different combinations of these variables, Kelly speaks in the language of research but, as specified elsewhere (Kelly, 1987; Trickett et al., 1985), from an ecological perspective both research and intervention roles are in the service of system impact. Two contrasting examples serve to highlight the potential costs and benefits of consultation under differing ecological conditions. The first situation is that in which the consultant is trusted, powerful, and supported by the local setting. Kelly casts this situation as one in which "the community psychologist is alive and well in the land of Oz." He writes: "This is a rare and illusive condition where all resources and influences are present and active on the community psychologist's behalf." While these circumstances may at first glance appear ideal, they have their potential costs as well. Under these conditions, the apparent freedom to influence accompanies a latent challenge; namely, the importance of guarding against complacency. "Where the environment offers no serious challenge to the existing preferred ways of thought or behavior of the consultant, the need to improvise, to innovate, lessens, and the threat of unintentionally supporting the status quo heightens ... comfort is unchallenging" (p. 11).

In contrast, Kelly describes the supportive context where both consultant trust and power are low as "how to be a white elephant and survive." He writes:

> This odd situation probably happens more than we care to think about,... This condition is probably the most tenuous for serious community-based inquiry, and represents the greatest potential for the community psychologist to respond prematurely and unnecessarily to fads in the latest research technology. The community psychologist under this condition can be caught up with trying to "sell" the research process to the community" (p. 13).

Thus, the environmental press under these ecological conditions pushes consultants to prove their expertise rather than, as in the previous example, becoming uncritical supporters of the status quo.

This condition also provides distinctive opportunities, however. Here, the consultant *must* attend to community dynamics as entry is negotiated and efforts at trust building begin. He or she must learn how to relate to varied constituencies to develop the resources and support necessary for the intervention. This necessary process allows the consultant to be of service to more diverse and potentially deviant segments of the setting more readily than might occur in a supportive context with *high* consultant trust and power.

Kelly (1974) outlines the contours of the tasks facing the consultant in each of the other sets of ecological circumstances involving conditions of high and low trust, power, and support. In each, the varying ecologies offer the consultant distinctive opportunities while concurrently posing distinctive problems. The overarching message, however, is that serving the goal of community development means being responsive to local conditions. Because local conditions vary across settings and over time, the consultative tasks themselves vary depending on the specific ecology of the setting hosting the consultation.

We now move from the hypothetical examples outlined by Kelly to real examples from the mental health consultation literature on how ecological influences impact on various aspects of mental health consultation. The intent is illustrative, to highlight some of the many ways that local ecology affects the activities of mental health consultants. The assumption is that attending to the context within which the consultation occurs provides the grist for making a systemic difference. Three areas are highlighted that correspond roughly to the three types of linkages comprised in the framework postulated by O'Neill and Trickett (1983): (1) linkages between the consultant and various individuals and groups in the host organization, (2) interpersonal and systemic dynamics operating with the host organization itself, and (3) linkages of the host organization to the broader community.

THE INDIVIDUAL IN CONTEXT: HUMAN DIVERSITY AS AN ECOLOGICAL INFLUENCE

This first section addresses how an ecological perspective orients the consultant to relationships with individuals and groups in the host organization. In this section, specific attention is paid to issues of human diversity. Here, an ecological perspective on individuals reminds us of the enduring socialization of individuals within the larger culture. It focuses attention on the transactions between individuals and the norms, values, and structures embodied by that larger culture. Most importantly, the ecological perspective highlights the importance of developing substantive knowledge about how culture, one's place in the social order (see Sarason, 1981), and the dominant structures of the larger society interact to affect individual behavior and adaptation. Human diversity, as used here, thus evokes the image of the sociocultural embeddedness of individuals and the ways in which the dominant culture defines and differentially responds to individuals (Trickett et al., 1994).

While the broad intent is to view all individuals within a sociocultural context, for purpose of this discussion, issues of race, gender, and cultural differences will serve as examples of how an ecological emphasis on human diversity can serve as a heuristic for consultation concerned with systemic impact. Gender, race, and cultural differences may be conceived as physical and/or psychological markers possessed by individuals. Some markers, particularly physically apparent ones, are readily identifiable, while others, such as sexual orientation and, in some instances, cultural differences, may be less visible or masked. The ways in which such markers are responded to by others in the broader culture (e.g., consultants, consultees, and the specific settings hosting the consultation) determine their influence on the psychology of individuals and the goals, processes, and outcomes of consultation (Duncan, 1995).

Precisely because the role of the consultant is one of having expertise in how to frame or structure the understanding of problems in a new light, the world view or underlying assumptions of the consultant are central to the consultation itself. The ecological world view involves (1) an appreciation of the various ways that markers shape the perspectives of individuals involved in the consultation, including, of course, the consultant himself or herself and (2) how factors in the setting—roles, norms, and values—interact with such markers to affect the consultation. A further implication of the ecological perspective is that individuals' perspectives of situations derive from multiple, rather than singular, markers. Thus, whites and blacks are also male and female, rich and poor, gay and straight, disabled and able-bodied, urban and rural, native and foreign-born.

The intent is not to define individuals solely or even primarily in terms of such markers. For some, being black, female, or a "good old boy" may characterize a basic sense of identity and a primary filter through which experience is processed; for others it may not. Nor is it to assert that in any particular consultation such markers may be a primary focus for the consultation (Conoley, 1994; Harris, Ingraham, & Lam, 1994). In a consultation involving issues of racial tensions, for example, the race of the consultant can be predicted to be a central dynamic in the consultation process. Where the consultation involves aiding teachers in dealing with issues of classroom differences, race may or may not be salient. The basic ecological thrust, however, is twofold: (1) on the level of the individual, to sensitize the consultant to some of the ways that one's sociocultural identity shapes one's world view, and (2) on the level of the setting where the consultation occurs, to develop an appreciation for how norms, values, and social structures may be experienced differently by individuals and groups of varied sociocultural identities.

HUMAN DIVERSITY AND CONSULTATION: ILLUSTRATIVE EXAMPLES

The literature in mental health consultation provides some, though not many, examples of how some of these sociocultural factors influence the process and outcome of mental health consultation. Three aspects of consultation will be used to provide illustrative examples: (1) consultative imperialism and unintended consequences, (2) intercultural relations and issues of entry, and (3) multicultural linkages between consultant, consultee, and client.

Consultative Imperialism and Unintended Consequences

The most striking illustrations of the importance of an ecological approach to human diversity in consultation involve instances where consultants enter into consultative relationships without considering the fit between their assumptions, belief systems, and modes of operation and those of the host setting. Such instances represent an implicit imperialism in which the consultative strategy is premised on cultural assumptions neither shared nor endorsed by the client. Such disregard for the cultural ecology of a setting may result in the arbitrary application of programs that are at best ineffective, and at worst disruptive or harmful (Aponte & Morrow, 1995).

Berlew and LeClere (1974) offer a frank and candid discussion of problems they encountered in a project to develop socioeconomic and human service resources on the island of Curacao. Here, the authors, who were white, native North Americans, describe their inattention to cultural differences between themselves and island residents:

> As Americans, we never really understood [the culture's] strange combination of the European and African. For example, when we described the existence of "powerful new change technologies" ... we inadvertently created a new basis for competition among groups. In a culture where power needs are exceptionally high, where the word of the expert is revered, and where belief in the occult is still alive, we described a "powerful new technology" and promised them control over it. Our failure to understand and deal with these issues more fully was clearly the weakest aspect of the intervention (p. 51).

Lack of understanding of how cultural factors may affect the processes and outcomes of consultation is by no means limited to consultants who work in countries other than their own. For example, King, Cotler, and Patterson (1973) report on a consultation with an elementary school consisting largely of Mexican-American students in a lower middle-class community near Oxnard, California. A behavior-modification program was chosen to reduce absenteeism among Mexican-American students, given that its rate at the school was twice as high as the rates at predominantly Anglo schools in the same district. The program involved offering prizes to parents and children if students attended school regularly. Students were reinforced on a daily basis with praise, a star next to their names, or two-cent candies. Results indicated the intervention to be generally unsuccessful, in fact, attendance rates actually decreased for experimental groups.

In interpreting their results, the authors concluded that one reason for the intervention's ineffectiveness was a lack of awareness about the Mexican-American students and families they targeted. First, past experience with Anglos had not inspired trust and was hard to overcome simply with relatively trivial reinforcers. Second, such reinforcement in and of itself might pale in importance to other realities of Chicano life. For example, the authors noted in their own initial explanation of the attendance problem that children were often absent due to being enlisted by their parents for child-care and other family responsibilities, including working to provide needed additional family income. Thus, the intervention, which may have proved more effective in other contexts, was poorly fitted to the cultural and socioeconomic realities of the Mexican-Americans it intended to serve.

A third example involves the response of the local school system to the murders of five children, all of them Southeast Asian refugees, by a deranged gunman on the playground of an elementary school in Stockton, California (Gross, 1989). While not a consultation per se, the case is an illustrative example of the potential incongruities between intervention modalities developed in one culture and the specific needs and desires of members of other cultures. The school was ethnically diverse, with a large number of Southeast Asians, especially Cambodian refugees. Signs of trauma were noted among many children. Here, the school was initially prepared to provide primarily crisis intervention and counseling services for children and their families. This seemed to be an appropriate intervention for white families, and service delivery problems here are cast mainly in terms of speed of response and resource availability.

In responding to the needs of the Southeast Asian families, concerns initially focused on whether enough translators could be recruited in order to facilitate psychological counseling. However, it quickly became apparent that the most formidable barriers to working with this group were cultural, rather than language-based. The idea of disclosing feelings of grief, anger, and anxiety was described as "uncomfortable" and "incomprehensible" to the Southeast Asians, who rely on informal networks (e.g., friends, relatives, monks) for support. Furthermore, the religious and cultural traditions of the Southeast Asians, and the Cambodian's particular history following the murderous reign of the Khmer Rouge, influenced the specific nature of their reactions to the deaths. Thus, the Southeast Asians were described as being less demanding than the white families, as well as less expressively angry. Many Cambodian children believed that the ghosts of their dead classmates still inhabited the schoolyard.

As a result, school officials fashioned their helping efforts in a more culturally congruent fashion. The principal of the school, Patricia Busher, was exceptionally responsive; she began by visiting a major housing project where the Cambodians lived, "bowing deeply in respect to the residents," and "promising the safety of their children." Furthermore, "she helped arrange a joint funeral for the children, as the parents requested, and a ceremony to rid the playground of ghosts" (Gross, 1989, p. 26). In their reaction to this tragedy, school officials were forced to attend to the culture of their students and their families in designing effective psychological interventions. This case is especially illustrative of the differential effects programs have across settings and populations, and how the success of any particular intervention is context dependent.

Intercultural Relations and Entry Issues

Entry into systems composed primarily of members of minority cultures may present particularly complex issues for consultants of differing backgrounds and statuses. Certain minority groups, for example, have historically been in conflict with the dominant culture, resulting in indifferent, suspicious, or hostile attitudes toward outsiders intending to "help" or "change" them. Everett, Proctor, and Cartwell (1983) summarize some of their experiences with Native Americans as follows:

> Throughout history, the nature of interventions experienced by American Indians has been that of attempts of various groups to change the customs, practices, and beliefs of the Indian population. As early as the 1600's, various religious groups attempted to persuade Indians to allow their children to be adopted by majority culture families. This purportedly was to enable the children to be reared in a "proper" or "superior" environment with the right attitudes and religious beliefs in order that they might be elevated from their savagery.... The federal government, under policy of Manifest Destiny, has intervened repeatedly, with disastrous results for Indians.... It should thus come as no surprise to find Indians today whose feelings toward mental health service providers range from caution to open hostility (p. 590).

Other cultures undoubtedly have similar issues with outsiders. As white consultants working in an elementary school in a black inner-city community, Gesten and Weissberg (1982) confronted skeptical attitudes on the part of blacks toward their efforts at intervention. The authors report having to address concerns about the use of children as guinea pigs for research, the drain on community resources the intervention might cause, and the level of commitment parents could expect from the consultants over the long haul. Obviously, such issues arise from a long history with the larger culture. They are real concerns resulting from instructive and painful experiences of community members that must be addressed by the consultant if the trust and support necessary for successful interventions is to be developed.

Thus, consultees who are members of minority groups may define entry issues differently than do their white counterparts. For example, Gibbs (1980) posits that in the initial phases of consultation, black consultees attend to the personal qualities of the consultant, as compared to whites who place more emphasis on the consultant's level of expertise and competence. Gibbs reports that in her experience as a black consultant with a white co-worker in a predominantly black elementary school, "White teachers tended to ask questions relating to the theory, methods, and goals of the project, while the Black teachers tended to ask questions or make comments about the motivation of the team and the impact of the project on the welfare of the school pupils" (p. 202). Furthermore, the importance of such issues may vary with time, as Gibbs points out that "Black teachers tended to respond to us in a very personal and non-task oriented way in the initial phase of the consultation, and became task oriented much later in the project; White teachers tended to be very task oriented initially, and developed personal relationships with us much later in the project, if at all" (p. 204).

Obviously, such issues also are important to consider when members of "minority" cultures are in the consultant role and "majority" norms and values predominate among consultees or at the level of the host setting. Frederick, Frettan, and Levin-Frank (1976) highlight this issue in an article entitled "Women Mental Health Consultants—Cutie Pies or Libbers?" that, while sounding dated in its terminology, resonates quite loudly with contemporary concerns regarding relationships between the sexes in the workplace. Here, a group of judges had requested consultation for a case from a local mental health center, which assigned two women. The judge's chamber is likened to a men's club, where the only females accustomed to entering the hall were two clerks who served coffee, delivered snacks, and took dictation. The female consultants encountered condescending and denigrating attitudes on the part of the judges. While the judges showed some inclination to utilize the consultants' expertise, interpersonal interchanges with the judges often left the consultants feeling devalued and disrespected. Thus, a crucial entry task in this setting was the need to establish an atmosphere of professionalism, respect, and collegiality. Eventually, the consultants report they were able to discourage such negative comments and actions, and to establish more appropriate and professional working relationships.

Individual prejudice and the norms and climate of the host setting will determine the specific human diversity issues that are evident early in any particular consultation. Invariably, consultants, consultees, and clients will view each other through the filters of their own backgrounds and statuses. An ecological approach to consultation acknowledges and values human diversity in society, and respects the powerful role of cross-cultural issues in shaping consultative relationships.

Consultation Involving a Variety of Multicultural Linkages

Issues of culture may be particularly salient in highly pluralistic environments where consultants must negotiate relationships with a variety of ethnic groups. Kinzie, Teoh, and Tan (1974) report on a group of psychiatrists who offered their services as consultants to a number of community agencies in Malaysia, which include doctors, clergy, and native healers. While it was considered important to establish relations with a broad range of caregivers, dilemmas arose that prevented successful contact with all groups. For example, in acknowledgment of the importance of native healers to indigenous Malaysians, the consulting team sought to establish contact with these helpers in order to broaden their influences. Not only were the native healers disinterested in collaboration, but the project staff felt it necessary to temper such interaction since it might have been looked upon with disfavor by Malaysian medical specialists who were implicitly skeptical about both native healers *and* psychiatrists. The greatest success for these consultants came in their work with members of a Christian Church counseling center. Here, consultants were involved with a group who shared their beliefs about mental health etiology and intervention, as well as a more general North American and European cultural background.

Yutiao and Kinzie (1975) report on a more successful series of consultations with Filipino boarding-home operators in Hawaii. As a reflection of a culture that values an extended family system and caring for others, Filipinos have assumed an important role in the care of the elderly in Hawaii. While there were cultural issues that were salient in establishing effective consultative relationships with these caregivers (e.g., "the persistence of folk medicine and folk theories of mental disorders in the Philippines"), such issues were compounded by the fact that in Hawaii these caretakers must deal with a particularly diverse population. As described by the authors, the Filipinos defined many of the problems they encountered with their clients along cultural and ethnic lines. For example, Japanese clients were perceived as dependent and passive, and Caucasians as aggressive, outspoken, and independent. Hawaiians, part Hawaiians, and Samoans, on the other hand, were perceived by the operators as more frequently having behavioral and sexual problems. This reportedly resulted in the operators feeling uneasy and angry, given Filipino cultural norms that typically discourage the expression of aggressive and sexual urges.

Here, an ecological approach directed specific attention to the cultural factors operating between consultant and consultee, and consultee and client. This led to an understanding of the Filipino's role in mental health aftercare, their attitudes toward mental health issues, and their interpretation of, and reaction to, the problems of their boarders. The result was the development of an orientation on the part of the boarding-home owners to view the problems of their residents through a mental health perspective, and to contact and utilize outside sources of help more readily. Thus, a cross-cultural approach on the part of the consultant is perceived as having the potential to create a rippling effect in the understanding between the consultee and others from diverse backgrounds.

The following two sections outline ecological influences operating at two broader levels: larger community influences as represented by rural–urban differences, and local setting effects, which both reflect larger community embeddedness and contribute distinctive variance to the consultation process. Both of these were selected to stress the importance of contextual factors in carrying out a consultative intervention.

LOCAL ECOLOGY AS A CONTEXTUAL INFLUENCE ON MENTAL HEALTH CONSULTATION

While individual differences along gender, ethnic, racial, and other lines provide one means for understanding the ecological context of consultative relationships, a second level of focus is on the aspects of the settings themselves that affect the processes, goals, and outcomes of consultation. Consultants concerned with systemic impact need to develop knowledge about the structure and dynamics of the organizations in which their work is conducted. Setting differences in structure and "climate" can and do affect interventions (Thomas, Gatz, & Luczak, 1997).

Open-system theory is one model that has been adopted to understand consultative impact at the systems level (se Miller, 1978; Katz & Kahn, 1978; Rice, 1969; Alderfer, 1976). One particularly useful concept from this broader literature is that of system boundaries. Alderfer (1981), as summarized in Smith and Corse (1986), describes the characteristics of organizations at each pole of this concept:

> Overbounded systems tend to have clear goals; be monolithic in their authority relations; be precise, detailed, and restrictive in role definitions, and be constrained and blocked in human energy. On the other hand, underbounded systems tend to have unclear goals, have multiple and competing authority structures, be imprecise and have inadequate connections among roles, and find difficulty in harnessing human energy (p. 255).

These differing degrees of system boundedness carry important differential implications for the task facing consultants. The authors continue:

> In systems that are well-organized, entry at one point, especially if the level has appropriate authority, may facilitate access to the whole system. In underorganized systems, or ones where portions are highly polarized, it may be necessary to use multiple entry strategies (p. 256).

There are a variety of other aspects of local settings that may affect the processes and goals of mental health consultation. For example, settings may be seen as having different kinds of "life cycles" (see Perkins, Nieva, & Ladler, 1982). Sarason (1972), for example, discusses how newly created settings inevitably reach a point where they must confront the unanticipated consequences and contradictions of their fundamental guiding assumptions. Presumably, both the goals of the consultation and the nature of the organizational issues relevant to the consultation may differ, depending on the current organizational phase of the setting. Kelly et al. (Chapter 7, this volume) highlight how differentiations in two generic aspects of settings—their structural components and their processes for accomplishing tasks—impact on the nature of potential interventions. And Moos (1974, 1975, 1979) has shown how the social climate of settings, in addition to their boundary relationships, structure, and processes, can vary. Moos' Social Climate Scales, developed to measure the social ecology of a wide variety of settings, have been used both to assess and change settings (see Pierce, Trickett, & Moos, 1972, for a prototypical example of this methodology).

The preceding represent some of the many potential aspects of the structure and climate of local settings that may influence mental health consultation designed to create systemic impact. Taken together, they suggest that local factors in the setting hosting the consultation affect the activities and goals of the consultants. With the notable exception of the organizational development literature in industrial/organizational psychology (see Argyris, 1970), however, most existing mental health consultation literature does not systematically employ such concepts, except as *post hoc* explanations of what happened in the consultation (see, however, Kelly & Hess, 1997). The following reports from the consultation literature do, however, clarify the fundamental assertion that local ecology influences mental health consultation.

ILLUSTRATIVE EXAMPLES OF THE IMPACT OF LOCAL ECOLOGY

For illustrative purposes, four different kinds of local influences are discussed: (1) local ecology and program implementation, (2) local ecology and the creation of unanticipated consequences, (3) within-setting group differences as an aspect of local ecology, and (4) organizational ideology as an ecological factor. Each of these areas adds richness to the ecological mindset underlying the present chapter.

Local Ecology and Program Implementation

Several reports in the literature suggest that consultants attempting to implement structured programs find that local ecology affects how such programs are implemented. Thus, any particular program or curriculum may be modified, adapted, and refined to meet the needs of each specific setting in which it is implemented. In many instances, these local impacts can be seen as representing positive adaptation on the part of the local setting.

For example, Cowen and his colleagues (Cowen, Spinell, Wright, & Weissberg, 1983; Cowen, Davidson, & Gesten, 1980) have evaluated the implementation of the Primary Mental Health Project, an early screening and instructional program for children, in which informal helpers provide direct service to at-risk children. Over time, the project was implemented in a wide variety of geographical areas with diverse racial and socioeconomic populations. In spite of extensive and standardized training by program staff, implementation varied widely from setting to setting across a number of program components. In a *post hoc* assessment of these trends in implementation, the authors stress the positive force of local ecology in shaping program goals and methods. They viewed such local adaptations as generally favorable outcomes that aptly reflected "the different pond ecologies (i.e., needs, perceived problems, resources, interests, and prior experiences of program personnel) of host systems" (Cowen et al., 1983, p. 125).

Other reports, however, focus on how local ecology may undermine, rather than refine or augment, program implementation. For example, Gutkin, Clark, and Ajchenbaum (1985) discuss the effect of organizational climate on parallel interventions in a pair of ecologically dissimilar schools. In this study, two doctoral students each served as a liaison from the central project to one of two primary schools. Each consultant was considered by supervisors and independent observers to be of equal ability, and each had similarly high satisfaction ratings from school staff. The authors emphasize that the key significance of the study was the marked differences in the processes and outcomes of the consultation in the two schools, consistent with their respective local ecologies.

In "School A," teachers were split along ideological lines; half were described as being older, more traditional, and having been at the school for a long period of time; the other half were portrayed as younger and more "progressive." The principal was described by staff as authoritarian, and they reported many conflicts with him. The organizational climate of School A is described by the authors as generally rigid, distant, and conflictive. "School B" had been designed to function using open-classroom and team-teaching concepts. It was described as having a collaborative problem-solving approach to issues, as exemplified in its use of a weekly staff meeting, devoted to discussing various school problems. The principal had handpicked his staff and was considered flexible, open, and interactive.

Not surprisingly, the consultant to School A met with a number of frustrating "obstacles" in attempting to develop the desired consultative relationship. In this authoritarian and conflict-prone climate, there was a virtually unshakable expectation for direct service to children, rather than indirect service to teachers. staff concerns focused more on specific "gripes" than on more general issues of school climate and leadership. The attitude towards the consultant often was characterized by either disinterest or suspicion that indirect service might signal weakness on the part of the teacher requesting it. Consistent with the prevailing level of mistrust and perceived need to protect themselves from additional scrutiny, the school staff associated the consultation with the authoritarian policies and procedures of the school principal.

In School B, however, staff were reported as comfortable with the idea of consultation, enthusiastic about indirect service delivery, and able to focus on child-related organizational issues. Little time was spent on interstaff difficulties, and there was greater emphasis on the consultative, rather than the direct-service, skills of the consultant. In general, the project was considered "successful" at each school, at least based on teacher ratings of the consultants' effectiveness. However, the two consultants faced highly different tasks, demands, and challenges as a function of each school's structure and social climate, and as such the authors attribute successes they were able to obtain to their consultant's ecological sensitivity, adaptability, and flexibility.

Local Ecology and the Creation of Unintended Consequences: Coupling with the Host Environment

As previously discussed, mental health consultation intended to create systemic impact must be concerned with the unintended consequences of its well-intentioned efforts. If the intervention is to "take hold" in the setting and be seen as a resource, then its multiple consequences need to be monitored. In the section above we have seen that the same program implemented in different settings may result in quite different processes and outcomes. Presumably, we may infer that these differences in program implementation may result in different unanticipated consequences as well. How consultative interventions are coupled with the host environment thus becomes a key topic in ecologically oriented consultation, for it requires the consultant to attend both to the nature of the local ecology and how to design an intervention that increases the likelihood of positive consequences.

A particularly compelling example of the ecological significance of this coupling process is provided by Ransen (1981). This study was an attempt to explain the short-term and long-term results of two conceptually similar intervention programs in institutions involved in residential care for the aged (Langer & Rodin, 1976; Schulz, 1976). Both programs sought to increase the amount of personal control residents perceived as having over their institutional lives, and both were successful in improving the physiological and psychological health of residents based on short-term evaluations. However, long-term effects differed markedly in the two programs. One study found positive effects on happiness, social interaction, and mortality rate for the experimental group in comparison to the control group at an 18-month follow-up. Results of the other study show a marked contrast: follow-up at 24, 30, and 42 months found the experimental group to be lower on indices of physiological and psychological health and higher on rates of mortality.

In an attempt to explain these discrepant findings, Ransen performed an analysis of differences in how the programs were structured in the two settings. Several differences emerged, including whether those implementing the intervention were insiders (e.g., staff vs. outside college students), the extent to which the ongoing social networks of residents were disrupted or kept intact, and whether a broad or narrow range of expectancies about institutional life were targeted. The tentative conclusion drawn from these analyses of long-term results was that the differential outcomes were a function of the ways in which programs were coupled with the two settings. In essence, the more congruent and embedded in the local ecology the program was, the greater its positive long-range impact. Programs take on new meanings and implications depending on how they are implemented. The ways in which such interventions can be implemented depends on the local ecology and the consultant's assessment of how to best utilize and enhance local resources as an intervention goal.

Within-Setting Group Differences as an Aspect of Local Ecology

In addition to focusing on differences between settings that impact on mental health consultation, any institution may also present the consultant with a variety of subgroups that differ among themselves in needs, resources, patterns of interaction, and orientation to consultation. Thus, assessment of the various subgroups in any particular setting represents an important component in the design of appropriate interventions.

Gabinet and Friedson (1981) describe how the provision of psychiatric case consultation differed in important ways across wards (e.g., orthopedics, obstetrics) in a large metropolitan hospital. Key issues here centered on responding to the different types of client populations, staff role relationships, hierarchical power structures, and attitudes toward psychiatry on each ward. For example, in orthopedics, where surgeons spend a minimal amount of time with patients on a daily basis and nurses are most affected by the effects of chronic pain on patients, there is a norm that supports nurse contact with the psychiatric consultant. This is not true on medical wards, where medical residents spend a lot of time on the ward and become deeply involved in total care; here, nurse contact with the consultant might be seen as an inappropriate overstepping of role boundaries. Even in cases where nurses are the first to be cognizant of a psychiatric problem, setting norms dictate an informal route to the consultant through the attending physician. In this setting, direct contact with nurses by the consultant might disrupt his or her relationship with the physician, to the detriment of the patient. Such concerns would not be relevant in orthopedics, where concern with overall functioning of the setting and the success of each consultation dictates attention to the effects of the consultant's action on the intraorganizational dynamics and role interdependence of various groups.

Ideology as a Dimension of Local Ecology

As consultants have expanded their activities, the types of organizations with which they interact have become increasingly diverse. While all organizations have cultures that impact on the consultation, some are more coherently founded on particular ideologies than are others. In such cases, the predominant ideology is a major factor in determining the structures, norms, policies, and attitudes of the setting, which in turn influence the nature of the consultant's entry into the setting and the quality of the ongoing consultative process.

In her work in an alternative public high school, Levy-Warren (1976) found that the particular ideology and organizational structure of the school were critical determinants of the consultation experience. The school was founded on a belief in the value of empowerment for teachers, students, and parents in the running of the school. During its early years, this ethic was translated into a kind of "radical individualism," where teachers and, indeed, students were granted considerable autonomy in how they structured their respective roles. One correlate of this was that there existed no real central authority with whom to negotiate issues of entry and to develop a consultative contract. No individual in the school could speak on behalf of the other teachers. Further, as is often the case in the early years of alternative settings, there existed a general suspicion of outsiders, which heightened the need for the consultant to visibly identify with the counter-cultural values underlying the creation of the school.

While all consultants must, over time, be able to generate a certain degree of trust in their relationship with the consultative setting, the strong ideological nature of this alternative school pushed the consultant to "show her colors" around values as a prelude to being willing to engage her skills as a consultant. Thus, the predominant ideology of the school, as reflected in its local ecology, influenced both the process and content of the consultation around different issues than are generally reported in the broader consultation literature (see Alpert, 1987; Gallessich, 1982).

Reinharz (1983) describes a consultation with a collective bakery in Massachusetts in which understanding ideological issues also played an important role in successful entry. For example, adaptation of the consultant to the local norms of this setting included forgoing a formal contract, as well as dressing informally for meetings. However, the most challenging task for the consultant was to mediate between the values of the workers as embodied in the norms and policies of the collective, and the organization's need to survive as a viable and profitable business. Here, the organization's commitment to certain values and methods of business conduct both defined its uniqueness and raised problems that the consultant was enlisted to address.

For example, while respect for the values of fairness, cooperation, and tolerance were important to the workers, they were often in direct conflict with the needs of the business to operate efficiently and manage costs. The collective had great difficulty developing a consensus around issues such as how to sanction workers or how to hold others in the community who used their facilities accountable for wear and damage. Sensitivity to the importance of setting ideology enabled the consultant to make such issues explicit to the consultees and to establish a framework for discussion in which conflicting needs and goals could be reconciled, while honoring their respective importance. In operating from a framework that emphasized the importance of attending to and respecting the local culture, and assisting the system in adapting to meet its own self-defined goals, the authors was able to optimize the prospects for a successful collaboration.

In these and other ways, the local ecology of a setting exerts its own influence over how consultation proceeds, regardless of whether or not its manifest goal involves systemic impact. Hence, consultation in general, but particularly consultants concerned with such impact, need a framework for understanding the settings in which they work.

COMMUNITY INFLUENCES ON MENTAL HEALTH CONSULTATION

An ecological perspective on mental health consultation also directs attention to the ways in which discrete settings hosting the consultation are themselves embedded in larger ecologies. These ecologies can influence consultative strategies and options in a variety of ways. For example, community norms may shape the kinds of interventions deemed thinkable, desirable, or permissible by the local setting and its members. Community size and heterogeneity may influence the network of ties between the setting hosting the consultation and other settings whose missions may be relevant to the consultative problem.

This section presents a third and final set of case examples, involving instances in which consultation has been affected by structures and processes operating at the level of the larger community. Such reports are somewhat infrequent, as research on mental health consultation has not paid consistent attention to how consultation in any particular setting is affected by the larger community in which it is embedded. Similarly, there are few conceptual frameworks for guiding the study of these processes.

One useful conceptual example for understanding the influence of communities on mental health consultation has been offered by Warren and Warren (1977). In their work on neighborhoods, they characterized different areas as being high or low on three dimensions of community structure and dynamics: interaction (the amount of contact between neighbors), identity (the extent to which community members perceive themselves as sharing common interests and values), and linkages (the number and quality of communication lines with other groups in the wider community). Any particular neighborhood can thus be characterized according to its profile across these three dimensions.

Attention to these qualities is considered useful in informing work with settings attempting to offer local mental health services. Imagine how certain cases requiring mental health intervention, such as child abuse, would need to be handled differently in neighborhoods varying along these dimensions. For example, a neighborhood high on identity and interaction and low on linkages is described by Warren and Warren as "parochial"; it is characterized as having a strongly homogenous character and as being assertive of its independence from the larger community. This neighborhood might attempt to draw largely on its own resources to prevent instances of child abuse and to intervene on its own terms with families who are suspected of such abuse. Contact with outside agents would tend to be avoided. In contrast, a neighborhood low on identity, interaction, and linkages is dubbed as "anomic," and is described as highly atomized and isolated. Such a neighborhood might be expected to show a lack of response to such problems. Treatment systems operating in this context would need to proceed quite carefully in maintaining, monitoring, and terminating such cases, given the dearth of indigenous community resources and absence of linkages to outside agencies.

COMMUNITY-LEVEL INFLUENCES ON MENTAL HEALTH CONSULTATION: RURAL–URBAN DISTINCTIONS

This section will provide several examples in which characteristics of the larger community or macrolevel culture impact on mental health consultation in discrete settings. Most of these examples are drawn from case studies of consultations conducted in rural areas. These are clear and illustrative examples of the role of community-level processes, such as, using one broad distinction, that between rural areas and their urban counterparts. It should be noted that while we are highlighting this variable, no monolithic conception of rural areas is implied and no single consultative approach to work in such areas is advocated. However, certain trends have been noted in the literature on rural consultation that show how the specific goals and processes of consultation can be shaped and constrained by environmental realities (Brogden & Cara, 1995; Field, Allness, & Knoedler, 1980; Harley, Rice, & Dean, 1996). Three areas will serve as examples for the many kinds of potential community influences on the consultant role: (1) the nature and definition of resources, (2) the visibility of the consultant, and (3) the density of the community network.

The Nature of Community Resources

One commonality among rural settings that sets them apart from some more densely populated areas is the extent to which they lack a variety of specialized resources. Like Barker's conception of small schools as contrasted with large ones (Barker & Gump, 1964), rural communities are likely to include fewer formalized roles and use a wider range of informal skills and knowledge of local citizens to accomplish necessary tasks. Further, rural areas often have a narrower base of economic resources, have populations with lower levels of formal education, and lack sufficient numbers of medical and mental health professionals (Dubois, Nugent, & Broder, 1991). Such conditions, though clearly variable from place to place, may offer significant and powerful informal resources to the consultant, as well as provide a number of formidable obstacles. However, consultative models developed for work in contexts with more explicitly defined and formalized resources do not necessarily guide the consultant to value and utilize other types of resources that may be present, and do not offer strategies for redefining consultation in the context of local realties.

For example, Laosa, Burstein, and Martin (1976) report on an effort they undertook to develop, through the training of paraprofessionals, mental health services for Chicanos in a rural area of southern Texas. The consultants here employed what they describe as a "classical 'Caplanian' conceptualization" of consultation, which would lead them from clinically oriented work to indirect service. Specifically, the authors intended to use direct service as a good faith effort that would provide a foundation for case-centered consultation. However, to the disappointment of the authors, the intended shift never occurred. While a number of other factors played a role in shaping their ongoing efforts, the authors concluded that the lack of direct service resources (e.g., psychotherapeutic, scholastic, and managerial) in the immediate community required them to redefine their role in ways they had not anticipated.

Curry, Anderson, and Munn (1980) report a similar experience in their consultation with child-development centers serving mentally retarded youngsters in rural north-central North Carolina. Mazer (1976), in recounting his experiences as a practicing psychiatrist in Martha's Vineyard, notes that even in this ostensibly more circumscribed role, he was required to use a broader and more flexible range of psychiatric skills than he would have in a metropolitan or suburban area. He attributes this to the absence in this context of a wide array of more specialized resources that would be present in larger cities, and emphasizes that "in a small community [the consultant] represents a public resource and must be prepared to respond to the manifold problems present" (Mazer, 1976, p. 226). Thus, the point there is not that consultation in all rural areas will require the consultant to perform direct services, but rather that the potential lack of manifest and specialized resources in such settings may demand a more flexible and diverse repertoire of consultant skills. While the operational goal remains the creation of resources, attention to ecological realities provides a cue to an appropriate starting point.

The Visibility of the Consultant

While the nature and availability of resources in rural areas requires the consultant to employ a more flexible repertoire of skills in the service of community development, the ecology of rural life may also force the consultant to develop different types of consultative relationships. One key issue is that, given their small size and informal communication networks, rural communities are quite efficient in developing a public portrait of the mental health professional. Here, the consultant is well advised to be aware of how his or her style, values, and demeanor meet with local norms (Kahn, 1970). For example, Berry and Davis (1978) note that:

> There is an effective word of mouth network among rural citizenry that reports all the activities of the mental health worker.... Rural mental health professionals must be concerned about their image in the community because local people will judge them on the basis of (personal factors) and this judgment will color their response to the professional's service (p. 677).

The issue has direct implications for the entry of the consultant into the host setting, and for a successful integration into local networks. For example, given the consultants visibility, people in rural areas may place more importance initially on the personal qualities of the consultant. Thus, consultants prone to selling themselves on their professional qualifications and the potential worth of their program may be frustrated in trying to gain entry and build trust with consultees. Some authors indicate that a more adaptive approach might be to focus on interpersonal interactions, especially during the preliminary stages of the consultation. Jeffrey and Reeve (1978) assert that "during the early stages ... a joint fishing trip with other agency workers is likely to be more productive than displays of imaginative programming or esoteric prowess" (p. 57).

Again, attention to local climate moves the consultant to depart from models developed in other types of contexts that rely on technical expertise and professional qualifications to establish credibility and develop collaborative working relationships. In the communities described above, cultural norms for personal interactions and the development of professional relationships orient the consultant to adopt a more personally-oriented entry strategy and to be sensitive to community concerns regarding trust and acceptance.

Density of Community Networks

In addition to special resource needs and social norm demands, a third aspect of rural settings that informs the process of consultation is the tight interconnection between various community groups and factions. The principle of interdependence is especially salient here, as well as the impact of local history in determining roles and relationships. In such densely bound communities, the mere presence of a consultant may create rippling effects across various segments of the population. For instance, natural or informal helping networks may be threatened by the introduction of new mental health professionals and their services into their community (Jeffrey & Reeve, 1978). Several authors have noted the salience of informal helpers in rural areas and the importance of attending to and preserving such ties to minimize disruption of the community, to reduce the sense of intrusion on the part of natural helpers, and to facilitate the implementation of any particular program (Bergstrom, Hill, & Miller, 1984; Field et al., 1980).

Other types of connections, such as those along political or economic lines, may also be important. These linkages, some of which may be readily apparent, and others that may surface only after a considerable period of time, possess the potential to facilitate and/or inhibit the consultative process. While such dynamics are not unique to rural areas, the relatively closed nature of such systems and the longstanding awareness of historical relationships and political dynamics lend an intensity to such interactions that is less likely to be "cooled out" than may be possible in more diffuse networks.

Thus, Laosa et al. (1976), in the study previously cited, report that, although they enjoyed good rapport with the consultees, relationships between these individuals, who were Chicanos, and economic officials, who were white, were strained due to the former's recent rise to dominance in local government. While Chicanos were described as distrustful and cynical about the business leaders' interest in providing economic resources, the latter group is characterized as having become isolated following its electoral defeat and reluctant to become involved. As a result, the base of community participation was narrowed and the efforts of the program to achieve self-sufficiency were compromised. Here community-level political dynamics, while outside the immediate context of the consultant/consultee relationship, presented potent forces that impacted and shaped the nature of the consultative process.

Berlew and LeClere (1974) were also caught in the tensions between various community factions on the Caribbean island of Curacao. These tensions determined the course of consultation. Labor unrest had resulted in striking and rioting, and the island's Chamber of Commerce approached the consultants to aid in promoting grass-roots economic development by encouraging Antilleans (island residents) to initiate business activity. However, input from various community leaders, initially encouraged by the Chamber, resulted in an expansion of the project's goals to include education and social benefits, as well as business-oriented efforts. While this promoted a personal investment in the project by community leaders, and resulted in goals that presumably reflected community needs, one consequence was the withdrawal of moral and economic support by the Chamber. The authors conclude that their decision to redefine their efforts resulted in a realignment of loyalties along the political lines operating within the broader culture of the island, thus enhancing the program's immediate relevance to the local community, but ultimately threatening its base of economic and material support.

Such intergroup dynamics do not, of course, occur only in rural or geographically bound areas. Indeed, in all the examples cited above, we see similarities to many cases that occur in a variety of communities with similar characteristics (i.e., low levels of resources, higher needs for establishing personal trust and acceptance, or the presence of dense and highly charged intergroup conflicts). The critical importance of the above examples is that they guide the consultant to undertake environmental reconnaissance regarding consultant-level dynamics and norms. Taken together, they provide a compelling rationale for the importance of attending to these broader contextual issues because they affect the opportunity for mental health consultation to create systemic impact.

INTERCULTURAL ISSUES IN ADAPTATION TO HIGH SCHOOL: A BRIEF ECOLOGICAL EXAMPLE

While the preceding examples highlight some of the many ways in which issues of social ecology, at varying levels of analysis, may affect consultative success, most were not developed with an ecological perspective in mind. Trickett and Birman (1990) provide an example of a consultative intervention focusing explicitly on an ecological approach to issues of cultural diversity. The setting was a public high school serving 2200 students, 20% of whom were from foreign countries. The first step in the consultation was to develop a collaborative process with the school to outline the dimensions of the problems facing both the foreign-born students and the school itself. Thus, the emphasis was on the interaction between the students and the norms, structures, and policies of the school. Next was the development of a process for gathering data to (1) build an empowering relationship with various groups in the school, (2) develop a multilevel conception of the problems facing foreign-born students, and (3) assess the school in terms of its manifest and latent resources relevant to the education of foreign-born students. This process included building relationships with a variety of formal and informal student and teacher groups, gathering data on various aspects of the school structure and "climate" as perceived by these various groups, and finding out who in the school had ideas and energy to work on issues of relevance to foreign-born students.

On the bases of these various activities, many kinds of information emerged that aided in understanding the contexts in which many students function. For example, many Hispanic students had to support themselves by working long hours after school and on weekends. Some went directly from school to work, arriving home late at night to study. Because of their necessary schedules, they were often tired at school, sometimes dozed in class, and did not have time for homework. In class, because of their difficulty in understanding the English-speaking teacher, they would turn to other Hispanic students to help them understand what the teacher was saying. Teachers, however, viewed this behavior from a quite different perspective. Being unaware of their jobs and schedules, the teachers often interpreted their classroom behavior as not caring about school and preferring to socialize with other Hispanics instead of paying attention in class. In turn, Hispanic students expressed anger at how teachers interpreted their behavior.

Further information at another level of analysis provided additional data of relevance to understanding the school ecology in which these students functioned. For example, this school was experiencing the larger national *Zeitgeist* for excellence and accountability in public education. Teachers were under increasing pressure from the county to produce students who performed well on standardized tests of achievement. Since knowledge of English is a prerequisite for performing well on such tests, and many foreign-born students were deficient in English, teachers viewed themselves as caught between the needs of these students and the externally imposed criteria of accountability. These pressures increased the tendency of teachers to express prejudicial or negative attitudes toward foreign-born students, not necessarily because of personal prejudice, but rather as a reaction to policies that made these students an easy target for system-induced frustrations.

From these and other data came ideas about how to better conceptualize the problems facing foreign-born students and the school. Thus, data on the dynamics of teacher–student interactions provided an alternative to the person-blame attributions teacher made about students. Such data increased the empathy of teachers for the complexity of the situation facing themselves and the foreign-born students they teach. In addition, defining the situation as partly policy-generated helped create energy to intervene at the level of county policy, in addition to attending to classroom issues. An in-service training meeting, designed in collaboration with ESOL teachers (English for Speakers of Other Languages), the principal, and external school-system resources helped consolidate the implications of the findings, validated the collaborative process, and helped identify salient resources in the school for designing future activities. For example, the principal of the school has increased his interest in finding additional school-system resources for aiding foreign-born students, and has supported further research on their experience in the school.

To conclude, an ecological approach to human diversity focuses not only on how multiple cultural identities and accompanying social attitudes are expressed in consultative interventions; it supports the active promotion and acceptance of such diversity as a resource for the development of settings. As stated by Moore, Nagata, and Whatley (1984), such diversity is an ideology that "specifically suggests that cultural groups in a given larger society should be allowed, even encouraged, to retain their unique identity *along with* their membership in the larger social framework" (p. 238; emphasis added). In the spirit of ecology, human diversity represents a contextualization of individual experience in transaction with the norms, attitudes, structures, and power dynamics of the broader culture. This level of ecological influences outlined in previous sections, and further concertizes how the ecological context influences consultation process and outcome.

SUMMARY

One potential contribution of community psychology to mental health consultation lies in its concerns with increasing the systemic impact of the consultant. This emphasizes the *community* of community psychology. Accomplishing this task requires the elaboration of both concepts and knowledge about the nature of the social context where the consultation occurs, and a general set of values to guide the work. Kelly's ecological metaphor has been proposed as one approach to this task. Undergirded by the values of empowerment and human diversity, and propelled by the goal of community development, the ecological metaphor focuses explicit attention on how the consultant can assess the social context in terms of its requirements for adaptation, resources, interdependence among its various components, and history. These aspects of the setting represent the building blocks for consultative interventions whose goal is to conserve and increase the resourcefulness of the setting for current and future problem-solving.

Three areas of the mental health consultation literature were selected as examples of how the ecological context has been shown to influence the activities and goals of consultants. While the vast majority of literature in mental health consultation does not focus on either the goal of community development or the ways in which ecological factors affect consultation, rural/urban factors, factors in the structure and climate of local settings, and the social meanings of race, gender, and culture were nominated as illustrative areas of ecological influence. Mental health consultation, as approached from an ecological perspective, involves the continuing quest to understand how the role of consultant can serve community goals. Knowledge of, and caring about, the social context where consultation occurs are central to this task.

REFERENCES

Agyris, C. (1970). *Intervention theory and methods.* Reading, MA: Addison-Wesley.

Alderfer, C. P. (1979). Change processes in organizations. In M. D. Dunnette (Ed.), *Handbook of industrial and organizational psychology* (pp. 1591–1638). Chicago: Rand-McNally.

Alderfer, C. P. (1981). The methodology of diagnosing group and intergroup relations in organizations. In H. Meltzer & W. R. Nord (Eds.), *Making organizations humane and productive: A handbook for practitioners* (pp. 355–371). New York: Wiley.

Alpert, J. L. (Ed.). (1982). *Psychology consultation in educational settings.* San Francisco: Jossey-Bass.

Aponte, J. F., & Morrow, C. A. (1995). Community approaches with ethnic groups. In J. F. Aponte & R. Y. Rivers (Eds.), *Psychological interventions and cultural diversity* (pp. 128–144). Boston: Allyn & Bacon.

Barker, R. G. (1968). *Ecological psychology.* Stanford, CA: Stanford University Press.

Barker, R. G., & Gump, P. U. (1964). *Big school, small school.* Stanford, CA: Stanford University Press.

Bergstrom, D. A., Hill, E. L., & Miller, L. S. (1984). Training for rural community psychology: A consultation and education practicum. *Journal of Rural Community Psychology, 5,* 19–31.

Berlew, D. E., & LeClere, W. E. (1974). Social intervention in Curacao: A case study. *The Journal of Applied Behavioral Science, 10,* 29–52.

Berry, B., & Davis, A. E. (1978). Community mental health ideology: A problematic model for rural areas. *American Journal of Orthopsychiatry, 48,* 673–679.

Brogden, J., & Cara, W. (1995). Using advanced communications and multimedia applications to provide real life benefits to remote rural areas. *Computers in Human Services, 12,* 141–150.

Bronfenbrenner, U. (1979). *The ecology of human development.* Cambridge, MA: Harvard University Press.

Caplan, G. (1959). *Concepts of mental health consultation: Their application in public health social work.* Washington, D.C.: Social and Rehabilitation Service, Children's Bureau.

Caplan, G. (1970). *The theory and practice of mental health consultation.* New York: Basic Books.

Conoley, J. C. (1994). You say potato, I .... *Journal of Educational and Psychological Consultation, 5,* 143–148.

Cowen, E. L., Davidson, E. R., & Gesten, E. L. (1980). Program dissemination and the modification of delivery practices in school mental health. *Professional Psychology, 11,* 36–47.

Cowen, E. L., Spinell, A., Wright, S., & Weissberg, R. P. (1983). Continuing dissemination of a school-based mental health program. *Professional Psychology: Research and Practice, 14,* 118–127.

Crocker, D. (1996). Innovative models for rural child protection teams. *Child Abuse and Neglect, 20,* 205–211.

Curry, J. F., Anderson, D. R., & Munn, D. E. (1980). A model for psychological consultation to rural development center. *Journal of Rural Community Psychology, 1,* 24–33.

Dougherty, A. M. (1995). *Consultation: Practice and Perspectives in School and Community Settings.* Pacific Grove, CA: Brooks/Cole.

Dubois, J. R., Nugent, K., & Broder, E. (1991). Psychiatric consultation with children in underserviced areas: Lessons from experiences in northern Ontario. *Canadian Journal of Psychiatry, 36,* 456–461.

Duncan, C. F. (1995). Cross-cultural school consultation. In C. L. Courtland (Ed.), *Counseling for diversity: A guide for school counselors and related professionals* (pp. 129–141). Boston, MA: Allyn & Bacon.

Everett, F., Proctor, N., & Cartwell, B. (1983). Providing psychological services to American Indian children and families. *Professional Psychology: Research and Practice, 14,* 588–603.

Field, G., Allness, D., & Knoedler, W. (1980). Application of the training in community living program to rural areas. *Journal of Community Psychology, 8,* 9–15.

Frederick, V., Frettan, N., & Levin-Frank, S. (1976). Women mental health consultants—cutie pies or libbers? *Psychiatric Opinion, 13,* 26–32.

Gabinet, L., & Friedson, W. (1981). The impact of ward dynamics on psychiatric consultation and liaison. *Comprehensive Psychiatry, 22,* 603–611.

Gallessich, J. (1982). *The profession and practice of consultation.* San Francisco: Jossey-Bass.

Gesten, E. L., & Weissberg, R. F. (1982). Setting up and disseminating programs for social problem solving. In J. L. Alpert (Ed.), *Psychological consultation in educational settings* (pp. 208–246). San Francisco: Jossey-Bass.

Gibbs, J. T. (1980). The interpersonal orientation in mental health consultation: Toward a model of ethnic variations in consultation. *Journal of Community Psychology, 8*, 195–207.

Grady, M. A., Gibson, M. J., & Trickett, E. J. (1981). *Mental health consultation: Theory research, and practice 1973–1978*. Washington, D.C.: Department of Health and Human Services, Government Printing Office.

Gutkin, T. B., Clark, J. H., & Ajchenbaum, M. (1985). Impact of organizational variables on the delivery of school-based consultation services: A comparative case study approach. *School Psychology Review, 14*, 230–235.

Harley, D. A., Rice, S., & Dean, G. (1996). Rural rehabilitation: A consortium for administration, coordination, and delivery of services. *Journal of Rehabilitation Administration, 20*, 109–117.

Harris, A. M., Ingraham, C. L., & Lam, M. K. (1994). Teacher expectations for female and male school-based consultants. *Journal of Educational and Psychological Consultation, 5*, 115–142.

Jeffrey, M., & Reeve, R. (1978). Community mental health services in rural areas: Some practical issues. *Community Mental Health Journal, 14*, 54–62.

Kahn, S. (1970). *How people get power: Organizing oppressed communities for action*. New York: McGraw-Hill.

Katz, D., & Kahn, R. L. (1978). *The social psychology of organizations*. New York: Wiley.

Kelly, J. G. (1968). Toward an ecological conception of preventive interventions. In J. W. Carter, Jr. (Ed.), *Research contributions from psychology to community mental health* (pp. 1–36). New York: Behavioral Publications.

Kelly, J. G. (1971). Qualities for the community psychologist. *American Psychologist, 26*, 897–903.

Kelly, J. G. (1974). *The community psychologist's role in community research: Creating trust and managing power*. Paper presented at the American Psychological Association, New Orleans, Louisiana.

Kelly, J. G. (1979). *Adolescent boys in high school: A psychological study of coping and adaptation*. Hillsdale, NJ: Lawrence Erlbaum Associates.

Kelly, J. G. (1986). Content and process: An ecological view of the interdependence of practice and research. *American Journal of Community Psychology, 14*, 581–589.

Kelly, J. G. (1987). An ecological paradigm: Defining mental health consultation as a preventive service. In J. G. Kelly & R. E. Hess (Eds.), *The ecology of prevention: Illustrative mental health consultation*. New York: Haworth.

Kelly, J. G., & Hess, R. (Eds.) (1987). *The ecology of prevention: Illustrating mental health consultation*. New York: Howard.

Kidder, M. G., Tinker, M., Mannino, F. V., & Trickett, E. J. (1986). Annotated reference guide to the consultation literature, 1978–1984. In F. V. Mannino, E. J. Trickett, M. F. Shore, G. Levin, & M. Kidder (Eds.), *Handbook of mental health consultation* (pp. 523–596). Washington, D.C.: U.S. Department of Health and Human Services, Government Printing Office.

King, L. W., Cotler, S. B., & Patterson, K. (1975). Behavior modification in a Mexican–American school: A case study. *American Journal of Community Psychology, 3*, 229–235.

Kinzie, J. D., Teoh, J. I., & Tan, E. S. (1974). Community psychiatry in Malaysia. *American Journal of Psychiatry, 131*, 573–577.

Langer, E. J., & Rodin, J. (1976). The effects of choice and enhanced personal responsibility for the aged: A field experiment in an institutional setting. *Journal of Personality and Social Psychology, 34*, 191–198.

Laosa, L. M., Burstein, A. G., & Martin, H. W. (1976). Mental health consultation in a rural Chicano community: Crystal City. *Aztlan, 6*, 433–453.

Levin, G., Trickett, E. J., & Hess, R. E. (1990). *Ethical implications for primary prevention*. New York: Haworth.

Levine, M., & Levine, A. G. (1970). *A social history of helping services*. New York: Appleton-Century-Crofts.

Levy-Warren, M. H. (1976). *The delicate balance: Consultation in an alternative inner-city high school*. Unpublished manuscript, Yale University.

Magnussen, D., & Endler, N. S. (Eds.). (1977). *Personality and the crossroads*. Hillsdale, NJ: Lawrence Erlbaum Associates.

Mannino, F. V., & Shore, M. F. (1975). The effects of consultation: A review of empirical studies. *American Journal of Community Psychology, 3*, 1–21.

Mannino, F. V., Trickett, E. J., Shore, M. F., Kidder, M. G., & Levin, G. (1986). *Handbook of mental health consultation*. Washington, D.C.: U.S. Department of Health and Human Services, Government Printing Office.

Mazer, M. (1976). *People and predicaments*. Cambridge: Harvard University Press.

Miller, J. G. (1978). *Living systems*. New York: McGraw-Hill.

Mills, R. C., & Kelly, J. G. (1972). Cultural adaptations and ecological analogies: Analysis of three Mexican villages. In S. E. Golann & C. Eisdorfer (Eds.), *Handbook of community mental health* (pp. 157–205). New York: Appleton-Century-Crofts.

Moore, T., Nagata, D., & Whatley, R. (1984). Training community psychologists and other social interventionists. In S. Sue & T. Moore (Eds.), *The pluralistic society* (pp. 237–253). New York: Human Sciences Press.

Moos, R. H. (1974). *Evaluating treatment environments: A social ecological approach.* New York: Wiley.

Moos, R. H. (1975). *Evaluating correctional community settings.* New York: Wiley.

Moos, R. H. (1979). *Evaluating educational environments.* San Francisco: Jossey-Bass.

O'Neill, P., & Trickett, E. J. (1983). *Community consultation.* San Francisco: Jossey-Bass.

Pearl, A., & Riessman, F. (1965). *New careers for the poor: The nonprofessional in human service.* New York: Free Press.

Perkins, N. T., Nieva, V. F., & Ladler, E. E. (1983). *Managing creation: The challenge of building a new organization.* New York: Wiley.

Pierce, W. D., Trickett, E. J., & Moos, R. H. (1972). Changing ward atmosphere through staff discussion of the perceived ward environment. *Archives of General Psychiatry, 26,* 35–41.

Ransen, D. L. (1981). Long-term effects of two interventions with the aged: An ecological analysis. *Journal of Applied Development Psychology, 2,* 13–27.

Reinharz, S. (1983). Consulting to the alternative work setting: A suggested strategy for community psychology. *Journal of Community Psychology, 11,* 199–212.

Rice, A. K. (1969). Individual, group, and intergroup processes. *Human Relations, 22,* 565–584.

Sarason, S. B. (1972). *The creation of settings and future societies.* San Francisco: Jossey-Bass.

Sarason, S. B. (1981). *Psychology misdirected.* New York: Free Press.

Schmuck, R., & Miles, M. (Eds.). (1971). *Organizational development in schools.* Palo Alto: National Press Books.

Schulz, R. (1976). The effects of control and predictability on the psychological and physical well-being of the institutional aged. *Journal of Personality and Social Psychology, 34,* 191–198.

Smith, K. K., & Corse, S. J. (1986). The process of consultation: Critical issues. In I. V. Mannino, E. J. Trickett, M. F. Shore, M. G. Kidder, & G. Levin (Eds.), *Handbook of mental health consultation* (pp. 247–278). Washington, D.C.: U.S. Department of Health and Human Services, Government Printing Office.

Stokols, D., & Altman, I. (Eds.). (1987). *Handbook of environmental psychology.* New York: Wiley.

Thomas, K. G., Gatz, M., & Luczak, S. E. (1997). A tale of two school districts: Lessons to be learned about the importance of relationship building and ecology on consultation. *Journal of Education and Psychological Consultation, 8,* 297–320.

Trickett, E. J. (1984). Towards a distinctive community psychology: An ecological metaphor for training and the conduct of research. *American Journal of Community Psychology, 12,* 261–279.

Trickett, E. J. (1986). Consultation as a preventive intervention. In J. G. Kelly & R. Hess (Eds.), *The ecology of prevention: Illustrating mental health consultation* (pp. 163–175). New York: Haworth.

Trickett, E. J. (1993). Gerald Caplan and the unfinished business of community psychology: A comment. In W. P. Erchul (Ed.), *Consultation in community, school, and organizational practice: Gerald Caplan's contributions to professional psychology.* Washington, SC: Taylor & Francis.

Trickett, E. J., & Birman, D. (1989). Taking ecology seriously: A community development approach to individually-based interventions. In L. Bond & B. Compas (Eds.), *Primary prevention in the schools* (pp. 187–204). Hanover, NH: University Press of New England.

Trickett, E. J., Kelly, J. G., & Todd, D. M. (1972). The social environment of the high school: Guidelines for individual change and organizational development. In S. Golann & C. Eisdorfer (Eds.), *Handbook of community mental health* (pp. 361–390). New York: Appleton-Century-Crofts.

Trickett, E. J., Kelly, J. G., & Vincent, T. A. (1985). The spirit of ecological inquiry in community research. In D. Klein & E. Susshind, *Knowledge-building in community psychology* (pp. 331–406). New York: Praeger.

Trickett, E. J., & Mitchell, R. (1992). An ecological metaphor for research and intervention in community psychology. In M. S. Gibbs, J. R. Lochenmeyer, & J. Sigal (Eds.), *Community psychology: Theoretical and empirical approaches,* 2nd ed. (pp. 12–28). New York: Wiley.

Trickett, E. J., Watts, R. J., & Birman, D. (1994). *Human diversity: Perspectives on people in context.* San Francisco: Jossey-Bass.

Vincent, T. A. (1987). Two into one: An ecological perspective on school consultation. In J. G. Kelly & R. Hess (Eds.), *The ecology of prevention: Illustrating mental health consultation* (pp. 283–233). New York: Haworth.

Warren, R. I., & Warren, D. I. (1977). *The neighborhood organizers handbook.* South Bend, IN: University of Notre Dame Press.

Yutiao, M., & Kinzie, J. D. (1975). Consultation with the Filipino boarding home: An after-care facility in Hawaii. *International Journal of Social Psychiatry, 21,* 130–136.

CHAPTER 14

Community and Neighborhood Organization

BILL BERKOWITZ

INTRODUCTION

Reasons for Concern

There are four compelling reasons why community psychologists should be directly concerned with community and neighborhood organization:[1]

1. Community organizing, through both the process and product of action, should ordinarily lead to personal empowerment, wellness, and increased competence for those involved; that is, to individual outcomes that are among the primary goals of our discipline.
2. Community organization, when successful, should also result in better communities; "better" in terms of the community's expressed needs. That is, there should be *bona fide* community accomplishments to point to and tangible improvements in place.
3. Scholarly reports (e.g., Berry, Portney, & Thomson, 1993; Fisher, 1985; Homan, 1994; Mattaini & Thyer, 1996; Mattesich & Monsey, 1997; Minkler, 1997; Mondros & Wilson; 1994; Mott, 1997; Wandersman & Florin, Chapter, 11, this volume; Wittig & Bettencourt, 1996) and popular accounts as well (e.g., Alinsky, 1971; Dyson & Dyson, 1989; Kahn, 1982; Medoff & Sklar, 1994) suggest that community organization does, in fact, lead to such positive outcomes, for both individuals and communities. Moreover, psychological research suggests that community organization may have additional personal and social consequences that we view as desirable: greater happiness

[1]The term "community organization" is often used alone in the text for reasons of economy. "Neighborhood organization" usually implies a somewhat smaller setting. The text material is meant to refer and apply to both equally.

BILL BERKOWITZ • Department of Psychology, University of Massachusetts Lowell, Lowell, Massachusetts 01854.

Handbook of Community Psychology, edited by Julian Rappaport and Edward Seidman. Kluwer Academic / Plenum Publishers, New York, 2000.

(Campbell, 1981; Diener, 1984), increased neighboring (Ahlbrandt, 1984), stronger social support networks (Pilisuk & Parks, 1986; Taylor, Repetti, & Seeman, 1997), and lower individual and community pathology (Aneshensel, 1992; Gesten & Jason, 1987; Heller, 1990; House, Umberson, & Landis, 1988; Kretzmann & McKnight, 1993; Naparstek, Biegel, & Spiro, 1982; Rodin, 1985).

4. Finally, in times of economic downturn or worse, community organization can stimulate cooperation and local self-reliance, at little or no cost, thus cushioning and protecting the community from outside adversity.

If tomorrow, for example, we could double or triple the existing levels of local organization in every community in the United States, we have every reason to believe that community life would be richer and more fulfilling for most of us, and more equitable for society as a whole. And so these reasons combined, one might think, should make community organization a dominant theme, or *the* dominant theme, in community psychology theory, training, research, and practice today.

However, it is not. Community organization is not dominant, nor even prominent. Consider the following:

• Articles on community or neighborhood organization rarely appear in either the *American Journal of Community Psychology* or the *Journal of Community Psychology*. Earlier content analyses of these journals have consistently found most studies focusing on formal institutional settings, in particular, clinics and schools (e.g., Lounsbury, Leader, Meares, & Cook, 1980; Novaco & Monahan, 1980). Informal examination of later volumes suggests that the situation has not appreciably changed.

• None of the current leading textbooks in community psychology (e.g., Heller, Price, Riger, Reinharz, & Wandersman, 1984; Levine & Perkins, 1997) contains a chapter on the topic, nor devotes more than a few pages to community or neighborhood organization as such.

• Those who do write and talk about community organization are not likely to be psychologists. The major academic texts in the field (e.g., Biklen, 1983; Brager, Specht, & Torczyner, 1987; Burghardt, 1982; Homan, 1994; Kettner, Daley, & Nichols, 1985; Minkler, 1997; Mondros & Wilson, 1994; Rothman, Erlich, & Tropman, 1995; Tropman, Erlich, & Rothman, 1995) have all been written from outside our discipline (one exception is Zander, 1990). As for the most notable popular books in the field, one looks to Bobo, Kendall, and Max's *Organizing for Social Change* (1991), written by professional community activists, Kahn's *Organizing* (1982), written by a union organizer/folksinger, or Alinsky's *Rules for Radicals* (1971), written by a former criminologist.

• And finally, the same argument applies to practice. Most community organizing in America is done by people who are neither psychologists or social science professionals. Community psychologists may do their share (or may not). But the most distinguished organizing, certainly that which has made the news—acting for the homeless, for toxic waste cleanups, for reproductive rights, for any social issue—has invariably been sparked and led by people without formal psychological training or background. One would be hard pressed to identify a single community psychologist who has initiated an organizing activity of remotely comparable impact.

Reasons for Neglect

Why so much mismatch between what could be and should be, and what is? The explanations lie close to the surface. Their very existence defines targets for change:

1. Community organizing within most social contexts has little direct economic payoff. There are no billable clients, no increased sales, no third parties to absorb the cost. The bottom line is not enhanced. We have few reimbursement mechanisms for service to a community; even if we had, those communities needing help the most can often afford it the least.

2. As a result, salaries for full-time organizers are painfully low. Offers of under $20,000 a year are still not uncommon, while community psychologists in academic or institutional settings can expect to earn double or triple that amount. Salaries are low too because organizers push against the status quo—society hesitates to pay people striving to change it.

3. Academics interested in community organization have minimal time for it, having other demands. There is more time if one is a researcher, but given its inherent complexity, community organization is hard to research, to isolate variables, to pinpoint effects. Yet doing community organization without doing research becomes a matter of "community service," which has not been favored historically by academic departments or tenure committees, and which, because of its built-in *ad hoc* and local nature, is unlikely to gain one much professional visibility in the field.

4. Potential community organizers in human service agencies also have time strictures, as most agency transactions are one-on-one, and there is frequently no particular mandate for, nor interest in, serving the broader community as such. Community organizing, moreover, may be seen as questioning the agency's established habits, challenging its internal structure, undercutting its community power, or all of these.

5. In any case, community organization is time-consuming, and often emotionally draining. Organizing activities tend to carry (or drag) on, largely because they are subject to forces beyond one person's influence. It is psychologically difficult to keep putting energy into a situation that one has little control over, where the outcome may not be known for some time, where one may win a very partial victory or lose outright, or where, even in victory, one's own precise contribution may be difficult to compute.

6. Finally, and ironically, most psychologists and many community psychologists have a limited community orientation. They are trained to work in the community or for it, but not to be part of it—there is a difference. They may be good at implementing their own community interventions, where they direct what's going on, but organizing is fuzzier, muddier, with more power sharing, more group decision-making, and more nonprofessionals wanting and needing control. Compared to (say) clinical practice, the psychologist here may be less powerful, less well prepared, and/or less favorably inclined to jump in.

Given this snapshot of community and neighborhood organization within the discipline, a reviewer might take on two primary tasks. One is to review the empirical evidence on community organization, and especially to indicate what principles and techniques seem to work best, so that one wishing to go out and organize will be guided by the highest quality data we can muster. The other is to advocate, to encourage organizing activity and applications, and unabashedly so, for in science, as in anything else, evidence alone may not prompt action. Put more plainly, community organization needs to be promoted and expanded, both from inside and outside the discipline, and to assist with this we will propose an agenda toward the end of this chapter. But first we should clarify our definitions.

Definition

Community organization means the intentional activities, begun by one person or a relatively small group, to bring community residents together, in a structured fashion, thus taking joint action to improve the local quality of life, generally in a lasting manner, both for the people organized and for the broader community.

The emphasis in this chapter is on geographic community rather than on broader vocational or avocational communities of interest; that is, on the communities that we live in and where we spend our time. And the emphasis here is on smaller communities, although similar principles may apply to larger ones. As a rule of thumb we'll be thinking of communities bounded by "easy walking distance"—in other words of neighborhood-sized communities or neighborhoods themselves.

These boundaries set, there are several points to note about our working definition:

First, community organization is an *active process*, with emphasis on both words. We're not examining the organization that already exists, but instead something moving in time, something deliberately superposed on the present structure, which may modify it or create an altogether new structure.

Second, there's generally a product involved. Some concrete result, some tangible outcome, event, or physical construction is supposed to emerge from the organizing work. Something demonstrable should happen that hadn't happened before. Community organization, then, is both process and product, and both the doing and the result may be valued.

Third, the product and the process both involve deliberate change from what previously existed. Most changes are not likely to please everyone, and so organizers incur a moderate-or-better risk of arousing opposition, weak or strong, passive or active, organized or not. Accordingly, community organization by its nature is likely to be controversial, which is perhaps another reason why it lies outside the mainstream.

Fourth, community organization, as the term is used here, is distinct from community intervention. Traditional interventions in psychology come from the top down; they require situational control. There is relatively little collaboration with, and sometimes minimal consent by, the intervention targets. Much of the purpose is research-oriented, either to find out whether a particular intervention "works" or to test some hypothesis; most interventions, as a result, have a strong evaluative component.

Community organizing, on the other hand, is more likely to be collaborative in both intent and implementation. The issue is usually one generated by the community rather than imported from outside. A larger group of established residents typically participates throughout. And while research on organizing effects is highly desirable, research in practice so far has generally played a secondary role—interest in practical outcome has exceeded interest in gathering and disseminating systematic data. Intervention and organization are similar but separate concepts, with overlapping but separable benefits and costs.

Models

Over and above this conceptualization, there are several different categories or models of community organization; while we won't dwell too long on taxonomy, a useful distinction is made by Rothman (1995; cf. also Fisher, 1985). In a nutshell, one may work to strengthen the community ties already in place (locality development), to import and develop new structures from the outside (social planning), or to focus community energy against external power sources (social action). All three models are useful, all have their strengths and weaknesses; nor are they mutually exclusive. When asked which type of community organizing we are describing and advocating, the answer is all of them. But given a choice of emphasis, one might focus on the first.

Locality development—or to substitute a livelier phrase, neighborhood-building actions—best reflect what people can do by and for themselves, without outside assistance; few relationships with agencies are required, while organized opposition is unlikely to be a factor. Neighborhood-building opportunities arise more frequently. The goals may be clearer; generating involvement may be easier. And neighborhood-building activities may, in many situations, be the least time-consuming, the least psychologically demanding, the least ideologically polarizing, and so the easiest to implement.

As a result, neighborhood-building actions are frequently the most energizing and the most empowering of people. The accomplishment may be smaller than in other organizing models, but the chances of goal attainment may be larger. Skills and attitudes may be taught to the greatest number; small successes may be built upon. And of no mean importance, the community psychologist has a convenient setting to work in, which could be just around the corner or down the street.

Granted, neighborhood building alone will sometimes not do the job. Those working with poor and disenfranchised groups in particular know that bolder and more forceful actions may also be required. The need for basic structural change cannot be overlooked. But given the present vacuum within the discipline, it may be sensible for community psychologists, as well as citizens, to start near home and move from there. For all three models, similar principles will apply (though for large-scale confrontational organizing others may need to be advanced). Our emphasis in this chapter, then, will be on these homelier kinds of organizing actions, which for better and worse are less glamorous, less encompassing, more common, and most likely to succeed.

Sources of Evidence

What works in community organization, and how do we know it? The sources of evidence need to be examined. The most instructive point about sources is that the bulk of them do not come from community psychology journals, nor from community psychologists, and frequently not from psychologists at all. In other words, *psychology does not have an established base of direct evidence from experimental or controlled field studies of community organization that informs us, with precision, as to what kinds of organizational attempts work best, when, and how.*

The current evidence is instead indirect and scattered. One part comes from experiments in social psychology (in leadership, group dynamics, persuasion, and interpersonal attraction in particular)—studies undertaken with narrower questions in mind, and which are of uncertain external validity (Rodin, 1985, p. 805). A second source derives from systematic observation or questioning by social scientists of community residents regarding their participation, relationships, desires, and satisfaction levels; these findings are generally limited to one point in time and space, and lack equivalent comparison groups.

A third and less formal body of data stems from observations and testimonies of community organizers themselves, often professionals, but not always. These take the shape of commercially published texts, homemade manuals, booklets, case studies, tip sheets, or memoirs. Finally, there is a mixed bag of newspaper stories, popular magazine articles, anecdotal accounts, current documents, and historical analyses, often rich in insight and lacking in systematization (for one systematic historical account, see Fisher, 1985). Whatever biases of observation, memory, or ideology may exist here, these last two classes of material probably constitute the bulk of the received wisdom about community organizing for most nonpsychologists.

Perhaps this patchwork is to be expected. Overall, what we have is a pattern of evidence that draws from multiple fields and disciplines, whose scientific quality ranges from laboratory study to banquet story, whose generalizability probably varies as well ("probably," since it's rarely been tested), and whose integration necessarily requires much inter- and extrapolation.

What is quite certain is that we lack a hard science of community or neighborhood organizing and will continue to lack one in the near future. There are simply too many variables to control; in any given natural setting, many will be uncontrollable. Yet a skillful integration will tell us a lot about community organization; our current knowledge can carry us far. If what we have at present more closely resembles a craft, that craftwork can be made more precise; it can move a shade closer into science. With intelligence and commitment, we should become more successful at forging the best tools for the job at hand, at sharpening our technique, and at refining our knowledge for the next generation.

Synthesizing the Evidence

So given these sources and their limitations, we can venture a first-draft synthesis of the empirical evidence on community and neighborhood organization. Our particular aim will be to list conditions associated with, and conducive to, successful organizing attempts. They are drawn from both individual and small-community levels of analysis. They are tendencies, lawful but not invariant, which need to be adapted, modified, and expanded to meet the individual case.

For expository purposes, we will divide these conditions into those pertaining to the organizer, the setting, the issue, and the communication itself. We will shape each factor into propositional form and number each in order, since short-form propositions may be easier to assimilate, and to accept or refute. Full citation of references for each proposition would be cumbersome and repetitive; we will not attempt them in every case. However, the more individual-level and social-psychological principles here in general draw extensively upon Cialdini (1993); Gilbert, Fiske, and Lindzey (1998); Karlins and Abelson (1970); Mattaini and Thyer (1996); Oskamp and Schultz (1998); Unger and Wandersman (1985); Weyant (1986); Zimbardo, Ebbesen, and Maslach (1977); and Zimbardo and Leippe (1991); while the principles of community setting and issue are derived in large part from Alinsky (1971); Biklen (1983); Bobo et al. (1991); Brager et al. (1987); Cunningham and Kotler (1983); Kahn (1982); Rothman (1974); Rothman et al. (1995); Tropman et al. (1995); and Warren and Warren (1977).

Once again, in considering, evaluating, and especially in applying these propositions, the reader ought to be deliberate, skeptical, and careful about overgeneralization; the practitioner ought also to be ready to customize principles to a particular situation and to report the results.

PROPOSITIONS

The Organizer

1. Organizers presumably derive many of their change-oriented values from their parents, insofar as parent–child attitudes are similar in many, but not all instances (reviewed in Kinder, 1998; Petty and Wegener, 1998; and Snyder and Cantor, 1998).

2. The childhood experiences of organizers, though, lack apparent commonality. Burns

(1978), in related research, reports on the diverse upbringings of national leaders. However, we lack comprehensive studies of organizers' childhood backgrounds.

3. No demographic characteristics seem to be reliable predictors of subsequent community- or neighborhood-organizing activity by individuals (Berkowitz, 1987; Fiske, 1987; Knoke, 1986; see also review by Wandersman and Florin, this volume). On the other hand, Vallance and D'Augelli (1982) have shown that "natural helpers" tend more often to be younger, better educated, and newer to their community settings. These differences remain to be reconciled.

4. Compared to other citizens, organizers tend to have smaller amounts of family or other outside obligations (Berkowitz, 1987). This applies especially to organizers making long-term commitments or grappling with bigger issues, and also while active organizing is occurring. Organizing takes time, and organizing attempts will be more fruitful if that time has fewer competitors. In the words of Alinsky: "The marriage record of organizers is with rare exceptions disastrous" (1971, p. 65). He means full-time and fully extended organizers, but the point is clear.

5. The documented evidence for common personality characteristics among successful organizers is weak. In the popular literature, Alinsky (1971) cites curiosity, irreverence, imagination, and humor, plus personal organization, vision, a strong ego, and an open mind as primary attributes, but does not attempt verification. Kahn (1982) also lists a number of organizer virtues, yet nevertheless states, "There is no one type of person that makes the best leader" (p. 22).

6. One can be a highly successful organizer without professional training. A confirming research example comes from Wandersman and colleagues' studies on neighborhood participation, where organizers were typically resident volunteers or students, yet where contact with these organizers proved to be the most significant variable influencing neighborhood involvement (Rich & Wandersman, 1983). The personal qualities of the organizer may be a determining factor here.

7. At the same time, organizers can be trained. A dozen or more free-standing organizing training schools and institutes across the country attest to this (see Fischer & Schwartz, 1995, sections 7 and 9), even though their training effects are not routinely evaluated. More precisely, Florin and Wandersman (1990), through the Block Booster Project in New York City, have shown that block leader training can extend block-association life expectancy. Fawcett and his associates (Fawcett, Seekins, Whang, Muiu, & Suarez de Balcazar, 1984; Seekins, Fawcett, & Mathews, 1987) have also developed convincing training programs in leadership and advocacy skills for ordinary citizens, as has Glidewell (1986) for negotiation skills. A starting commitment to give training in organizing techniques, plus the clear specification of training outcome goals, would undoubtedly yield more successful results along these lines.

As can be seen, we know relatively little about the relationship between the personal attributes of the organizer and organizing success. The qualities of a successful organizer do appear setting-specific to a substantial degree. The situation may be akin to related fields such as leadership, where "there do not appear to be broad and invariant characteristics that generally distinguish leaders from nonleaders" (Hollander, 1985, p. 516), and altruistic behavior, where evidence for personality correlates of altruism is inconclusive at best (Batson, 1998).

On the other hand, one may still suspect some uniform personality core. In a series of interviews with particularly successful grass-roots program-starters, Berkowitz (1987) identified enthusiasm (in the sense of passionate, consuming enthusiasm) and "traditional virtue" (commitment, hard work, persistence, considerateness, confidence, willingness to risk, tolerance for criticism, optimism) as linking personality characteristics. Bass and Stogdill's *Handbook of Leadership* reveals a similar listing (1990). These qualities are hardly novel, and not necessarily causal, but they are stimulants to further investigation. Quantitative studies of organizer personality characteristics have, to my knowledge, not appeared in psychology journals—this is a research gap.

The Setting

Setting is a larger scale, higher order variable, and we shift here from an individual to a group or neighborhood level of analysis. Setting qualities divide easily into structural and functional aspects, as below.

Structural Qualities

Other things equal, an organizational attempt is more likely to be successful:

8. The smaller the physical boundaries of the setting. Fewer independent units then need be brought into concert; this is a simple systems principle (Miller, 1978). As a rule, it is easier to organize something on your block than in your neighborhood, and in your neighborhood than in the entire community.

9. The greater the population density of the setting. In denser settings, informal communication networks are more likely to exist, the linkage generally being density → proximity → contact opportunity → establishment of communication channels. Normally, it's easier to organize the residents of an apartment building than the same number of people spread over the countryside.

10. The more time people spend within the setting. Time spent will also lead to contact opportunity and communication channel development, and this pathway may bend back on itself, for good communication can, in turn, lead to more time spent. But in any event, it should be harder to organize a stereotypical bedroom community than one where people are physically in the community for longer periods, and more visible to each other.

11. The more people are known within the setting. Note that the propositions in this section are interconnected: more people, for example, will typically be known in settings that are smaller, denser, and more often frequented. And other derivations follow (cf. Pilisuk & Parks, 1986): given open channels, more informal interaction should then take place. Informal interaction predicts participation, which leads back to more informal interaction (Jeffres & Dobos, 1984; Unger & Wandersman, 1983); this self-enhancing loop should make formal organizing easier. Some limits may exist here, for open channels may also facilitate the development of customs and behavior patterns that are resistant to change.

12. The more homogeneous the socioeconomic, cultural, and religious backgrounds of people within the setting. Ahlbrandt (1984), for example, has shown that strong local church structures make organizing easier. Homogeneity leads to more preexisting interpersonal ties and less diversity of opinion. Fewer people will need to be convinced and more are likely to show support if the issue is relevant and the appeal is right (Guest & Oropesa, 1984; Unger & Wandersman, 1982).

13. The stronger the presence of certain demographic factors within the setting, which include residents who are (a) suburban (Fischer, 1982), (b) older, (c) married, (d) female, (e) homeowners, and (f) living in smaller households (Florin & Wandersman, 1984, for b

through f), and also residents who (g) have lived longer in the area (Wandersman, Jakubs, & Giamartino, 1980; but cf. also Fischer, 1982; Vallance & D'Augelli, 1982), and (h) have children living at home (Unger & Wandersman, 1982). These factors influence either participation in block associations (b through g), or neighboring in general, both of which should facilitate organizational attempts by others.

14. The closer the socioeconomic level of the neighborhood approaches a middle range. Burghardt (1982) notes that low-income settings are difficult to organize, for residents may have little cooperative experience and low expectations of success. His argument is supported by Ahlbrandt (1984), Checkoway and Van Til (1978), Rothman (1974), and Unger and Wandersman (1982), even though numbers of low-income community groups may be expanding (Dreier, 1996). On the other hand, very wealthy settings might be harder to organize, too, residents being more able to use their wealth as a buffer against intrusion (these settings also being less dense). The overall income-organizing relationship appears to be curvilinear.

15. The greater the amount of tangible resources within the setting. Resources commonly divide into money, people, talent, contacts, and time, and to that extent this proposition overlaps with several of those above. These resources, though, must be mobilized.

Functional Qualities

Turning more toward more functional variables—those having more to do with dynamic attributes of the setting and its residents than upon underlying physical or social structure—an organizing attempt should be more successful:

16. The more visible, extensive, active, powerful, and formalized the existing leadership patterns within the setting. Strong existing leadership can create a climate of opinion, and then can diffuse it. This can also work to the organizer's disadvantage, but more frequently leadership can be leveraged to do much of the organizer's work.

17. The more established the norms for community participation within the setting (see, in a related context, Foss, 1986).

18. The more visible the presence of persons who model participation (D'Augelli & Vallance, 1982) and, as a corollary, the more opportunities for participation there are, through varied organizational roles.

19. The more lengthy, eventful, and successful the past history of people acting together for a common cause within the setting (Fisher, 1985). In other words, groups with a track record, that is, with a reinforcement history of successful organizing, are those more likely to organize again.

20. The greater the perception of collective competence, power, cohesion, and solidarity by the residents in the setting themselves, over and above the more behavioral criteria in proposition 19. This is particularly important when organizing is geared to move against some outside force.

21. The greater the perception of competence, power, cohesion, and solidarity of the residents in the setting by that same outside force. According to Alinsky: *"Power is not only what you have but what the enemy thinks you have"* (1971, p. 127, emphasis in original).

Other psychodynamic attributes pertain more explicitly to the individual residents in the setting, rather than to the setting as a whole. That is, an organizing attempt should yield better results the more that individuals (though not necessarily groups in aggregate) possess the following inner qualities:

22. A sense of personal well-being.

23. A sense of personal duty.

24. A sense of personal competence.
25. Valuation of one's own skills.
26. Expectancy that participation will lead to success.
27. Feelings of rootedness and integration within the setting.
28. Valuation of one's block or community.
29. Commitment to one's block or community.
30. A psychological sense of community.

These cognitive and affective variables—again, interrelated—variously predict participation, neighboring, and block-association membership (Ahlbrandt & Cunningham, 1979; Florin & Wandersman, 1984; Wandersman & Florin, 1984). Wandersman and Florin argue that cognitive intrapsychic factors predict these behaviors (and so, presumably, ability to become organized, as contrasted with organizing ability) better than the demographic variables previously cited. Their chapter on citizen participation in this volume elaborates on their position and reviews other internal and external factors associated with higher levels of citizen activity.

Note, however, that two other predictors from Florin and Wandersman's research are:

31. The perception of a moderate degree of problems on the block.

32. Some degree of dissatisfaction with current block conditions, though paired with apparent overall setting satisfaction. The point is that complete satisfaction with the community is a disincentive to organizing.

33. The better the fit between the setting variables in this section and the organizer variables already listed. Setting and organizer effects have separate weight, but also interact. In this case we are looking for facilitating interactions, ones where organizer and setting match up well and enhance each other. So, for example, a charismatic leader may be more effective in settings where little prior organization has taken place (Bass, 1985), but less effective elsewhere.

We cannot list all interactions or best fits here, partly because of space limitations, partly because optimal interactions will themselves change through the organizing life cycle, and partly because many interactions are unknown and need to be researched. But the interactional theme has been independently noted by commentators from several different disciplines (Alinsky, 1971; Burns, 1978; Hollander, 1985; Snyder & Cantor, 1998), and it will recur later.

The Issue

34. An organizational attempt is more likely to be successful, and is more probable to begin with, if there is an issue around which to organize. An issue defines the purpose of the intervention and focuses the organizing activity. Sometimes the issue already exists, sometimes overwhelmingly so; other times the issue may need to be created and marketed, which is more difficult, although possible, to do. In either case, there are issue characteristics that generally will facilitate organizing success, and these include:

35. A simple issue, as contrasted with one that is complex and many-sided. "Simple," however, does not imply "trivial" (see proposition 36).

36. An important issue, one which is salient for the residents in the setting, and strongly felt (Kahn, 1982).

37. A proximate issue, one impinging directly on its targets in both time and space. An issue that is alive now, and nearby (Rothman, Erlich, & Teresa, 1976).

38. A specific issue (Alinsky, 1971; Rothman et al., 1976), one with clear behavioral referents. Simple, salient, proximate, and specific issues—school busing, traffic lights, trash dumping, rent control—are easier to visualize, possible outcomes are easier to foresee, and linkages to action are more apparent.

39. A threatening issue, one in which there is a perceived likelihood either that (a) some positively valued element of the setting will be reduced or removed, or that (b) some negatively valued element will be introduced. Threats *do* mobilize people; crises (urgent and strong threats) mobilize them even more. The stronger the threat, the stronger the pressure to restore inner equilibrium by taking outward action.

40. An immediate issue, that is, one in which action must be taken before a rapidly approaching deadline. Immediate issues, by their nature, also entail shorter time commitments. Rothman (1974) points out that this, and the other issue qualities above, may be especially relevant for low-income groups.

41. A quickly resolvable issue, in the sense that the time period between action and outcome is seen as short. As in reinforcement theory, when positive reinforcement is expected to follow more closely upon response, the probability of response will be higher.

42. A winnable issue, meaning the chance that the requested action will lead to desired consequences is seen to be high. This will depend upon available resources within the setting (proposition 15), as well as upon obstacles outside of it, be they legal, financial, or political. Winnability is in large part a matter of perception, and one that applies to both the organizer and the organized. Both will work harder if success is seen as likely; such perception, of course, can be self-fulfilling.

43. An issue that suggests low personal obligation for a potential recruit. This may not always be possible, but to the extent that the previously characterized issues can be won with modest personal expense, it is an advantage.

44. An issue where the obstacles, if they exist at all, can be personalized. Giving a face to the opposition, isolating and targeting the enemies, can unify present and potential supporters and provide them with a superordinate goal. If the opposition is also seen as vulnerable, so much the better (Brager et al., 1987, chap. 16).

45. An issue chosen by the people affected, as contrasted with one imposed or introduced from the outside, in the absence of a particular threat (Brager et al., 1987, chap. 6).

46. Finally, an issue that offers more than material incentives to the people—instead one which promotes competence, confidence, and personal development (Fisher, 1984) and which unites people and builds upon their sense of community (Kahn, 1982).

Interactions and qualifications regarding these propositions again occur. When an issue is very important, for instance, people may accept a lower likelihood of success. With a record of accomplishment, residents may seek out more challenging issues, even with obstacles attached. But when the above issue conditions exist, or most of them, residents will frequently organize with little additional stimulus.

Successful organization is possible even if no issue is simmering, or imported for the occasion. People can come together for mutual support, to gain information, to be entertained, or simply for a good time. Such gatherings work better when there is prior common identification—block residence, for example, or school, church, or work connections—and when food and drink are available as generalized reinforcers. Though motivation for these occasions may be primarily social, they can also be used as vehicles for low-key issue organizing.

The Communication

In addition to organizer, setting, and issue variables, organizing success will turn upon who says what and how. These are communication characteristics. They commonly subdivide into those belonging to the communicator, the format, and the message content, and we will follow that arrangement here.

The communication principles themselves come mainly from laboratory and field studies in social psychology, many of which are "senior citizens" of that literature by now—they aren't new. They are discussed in standard social psychology texts, in recent specialized accounts (e.g., Cialdini, 1993; Zimbardo & Leippe, 1991), in recent reviews such as Cialdini and Trost (1998), Petty and Wegener (1997), and Petty, Wegener, and Fabrigar (1998), as well as in older books such as Karlins and Abelson (1970) and Zimbardo, Ebbesen, and Maslach (1977). Readers are referred there for most original sources and accompanying detail and caveats. However, since most community psychologists are on unfamiliar ground here, having entered the field through a different gateway, it pays to summarize these principles, if only briefly.

The Communicator

The organizer variables described previously are dispositional, qualities of the person; while the communicator variables described here are situational, relating to the particular setting and audience at hand. Given that distinction, an organizing attempt will be more successful the more the communicator of the organizing message is, or is seen as:

47. Credible, or believable, both in general and on the particular issue. Credibility will, in turn, depend on perceived qualifications and past performance.
48. Sincere, with no apparent concealed motive. If communicator self-interest will be obvious to the listener, it should be mentioned openly.
49. Knowledgeable on the issue. Expertise is generally an asset, but the expertise must be perceived as relevant to *this* setting and *this* issue, or it can become counterproductive (see below).
50. Powerful, in the sense of having a formal leadership role within the setting or outside of it.
51. Similar to the audience in background and values. Similarity increases liking, which in turn increases message acceptance.

Once again, these variables overlap; a formally powerful communicator, for example, will tend to be seen as more credible. The variable loadings will change with the situation; on more technical issues, for instance, expertise may carry more weight. Furthermore, their relationships to organizing success and outcome may not always be direct—too much expertise, communicated heavy-handedly, is distancing and can backfire. The ideal communicator will have the right credentials and a highly regarded character, but will still be "one of us"; he or she will be one of us writ large.

The Format

52. Personal communication is generally more effective than less personal forms. Supporting evidence comes from the fund-raising literature, where personal requests in soliciting donations are consistently recommended (e.g., Warner, 1992), and from surveys of volunteers—when asked how they got started, the most frequent response is commonly "someone asked me" (Hodgkinson & Weitzman, 1994). Personal appeals are harder to turn down. And in particular:
53. An organizing attempt will be more successful when the communication is face-to-

face. Some direct evidence comes from Rich & Wandersman (1983), who found that 62% of residents personally contacted by an organizer subsequently joined a block organization, compared to only 10% of those who were not. Moreover, the training or personal style of the organizer there seemed not to matter; face-to-face contact was apparently the key variable. Such contact in general can be multiplied by block representatives, or by division of territory among a core group.

54. When face-to-face contact is not feasible, person-to-person contact over the telephone would appear to be the next best choice. Other things equal, a given telephone call from a community member, especially a credible one, will probably be more impactful than a mailed communication, although both together may be more effective than either one taken singly.

55. Format variables associated with effective mailed communications appear to include: (a) first-class (and commemorative) stamps; (b) use of color in paper and design; (c) personalized content (handwritten, for example, but not computer-generated, as in "We know that you, Mr./Ms. Reader ..."); (d) handwritten or typed addressing, instead of mailing labels; and (e) perceptual contrast and novelty in the overall mailing package. Some of the existing literature is reviewed by Alreck and Settle (1994), Bailey (1994), Dillman (1991), and Simon (1993). The separate impacts of the factors above have been incompletely researched and may be slight, though conceivably additive and cost-effective, especially for local mailers and recipients.

Mailed communications can work well. So can other print forms such as handed-out flyers (Geller, Johnson, & Pelton, 1982), and, despite earlier skepticism, larger scale media campaigns (Roberts & Maccoby, 1985). Particular format choices (face-to-face, phone, mail, or other), like other choices, will and should be governed by available time, resources, and money, as well as by empirical data. Again, formats can be combined, or "sandwiched" (as in call—mailing—call). But in general, personal, face-to-face contact is probably more practical in community and neighborhood settings than is generally realized, and has the added potential advantage of increasing the commitment of the contactor as well as the contactee.

The Message Content

An organizing attempt will be more successful to the extent that the content of the message:

56. Is planned in advance, to meet the needs of the particular audience (Vernon & D'Augelli, 1987).

57. Enters the perceptual system of the audience, so that it gets attention. An organizing message must first be perceived before it can be comprehended and acted upon. Factors determining such perception are the same as those for any stimulus: intensity, duration, novelty, and contrast, all relative to other messages of similar category.

58. Is repeated. This is the well-documented principle of exposure effect, which suggests that repetition increases liking for, and attraction to, a stimulus.

59. Has, or is made to seem as though it has, high importance or salience for the target group.

60. Utilizes one or more motivational appeals, which may include: (a) authority (formal power of the communicator); (b) expertise; (c) reference group norms; (d) membership group norms, or peer pressure, possibly accompanied (as also for reference group appeals) by descriptions of salient models who have benefitted from acting upon the message; (e) fear, including threats to physical security, material wealth, or emotional well-being, especially if

the issue is salient and fear-reducing action opportunities are made explicit; (f) the desire of people to help others when they can; (g) reciprocity, stated or implied; (h) consistency of the proposed action with other audience actions or beliefs; or, conversely, the inconsistency of failing to act juxtaposed with those same behaviors or cognitions; (i) abstract values, such as patriotism, honesty, duty, intelligence, good citizenship, or underlying moral principles; and (j) personally relevant motives of particular audience members (e.g., approval, status, power, self-esteem, social attractiveness).

61. Provides a variety of different appeals, to different motives and segments within and among audience members, especially if the audience is heterogeneous. The appeals should be custom-fitted, in this sense. Recall Alinsky's classic organizing aphorism: *"Never go outside the experience of your people"* (1971, p. 127, emphasis in original).

62. Employs positively reinforcing stimuli concurrently with the message, which may include nonverbal stimuli such as smiling and eye contact, verbal stimuli such as humorous remarks or expressions of respect, or material stimuli such as refreshments or pleasant surroundings (as in neighborhood picnics, get-togethers, and the like).

63. Employs mild distractors concurrently with the message, which can include any of the positively reinforcing stimuli specified directly above.

64. Requests an action step. Normally, the audience or target group should be asked to do something, even if no more than to pay attention. The proposed action, to begin with, should be (a) clear, (b) specific, (c) immediate (sooner, rather than later), (d) realizable (possible and feasible for the respondent to do), and (e) beneficial, in the sense of presenting understandable, tangible, and believable benefits for engaging in the proposed action or, conversely, costs for not engaging in it or for taking an opposing course. The recommended action may effectively be accompanied by explicit provision of reasons for acting, by descriptive bridging steps between request and execution (as in, "Do you think you might make a call or two?"), or by deadline statements, especially if the proposed benefits are scarce, the costs are severe, or the probability of either benefit or cost is likely (Cialdini, 1993).

Note that these desired characteristics for action steps parallel desired qualities for issues themselves (cf. propositions 35–42). But there are two others, which deserve separate enumeration:

65. Requests action of a size corresponding to the audience's knowledge of, concern about, and prior support for, the issue. When these measures are low, the requested step should be small; when higher, they should be larger. Note that larger requests in general seem to be more effective in producing attitude, rather than behavioral, change.

This is a delicate and still somewhat controversial area within the social-psychological literature, which has documented evidence both for the success of small initial requests [the foot-in-the-door technique; the proposed pilot, trial, or demonstration study (Freedman & Fraser, 1966; Rothman et al., 1976)], and also for larger ones [the door-in-the-face technique, i.e., requesting a large action first, and then scaling down the request as necessary (Cialdini, 1993)].

The delicacy lies in not wanting to ask for too much, nor for too little. A resolution here is to request action proportional to perceived audience investment in the issue and to ability to respond, and to err, if at all, on the side of modesty, of generating some response; for any action taken is likely to strengthen attachment to the cause ("ownership," in the community organization literature). Given some uncertainty, it may be possible to offer the respondent a menu of graded choices and request self-selection. In this regard, legitimizing even the most modest actions can sometimes be used to advantage, as in studies where an "even a penny will help" appeal has increased the percent of contribution compliance (Cialdini & Schroeder, 1976; Weyant, 1984).

66. Requests, if only implicitly, making a commitment to perform the action, preferably a public one that is or can be made known to others (e.g., Foss, 1986). Commitments in general will foster compliance, and compliance will, in turn, strengthen commitment. Commitment effects do not always appear (Burn & Oskamp, 1986; Katzev & Johnson, 1984), and mild commitments may be at least as effective as strong ones (Shippee & Gregory, 1982). However, research suggests that, in general, some commitment, and some action, should be elicited, no matter how small.

67. Anticipates and publicly acknowledges the possible sources of resistance to action, and provides customized arguments to overcome them, especially if resistance is believed to be strong, the issue important, and the audience intelligent.

68. Does not promote reactance, and thus generate a boomerang effect, by impinging upon the perceived freedom of the target group to choose. In clean-up campaigns, for example, strong anti-littering directives have sometimes been shown to increase littering instead (Reich & Robertson, 1979). Both ethically and practically, the message and the request can and should be convincing and forceful, but also openly respectful of the recipient's right and ability to decide.

69. Summarizes and encapsulates the message and the recommended action in an attractive and easy-to-remember manner, as in an aphorism, slogan, symbol, or pictorial device.

70. Is timed to occur directly before the prime opportunity to act (as in voting, demonstrations, etc.), though this need not, and ordinarily should not, preclude prior communications.

71. Reinforces (for example, thanks) the recipient after the message and recommendation are presented. The reinforcement should be attached to consideration of the recommendation content (thus maintaining recipient choice), rather than to expected compliance with it.

72. Inoculates the recipient against possible subsequent attempts by others to sway opinion or action in a different direction. This may be done, for instance, by presenting weak forms of opposing arguments and then refuting them.

73. Maintains the anticipated new belief or action with subsequent communications, designed as prompts, reminders, or "booster shots," to keep motivation and action potential high (Ferrari, Barone, Jason, & Rose, 1985; Geller et al., 1982; Oskamp & Schultz, 1998). It helps if the likelihood of these prompts occurring is established in advance.

74. Finally, evaluates the impact of the message and of the communication in general, because optimum effect in a given situation will call for a unique constellation of these message variables, operating at different intensities, frequencies, and durations. Evaluation is needed to pinpoint possible sources of success or failure, and to provide a basis for adjusting variable settings.

Evaluating the Evidence

Space limits oblige us to pause here and evaluate the information presented so far. Perhaps the key evaluative question is one of utility: How useful are these propositions to someone, community psychologist or otherwise, who actually intends to go out and do community organization on real streets, starting tomorrow, or else might some day do so?

It's hard to put a figure on it, but a best guess is that the propositions are more than marginally useful, and are as useful as any summation of empirical, derivative, and methodologically flawed data might be expected to be. Community psychology can with evidence and confidence point to circumstances that will aid and abet the community organizer, and which will favor most organizing efforts. That achievement should not be taken lightly. Community organization has a foundation of experience-based psychological principles. These principles help.

But the limits of these principles, and of present knowledge, should not be taken lightly either. To review: the principles in general are often inadequately documented, and are of largely untested generality, of unknown component weightings, imperfectly descriptive of nonlinear and interactional relationships, and atheoretical as well. In addition, they are incomplete, in two senses of the word.

In one sense, they are incomplete because the principles have not yet drawn fully from the full range of behavioral science knowledge. Other literatures within psychology could contribute additional propositions, and extensively so; these include social learning, social support, behavior modification, mass communication, and organizational development, to cite a few. The same applies to areas often considered outside academic psychology *per se*—public relations, graphic design, fund-raising, lobbying, and business administration, among others. None of these areas has been more than mentioned here.

In a second sense, these propositions are incomplete also because they do not tell the fledgling (or experienced) community organizer what to *do* when he or she walks out the door. What issue to choose? What tactics? Whom do you contact first? What do you say? What do you wear? For that kind of information, we must go beyond the formal research evidence and into the many volumes of advice that have been written by seasoned community organizers for greener ones. Their words are thoughtful, heartfelt, and forged by experience. But are they true?

To pick one from thousands of examples, Si Kahn's advice on organizing door-to-door:

1. Introduce yourself.
2. Ask if you can come in.
3. Talk about something you know they're interested in.
4. Find something in the home to talk about.
5. Talk to parents and kids together.... (Kahn, 1982, p. 116).

These points make sense. Yet wise as Kahn and others like him may be, they do not provide verifying data of the kind psychologists are used to. What evidence exists here is based upon personal experience, observation, testimony, and case study analysis. The evidence is empirical, but not systematic, nor experimental. There are no controls, no probability samples, no tested hypotheses, and no independent validity checks.

The case can be made that statements such as "introduce yourself," "ask if you can come in," and the like should not be judged only by precise evidential criteria. They are not hypotheses to be tested, but rather statements of common sense, meant mainly as reminders and as confidence-boosters; they are "beyond evidence" by their intent. In one variation of this argument, the first truth about community organization is that the best organizers move by intuition and feel. The second truth is that community organization is too subtle, too finely textured, and too elusive to be codified. You have to get your feet wet; you learn on the job.

But as psychologists, part of our job is to codify. As scientists, our standards of evidence should, in fact, be higher. Intuition is important, but intuitions are codes telescoped and internalized. Our codified knowledge now is flawed, yet is precious at the same time. It will not ensure victory, but it can give a winning edge. The codification we have is better than that of, say, 20 years ago, when community psychology was adolescent in years and stature. Now, as a young adult, perhaps right on schedule, there is the promise for further maturation. That's one next step among others, and it leads us into a section headed "Agenda."

AGENDA

Coming out of the community organization literature and going back to America heading into the twenty-first century, we run up against the need to link one to the other. The issue of linkage, of connecting our knowledge to the brightness and jumble and pulse of the world around us, defines our agenda. And it will take barely a moment to realize that that agenda is imposing, enormous, a lifetime's work at least. Because right now the linkages are tenuous and poorly appreciated, and the hard prospect is that we and our successors will be working far past the year 2000 before the psychology of community organization is given away as it should be given.

The agenda is enormous because well-chosen and well-designed research on untested and unsettled issues of community organization will continue to be essential; because retrieval and integration of accumulating evidence from inside and outside the discipline will be called for; because that integrated evidence will require dissemination; because dissemination must be accompanied by more vigorous application than in the past; and lastly because the need, and possibly also the desire, for community and neighborhood organization by citizens themselves is likely to grow, since less public money to start and maintain local services will probably be available, and also since any economic slowdown will force even more development of home-grown resources. The chances are excellent that increased community and neighborhood organization will become vital—perhaps crucial—to the maintenance of community life as we know and value it.

So we will need successive new waves of research, integration, dissemination, and application, and we will keep on needing them. These points are separately elaborated below. The bright side of this agenda is that many choices exist. The cafeteria of opportunity is open round the clock. The community psychologist/community organizer of the future will not go hungry for things to do, and won't be bored.

Research

Research in community organization should focus on content areas where we expect maximum applied yield. This means, first of all, studies of *practical persuasion*, in *natural settings*, where we analyze very concretely the content and the outcomes of real community-organizing actions, and the best ways to encourage people to take Step X.

Community psychology is still short on research in which people are studied making and carrying out actual decisions in their own neighborhoods and community settings, in vivo, not to mention research where residents have input and control over what's going on. It's not just the importance of being right at the scene; it's also that the operating principles may be somewhat different there. That is, local residents will have *ongoing* relationships with each other; the local organizer will need to be effective not only today, but also tomorrow and the day after; the appropriate techniques and qualities to sustain credibility and impact may then vary. Specifically, one may need to proceed more slowly, more cautiously, more gently, and more respectfully of people and their choices. This statement itself needs verification.

Some examples of research needed: What precise organizing techniques and styles are optimally and demonstrably effective in encouraging people to go to a meeting, sign a petition, speak at a hearing, ring a doorbell, write a letter, or get out and vote? What scripts and strategies work best on the phone? What specific appearance and content will prompt people to open, read, and heed a letter, flyer, or brochure? Here are fertile grounds for experimentation.

On a different tack, what kinds of people make the best organizers? The key personality and stylistic variables remain unclear. Though many types of people can excel at organizing, some will excel more than others (and some will step forward sooner than others), and what separates the A's from the B's.

And how, and how well, can organizers be trained? If we are to seriously consider training students to make community organization (however labelled) their careers, our present curricula must be reevaluated. What training modules or programs can be *demonstrated* to work? And if personality/stylistic attributes are important, can one, or *how* can one, train for them, draw them out, or at least encourage them? In current management talk, for example, there is much mention of "visionary" or "transformational" leadership (Bass, 1985; Pfeffer, 1998; Wilpert, 1995), which sounds like something we would want in the nonprofit sector too. So how could we, in full seriousness, train our students to be visionary leaders?

Finally on this short list, if we are interested in community organization as outcome as well as input, we ought to be looking at how well organized a community is, while seeking some scale or device with indicator values that are sensitive to particular organizing actions and measurable over extended time. How will those actions affect the measured level of organization? If "highly organized" communities are desired, how do we get there?

Several recent research directions allow for optimism. Fawcett and colleagues (Fawcett et al., 1982; Fawcett et al., 1984; Seekins, Mathews, & Fawcett, 1984; Seekins et al., 1987) have embarked upon an ambitious and multipronged program of behavioral technology, which, for example, has taught citizens to write "letters to the editor," form skills exchanges, and shape local human service agendas. The participation-building research of Wandersman and his co-investigators has been cited extensively elsewhere. D'Augelli and associates, in one of the rare lines of work dealing with rural populations (D'Augelli & Ehrlich, 1982; D'Augelli & Vallance, 1982), have indicated that helping ability can be further trained. A variety of scales on sense of community or neighborhood cohesion, at least tangentially related to degree of community organization, have been developed (e.g., Buckner, 1988; Chavis, Hogge, McMillan, & Wandersman, 1986; Glynn, 1986; see also the reviews in McMillan, 1996; McMillan & Chavis, 1986; and Puddifoot, 1996). Moreover, in one of the very few research studies ever to evaluate the effects of a specific organizing action, Steiner and Mark (1985) demonstrated that a particular organizing campaign reduced passbook savings account holdings in a targeted bank. More studies evaluating organizing attempts like this are guaranteed a warm welcome.

These research directions, and others like them, of course need red carpets. Research programs, as compared to one-shot studies, need special salutes. In encouraging both, we must also tolerate diversity of method. The experimental model, powerful and valuable as it is, will not always be applicable to, or available for, particular community organizing activities: ethics may not allow it, residents may not permit it, and a given campaign may be history by the time the researcher hears of it. The community psychologist must accordingly learn to appreciate and utilize the full spectrum of observational, historical, and qualitative methods, and to value them for what they can reveal, while not harping on what they can't.

Open arms need not mean indiscriminate embraces. The goal will be to supply the strongest evidence possible, given the situation. But given the situation, eclecticism applies. A student of community organization must be rigorous and selective, but also omnivorous.

Integration

Integration must follow research. The research, done and published, cannot just remain squashed between journal covers. Community organization really does cut across established disciplinary turf, and so we especially need formats and mechanisms for pulling diverse materials together. What should these be?

A full generation ago, the behavioral scientists Bernard Berelson and Gary Steiner published a distinguished and now nearly-forgotten book called *Human Behavior* (1964), in which they attempted to synthesize all known scientific information about behavior into a 700-page compendium of propositions. Ten years later, Jack Rothman published a related itemization of principles limited to social change (Rothman, 1974). Neither of these groundbreaking efforts has been repeated; both should be.

The time is right for a detailed propositional review of community organization (and community psychology, for that matter), going well beyond that given here. In that review, empirical principles would be thoroughly researched, compiled, organized, numbered, and displayed, together with statements as to the extent and quality of their supporting evidence. We would then have a manual of principles to serve as a field guide for practitioners, a teaching tool for instructors, and a hypothesis-generator for the theoretically-oriented. Such a manual would be revised on a regular basis, reflecting changes in the knowledge base.

We'd then be approaching "the state of the art." Alternatively, or in addition, we might develop something like an "Applied Community Psychology Annual," or an "Advances in Community Organization" series, the latter again with an interdisciplinary focus. These efforts begin when someone takes the first step. And that someone will have two major advantages over his or her predecessors—computerized information-search capacity, plus previous models to draw upon.

Dissemination

After integration comes dissemination. Once again, this goes beyond publication in academic journals. A general-audience book like Si Kahn's *Organizing* has sold over 20,000 copies (McGraw-Hill, personal communication); sales of this volume will not come close. There are good reasons why, but these figures must still be faced squarely. Any solid evidence on community organization, or any proposed inventory, must get out to practitioners, and general readers as well, so that it can be used.

Much of science is communication, and community psychologists, of all people, have not done a particularly good job at communicating to the general public. Few community psychologists have visibility outside the profession. We are not media stars or starlets, not household words; few of us are professionally known even in our own neighborhoods. And it's not that all of us should be, but rather that major opportunity awaits. Melton (1987), writing about psycholegal knowledge, makes the obvious but telling point that utilization is more likely when conscious attempts are made to disseminate; juvenile court judges, for example, will not read *AJCP*, but they might read *Time*, and they will read their state bar association newsletter. The implications for community psychology should be clear.

Publicizing and marketing our findings may be central to disciplinary effectiveness. One recent study of landmark private-sector product innovations (Nayak & Ketteringham, 1986), notes that success is attributable not only to great ideas, but also to great promotion. Likewise, maybe, for our innovations too. It is possible and desirable for community psychology in general and community organization in particular to be popularized without being trivialized, to be commercial without being sensational. And while this can come about through media coverage (and also coverage in our own introductory psychology texts; Cook, 1987), it can happen too through conscious partnerships with those we are serving (Chavis & Wandersman, 1986; Fawcett, 1990), so that they will become enmeshed in the work and, with training and inspiration from us, be able to carry it on.

But as things stand now, community psychologists (including the community-organization-minded among us) have done very little to promote their work to the outside world. As a result, the general public has little idea what community psychology is or can do; until this changes, that puzzlement will surely remain.

Application

Once disseminated, the research findings must be applied, so that they impact upon daily life. This is the practitioner's part of the agenda. The purpose of application should be to do good works—good enough and powerful enough so that strangers will take notice. Skillful applications should call attention to themselves; they should touch everyday people in pleasing and unexpected ways.

The list of possible settings for application is very long, much longer than we can deal with here. There is hardly an area of social life where community organization does not tie in. Suffice it to say that if an organization in the community exists, or should exist, community organization principles apply to it. Applications in many of these settings are considered in later chapters of this volume. But several equally important areas of application have been less frequently examined. We can give two illustrations.

The first of these is local government. If the question is how might the community psychologist apply community organization principles to strengthen local government, some answers are that he or she might organize voter registration or get-out-the-vote campaigns, consult to candidates running for local office, run for local office directly, draft and lobby for the passage of local legislation, work with local officials to expand citizen input into planning, recruit citizens for commissions and boards, consult and/or serve on those boards, and conduct workshops for municipal leaders. More generally, given an opening, the community psychologist can help bring community building toward the top of local government's agenda, which is exactly where it should be. Good government requires organized citizen action: the relationship between government and citizen should be not only agreeable and cooperative, but also symbiotic.

Neighborhood organizations themselves are another example. Imagine community psychologists and neighborhood organizations as natural allies. The alliance once established, the community psychologist can then apply community organizational principles to teach the organization how to assess community needs; design publicity; recruit and keep members; fix goals; set agendas; run meetings; design projects that will capture neighborhood attention; raise money for, trouble-shoot, and evaluate these projects; join forces with other neighborhoods; and obtain services from institutions. The psychologist might also sow seeds for an organization when one is lacking, perhaps by aligning with and influencing natural helping networks, perhaps by starting the organization oneself (Dreier, 1996; Saegert & Winkel, 1996; Watts, 1993; Wicker & Sommer, 1993).

This particular application is important because of the very reasons stated at the beginning of the chapter: Of all the settings where our disciplinary values and skills can be instilled, neighborhood and community organizations are among the easiest, while the rewards for both giver and recipient are among the highest. Externally-funded projects like Block Booster have worked successfully in New York, but the potential and need for low-cost neighborhood applications remain throughout the country. Such applications could easily become part of our graduate programs through evening courses for community leaders, field placements for graduate students, cross-disciplinary institutes, and multiagency collaboratives. Here would also be a next-door research laboratory, an excellent way to improve "town–gown" relations, and another area for symbiosis.

These types of applications, and other reported intentional applications of community organization principles, are relatively rare. Applied studies in the professional literature where the primary intent is to create some social benefit tend to be narrower in scope, e.g., on littering, donating blood, wearing a seat belt. At this point, we need to widen the sights, to work directly for social good on a larger scale. The way to do this is to start doing it, for few precedents are on file. The bonus, though, is that through such applications hypotheses can be tested and new propositions advanced. Application and research here combine.

Within all of this agenda, on the continuum from research, through integration, through dissemination and application, there is plenty of room to operate. Wide open spaces are the rule. Discovery, synthesis, communication, and action are all essential links in the loop. It is legitimate to step in anywhere, but it is important to step in somewhere. The first tasks for the community psychologist who sees the value of community organization are to plan one's entrance, take the step, and wave others on to follow.

CONCLUSIONS

The research and applied components we have been separately discussing fold together into a larger agenda, and that agenda is moral. Much debate in behavioral science has centered around the ethics of action, the "whens" and the "hows." The ethics of inaction have been less well-addressed. But there may be, especially in community and neighborhood organizing, some ethical injunction *to* intervene, in proper ways. Failure to act may be morally at fault. We come face-to-face with obligation and duty, those persistent callers.

To the extent that community and neighborhood organization embody our underlying disciplinary values and goals, the community psychologist may incur some obligation to foster them both. If local community and neighborhood organization will become increasingly essential in the United States and beyond, the community psychologist may have some duty to get personally involved, at least from a distance, and maybe up close. If we support a value shift in American society away from private pursuits and back toward public life, then community psychology, and community psychologists, should help bring about that shift. It, and we, should take a leadership role. To do so will require a different mindset, different talents, and a different order of willpower than that to which we've become accustomed. The question is from where the generative energy will come.

It may not come; we may fail to meet that challenge. As before, we may choose to, or need to, settle for knowledge gains through slow accretion, hoping that supply outruns demand. But maybe, just possibly, there could be some breakthrough idea on the horizon to turn our thinking around, even though odds might be against it. To look for a breakthrough, though, could help make it happen. At any rate, there's no harm in speculating on what such an idea might be.

Though we've not been able to weight the components of organizational success, I have personally come to believe that despite the importance of setting, issue, message variables, and the like, success lies fundamentally within the individual actor. I have seen too many triumphs that shouldn't have happened, were it not for some untutored citizen-turned-organizer who passionately wanted otherwise. We have few better words than "spirit" to explain those triumphs. Most of us have that same spirit tucked inside, the potential for extraordinary community accomplishment. If a breakthrough is possible, it may be connected with turning in upon one's self, in ways we do not normally consider as community psychologists. It may have to do with contemplating one's inner resources, marshalling them, strengthening them, or, saying it aloud, developing one's spiritual nature. (cf. Jason, 1997).

If asked to name the greatest community organizers in human history, we might name no better than our greatest spiritual leaders, the founders of world religions: Moses, Buddha, Jesus, Mohammed, among others. Their organizing ability derived from intense spiritual exploration and struggle, as well as periods of voluntary retreat from the world. But these are the people whose organizational accomplishments have endured for centuries and will endure when we are gone. However brilliant Saul Alinsky was, the Sermon on the Mount will outlive *Rules for Radicals*.

To put it differently, it may be that to organize most effectively, to create and execute and sustain a vision that will embrace strangers and help them embrace each other, one ought to explore one's self more fully. It may seem ironic that by going inside, one begins to appreciate, in ways not appreciated before, the community of all beings. Yet it may be true that acting on that basis, grounded and centered, yields impacts not previously achieved. We have no operational definitions, no empirical analyses, for terms like "grounding" or "centering": we could aim for them.

Spirituality may be a "personality variable," but, in any case, it is an unexamined one, particularly in its relationship to social change. It's a positive sign that a chapter on religious life is appearing in this volume. Another provocative (and moving) discussion linking spirituality to action may be found in a recent popular book by Dass and Gorman (1985); one of their vignettes brings out the point suggested here. In it, a Western student of meditation meets a Thai monk who was curing heroin and opium addicts, in ten days for $15, within a monastery he had built himself:

> When we met him, my most immediate reaction was that I was shaking hands with an oak tree.... As I hung out with him longer I began to realize that his mind was so centered and one-pointed that his being was stronger than their addiction. Somehow he conveyed to those addicts a sense of their non-addiction that was stronger than their addiction. And I saw that his commitment was so total, that he wasn't just someone using a skill. He had died into his work. He *was* the cure.... I returned to meditation with renewed vigor (pp. 95–96).

All this could be a false trail—simply the natural turning inward of the mind as one grows older. Or it could be that spiritual concern is a defense, a kind of coping mechanism for having to organize over and over and yet again, for not being able to do more in this world. Or possibly this is just a grasping for something new, something merely to "introduce drama and adventure into the tedium of middle-class life" (Alinsky, 1971, p. 195). We lack enough data to know what is true.

Having followed traditional approaches, we are wiser about community organization than we have been before. By continuing along the same lines, we can become wiser still. Nature will yield; persistence pays off. And yet, to think of ourselves as being that oak tree, as developing that one-pointed consciousness, then focusing it to heal community and self....

This approach seems so foreign, so far away from home. But might not its promise be worth pursuing?

REFERENCES

Ahlbrandt, R. S., Jr. (1984). *Neighborhoods, people, and community*. New York: Plenum.

Ahlbrandt, R. S., Jr., & Cunningham, J. V. (1979). *A new public policy for neighborhood preservation*. New York: Praeger.

Alinsky, S. (1971). *Rules for radicals: A practical primer for realistic radicals*. New York: Random House.

Alreck, P. L., & Settle, R. B. (1994). *The survey research handbook*, 2nd ed. Homewood, IL: Richard D. Irwin.

Aneshensel, C. S. (1992). Social stress: Theory and research. *Annual Review of Sociology, 18*, 15–38.

Bailey, K. D. (1994). *Methods of social research*, 4th ed. New York: Free Press.

Bass, B. M. (1985). *Leadership and performance beyond expectations*. New York: Free Press.

Bass, B. M., & Stogdill, R. M. (1990). *Bass and Stogdill's handbook of leadership: Theory, research, and managerial applications*, 3rd ed. New York: Free Press.

Batson, C. D. (1998). Altruism and prosocial behavior. In D. T. Gilbert, S. T. Fiske, & G. Lindzey (Eds.), *Handbook of social psychology*, Vol. 2. 4th ed. (pp. 282–316). New York: McGraw-Hill.

Berelson, B., & Steiner, G. A. (1964). *Human behavior: An inventory of scientific findings*. New York: Harcourt, Brace & World.

Berkowitz, B. (1987). *Local heroes*. Lexington, MA: Lexington Books.

Berry, J. M., Portney, K., & Thomson, K. (1993). *The rebirth of urban democracy*. Washington, D.C.: Brookings Institution.

Biklen, D. (1983). *Community organizing: Theory and practice*. Englewood Cliffs, NJ: Prentice-Hall.

Bobo, K., Kendall, J., & Max, S. (1991). *Organizing for social change: A manual for activists in the 1990s*. Cabin John, MD: Seven Locks Press.

Brager, G. A., Specht, H., & Torczyner, J. L. (1987). *Community organizing*, 2nd ed. New York: Columbia University Press.

Buckner, J. C. (1988). The development of an instrument to measure neighborhood cohesion. *American Journal of Community Psychology, 16*, 771–791.

Burghardt, S. (1982). *Organizing for community action*. Beverly Hills, CA: Sage.

Burn, S. M., & Oskamp, S. (1986). Increasing community recycling with persuasive communication and public commitment. *Journal of Applied Social Psychology, 16*, 29–41.

Burns, J. M. (1978). *Leadership*. New York: Harper & Row.

Campbell, A. (1981). *The sense of well-being in America: Recent patterns and trends*. New York: McGraw-Hill.

Chavis, D. M., Hogge, J. M., McMillan, D. W., & Wandersman, A. (1986). Sense of community through Brunswik's lens: A first look. *Journal of Community Psychology, 14*, 24–40.

Chavis, D. M., & Wandersman, A. (1986). Roles for research and the researcher in neighborhood development. In R. Taylor (Ed.), *Urban neighborhoods: Research and policy* (pp. 215–247). New York: Praeger.

Checkoway, B., & Van Til, J. (1978). What do we know about citizen participation?: A selective review of research. In S. Langton (Ed.)., *Citizen participation in America: Essays on the state of the art* (pp. 13–24). Lexington, MA: Lexington Books.

Cialdini, R. B. (1993). *Influence: Science and practice*, 3rd ed. New York: HarperCollins.

Cialdini, R. B., & Schroeder, D. A. (1976). Increasing contributions by legitimizing paltry contributions: When even a penny helps. *Journal of Personality and Social Psychology, 34*, 599–604.

Cialdini, R. B., & Trost, M. R. (1998). Social influence: social norms, conformity, and compliance. In D. T. Gilbert, S. T. Fiske, & Lindzey (Eds.), *Handbook of social psychology*, Vol. 2. 4th ed. (pp. 151–192). New York: McGraw-Hill.

Cook, J. R. (1987). Undergraduate education in community psychology: A call for action. *The Community Psychologist, 21*, 4–6.

Cunningham, J. V., & Kotler, M. (1983). *Building neighborhood organizations*. Notre Dame, IN: University of Notre Dame Press.

Dass, R., & Gorman, P. (1985). *How can I help?: Stories and reflections on service*. New York: Knopf.

D'Augelli, A. R., & Ehrlich, R. P. (1982). Evaluation of a community-based system for training natural helpers. II. Effects on informal helping activities. *American Journal of Community Psychology, 10*, 447–456.

D'Augelli, A. R., & Vallance, T. R. (1982). The helping community: Issues in the evaluation of a preventive intervention to promote informal helping. *Journal of Community Psychology, 10,* 199–209.

Diener, E. (1984). Subjective well-being. *Psychological Bulletin, 95,* 532–575.

Dillman, D. A. (1991). The design and administration of mail surveys. *Annual Review of Sociology, 17,* 225–249.

Dreier, P. (1996). Community empowerment strategies: The limits and potential of community organizing in urban neighborhoods. *Cityscape, 2,* 121–159.

Dyson, B. C., & Dyson, E. U. (1989). *Neighborhood caretakers: Stories, strategies, and tools for helping urban community.* Indianapolis, IN: Knowledge Systems.

Fawcett, S. B. (1990). Some emerging standards for community research and action: Aid from a behavioral perspective. In P. Tolan, C. Keys, F. Chertok, & L. Jason (Eds.), *Researching community psychology: Issues of theory and practice.* Washington, D.C.: America Psychological Association.

Fawcett, S. B., Fletcher, R. K., Mathews, R. M., Whang, P. L., Seekins, T., & Nielsen, L. M. (1982). Designing behavioral technologies with community self-help organizations. In A. M. Jeger & R. S. Slotnick (Eds.), *Community mental health and behavioral ecology: A handbook of theory, research, and practice* (pp. 281–302). New York: Plenum.

Fawcett, S. B., Seekins, T., Whang, P. L., Muiu, C., & Suarez de Balcazar, Y. (1984). Creating and using social technologies for community empowerment. *Prevention in Human Services, 3,* 145–171.

Ferrari, J. R., Barone, R. C., Jason, L. A., & Rose, T. (1985). The effects of a personal phone call prompt on blood donor commitment. *Journal of Community Psychology, 13,* 295–298.

Fischer, C. A., & Schwartz, C. A. (Eds.) (1995). *Encyclopedia of associations* (30th ed., Vol. 1, Part 2, Secs. 7 & 9). Detroit: Gale Research.

Fischer, C. S. (1982). *To dwell among friends: Personal networks in town and city.* Chicago: University of Chicago Press.

Fisher, R. (1984). Neighborhood organizing: Lessons from the past. *Social Policy, 15,* 9–16.

Fisher, R. (1985). *Let the people decide: Neighborhood organizing in America.* Boston: G. K. Hall.

Fiske, S. T. (1987). People's reactions to nuclear war: Implications for psychologists. *American Psychologist, 42* 207–217.

Florin, P. R., & Wandersman, A. (1984). Cognitive social learning and participation in community development. *American Journal of Community Psychology, 12,* 689–708.

Florin, P. R., & Wandersman, A. (1990). An introduction to citizen participation, voluntary organizations, and community development: Insights for empowerment through research. *American Journal of Community Psychology, 18,* 41–54.

Foss, R. D. (1986). Using social psychology to increase altruistic behavior: Will it help? In M. J. Saks & L. Saxe (Eds.), *Advances in applied social psychology,* Vol. 3 (pp. 127–151). Hillsdale, NJ: Erlbaum.

Freedman, J. L., & Fraser, S. C. (1966). Compliance without pressure: The foot-in-the-door technique. *Journal of Personality and Social Psychology, 4,* 195–202.

Geller, E. S., Johnson, R. P., & Pelton, S. L. (1982). Community-based interventions for encouraging seat belt use. *American Journal of Community Psychology, 10,* 183–195.

Gesten, E. L., & Jason, L. A. (1987). Social and community interventions. *Annual Review of Psychology, 38,* 427–460.

Gilbert, D. T., Fiske, S. T., & Lindzey, G. (Eds.). (1998). *Handbook of social psychology* (4th ed.). New York: McGraw-Hill.

Glidewell, J. C. (1986). *Psychosocial empowerment in community action.* Unpublished manuscript, Vanderbilt University. Cited in Gesten, E. L., & Jason, L. A. (1987), Social and community interventions. *Annual Review of Psychology, 38,* 427–460.

Glynn, T. J. (1986). Neighborhood and sense of community. *Journal of Community Psychology, 14,* 341–352.

Guest, A. M., & Oropesa, R. S. (1984). Problem-solving strategies of local areas in the metropolis. *American Sociological Review, 49,* 828–840.

Heller, K. (1990). Social and community interventions. *Annual Review of Psychology, 41,* 141–168.

Heller, K. (1992). Ingredients for effective community change: Some field observations. *American Journal of Community Psychology, 20,* 143–163.

Heller, K., Price, R. H., Reinharz, S., Riger, S., & Wandersman, A. (1984). *Psychology and community change* (2nd ed.). Homewood, IL: Dorsey.

Hodgkinson, V. A., & Weitzman, M. S. (1994). *Giving and volunteering in the United States: Findings from a national survey* (4th ed.). Washington, D.C.: Independent Sector.

Hollander, E. P. (1985). Leadership and power. In G. Lindzey & E. Aronson (Eds.), *Handbook of social psychology,* Vol. 2. 3rd ed. (pp. 485–537). New York: Random House.

Homan, M. S. (1994). *Promoting community change: Making it happen in the real world.* Pacific Grove, CA: Brooks/Cole.

House, J. S., Umberson, D., & Landis, K. R. (1988). Structures and processes of social support. *Annual Review of Sociology*, *14*, 293–318.

Jason, L. A. (1997). *Community building: Values for a sustainable future*. Westport, CT: Praeger.

Jeffres, L., & Dobos, J. (1984). Communication and neighborhood mobilization. *Urban Affairs Quarterly*, *20*, 97–112.

Kahn, S. (1982). *Organizing: A guide for grassroots leaders*. New York: McGraw-Hill.

Karlins, M., & Abelson, H. I. (1970). *Persuasion: How opinions and attitudes are changed.* (2nd ed.). New York: Springer.

Katzev, R. D., & Johnson, T. R. (1984). Comparing the effects of momentary incentives and foot-in-the-door strategies in promoting residential electricity conservation. *Journal of Applied Social Psychology*, *14*, 12–27.

Kettner, P., Daley, J. W., & Nichols, A. W. (1985). *Initiating change in organizations and communities: A macro practice model*. Monterey, CA: Brooks/Cole.

Kinder, D. R. (1998). Opinion and action in the world of politics. In D. T. Gilbert, S. T. Fiske, & G. Lindzey (Eds.), *Handbook of social psychology*, Vol. 2. 4th ed. (pp. 778–867). New York: McGraw-Hill.

Knoke, D. (1986). Associations and interest groups. *Annual Review of Sociology*, *12*, 1–21.

Kretzmann, J. P., & McKnight, J. L. (1993). *Building communities from the inside out: A path toward finding and mobilizing a community's assets*. Chicago: ACTA Publications.

Levine, M., & Perkins, D. V. (1997). *Principles of community psychology: Perspectives and applications* (2nd ed.). New York: Oxford University Press.

Lounsbury, J. W., Leader, D. S., Meares, E. P., & Cook, M. P. (1980). An analytic review of research in community psychology. *American Journal of Community Psychology*, *8*, 415–441.

Mattaini, M. A., & Thyer, B. A. (Eds.). (1996). *Finding solutions to social problems: Behavioral strategies for change*. Washington, D.C.: American Psychological Association.

Mattesich, P., & Monsey, B. (1997). *Community building: What makes it work: A review of factors influencing successful community building*. St. Paul, MN: Amherst H. Wilder Foundation.

McMillan, D. W. (1996). Sense of community. *Journal of Community Psychology*, *24*, 315–325.

McMillan, D. W., & Chavis, D. M. (1986). Sense of community: A definition and theory. *Journal of Community Psychology*, *14*, 6–23.

Medoff, P., & Sklar, H. (1994). *Streets of hope: The fall and rise of an urban neighborhood*. Boston: South End Press.

Melton, G. B. (1987). Bringing psychology to the legal system: Opportunities, obstacles, and efficacy. *American Psychologist*, *42*, 488–495.

Miller, J. G. (1978). *Living systems*. New York: McGraw-Hill.

Minkler, M. (Ed.) (1997). *Community organizing and community building for health*. New Brunswick, NJ: Rutgers University Press.

Mondros, J. B., & Wilson, S. M. (1994). *Organizing for power and empowerment*. New York: Columbia University Press.

Mott, A. H. (1997). *Building systems of support for neighborhood change*. Washington, D.C.: Center for Community Change.

Naparstek, A. J., Biegel, D. E., & Spiro, H. R. (1982). *Neighborhood networks for humane mental health care*. New York: Plenum.

Nayak, P. R., & Ketteringham, J. M. (1986). *Breakthroughs!* New York: Rawson Associates.

Novaco, R. W., & Monahan, J. (1980). Research in community psychology: An analysis of work published in the first six years of the *American Journal of Community Psychology*. *American Journal of Community Psychology*, *8*, 131–145.

Oskamp, S., & Schultz, P. W. (1998). *Applied social psychology*, 2nd ed. Upper Saddle River, NJ: Prentice Hall.

Petty, R. E., & Wegener, D. T. (1998). Attitude change: Multiple roles for persuasion variables. In D. T. Gilbert, S. T. Fiske, & G. Lindzey (Eds.), *Handbook of social psychology*, Vol. 1. 4th ed. (pp. 323–390). New York: McGraw-Hill.

Petty, R. E., Wegener, D. T., & Fabrigar, L. R. (1997). Attitudes and attitude change. *Annual Review of Psychology*, *48*, 609–647.

Pfeffer, J. (1998). Understanding organizations: conflicts and controversies. In D. T. Gilbert, S. T. Fiske, & G. Lindzey (Eds.), *Handbook of social psychology*, Vol. 2. 4th ed. (pp. 733–777). New York: McGraw-Hill.

Pilisuk, M., & Parks, S. H. (1986). *The healing web: Social networks and human survival*. Hanover, NH: University Press of New England.

Puddifoot, J. E. (1996). Some initial considerations in the measurement of community identity. *Journal of Community Psychology*, *24*, 327–336.

Reich, J. W., & Robertson, J. L. (1979). Reactance and norm appeal in anti-littering messages. *Journal of Applied Social Psychology*, *9*, 91–101.

Rich, R. C., & Wandersman, A. (1983). Participation in block organizations. *Social Policy*, *14*, 45–47.

Roberts, D. F., & Maccoby, N. (1985). Effects of mass communication. In G. Lindzey & E. Aronson (Eds.), *Handbook of social psychology*, Vol. 2, 3rd ed. (pp. 539–598). New York: Random House.

Rodin, J. (1985). The application of social psychology. In G. Lindzey & E. Aronson (Eds.), *Handbook of social psychology*, Vol. 2, 3rd ed. (pp. 805–881). New York: Random House.

Rothman, J. (1974). *Planning and organizing for social change: Action principles from social science research.* New York: Columbia University Press.

Rothman, J. (1995). Approaches to community intervention. In J. Rothman, J. L. Erlich, & J. Tropman (Eds.), *Strategies of community intervention*, 5th ed. (pp. 26–63). Itasca, IL: F. E. Peacock.

Rothman, J., Erlich, J. L., & Teresa, J. G. (1976). *Promoting innovation and change in organizations and communities.* New York: Wiley.

Rothman, J., Erlich, J. L., & Tropman, J. E. (Eds.). (1995). *Strategies of community organization: Macro practice*, 5th ed. Itasca, IL: F. E. Peacock.

Saegert, S., & Winkel, G. (1996). Paths to community empowerment: Organizing at home. *American Journal of Community Psychology, 24*, 517–550.

Seekins, T., Fawcett, S. B., & Mathews, R. M. (1987). Effects of self-help guides on three consumer advocacy skills: Using personal experience to influence public policy. *Rehabilitation Psychology, 32*, 29–38.

Seekins, T., Mathews, R. M., & Fawcett, S. B. (1984). Enhancing leadership skills for community self-help organizations through behavioral instruction. *Journal of Community Psychology, 12*, 155–163.

Shippee, G., & Gregory, W. L. (1982). Public commitment and energy conservation. *American Journal of Community Psychology, 10*, 81–93.

Simon, J. L. (1993). *How to start and operate a mail-order business*, 5th ed. New York: McGraw-Hill.

Snyder, M., & Cantor, N. (1998). Understanding personality and social behavior: A functionalist strategy. In D. T. Gilbert, S. T. Fiske, & G. Lindzey (Eds.), *Handbook of social psychology*, Vol. 1. 4th ed. (pp. 635–679). New York: McGraw-Hill.

Steiner, D. D., & Mark, M. M. (1985). The impact of a community action group: An illustration of the potential of time series analysis for the study of community groups. *American Journal of Community Psychology, 13*, 13–30.

Taylor, S. E., Repetti, R. L., & Seeman, T. (1997). Health Psychology: What is an unhealthy environment and how does it get under the skin? *Annual Review of Psychology, 48*, 411–447.

Tropman, J. E., Erlich, J. L., & Rothman, J. (Eds.). (1995). *Tactics and techniques of community intervention*, 3rd ed. Itasca, IL: F. E. Peacock.

Unger, D. G., & Wandersman, A. (1982). Neighboring in an urban environment. *American Journal of Community Psychology, 10*, 493–509.

Unger, D. G., & Wandersman, A. (1983). Neighboring and its role in block organizations: An exploratory report. *American Journal of Community Psychology, 11*, 291–300.

Unger, D. G., & Wandersman, A. (1985). The importance of neighbors: The social, cognitive, and affective components of neighboring. *American Journal of Community Psychology, 13*, 139–169.

Vallance, T. R., & D'Augelli, A. R. (1982). The helping community: Characteristics of natural helpers. *American Journal of Community Psychology, 10*, 197–205.

Vernon, C. L., & D'Augelli, A. R. (1987). Community involvement in prevention programs: The use of a telephone survey for program development. *Journal of Community Psychology, 15*, 23–28.

Wandersman, A., & Florin, P. (1984). Community psychology and the questions of participation. *Citizen Participation, 5*, 7, 8, 20.

Wandersman, A., Jakubs, J. F., & Giamartino, G. (1980). Community and individual difference characteristics as influences on initial participation. *American Journal of Community Psychology, 8*, 217–228.

Warner, I. R. (1992). *The art of fund raising* (3rd ed.). Farmington Hills, MI: Taft Group.

Warren, R. B., & Warren, D. I. (1977). *The neighborhood organizer's handbook.* Notre Dame, IN: University of Notre Dame Press.

Watts, R. J. (1993). "Resident research" and community psychology. *American Journal of Community Psychology, 21*, 483–486.

Weyant, J. M., (1984). Applying social psychology to induce charitable donations. *Journal of Applied Social Psychology, 14*, 441–447.

Weyant, J. M. (1986). *Applied social psychology.* New York: Oxford University Press.

Wicker, A. W., & Sommer, R. (1993). The resident researcher: An alternative career model centered on community. *American Journal of Community Psychology, 21*, 469–482.

Wilpert, B. (1995). Organizational behavior. *Annual Review of Psychology, 46*, 59–90.

Wittig, M. A., & Bettencourt, B. A. (Eds.) (1996). Social psychological perspectives on grassroots organizing. *Journal of Social Issues* [special issue] *52*, 1–220.

Zander, A. (1990). *Effective social action by community groups.* San Francisco: Jossey-Bass.

Zimbardo, P. G., Ebbesen, E. B., & Maslach, C. (1977). *Influencing attitudes and changing behavior: An introduction to method, theory, and applications of social control and personal power*, 2nd ed. Reading, MA: Addison-Wesley.

Zimbardo, P. G., & Leippe, M. R. (1991). *The psychology of attitude change and social influence*. New York: McGraw-Hill.

CHAPTER 15

The Creation of Alternative Settings

CARY CHERNISS AND GENE DEEGAN

> It must be considered that there is nothing more difficult to carry out, nor more doubtful of success, nor more dangerous to handle, than to initiate a new order of things.
>
> NICCOLO MACHIAVELLI, *The Prince*

This quote from Machiavelli captures the spirit of much that has been written about the creation of alternative settings. There are no data on the incidence of failure in the creation of alternatives, but the literature on this topic implies that it is quite high. New settings usually begin with great expectations, but hope frequently gives way to disillusionment within a relatively short time (Sarason, 1972). Nevertheless, there have been some notable exceptions: alternative settings that not only survived, but remained true to their original spirit. What, then, are the factors that influence the ultimate success or failure of alternative settings? If the creation of alternative settings is to be a viable intervention strategy in community psychology, this is a crucial question to address.

Thus, the focus of this chapter is on factors associated with success. Most previous works on alternative settings have not been primarily concerned with how one might maximize success. Instead, they have sought to describe alternative settings and identify distinctive problems and processes. However, even though the empirical base for the creation of alternative settings is a limited one, there has been enough research to provide some guidance. Because individuals will continue to create alternative settings, it seems better to develop guidelines based on systematic research, however limited it may be, than allow setting creators to proceed in ignorance.

CARY CHERNISS AND GENE DEEGAN • Graduate School of Applied and Professional Psychology, Rutgers University, Piscataway, New Jersey 08854.

Handbook of Community Psychology, edited by Julian Rappaport and Edward Seidman. Kluwer Academic / Plenum Publishers, New York, 2000.

DEFINITION AND SCOPE OF THE PROBLEM

Before considering what factors contribute to creating a successful setting, it might be helpful to define what is meant by "the creation of alternative settings," and place it in the context of this volume. Those who wish to make social systems more just and responsive have several intervention strategies from which to choose. They can work collaboratively within a system as consultants or members of the system, using information and persuasion to effect change. Or they can assume a more adversarial stance. In either case, the focus is on changing existing systems; the consultant or activist takes the system as it is and attempts to make it better. Creators of alternative settings take a radically different approach. In creating an alternative, one chooses to abandon or ignore existing institutions.

Using Sarason's (1972) very broad definition, the creation of settings can occur at any of several different levels. He defines the creation of a setting as "any instance in which two or more people come together in new relationships over a sustained period of time in order to achieve certain goals" (Sarason, 1972, p. 1). Thus, new settings can include a marriage, a group, a new program within an existing organization, or a new organization. Settings also can be found at higher levels: communities (e.g., a commune or a planned "new town") or even societies. In fact, one of Sarason's favorite examples is the original constitutional convention in 1787, which created a new, national political system. Using Sarason's broad definition, alternative settings thus can vary greatly in size and level. They also can vary in scope (e.g., a commune, which encompasses all aspects of life, versus a bakery, which is merely a workplace for its staff and a store selling one type of food for its customers).

Given the great breadth of community psychology, Sarason's very general definition may be appropriate, for community psychologists seek to work on many different levels and address many different aspects of community life. However, in practice, the creation of alternative settings in community psychology has usually involved either groups (e.g., self-help groups or block clubs) or formal organizational settings. In fact, much of the literature on this topic has been limited to human service and educational settings. Thus, in this chapter we will try to adopt a middle course: the domain will include more than just human-service programs, but no claim will be made that the conclusions will encompass intimate relationships (such as marriage), informal groups with little or no task focus, or very large systems (such as societies). What we write about the creation of alternative settings will apply primarily to relatively permanent groups created to achieve a specific purpose, organizational settings, and relatively small, circumscribed communities.

Having defined "setting," the next term that needs to be considered is "alternative." New settings are not necessarily *alternative* settings. One definition of what constitutes a true alternative was developed by Kanter and Zurcher (1973): "Alternative [settings] are radically different ways of perceiving, enacting, and experiencing work, religion, family, politics, education, leisure, therapy, and other basic relationships and life activities" (p. 173). In other words, an alternative setting is meant to be an alternative to something else. It is a protest, a reaction, an attempt to find a better way, a rejection. (Community psychology itself thus began as an alternative setting—an alternative to clinical psychology.)

In the 1960s, when community psychology emerged and the term "alternative setting" became popular, most alternative settings were progressive, democratic, antiprofessional, and antibureaucratic. But in the last two decades, we have seen the emergence of fundamentalist religious cults, communes, and even societies (e.g., Iran). These alternative settings are reactionary, authoritarian, and antihumanistic. Yet they, too, are alternative settings as defined by Kanter and Zurcher, even though they clearly differ from progressive alternatives in many important ways.

Another problem with many definitions of alternativeness is that they imply a categorical construct: a setting either is, or is not, an alternative. Yet there are many settings that fall somewhere on a continuum between alternative and traditional. For instance, both a quality circle for teachers in an elementary school and a social support group for parents of young children are intended to fill gaps or correct deficiencies left by existing institutions; both are new, innovative types of settings. But do they represent "radically different ways of perceiving ..."?

These examples suggest that alternativeness actually is a continuous construct; it also seems to be a multidimensional one. A setting can be alternative in terms of its *organizational structure* (e.g., antibureaucratic or collective), *goals* (e.g., serving a target population not served by traditional settings), *ideology* (e.g., a new religious group), or *technology* (e.g., the first behavior modification program for autistic children). A traditional–alternative continuum can be defined for each of these dimensions, and any particular setting can be placed somewhere on each continuum. Many alternative settings actually may fall on different points of the continuum for each dimension. In other words, a given setting may be more nontraditional in its structure, but more traditional in its goals.

This discussion of the problems involved in defining alternativeness is relevant for the ensuing sections of this chapter. The research on the creation of alternative settings has been done on settings that vary in ideology and values, as well as in where they fall on the various dimensions. In general, the research has dealt with relatively unambiguous cases: progressive, antibureaucratic, and antiprofessional settings that clearly would fall on the nontraditional end of the continuum for virtually all of the dimensions. It is not clear to what extent the results of this research apply to settings that are more traditional on some of the dimensions.

There also is some ambiguity inherent in the term "creation." Sarason, in the definition presented above, refers to two or more people "coming together." A somewhat more elaborate definition was suggested by Van de Ven, Hudson, and Schroeder (1984, p. 95): "Organizational creation is a collective, network-building achievement that centers on the inception, diffusion, and adoption of a set of ideas among a group of people who become sufficiently committed to these ideas to transfer them into a social situation." Whatever definition one adopts, ambiguity results because there is a fine line between creating a new setting and changing an existing one. For instance, imagine a couple that marries, and then some time later they decide to start a family by having a child. Is the birth of the child a change in the existing setting that was created when the couple married, or, as the phrase "starting a family" implies, is the child's birth really the creation of a new setting?

Although we are regarding setting creation and setting change as distinctly different intervention strategies in this volume, in reality we are usually dealing with intervention strategies that lie on a continuum between these two extremes. If this is the case, much of what is said about the creation of settings may also apply to some instances of planned change of existing settings. On the other hand, some of the conclusions that have emerged from the study of the creation of distinctly new, separate settings may not apply to the creation of settings within existing systems, where it is not clear whether we are dealing with setting creation or organizational change. But having considered some of the ambiguities and attendant problems inherent in trying to define "the creation of alternative settings," we now can consider how this area emerged as a central concern in community psychology.

THE EMERGENCE OF SETTING CREATION AS A PROBLEM

Like many problems in the social sciences, the creation of alternative settings has been rediscovered many times over the ages. For instance, Plato's *Republic* could be seen as an early (and still relevant) attempt to understand and improve on the process by which social systems emerge. However, as Sarason (1972) noted, many of the works in the utopian tradition have not really examined the creative process in a systematic, empirical way. Most utopian works, from Plato to Skinner, have presented ideal designs for social systems, describing in great detail how they should function, but not indicating how one might "get from here to there."

A more empirical tradition has been the sociological research on social movements, communes, and voluntary organizations. Long before community psychologists became involved with alternative settings, sociologists were studying the dynamics and problems of these types of settings. But it was Seymour Sarason's seminal work, *The Creation of Settings and the Future Societies* (1972), that marked the emergence of this topic as a major concern in community psychology.

Sarason's interest in the creation of settings grew out of his earlier work with other intervention strategies. During the early 1960s, Sarason and his colleagues at the Yale Psycho-Educational Clinic had worked as consultants in a number of community settings (Sarason, Levine, Goldenberg, Cherlin, & Bennett, 1966). Initially, the focus of their consultation was individual "cases," but they soon became involved in organizational change efforts as well. They found that many of the settings in which they worked were plagued by "organizational craziness," i.e., poor communication, inefficient and irrational problem-solving processes, cumbersome bureaucratic procedures, interpersonal and intergroup conflict, low morale, an excessive preoccupation with protecting one's own interests, etc. They came to believe that these destructive organizational processes adversely affected individual well-being and made it nearly impossible to treat, much less prevent, psychological problems in these settings.

As Sarason and his group became more deeply involved in organizational change efforts, they discovered that the amount of time and effort necessary to effect change in even a relatively small social system was considerable. Employing the same economic logic used by Albee (1959) in his earlier critique of traditional psychotherapy as a vehicle of individual change, Sarason concluded that organizational consultation was similarly limited as an intervention strategy: There simply were too many organizations needing help, too few organizational consultants to help them, and little hope of ever having enough trained personnel to "catch up." Sarason then concluded that the idea of prevention was as applicable to settings as it was to individuals. He became convinced that it ultimately would make more sense to prevent organizational craziness than to treat it, and the best way to prevent it would be to create new settings in ways that would make them resistant to the self-destructive processes found in too many established settings.

Of course, there are many other appealing reasons for creating alternative settings. Alternative settings can meet needs not currently being met by existing institutions, and can provide greater choice and diversity within a society. Creating an alternative setting also is a strategy for empowering people. Further, alternative settings can have a radiating effect by providing "demonstrations of new social forms that others can adopt if they so choose" (Reinharz, 1984, p. 329).

As Sarason began to systematically study his own experiences in creating new settings, as well as those of others, he soon became convinced of three things. First, creating a new setting was very different from managing or even changing a setting that already existed. Second, the process of creating a new setting was filled with difficulties and perils. In fact, he came to see how many of the problems that plagued "mature" settings really had their roots in the earliest periods of a setting's history: How a setting was created seemed to affect how it subsequently developed. Third, there were no "conceptual roadmaps" to help creators of new settings effectively deal with the problems they faced. Thus, in order to reduce the incidence of organizational craziness, Sarason believed that community psychologists needed to intervene early during the creation phase. Also, in order to do a better job of creating new settings, community psychologists needed to help develop a new science and art of setting creation.

Although Sarason's thinking broke much new ground, there had been earlier intimations of many of his basic notions, even within psychology. For instance, in a book describing the creation of an innovative treatment program in a traditional mental hospital, Colarelli and Siegel (1966) concluded by proposing that psychologists become "social systems architects." However, Sarason's work was the first within community psychology to place the creation of settings in the context of the field's other major intervention strategies. Also, it made a significant start in developing a more systematic set of guiding principles for the creation of new settings, and inspired several more works on the topic (e.g., Cherniss, 1972; Goldenberg, 1971; Perkins, Nieva, and Lawler, 1983; Trickett, 1991). Together, these empirical and theoretical efforts have provided a rich source of insights on how to create more successful alternative settings.

CHARACTERISTICS OF ALTERNATIVE SETTINGS

The creation of alternative settings can be a particularly difficult and discouraging intervention strategy. Establishing an alternative setting often is a lengthy, frustrating process, and even after a new setting becomes operational, many potential problems and pitfalls remain. In fact, one of the findings to emerge from research on alternative settings is that many do not survive beyond the first year or so, and those that do often lose their "essence" and become more like traditional settings as time passes (Rappaport, Seidman, & Davidson, 1979).

New alternative settings often *do* have many positive features. In the earliest stages, alternatives tend to be less bureaucratic: there is a sharper focus on the guiding purposes of the setting; there are few, if any rules; and roles are largely undifferentiated and fluid. The climate tends to be characterized by high energy and good will. Member rewards tend to be nonmonetary, e.g., ideological commitment, social contact, personal growth, and autonomy. Influence tends to be shared widely among a closely knit, cohesive core group (Holleb & Abrams, 1975; Jason & Kobayashi, 1995; Perkins et al., 1983; Trickett, 1991).

On the other hand, alternative settings often manifest various shortcomings, even during the early stages. Such settings tend to be "underbounded" (Alderfer, 1980; Trickett, 1991)—role obligations are fragmented and unclear, and responsibility for specific tasks is diffuse. As a result, efficiency and productivity suffer. The quality of care may be much more uneven in these sorts of settings. Important work often does not get done, and "public relations" frequently are handled poorly. Also, there typically is little or no money available for securing necessities, decision-making procedures are obscure, and interpersonal conflicts and power struggles seem to emerge relatively soon after the new setting becomes operational. Finally, the commitment of setting members often is uncertain and difficult to sustain, and workers seem to be more likely to experience burnout (Holleb & Abrams, 1975; Reinharz, 1984).

In addition to these internal problems, new alternative settings also tend to encounter indifferent, if not hostile, external environments. External relations tend to be problematic in new alternative settings, in part because alternatives challenge traditional settings. Thus, it is not unusual for alternative settings to encounter legal barriers, social ostracism, and even violence. Funding also can be particularly difficult to obtain for these kinds of settings (Reinharz, 1984). Yet, unless they can become totally autonomous and self-sufficient, new alternative settings depend to some extent on the institutions they challenge.

Some sort of compromise and accommodation with the external world thus is almost inevitable, and the negotiation process represents yet another threat to an alternative setting. The alternative may compromise too little and find itself driven out of business, or it may compromise too much and lose its distinctiveness. For instance, mutual aid and self-help groups gain legitimacy and expertise when they collaborate with professionals, but the professionals quickly may come to dominate these programs. When this happens, the alternatives may lose the qualities that make them uniquely helpful to their members (Cherniss & Cherniss, 1987).

Even when new alternative settings are able to preserve their distinctiveness, they eventually may become victims of their own success. As alternative settings grow and establish legitimacy, traditional settings may adopt some features of the alternatives in order to maintain their competitive advantage. When this happens, resources that might have gone to the alternative instead will go to the traditional setting, which usually can offer more stability and legitimacy.

Thus, it is not surprising that, over time, alternative settings that survive tend to change in character. They often become more formal, more differentiated, and more bureaucratic. Power comes to be exercised by a small, select group of people. Roles become more clearly defined and rigid, while communication is less open. The initial core group begins to split into different factions; a formal hierarchy is set up. Personal growth or social support become less important rewards for setting members, and monetary remuneration becomes more important. In other words, alternative settings over time come to resemble traditional settings.

This pattern of change has been noted by a number of researchers (e.g., Holleb & Abrams, 1975; Perkins et al., 1983; Sarason, 1972; Trickett, 1991) and is consistent with classical organizational theory. For instance, Weber (1947) proposed that charismatic organizations eventually become bureaucracies, and Michel's "Iron Law of Oligarchy" stated that, in any form of government, power eventually comes into the hands of a small group of people (Reinharz, 1984).

Greiner (1972) has proposed a general principle of organizational evolution that seems to explain why so many alternative settings become more bureaucratic and traditional over time. He rejects the popular view that new settings change over time because they are "co-opted," or undermined by external forces in their environment. Instead, he suggests that the distinctive characteristics of the initial stage create tension and conflict that increase over time. In their effort to reduce these strains, members of the setting tend to adopt changes that make the setting more differentiated, hierarchical, and bureaucratic.

For instance, the informal communication and decision-making processes characteristic of the first stage tend to require considerable amounts of time, which leads to frustration and impatience (Mansbridge, 1973; Trickett, 1991). Over time, more formal and hierarchical patterns may emerge in order to increase efficiency. As another example, interpersonal conflicts tend to increase in frequency and disruptiveness over time because there are neither adequate organizational mechanisms nor individual competencies for dealing with such conflicts in the early period. Setting members gradually begin to create rules as a way of reducing conflict, and the setting then becomes more bureaucratic. As this occurs, workers become less satisfied with receiving little or no pay, and monetary rewards become more important (Reinharz, 1984).

When the early problems of alternative settings come to be attributed to "a lack of resources," as frequently happens, another force pushing the setting toward bureaucracy may become activated. Members of the setting begin to feel that if they could secure more resources (physical space, money, equipment, clients, skilled staff), the setting would function better and satisfaction would increase. Attempts then are made to secure more resources from the environment. But outside support brings with it new demands: bookkeeping requirements, compliance with externally imposed rules, and other forms of accountability. Thus, many of the characteristic problems found in new alternative settings seem to generate forces that eventually undermine their distinctiveness. The settings may survive, but their potential to provide a true alternative is lost.

Fortunately, not all alternative settings fail or lose their distinctiveness with the passage of time. For instance, Alcoholics Anonymous has retained many of its original organizational characteristics for over 50 years, and some religious communes created in the last century persisted in their original form for nearly a century (Holloway, 1966; Kanter, 1972). However, there clearly are forces within alternative settings, as well as in their environments, that threaten their survival. This state of affairs calls into question their efficacy as an intervention strategy. Unless creators of alternative settings are able to find ways of dealing with these forces, their efforts are bound to fail. Fortunately, research on the creation of alternative settings has suggested a number of actions that seem to promote success.

THE CREATIVE PROCESS: GUIDELINES FOR INTERVENTION

Previous research on the creation of alternative settings can be a rich source of guidelines for those who wish to use this strategy. This research has examined both successes and failures, and has involved a variety of different kinds of settings. And, to a surprising degree, the conclusions tend to converge. Although we are a long way from a "science" of setting creation, it is possible to identify a large number of empirically based guidelines for the creation of alternative settings.

External Relations

As noted in the previous section, alternative settings often have problematic relations with their environment. Hostility and resistance from external groups represents a major source of difficulty. Such resistance can be particularly frustrating because creators of new settings usually have limited control over external factors. However, the research does suggest a number of ways in which new settings can promote a more positive response from their environment.

The first guiding principle is that one should identify potential sources of conflict and opposition before they emerge and create difficulty. One specific way of doing this is to examine a new setting's "prehistory" (Sarason, 1972). According to Sarason, resistance can begin during a new setting's prehistory for any one of a number of reasons. First, the idea for any new, alternative setting contains within it a criticism of existing settings. Those settings that are being challenged are one potential source of opposition.

Second, new alternative settings are in competition with older settings for scarce resources. Any existing setting that may lose resources to a new setting represents another potential source of opposition. Third, any individual or group that was denied a voice in the creation of a new setting also may become a source of opposition later. Finally, even when other individuals and groups have had a voice in the process, there often will have been some heated debates about whether the new setting should be created and what form it should take. Those who "lost" important debates may become adversaries in the future.

Thus, a new setting's prehistory can provide many clues about where opposition may arise. Creators of new settings should devote a considerable amount of thought and effort to the process of identifying potential sources of opposition. Part of this effort should be directed towards cultivating key informants who can help the creators develop an adequate understanding of a new setting's precursors (Goldenberg, 1971).

Identifying potential sources of resistance is useful, but what should one do once they are identified? The most frequent recommendation found in the literature is that one should "involve" potentially resistant outsiders as early as possible (Bartunek & Betters-Reed, 1987; Goldenberg, 1971; Reinharz, 1984). As Goldenberg put it, in order to maintain control over a setting, its creators must share control with others. Ideally, one should involve outside groups early, in the planning process, even before the new setting has come into existence (Bartunek & Betters-Reed, 1987). This involvement should be more than tokenism: Goldenberg (1971) found that attempting to "convert" community groups was less effective in winning their support than trying to learn from them. The most effective approach was to involve outsiders in concrete ways; for instance, an important member of one community organization was enlisted to build a carpentry shop in the basement of a new residential program for inner-city youth (Goldenberg, 1971). Reinharz (1984) has suggested two other methods for involving outsiders: share board members with "mainstream" agencies, and seek out formal consultation from mainstream organizations and individuals (e.g., professionals).

The staff of another new alternative setting tried to involve others in their program, while also seeking ways of becoming involved in other programs in the community (Sarason, Zitnay, & Grossman, 1971). A considerable amount of staff time was set aside to help other agencies and groups develop their own programs. Such a practice helped to win the support of external settings that might have opposed the new program. A similar tactic was used by the community residential alternative described by Goldenberg (1971): any member of the community was allowed to use the center's facilities free of charge. In all of these cases, the underlying principle that was used seems to be one of reciprocity, or "resource exchange." Giving and getting help from potential adversaries seems to be a particularly effective way of reducing resistance.

However, the ultimate effectiveness of any tactic for gaining support probably will depend on one's attitudes towards external groups. For instance, the staff in one program worked hard to adopt a positive attitude even towards those groups (e.g., the police) whom they initially perceived in negative ways (Goldenberg, 1971). By setting aside the stereotypes they had about these groups, they found that they could more effectively develop collaborative relationships with them. Unfortunately, those who create new alternative settings often adopt a superior, if not hostile, attitude towards outsiders (Sarason, 1972). Such an outlook, though understandable in some cases, most likely will increase opposition.

On the other hand, even having the most benevolent attitude towards external groups may not be sufficient for securing their support. Bartunek and Betters-Reed (1987) found that involving outside groups in the planning process was not effective if the "social climate" was particularly negative. For instance, those who have attempted to establish community residential programs for "undesirables" in middle-class neighborhoods have sometimes found that trying to inform and involve the neighbors early in the process just gave them the extra time and information necessary to effectively block establishment of the new program. Thus, in some cases, a covert entry strategy may be a more effective way of dealing with external resistance. More research is needed to determine when collaborative strategies are indicated.

Until now we have considered the best ways to deal with potentially hostile groups in the external environment. Yet the environment can contain friends as well as adversaries. Even if many outside groups remain hostile, alternative settings can enhance their chances of success by forming ties with other alternatives that share many of their goals and ideologies. Such linkages can include mutual funding arrangements, information exchanges, and lobbying efforts (Reinharz, 1984).

Although external relations always play a significant role in the creation and development of alternative settings, creators sometimes can increase or decrease the setting's independence from outside influence. Cherniss (1972) found that successful new settings were more autonomous than unsuccessful ones. Trickett (1991), however, found that an alternative setting that initially enjoyed considerable autonomy eventually needed to become less isolated in order to increase its legitimacy and support. He concluded that, during the initial phase, a new setting should maximize its independence, but over time it should seek to achieve a rapprochement with outside groups and institutions.

In conclusion, dealing with external relationships can be particularly difficult because it is one of the most "political" aspects of the creation of settings, and those who create alternative settings tend to be visionaries with little interest in, or patience for, "politics" (Sarason, 1972). In fact, it sometimes is a disdain for dealing with political issues that leads one to create an alternative setting, rather than try to change an existing one. Yet one really cannot avoid political realities in the creation of settings. Those who are willing to confront them are more likely to succeed: for instance, Trickett (1991, p. 191), in his study of an alternative high school, found that success was enhanced by the staff's willingness and ability to "read the environment," sizing up potential sources of support and opposition, and to "accommodate to broader school system pressures in a way that preserved the school's integrity." Although it can be difficult for the creators of new settings to deal with the political aspects of external relations, there are a number of useful guides available to help them (e.g., Brager & Holloway, 1978).

Leadership

Leadership is one of the most controversial issues for those who create alternative settings. Many alternatives are intended to be democratic and non-authoritarian. In such settings, the concept of leadership seems to be antithetical to the basic goals and ideology (Trickett, 1991); however, empirical research on alternative settings suggests that leadership emerges and plays an important part in their creation, even when members of the setting try to ignore it.

According to Sarason (1972), there is always an originator or founder of a new setting, a proposition supported by the research of Bartunek and Betters-Reed (1987). There can be more than one founder, but there probably are never more than two or three real leaders in the creation of any new setting. In the vast majority of cases, there is a single dominant figure who either is the recognized leader from the beginning, or emerges very early as the informal leader. Inequalities in expertise, personal attractiveness, verbal skill, self-confidence, access to information, and interest make the emergence of leadership inevitable in new alternative settings, even those with collectivist ideologies (Mansbridge, 1973).

Leaders strongly influence the creation of new alternative settings by their actions, but their actions are in turn shaped by their perceptions, motives, and feelings. Sarason (1972) has suggested that these aspects of the leader, which he refers to as the "phenomenology of leadership," are frequently the source of difficulty in new settings. Specifically, Sarason has emphasized four problems related to the leader's thoughts and feelings. The first concerns the leader's self-confidence: insecure leaders who fear failure are more likely to act in self-defeating, destructive ways. Sarason has identified several factors that might influence the leader's fear of failure, such as previous experience in creating settings and whether the leader's career and livelihood are dependent on the new setting's success.

A second problem concerns the leader's sense of superiority and parental-like attitude towards other members. Leaders with this outlook tend to be overly protective of others, reluctant to express self-doubts, and insufficiently concerned with their own limitations and needs for self-development (Sarason, 1972). Also, this sense of superiority becomes increasingly detrimental over time as setting members become more self-confident and desire increased independence.

A third and related problem concerns the leader's possessiveness and sense of ownership. Leaders tend to think of new settings as *their* settings, and this attitude can exacerbate internal conflict. It also can impede the development of positive linkages with the external environment.

One other potential leadership problem is lack of sustained commitment beyond the initial stage. Other writers (e.g., Greiner, 1972) have noted that those who create new settings often are pioneers and visionaries who lack the personal attributes required for managing established settings. There is also a tendency for the original leaders to become frustrated or bored with the project and lose their enthusiasm long before they actually depart. During this interim period, during which the original leaders still are involved formally but have withdrawn psychologically, they may act in ways that have a particularly destructive impact on their settings.

In addition to these phenomenological aspects of leadership, there can be other kinds of leadership problems as well. Leadership in groups and organizations has received extensive study in social and organizational psychology during the last 30 years, and much of what has been learned about effective leadership in established settings probably applies to new, alternative settings as well.

Perhaps the most studied topic concerns leadership style. A number of investigations have identified two particularly important dimensions of leadership style: task-oriented and people-oriented (Stogdill, 1974; Bass, 1981). Task-oriented leaders emphasize productivity, order, and organization. People-oriented leaders are especially concerned about the needs and feelings of their followers, and thus emphasize friendliness, empathy, and support. Most leaders tend to favor one of these dimensions in their interactions with followers. (Some leaders, of course, emphasize both or neither.)

There continues to be debate concerning whether there is one best style for all situations. Yet in most settings, the optimal leadership style seems to be one that combines both orientations. Thus, new alternative settings presumably will be more likely to succeed if they are created and led by individuals who emphasize both task and people dimensions.

A final problem relating to leadership, which has been noted especially in the research on new settings, concerns the first leader's departure. No matter how long the original leaders remain, their departure often sets off considerable turbulence within the setting. Anxiety, self-interest, and conflict tend to increase at this time, posing a real threat for the continued vitality of the setting (Sarason, 1972).

These problems of leadership in alternative settings pose significant challenges. Fortunately, research has identified a number of promising means of preventing or minimizing these problems. Perhaps the most basic recommendation is that those who create alternative settings acknowledge the existence of leadership and become aware of the pitfalls that we have identified here. As suggested above, there is a tendency for members of new alternative settings to deny the presence of leadership, or to assume that if they are truly committed to a collective structure, leadership will not emerge.

Once leadership and its attendant problems are recognized, there are many ways of addressing them. Leaders, of course, carry a particular responsibility for dealing with these problems. New alternative settings are more likely to fare well if their leaders are open and honest with themselves, while encouraging candor and independence in followers. But new settings need not rely just on the personal virtues of their leaders, for there are formal structures that can help leaders to act in more constructive ways. One commonly used mechanism found in alternative settings is the practice known as "mutual criticism." This refers to having regularly scheduled meetings in which individual members of the setting receive constructive evaluative feedback from the rest of the group (Holloway, 1966; Riger, 1984). This type of practice can take different forms and labels; for instance, in Goldenberg's (1971) alternative setting, it was called "sensitivity training." Whatever the form, however, mutual criticism seems to be one way in which the problems of leadership in alternative settings can be managed effectively.

A somewhat different mechanism for helping leaders and followers to deal with problems of leadership is the "external critic." Sarason, Zitnay and Grossman (1971) report on how a group of outsiders from a local university met regularly with the staff of an alternative setting for mentally retarded individuals. The purpose of these meetings was to help the members of the setting to critically examine the relationship between the stated values of the setting and actual practice. Trickett (1991) studied an alternative high school in which an outside evaluation team served a similar function during the initial years of the setting. The external critic concept thus combines elements of both organizational consultation and program evaluation, but it is unique in that the external critic is continuously involved with the setting from its inception.

Another mechanism that has proved helpful is to make the tenure of the initial leader time-limited. This practice was adopted in the alternative residential program for youth described by Goldenberg (1971). All of the staff and the funding agency agreed that the first director of the program would serve in that position for just six months. Also, his successor (one of the other staff) was selected at the outset. This arrangement served many purposes. It helped to minimize staff dependency on the first leader, gave the first leader more opportunity to experiment and take risks, limited the leader's possessiveness, reduced the psychological distance between staff and leader, and minimized the disruption accompanying change in leadership. The importance of planned succession was reinforced by the study of a less successful alternative setting (Perkins et al., 1983). In this case, the unplanned departure of the first leader seemed to contribute to many of the setting's subsequent problems.

Thus, leadership and its vicissitudes seem to be another important aspect of the creation of alternative settings. Creators of new settings seem to be more successful when they are more aware of the common problems associated with leadership and develop mechanisms for dealing with them.

The Planning Process

Another set of issues that seems to be critical for the ultimate success of new settings involves the planning process. Much of the important planning for a new setting occurs long before it becomes operational. It is during this "pre-birth" or "before-the-beginning" phase that significant actions occur, actions that will fundamentally affect the ultimate fate of the new setting (Bartunek & Betters-Reed, 1987; Sarason, 1972).

Previous research on the creation of alternative settings has identified several aspects of the planning process that seem to affect outcomes. One of the most basic involves the extent to which the creators of a new setting adequately explore the "universe of alternatives" (Sarason, 1972). Bartunek and Betters-Reed (1987) found that more successful settings were the products of a particularly creative and thorough initial exploration of ideas. New alternative settings usually represent a solution to a set of problems. There is a tendency for creators of new settings (like all problem-solvers) to move too quickly through the initial problem-exploration phases of the process, prematurely locking in on a particular solution. Thus, one guideline for the planning process is to adequately explore various aspects of the problems being addressed, and to consider a variety of strategies for dealing with them before moving into the implementation phase.

A second important aspect of the planning process concerns one's time perspective. Many new alternative settings founder because their creators have an unrealistic time perspective (Cherniss, 1977; Sarason, 1972). Usually they underestimate the amount of time required for certain tasks to be accomplished. When they encounter unexpected delays, frustration mounts and undermines the sustained commitment necessary for success.

Several studies have emphasized the importance of adequate planning time before the setting becomes operational (e.g., Cherniss, 1998). For instance, the founders of the setting described by Goldenberg (1971) spent much time in team-building and planning before their residential youth center opened, and this opportunity to anticipate problems and develop a cohesive group seemed to help make the program more adaptable when the doors opened. In another case, Perkins et al. (1983) concluded that the lack of preplanning time for the management team was one of the factors contributing to the difficulties encountered in a new, "high-involvement" work organization.

One reason that preplanning time is so important is that, when a new setting becomes operational, the members quickly become overwhelmed with a myriad of "housekeeping" tasks. Once the setting's members are preoccupied with system maintenance, it is difficult for them to step back and reflect on governance issues, the relationship between values and practice, and other fundamental matters (Sarason, 1972; Kelly, 1987). An extended preplanning period, when there are no demands for producing a product or providing a service, can make it easier to adequately consider the important issues.

Another planning issue relates to the goodness of fit between different components of a new setting, such as the goals and the organizational structure. The founders of many new alternatives often do give considerable thought to certain aspects of the structure, but sometimes they overlook other important aspects. For instance, both Bartunek and Betters-Reed (1987) and Sarason (1972) comment on the importance of physical buildings. Bartunek and Betters-Reed (1987) discovered that founders of new settings sometimes lose sight of the original values and purposes when it comes time to select or design a new building. Sarason suggests that constructing new buildings often is a costly "distraction" that greatly complicates the planning process. He also believes that it often is unnecessary for new buildings to be constructed.

The fit between technology and structure is also important. For instance, Perkins et al. (1983) found that a new work organization faltered because some of the innovative organizational structure was inappropriate for the technology and its requirements.

Selection processes are another aspect of an organization that frequently do not receive adequate attention in alternative settings. Goldenberg (1971) and Sarason et al. (1971) described two alternative human-service programs that consciously recruited staff who were dissatisfied with traditional settings and who seemed to be risk-takers. They believed that people with these qualities were needed to make their new programs true alternatives, and that special care had to be taken to insure that the staff who were asked to join the programs possessed those characteristics.

Another planning problem that has plagued many alternative settings is that abstract principles often are not translated into concrete structures for regulating daily activity. Kanter (1972) found that successful communal settings were more likely to develop extensive and elaborate rules for daily living based on the general ideology. Perkins et al. (1983) believed that failure to do this in a participative work experiment contributed to its demise. The lesson here seems to be that good intentions and lofty values often are not enough; alternative settings are more likely to succeed when many specific, structured activities are designed to infuse the new setting with its founders' values.

The socialization and training of new members is another issue that sometimes is neglected in planning alternative settings (Bartunek & Betters-Reed, 1987; Perkins et al., 1983). Those who directly participate in the creation of an alternative setting possess a unique understanding and commitment. Those who join the setting later have not participated in this unique experience, and therefore they usually do not automatically share the same outlook. For them to develop the same commitment and identification with the setting, special orientation and socialization programs can be helpful.

More specific skill training may also be helpful. For instance, Perkins et al. (1983) believed that managers in a new, high-involvement work setting had difficulty implementing participative decision-making because they lacked experience and training in the skills required for this kind of management style. Kelly (1987) reached a similar conclusion in his study of two alternative social movement organizations. Trickett (1991) found that the ideology and structure of an alternative high school required special competencies for both teachers and students that many did not possess at the outset. This is the case with many alternative settings, whose unusual organizational structures often require special competencies that setting members may not possess when they join. Thus, identification of, and adequate training in, those required competencies may be helpful.

The last planning issue that deserves attention concerns resources. Bartunek and Betters-Reed (1987) found that many new settings faltered because their planners never adequately estimated the resources (personnel, space, material resources, and clientele, as well as money) that would be necessary for the setting's operation. Sarason (1972) observed that when setting members first realize that their resources are inadequate, they usually experience considerable stress, which often is followed by an increase in conflict, dependency, and alienation. Too often, the response tends to be a frantic effort to acquire traditional types of resources (e.g., grants), which are always limited and usually impose unknown demands and constraints on the setting. Sarason urges a more innovative and creative approach to resource generation in new settings, such as finding untapped volunteer talent in the local community, or adopting "bartering" arrangements with other groups (Sarason & Lorentz, 1979).

Another solution to the problem, suggested by Greiner (1972), is simply to decide at some point that the setting will not grow, thus limiting the amount of resources that are necessary to maintain the setting's viability. Unfortunately, Sarason (1972) has found that there is a strong tendency in all settings to regard growth as desirable. Nevertheless, a no-growth policy is another mechanism for dealing with the problem of limited resources.

Many of the points that have been made about the planning process suggest the need for a much more careful and reflective approach than usually occurs in the creation of alternative settings. On the other hand, Trickett (1991) has argued that in order to generate the hope, energy, and spontaneous creativity needed for success, it is better not to have too much critical scrutiny and debate at the outset. However, a number of social theorists have argued that a certain amount of order and organization seem to be necessary for spontaneous self-expression to flourish (e.g., May, 1975; Moos, 1974). Also, as noted earlier, a common problem of new alternative settings is that they tend to be "underbounded" (Alderfer, 1980; Frank, 1982; Perkins et al., 1983; Trickett, 1991); while many established settings become stifled by too much structure, new alternative settings often suffer from just the opposite problem. A careful and thoughtful approach to the planning process is one way of insuring that there will be the right kind of structure in new alternative settings.

Group Dynamics: Conflict vs. Commitment

Alternative settings tend to emphasize close, intense interpersonal relationships among their members (Mansbridge, 1973). Such relationships are one of the strengths of these kinds of settings. They provide a strong sense of community, which is a major source of gratification for the group's members. However, these relationships also can be a source of stress. When dissension develops within the membership, the survival of the setting is in jeopardy.

A basic way to reduce dissension is to anticipate the sources of conflict ahead of time and create mechanisms for resolving them *before they arise* (Bartunek & Betters-Reed, 1987). One potentially useful way of reducing dissension before it ever arises involves the way new members are recruited. According to Sarason (1972), there is a tendency for creators of settings to present an overly positive view of the way things will be. When reality falls short, disillusionment and resentment can become festering sources of later conflict. An obvious method for dealing with this problem is to provide more realistic "previews" of the problems to be expected in developing the new setting (cf. Wanous, 1980).

Another potential vehicle for preventing dissension involves the criteria used in selecting new members. Sarason (1972) found that compatibility in interpersonal styles among the leader and core group rarely is considered when members of a new setting are selected. Goldenberg (1971) described one successful alternative setting in which this issue was considered. All of the original members of the new setting, with one exception, were individuals who had worked together before in similar programs; only those who seemed likely to work well together were encouraged to participate in the new program.

However, even when recruitment and selection are designed to minimize divisiveness, disruptive internal dynamics may develop over time. One such dynamic involves the emergence of status differences (Sarason, 1972). Status hierarchies can form on the basis of many different factors, including the order in which core group members were chosen (those who joined the group earlier are likely to assume higher status within the group); differential influence with the leader; inequality in expertise, personal attractiveness, self-confidence, access to information, or interest; and race and social class. Whatever the source, unacknowledged differences in status among members of a setting can be a major source of resentment and dissension.

Even when status differences between individuals are minimized, there is still a tendency for subgroups and factions to develop over time (Sarason, 1972). Such differentiation is a natural part of the process of growth in social organizations (Greiner, 1972). As settings grow, they tend to develop specialized, functional subgroups. For instance, a single, all-purpose "coordinating committee" may not be able to handle all of the functions of a voluntary organization as it expands; thus, different subcommittees dealing with membership, fund-raising, program, and publicity will begin to evolve. Over time, the members of these committees may identify more strongly with their own subgroup than with the organization as a whole. When this occurs, the situation is ripe for the development of factionalism.

Factions also can form around substantive conflicts. Perhaps the most basic and pervasive one to be found in alternative settings concerns the conflict between ideological purity and pragmatism (Riger, 1984). Those who tend to take the same sides on this issue are likely to form factions that eventually can divide and weaken the organization. For instance, Reinharz (1984) described a bakers' collective in which the staff were bitterly divided into "business types" and "social change types."

Conflicts also can occur over a multitude of other issues in new alternative settings. Reinharz (1984) identified several, including reluctance on the part of members to take on unpopular jobs, a member who wants to spend a great deal of time performing a superfluous task, and a member who does not perform well. Even in alternative settings where there initially is a high degree of commitment and cooperation, such issues are likely to arise at some later point. Dealing with these problems can be especially difficult in alternatives because the initial good will and antibureaucratic ethos make it difficult for setting members to anticipate such problems and develop means of resolving them ahead of time.

Thus, a key idea concerning the problem of interpersonal conflict involves the importance of planning and prevention. Too often, less-than-optimal, informal norms for dealing with interpersonal strife evolve over time in a reactive fashion (Sarason, 1972). The resultant procedures may prove to be effective, but usually this reactive approach is less successful than one in which the procedures are developed ahead of time through a deliberative planning process.

Sarason (1972) has attempted to capture the essence of this more rational, preventive approach to dealing with interpersonal problems by focusing on what he calls the setting's "constitution." The constitution consists of the setting's governing rules: how decisions are to be made, how conflicts are to be dealt with, how tasks are to be allocated, sanctions for failure to fulfill one's responsibilities, procedures for resolving grievances, and so on. Sarason's research has suggested that almost all settings have a constitution, but it usually is informal and implicit. Research on the creation of new settings suggests that success is more likely if the founders consciously and deliberately develop the constitution ahead of time, preferably during the preplanning process (Bartunek & Betters-Reed, 1987; Perkins et al., 1983).

Research on new settings has identified a number of different mechanisms that have proved useful for dealing with the sources of conflict that we have considered, and many of these practices could become part of any new setting's constitution. Some of the mechanisms that might prove useful have already been noted in this and previous sections (e.g., regular, sanctioned mutual criticism; external critics; and more realistic previews during recruitment of members). Yet many others could be noted.

For instance, the community residential program described by Goldenberg (1971) not only used sensitivity training, as described previously, but also kept transcripts of its meetings; these transcripts were studied frequently in order to gain some insight and perspective on the setting's internal dynamics. This program also used what they referred to as "horizontal structure," which meant that every staff member (including the cook and secretary) carried a caseload and had complete responsibility for all decisions affecting his or her clients, roles were exchanged on a regular basis so that every staff member performed every role at least once each month, and decisions were made democratically. This horizontal structure was created in order to minimize status differences and to improve communication and understanding between members of the setting. Outcome data on staff commitment and turnover, as well as client improvement, suggest that these mechanisms for promoting organizational health worked well.

Several of these same mechanisms were utilized in a larger program, the Central Connecticut Regional Center, which was an alternative setting developed to serve mentally retarded individuals and their families (Sarason et al., 1971). Because this program was larger and more differentiated, there was an even greater danger of fragmentation and factionalism. To combat these tendencies, staff were assigned to work in more than one program, and no formal professional departments were created.

Riger (1984), based on her study of feminist movement organizations, has suggested several other helpful practices for promoting a healthy internal climate in alternative settings. These include distributing skills and knowledge equally among members of the setting; keeping the setting small; explicitly valuing participation over efficiency; emphasizing interpersonal rewards rather than monetary ones; and making sure that networks of friendship, expertise, and support do not overlap. (This last mechanism is designed to insure that informal sources of power do not become centralized.) Yet another potentially helpful practice, utilized in an alternative human service program described by Reinharz (1984), was a rule that paid staff could work there for only one year.

Another potentially useful way to conceptualize the internal problems of alternative settings is to see them as both threats to commitment and as reflections of a lack of commitment on the part of setting members. Thus, mechanisms that enhance commitment may reduce dissension and factionalism. Kanter (1972) has extensively studied the commitment mechanisms used in numerous communal settings, and many of these could be adopted by other alternatives. These mechanisms include requiring that members make personal sacrifices and cut off ties with outside interests, reducing individuality, enhancing identification with the collective through physical and financial investment, regular contact and sharing, and development of a strong ideology.

A somewhat different approach to fostering commitment and identification with the setting was adopted in the alternative human service programs described by Goldenberg (1971) and Sarason et al. (1971). In both of these settings, the self-development of the staff and the health of the organization were considered to be two of the most important priorities. One way of operationalizing this philosophy was to require that a staff member's interests and skills be used as the primary factors in determining his or her duties. Also, all staff were given time to develop a special program based on what *they* found stimulating and enjoyable. In addition, innovation and experimentation were encouraged, and various practices were set up to provide emotional support to staff. By supporting staff and providing opportunities for self-actualization through the job, these programs hoped to reduce individual alienation and promote a positive social climate.

In conclusion, it should be clear that no single mechanism for promoting positive interaction and personal commitment in alternative settings is either necessary or sufficient. Each alternative setting faces unique circumstances requiring unique responses. Also, no matter what formal procedures are developed for dealing with interpersonal conflicts, setting members must believe in and support open discussion of such problems. A common tendency found in new alternative settings is a reluctance to "rock the boat" (Reinharz, 1984; Sarason, 1972). But unless the setting's members are willing to confront one another openly about interpersonal problems, no formal mechanism can be very effective.

However, positive attitudes by themselves are probably not enough. Formal rules and procedures also seem necessary to minimize factionalism, promote individual commitment and satisfaction, and facilitate constructive response to conflict. New alternative settings may be less likely to develop such practices, partly because they are new and partly because their ideologies often favor spontaneity and informality. But the examples we have considered suggest that the development of formal structures for regulating group life need not be incompatible with the values of alternative community settings.

THE CREATION OF ALTERNATIVE SETTINGS IN A LARGER CONTEXT

We have considered some of the characteristic problems of new alternative settings, as well as practices that might prevent or mitigate them. However, we should also consider some more fundamental questions that are raised by the use of setting creation as a social change strategy. For in choosing to create an alternative setting, one also chooses not to utilize another intervention strategy, such as changing existing settings through consultation or community organizing. Although we have noted that there are many advantages associated with setting creation as a strategy, there also are some limitations.

First, alternative settings usually are limited in the number of people they can benefit. Second, while one rationale for creating alternatives is so that they can catalyze change in traditional settings by serving as models, this outcome by no means is assured. For instance, Colarelli and Siegel (1966) described an alternative treatment program created on a ward of a state mental hospital. The program was carefully evaluated and proved to be highly successful on every single outcome criterion measured. But the guiding principles and practices never spread to other wards in the hospital, and the program itself was eventually eliminated because it was "just an experiment."

A third potential limitation of setting creation is that the establishment of alternatives may discourage the larger community from assuming responsibility for certain problems. For instance, if an alternative setting is created to deal with a certain population, established institutions can justify inaction in that area by pointing to the alternative program as evidence that "something already is being done about that."

The last limitation is perhaps the one most often mentioned in the literature: creating alternative settings diffuses energy that might be directed towards changing established settings. Thus, rather than promoting social reform, the creation of alternative settings actually might impede it.

Faced with these potential limitations, one either could abandon the creation of alternative settings as an intervention strategy or choose to ignore the potential shortcomings and create alternative settings anyway. But a more valid and useful response might be to explore how, in creating alternatives, one might overcome the limitations we have noted. There have been some alternative settings that have avoided many of the potential drawbacks. One well-known example is Alcoholics Anonymous. Whatever one may think about AA's philosophy and practices, it has managed to overcome most of the limitations associated with alternative settings: AA has survived for over 50 years, it is open to anyone who wants to join, it has influenced the lives of thousands of people around the world, and it has had a significant impact on many other treatment programs.

Thus, a critical question for future research is: What are the factors that lead to the kind of organizational success achieved by alternative settings such as AA? In other words, what has enabled these alternatives to survive, grow, serve large groups of people, and influence the larger society without excessively diluting their original principles? We believe that many potential leads for studying this question have been presented in this chapter.

In conclusion, many of the issues considered in this chapter point to the importance of the larger social context. The creation of an alternative setting, even a small and limited one, is always affected by social and historical forces that transcend the setting itself. For instance, during certain periods in this country's history, the *zeitgeist* has been especially ripe for the creation of alternative settings (Chambre, 1995). Assuming that the creation of alternative settings is a strategy that we wish to encourage, it is important to learn more about the political and economic factors that favor setting creation. Such research eventually might have some practical utility, for it could suggest concrete changes in social policies (e.g., laws, administrative rules and regulations, funding mechanisms, and educational practices) that would promote the creation of viable, constructive alternatives. For like so many other issues in community psychology, the creation of alternative settings ultimately relates to matters of social policy, to questions of how we wish to live and what kind of society we wish to be.

REFERENCES

Albee, G. W. (1959). *Mental health manpower trends.* New York: Basic Books.

Alderfer, C. P. (1980). Consulting to underbounded systems. In C. P. Alderfer & C. L. Cooper (Eds.), *Advances in experiential social processes*, Vol. 2 (pp. 267–295). New York: Wiley.

Bartunek, J. M., & Betters-Reed, B. L. 1987). The stages of organizational creation. *American Journal of Community Psychology, 15*, 287–304.

Bass, B. M. (1991). *Stogdill's handbook of leadership*, rev. ed. New York: Free Press.

Brager, G., & Holloway, S. (1978). *Changing human service organizations: Politics and practice.* New York: Free Press.

Chambre, S. M. (1995). Creating new nonprofit organizations as a response to social change: HIV/AIDS organizations in New York City. *Policy Studies Review, 14*, 117–126.

Cherniss, C. (1972). *New settings in the university.* Unpublished doctoral dissertation, Yale University, New Haven, CT.

Cherniss, C. (1977). Creating new consultation programs in community mental health centers: Analysis of a case study. *Community Mental Health Journal, 13*, 133–141.

Cherniss, C. (1998). *The problem of teacher burnout in educational reform efforts.* Paper presented at the Annual Convention of the American Psychological Association, San Francisco, CA, August 18.

Cherniss, C., & Cherniss, D. (1987). Professional involvement in self-help groups for parents of high-risk newborns. *American Journal of Community Psychology, 15*, 435–444.

Colarelli, N. O., & Siegel, S. M. (1966). *Ward H: An adventure in innovation.* New York: Van Nostrand.

Frank, S. J. (1982). *Advocacy for community-based organizations: Definition deficits, boundary binds, and measurement messes.* Paper presented at the Annual Convention, American Psychological Association, Washington, D.C.

Goldenberg, I. I. (1971). *Build me a mountain: Youth, poverty, and the creation of new settings.* Cambridge, MA: MIT Press.

Greiner, L. E. (1972). Evolution and revolution as organizations grow. *Harvard Business Review, 50(4)*, 37–46.

Holleb, G. P., & Abrams, W. H. (1975). *Alternatives in community mental health.* Boston: Beacon.

Holloway, M. (1966). *Heavens on earth: Utopian communities in America*, 1680–1880. New York: Dover.

Jason, L. A., & Kobayashi, R. B. (1995). Community building: Our next frontier. *Journal of Primary Prevention, 15*, 195–208.

Kanter, R. M. (1972). *Commitment and community: Communes and utopias in sociological perspective.* Cambridge, MA: Harvard University Press.

Kanter, R. M., & Zurcher, L. A. (1973). Concluding statement: Evaluating alternatives and alternative valuing. *Journal of Applied Behavioral Science, 9*, 381–397.

Kelly, J. G. (1987). *Preserving the efficacy of policy reform organizations: Reflections from two case studies.* Paper presented at the First Biennial Conference on Community Research and Action. Columbia, SC, May 20–22.

Mansbridge, J. J. (1973). Time, emotion, and inequality: Three problems of participatory groups. *Journal of Applied Behavioral Science, 9*, 351–367.

May, R. (1975). *The courage to create*. New York: Norton.

Moos, R. H. (1974). *Evaluating treatment environments: A social ecological approach*. New York: Wiley.

Perkins, D. N. T., Nieva, V. F., & Lawler, E. E., III. (1983). *Managing creation: The challenge of building a new organization*. New York: Wiley.

Rappaport, J., Seidman, E., & Davidson, W. S. (1979). Demonstration research and manifest versus true adoption. In R. F. Munoz, L. R. Snowden, & J. G. Kelly (Eds.), *Social and psychological research in community settings* (pp. 101–131). San Francisco: Jossey-Bass.

Reinharz, S. (1984). Alternative settings and social change. In K. Heller, R. H. Price, S. Reinharz, S. Riger, & A. Wandersman (Eds.), *Psychology and community change* (2nd ed., pp. 286–336). Homewood, IL: Dorsey Press.

Riger, S. (1984). Vehicles for empowerment: The case of feminist movement organizations. *Prevention in Human Services, 3*, 99–118.

Sarason, S. B. (1972). *The creation of settings and the future societies*. San Francisco: Jossey-Bass.

Sarason, S. B., Levine, M., Goldenberg, I. I., Cherlin, D. L., & Bennett, E. M. (1966). *Psychology in community settings: Clinical, vocational, educational, and social aspects*. New York: Wiley.

Sarason, S. B., & Lorentz, E. (1979). *The challenge of the resource exchange network*. San Francisco: Jossey-Bass.

Sarason, S. B., Zitnay, G., & Grossman, F. K. (1971). *The creation of a community setting*. Syracuse, NY: Syracuse University Press.

Stogdill, R. M. (1974). *Handbook of leadership: A survey of theory and research*. New York: Free Press.

Trickett, E. J. (1991). *Living an idea: Empowerment and the evolution of an alternative high school*. Boston: Brookline Books.

Van de Ven, A. H., Hudson, R., & Schroeder, D. M. (1984). Designing new business startups: Entrepreneurial, organizational, and ecological considerations. *Journal of Management, 10*, 87–107.

Wanous, J. P. (1980). *Organizational entry*. Reading, MA: Addison-Wesley.

Weber, M. (1947). *The theory of social and economic organization*. New York: Free Press.

CHAPTER 16

Action-Oriented Mass Communication

ALFRED MCALISTER

Ideas about the effects of the mass media in the United States have changed during the history of communication research and three stages have been identified (Roberts and Maccoby, 1985; Flora, Maibach, and Maccoby 1989). Initially, mass media messages were considered almost omnipotent in altering behavior (Katz and Lazarsfeld, 1955). Later, the mass media were considered virtually incapable of producing independent effects (Klapper, 1960). The earlier excessive claims of large effects spurred overzealous public communication campaigns, which failed to meet expectations (Bauer, 1964; Hyman and Sheatsley, 1947; Lazarsfeld and Merton, 1948). As theories about communication and behavior have merged in the analysis of phenomena such as the diffusion of innovation (Rogers, 1983; Bandura, 1986), the most recent trend is toward the belief that mass media messages have little direct effect and that their greatest influence is indirect and largely dependent on interpersonal influences and environmental circumstances. Even small direct effects, such as shifts of a few percentage points in consumer preferences, are of great commercial value and similar changes in health-related behaviors may have enormous absolute significance in a population of millions (Puska et al., 1985b). Contemporary research and accompanying developments in theory have shown that when campaigns combine community-based interpersonal communication with mass media messages the effects can be substantial (McAlister, Ramirez, Galavotti, and Gallion, 1989; Ramirez and McAlister, 1988; Flora, Maccoby and Farquhar, 1989; Bracht, 1990; Rice and Paisley, 1981). An agreed-upon effect of mass communication is "agenda-setting" (McCombs and Shaw, 1972; McCombs, 1981). Mass media powerfully influence the topics that receive attention in formal and informal social gatherings. But how people actually behave with regard to a particular topic of discussion depends on that interpersonal communication more than on the media messages (Atwood, Sohn & Sohn, 1976). The concept of knowledge- and communications-effects gaps (Gaziano, 1983; Shingi & Mody, 1976) is also important, as it highlights the disproportionate acquisition of knowledge and power by advantaged socio-

ALFRED MCALISTER • School of Public Health, University of Texas, Houston, Texas 77225.

Handbook of Community Psychology, edited by Julian Rappaport and Edward Seidman. Kluwer Academic / Plenum Publishers, New York, 2000.

economic groups, while the less powerful receive little really useful information during heavy consumption of media entertainment and diversion (Ettema & Kline, 1977).

The challenges for action-oriented community psychologists include setting an agenda and, in many cases, reversing or reducing gaps in the knowledge and competence of higher and lower social classes. By using existing formats and channels, media campaigns can engage learning processes by providing role models for innovation or maintenance of positive actions and lifestyles. This chapter presents a guide for community psychologists interested in the use of mass media and interpersonal communication to influence behavior in a community setting. First, major theoretical notions to guide communication design will be briefly reviewed. Then, essential skills for publicity, production, and coproduction will be outlined and illustrated by health promotion projects that reduced cigarette smoking and other risk factors for chronic disease on the Mexican border (McAlister, Ramirez, Amezcua, Pulley, Stern, & Mercado, 1992) and in Finland (Puska, Salonen, Koskela, McAlister, Kottke, Maccoby, & Farquhar, 1985b) and by urban AIDS prevention campaigns (O'Reilly and Higgins, 1991; Center for Disease Control and Prevention, 1996; Pulley, McAlister, Kay, & O'Reilly, 1996). Illustrative material is also drawn from successful efforts to reduce drunk driving (J. Winsten, personal communication) and child abuse, to increase literacy and family planning in Mexico (Sabido, 1981), and to increase citizen lobbying against nuclear weapons (McAlister, 1991).

THEORETICAL LEARNING PROCESSES

Most theorists believe that the functions of mass media and interpersonal communication can be complementary (Chaffee, 1982; Bandura, 1986, 1997; Reardon and Rogers, 1988; Green and Kreuter, 1991). A useful framework for considering these functions in a communication campaign is shown in Table 1, which based on McGuire's (1972, 1984, 1989) "information processing" model, its elaboration by Flay et al., (1980, 1990), and Ray's (1973) concept of hierarchy of effects. The table presents the correspondence of learning processes with characteristics of mass media communication and features in the community setting that support that communication. For communication to be most effective, the media messages must be combined with favorable interpersonal influence. Thus the learning process requires both well-designed communication messages and favorable community factors. These community factors can, to a certain extent, be influenced by community mobilization, organization, and training. The mass communication message can be designed not only to facilitate individual behavioral change but also to help organize individuals to influence their environment collectively (McAlister, 1991).

Effective communication requires consideration of each processing step in the model outlined above, from exposure to the message to maintenance of the new behaviors. *Exposure* depends mostly upon the choice of the media channels for the message. The channels that people receive depend upon the group and setting they are part of and the choices they are given. *Attention* depends on the perceived importance and relevance of the message. This can be enhanced by supportive interpersonal contacts and by reactions from opinion leaders. For easy *comprehension*, messages should use simple concepts and familiar analogies.

Comprehension can be greatly improved if there is some possibility for personal discussion and feedback (Sheffield and Maccoby, 1961). There is a rich body of literature on *persuasion* (McGuire, 1989), which emphasizes attributes (e.g., credibility, attractiveness) of the source, the nature of the message (cognitive and emotional components), and the anticipation of receiver reactions and counterarguments (Festinger and Maccoby, 1964). A major consid-

TABLE 1. Media and Interpersonal Influences on Processes of Attitudinal/Behavioral Change

Learning process	Features of media messages	Supportive community factors
1. Exposure to information	Channel selection, timing, positioning	Subculture, social setting, media availability
2. Attention	Message relevance, novelty, drama, humor, suspense	Interests of family and significant others
3. Comprehension (knowledge)	Simple concepts, illustration and analogy	Opportunity for discussion and feedback, question-and-answer sessions
4. Belief/affective valence (attitude)	Expertise and trustworthiness of source, refutation of counter-arguments, social models displays of affective emotional responses	Perceived normative support, primary and reference groups, conformity pressures opinion leaders
5. Decision (intention)	Displayed balance of incentives	Group decision-making, public commitment
6. Skill	Step-by-step modeling demonstrations, guides for practice and feedback (self-tests)	Direct demonstration guided practice, feedback, positive support: sympathy, encouragement, advice assistance
7. Action	Modeling, cuing stimuli, scheduling and record-keeping aids, deadlines	Actions of and encouragement from significant others, cues, access and availability, organizational support in environment
8. Persistence/ maintenance	Models of persistence, reminders, displays of long-term goals	Consequences of the behavior, social support

eration distinguishes between acquisition and *performance* of behaviors learned from observation (Bandura, 1986). Whether the audience is able to respond to the message may depend upon the skills they have to put their intentions into action and on their social support for doing so (Green and Kreuter, 1991). Actual consequences carry the greatest weight, while behaviors or opinions without noticeable consequences (i.e., some product or candidate choices) may be sustained by repetitive messages and positive affective displays from attractive models (Bandura, 1986). The information-processing model is more thoroughly explicated by Flay and Burton (1990). One issue worth noting concerns the extent to which learning processes result in predictable stages of change (DiClemente and Prochaska, 1982). As Ray (1973) demonstrated, attitude change often follows behavior change—especially when choices are determined by minimal influences such as shelf placement or receiving a product sample from a friend. The bicausal relationship between attitudes and behavior is well known (Green, 1970; Kelman, 1961). Many behaviors are adopted without the use of information or decision-making, with reasons or attitudes supplied after the act. But when change does occur in stages, as in self-control of addictive behaviors, communication planned to support learning processes outlined in Table 1 may significantly enhance change.

The diffusion of innovation can be accelerated by combining mass media modeling with networks for interpersonal support and reinforcement (McAlister, 1991). *Social modeling* is an observational or imitative learning process in which the words, emotional responses, and other behaviors of models are reproduced or approximated by observers (Bandura, 1977). Modeling processes underlie the influence of communication in all processes and steps of the preceding framework. Numerous studies have examined the attributes of message sources (social models) who are effective in influencing change in attitudes, beliefs, decision-making, and the acquisition of new patterns of behavior in other people (McGuire, 1989). Popular models in television or other mass media are particularly influential in all stages of learning. Factors such as attractiveness, perceived social competence, perceived expertise, and trustworthiness contribute to the power of specific models. Powerful influences on beliefs and decisions occur when observers perceive similarities between models and themselves, as when they report that they "identify" with public figures or dramatic characters in the mass media. However, many social change objectives involve more than a decision to change and may require a person to learn challenging new skills of self-control and lifestyle management. Skill acquisition, which is facilitated by the demonstration of complex sequences in a gradual, step-by-step process, is accomplished through modeling when different parts of an action sequence are explicitly identified and repeated by a model (Bandura, 1986). Learning is also facilitated when models show realistic standards for self-reinforcement. This is particularly important in the trial-and-error learning of the type associated with difficult tasks.

Modeling is a concept with obvious applications in the construction of mass communication campaigns. People are naturally interested in details of relevant experiences of other people, and this interest provides the support for our vast industries of communication. Much dramatic entertainment, from children's cartoons to cinema, performs explicit modeling functions, as do myths and parables. News and various real or simulated documentary information provides the most relevant information about real experiences, as shown by the vast audiences for television news and the growing popularity of talk shows revealing intimate personal information about habits and standards of behavior. As will be shown in the following sections, these existing mass media formats provide natural opportunities for the guided application of theoretical concepts about modeling information and its effects on behavior.

According to social cognitive theory (Bandura, 1977, 1986, 1997), the imitation of modeled behaviors is largely controlled by the reactions and support from persons in the immediate social environment. This has led to investigation of community-based training and organizational activities to multiply the effects of the mass media by harnessing the power of interpersonal communication in informal social networks (McAlister, 1991). Study of the enhancement of mass media effects through community organization has broad theoretical implications in social program planning (e.g., Colletti and Brownell, 1982). Media and community activities can be specifically designed to interact with each other (McAlister, 1991). The primary theoretical function of the media materials is to model the desired behaviors, while the primary role of community networking and organization is to reinforce imitation of those behaviors and to change environments to facilitate performance (McAlister et al., 1980, 1982). The recruitment and deployment of indigenous change agents, has been demonstrated in political organization, agricultural and other economic innovations, and in numerous programs to promote preventive medical care (Rogers, 1983; Puska et al., 1986). Depending upon circumstances, organized social change campaigns may apply different conceptual models for involving community members in goal-setting and environmental change through political and economic processes of empowerment (Bracht, 1990; Olson, 1965), as discussed more thoroughly in other chapters in this volume.

PRACTICAL SKILLS

There are three main ways to use mass media that, although not mutually exclusive, involve different skills, costs, and degrees of control over the content, timing, frequency, and intensity of messages. The following sections describe and illustrate skills for public relations (or publicity), production, and coproduction, with an additional section briefly sketching how community organization and networking can supplement media campaigns.

Publicity

Almost any organization that sells a product, provides a service, or promotes a value is interested in being in the news. The main advantage of this kind of communication is its cost, which is only the time and work involved in establishing and maintaining good working relations with media outlets and providing supportive materials. Press packets and news releases that contain complete information about the event or project being publicized are effective because they reduce the workload of reporters and editors. The disadvantage of publicity is that it is controlled by the media outlet; your message can be ignored, distorted, and, worse of all, it can be turned into negative publicity. Major forms of free media exposure include news and feature stories, the editorial page in newspapers, and broadcast (radio and TV) editorials, news, features, and talk shows.

When the objective is to sway public opinion on clearly defined issues, *media advocacy* techniques can be used to forcefully present a point of view (Wallack, 1990a, 1990b). At the simplest level, it is not difficult to get a letter to the editor published, especially in a small-town newspaper. It is best to refer to a recent letter, editorial, or news story, and to make a clear point, state a fact, or offer an opinion. A "Guest Viewpoint" type column requires some telephone and/or face-to-face negotiation with the editor or associate editor, but may be quite feasible for newsworthy issues. Inquire in advance about maximum length, and be prepared to edit yourself or be edited for brevity. For a news story, editors and reporters need to be alerted about important events that they do not routinely cover. A press release, suitable for publication as written, should be accompanied by telephone calls to bring it to the attention of key editors. News conferences are difficult to arrange, and must include significant new information that, if possible, is related to issues already in the news. For example, agencies with information about HIV testing find it easy to convey information about their services when a public figure reports infection. News packets may be prepared in advance and distributed when opportunities arise for linkage with random news events. Celebrity visits and endorsements by public officials can also attract reporters. Reports of data, especially on changes in the magnitude of public threats, are also attractive, as are opinion or behavior surveys if they reveal something unexpected or controversial.

A feature story is like a news story, but it is usually longer and written or produced in a less formal style. It often takes the form of an interview and contains references to anecdotes, emotions, human interest, and local color. Many times newspaper feature stories are accompanied by relevant photographs of people or events. Sunday papers and "Health" or "Lifestyle" sections in the papers are the most likely places to get a feature story published. It can be prepared by a reporter assigned to it by the editor, it can be written by a freelance writer who will sell it to the paper or magazine, or it can be written by you or someone in your organization. Feature stories in broadcast media may be used to provide a kind of behavioral journalism in which real case studies are used to display modeling information for skill acquisition or in which personal stories are intended to influence opinions on a given topic. Because such a story is not considered to be "hard" news, it may not be necessary to present different points of view or to link the story to current events. This has been called "soft path" media advocacy (Department of Health and Human Services, 1988). Stories provided by people who overcome barriers in accomplishing personal or collective change may be edited with guidance from theories of behavioral change in order to emphasize processes that are believed to be influential in promoting imitation of the models that are presented.

News and features in broadcast media involve the presence of cameras and microphones. Any action or movement, such as a demonstration, or a presentation of charts, slides, or clips, should be carefully rehearsed beforehand to make sure that it goes smoothly, because, with the exception of feature stories, there are seldom retakes at events and news conferences. Research on local media outlets should yield information about programs that will invite guests to present issues and concerns of interest to the community. If the host or producer is contacted well in advance, they may be convinced to present guests they think will be of interest to their audience. This can provide another opportunity to present behavioral modeling.

In a study by the Center for Health Promotion Research and Development, School of Public Health, University of Texas Houston Health Science Center and sponsored by the National Cancer Institute, a media intervention was used in tandem with community organization to promote smoking cessation and risk reduction for chronic disease in south central Texas (Ramirez and McAlister, 1988; Amezcua et al., 1990; McAlister et al., 1992). The media activities for this research project consisted almost entirely of publicity. In all four program sites, the media campaign began with a local press conference and news release providing data on local mortality (number of deaths) attributable to smoking and other major behavioral risk factors for disease and injury. At the press conference appeal was made to the community to become involved in fighting these "killers" (risk factors). Appearances by local officials, such as the mayor and county judges, with project staff from the state university, increased the perceived newsworthiness of these press conferences. Because numerous contacts were made with reporters and editors prior to the event, it was extensively covered by the local press.

Following the press conferences, social models for the selected health behaviors (e.g., smoking cessation) were recruited and featured in radio and television news and talk shows, and in newspaper feature stories in a format that has been termed "behavioral journalism" (McAlister, 1995). The negotiations, during which individual media outlets agreed to participate on a regularly scheduled basis, were completed in advance of the press conference. Under these agreements, project staff were responsible for finding and preinterviewing the social models, assisting in scheduling of taping (broadcast) and photography (print), and providing background material for relevant health or behavioral issues. Some media outlets agreed to participate with no additional incentive, while others asked for modest reimbursement through purchase of advertising space or for staff time for taping of broadcast segments. Project control of content varied across sites and media. In one town, newspaper role model stories were written by project staff and run without editing. Generally, however, project staff provided the model, and an outline of that person's story and points to be emphasized, to the reporter who then assumed creative control of the feature. One example of this more common process is a newspaper story published in a Spanish language newspaper for the Eagle Pass intervention site. The topic to be covered was behavioral techniques for smoking cessation. A role model was found who had used the techniques of making a list of reasons to stop smoking and asking for social support from significant others. Project staff arranged an interview between this person and newspaper staff in a supermarket parking lot, provided a short biosketch and list of questions to elicit the role model's story, and specifically requested that attention be paid to the role model's technique of listing and reviewing his reasons to quit smoking. The resulting story included a large photograph of the role model reading from his list, which modeled an important skill in urge management. The story also described the social support he received from his friends and family.

In the community in which the most intensive media activity occurred, two cable television stations, two radio stations, and two newspapers featured distinct Spanish language role model stories each week. In addition, regional media that was received by all the research sites typically consisted of weekly role models in one English and one Spanish television station, and in one English language newspaper. The result was that over a four-year period, 94 English- and 258 Spanish-language modeling displays were featured in television news, a total of 379 news stories were printed about role models, and more than 1,000 radio messages provided similar information (McAlister et al., 1992). This level of media involvement over time was facilitated by a careful cultivation of media contacts and by a rotating schedule of topics (tobacco, AIDS, nutrition, cancer screening, alcohol and drug abuse, safety). It was also helpful to offer exclusive rights to campaign features within a given medium, feature cross-promotions between media, and mobilize community participation in promoting the media campaign. Five years of follow-up in panels of heavy smokers from study and comparison communities yielded evidence of increased cessation in the study area (McAlister et al., 1992). Subsequent studies indicate effects on cancer screening (McAlister, Fernandez-Esquer, & Ramirez et al., 1995; Ramirez, McAlister, & Gallion et al., 1995).

Production

When free publicity is not focused or specific enough to do the job, it may be necessary to consider producing your own materials. Both radio and TV stations will broadcast free public service spots on behalf of nonprofit organizations. *Free Speech Messages* are statements of opinion, while *Public Service Announcements* refer to less controversial events or services. The rules about content, format, length (10, 30, or 60 seconds) vary from station to station, and with the specific rules of each media outlet in your area. As a general rule, a programming director will schedule the available PSAs around time slots that have not been sold for commercial advertisements. This means that you cannot control directly when and how often your message will air. The better the professional broadcast quality of a spot, the better its chances are to be selected for broadcast. However, production can be a very expensive endeavor, especially when dealing with audiovisual media, such as television. For maximum effectiveness, the production process should involve as much professional involvement as possible, including expertise in technical and artistic skills. In addition, the development process from conception to final production may need to include story boards, scripts, prototypes, rehearsals, pilot tests, and field tests before final production and reproduction. It is often possible to raise money for professional production or to procure voluntary assistance from an advertising agency or production company. For example, a campaign in Houston to reduce child abuse (*Houston Chronicle*, 1992) was selected by a local advertising association to receive free help in production of spot announcements for radio and television. Public service announcements to promote a hotline for parents with substance abuse and potential child abuse problems were produced with high standards of creative and technical expertise, including a "catch" phrase ("abuse is abuse") and engagingly paced jump-editing, which made the message competitive with similarly crafted commercial ads. The spots were based on the social modeling concept and drawn from real case studies and interviews with clients and staff at the crisis center. The advertising agency was delighted to use the real story as content for its creative "packaging" skills. Messages were selected to model decision-making processes and how clients overcame perceived barriers to seeking help. For example, one spot was edited to evoke an emotional response by a sequence of concerned facial expressions and jerky movements, followed by a more naturally timed close-up of a parent and child hugging (mimicking the technique in dramatic ads for a product to alleviate gastric discomfort). The audiotrack carried these words: (*Male voice*) "I woke up this morning, and I see this hole in the wall where I had thrown a bottle. I look at my kids and I see the scared look in their eyes. And I wonder what I had done last night." (*Female voice*) "I almost abandoned my son because I was crazy from alcohol. I can't take care of him. I'm scared I'll have to give him up. But I know I can't be a mother unless I do something about my drinking." (*Narrator*) "If you are drinking or drugging, you are not the only one who gets hurt. Get help." These PSAs were well-placed by television stations in Houston because they were of a quality comparable to other content in prime or near prime-time periods. Each such ad placement produced a noticeable increase in calls to the hotline (*Houston Chronicle*, 1992).

With small items, such as leaflets, fliers, and posters, this production can be much less expensive, often feasible for in-house resources in the small social service agencies where many community psychologists practice. An important characteristic of print media and some other materials such as audio- or videotapes is that they can be distributed through interpersonal networks. Although mailings or distribution racks may disseminate a high volume of materials, interpersonal transmission (handing it out directly) provides an opportunity for engaging encouragement and reinforcement processes that directly influence behavioral and attitudinal change. Many organizations use newsletters to keep members, constituencies, and key decision-makers and opinion-makers informed of recent developments in their field of interest. Newsletters may also provide modeling stories and testimonials. Having a professional-looking newsletter adds credibility to an organization. Layout and design, choice of size and format, and overall appeal can be determining factors in its effectiveness as a communications tool. A single page leaflet can contain facts, background information, tips about resources, suggestions for activities or practices, and specific information about the agency or organization that produced it. Leaflets also provide opportunities to present models for skill acquisition or attitude change. Visual appeal is an important factor in the effectiveness of a leaflet; artistic and technical experience greatly improve the final product when there is a need to present more information. A brochure or booklet is a relatively inexpensive means of communicating information. One should always first collect similar material from other agencies, groups, and organizations to see if there is already a product that could be used intact or with minor modifications.

Posters are another print medium that can be very effective in publicizing an event, presenting a role model or a simple concept or idea. Posters that are produced to publicize a specific event are soon outdated. Others contain messages of a more long-lasting appeal and currency, and can be displayed on a more or less permanent basis. Specific projects and campaigns can be publicized using a common logo, motto, or visual image that can be reproduced in leaflets, posters, buttons, t-shirts, billboards, bumper stickers, and stick-on labels.

In a recent CDC AIDS prevention demonstration project (O'Reilly and Higgins, 1991; MMWR, 1996; Pulley et al., 1996), five sites across the United States are producing their own media materials to be distributed by community "networkers" to reach such "hard-to-reach" at-risk groups as injection drug users (IDUs), the female sex partners of IDUs (FSP), prostitutes, street youth, and men who have sex with men but are not part of the gay community. The content of the material to be disseminated, and the groups to be reached, in part preclude the use of mass media, which would be unlikely to devote coverage to techniques of cleaning injection equipment with bleach, or negotiating condom use with sex clients. Materials are tailored to the stages of change (DiClemente and Prochaska, 1982) most prevalent in the intended audience, and are designed to provide peer modeling of risk-reduction behavior and factual information about HIV. Attractive packaging, the inclusion of other topics of interest to the audience, and the efforts of the indigenous distribution network help capture the attention of the intended audience. In a technique termed *behavioral journalism* (McAlister, 1996), indigenous role models are used to create believable stories and increase perceived similarity by the audience, although the names are usually changed, and photographs of models are used to shield the identity of individuals engaged in illegal or private behaviors. Composite role model stories are often used, taking parts of different individuals' stories and weaving them together to create a story that is more tightly focused on attitudes or skills that formative qualitative and quantitative research and/or theory suggest are most important in facilitating behavior change.

It is important to be familiar with the intended content and audience before beginning the production process. Extensive formative research was conducted for the demonstration projects to better understand the audience, examine their current media use and reading level, and identify access points for distribution (Pulley et al., 1996). Based on this research, mock-ups of material were prepared and pretested, and when necessary these steps were repeated until a product acceptable to both the project and the audience was developed. In a site where the project sought to reach street youth, it was found that gum cards were kept and traded, so a card format, with a role model picture on one side and role model story and resource information on the other, was produced. In another site focusing on female sex partners of IV drug users, tabloids and romances were the reading materials of choice, so a newsletter was developed to present role model stories written in a romance/true confession format. HIV facts, tips on child rearing, and a calendar of local events are also regularly included in this publication. A specific example of the development process is a series of comic strips produced by the Dallas site. Based on feedback from focus groups suggesting that materials should be "fun, fast," and short enough to be easily remembered, the decision was made to include a comic strip with a gag line in project materials. Real situations and dialogue elicited from audience members were selected to match hypothesized predictors of behavior change. For example, it is hypothesized that among the most important predictors for condom use are perceived pleasantness for men and anticipated self-efficacy for women (e.g., knowing how to get a man to agree to use a condom). One strip depicts a woman convincing her partner to use a condom by resisting his counterargument and telling him "I'll just have to be creative and show you how fun this can be." The closing frame shows the man with an obvious look of pleasure on his face exclaiming, "oooooohh!" followed by the advice to "Have fun! Let your partner put it on for you!" These comic strips are featured in volunteer-distributed materials that include condoms. In a quasiexperimental evaluation study, this form of community education appears to be effective in promoting consistent condom use among persons with multiple sexual partners. In the experimental communities, consistent condom use for vaginal sex increased from 23% to 36%, but decreased slightly in the comparison communities (Center for Disease Control and Prevention, 1996).

An important step in producing these materials was the pretesting form and content. Some steps, such as checking the reading level of materials can be done by project staff, while others require community input. Focus groups (Department of Health and Human Services, 1989) and/or individual interviews with audience members and community leaders are important to elicit feedback on the acceptability of the materials, preferences in styles and formats, comprehension, credibility, and perceived personal relevance. Acceptability can be determined by asking if elements of materials are attractive or offensive. Preferences can be judged by presenting a variety of examples from which the participants may choose text, graphics, and titles. It is also a good idea to ask participants to compare project generated mockups with a selection of competing materials, such as brochures or posters produced for your topic area by other organizations, and popular print media, to provide an indication of how your materials will compete for attention. Comprehension can be explored by asking audience members to paraphrase the message or main idea. More detailed information on pretesting can be found in Windsor et al. (1984), Department of Health and Human Services (1989), Flay (1987b), Basch (1987), and Palmer (1981).

Coproduction

Coproduction involves pooling the resources of two or more organizations that share a common goal or concern, and that will benefit equally from the partnership. This is the most effective strategy for generating high-budget communication without paying commercial production rates. Of particular importance is the coproduction of films and television programs, especially when the partner is a local television station or a networker. This is possible if the issue or concern is perceived to be a benefit to the public at-large, as is the case with personal security and health issues, education, and issues involving children and the family. In a coproduction, the community psychologists' organization provides the content expertise, and the media partner provides the talent, equipment, technicians, studio, and broadcast time. To ensure optimal exposure, time can be bought at the regular rate for a specific time slot, with the station matching it with donated time. Coproduction can be an effective tool for conveying modeling information to improve skills and influence attitudes.

Documentary

Credible documentary or journalistic formats can investigate how and why people change, either individually or collectively, and thus provide social modeling information to accelerate diffusion of new behaviors. The North Karelia Project in Finland illustrates an effective coproduction arrangement in which behavioral scientists originated and shaped the content of a major documentary television series as part of a cardiovascular disease prevention campaign (McAlister et al., 1980; Puska et al., 1987).The series, titled *Keys to Health*, has been presented eight times in varying forms since 1978. The format was based on a small-scale laboratory study (McAlister, 1976; Flay, 1987a) in which would-be exsmokers were randomly assigned to live or televised behavioral counseling with volunteer facilitators assisting those viewing the televised material. In the live counseling condition the television camera was treated as a member of the group and viewers in the televised condition were explicitly instructed by the counselor (via television) and facilitator to imitate the learning experiences they observed among those who received the counseling directly. Quit rates were the same among live and televised counseling groups. This type of televised behavioral counseling was previously reported by Ferstl, Jockusch, and Brengelmann (1975).

In the Finnish series, the studio group was selected from volunteers seeking to stop smoking and, in other years, to also lose weight, reduce blood pressure, and cholesterol, or increase exercise and improve stress-coping. The studio group members were chosen from the volunteers who were judged to be adequately prepared to make a serious change attempt. After that, the main selection criteria were personal attributes, such as occupation, appearance, and manner of speech, that might increase attractiveness and perceived similarity to the different population segments that were to be reached in North Karelia. In a typical program, behavioral instruction from professional health educators and nutritionists was combined with directed group discussion in the studio and taped segments illustrating how instructions were put into action at home, work, or place of leisure. The number of broadcasts ranged from eight to fifteen over 6 to 12 months, with each segment lasting 30 to 45 minutes. The behavioral counseling was based on established techniques (e.g., Pechacek and McAlister, 1980), with a strong emphasis on problem-solving skills for relapse prevention. Thus, for example, group members learned relaxation techniques and demonstrated their use in actual stress situations.

The National Public Health Institute provided primary content expertise and leaders for the studio groups, while the TV2 network provided professional leadership for the production as well as studio facilities, broadcast time, and all of the other technical support that was needed. The popularity and impact of these programs, which were supported by grassroots volunteers in North Karelia (presented later), have been amply documented (Puska, Wiio, & McAlister, 1985a; Puska et al., 1986; Puska, McAlister, & Niemensivu, 1987). For example, the effects of one program about weight loss that was viewed by 15–20% of the population in Finland was assessed in a 6-month follow-up survey of viewers, among whom 4–7% reported that they maintained an average loss of 7–11 pounds of body weight. This extrapolates to more than 50,000 cases of medically significant weight loss in Finland's population of 3 million. The programs have been especially helpful in reducing knowledge gaps, as exposure and attention to the *Keys to Health* broadcasts was two to three times higher among people without the equivalent of a high school education than among those with more education. The most recent series was jointly produced as a binational project of Finnish and Estonian television networks and attracted a very large audience in both countries. While changes in health behavior were the objectives of the public health agencies, the broadcasters were motivated and rewarded by the programs' popularity and audience satisfaction. This type of documentary group counseling format for smoking cessation has also been demonstrated in Houston, Los Angeles, and Chicago, largely through arrangements with producers of news features for local television stations (Flay, 1987a). The studio group counseling technique is well-suited for emerging talk-show formats in daytime television and deserves increasing attention as a vehicle for planned social change. Contemporary talk-shows such as Oprah Winfrey's often jointly interview real people and experts to provide explicit guidance for audience members with problems similar to their guests. This approach has an enormous potential for diffusing behavioral counseling and self-initiated changes, particularly to groups without access to or inclination toward professional help.

Coproduced television documentary material can also be useful in influencing grassroots political behavior such as communication with members of Congress (McAlister, 1991). This is illustrated by the one-hour broadcast program *Thinking Twice*, which was produced in 1982 through a collaboration between several arms control groups, the Public Interest Video Network (Washington, D.C.), and the Public Broadcasting System, with major support from private foundations. The broadcast combined two kinds of social modeling. During the first half-hour, a middle-class southern family was followed as they learned about issues such as the cost of nuclear weapons and whether a nuclear war could be won without unacceptable costs. By the end of this part of the broadcast, which covered a month-long learning experience by the featured family, they had decided that the risk of war must be reduced and were asking what they could do to help. The next half-hour provided brief views of the opinions and work of volunteer and professional arms control activists, who were explicitly presented as possible role models for the featured family and the viewing audience. To provide balance, the role models included people trying, for example, through congressional letter-writing campaigns, to stop production of nuclear weapons and others who favored more weapons and peace through strength. The program ended with encouragement for the audience to get involved and an 800 number for more information. The program was carried by most PBS affiliates. In several congressional districts, the program received promotional assistance from local volunteers and served as a way of recruiting more participants in grassroots activities. In the two southern congressional districts that were of greatest interest, local PBS affiliates did not broadcast the program from the original satellite feed, but presented it later after viewer demand was expressed by local activists. Such organized expressions of viewer interest may be crucial for influencing gatekeepers for important media channels in both the public and private sectors. Although the specific contribution of the *Thinking Twice* broadcast cannot be separated from other influences, it was seen by participants as a helpful part of their citizen lobbying campaign both for increasing awareness or "agenda-setting" and for activation of the letter-writing campaign. The lobbying effort promoted by the *Thinking Twice* broadcast succeeded in at least partly influencing two powerful southern congressmen from Texas and Mississippi to join successful votes against bills to appropriate tax money to build one hundred MX or "peacekeeper" missiles (McAlister, 1991). After a protracted battle in Congress, fifty missiles were finally produced at a cost of approximately $100,000,000 each, with a total cost of several billion dollars lower than President Reagan had demanded.

Entertainment

Another coproduction approach involves efforts to influence the content of popular entertainment through various arrangements with scriptwriters and producers as discussed by Rogers (1983) and Bandura (1986). The best-known example is the Mexican television dramatic series reported by Sabido (1981), which engaged millions of viewers' attention for actors' modeling of specific opinions and behaviors related to family planning and other health and social issues. As described by Bandura (1986), the programs were guided by behavioral science principles and designed to meet social objectives, while being produced through collaboration with mainstream professional talent and production and broadcasting resources. The soap opera format was used, with highly popular performers cast in key roles. One campaign to increase literacy followed characters as they learned about where to get help with reading and what the benefits would be. Enrollment in literacy programs increased eightfold in the year of the first soap opera series. In a later series, to increase use of family planning services, a young woman was the focus of dramatic attention as she learned to gain more control over her life through services and assistance from a family planning center. Information about local resources was provided at the end of some programs and large increases in the use of services and in sales of contraceptives were observed during and after the series. For both the literacy and family planning campaigns, the soap operas were combined with local networks of educators and service providers who encouraged attention and reinforced responses to the modeling displays by the characters in the soap operas.

In the United States, this approach has been most notably applied by the Center for Health Communication at the Harvard School of Public Health in campaigns to reduce drunk driving by promoting the concept of a "designated driver" (Winsten, 1992). After meetings and discussions with the Harvard team, scriptwriters for a number of popular television series agreed to insert subplots explicitly modeling the designated driver concept. Over several years, this has yielded more than 140 primetime episodes in which the behavior has been displayed. The campaign appears to have been responsible for widespread diffusion of the designated driver innovation, with 37% of a national sample reporting the behavior in 1991.

These kinds of partnerships with scriptwriters in commercial entertainment may be highly productive, but results are unreliable when the profit motive is involved. For example, the author of this chapter resigned from such a partnership with a major Hollywood production house when a carefully scripted show on stress control was used to promote a medically questionable gadget (gravity-boots) as part of a national sales campaign. When coproduction involves unequal partnerships with private enterprise, entertainment and commercial value may be expected to outweigh other potential social benefits. Even when stakes are smaller, when artists collaborate with social engineers, it is necessary to make compromises that balance form and function creatively to maximize overall satisfaction with the product.

Organizing Interpersonal Networks

In the preceding illustrations of mass media communication approaches, it is important to note that an interpersonal networking component was included in each case. Local support for the Mexican soap operas came from the staff and outreach workers at education and health centers, who promoted and reinforced the programs in villages and neighborhoods. Local volunteers were important in the *Thinking Twice* program and critical for assuring that the show was broadcast in the campaign areas. In the North Karelia Project in Finland, a network of several hundred local volunteers was trained to encourage attention to and imitation of the televised studio models. The training in each village consisted of a preview of the television series, and a discussion of its benefits. Leaders performed specific role plays of how to talk about the program to relatives, neighbors, coworkers, and other members of natural networks. In the *Salud* campaign on the Mexican border and in the Centers for Disease Control studies of HIV prevention, peer volunteers and other networkers (store clerks, bartenders) participate by learning how to encourage and reinforce imitation of role models in media materials, while maintaining purely positive communication, that is, without blaming or punishing persons who are unwilling or not interested. In all of the case studies, these interpersonal networks function for communication and for organized social/institutional change, as most obviously evident in the *Thinking Twice* campaign to increase citizen lobbying against nuclear weapons. Although they may come about very slowly, environmental and socioeconomic changes that result from grassroots efforts, combined with expert leadership and effective mass communication, can be very significant. A good example comes from the Finnish study, where the partial conversion of meat and dairy production to fish and berry cultivation has been accomplished by volunteers associated with the project in North Karelia (Kuusipalo, Mikkola, Moisio, & Puska, 1988). In the *Salud* project, organized members of the communication networks have successfully sponsored anti-smoking ordinances and the creation of a new chapter of the American Cancer Society (Amezcua et al., 1990).

After a pioneering three-community study near Stanford found that even the best mass communication effort may be ineffective without a supporting campaign of interpersonal communication (Maccoby, Farquhar, Wood, & Alexander, 1977), Maccoby challenged students to describe how necessary functions of interpersonal contact can be accomplished with the lowest possible cost and greatest possible cultural sensitivity by designing them to interact with the influences of a mass media campaign. At the same time, social critics such as Ivan Illich were using the Stanford project to assail the disempowering nature of expert-devised messages constructed by highly paid social marketing professionals to manipulate perceptions of the health attributes of consumer products (Illich, 1976). It may be argued that effective mass communication combined with well-led peer volunteer networks can reach more people and influence more long-lasting change than the one-on-one or group education, counseling, and therapy that is the core of the profession of psychology. If messages are based on real peer role models and delivered or supported by a network of peers, the audience is the source of the messages and control over their interpretation is decentralized by the breadth of participation in supportive social networks. If the problem or approach is not a priority for the community, widespread grassroots interest and participation will not be achieved. In the Mexican border study, direct individual and group counseling was not more effective in promoting smoking cessation than the peer modeling media and peer volunteer program that was delivered to the entire community at a relatively low cost ($30–50,000 per year) (McAlister et al., 1992). Randomly selected panels of cigarette smokers were followed for four years to compare responses to different types of communication. Personal and group counseling did not significantly add to the effect of a combined media campaign and peer communication network (McAlister et al., 1980).

In organizing the interpersonal component of a communication plan, community analysis and ethnographic data may be used to prepare plans for systematic involvement of formal systems, informal networks, and geographic units as channels of access to a community (O'Reilly and Higgins, 1991). Charts can be drawn that tentatively map an access plan, with final plans based on input from local advisors and volunteers. Results of this community analysis process, which can identify points of access into subculture networks, provides the starting point for networking and organization. For example, to reach IV drug users, the staff needs to build extensive contacts with current or former IV drug users (peers) and with other individuals who have regular contact with IV drug users (interactors) who know and are accepted by them. The possible sources for volunteer networks include health care organizations, the criminal justice system, social welfare agencies, political organizations, neighborhood or cultural organizations, laundromat supervisors, liquor store clerks, and bartenders. Peer volunteers may be drawn by canvassing residents of housing units and persons found at street "hang-outs."

Minimal responsibilities of network participants may include regular distribution of information and media material packages, encouraging emulation of mass media role models, verbally conveying basic messages, and providing referral to services or additional information sources. Networkers may provide personalized words of encouragement to persons they know as part of their everyday routine. The quality of performance may be variable, but many can provide significant social reinforcement with active and frequent encouragement (Puska et al., 1986). Some persons may also accept responsibility for recruiting, training, and managing other volunteers, or for advocacy roles such as the organization of citizen lobbying.

As community psychologists explore possible objectives for advocacy and environmental or regulatory change with network participants and local leaders (Bracht, 1990; Rice and Paisley, 1981; Olson, 1965), a critical task is the establishment of a sense of individual and collective self-efficacy (Zimmermann & Rappaport, 1988). A general recommendation is to start small, with clearly attainable goals. Participation in a communication campaign network accomplishes this by providing a realistic first step toward more ambitious long-term goals. Although institutional rules or political considerations may limit formal agency involvement in controversial issues, self-perpetuating advocacy and environmental change activities can be sparked by impartial education and disinterested training. Other chapters in this volume provide more detailed treatments of community networking and organization.

SUMMARY AND CONCLUSIONS

The available tools for mass communication can be used most effectively if theory is considered in the design and planning of specific materials and events. The communication-to-behavior-change process is complex and multistepped. Any single message can be expected only to produce a small, incremental effect. The most powerful theoretical concept for engaging multiple learning processes is social modeling. As illustrated in the case studies, stories about real people can effectively convey decision-making, skill-acquisition, and other cognitive and behavioral content that may lead to action. By featuring stories about real people, campaigns in the case studies achieved low production costs and, in some instances, were able to have their material treated as news. The case studies also illustrate the importance of simultaneously organizing interacting media and interpersonal communication, either through existing networks or through an organization that is created to cope with the specific problem at hand. The critical component in interpersonal communication appears to be the provision of directive encouragement and social reinforcement. When combined with media messages which model the behaviors that are being encouraged, low-cost efforts based on the voluntary participation of natural leaders may be capable of significantly influencing diverse forms of social action.

The case studies that were described in this chapter were drawn primarily from the field of public health, a growing practice area for interdisciplinary work by community psychologists. Useful tools for social change have been developed and demonstrated to have some positive effects on consensus public health problems such as hypertension or (to some degree) cigarette smoking. At the same time, the scope of public health has expanded to include almost purely behavioral problems such as violence (National Research Council, 1993; Velez, McAlister, & Hu, 1997) and intergroup relations (McAlister, 1997; Liebkind & McAlister, 1999), which are among the traditional concerns of community psychology.

As action-oriented psychologists follow the pioneering example of leaders such as Nathan Maccoby (1980) by increasingly embracing the public health perspective which seeks to influence whole populations, they will find that well-directed communication programs may have much more impact than legions of professional health educators, behavioral counselors, and psychotherapists. The present political economy of health services in the United States favors client-oriented, fee-for-service activity, but increasing understanding and effectiveness of community-level approaches may eventually lead them to be highly valued as well (Farquhar, 1978). As communicators and organizers with theoretical concepts and practical skills, community-oriented psychologists may provide leadership in many areas of social change, as they have in the public health projects described here.

ACKNOWLEDGMENTS. This chapter is dedicated to Nathan Maccoby (1912–1992) in appreciation for his leadership and inspiration for generations of scholars in psychology, communication, and public health. The author wishes to thank LeaVonne Pulley, Ph.D., Kipling Gallion, M.S., and Renato Espinoza, Ph.D., M.P.H. for their assistance in the preparation of this chapter.

REFERENCES

Amezcua, C., McAlister, A., Ramirez, A., & Espinoza, R. (1990). Health promotion in the Mexican American community: *A su salud*. Neil Bracht (Ed.) In *Organizing for community health promotion: A handbook*. Newbury Park, CA: Sage.

Atwood, L. E., Sohn, A., Sohn, H. (1976). *Community discussion and newspaper content*. Paper presented at the annual meeting of the Association for Education in Journalism, College Park, MD.

Bandura, A. (1977). *Social learning theory*. Englewood Cliffs, NJ: Prentice-Hall.

Bandura, A. (1986). *Social foundations of thought and action*. Englewood Cliffs, NJ: Prentice-Hall.

Bandura, A. (1997). *Self-efficacy: The exercise of control*. New York: W.H. Freeman.

Bauer, R. (1964). The obstinate audience: The influence process from the point of view of social communication. *American Psychologist, 19*, 319–328.

Bracht, N. (1990). *Organizing for Community Health Promotion*. Newbury Park, CA: Sage.

Centers for Disease Control and Prevention. (1995). Community level prevention of HIV infection among high-risk populations: Methodology and preliminary findings from the AIDS Community Demonstration Projects. *MMWR Supplement*.

Centers for Disease Control and Prevention. (1996). Community-level prevention of HIV infection among high-risk populations. MMWR Recommendations and Reports, May 10, Vol. 45 (10(RR-6), 1–24.

Chaffee, S. (1982). Mass media and interpersonal channels: competitive, convergent or complementary. In G. Gumpert and R. Cathcart (Eds.), *Inter/Media: Interpersonal communication in a media world* (pp. 57–77). New York: Oxford University Press.

Colletti, G., Brownell, K. D. (1982). Self-change and therapy change of smoking behavior: a comparison of processes of change in cessation and maintenance. *Addictive Behaviors, 7*, 133–143.

Ettema, J., Kline, F. (1977). Deficits, difference and ceilings: Contingent conditions for understanding the knowledge gap. *Communication Research, 4*, 179–202.

Farquhar, J. W. (1978). The community-based model of lifestyle intervention trials. *American Journal of Epidemiology, 108*, 103–111.

Ferstl, R., Jockusch, U., & Brengelmann, J. C. (1975). Die verhaltenstherapeutische Behandlung des Ubergewichts. *Internationales Journal fur Gesundheitserziehung, 18*, 119–136.

Festinger, L., and Maccoby, N. (1964). On resistance to persuasive communications. *Journal of Abnormal and Social Psychology, 68*.

Flay, B. R., Ditecco, D., & Schlegel, R. P. (1980). Mass media in health promotion. *Health Education Quarterly, 7*, 127–143.

Flay, B. R. (1987a). Mass media and smoking cessation: A critical review. *American Journal of Public Health, 77*(2), 153–160.

Flay, B. R. (1987b). Evaluation of the development, dissemination, and effectiveness of mass media health programming. *Health Education Research, 2*, 123–130.

Flay, B. R., Burton, D. (1990). Effective mass communication campaigns for public health. In Atkin, C., and Wallack, L. (Eds.) *Mass Communication for Public Health*. Newbury Park, CA: Sage.

Flora, J., Maccoby, N., & Farquhar, J. (1989). Communication campaigns to prevent cardiovascular disease: The Stanford community studies. In R. Rice & C. Atkins (Eds.), *Public Communication Campaigns*, 2nd ed. (pp. 233–252). Newbury Park, CA: Sage.

Flora, J., Maibach, E., & Maccoby, N. (1989). The role of media across four levels of health promotion intervention. *Annual Review of Public Health, 10*, 181–201.

Gaziano, C. (1983). The knowledge gap: An analytical review of media effects. *Communication Research, 10*, 447–486.

Green, L. W. (1970). Should health education abandon attitude-change strategies: Perspectives from recent research. *Health Education Monograph, 1*, 24–48.

Green, L. W., & Kreuter, M. W.(1991). *Health promotion planning: An educational and environmental approach*, 2nd ed. Mountainview, CA: Mayfield.

Houston Chronicle, (April 24, 1992). Alcohol, hard drugs linked to child abuse, p. 7.

Hyman, J., Sheatsley, P. (1947). Some reasons why information campaigns fail. *Public Opinion Quarterly*, pp. 448–466.

Illich, I. (1976). *Medical nemesis: The expropriation of health*. New York: Pantheon.

Katz, E., & Lazarsfeld, P. (1955). *Personal influence: The part played by people in the flow of mass communications*. New York: Free Press.

Kelman, H. C. (1961). Processes of opinion change. *Public Opinion Quarterly, 25*, 57–61.

Klapper, J. T. (1960). *The effects of mass communication*. New York: Free Press.

Kuusipalo, J., Mikkola, M., Moisio, S., Puska, P. (1988). The East Finland berry and vegetable project: A health-related structural intervention programme. *Health Promotion, 1*, 385.

Lazarsfeld, P., Merton, R. (1948). *Mass communication, popular taste, and organized social action*. Reprinted in W. Schramm and D. Roberts (Eds.), (1977) *The process and effects of Mass Communication* (pp. 554–578). Urbana: University of Illinois Press.

Liebkind, K., & McAlister, A. (1999). Extended contact through peer modeling to promote tolerance in Finland. *European Journal of Social Psychology, 29*, 765–780.

Maccoby, N. (1980). Promoting positive health-related behavior in adults. In L. A. Bond and J. C. Rose (Eds.), *Primary prevention of psychopathology: Competence and coping in adulthood*. Proceedings of Fourth Vermont Conference, University Press of New England, Hanover, NH.

Maccoby, N., Farquhar, J. W., Wood, P., & Alexander, J. (1977). Reducing the risk of cardiovascular disease: effects of a community-based campaign on knowledge and behavior. *Journal of Community Health, 3.*

McAlister, A. (1976). Toward the mass communication of behavioral counseling. Unpublished doctoral dissertation, Stanford University, Stanford, CA.

McAlister, A. (1991). Population behavior change: A theory-based approach. *Journal of Public Health Policy, 12*, 345–361.

McAlister, A. (1995). Behavioral journalism: Beyond the marketing model for health communication. *American Journal of Health Promotion, 9*, 417–420.

McAlister, A. (1997, October 15–17). Improving intergroup relations through students' behavioral journalism. Paper presented at Carnegie Corporation meeting on Research to Improve Intergroup Relations among Youth. New York.

McAlister, A. L., Fernandez-Esquer, M. E., Ramirez, A. G., Trevino, F., Gallion, K. J., Villareal, R., Pulley, L., Hu, S., Torres, I., & Zhang, Q. (1995). Community level cancer control in a Texas *barrio*: Part II: Baseline and preliminary outcome findings. *Journal of the National Cancer Institute Monograph, 18*, 123–126.

McAlister, A., Puska, P., Koskela, K., Pallonen, U., & Maccoby, N. (1980). Mass communication and community organization for public health education. *American Psychologist, 35*, 375–379.

McAlister, A., Puska, P., Salonen, J. T., Tuomilehto, J., Koskela, K. (1982). Theory and action for health promotion: Illustrations from the North Karelia Project. *American Journal of Public Health, 72*, 43–50.

McAlister, A., Ramirez, A., Amezcua, C., Pulley, L., Stern, M., & Mercado, S. (1992). Smoking cessation in Texas–Mexico border communities: A quasi-experimental panel study. *American Journal of Health Promotion, 6*, 274–279.

McAlister, A., Ramirez, A., Galavotti, C., & Gallion, K. (1989). Anti-smoking campaigns: Progress in the application of social learning theory. In R. E. Rice and C. Atkins (Eds.) *Public communication campaigns*, 2nd ed. Newbury Park, CA: Sage.

McAlister, A., & Velez, V. (1999). Behavioral sciences concepts in research on the prevention of violence. *Pan American Journal of Public Health, 5*, 316–321.

McCombs, M. & Shaw, D. (1972). The agenda setting function of mass media. *Public Opinion Quarterly, 36*, 176–187.

McCombs, M. (1981). The agenda-setting approach. In D. D. Nimmo & K. R. Sanders (Eds.), *Handbook of political communication* (pp. 121–140). Beverly Hills, CA: Sage.

McGuire, W. J. (1972). Attitude change: The information-processing paradigm. In McClintock, C. (Ed.), *Experimental Social Psychology*. New York: Holt, Rinehart and Winston.

McGuire, W. J. (1984). Public communication as a strategy for inducing health promoting behavioral change. *Preventive Medicine, 13*, 299–319.

McGuire, W. J. (1989). Theoretical foundations of campaigns. In R. Rice and C. Atkins (Eds.), *Public communication campaigns*, 2nd ed.) (Pp. 43–66). Newbury Park, CA: Sage.

Meyer, A., Nash, J., McAlister, A., Farquhar, J., Haskell, W., & Wood, P. (1980). Skills training in a cardiovascular health education campaign. *Journal of Consulting and Clinical Psychology, 48*, 129–142.

National Research Council. (1993). *Understanding and preventing violence*. Washington, D.C. National Academy Press.

Olson, M. (1965). *The logic of collective action*. Cambridge, MA: Harvard University Press.

O'Reilly, K. R., Higgins, D. L. (1991). AIDS community demonstration projects for HIV prevention among hard-to-reach groups. *Public Health Reports, 106*, 714–720.

Palmer, E. (1981). Shaping persuasive messages with formative research. In R. E. Rice, and J. W. Paisley (Eds.), *Public Communication Campaigns*. Beverly Hills, CA: Sage.

Pechacek, T., & McAlister, A. (1980). Strategies for modification of smoking behavior: Treatment and prevention. In J. Ferguson and B. Taylor, (Eds.), *The Comprehensive Handbook of Behavioral Medicine*, Vol. 3. New York: Spectrum.

Pulley, L., McAlister, A., Kay, L., & O'Reilly, K. (1997). Prevention campaigns for hard-to-reach populations at risk for HIV infection: Theory and implementation. *Health Education Quarterly, 23*, 488–496.

Puska, P., Wiio, J., McAlister, A., & Koskela, K. (1985a). Planned use of mass media in national health promotion: The "Keys to Health" TV program in 1982 in Finland. *Canadian Journal of Public Health, 76*, 336–342.

Puska, P., Salonen, J. T., Koskela, K., McAlister, A., Kottke, T. E., Maccoby, W., & Farquhar, J. W. (1985b). The community-based strategy to prevent coronary heart disease: Conclusions from the ten years of the North Karelia project. *Annual Review of Public Health, 6*, 147–193.

Puska, P., Koskela, K., McAlister, A., Mayranen, H., Smolander, A., Moisio, S., Viri, L., Korpelainen, V., & Rogers, E. M. (1986). Use of lay opinion leaders to promote diffusion of health innovations in a community programme: Lessons learned from the North Karelia Project. *Bulletin of the World Health Organization, 64*(3), 437–446.

Puska, P., McAlister, A., Niemensivu, H. O., Piba, T., Wiio, J., & Koskela, K. (1987). *Keys to Health*: Television format for national public health promotion. *Public Health Reports, 102*, 263–269.

Ramirez, A., & McAlister, A. (1988). *A su salud. Preventive Medicine, 17*, 608–621.

Ramirez, A. G., McAlister, A., Gallion, K. J., Ramirez, V., Garza, I. R., Stamm, K., de la Torre, J., & Chalela, P. (1995). Community-level cancer control in a Texas *barrio*: Part I: Theoretical basis, implementation and process evaluation. *Journal of the National Cancer Institute Monograph, 18*, 117–122.

Ray, M. L. (1973). Marketing communication and the hierarchy-of-effects. In P. Clarke (Ed.), *New models for communication research.* Beverly Hills, CA: Sage.

Reardon, K., & Rogers, E. (1988). Interpersonal versus mass media communication: A false dichotomy. *Human Communication Research, 15*, 284–303.

Rice, R. E., and Paisley, W. J. (Eds.) (1981). *Public communication campaigns.* Beverly Hills, CA: Sage.

Roberts, D., & Maccoby, N. (1985). Effects of mass communication. In G. Lindzey & E. Aronson (Eds.), *The handbook of social psychology*, Vol. II. 3rd ed. (pp. 539–598). New York: Random House.

Rogers, E. (1983). *Diffusion of innovations.* 3rd ed. New York: Free Press.

Sabido, M. (1981). *Towards the social use of soap operas.* Mexico City, Mexico: Institute for Community Research.

Sheffield, F. D., & Maccoby, N. (1961). Learning complex sequential tasks from demonstration and practice. In A. A. Lumsdaine (Ed.), *Student response in programmed instruction.* Washington, D.C.: National Academy of Sciences–National Research Council Publication 943.

Shingi, P. M., & Mody, B. (1976). The communication effects gap: A field experiment on television and agricultural ignorance in India. *Communication Research, 3*, 171–190.

U.S. Department of Health and Human Services. (1988). *Media strategies for smoking control: Guidelines.* From a consensus workshop conducted by The Advocacy Institute for the National Cancer Institute, Washington, D.C., January 14–15.

U.S. Department of Health and Human Services. *Making health communication programs work: A planner's guide.* Office of Cancer Communications, National Cancer Institute, NIH Publication No. 89-1493, April 1989.

Velez, L., McAlister, A., & Hu, S. (1997). Measuring attitudes related to violence in Colombia. *Journal of Social Psychology, 137*, 1533–1534.

Wallack, L. (1990a). Improving health promotion: Media advocacy and social marketing approaches. In C. Atkin, L. Wallack (Eds.), *Mass communication and public health: Complexities and conflicts* (pp. 147–163). Newbury Park, CA: Sage.

Wallack, L. (1990b). Media advocacy: Promoting health through mass communication. In K. Glanz, F. Lewis, & B. Rimer (Eds.), *Health behavior and health education: Theory and practice* (pp. 370–386). San Francisco: Jossey-Bass.

Windsor, R. A., Baranowski, T., Clark, N., & Cutter, G. (1984). *Evaluation of Health Promotion and Education Programs.* Palo Alto, CA: Mayfield.

Zimmermann, M. A., & Rappaport, J. (1988). Citizen participation, perceived control and psychological empowerment. *American Journal of Community Psychology, 16*, 725–750.

CHAPTER 17

Social Policy and Community Psychology

DEBORAH A. PHILLIPS

> By and large it is the objective of social policy to build the identity of a person around some community with which he is associated. Social policy is that which is centered in those institutions that create integration and discourage alienation
>
> Boulding, 1976, p. 15.

> Part of what is meant by social policy is a system of knowledge and beliefs—ideas about the causes of social problems, assumptions about how society works and notions about appropriate solutions. A policy, then, might be described as a grand story: a large and loose set of ideas about how society works, why it goes wrong, and how it can be set right
>
> Cohen & Garet, 1975, p. 21.

> It has not gone unnoticed that the wonders of science and technology have had little or no effect on society's capacity to help its members feel less alone in the world, to enjoy a sense of community, and to help them cope with anxiety about death
>
> Sarason, 1978, p. 378.

> Community competence building is one response to the theory that inequality, alienation, dependence, and helplessness are attributable to lack of participation and self-determination
>
> Levine & Perkins, 1987, p. 335.

Policy applications are a natural, albeit underexplored, extension of community psychology, as illustrated by these opening quotes. This is the guiding premise of this chapter. Preceding chapters have examined the traditions, theories, methods, and empirical repertoire of community psychology. Here, we examine policy as an arena in which community psychology applies its expertise to the goal of social change.

The enduring controversy that surrounds acceptance of policy involvement as a fully legitimate undertaking of psychologists provides the departure point. The "culture of policy" and its implications for assessing psychology's impact on social policy are then discussed. This entails reviewing the meaning of "utilization" and raising several issues about the dissemination of research to policymakers. The relation between community psychology and social policy is then examined directly, with an emphasis on several characteristics of the

---

DEBORAH A. PHILLIPS • Institute of Medicine, National Research Council, Washington, D.C. 20418.

Handbook of Community Psychology, edited by Julian Rappaport and Edward Seidman. Kluwer Academic / Plenum Publishers, New York, 2000.

discipline that make it particularly suitable for policy applications. The chapter concludes with a discussion of opportunities and challenges that will affect the future shape and strength of the association between community psychology and social policy.

In the "levels of analysis" framework of this handbook, this chapter will be viewed by most as focusing on the most distal layer of environmental influence, the macrosystem, which encompasses a culture's ideologies and their expression in institutional structures and policies (Bronfenbrenner, 1979; Seidman, 1981). The construction of policy, however, entails consideration of all levels in the search for fruitful points of intervention. Moreover, while social policy is most often conceptualized as a top-down process, we will see that it frequently emanates from the bottom up, and is most often the product of a dynamic interplay between localized influences and national priorities.

The subject of this chapter, social policy, has wide latitude. It encompasses decision-making through both private and public mechanisms occurring in city councils, hospitals, small businesses, community organizations, universities, courts, and state legislatures. Environmental and economic issues, as well as distinctly social issues, are included because they too have extensive social implications. With this vast scope, this discussion is kept manageable by restricting its emphasis to policy that is constructed through public laws and the regulations that accompany these laws. Other chapters address the related strategies of neighborhood advocacy, media campaigns, and judicial policymaking.

THE UNEASY RELATIONSHIP

Efforts to forge a comfortable and effective relation between community psychology and public policy have a heritage that is steeped in controversy. Psychologists, at best, have an ambivalent attitude toward their role in the formulation and implementation of public policy. Cautionary tales of being reduced to political handmaidens, and thus stripped of scientific credibility, stand alongside scathing critiques of ill-informed social policies that proceeded in ignorance of scientific expertise (Atkinson, 1977; Robinson, 1984).

These two wishes, to be used and not to be used, are interwoven throughout the articles and reports that record the debate over the science–policy alliance. As several have noted (McCall, 1996; Reppucci, 1985; Zigler, 1980), this controversy reflects the longstanding dichotomy between basic versus applied research projected onto the policy arena. The logical positivist roots of psychology, and the accompanying myth of value-neutral science, are entrenched in the priorities of the discipline. Theoretically guided basic research and social-policy applications mark the distant poles of the accompanying spectrum of acceptable activities for psychologists (Friedrich-Cofer, 1986; Kiesler, 1980; Kelly, 1986). It is the rare psychologist who recognizes that heavily theoretical research often carries profound implications for social policy (see, e.g., Ruble & Thompson, 1992).

The Contemporary Dilemma

Some constructive movement can be deciphered, however, from internecine disputes over whether psychologists should apply their expertise to policy issues to discussions of the conditions under which they either have a responsibility to contribute or are most likely to make an effective contribution to policymaking. This progress is, in part, attributable to growing recognition of the fact that psychological research (even in the absence of psychologists) is used and has historically been used, in the development of public policies (DeLeon,

O'Keefe, Vandenbos, & Kraut, 1982; Korten, Cook, & Lacey, 1970; Lorion, Iscoe, DeLeon, & VandenBos, 1996; McCall & Weber, 1984; Sigel, 1998; Zigler, Kagan, & Hall, 1996). This question of utilization is explored in detail later; here it suffices to point to policy in the areas of early intervention, desegregation, and deinstitutionalization to illustrate the foundation of psychological evidence on which some of the most expansive national policies are based—for better or for worse.

Acknowledging that psychological information is used for policy purposes then shifts the debate from one of involvement versus noninvolvement to one of deciding whether psychologists should guide or distance themselves from the policy uses of their knowledge base. The alternatives posed in response to this contemporary dilemma regarding the psychology–policy interface vary along two dimensions: (1) the nature of the issues on which psychologists should seek policy involvement, and (2) the amount of institutional weight that should accompany efforts to link science to policy. While one could argue that all public policies have social impacts, and thus require social scientific input, no one in the psychological mainstream has suggested that the issues appropriate to the policy involvement of psychologists are unlimited. The boundaries of involvement vary, however, with the orientation of the particular individual who is drawing the line. Different psychologists navigate their relation to policy in different ways, juggling the scientific goals of objectivity, reliability, and validity, while valuing the action goal of applying science to social change (Kelly, 1986).

At one end of the spectrum, Robinson (1984) and Kimble (1982) draw the line where professional guild interests end and broader social issues begin. The American Psychological Association's (APA) advocacy positions on the Equal Rights Amendment, gay rights, and abortion are specifically cited by Robinson as extending far beyond the limits of appropriate policy involvement. From this vantage point, policies affecting federal research support, inclusion of psychological services in federal health insurance legislation, and regulations governing animal research constitute more appropriate targets for involvement.

At the other end of the spectrum is the 1984 statement of the APA Task Force on Psychology and Public Policy (American Psychological Association, 1984): "The formulation of policy stances on issues related to psychology and human welfare are not only legitimate, but demanded by our avowed commitment to public well-being.... It might, indeed, be improper to have knowledge important to societal concerns and fail to put forward that knowledge." Even those who have adopted this broad pro-involvement stance acknowledge that there is a point "at which psychological expertise ends and personal values begin" (Reppucci, 1985, p. 127). As George Miller (1969) cautioned in his 1969 APA Presidential Address, "Let us by all means do everything we can to promote human welfare, but let us not forget that our real strength in that cause will come from our scientific knowledge" (p. 1065).

The second dimension that characterizes contemporary approaches to the psychology–policy interface addresses our dual roles as scientists and citizens. Our discipline is both an identifiable subfield of the social sciences and a collection of individuals that comprise widely differing perspectives and opinions. These distinctions capture the amount of institutional weight that is thrust behind policy involvement, ranging from none (the individual citizen) to the total collective weight of the scientific society. The poles of this dimension range from Atkinson's (1977) admonition that, "there is no reason why psychologists should not advocate political viewpoints, but they should advocate them only as citizens" (p. 207) to Bevan's (1976) call for "a social commitment for science" in which the scientific societies are going to have "not only to preach but also to practice" (p. 490).

The motivation for the more activist, institutional stance toward policy involvement derives largely from a belief that the future viability of psychology, reliant as it is on public funding, depends on the public relevance, knowledge about, and acceptance of our work

(APA, 1984; Bevan, 1976, 1982; Bevan & Kessel, 1994; Lorion et al., 1996; Miller, 1969). Psychology is not only an informant for policy development, but also the beneficiary of policy decisions—a perspective that was brought into sharp focus in 1981 when the Reagan Administration proposed substantial funding reductions for social science research galvanizing scientific communities to increase their Washington presence. Others have argued that science and policy are engaged in a reciprocal relationship, with a shared interest in social issues (Bronfenbrenner, 1974; Cairns & Cairns, 1986; Garner, 1972; Zigler et al., 1996). As Prewitt (1983) notes, "A large share of social scientific resources has always been directed to issues, problems, and questions suggested by the contemporary political-social agenda. What is on the mind of the society is, not surprisingly, what is on the mind of those who study society" (p. 297).

The Two Worlds of Science and Policy

Reciprocity, however, does not presume that scientific and policy endeavors are inherently compatible. The literature that examines the science–policy relation is, in fact, replete with colorful descriptions of the two worlds of science and policy. Among the most entertaining and lucid descriptions is that provided by March (1979):

> Science presumes a process by which alternative theories are evaluated systematically against available data within a framework shared by "reasonable" people in order to rank ideas in terms of their plausibility.
>
> Politics presumes a process by which alternative policies are compared on the basis of the power of the people supporting them in order to rank programs in terms of their acceptability. On the surface, one process attempts to reduce subjectivity through standardized procedures designed to assure verifiable knowledge; the other attempts to organize subjectivity through a set of bargains designed to assure social stability. One process seeks data; the other seeks allies. The prototypic scientist engages in an experiment; the prototypic politician engages in a logroll (p. 29).

Other commentators on the science–policy interface have emphasized disparities between (1) the time-consuming process of accumulating data and the immediacy of policy issues (Coleman, 1978; Lynn, 1978; Seidman, 1981), (2) the inherent inconclusiveness of research and politicians' demands for one "best answer" (Kiesler, 1980; MacRae, 1976; Weiss, 1978), (3) the rationality of the laboratory and the passionate, manipulative climate of policy settings (Bevan, 1976), and (4) the person-centered orientation of psychological research and the sociocultural basis of the problems addressed by policy (Reppucci & Kirk, 1984; Sarason, 1978, 1981).

Each of these distinctions has a solid bearing in reality. Their interpretation, however, either as irreconcilable differences or as challenges that suggest specialized training for the scientist, is a matter of personal taste. The orientation of this chapter is one of acknowledging the challenge, and concluding with Reppucci (1985) that "for psychology to be effective in the realm of policy, it must be carefully attuned to the culture of policy, as well as to its own theories and data" (p. 146).

THE CULTURE OF POLICY

Misconceptions of the policy process are among the most frequently mentioned causes of failed attempts to develop more constructive relations among psychologists and policymakers (Cohen & Garet, 1975; Weiss, 1984). Reppucci (1985), for example, links the success with which psychologists contribute to social policy to their sensitivity to the special demands and perspectives of those who operate in the policy realm. Even March (1979), following on the heels of the comments quoted above, notes that there is no virtue in ignorance about the conduct of policy. As we will see in the following, an appreciation of the culture of policy is also essential to the task of assessing the effectiveness of the psychology–policy alliance.

Characteristics of the Process

Weiss (1983) states that every policy is part information, part ideology, and part drama. As with any good drama, the plot of specific policies unfolds over time. The cast of characters is diverse, encompassing starkly differing perspectives, ideological positions, and institutional roles. The construction of policy takes place in a social and value context that creates systematic biases favoring some interests, promoting certain types of action, and affecting whether some issues get on the political agenda at all (Marmor, 1983). And the "product" of public policymaking is better described as a calculated risk than as a solution. A few of these characteristics of the culture of policy are now examined in somewhat more detail.

Policy as the Art of the Possible

Multiple factors, such as re-election pressures, the need to forge coalitions, unassailable values, and prior policy decisions, place limits on what is considered and what can be accomplished through the channels of public policymaking. Today, budgetary pressures constitute a particularly salient boundary within which policies at all levels of government are considered. Proposals that can claim cost-effectiveness or that offset spending increases with budget cuts take precedence.

Political philosophers (Lindblom, 1959; Marmor, 1983) have emphasized how these practical pressures and institutional constraints foster expedient responses to issues and, accordingly, marginal change. In response to media reports of sexual abuse in child-care settings during the mid-1980s, for example, criminal records checks of child-care workers, rather than policies directed at enhancing their compensation and status, emerged as the salient federal policy response. Responses to the wave of public school shootings by school-age children in the mid-1990s were greeted with calls for reducing the age at which children can be tried as adults and enhancing the presence of law enforcement officials in public schools, rather than with a serious look at either gun control laws or preventive interventions for troubled children and families. Investments in genuinely restructuring or redistributive policies are highly unusual. Politicians prefer feasible, short-term responses rather than longer-term approaches that often have less apparent or immediate links to the pressing problem.

Policy as Bidirectional

Prevailing conceptions of policymaking assume a hierarchical process in which federal or state objectives are ultimately translated into a course of action that is implemented at the local or recipient level. Elmore (1980, 1983) proposes an alternative conception that runs in the opposite direction. Policymaking is sparked not by a statement of intent from the top, but with a behavior or event at the immediate, local level that attracts the attention of government decision-makers.

In practice, both occur. Policymaking is bidirectional. Elected officials are acutely sensitive to problems that affect their constituents. Thus, a letter complaining about a Social

Security underpayment from an elderly constituent in one Congressman's district spawned a national press conference and series of procedural changes in the Social Security Administration. Sometimes a local event is so compelling as to redirect the national policy agenda: professional basketball player Len Bias's cocaine-related death resulted in federal drug legislation authorized at $4 million. At the same time, the recent overhaul of the national welfare system follows more closely the top-down perspective on policymaking, although many of the changes made at the federal level in 1996 had already been implemented by selected state governments.

Policy as a Moving Target

This characterization of policy has two aspects. The first is temporal: public policies are constructed over time. The second is organizational: the course of a given policy, from identification of an issue to the enactment of a policy, involves a multitude of decision points that rarely occur in an orderly sequence. Policy formulation, therefore, cannot be approached as a discrete decision, or even as a predictable chain of events. It is more appropriately portrayed as a cumulative product that is shaped as it moves in and out of different levels of policymaking (Hayes, 1982). Each step toward the enactment of a policy alters the climate in which subsequent steps are considered (Hayes, 1982; Marmor, 1983). The trajectory of the policy process changes from day to day, sometimes from minute to minute, and it is riddled with feedback loops.

Public policy also repeats itself over time. Seldom are policy problems decisively resolved (Sarason, 1978). Broad social concerns, such as welfare reform, crime prevention, school reform, unemployment, and health and mental health policy are revisited again and again as legislation is reauthorized, social ills recapture the attention of the media, and prior policies fail. Thus, while some observers of the policy process have lamented the disparity between the presumed now-or-never time constraints of policymaking, and the gradual, cumulative process of research (Maccoby, Kahn, & Everett, 1983), it is just as appropriate to characterize both policymaking and research as processes that continually modify prior conclusions and decisions.

Policy as Conflict Resolution

Bauer (1966) distinguishes the rational decision-making model that many psychologists bring to policymaking from the conflict-resolution model that more adequately fits the political tasks of mediating among competing interests and stakeholders, balancing contradictory values, and forming coalitions among unlikely, if not antagonistic, groups. Negotiation, rather than optimization, is the apt metaphor for policymaking (Bauer, 1966; Nelson, 1977). Few issues that find their way onto the public agenda have one-sided or clear-cut resolutions. As a consequence, the policy that emerges from Weiss's interplay of information, ideology, and drama is more likely to resemble a series of compromises that the involved parties can "live with" than a decision that all view as a solution.

Among the thorniest conflicts are those that involve value choices. A central dilemma facing policymakers concerns "implementing the values of the citizenry on a given issue without unduly compromising other values on other issues" (Bauer, 1966, p. 934). Often, conflicting values collide in the context of a single policy debate. Several contemporary issues provide examples: (1) Should federal policy be designed to protect the civil rights of citizens with AIDS or to protect public health in instances, for example, when AIDS testing is proposed for health workers? (2) Should public welfare programs be designed to enable impoverished, single mothers of young children to stay home—the original intent of the federal Aid to Dependent Children program—or should benefits be tied to mandatory participation in education, job training, and employment programs that may alleviate welfare dependency—the new thrust of welfare reform? (3) Should the process by which children in foster care are either returned to their parents or released for adoption be sped up in order to promote permanent placements for children, or should it be slowed down to protect the rights of parents who may need extended periods of time to overcome the problems that led to their loss of custody?

ASSESSING EFFECTIVENESS

Discussions of the utilization of scientific information in public policy are often introduced with laments about underutilization, ineffective attempts to influence policy, and misuses of research. Assessments of effectiveness, however, are profoundly affected by assumptions about the policy process and expectations regarding the role of scientific information in this process. Thus, evaluation of effectiveness must begin with a discussion of what research utilization means.

The Meaning of Utilization

Early efforts to trace the utilization of research in public policymaking sought evidence of direct links between specific research conclusions and specific policy decisions (Deitchman, 1976; Goodwin, 1975; Horowitz, 1971). This orientation assumed a rational, linear model of policymaking, with research data interjected between problem definition and choice of policy, or between program implementation and evaluation-guided refinement. The literature was preoccupied with immediate and concrete uses of social science, and the consensus that emerged was not encouraging. A conspicuous gap was revealed between scientific knowledge and its use in public decision-making. The theme was one of neglect, not illumination: "On the whole, for all that it taught those involved, the impact of the research on the most important affairs of state was, with few exceptions, nil" (Deitchman, 1976, p. 390).

Faced with a preponderance of evidence that suggested *non*utilization of social science, those studying the contribution of research to policymaking began to search for more subtle and indirect paths from science to policy (Weiss, 1977; Lynn, 1978; Rein & White, 1977; Caplan & Nelson, 1973; Glaser & Taylor, 1973; Rich, 1977). A distinction was drawn between instrumental (having direct and concrete effects on specific policies) and conceptual (having diffuse effects on how a policymaker thinks about an issue) uses of science. Appreciation grew for the fact that expecting a one-to-one correspondence between research and policy was unrealistic. A new perspective on the science–policy relation took shape: Research rarely generates noncontroversial results, let alone once-and-for-all truths, political power is diffuse, and the pathway from problem to policy or from program to refinement is convoluted.

Accordingly, utilization was redefined to include effects on how policymakers conceptualize a policy issue, on which issues are viewed as appropriately placed on the public agenda (and which are not), on the assumptions that are made about the causes of problems, and thus on which policy responses are considered. Research came to be viewed, generally, as shifting the frame of reference within which policymakers select, define, and respond to social issues.

Weiss (1984), for example, looks for instances where research has "laid down a sedimentation of ideas, concepts, generalizations, and findings that affect the way in which people look at programs" (p. 176). She refers to this as the "enlightenment" function of social research (Weiss, 1977, 1978). Others (Cohen & Garet, 1975; Goodwin, 1973; Rein & White, 1977) have also highlighted the role of research in altering the context or climate within which policy is shaped.

Several features of the "enlightenment function" are worth noting. First, it does not seek immediate uses of research, but rather expects that influence occurs over time as scientific evidence percolates with other ideas, policy proposals, and sources of factual information. Second, an accumulated record of research that converges on an issue (e.g., effects of television viewing on violence, the validity of eyewitness testimony, the psychological effects of environmental contaminants, the importance of school size and organization), rather than single studies, constitute the "dependent variable" for which effects are sought. Third, the "enlightenment" orientation does not presume, as did the more utilitarian definitions, that utilization is enhanced when research adapts to the assumptions, goals, and political constraints of decision-makers. To the contrary, the enlightenment model sees a role for research as "social criticism" (Weiss, 1984). Prewitt (1983) similarly observes that "social science makes its most profound contribution to policymaking when it subverts rather than tries to accommodate itself to preexisting policy premises" (p. 294).

Ultimately, research may make its most significant contribution not when it produces answers to existing policy questions, but rather when it leads policymakers to conceive of social issues and problems in new ways. It is the nature of the policy debate, more than the fate of specific policies, that appears to provide the most fertile territory for scientific influence. The effect, however, is frequently to make the problem-framing more complex than originally cast by policymakers.

Utilization of Research

The second wave of studies on utilization, based on the enlightenment model, provided more optimistic conclusions than those of the early research in this area. Policymakers in many fields, at all levels of government, and in both executive and legislative positions report that they rely on social research. Caplan, Morrison, and Stambaugh (1975), for example, reported that 82% of federal policymakers in upper-echelon executive branch positions responded "yes" to the question, "Can you think of instances where a new program, a major program alternative, a new social or administrative policy, legislative proposal, or a technical innovation could be traced to the social sciences?"

When asked to identify specific examples, however, policy decision-makers typically revert to citing broad generalizations—early intervention is more effective than later intervention; unemployment is associated with increased child abuse; and the social science concepts such as work-related stress, upward mobility, deinstitutionalization, the working poor. Policymakers further indicate that they draw upon this knowledge as they select issues for attention, conceptualize these issues, consider solutions, and enlist support for their positions (Alkin, Daillak, & White, 1979; Caplan, Morrison, & Stambaugh, 1975; Knorr, 1977; Weiss & Bucuvalas, 1977).

In this context, it is important to note that policymakers tend to obtain research indirectly and in heavily predigested form. At its most systematic, executive agencies, advocates, staff, and others summarize results across multiple studies and present key findings in pithy summaries. As research is recounted and filtered time after time, the resemblance of the final message to the original findings can be seriously obscured. It is no wonder that policymakers report generalities when called upon to support their claims that research has been used.

This is not to say that examples in which a specific program of research had a decisive effect on a specific policy decision cannot be found. In 1982, the Department of Labor issued revised regulations for the Child Labor Law that extended the allowable hours of employment of minors, largely at the urging of amusement-park owners. The Labor Standards Subcommittee in the U.S. House of Representatives held a hearing on the proposed changes, with psychologist Ellen Greenberger as a key witness. Greenberger and her colleagues had extensively studied the psychosocial effects of child employment (Greenberger & Steinberg, 1986). Their data, as presented to the subcommittee, demonstrated that detrimental effects, including increased use of cigarettes and marijuana and decreased involvement in the family and in school, emerged at exactly the shift in hours of employment (from less than 15 hours to 15 hours or more per week) being proposed by the Administration (Greenberger, 1983). As Greenberger testified, the disinterested stares of the Republican subcommittee members changed visibly to looks of surprise, and then dismay, as they realized that Greenberger's research single-handedly discredited the proposed regulatory changes. Subsequent to the hearing the administration withdrew the draft changes. These dramatic instances of a research-driven about-face on public policy are, however, extremely rare.

The Weiss and Bucuvalas study of utilization (1977) is of particular interest because the substantive area from which they drew their sample of research was mental health, and their respondents were federal, state, and local level decision-makers in executive agencies (e.g., Alcohol, Drug Abuse, and Mental Health Administration; Department of Health, Education, and Welfare; National Institute of Mental Health), state departments of mental health, and administrative positions in local mental health centers, hospitals, and associated service agencies. The study was designed to examine not only whether research is used by these decision-makers, but what characteristics make some studies more useful than others.

The results suggested that the perceived relevance of the research to pending decisions and to decision-makers' concerns triggered attentiveness. Trust in the research was then enhanced when it was viewed as both technically sound and supportive of the decision-maker's basic assumptions about how the world works. Research quality is important primarily because it reduces the chances that the decision-maker can be "blindsided" by an opponent armed with a critique of the research or a better study.

Once relevance and trust were established, reliance on research as a guide for action was fostered by two seemingly contradictory factors. The first is compatibility of the results with the decision-maker's personal positions, prior knowledge, and values. Problem-oriented research is used when the decision-maker is comfortable with its conclusions and when it can guide incremental changes in existing policies and programs. The second is the degree to which the results challenge prevailing assumptions, imply new directions for policy, and raise new issues or perspectives. Decision-makers give tremendous weight to research that suggests innovative ideas, can contribute to new directions for policy, and can identify the politician or program director as a creative leader (see Table 1). It is this finding that led Weiss to adopt the phrase "enlightenment" to portray her model of research utilization. Of course, utilization, even in the enlightenment sense, does not imply appropriate nor effective use to "promote human welfare." Enlightenment, in other words, does not imply enlightened: "Many of the notions and generalizations that gain currency are important new ways of thinking about policy, but many are unverified, inadequate, partial, oversimplified, or wrong" (Weiss, 1977, p. 17). Research can be used selectively as political ammunition to lend a "veneer of

TABLE 1. **Effects of Research Characteristics on Appropriate Uses: Standardized Regression Coefficients for Appropriateness of Uses Regressed on Research Characteristics**

Appropriate uses	Research quality	Conformity to user expectations	Action orientation	Challenge to status quo	R(2)
Raising an issue to the attention of government decision-makers	.06	.10	.23	.34	.26
Formulating new government policies or programs	.06	.18	.21	.39	.32
Evaluating the merit of alternative proposals for action	.14	.10	.27	.29	.30
Improving existing programs	.06	.16	.34	.33	.38
Mobilizing support for a position or point of view	.25	.09	.20	.28	.30
Changing ways of thinking about an issue	.25	−.01	.18	.40	.36
Planning new decision-relevant research	.16	−.06	.16	.31	.20

Note: 284 is the lowest *N* for a simple correlation. Most of the correlations are based on larger *N*s, average about 295 of 310 cases.
Source: Reprinted with permission from C. Weiss (1977), *Using social research in public policy making*. (p. 255). Lexington, MA: Heath.

legitimacy" to predetermined positions (Cohen & Garet, 1975; Lynn, 1978; Weiss, 1977), as a ploy to defer action on a policy while "more research" is conducted (Rein & White, 1977; Weiss, 1978), and as a symbolic act intended merely to create the appearance that "something is being done" (Lynn, 1978). Others have noted that research "tends not to simplify problems but to reveal new complexities" (Weiss, 1987, p. 277), which can aggravate cynicism about centralized, governmental responses to social problems (Cohen & Garet, 1975; Elmore, 1983).

A Word about Dissemination

Reppucci (1985), in asking "which psychologist should give what psychology to whom?" (p. 129), directed attention to the critical, but largely neglected, question of dissemination. "Dissemination tends to be nobody's job" (Weiss, 1978, p. 57). Utilization is, of course, dependent upon dissemination, making its neglect among psychologists an obvious culprit when policies defy the drift of research. Rectifying this situation requires determining how policymakers obtain scientific information, and then capitalizing on these accustomed channels of communication.

Unlike the evidentiary procedures of the legal system, there are few systematized, institutional mechanisms for bringing social science knowledge to legislative or administrative policymakers. There is also no equivalent in public policy to a "search" for evidence (Weiss, 1987). On the other hand, information acquisition is neither halfhearted, nor haphazard.

Institutional demands are extremely powerful determinants of policymakers' exposure to social science. Members of Congress, for example, devote an average of 11 minutes a day to reading (Weiss, 1987). Numerous implications follow from this startling fact: Results that are distilled in usable chunks of information, oral communication, sustained personal contact, and repeated messages are essential. In the process, the two goals of maximizing comprehension and minimizing the potential for distortion of results must be kept in mind (Koretz, 1982). Trust is as essential a commodity as expertise in determining to whom, among the constant press of people, policymakers and their staff will listen. Researchers who have engaged policymakers *in two-way* discussions of their evidence over extended periods of time enhance their chances of policy impact (Glaser & Taylor, 1973).

Individuals in intermediary, or "research brokerage," (Sundquist, 1978) roles often intervene between scientific data and policymakers. The popular media, with its high public profile and impact in shaping the public agenda, has a vast influence on what policymakers hear, attend to, and use. Those who inform decision-makers—their staff, advocacy organizations, interest groups—are pivotal, intermediary players in the dissemination process. In the policy arena, it does not necessarily pay to "go to the horse's mouth." Scientific information may, in fact, travel faster along indirect routes. In this regard, growing appreciation of the influential role of "issue networks" (Heclo, 1978; Takanishi & Melton, 1987; Weiss, 1987), which consist of key individuals who are intensely involved in policymaking on an issue and whose expertise is widely sought, is significant. These networks often provide the mechanism for shepherding research-based information between scientists and policymakers, thereby fostering both the policy-relevance of research and the research-relevance of policy.

Timing is also central to effective dissemination. As a policy evolves, there are periods of greater and lesser receptivity to new information. Maximum openness to empirical information is likely when a legislator is establishing a policy agenda, identifying and examining responses to a new issue, or otherwise not yet committed to a particular issue or hardened position (Weiss, 1987). Research may also be particularly effective when it offers an unexpected way around a deadlocked policy debate (Hayes, 1982). For example, a temporary impasse in efforts to construct federal daycare standards, in which supporters of stringent staff–child ratio requirements were set against opponents of costly provisions (such as stringent ratios), was resolved when results of the National Day Care Study (Ruopp, Travers, Glantz, & Coelen, 1979) revealed that classroom (group) size, rather than staff/child ratio, was the most potent predictor of positive developmental outcomes for children in daycare. This offered the pro-developmentalists a way to support quality without insisting on stringent ratios, and offered their cost-conscious opponents a way to support quality (group size is a low-cost criterion of quality) without spending huge sums of public money.

Finally, despite this attempt to describe some generalities about dissemination, it is critical to recognize that policymakers in different positions obtain scientific information through different routes. Saunders and Reppucci (1977), for example, found that superintendents of juvenile correctional facilities, directors of institutions for the mentally retarded, and principals of elementary schools relied differentially upon written versus "word of mouth" communication and internal versus external sources of expert information. Melton (1987a) similarly discovered that juvenile judges and juvenile probation officers read different professional journals. Effective dissemination, therefore, requires a certain degree of tailoring to the audience of policymakers whose attention is sought.

PUBLIC POLICY AND COMMUNITY PSYCHOLOGY

Community psychology shares it origins with the civil rights movement, the war on poverty, and the community mental health movement. This is no accident. Prior responses to mental illness, poverty, discrimination, crime, and other social ills were held up to public scrutiny and found lacking. The time was ripe for new perspectives and approaches to enduring problems. Social reform, rather than individual remediation, and empowerment, rather than treatment, provided the new lens through which prevailing issues were examined by both the maverick group of psychologists who convened at Swampscott in 1966 (Bennett, Anderson, Cooper, Hassol, Klein, & Rosenblum, 1966) and political leaders of the time.

Shared history does not assure a happy alliance. But, as implied by the quotes that began this chapter, community psychology is intimately related to political action, and thus to public policy. The association derives from multiple sources: (1) the multilevel orientation toward framing issues, (2) the explicit attention to the values inherent in social research, (3) the emphasis on empowerment models of intervention, (4) the reliance on collaborative research methods, and (5) contemporary policy issues.

Framing Issues and Identifying Responses: Levels of Analysis

We have seen that public policy is fundamentally a process of construing problems and constructing responses, albeit cast within a value-laden, adversarial, and emotion-charged context. Further, policy deals in interaction terms (Brim & Phillips, 1988): When, where, and with whom to intervene? The same may be said of community psychology, which is defined as much by a multifactorial orientation to issues as by a core of substantive knowledge. This orientation, expressed in the levels of analysis theme of this volume, is the basis for community psychology's most constructive contribution to public policy.

As Rappaport (1977, 1987), Reppucci (1985, 1987), Sarason (1978, 1981), Seidman (1981, 1991), and others have noted, public policy deals with complex problems that are encircled by multiple layers of influence and causation. Each layer suggests a distinct perspective on the problem being addressed. The perspective that gains popularity within the policy arena dictates and constrains the nature and form of the policy response: Which premises for government involvement are invoked? Which value questions are raised? Which constituencies become involved and which coalitions are formed? Which policy structures and players come to shape the course of the policy?

Child care, for example, may be viewed as a response to poor children's inadequate preparation for school (as with Head Start) or as a necessary support for poor parents' efforts to obtain and sustain employment (Phillips, 1991; Phillips & Zigler, 1987). Both approaches enlist child care in efforts to reduce poverty and promote productivity. Yet they differ dramatically with respect to their policy priorities. The Head Start approach is preventive in focus. The adequacy with which children's developmental needs are met is central to the policy's success and thus the quality of the services provided is a salient consideration. In contrast, child care that is linked to welfare reform serves primarily to remove one impediment to mothers' participation in job training. The primary goal of welfare reform is to reduce welfare costs, thus creating a strong incentive to trade-off child-care quality for policies that will provide as much care as possible at the lowest cost. In fact, recent evidence regarding the effects of the last decade's substantial expansion in public child-care expenditures, most of which was tied to efforts to enhance employment among poor families, suggests that while the supply of child care has been positively affected, the quality of that care may actually have declined (Whitebook, Howes, & Phillips, 1998).

Community psychology brings to this haphazard process the tools for analyzing policy issues from a multilevel, ecological perspective. This perspective, developed largely within the specialities of developmental, lifespan, and community psychology, is explicitly designed to expand the scope and context within which social issues are considered (Baltes, Lindenberger, & Staudinger, 1998; Bronfenbrenner, 1979, 1986; Bronfenbrenner & Morris, 1998; Elder, 1998; Garbarino, 1982; Goodwin, 1973; Goodstein & Sandler, 1978; Kelly, 1968;

Rappaport, 1977; Reppucci, 1987; Seidman, 1991). It replaces a view of problems as residing exclusively within individuals (e.g., poverty derives from lack of individual initiative, teenage pregnancy is a result of individual failures to contracept competently, pervasive individual testing is the answer to AIDS), with a view of problems as multiply determined, dynamic, historically located, and of a relational nature (Seidman, 1981).

As such, the ecological approach has the potential to redirect narrowly conceived policies focused on individual change. By attending to multiple layers of influence, this approach increases the chances of identifying unintended consequences of intervening at one point rather than another, and may advance policies that intervene simultaneously at several points. The ecological perspective also explicitly recognizes that people are embedded in a policy and historical context, as well as in the more immediate contexts of their families, support networks, and communities. It therefore directs attention to the ways in which specific policies at specific historical moments alter the incentives, perceptions, and supports that constitute the broad frameworks of individual lives.

One prominent social problem, domestic violence, is used here to illustrate the levels-of-analysis approach to public policy issues. Domestic violence has emerged as a major social, health, and law-enforcement issue that contributes to a broad array of fatal and nonfatal injuries and medical and psychiatric disorders each year (National Research Council, 1998). Interventions to address domestic violence, ranging from mandatory arrest policies to community-wide public education initiatives, have proliferated in recent years.

Table 2 presents a range of potential responses, organized by level of analysis within an ecological framework. The framework begins at the level of the individual, defined in this case

TABLE 2. Domestic Violence: Levels of Policy Response

Level of analysis	Problem definition	Policy response
Individual	Men and women who abuse their spouses have unaddressed mental health and substance abuse problems	Individual mental health and substance-abuse services (sometimes court-mandated)
Microsystem	Domestic violence arises from dysfunctional family interaction dynamics	Family or couples counseling; mental health services for children who witness domestic violence
Mesosystem	Couples experiencing domestic violence are not embedded in a system of supports and social controls that can prevent and ameliorate domestic violence	Protective orders; battered women's shelters; health care services
Exosystem: Social networks	Adults who are isolated from social supports are more likely to engage in domestic violence and to continue such violence undetected	Group counseling programs for couples; peer support groups for battered women; reporting requirements
Exosystem: The economy	Poverty places stresses on couples that can erupt in domestic violence and creates dependency on abusive partners	Income support, minimum wage, welfare-to-work, and housing policies
Macrosystem	Social, cultural, and gender norms that portray acceptable violent behavior and reinforce power imbalances between men and women create a social environment that tolerates domestic violence	Public education campaigns; communitywide domestic violence prevention programs, gender equity policies

Note: This materials draws on the 1998 report of the National Research Council and the Institute of Medicine, *Violence in Families: Assessing Prevention and Treatment Programs.*

as the perpetrator or victim of abuse, and traces alternative problem definitions and responses through the four embedded systems defined by Bronfenbrenner (1979): (1) the microsystem, which represents any immediate setting containing the abuser, victim, or other family members (e.g., the family setting); (2) the mesosystem, which captures interrelationships among microsystems (e.g., the home–social-services interface); (3) the exosystem, which contains formal and informal societal structures that do not contain the abuser or victim, but impinge directly on their behavior (e.g., surrounding social networks); and (4) the macrosystem, which encompasses prevailing values and organizational patterns that broadly characterize a culture (e.g., social norms regarding gender roles).

As can be seen, differing definitions of the nature of the problem dictate distinct levels of intervention and types of policies. Does the "problem" reside with the individual abuser, with social norms about violence, or both? Who is responsible—the abuser, the victim, the surrounding community—for addressing the problem? The range of responses is vast, spanning from individual mental health counseling to gender equity policies. Moreover, policies that intervene at one level may defeat the intent of policies that intervene at other levels. For example, the goal of improving the mental health of abusers may be attenuated by efforts aimed at mandatory reporting and sentencing that imply that abusers are unlikely to change absent strong community sanctions against domestic violence.

The mesosystem is an especially interesting domain insofar as domestic violence has emerged as a major health and law-enforcement issue, and, more traditionally, as a social-services issue. As a result, initiatives, often at the community level, to mobilize interactions among institutional settings that have operated quite independently are proliferating (see National Research Council, 1998). These include forming domestic violence units in the prosecutor's office, launching treatment programs for abusive husbands in probation departments, training health-care professionals to identify and refer family-violence victims, and establishing fatality review teams that are composed of representatives of multiple agencies.

This capacity to stretch the boundaries and premises that guide public policy has been identified by some as the source of psychology's greatest impact on society. Rappaport (1981, 1987), using the metaphor of "unpacking," urges psychologists to pursue and articulate paradoxical definitions of social problems (e.g., Head Start both compensates for parenting that is labeled "inadequate" and empowers the parents of poor children), and to facilitate consideration of multiple solutions to social problems. Divergent, rather than singular, resolutions to complex problems should be revealed. This is precisely the "enlightenment" function that Weiss (1977) found to predict policymaker's attention to social science data.

Acknowledgment of Values

Public policy is a value-laden arena. Decisions affecting maintenance of life supports for severely handicapped infants, disclosure of hazard information to consumers, use of federal funds for abortion, and eligibility of homosexuals for public adoption subsidies are commonplace. Ethical dilemmas necessarily accompany the selection of issues for policy attention (what is a private vs. a public problem?), the allocation of public resources (who wins, who loses?), and the design of interventions (who is eligible and who is not?).

Preparation for the dilemmas that arise when facts and values collide is a prerequisite for psychologists who seek to apply their knowledge and skills to public policy. Policymakers operate in a partisan, adversarial climate, and are unaccustomed to information that arrives in the form of objective advice. As Schick has noted, "The objective analyst finds a communication gulf right away with most committee staff because there is no room for neutrality" (1977, p. 117, cited in Weiss, 1984). Sarason has warned (1981): "In the chasm between your scientific findings and solutions, on the one hand, and the realm of human affairs, on the other hand, there is a mine field of values for the traversing of which your science provides no guide" (p. 373).

Community psychology, perhaps as a result of studying such thorny issues as abortion, discrimination, and mental health, has come closer than most other specialities of psychology to explicitly acknowledging that values infiltrate science. Community psychologists, as a consequence, may be more accustomed to examining the assumptions that guide their own work. Indeed, several of the seminal articles in this field (Cowen, 1977; Kelly, 1986; Price, 1989; Rappaport, 1981; Sarason, 1981; Trickett, 1984) have explicitly addressed the value frameworks that guide the field, including an emphasis on disenfranchised or "high-risk" groups (e.g., the poor, the institutionalized, the homeless, the unemployed), the promotion of empowerment and self-help, the design of natural support systems as opposed to institutional or professional ("expert–client") interventions, and respect for individual autonomy and diversity.

While considered a liability in scientific circles, forthrightness about value assumptions may, in fact, facilitate effective interaction in policy circles (Weiss, 1983). Sarason (1981), for example, has suggested that being "true to your values" may provide the most dependable guide for psychologists who enter the policy arena. Judge David Bazelon (1982) takes this one step further, criticizing psychologists for their "sins of nondisclosure." He urges that scientists share with policymakers the limitations of their data, competing hypotheses, and the values that guide their interpretations.

None of these experts is suggesting that scientists blur the boundaries between their data and their values any more than is inevitable. To the contrary, calls for methodological rigor often accompany calls for disclosure and relevance (Cairns & Cairns, 1986; Campbell, 1969; Garner, 1972; Scarr, 1985). Moreover, stating the limitations and ambiguities in research may serve to minimize the potential for distortion of results. Koretz (1982), for example, discusses the uncertainties inherent in probabilistic research, and then specifies three limitations that characterize evaluation research: (1) most evaluations address a subset of program goals, (2) most evaluations do not sample a truly representative sample of program types or beneficiaries, and (3) few evaluations are designed to inform questions of differential effectiveness within a federal program. The challenge facing the psychologist who ventures into the policy arena is essentially one of becoming self-conscious about the values, assumptions, and constraints that have affected one's work.

The Theory of Empowerment

Community psychology has been instrumental in advancing empowerment models of social intervention (Albee, 1980; Iscoe, 1974; Levine, 1982; Rappaport, 1981, 1987; Chapter 1, this volume). To empower people (Berger & Neuhaus, 1977) is to enhance their ability to control their own lives; this requires policies that approach recipients as competent citizens, rather than as victims. Thus, empowerment encompasses both personal control and political action. Rappaport states "empowerment conveys both a psychological sense of personal control or influence and a concern with actual social influence, political power, and legal rights" (1987, p. 121).

Public policies concerning human services typically defy the empowerment orientation.

Instead, they tend to have a disparaging and compensatory thrust. We have remedial policies targeted to individuals and families for whom something, by definition, has gone wrong, rather than policies that aim to prevent the onset of problems, sustain benefits, or build competencies (Grubb & Lazerson, 1982; Steiner, 1981). Taking the child-care example discussed earlier, both the compensatory education and welfare-reform justifications for public expenditures on child care assume that the recipient families are not competent to provide adequate home environments, sustain employment and, thus, be self-sufficient. The alternative approach would cast child care as a fully legitimate and essential part of enabling families to combine parenting and employment roles. The public interest in strong families and a productive economy, rather the child-welfare model of compensating for individual families' deficiencies, would provide the empowerment-based rationale for a public role in child-care provision (Phillips & Zigler, 1987).

As seen from this example, human-service policies also tend to portray the failures and inadequacies of recipients in individual, personal terms, thus diverting attention from societal and systemic causes of problems (Ryan, 1971). This individualistic, deficit approach to human services derives in large measure from the tremendous reluctance in our society to replace private responsibility for "personal" needs, such as child care, health care, housing, and employment, with policies that legitimate public responsibility. Public responsibility is approved only as a last resort when private mechanisms are deemed inadequate (Grubb & Lazerson, 1982).

The disparity between the empowerment orientation of community psychology and the deficit orientation of most human-service policies represents a classic test case for the enlightenment role of research. As Rappaport (1981) has noted, this will force attention to intervening, or mediating, structures—the neighborhood, churches, and self-help groups—that stand between individuals and large institutional structures that often confound opportunities for personal competence and self control.

A final example of how community psychology can be used to empower the recipients of public policies is demonstrated in the work of Brody and colleagues (Brody, 1985; Brody, Fleishman, & Galavotti, 1986). In their efforts to elucidate the psychological impacts of locating a nuclear waste dumpsite in an agricultural community in Texas, public opinion surveys were used not only to assure systematic public input into a policy decision, but also to lend an independent voice to a broader and more representative spectrum of the affected community. This approach (see also Fawcett, Seekins, Whang, Muiu, & Suarez de Balcazar, 1984) serves the dual functions of empowering the local community and expanding the knowledge base about how people and communities cope with environmental threats.

Collaborative Research Methods

The methods, as well as the basic orientations, of community psychology lend it relevance to policy issues. Reppucci (1985) speculated that "research which is formulated and undertaken in natural environments within a theoretical framework may be more directly relevant to public policy issues than theoretical research which is conducted in the artificial environment of the laboratory" (p. 24). In practice, public policies are social experiments—Head Start, welfare reform, deinstitutionalization (Cohen and Garet, 1975). Research that closely approximates this model of testing theory in a public arena is likely to be more immediately understandable to policymakers, and potentially more meaningful to them as a consequence.

Lewin (1947) formulated a social-action research model with the goal of stimulating the application of social science to solving major social problems while, at the same time, enhancing the creativity of theoretical and methodological research. Reciprocity, sustained feedback, immersion in community problem-solving, and collaboration between researchers and practitioners lie at the heart of action research (Ketterer, Price, & Polister, 1980; Trickett, 1984). The study of people in context is a hallmark of community psychology (Kelly & Hess, 1986; Trickett, Kelly, & Vincent, 1985). Contemporary methods in community psychology have retained the emphasis on collaboration, longitudinal study, and a participatory style of research (Kelly, 1986; Levine & Perkins, 1987). Asymmetrical professional–client models of intervention are rejected in favor of models that approach recipients as partners and researchers as participants (Connell, Kubish, Schorr, & Weiss, 1995; National Research Council, 1998; Rappaport, 1987).

These methodological orientations offer community psychologists several advantages in the policy arena. First, stories rather than statistics tend to stimulate public policymaking. Contrary to top-down models of policy development, human-interest anecdotes, and concrete examples of how programs really work (or don't work), the so-called "ordinary knowledge" (Lindblom & Cohen, 1979), are among the most influential starting points for public policy. The demands of action research, including immersion in the daily experiences of people and hands-on knowledge about community structures, yield substantial ordinary knowledge in the process of acquiring scientific data. Armed with both stories and statistics, community psychologists can be influential shapers of the policy agenda.

Second, the multiple perspectives that are encompassed in studies that employ the action research model offer policymakers a valuable glimpse at the concerns that diverse groups will bring to a policy issue. Recent work in the evaluation field calls for efforts to systematically explore the "theories of change" that are held by various designers and participants involved in community interventions as a first step in planning a program of research tied to such programs (Weiss, 1995). Third, as Elmore (1983) states

> The critical juncture in social problem-solving is at the boundary between broad (funding formulas, assignment of responsibilities, rules) and fine (individual skills, interpersonal communication and commitment) structures of action. It is in these transactions that policy is or is not made intelligible. Hence, the success of policies in "solving" social problems is determined less by the context of the policies themselves than by the capacity of the organizations that implement them (p. 233).

Community psychologists' firsthand knowledge of the organizations that are responsible for policy implementation can provide critical insights into impediments, unintended consequences, and points of leverage as they seek to apply research to public policymaking.

Contemporary Issues

Many of the major issues commanding national policy attention are of obvious relevance to community psychologists, including health care reform, crime prevention, urban renewal, education reform, and early intervention. However, issues that at face value may appear quite far removed from the concerns of community psychologists often have far-reaching effects on people and communities. Highway speed-limit regulations and handgun control legislation have direct impacts on child safety, for example. Tax legislation can have profound effects on income redistribution. Environmental protection and hazardous-waste laws have vast human implications. Brody and colleagues (Brody, Fleishman, & Galavotti, 1986) have cogently demonstrated the association between a federal decision about the location of a nuclear waste dumpsite and family relations, the community economy (and thus jobs and family income), and stress and physical symptomatology. Similarly, Levine (1982) has drawn attention to the devastating personal, family, and community impacts of toxic contamination at Love Canal.

Increasingly, the human dimensions of these ostensibly non-human and nonsocial policies are receiving the attention of policymakers. The human impact of workplace technologies, the community effects of toxic contamination, and the family effects of economic disruption provide examples of less conventional topics in which community psychologists and politicians now share interest.

FUTURE OPPORTUNITIES AND DILEMMAS

Community psychology grew out of a serious commitment to more reasoned, careful, and effective public policies. The ecological, social-action orientation of this subdiscipline lends it a special comparability with the processes, orientations, and issues that characterize public policymaking. Yet, the presence of community psychology (and of psychology in general) in the legislative policy arena, while clearly discernable, has not been prominent (DeLeon, 1986; Kiesler, 1980; Reppucci, 1985; Sarason, 1983). This is attributable, in part, to some continuing resistance within the mainstream of psychology to political involvement; to the traditional emphasis in community psychology on local issues, community-level interventions, and, more recently, legal policy; and to genuine impediments to the effective involvement of scientists in the policy arena.

Community research, like all research, enters a crowded arena in the policy sphere. While this means that research is rarely determinative, a fact that may assuage the concerns of those who believe science and politics should not mix, it also implies that without careful attention to dissemination and a persistent presence, the influence of psychological research will be severely attenuated. Many of the issues central to the community discipline, such as homelessness, teenage pregnancy, violence and crime, and school reform, are framed in the context of highly value-laden debates. This raises the volume and the heat to which community psychologists who enter the policy arena will be subjected. Policies geared toward prevention and empowerment face an uphill battle given the pressures to demonstrate immediate responses to problems and the "last-resort" mentality of many government policymakers (Brim & Phillips, 1988).

Closer to home, a central challenge involves removing the structural barriers within academic psychology to "giving psychology away" (Kelly, 1984; Melton, 1987a; Miller, 1969; Task Force on Psychology and Public Policy, 1986). These include expanding the reward structure to give credit for public service, publication of research in nonscientific outlets, and sabbaticals and fellowships spent in policy positions. Brody (1986) highlights the essential task of "bringing in more troops," and thus raises serious questions about training community psychologists to be conversant with policy issues and processes (see Doyle, Wilcox, & Reppucci, 1983). The involvement of policy experts as partners in the design, conduct, and interpretation of research poses an additional challenge.

Clarifying policy roles for community psychologists that will promote effective exchanges among scientists and policymakers is also essential (Reppucci, 1985; Task Force on Psychology and Public Policy, 1986). Along these lines, the value of placing individuals in "brokering" roles that bridge the scientific and policy worlds needs to be recognized. They demand a blend of technical expertise, substantive knowledge, and political judgment. Scientists are hired to fill them largely as a result of their technical and disciplinary expertise, and are retained because of their skill in translating this expertise into policy implications. These roles are among the most sought-after nonacademic positions in our field. For example, a recent interview with 59 of the more than 60 Congressional Science and Executive Branch Fellows sponsored by the Society for Research in Child Development between 1978 and 1994 revealed that only 25 are now in academic positions, with the remaining 34 in a wide variety of nonacademic positions (Thomas, 1997). These positions have included Executive Director of the National Committee for the Prevention of Child Avuse; the President of the Foundation for Child Development; Director of the Board on Children, Youth, and Families at the National Research Council; administrative officers for Child, Youth, and Family Policy, Health Policy, and Office of Ethnic Minority Affairs at the American Psychological Association; Staff Director for Human Resources with the Ways and Means Committee of the U.S. House of Representatives; and Director of Public Policy with the Child Welfare League of America.

The day-to-day demands of these positions interweave science, personal judgment, and advocacy. Congressional Science Fellows, for example, are called upon to find academic witnesses for congressional hearings (largely a "scientific" task), to write briefing memos *with recommended actions* on proposed legislation (a technical and political task), and to write inflammatory partisan speeches (a purely political task). Clearly, the dilemmas that have been portrayed here between demands for answers and the limits of data, and between being scientific and being partisan, constitute everyday issues for psychologists in policy positions—a reality that training programs must take into account (Phillips, 1983).

What does community psychology, and psychology in general, stand to gain from moving into the public arena? In Bronfenbrenner's words "science needs policy—needs it not to guide our organizational activities, but to provide us with two elements essential for any scientific endeavor—vitality and validity" (Bronfenbrenner, 1974, p. 1). Psychologists presently involved in policy activities, and policymakers who have benefitted from interactions with these psychologists, will create pressures for our discipline to reconcile its two wishes for non-involvement and influence. Scarce research support and competition for jobs will compel greater integration of policy work and policy issues within psychology's central mechanisms for communication and training. Moreover, pressing social problems will not disappear, thus continuing to confront psychologists with the challenge of promoting human welfare. It is the premise of this chapter that these pressures for change present opportunities rather than annoyances. As the Task Force on Psychology and Public Policy concludes (1986), the challenges invite us "to do what (we) do best: facilitate growth in psychological knowledge and its application in the world of which psychology becomes a continually larger part" (p. 920).

REFERENCES

Albee, G. W. (1980). A competency model to replace the deficit model. In M. Gibbs, J. Lachenmeyer, & J. Sigal (Eds.), *Community psychology: Theoretical and empirical approaches*. New York: Gardner.

Alkin, M. L., Daillak, R., & White, P. (1979). *Using evaluations: Does evaluation make a difference?* Beverly Hills: Sage.

American Psychological Association. (1984). Task Force on Psychology and Public Policy *Final Report*. Washington, D.C.: Author.

Atkinson, R. C. (1977). Reflections on psychology's past and concerns about its future. *American Psychologist, 32*, 205–210.

Baltes, P. N. B., Lindenberger, U., & Staudinger, U. M. (1998). Life-span theory in developmental psychology. In W. Damon (Ed.), *Handbook of child psychology* (5th ed, pp. 1029–1144). New York: Wiley.

Bauer, R. A. (1966). Social psychology and the study of policy formation. *American Psychologist*, 933–942.

Bazelon, D. (1982). Veils, values, and social responsibility. *American Psychologist, 37,* 115–121.

Bennett, C. C., Anderson, L. S., Cooper, S., Hassol, L., Klein, D. C., & Rosenblum, G. (1966). *Community psychology: A report of the Boston conference on the education of psychologists for community mental health.* Boston: Department of Psychology, Boston University.

Berger, P. I., & Neuhaus, R. J. (1977). *To empower people: The role of mediating structures in public policy.* Washington, D.C.: The American Enterprise Institute.

Bevan, W. (1976). The sound of the wind that's blowing. *American Psychologist, 31,* 481–491.

Bevan, W. (1982). A sermon of sorts in three parts. *American Psychologist, 37,* 1303–1322.

Bevan, W., & Kessel, F. (1994). Plain truths and home cooking: Thoughts on the making and remaking of psychology. *American Psychologist, 49,* 505–509.

Boulding, K. E. (1976). The boundaries of social policy. In J. E. Tropman, M. Bluhy, R. Lind, W. Vasey, & R. A. Croxton (Eds.), *Strategic perspectives on social policy* (pp. 11–21). New York: Pergamon.

Brim, O. G., & Phillips, D. A. (1988). The life-span intervention cube. In E. M. Hetherington, R. M. Lerner, & M. Perlmutter (Eds.), *Child development in life-span perspective* (pp. 277–298). New York: Erlbaum.

Brody, J. G. (1985). New roles for psychologists in environmental impact assessment. *American Psychologist, 40,* 1057–1060.

Brody, J. G. (1986). Community psychology in the eighties: A celebration of survival. *American Journal of Community Psychology, 14,* 139–145.

Brody, J. G., Fleishman, J., & Galavotti, C. (1986). *Community responses* presented at the Annual Convention of the American Psychological Association, Washington, D.C., August.

Bronfenbrenner, U. (1974). Developmental research, public policy, and the ecology of childhood. *Child Development, 45,* 1–5.

Bronfenbrenner, U. (1979). *The ecology of human development: Experiments by nature and design.* Cambridge, MA: Harvard University Press.

Bronfenbrenner, U. (1986). Ecology of the family as a context for human development: Research perspectives. *Developmental Psychology, 22,* 723–742.

Bronfenbrenner, U., & Morris, P. A. (1998). The ecology of developmental processes. In W. Damon (Ed.), *Handbook of child psychology* (5th ed., pp. 993–1028). New York: Wiley.

Cairns, R. B., & Cairns, B. D. (1986). On social values and social development: Gender and aggression. In L. Friedrich-Cofer (Ed.), *Human nature and public policy: Scientific views of women, children, and families.* (pp. 177–201). New York: Praeger.

Campbell, D. (1969). Reforms as experiments. *American Psychologist, 24,* 409–429.

Caplan, N., Morrison, A., & Stambaugh, R. J. (1975). *The use of social science knowledge in policy decisions at the national level.* Ann Arbor: Institute for Social Research, University of Michigan.

Caplan, N., & Nelson, S. D. (1973). On being useful: The nature and consequences of psychological research in social problems. *American Psychologist, 28,* 199–218.

Cohen, D. K., & Garet, N. S. (1975). Reforming educational policy with applied social research. *Harvard Educational Review, 45,* 17–43.

Coleman, J. S. (1978). The use of social science research in the development of public policy. *Urban Review, 10,* 197–202.

Connell, J. P., Kubisch, A. C., Schorr, L. B., & Weiss, C. H. (Eds.). (1995). *New approaches to evaluating community initiatives: Concepts, methods, and contexts.* New York: The Aspen Institute.

Cowen, E. G. (1977). Baby steps toward primary prevention. *American Journal of Community Psychology, 5,* 1–22.

Deitchman, S. (1976). *The best-laid schemes: A tale of social research and bureaucracy.* Cambridge, MA: MIT Press.

DeLeon, P. H. (1986). Increasing the societal contribution of organized psychology. *American Psychologist, 41,* 466–474.

DeLeon, P. H., O'Keefe, A. M., Vandenbos, G. R., & Kraut, A. G. (1982). How to influence public policy. A blueprint for action. *American Psychologist, 37,* 476–485.

Doyle, J. B., Wilcox, B. L., & Reppucci, N. D. (1983). Training for social and community change. In E. Seidman (Ed.), *Handbook of social intervention* (pp. 615–638). Beverly Hills: Sage.

Elder, G. H. (1998). The life course and human development. In W. Damon (Ed.), *Handbook of child psychology* (5th ed., pp. 939–992). New York: Wiley.

Elmore, R. (1980). Backward mapping: Implementation research and policy decisions. *Political Science Quarterly, 94,* 601–616.

Elmore, R. F. (1983). Social policymaking as strategic intervention. In E. Seidman (Ed.), *Handbook of social intervention* (pp. 212–236). Beverly Hills: Sage.

Fawcett, S. B., Seekins, R., Shang, P. W., Muiu, C., & Suarez de Balcazar, Y. (1984). Creating and using technologies for community empowerment. *Prevention in Human Services, 13,* 145–171.

Friedrich-Cofer, L. (Ed.) (1986). *Human nature and Public Policy: Scientific views of women, children, and families.* New York: Praeger.

Garbarino, J. (1982). *Children and families in the social environment.* New York: Aldine.

Garner, W. R. (1972). The acquisition and appliation of knowledge: A symbiotic relation. *American Psychologist, 27*, 941–946.

Glaser, E. M., & Taylor, S. H. (1973). Factors influencing the success of applied research. *American Psychologist, 28*, 140–146.

Goodstein, L. D., & Sander, I. (1978). Using psychology to promote human welfare: A conceptual analysis of the role of community psychology. *American Psychologist, 33*, 882–892.

Goodwin, L. (1973). Bridging the gap between social research and public policy. *Journal of Applied Behavioral Science, 9*, 85–114.

Goodwin, L. (1975). *Can social science help resolve national problems?* New York: Free Press.

Greenberger, E. (1983). A researcher in the policy arena: The case of child labor. *American Psychologist, 38*, 104–111.

Greenberger, E., & Steinberg, L. (1986). *When teenagers work: The psychological and social costs of adolescent employment.* New York: Basic Books.

Grubb, W. N., & Lazerson, M. (1982). *Broken promises: How Americans fail their children.* New York: Basic Books.

Hayes, C. (1982). *Making policies for children: A study of the federal process.* Washington, D.C.: National Academy of Sciences.

Heclo, H. (1978). Issue networks and the executive establishment. In A. King (Ed.). *The new American apolitical system* (pp. 87–124). Washington, D.C.: American Enterprise Institute.

Horowitz, I. L. (Ed.). (1971). *The use and abuse of social science.* New Brunswick, NJ: Transactionbooks.

Iscoe, I. (1974). Community psychology and the competent community. *American Psychologist, 29*, 607–613.

Kelly, J. G. (1968). Toward an ecological conception of preventive intervention. In J. Carter (Ed.), *Research contributions from psychology to community mental health* (pp. 76–100). New York: Behavioral Publications.

Kelly, J. G. (1984). Interpersonal and organizational resources for the continued development of community psychology. *American Journal of Community Psychology, 12*, 313–317.

Kelly, J. G. (1986). Context and process: An ecological view of the interdependence of practice and research. *American Journal of Community Psychology, 14*, 581–589.

Kelly, J. G., & Hess, R. (Eds.). (1986). *The ecology of prevention: Illustrating mental health consultation.* New York: Haworth.

Ketterer, R., Price, R., & Politser, P. (1980). The action research paradigm. In R. Price, & P. Politser (Eds.), *Evaluation and action in the social environment.* New York: Academic.

Kiesler, C. (1980). Psychology and public policy. In L. Bickman (Ed.), *Applied Social Psychology Annual*, Vol. 1. Beverly Hills, CA: Sage.

Kimble, G. A. (1982). *The limits of advocacy.* Unpublished manuscript.

Knorr, K. D. (1977). Policymakers' use of social science knowledge: Symbolic or instrumental? In C. Weiss (Ed.), *Using social research in public policymaking* (pp. 165–182). Lexington, KY: D.C. Heath.

Koretz, D. (1982). Developing useful evaluations: A case history and some practical guidelines. In L. Saxe & D. Koretz (Eds.), *New directions for program evaluation: Making evaluation research useful to Congress* (No. 14, pp. 25–50), San Francisco: Jossey-Bass.

Korten, F. F., Cook, S. W., & Lacey, J. I. (1970). *Psychology and the problems of society.* Washington, D.C.: American Psychological Association.

Levine, A. G. (1982). *Love Canal: Science politics, people.* Lexington, MA: Lexington Books.

Levine, M., & Perkins, D. V. (1987). *Principles of community psychology.* New York: Oxford University Press.

Lindblom, C. E. (1959). The science of muddling through. *Public Administration Review, 19*, 79–88.

Lindblom, C. E., & Cohen, D. (1979). *Usable knowledge: Social science and social problem solving.* New Haven, CT: Yale University Press.

Lorion, R. P., Iscoe, I., DeLeon, P. H., & VandenBos, G. R. (Eds.). (1996). *Psychology and public policy: Balancing public service and professional need.* Washington, D.C.: American Psychological Association.

Lynn, L. E. (1978). The question of relevance. In L. E. Lynn (Ed.), *Knowledge and policy: The uncertain connection.* (pp. 12–22). Washington, D.C.: National Academy of Sciences.

Maccoby, E. E., Kahn, A. J., & Everett, B. A. (1983). The role of psychological research in the formation of policies affecting children. *American Psychologist, 38*, 80–84.

MacRae, D. (1976). *The social function of social science.* New Haven: Yale University Press.

March, J. G. (1979). Science, politics, and Mrs. Gruenberg. In *The National Research Council in 1979* (pp. 27–36). Washington, D.C.: National Academy of Sciences.

Marmor, T. R. (1983). Competing perspectives on social policy. In E. Zigler, S. L. Kagan, & E. Klugman (Eds.),

Children, government and families: Perspectives on American social policy (pp. 35–56). Cambridge: Cambridge University Press.

McCall, G., & Weber, G. (1984). *Social science and public policy: The roles of academic disciplines in policy analysis.* Washington, NY: Associated Faculty Press.

McCall, R. B. (1996). The concept and practice of education, research, and public service in university psychology departments. *American Psychologist, 51,* 379–388.

Melton, G. B. (1987a). Bringing psychology to the legal system. *American Psychologist, 42,* 488–495.

Melton, G. B. (1987b). Adolescent abortion: Psychological perspectives on public policy. *American Psychologist, 42,* 69–72.

Miller, G. A. (1969). Psychology as a means of promoting human welfare. *American Psychologist, 24,* 1063–1075.

National Research Council (1998). *Violence in families: Assessing prevention and treatment programs.* R. Chalk & P. A. King (Eds.). Washington, D.C.: National Academy Press.

Nelson, R. (1977). *The moon and the ghetto.* New York: W.W. Norton.

Phillips, D. (1983). *Improving the connections between child development and social policy.* Invited presentation before the Conference on Training and Research in Child Development and Social Policy, Vanderbilt Institute for Public Policy Studies, Nashville, TN.

Phillips, D. (1986). The federal model child care standards act of 1985: Step in the right direction or hollow gesture? *American Journal of Orthopsychiatry, 56,* 56–64.

Phillips, D. (1991). With a little help: Children in poverty and child care. In A. Huston (Ed.), *Children in poverty: Child develoment and public policy* (pp. 158–189). Cambridge: Cambridge University Press.

Phillips, D., & Zigler, E. (1987). The checkered history of federal child care regulation. In E. Rothkopf (Ed.), *Review of reserach in education, Vol. 14* (pp. 3–41). Washington, D.C.: American Educational Research Association.

Prewitt, K. (1983). Subverting policy premises. In D. Callahan & B. Jennings (Eds.), *Ethics, the social sciences and policy analyses.* New York: Plenum.

Price, R. (1989). Bearing witness. *American Journal of Community Psychology, 17,* 151–167.

Rappaport, J. (1977). *Community psychology: Values, research and action.* New York: Holt, Rinehart, & Winston.

Rappaport, J. (1981). In praise of paradox: A social policy of empowerment over prevention. *American Journal of Community Psychology, 9,* 1–26.

Rappaport, J. (1987). Terms of empowerment/exemplars of prevention: Toward a theory for community psychology. *American Journal of Community Psychology, 15,* 121–148.

Rein, M., & White, S. H. (1977). Policy research: Belief and doubt. *Policy Analysis, 3,* 239–272.

Reppucci, N. D. (1985). Psychology in the public interest. In A. M. Rogers & C. J. Scheier (Eds.), *The G. Stanley Hall Lectures Series,* Vol. 5. (Pp. 125–126). Washington, D.C.: American Psychological Association.

Reppucci, N. D. (1987). Prevention and ecology: Teen-age pregnancy, child sexual abuse, and organized youth sports. *American Journal of Community Psychology, 15,* 1–22.

Reppucci, N. D., & Kirk, R. (1984). Psychology and public policy. In G. McCall & G. Wever (Eds.), *Social science and public policy: The roles of academic disciplines in policy analysis* (pp. 129–158). Port Washington, NY: Associated Faculty Press.

Rich, R. F. (1977). Use of social science information by federal bureaucrats: Knowledge for action versus knowledge for understanding. In C. Weiss (Ed.), *Using social science research in public policy making* (pp. 199–212). Lexington, MA: D.C. Heath.

Robinson, D.N. (1984). Ethics and advocacy. *American Psychologist, 39,* 787–793.

Ruble, N. D., & Thompson, E. P. (1992). The implications of research on social development for mental health: An internal socialization perspective. In D. N. Ruble, P. R. Costanzo, & M. E. Oliveri (Eds.), *The social psychology of mental health: Basic mechanisms and applications.* (pp. 81–125). New York: Guilford.

Ruopp, R., Travers, J., Glantz, F., & Coelen, C. (1979). *Children at the center: Final report of the National Day Care Study.* Boston: Abt Associates.

Ryan, R. (1971). *Blaming the victim.* New York: Random House.

Sarason, S. B. (1978). The nature of problem-solving in social action. *American Psychologist, 33,* 370–380.

Sarason, S. B. (1981). *Psychology misdirected.* New York: Free Press.

Sarason, S. B. (1983). Psychology and public policy: Missed opportunity. In R. Felner, L. A. Jason, J. N. Moritsugu, & S. S. Farber (Eds.), *Preventive psychology: Theory, research, and practice* (pp. 245–250). New York: Pergamon.

Saunders, J. T., & Reppucci, N. D. (1977). Learning networks among administrators of human service institutions. *American Journal of Community Psychology, 5,* 269–276.

Scarr, S. (1985). Constructing psychology: Facts and fables for our time. *American Psychologist, 40,* 499–512.

Seidman, E. (1981). The route from the successful experiment to policy formation. In R. Roesch & R. Corrado (Eds.), *Evaluation and criminal justice policy* (pp. 81–102). Beverly Hills: Sage.

Seidman, E. (1991). Social regularities and prevention research: A transactional model. In P. Muehrer (Ed.), *Concep-*

tual research models for preventing mental disorders (pp. 145–164). Rockville, MD: National Institute of Mental Health.

Sigel, I. E. (1998). Practice and research: A problem in developing communication and cooperation. In W. Damon (Ed.), *Handbook of child psychology*, (5th ed., pp. 1113–1132). New York: Wiley.

Steiner, G. Y. (1981). *The futility of family policy.* Washington, D.C.: The Brookings Institution.

Sundquist, J. L. (1978). Research brokerage: The weak link. In L. E. Lynn (Ed.), *Knowledge and policy: The uncertain connection* (pp. 126–144). Washington, D.C.: National Academy of Sciences.

Takanishi, R., & Melton, G. B. (1987). Child development research and the legislative process. In G. S. Melton (Ed.), *Reforming the law: Impact of child development research* (pp. 86–101). New York: Guilford.

Task Force on Psychology and Public Policy, American Psychological Association (1986). Psychology and public policy. *American Psychologist, 41,* 914–921.

Thomas, N. (1997, March). *A review of SRCD's Congressional Science and Executive Branch Fellowship Program: Interviews with past fellows.* Unpublished document prepared for the SRCD Committee on Social Policy, University of Michigan, Ann Arbor.

Trickett, E. J. (1984). Toward a distinctive community psychology: An ecological metaphor for the conduct of community research and the nature of training. *American Journal of Community Psychology, 12,* 261–280.

Trickett, E. J., Kelly, J. G., & Vincent, T. (1985). The spirit of ecological inquiry in community research. In E. Susskind & D. E. Klein (Eds.), *Community research: Methods, paradigms, and applications* (pp. 283–333). New York: Praeger.

Weiss, C. (1977). Research for policy's sake: The enlightenment function of social research. *Policy Analysis, 3,* 531–545.

Weiss, C. (1978). Improving the linkage between social research and public policy. In L. Lynn (Ed.), *Knowledge and policy; the uncertain connection* (pp. 23–81). Washington, D.C.: National Academy of Sciences.

Weiss, C. (1983). Ideology, interests, and information. The basis of policy positions. In D. Callahan and B. Jennings (Eds.), *Ethics, the social sciences and policy analysis* (pp. 213–245). New York: Plenum.

Weiss, C. (1984). Increasing the likelihood of influencing decisions. In L. Rutman (Ed.), *Evaluation research methods: A basic guide* (pp. 159–190). Beverly Hills, CA: Sage.

Weiss, C. (1987). The circuitry of enlightenment. *Knowledge: Creation, Diffusion, and Utilization, 8,* 274–281.

Weiss, C. H. (1995). Nothing as practical as good theory: Exploring theory-based evaluation for comprehensive community initiatives for children and families. In J. P. Connell, A. C. Kubisch, L. B. Schorr, & C. H. Weiss (Eds.), *New approaches to evaluating community initiatives: Concepts, methods, and contexts.* New York: The Aspen Institute.

Weiss, C., & Bucuvalas, M. J. (1977). The challenge of social research to decision making. In C. Weiss (Ed.), *Using social research in public policy-making* (pp. 213–234). Lexington, MA: Heath.

Whitebook, M., Howes, C., & Phillips, D. (1998). *Worthy work, unlivable wages: The national child care staffing study, 1988–1997.* Washington, D.C.: Center for the Child Care Workforce.

Zigler, E. (1980). Welcoming a new journal. *Journal of Applied Developmental Psychology, 1,* 1–56.

Zigler, E., Kagan, S. L., & Hall, N. W. (Eds.). (1996). *Children, families, and government: Preparing for the 21st century.* New York: Cambridge University Press.

CHAPTER 18

Dissemination of Innovation as Social Change

JEFFREY P. MAYER AND WILLIAM S. DAVIDSON II

For community psychology, the phrase "dissemination of innovation" implies the use of new social programs or social policies. As such, it also implies the potential for broad-scale change. It typically addresses how individuals and organizations can improve their approach to particular problems. Hence, for community psychologists interested in promoting human welfare, this paradigm offers an approach to the study and creation of social change (e.g., Rappaport, 1977; Fairweather & Davidson, 1986). If solution of a social problem is the goal of an innovation, then dissemination and implementation of that innovation on a wide scale may mean that important steps have been accomplished (Fairweather & Tornatzky, 1977).

Such an approach is not specific or unique to community psychology, but has been applied within a variety of disciplines. Other labels for this approach include research, development, and dissemination (House, Kerins, & Steele, 1972), knowledge utilization (Havelock, 1973), diffusion of innovation (Radnor, Feller, & Rogers, 1978), and technological innovation (Tornatzky, Eveland, Boylan, Hetzner, Johnson, Roitman, & Schneider, 1983). The use of this paradigm has occurred in fields as diverse as political science (Pressman & Wildavsky, 1973); sociology (Ryan & Gross, 1943); agriculture (Havelock, 1973); and public health (Green & Johnson, 1996); and has been applied to numerous social problems, including youth violence (Thomas, 1998); HIV/AIDS prevention (Dearing, 1994); poor nutrition (Harveyberino, Ewing, Flynn, & Wick, 1998), adolescent drug, alcohol, and tobacco use (Laflin, Edmundson, & Moore-Hirsch, 1995; Brink, Levenson, & Gottlieb, 1991); and citizen action against nuclear weapons (McAlister, 1991). Other recent reviews include chapters by Parcel, Perry and Taylor (1990); Oldenberg, Hardcastle and Kok (1997); Portnoy, Anderson, and Eriksen (1989); and Basch, Eveland, and Portnoy (1986).

For community psychologists, the dissemination of innovation is typically viewed in the specific context of social innovations such as social programs or policies. These "social technologies" represent new approaches designed for the solution of particular social prob-

JEFFREY P. MAYER • Department of Community Health, School of Public Health, St. Louis University, St. Louis, Missouri 63108. WILLIAM S. DAVIDSON II • Department of Psychology, Michigan State University, East Lansing, Michigan 48824.

Handbook of Community Psychology, edited by Julian Rappaport and Edward Seidman. Kluwer Academic/Plenum Publishers, New York, 2000.

lems. Dissemination has as its goal the creation of positive social change. This chapter is concerned with applications of the dissemination of innovation paradigm to the improvement of human and community functioning. The dissemination of innovation can be thought of as a specific approach to influencing social policy, one of several delineated by Phillips (Chapter 17, this volume). The dissemination of innovation, as it has been approached by community psychologists, is unique in two ways relative to other social policy approaches. First, the dissemination of innovation involves systematic approaches that are active in style and involve the intentional of spread of the innovation. This is to be contrasted to investigations of other approaches that involve the naturally occurring spread of social programs. As seen later in this chapter, active interpersonal, group, and organization tactics are involved in the dissemination of innovations. Second, this approach has typically involved the dissemination of particular specifiable social-program models. While the dissemination of innovations can and has (in other fields) involved multiple levels of behavior, including policies, procedures, and personnel, as practiced within the field of community psychology it has typically involved the dissemination of particular social programs.

Fairweather and colleagues (Fairweather, 1972; Fairweather & Tornatzky, 1977; Fairweather, Sanders, & Tornatzky, 1974; Fairweather & Davidson, 1986; Rappaport, 1977; Tornatzky, Fergus, Avellar, Fairweather, & Fleischer, 1980) are primarily responsible for introducing the notion of dissemination of innovation as a social-change process to community psychology. For this group, the dissemination of innovation is embedded in Fairweather's framework of experimental social innovation (Fairweather & Davidson, 1986). This overall theory of social change describes an incremental process involving four sequential steps ending in the dissemination of innovations.

While not necessarily dependent on the overall experimental social-innovation model of social change, it is best to understand how the dissemination of innovation fits within the four-phase model of social change: (1) the *creation of innovative models* designed to solve a specific social problem; (2) a *scientifically credible evaluation* of the effectiveness of the innovation; (3) *limited replication* of the model, assuming a positive assessment of its effectiveness; (4) an *active dissemination* or purposeful attempts to have the program implemented on a large-scale fashion. These four phases represent a dynamic process, with each phase dependent on previous steps. Failure at any phase necessitates reverting to prior phases.

The dissemination-of-innovation phase itself consists of three components—adoption, implementation, and institutionalization. *Adoption* involves the host setting's decision to use an innovative social program. *Implementation* is the actual use of the program. Finally, *institutionalization or routinization* (Yin, 1978) of the innovative social program takes place when a new social program moves to the status of being part of business as usual.

DEVELOPMENTAL PERSPECTIVES ON INNOVATION

Within a dissemination framework, it is assumed that the impetus for innovation and change stem from a basic dissatisfaction with a current practice, policy, or program (Barnett, 1953; Lapiere, 1965). Because institutions and organizations are notorious for maintaining the *status quo* and resisting change (Coch & French, 1948; Mirvis & Berg, 1977; Frank & Hackman, 1975), action-oriented steps to facilitate the adoption and implementation of social problem-solving innovations are other critical aspects of the process of dissemination. Although dissatisfaction with the prevailing situation is a necessary condition, it is not enough to create the needed change. Change also requires active efforts to facilitate adoption, implementation, and routinization. Before delving into this chapter's primary aim, we describe a developmental perspective on dissemination.

Many theorists have offered descriptions of the innovation process as a series of successive events, or stage models (Beyer & Trice, 1978; Ettlie, 1980; Guba, 1968; Fairweather, Sanders, & Tornatzky, 1974; Rogers, 1983; Yin, 1978; Zaltman, Duncan, & Holbek, 1973). Basic to stage-model conceptualizations is the developmental notion that dissemination is a set of progressive steps or phases, or classes of decisions and actions, that are temporal and ordered, and are necessary precursors to the ultimate adoption decision or innovation implementation.

Stage models offer a descriptive heuristic within which community psychologists think about the social change process. At the moment there is little empirical support for these models. It is not clear that real-world decision processes proceed in such a rational and ordered manner. For example, Eveland, Rogers, and Klepper (1977) suggested that innovation can occur with little awareness on the part of key actors in the process. This possibility is supported by other organizational psychologists who have noted the haphazard and serendipitous nature of decision processes (Cohen, March, & Olsen, 1972), and the fact that decisions are rarely rational, centrally controlled, or organization-wide. Weick's (1976) notion of the "loosely-coupled" functioning of organizational subsystems (Weick, 1976) further suggests that small units within organizations can operate relatively autonomously with regards to many decisions.

These caveats aside, stage models provide a useful schema for organizing theoretical notions and past research in the area. In addition, they can be useful in that they suggest that for different stages, different explanatory factors and dissemination strategies may be pertinent and/or effective (Parcel, Taylor, Brink, & Gottlieb, 1989). For example, Goodman, Tenney, Smith, and Steckler (1993) report that principal and superintendent behaviors were influential during the adoption and routinization stages, whereas teacher behaviors were critical during the implementation stage in a program to disseminate tobacco-prevention programs to schools. In a related finding, Brink and colleagues (1995) found it effective to match messages about the innovation with a particular stage. For example, based on theory and findings from prior research reviews, the relative advantage and compatibility of the innovation were emphasized during the adoption stage, while trailability and observability were to be emphasized during the implementation stage.

A useful distinction concerning stage models of the innovation process was provided by Tornatzky, Eveland, Boylan, Hetzner, Johnson, Roitman, and Schneider (1983). They sought to derive an explicit difference between source-centered models and user-centered models. *Source-centered* models embody the viewpoint of the developer of the innovation, that is, the stages reflect the perspective of the developer of the innovation. Such models enumerate the phases necessary to convince an organization or individual to adopt an innovation; they often have a research and development flavor. On the other hand, *user-centered* models reflect the viewpoint of the innovation adopter, that is, those individuals or organizations that may ultimately make use of the new program. Both *source-centered* and *user-centered* models detail the process of activity within organizations who are considering implementing an innovation. Source-centered models begin with innovation creation and basic and applied research, and end with active dissemination efforts by the developer, usually ceasing at the point of adoption; user-centered models begin with awareness of the innovation and end with routinization of the innovation.

To date, research on the dissemination of innovations has been predominantly concerned with events prior to and including the adoption decision (Blakely et al. 1987). Innovation was assumed to imply increased effectiveness, the so-called "pro-innovation bias" (Rogers, 1983, 1993; O'Neil, Pouder, & Bucholtz, 1998; Smith, Zhang, & Colwell, 1996). It has often been assumed that innovations were immutable technologies that were easily transportable and transplantable. Given this conception, the major focus of research has been on the adoption phase of spreading innovations. Hence, the latter part of the innovation process, those stages describing actual implementation, has remained largely a mystery. Recent efforts in the current decade have begun to unravel postadoption processes.

This chapter will be primarily devoted to the latter parts of the innovation process because reviews on the adoption process already exist (Greer, 1977; Rogers, 1983; Cockerill & Barnsley, 1997). This chapter will also focus on adoption and implementation of social programs rather than physical technologies. This focus was selected because community psychologists legitimately have an interest in the implementation of new social programs. Hence, simple and relatively discrete innovations by individual actors, such as new medical procedures by physicians (Menzel, 1960) or agricultural techniques by farmers (Ryan and Gross, 1943), are of minimal interest. However, before turning to treatments of the implementation and routinization of complex social programs and policies, attributes of innovations and characteristics of adopters will briefly be considered.

PROPERTIES OF INNOVATIONS AND INNOVATORS

Research focusing on the adoption decision has been characterized by two major streams of inquiry. One employed the adopting organization or individual as the focus. The second focused on the dimensions of the innovation itself. Although the great majority of research studies involved the individual as the unit of analysis, some more recent investigations have examined the organizational correlates of innovation adoption.

Characteristics of Adopters

The first stream of research measured variables primarily focused on attributes of adopters. This line of inquiry explored concerns for the personality and sociodemographic characteristics of individuals, as well as dimensions of organizations, that distinguished early adopters from later adopters and non-adopters. Classic innovation theory posited an initially slow rate of adoption in a population, followed by a period of much more rapid adoption among the majority, with a slowing near the end of the process as only the more recalcitrant members of the population remained as non-adopters (Rogers, 1983; Green & McAlister, 1984). Early adopters have been labeled "innovation champions" since they often serve as opinion leaders and/or role models to later adopters (Chakrabati, 1972; Backer & Rogers, 1998).

At the individual level of analysis, Rogers and Shoemaker (1971) and Rogers (1983) reviewed a large number of studies (over 1,500) concerning the characteristics of individuals who adopt innovations. Many of the studies involved the adoption of agricultural innovations or medical technologies in less-developed countries. In general, adopters were found to be characterized by: (1) more years of education, (2) higher social status, (3) greater intelligence and empathy, (4) higher achievement motivation, (5) greater likelihood of participating in social networks, (6) greater likelihood of holding opinion leadership roles, and (7) greater likelihood of having contact with national networks. Despite these findings, important caveats to relying on high SES individuals as opinion leaders in active dissemination campaigns have been noted (Lindbladh, Lyttkens, Hanson, & Ostergren, 1997).

At the organizational level of analysis, the early work of Burns and Stalker (1961) described two kinds of organizations—organic and mechanistic. Organizations that possessed "organic" structures are more flexible, decentralized in their decision-making process, and fluid. "Mechanistic" structures are seen as more inflexible, centralized in their decision-making, and formal. This early theoretical formulation predicted that organic organizations were more likely to be innovative. Subsequent research provided empirical support for these notions (Thompson, 1967; Lawrence & Lorsch, 1967; Litwak, 1961; Witte, 1993). Additional research examined the relation between key structural variables, such as formalization, complexity, and centralization with organizational innovativeness. Innovativeness has been positively linked to complexity (Hage & Aiken, 1970; McCormick, Steckler, & McLeroy, 1993) and extra organizational resources (Cyert & March, 1963), but negatively linked to formalization and centralization (Aiken & Hage, 1971; Hage & Dewar, 1973; Shepard, 1967; Rothman, 1974), although some exceptions to these general findings exist (Scheirer, 1990). For a more detailed discussion of these issues, the reader is referred to Zaltman, Duncan, and Holbek (1973).

Characteristics of Innovations

The second line of research has primarily involved assessment of aspects of the innovation itself. There have been a number of key concepts in studying the characteristics of innovations. *Relative advantage* is the extent to which the innovative program or policy appears to be an improvement over existing practice. The key concept is the comparative effectiveness. A second concept, *trialability*, is the degree to which the innovation appears easy to implement. A third concept is the *relative and absolute cost* of the innovation. Budget realities are thought to be major constraints on contributors to the dissemination of innovation. A fourth concept is the *observability* of the innovation. Both the ease of observation and the degree to which innovations become noticed are important dimensions. Finally, the innovation's *communicability* is thought to be an important dimension. The degree to which an innovation is easy to describe is the core aspect of this concept.

As was the case in studying the characteristics of adopters, research on the characteristics of innovations almost exclusively utilizes the individual level of analysis. Methodologically, it has typically involved surveys of potential adopters who were asked about the hypothetical adoption and characteristics of a new social program or policy. Although several useful generalizations have been offered by Rogers (1983) and others (Kivlin & Fliegel, 1967; Ascione et al., 1987; Cummings, Jaen, & Funch, 1984), the relationships have exhibited instability and inconsistency, and little standardization has existed in how attributes and adoption have been operationalized.

Tornatzky and Klein (1982) reviewed 75 studies of the relation between innovation attributes and adoption. They employed formal meta-analytic techniques to assess the consistency of the direction of attribute–adoption relationships (although effect size was not considered), and provided an analysis of the methodological state of the literature. Their major methodological criticisms of this literature included lack of predictive designs, unreplicability of measurement, predominance of case studies dealing with only a single adopter or a handful of adopters and a limited number of innovation attributes, and excessive focus at the individual level of analysis. Of the 20 different characteristics of innovations which Tornatzky and Klein reviewed, only compatibility, relative advantage, and complexity exhibited a consistent relationship with adoption. In other words, innovations that were more compatible with existing practice were seen as relatively more advantageous, relatively simple (versus complex), and more often adopted.

Recently, some authors have advocated preemptively incorporating positive attributes into innovations during design and development to hasten their later rapid dissemination (Bartholomew, Parcel, & Kok, 1998; Howze & Redman, 1992). This perspective argues for creating innovative programs with the qualities of high relative advantage, low complexity, high compatibility, and so on, at the outset, thereby reducing potential difficulties during the adoption and implementation stages. Although the intransigence of many social problems may preclude making all innovative interventions simple, easily communicated, and trialable, etc., consideration of dissemination at an early part of the process may ultimately lead to greater success in having effective innovations become widely employed.

Critique

Several criticisms of this research have been offered. One major criticism has been offered by Downs and Mohr (Mohr, 1982; Downs & Mohr, 1976, 1979; Downs, 1978). They suggest that the enormous variability and instability reported by research on the relationships between adopter characteristics, innovation characteristics, and adoption occurs in large part because these relationships are specific to a particular pairing of an innovation attribute and an organization. They suggest that the proper methodological relationship is what they call the "innovation decision design," wherein a specific innovation attribute is studied in relation to a specific organization. They argue that generalizable relationships involving secondary attributes simply do not exist. This criticism essentially attacks the entire body of research reviewed above.

A second criticism concerns poor operationalization of the criterion in innovation research. Frequently, the measurement of adoption is a simple "yes–no" dichotomous variable. Several analysts have questioned how well dichotomous measures of adoption capture the richness of subsequent innovative activity, or lack of it, particularly when considering complex innovations within organizations (Downs & Mohr, 1976; Eveland, 1979). Does a verbal decision to adopt imply appropriate and continued use of an innovation? If a commitment or formal decision to adopt is made, are the actions of implementation automatically carried out?

Additionally, there exist no standard or commonly used measures of adoption. Hence, what one investigator has measured and labeled may be entirely different from another. Many investigators have employed a criterion variable labeled "success," but how this has been defined has varied from staff perceptions concerning innovation goal attainment (Berman & McLaughlin, 1978), to detailed observation of social-program components (Hall & Loucks, 1978). Verbal intention of using an innovation has been confused with actual use, and actual use has been confused with innovation effectiveness or consequences. This creates obvious problems when attempting to discern a general theory of innovation process.

A final criticism of innovation attribute research involves specification of the unit of analysis. From an organizational perspective, whose responses constitute the organizational response? Simple aggregation of individual responses may not always be appropriate because innovation may be the product of smaller groups within the organization whose perceptions and actions are critical. These smaller groups may include the dominant coalition (Hage, 1980), the change agent group (Fairweather, Sanders, & Tornatzky, 1974), or top management (Perry & Kraemer, 1980).

What should be clear from this discussion is that there is not strong consensus about what is known in this field. The debates about research design, criterion measurement, and unit of analysis problems reflect differing points of view about the process and the proper means of investigation. The field awaits future research to integrate the divergent points of view or offer alternative, more satisfactory, explanations. This should not be viewed as a source of undue pessimism. At the organizational level, this area of investigation is really only a little over two decades old, a relatively short period of time for unambiguous results.

IMPLEMENTATION AND POST-ADOPTION ACTIVITY

From the perspective of the community psychologist, adoption is only a prelude to implementation. It is useful to consider two components of postadoption activity. The first has been called implementation, which refers to the degree to which the innovation is put into use within the organization. We will limit our discussion to what has been commonly labeled "program implementation" (Scheirer, 1982), or "micro-implementation" (Berman, 1978), rather than to policy or macro-implementation (Pressman & Wildavsky, 1973; Nelson & Yates, 1978; Williams, 1975). This means we will limit our discussion to the implementation of specific program models as new approaches to social problems or alternatives to prior practice. This is in contrast to broad policy implementation that may include, but not be limited to, program implementation. As we will see shortly, confusion of the two has fueled a largely unnecessary debate about how to measure innovation, as well as the actual nature of implementation.

The second component of postadoption activity is what has been called routinization or institutionalization. It has also been labeled incorporation, durability, persistence, or sustaining ability by various authors. Routinization comes after implementation, and therefore might be considered the final stage of the innovation process. It refers to the degree to which the innovation becomes accepted by the organization and becomes an integral part of "standard operating procedures." It also implies longevity or continued use of an innovation long after initial implementation (Yin, 1978; Goodman & Steckler, 1989; Glaser & Backer, 1980).

The desire to successfully implement effective programs spans across many human service areas. Federal and state agencies have developed programs with the specific mission of disseminating exemplary projects. For example, the United States Department of Education developed the National Diffusion Network (Raizen, 1979; Emrick, 1977), and the National Institute of Justice developed the Exemplary Projects Program (Ellickson and Petersilia, 1983; Mayer and Blakely, 1984). Brink et al. (1991) describe a campaign to disseminate tobacco prevention programs to all elementary schools in Texas. Chapko (1991) discusses an effort to spread preventive technology to all dentists in the State of Washington. These broad federal and state programs are underpinned by the "linking agent" concept, which suggests that successful dissemination only occurs when a planned, active effort is in place that connects the resource system (e.g., the innovation developer) with the user system (Havelock, 1973; Dijkstra & Parcel, 1993; Monahan & Scheirer, 1988; Scheirer, 1990). Hence, the goal of these programs is to promote the adoption of innovations that have gone through rigorous demonstration and evaluation efforts, and which have been found to have positive effects.

A related concern in program evaluation revolves around the "integrity" or "strength" of treatment (Sechrest & Redner, 1978; Boruch & Gomez, 1977; Leonard & Lowery, 1979). Originally cited in the context of trying to explain why evaluation study results are frequently null or inconsistent, it was argued that inappropriate emphasis was placed on outcome, with little attention to the "black box" of the program itself (Leonard & Lowery, 1979; Davidson, Redner, & Saul, 1983). Charters and Jones (1973) suggested that many educational evaluations yield no encouraging results because program elements may not be implemented at all, resulting in an evaluation study of "non-events." Tornatzky (1982) indicated that the field of program evaluation should be just as concerned with the "robustness of programs," meaning their endurance over repeated replication, as with the statistical robustness of findings. Data concerning the degree of implementation of evaluated programs is critical for subsequent utilization and for good policy decisions. Measurement of programs will need to be more than a dichotomous judgement, and involve more detailed assessment of individual components and process.

In studying implementation, it is also important to determine if the innovation is actually used by the clients of the implementing organization over time. Without continued use of innovations, or with their continued but "reinvented" use, benefits for the target population may be non-existent or severely diluted (Hall & Loucks, 1978; Tornatzky, Fergus, Avellar, & Fairweather, 1980). Routinization is also important because the longer the innovation survives, the longer potential benefits to clients will continue (Mayer, Blakely, & Davidson, 1986), at least until newer problems gain priority over older ones (Green, 1989). Community psychologists interested in systemic change should find this a particularly germane issue.

MEASURING IMPLEMENTATION

Because little precedent exists, methods for reliably and validly recording implementation activity are still emerging. All commonly used methods of data collection (i.e., observations, interviews, questionnaires, coding of archives) are possible, and all actors involved in the innovation process (i.e., developers, users, change agents, clients) are potential candidates from whom to gather information. Some investigators have attempted to measure innovation processes common to all innovations. For example, investigators at the Centers for Teacher Education at the University of Texas have developed a "levels of use" measure for many educational innovations (Loucks, Newlove, & Hall, 1975). Others have attempted to assess the degree of implementation of a single specific social-program innovation (Owens & Haenn, 1979; Leithwood & Montgomery, 1980).

Scheirer and Rezmovic (1983) conducted a review of 75 projects that involved measuring implementation in nine content areas. They reported a descriptive analysis and provided recommendations for future measurement work. The recency of the field was demonstrated by the fact that over half of the reviewed studies had been published after 1979, and this was in 1982! The predominant data collection method was personal interview. Reliability and/or validity assessments were performed for less than a quarter of the studies, and only a third collected data at more than one point in time.

Perhaps the most crucial problem in implementation measurement concerns explicit specification of the innovation prior to actual fieldwork, a problem that occurs when the study of macro- and micro-implementation becomes confused. If an innovation is a policy, that is, a general provision of direction to an organization, but with no particular programmatic focus, it is impossible to delineate the innovation in clear and precise terms. Hence, measuring a policy innovation is quite different from measuring a complex technology possessing both material and social components. Not making clear at the outset the nature of the innovation, and possibly trying to measure aspects of an innovation that elude measurement have been the primary sources of the problem. Various analysts have labeled this imbroglio "specification failure" (Hollisfield and Slavin, 1983) or "task specificness" (Yin, 1979).

FIDELITY VERSUS ADAPTATION AND REINVENTION

Fidelity of implementation concerns the degree to which an innovation is implemented in a manner similar to the original demonstration model. There has been a great deal of controversy concerning the desirability of such duplication (Datta, 1981; Charters & Pellegrin, 1973; Fullan & Pomfret, 1977). Advocates of high fidelity conceptualize innovations as consisting of a number of well-specified program components that should be closely matched at replication sites. If not, program effectiveness could be diluted (Calsyn, Tornatzky, & Dittmar, 1977; Hall & Loucks, 1978).

Adaptation, in a sense, is the converse of fidelity. It refers to modification or change in the innovative social model. Other analysts have used the term "reinvention" to capture the forces of interaction between innovation and organization that shape adaptation (Rice & Rogers, 1979; Larsen & Agarwala-Rogers, 1977; Brunk & Goeppinger, 1990; Paine-Andrews, Murray, Fawcett, & Campuzano, 1996). Others have attempted to distinguish between the deletion of components, the modification of components, or the addition of new components (Palumbo, Maynard-Moody, & Wright, 1984; Mayer, Blakely, & Davidson, 1986).

Proponents of the adaptation perspective suggest that differing organizational environments and needs almost always demand local modification. They claim that higher levels of program flexibility and modification lead to greater user sense of program ownership, and therefore effectiveness and routinization. For example, Berman and McLaughlin's (1978) influential study of educational-program dissemination found three patterns of implementation. The first, *cooptation*, involved an organization adopting an innovation without any co-occurring changes in the rest of the organization. This could involve adopting innovations completely congruent with the organizations functioning, or could be additions to existing organizations that did not alter their overall operation. The second, *mutual adaptation*, involved an organization adopting an innovation with co-occurring changes in the organization itself and alterations of the original innovation. This type of implementation required alterations in organization functioning, but also involved modifications in the innovative model. Finally, Berman and McLaughlin (1978) observed *nonimplementation*. Because mutual adaptation was the only mode under which successful and long-term change occurred, these analysts concluded that high fidelity is uncommon, and that changes in both the innovation model as well as the organization are necessary.

Middle-ground positions have also been proposed. Hall and Loucks (1978) argued that adaptation or reinvention was acceptable up to a "zone of drastic mutation," beyond which continued dilution compromised the program's integrity and effectiveness. In other words, certain "configurations" of components may be more acceptable or unacceptable than others, resulting in partial implementation. Berman (1981) proposed a contingency model of implementation, suggesting that the fidelity perspective is likely to function best with structured and well-specified innovations, while the adaptation perspective is more appropriate for looser, policylike innovations. However, many situations are so complex that some combination of the two strategies might prove to be most successful, requiring careful replication of important program ingredients with adaptation of other ingredients necessary to make the program palatable to local users.

In a recent *American Journal of Community Psychology* article, Bauman, Stein, and Ireys (1991) argue that while reinvention of the operational components of programs is inevitable, fidelity to the innovative program model's theory base is what is most critical. This perspective suggests that it is appropriate to modify or even replace procedural aspects of replicate programs, as long as these reinventions target the same theory-based intermediate outcomes with a similar level of effort as the demonstration program, so that ultimate outcomes will not be comprised. Miller, Klotz, and Eckholdt (1998) provide a recent example from HIV prevention. In this replication study, although significant operational reinvention of the program model was reported, positive changes in both theory-based mediators and unprotected sexual behaviors were maintained, similar to the effects obtained during the original demonstration-project evaluation.

A large-scale study conducted at the Center for Innovation Research at Michigan State University examined the active dissemination of three educational and four criminal justice innovations among a purposeful, nationwide sample of organizations (Mayer, Blakely, & Davidson, 1986; Blakely, Mayer, Gottschalk, Schmitt, Davidson, Roitman, & Emshoff, 1987; Roitman & Mayer, 1982; Roitman, Gottschalk, Mayer, & Blakely, 1983). The seven innovations were remedial reading, experiential education, alternative school, jury management, juvenile diversion, work release, and community crime prevention. Each of the innovations had been the subject of active dissemination efforts by the federal government. During site visits to 70 organizations (10 had adopted each of the 7 innovative programs), measures of fidelity, reinvention, routinization, and effectiveness were collected. The 70 were selected from over 200 that had been identified in a phone survey of potential adopters of the innovations. These organizations included schools, courts, police departments, prisons, and community agencies.

The findings from this large study indicated that relatively high fidelity to the developer model was the norm. In other words, when replicates of innovative programs occurred, they were typically similar to the original innovative model. In addition, fidelity and reinvention were positively related to effectiveness. Replicates that showed a relatively strong resemblance to the original prototype were more likely to produce the desired outcomes. "Modification" reinvention was not related to effectiveness, but "addition" reinvention was. Replicate programs that went beyond the original model (i.e., added new components) were more likely to produce desired outcomes than those that only modified the original prototypical program. Although others had suggested that program users made positive additions to social models (Palumbo, Maynard-Moody, & Wright [1984] discussed "constructive adaptation"), and that high fidelity produced effectiveness (Scheirer, 1982; Heck, Steigelbauer, Hall, & Loucks, 1978), empirical evidence making these links in a multiinnovation, multiorganizational sample that had not previously existed.

Although most innovation-process research has been correlational in nature, there are several exceptions. Fairweather, Sanders, and Tornatzky (1974) conducted a national study to investigate methods to disseminate a mental health innovation. The "Lodge" program was demonstrated effective in maintaining a useful community role for chronic patients. Employing a two-phase experimental design with 255 psychiatric hospitals across the country, it was found that action-oriented approaches were critical to institute actual efforts by hospitals to implement the community lodge. Although relatively few hospitals adopted the program, hospitals that received "action consultation" were more likely to adopt, and then go on to implement, the program than were hospitals who only received a "written manual." Also important to eventual implementation were the efforts of small, cohesive groups of internal change agents identified as a part of process evaluation data analysis. A second round of active dissemination efforts with hospitals that did not adopt during the first experiment produced additional adopters, and reinforced earlier findings that action consultant approaches create greater change (Tornatzky, Fergus, Avellar, & Fairweather, 1980).

Stevens and Tornatzky (1979) reported on a randomized experiment to examine methods of disseminating program-evaluation methodology to substance-abuse agencies. The two-by-two design contrasted group and private organizational consultations and on-site versus telephone modes of communication. Each of 40 agencies involved in the experiment were contacted at a five-month follow-up to assess the extent and quality of evaluation activities. Main effects existed for both independent variables favoring on-site/group approaches.

In a quasi-experiment involving 128 intervention and 38 comparison schools, Parcel and colleagues (Parcel et al., 1995; Brink et al., 1995) evaluated a statewide effort to disseminate tobacco prevention programs. The dissemination intervention was grounded in social learning theory as well as concepts from dissemination of innovation. Hence, in addition to messages emphasizing the high relative advantage, high compatibility, and low complexity of the tobacco prevention program, the dissemination campaign included interpersonal and video components that operationalized observational learning, outcome efficacy, and self-efficacy. At 2-year follow-up, 56% of the intervention schools and only 10% of the comparison schools had adopted the program. These results were maintained when adjusted for baseline values of the theory-based covariates (e.g., relative advantage, teacher self-efficacy to implement the program). This study is noteworthy for its large scope involving essentially all school districts in Texas, and for its active utilization of innovation attribute concepts in the design of the intervention.

ROUTINIZATION

Studies of routinization attempt to discover the process and associated factors by which innovations become integrated into the ongoing procedures of a setting. Yin (1977) studied the "life history" of six innovations implemented in a diverse sample of municipal bureaucracies. The retrospective design required that organizational incumbents recall critical events in the innovation's development. The major conceptual advance of this study was to view routinization as the survival of an innovation through a series of passages and cycles. Cycles refer to events that can occur repeatedly (such as survival of equipment or personnel turnover, or another budget period), while passages imply events that occur only once (such as transition to support of local funds, or incorporation into organizational rules of governance). Operationalized as the number of passages and cycles that had been survived, three stages of routinization were hypothesized—improvisation, expansion, and disappearance. Improvisation reflected a marginal degree of routinization, while the disappearance stage implied total integration (i.e., disappearance into routine). Yin has studied several examples of purposeful federal dissemination efforts. The results of his work in this area has suggested several things. It appears that internal factors, such as organizational and budget considerations, are more important predictors of continued use than are external factors, such as relationships to national groups. Yin concluded that the federal investment in active dissemination activity was well spent, and that a substantial proportion of the disseminated innovations were routinized. He concluded that municipal bureaucracies were not as resistant to change as was commonly thought to be the case.

Tornatzky, Fergus, Avellar, and Fairweather (1980) examined the survival of three mental health innovations within a sample of psychiatric hospitals. Their methodology involved a case study approach in which dichotomous data concerning survival through each passage and cycle was collected. While the innovations had substantial success in negotiating the cycles, they experienced difficulty with the passages. The authors concluded that the studied innovations had stood the "initial test of temporal survival," but had not achieved "organizational legitimacy."

Glaser and Backer (1977) argued that local adaptation of innovations would promote routinization to the extent that it countered the "not invented here" syndrome, and would provide users with a "sense of ownership" and investment in the program. To support these notions, Glaser and Backer (1980) compared six terminated innovations with four others that had survived. Programs that continued successfully helped in closing performance gaps, experienced substantial reinvention, and had high levels of staff involvement in decision-making.

Berman and McLaughlin (1977) investigated the continuation of educational innovations two years following the termination of federal financial support. Unlike Yin (1977), these analysts discovered that long-term use of innovative programs was rare. Most organizations formally eliminated the innovation with only traces of innovative teacher behavior remaining (labeled isolated continuation), or they continued use of the innovation in name only (*pro forma* routinization). Routinization was positively associated with more ambitious and complex innovations, high-quality training and staff support, and a large degree of teacher participation in decision-making.

In an extension of Yin's work, Goodman and Steckler (1989) add the concept of niche saturation to the passages and cycles, and embed all three concepts within the organizational subsystems (i.e., production, maintenance, support, adaptive, and managerial) described by Katz and Kahn (1978). Niche saturation is defined as an institutionalized program's "maximum feasible expansion" within the host organization, and in Goodman and Steckler's framework reflects the third and final phase of institutionalization occurring after attainment of the passages and cycles. In a school production subsystem, for example, niche-saturation criteria would be satisfied if all classrooms in a school that could possibly employ an innovative curriculum actually did so, regardless of the length of time the curriculum had been used in a smaller number of classrooms. In multiple case studies of both school (Steckler, Goodman, McLeroy, Davis, & Koch, 1992) and community (Steckler & Goodman, 1989; Goodman & Steckler, 1989) health-promotion programs, these investigators contrasted low and highly institutionalized programs, and offered a set of prescriptions for enhancing program longevity and incorporation. Moreover, they developed a quantitative measure of institutionalization with eight subscales assessing cycle and niche saturation for four Katz and Kahn subsystems. This measure exhibited good internal consistency, and was significantly related to years of program operation and perceived permanence (Goodman, McLeroy, Steckler, & Hoyle, 1993).

CONCLUSIONS

It should be obvious from this chapter that the current state of knowledge about the dissemination of innovations is filled with many questions. There have been questions of definition, level of analysis, and research design. Yet there are, at this juncture, some tentative conclusions that can be drawn that have pertinence to community psychology and future directions for the field.

Dissemination of innovation, as a paradigm, offers a valuable framework to community psychologists for conceptualizing social change. While distinct from broader considerations of social policy change, the dissemination of innovation has an important and distinct tradition within the field (Davidson & Fairweather, 1986; Rappaport, 1977).

It is often assumed that a natural motivation occurs out of a dissatisfaction with the *status quo*, but the investigation of dissemination of innovations has revealed that resistance to change is common and entrenched, and implementation following adoption is not automatic. Community psychology needs to understand these processes. This understanding will have implications for our theoretical perspectives on the change process and on the professional roles thought appropriate for the field.

Although a large literature exists concerning innovation adoption of simple technologies by individuals, community psychologists are more legitimately concerned with the adoption and postadoption implementation of complex interventions and programs in organizations and communities. Research concerning characteristics of individual adopters suggests that early use of innovation is associated with a set of roles, and demographic and personality variables, such as cosmopoliteness, opinion leadership, and boundary spanning. Further, particular patterns of organizational structure are associated with innovation. Innovation is more likely in organizations that are organic and nonbureaucratic; it is less likely to occur in organizations that are highly formalized and centralized. However, we know considerably less about the characteristics of organizations that lead to effective implementation of innovations or the extent to which innovation longevity relates to effectiveness (Rappaport, Seidman, & Davidson, 1977; Seidman, 1983). Innovations with the secondary attributes of compatibility, relative advantage, and complexity are more likely to be adopted by individuals and organizations. However, problems in criterion operationalization, selection of the appropriate unit of analysis, idiosyncratic measurement, and the predominance of case studies inhibit the founding of a generalizable theory of attribute–adoption relationships.

The study of the implementation and routinization of innovation has proceeded only in very recent times, and can be characterized as emerging. Despite the paucity of research, it is an important area of inquiry for improving the quality of conclusions reached in program evaluation studies, and is critical if the potential benefits offered by new demonstration programs eventually are to accrue to a broad population. In this context, the fidelity-adaptation debate continues, although a better understanding of the context of particular studies has cleared away a considerable amount of ambiguity and lack of consistency in findings. The contingency perspective suggests that a fidelity approach best matches microimplementation, and an adaptation approach best matches macroimplementation. This is an example of where confusion between the dissemination of innovative social problem-solving interventions and more general social policy change has obfuscated our understanding of two different phenomena. More recently, the concept of fidelity itself has been broadened to include adherence to the prescribed theory base of interventions as well as the operational components of programs (Bauman, Stein, & Ireys, 1991).

Reinvention is not the simple lack of fidelity. Recent research has suggested that creative and additive reinvention may contribute to, rather than distract from, implementation. Further, reinvention may play a role in increasing innovative program effectiveness. Having said this, it appears to be the case that a moderate positive relationship exists between degree of implementation and the effectiveness of a social program. Although additional research is needed, it seems prudent to promote high-fidelity replication of well-specified social models (Blakely et al., 1987; Mayer, Blakley, & Davidson, 1986).

Finally, findings concerning the extent of routinization of innovations vary greatly from study to study. They suffer from the retrospective nature of all of the data available on this topic. It seems that the likelihood of continued use and integration of innovations increases as certain key events, such as annualized budgeting, equipment and personnel turnover, inclusion in organizational governance, and the like occur. Recent conceptual and measurement advances (Goodman, McLeroy, Steckler, & Hoyle, 1993) may spur more research and greater understanding of institutionalization.

In many ways we end where we began. The dissemination of innovation describes a domain of practice and research of concern to community psychology. As such it is a relatively new arena for social scientists generally and community psychologists specifically. The dissemination of innovation represents a domain of professional and scientific challenge critical to the field as it continues to expand its horizons. Included are many issues to which the community psychologist brings an important perspective. The dissemination of innovation represents an important avenue for social change involvement that holds the promise of expanding professional boundaries, encouraging an interdisciplinary perspective, demanding an action orientation, and crying out for high-quality investigation. These are the challenges that this field needs to address.

REFERENCES

Aiken, M., & Hage, J. (1971). The organic organization and innovation. *Sociology, 5*, 563–582.

Ascione, F. J., Kirking, D. M., Wenzloff, N. J., Foley, T. A., & Kwok, D. K. (1987). Effect of innovation characteristics on pharmacists' use of written patient medication information. *Patient Education & Counseling, 9*, 53–64.

Backer, T. E., & Rogers, E. M. (1998). Diffusion of innovations theory and work-site AIDS programs. *Journal of Health Communication, 3*, 17–28.

Baldridge, J. V., & Burnham, R. A. (1975). Organizational innovation: individual, organizational and environmental impacts. *Administrative Science Quarterly, 20*, 165–176.

Barnett, H. G. (1953). *Innovation: The basis of cultural change.* New York: McGraw-Hill.

Bartholomew, L. K., Parcel, G. S., & Kok, G. (1998). Intervention mapping: A process for developing theory and evidence based health education programs. *Behavior, 25*, 545–563.

Basch, C. E., Eveland, J. D., & Portnoy, B. (1986). Diffusion systems for education and learning about health. *Family and Community Health, 9*, 1–26.

Bauman, L. J., Stein, R. E., & Ireys, H. T. (1991). Reinventing fidelity: The transfer of social technology among settings. *American Journal of Community Psychology, 19*, 619–639.

Berman, P. (1978). The study of macro- and micro- implementation. *Public Policy, 26*, 157–184.

Berman, P. (1980). Thinking about programmed and adaptive implementation: Matching strategies to situations. In D. Mann and H. Ingram (Eds.), *Why policies succeed or fail.* (pp. 205–227). Beverly Hills, CA: Sage.

Berman, P., & McLaughlin, M. W. (1978). *Federal programs supporting educational change: Implementing and sustaining innovations.* Santa Monica, CA: Rand Corporation. R-1589/8-HEW.

Beyer, J. M., & Trice, H. M. (1978). *Implementing change: Alcoholism policies in work organizations.* New York: Free Press.

Blakely, C. H., Mayer, J. P., Gottschalk, R. G., Schmitt, N., Davidson, W. S., Roitman, D. B., & Emshoff, J. G. (1987). The fidelity-adaptation debate: Implications for the implementation of public sector social programs. *American Journal of Community Psychology, 15*, 253–268.

Boruch, R. F., & Gomez, H. (1977). Sensitivity, bias and theory in impact evaluations. *Professional Psychology, 8*, 411–434.

Brink, S. G., Levenson-Gingiss, P., & Gottlieb, N. H. (1991). An evaluation of the effectiveness of a planned diffusion process: The Smoke-Free Class of 2000 Project in Texas. *Health Education Research, 6*, 353–362.

Brink, S. G., Basen-Engquist, K. M., O'Hara-Tompkins, N. M., Parcel, G. S., Gottlieb, N. H., & Lovato, C. Y. (1995). Diffusion of an effective tobacco prevention program: Part 1: Evaluation of the dissemination phase. *Health Education Research, 10*, 283–295.

Brunk, S. E., & Goeppinger, J. (1990). Assessing reinvention of community-based interventions. *Evaluation and the Health Professions, 13*, 186–203.

Burns, T., & Stalker, G. M. (1961). *The management of innovation.* London: Tavistock.

Calsyn, R., Tornatzky, L. G., & Dittmar, S. (1977). Incomplete adoption of an innovation: The case of goal attainment scaling. *Evaluation, 4,* 128–130.

Chakrabati, A. K. (1974). The role of champion in project innovation. *California Management Review, 17,* 58–62.

Chapko, M. K. (1991). Time to adoption of an innovation by dentists in private practice: Sealant utilization. *Journal of Public Health Dentistry, 5,* 144–151.

Charters, W. W., & Jones, J. E. (1973). On the risk of appraising non-events in program evaluation. *Educational Researcher, 12,* 5–7.

Charters, W. W., & Pellegrin, R. J. (1973). Barriers to the innovation process: Four case studies of differential staffing. *Educational Administration Quarterly, 17,* 1–25.

Coch, L., & French, J. R. (1948). Overcoming resistance to change. *Human Relations, 15,* 512–533.

Cockerill, R., & Barnsley, J. (1997). Innovation theory and its applicability to our understanding of the diffusion of new management practices in health care organizations. *Healthcare Management Forum, 10,* 35–38.

Cohen, M. D., March, J. G., & Olsen, J. P. (1972). A garbage-can model of organizational choice. *Administrative Science Quarterly, 17,* 1–25.

Coombs, J. A., Silversin, J. B., & Drolefte, M. E. (1980). Policy research related to the diffusion of medical; technologies. *Journal of Dental Education, 44,* 520–525.

Cummings, K. M., Jaen, C. R., & Funch, D. P. (1984). Family physicians' beliefs about screening for colorectal; cancer using the stool guaiac slide test. *Public Health Reports, 99,* 307–312.

Cyert, R. M., & March, J. G. (1963). *A behavioral theory of the firm.* Englewood Cliffs, NJ: Prentice-Hall.

Datta, L. E. (1981). Damn the experts and full speed ahead. *Evaluation Review, 55,* 5–32.

Davidson, W. S., Redner, R., & Saul, J. (1983). Research modes in social and community change. In E. Seidman (Ed.), *Handbook of social intervention* (pp. 99–118). Beverly Hills, CA: Sage.

Dearing, J. W., Meyer, G., & Rogers, E. M. (1994). Diffusion theory and HIV risk behavior change. In R. J. DiClemente, & J. L. Peterson (Eds.), *Preventing AIDS: Theories and methods of behavioral interventions* (pp. 79–93). New York: Plenum.

Dijkstra, M., de Vries, H., & Parcel, G. S. (1993). The linkage approach applied to a school-based smoking prevention program in The Netherlands. *Journal of School Health, 63,* 339–342.

Downs, G. W. (1978). Complexity and innovation research. In M. Radnor, I. Feller, and E. M. Rogers (Eds.), *The diffusion of innovations: An assessment* (pp. 1–21). Evanston, IL: Northwestern University.

Downs, G. W., & Mohr, L. B. (1976). Conceptual issues in the study of innovation. *Administrative Science Quarterly, 21,* 700–714.

Downs, G. W., & Mohr, L. B. (1979). Toward a theory of innovation. *Administration and Society, 10,* 329–408.

Ellickson, P., & Petersilia, J. (1983). *Implementing new ideas in criminal justice.* Santa Monica, CA: Rand Corporation.

Emrick, J. A. (1977). *Evaluation of the national diffusion network.* Menlo Park, CA: Stanford Research Institute.

Ettlie, J. E. (1980). Adequacy of stage models for decisions on adoption of innovation. *Psychological Reports, 46,* 991–995.

Eveland, J. D. (1979). Issues in using the concept of adoption of innovations. *Journal of Technology Transfer, 4,* 1–14.

Eveland, J. D., Rogers, E. M., & Klepper, C. M. (1977). *The innovation process in public organizations: Some elements of a preliminary model.* Ann Arbor: University of Michigan.

Fairweather, G. W. (1972). *Social change: The challenge to survival.* Secaucus, NJ: General Learning Press.

Fairweather, G. W., & Davidson, W. S. (1986). *An introduction to community experimentation: Theory methods and practice.* New York: McGraw-Hill.

Fairweather, G. W., Sanders, D. H., & Tornatzky, L. G. (1974). *Creating change in mental health.* New York: Pergamon.

Fairweather, G. W., & Tornatzky, L. G. (1977). *Experimental methods for social policy research.* New York: Pergamon.

Frank, L., & Hackman, J. R. (1975). A failure of job enrichment: The case of the change that wasn't. *Journal of Applied Behavioral Science, 11,* 413–436.

Fullan, M., & Pomfret, A. (1977). Research on curriculum instruction and implementation. *Review of Educational Research, 47,* 335–367.

Glaser, T., & Backer, T. (1977). Innovation redefined: Durability and local adaptation. *Evaluation, 4,* 131–135.

Glaser, T., & Backer, T. (1980). Durability of innovations: How goal Attainment scaling programs fared over time. *Community Mental Health Journal, 16,* 130–143.

Goodman, R. M., Tenney, M., Smith, D. & Steckler, A. (1992). The adoption process for health curriculum innovation in schools: A case study. *Journal of Health Education, 23,* 215–220.

Goodman, R. M., & Steckler, A. (1989). A framework for assessing program institutionalization. *Knowledge, 2,* 57–71.

Goodman, R. M., & Steckler, A. (1989). A model for the institutionalization of health promotion programs. *Family and Community Health, 11*, 63–78.

Goodman, R. M., McLeRoy, K. R., Steckler, A., & Hoyle, R. H. (1993). Development of Level of Institutionalization Scales for health promotion programs. *Health Education Quarterly, 20*, 161–178.

Green, L. W. (1989). Is institutionalization the proper goal of grantmaking? *American Journal of Health Promotion, 3*, 43–44.

Green, L. W., Johnson, J. L. (1996). Dissemination and utilization of health promotion and disease prevention knowledge: Theory, research and experience. *Canadian Journal of Public Health, 87*, (Suppl2), S11–S17.

Green, L. W., & McAlister, A. L. (1984). Macro intervention to support health behavior: Some theoretical perspectives and practical reflections. *Health Education Quarterly, 11*, 323–339.

Greer, A. L. (1977). Advances in the study of diffusion of innovation in health care organizations. *Milbank Memorial Fund Quarterly, 55*, 505–532.

Gross, N. G., Gianquinta, J. B., & Bernstein, M. (1971). *Implementing organizational innovations*. New York: Basic Books.

Guba, E. (1968). Diffusion of innovations. *Educational Leadership, 25*, 292–295.

Hage, J. (1980). *Theories of organization*. New York: Wiley.

Hage, J., & Aiken, M. (1970). *Social change in complex organizations*. New York: Random House.

Hage, J., & Dewar, R. (1973). Elite values versus organizational structure in predicting innovation. *Administrative Science Quarterly, 18*, 27–31.

Hage, G. E., & Loucks, S. F. (1978). *Innovation configurations: Analyzing the adaptation of innovations*. Presented at the American Educational Research Association, Toronto, Canada.

Harveyberino, J., Ewing, J. F., Flynn, B., & Wick, J. R. (1998). Statewide dissemination of a nutrition program: Show-the-Way to 5-A-Day. *Journal of Nutrition Education, 30*, 29–36.

Havelock, R. G. (1973). *Planning for innovation through dissemination and utilization of knowledge*. Ann Arbor: Center for Research on Utilization of Scientific Knowledge, University of Michigan.

Heck, S., Steigelbauer, S., Hall, G. E., & Loucks, S. F. (1981). *Measuring innovation configurations: Procedures and applications*. Austin: Research and Development Center for Teacher Education, University of Texas.

Hollisfield, J. H., & Slavin, R. E. (1983). Disseminating student team learning through federally funded programs. *Knowledge: Creation, Diffusion, Utilization, 4*, 576–589.

House, E. R., Kerins, T., & Steele, J. M. (1972). A test of the research and development model of change. *Educational Administration Quarterly, 8*, 1–14.

Howze, E. H., & Redman, L. J. (1992). The uses of theory in health advocacy: Policies and programs. *Health Education Quarterly, 19*, 368–383.

Johnston, J. (1982). Evaluation of curriculum innovations: A product validation approach. In R. Lehming, & M. Kane (Eds.), *Improving schools: Using what we know* (pp. 79–99). Beverly Hills, CA: Sage.

Katz, D., & Kahn, R. L. (1978). *The social psychology of organizations* (2nd Ed.) New York: Wiley.

Kivlin, J. E., & Fliegel, F. C. (1967). Differential perceptions of innovations and rate of adoption. *Rural Sociology, 32*, 78–91.

Laflin, M., Edmundson, E. W., & Moore-Hirsh, S. (1995). Enhancing adoption of an alcohol prevention program: An application of diffusion theory. *Journal of Primary Prevention, 16*, 75–101.

LaPiere, R. T. (1965). *Social change*. New York: McGraw-Hill.

Larsen, J. K., & Agarwala-Rogers, R. (1977). Reinvention of innovative ideas. *Evaluation, 4*, 136–140.

Lawrence, P. R., Lorsch, J. W. (1967). Differentiation and integration in complex organizations. *Administrative Science Quarterly, 12*, 1–47.

Leithwood, K. A., & Montgomery, D. J. (1980). Evaluating program implementation. *Evaluation Review, 4*, 193–214.

Leonard, W. H., & Lowery, L. F. (1979). Was there really an experiment? *Educational Researcher, 8*, 4–7.

Lindbladh, E., Lyttkens C. H., Hanson, B. S., & Ostergren, P. O. (1997). The diffusion model and the social-hierarchical process of change. *Health Promotion International, 12*, 323–330.

Lindblom, C. E. (1959). The science of muddling through. *Public Administration Review, 19*, 79–88.

Litwak, E. (1961). Models of bureaucracy which permit conflict. *American Journal of Sociology, 67*, 177–184.

Loucks, S. F., Newlove, B., & Hall, G. E. (1975). *Measuring levels of use of an innovation: A manual*. Austin: Research and Development Center for Teacher Education, University of Texas.

Mayer, J. P., & Blakely, C. H. (1984). *Implementation and outcome in criminal justice innovation*. Presented at the Academy of Criminal Justice Sciences, Chicago, IL.

Mayer, J. P., Blakel, C. H., & Davidson, W. S. (1986). Social program innovation and dissemination: A study of organizational processes. *Policy Studies Review, 6*, 273–286.

McAlister, A. L. (1991). Population behavior change, A theory-based approach. *Journal of Public Health Policy, 12*(3), 345–361.

McCormick, L. K., Steckler, A. B., & McLeroy, K. R. (1995). Diffusion of innovations in schools: A study of adoption and implementation of school-based tobacco prevention curricula. *American Journal of Health Promotion, 9,* 210–219.

Menzel, H. (1960). Innovation, integration and marginality: A survey of physicians. *American Sociological Review, 25,* 704–713.

Miller, R. L., & Eckholdt, H. M. (1998). HIV prevention with male prostitutes and patrons of hustler bars: Replication of an HIV preventive intervention. *American Journal of Community Psychology, 26,* 97–131.

Mirvis, P., & Berg, D. (1977). *Failure in organizational development and change.* New York: Wiley Interscience.

Mohr, L. B. (1969). Determinants of innovation in organizations. *American Political Science Review, 63,* 111–126.

Mohr, L. S. (1982). *Explaining organizational behavior.* San Francisco: Jossey-Bass.

Monahan, J. L., & Scheirer, M. A. (1988). The role of linking agents in the diffusion of promotion programs. *Health Education Quarterly, 15,* 417–433.

Nelson, R. R., & Yates, D. (1978). *Innovation and implementation in public organizations.* Lexington, MA: Lexington Books.

Oldenburg, B., Hardcastle, D. M., & Kok, G. (1997). Diffusion of innovations. In K. Glanz, F. M. Lewis, & B. Rimer (Eds.), *Health behavior and health education.* 2nd ed. (pp. 270–286). San Francisco: Jossey-Bass.

O'Neill, H. M., (1998). Patterns in the diffusion of strategies across organization: Insights from the innovation diffusion literature. *Academy of Management Review, 23,* 98–114.

Owens, T. R., & Haenn, J. F. (1979). *Assessing the degree of implementation of experience-based career education programs.* Portland, OR: Northwest Regional Educational Laboratory.

Paine-Andrews, A., Vincent, M. L., Fawcett, S. B., & Campuzano, M. K. (1996). Replication of a community initiative for preventing adolescent pregnancy. *Family and Community Health, 19,* 14–30.

Palumbo, D. J., Maynard-Moody, S., & Wright, P. (1984). Measuring degrees of successful implementation: Achieving policy versus statutory goals. *Evaluation Review, 8,* 45–74.

Parcel, G. S., O'Harra-Tompkins, N. M., Harrist, R. B., Basen-Engquist, K. M., McCormick, L. K., Gottlieb, N. H., & Eriksen, M. P. (1995). Diffusion off an effective tobacco prevention program: Part II: Evaluation of the adoption phase. *Health Education Research, 10,* 297–307.

Parcel, G. S., Perry, C. L., & Taylor, W. C. (1990). Beyond demonstration: Diffusion of health promotion innovations. In N. Bracht (Ed.), *Health promotion at the community level,* (pp. 229–251). Newbury Park, CA: Sage.

Parcel, G. S., Taylor, W. C., Brink, S. G., & Gottlieb, N. (1989). Translating theory into practice: Intervention strategies for the diffusion of a health promotion innovation. *Family and Community Health, 12,* 1–13.

Perry, J. L., & Kraemer, K. L. (1980). Chief executive support and innovation adoption. *Administration and Society, 12,* 158–177.

Portnoy, B., Anderson, D. M., & Ericksen, M. P. (1989). Application of diffusion theory to health promotion research. *Family and Community Health, 12,* 63–71.

Pressman, J. L., & Wildavsky, A. B. (1973). *Implementation.* Berkeley: University of California Press.

Radnor, M., Feller, J., & Rogers, E. M. (1978). *The diffusion of innovations: An assessment.* Evanston, IL: Northwestern University.

Raizen, S. A. (1979). Dissemination programs at the National Institute of Education. *Knowledge, 1,* 259–291.

Rappaport, J. (1977). *Community psychology: Values, research and action.* New York: Holt, Rinehart and Winston.

Rice, R. E., & Rogers, E. M. (1980). Reinvention in the innovation process. *Knowledge, 1,* 499–514.

Rogers, E. M. (1983). *Diffusion of innovations,* 3rd ed. New York: Free Press.

Rogers, E. M. (1993). Diffusion and reinvention of project D.A.R.E. In T. E. Backer, E. M. Rogers (Eds.), *Organizational aspects of health communication campaigns: What works?* (pp. 139–162). Newbury Park, CA: Sage.

Rogers, E. M., & Shoemaker, F. F. (1971). *Communication of innovations: A cross-cultural approach.* New York: Free Press.

Roitman, D., Gottschalk, R., Mayer, J. P., & Blakely, C. H. (1983). Implementation of social program innovations in public sector organizations. *IEEE Transactions on Engineering Management, 2,* 68–75.

Roitman, D., & Mayer, J. P. (1982). *Fidelity and reinvention in the implementation of innovations.* Paper presented at the American Psychological Association, Washington, D.C.

Rothman, J. (1974). *Planning and organizing for social change: Action principles from social science research.* New York: Columbia University Press.

Ryan, B., & Gross, N. C. (1943). The diffusion of hybrid seed corn in two Iowa communities. *Rural Sociology, 8,* 15–24.

Scheirer, M. A. (1982). *Program implementation: The organizational context.* Beverly Hills, CA: Sage.

Scheirer, M. A., & Rezmovic, E. (1983). Measuring the implementation of innovations. *Evaluation Review, 7,* 599–633.

Scheirer, M. A. (1990). The life cycle of an innovation: Adoption versus discontinuation of the fluoride mouth rinse program schools. *Journal of Health and Social Behavior, 31*, 203–215.
Sechrest, L., & Redner, R. (1978). Strength and integrity of treatments. In *Review of Criminal Evaluation Results* (pp. 19–62). Washington, D.C.: U. S. Department of Justice.
Shepard, H. A. (1967). Innovation resisting and innovation producing organizations. *Journal of Business, 40*, 470–477.
Smith, D. W., Zhang, J. J., & Colwell, B. (1996). Pro-innovation bias: The case of the Giant Texas Smoke Screen. *Journal of School Health, 66*, 210–213.
Steckler, A., & Goodman, R. M. (1989). How to institutionalize health promotion programs. *American Journal of Health Promotion, 3*, 34–43.
Steckler, A., Goodman, R. M., McLeroy, K. R., Davis, S., & Koch, G. (1992). Measuring the diffusion of innovative health promotion programs. *American Journal of Health Promotion, 6*, 214–224.
Stevens, W. F., & Tornatzky, L. G. (1979). The dissemination of evaluation: An experiment. *Evaluation Review, 4*, 339–354.
Thomas, S. B., Leite, B., & Duncan, T. (1998). Breaking the cycle of violence among youth living in metropolitan Atlanta: A case history of kids alive and loved. *Health Education and Behavior, 25*, 160–174.
Thompson, J. D. (1967). *Organizations in action*. New York: McGraw-Hill.
Tornatzky, L. G., Eveland, J. D., Boylan, M. G., Hetzner, W. A., Johnson, E. C., Roitman, D., & Schneider, J. (1983). *The process of technological innovation: Reviewing the literature*. Washington, D.C.: National Science Foundation.
Tornatzky, L. G. (1982). *Research on implementation: Implications for evaluation practice and evaluation policy*. Presented at Evaluation Research Society, Austin, TX.
Tornatzky, L. G., Fergus, E. O., Avellar, J. W., Fairweather, G. W., & Fleischer, M. (1980). *Innovation and social process*. New York: Pergamon.
Tornatzky, L. G., & Klein, K. J. (1982). Innovation characteristics and innovation adoption-implementation: A meta-analysis of findings. *IEEE Transactions on Engineering Management, 29*, 28–45.
Weick, K. E. (1976). Educational organizations as loosely coupled systems. *Administrative Science Quarterly, 21*, 1–19.
Williams, W. (1975). Implementation analysis and assessment. *Policy Analysis, 3*, 531–566.
Witte, K. (1993). Managerial style and health promotion programs. *Social Science and Medicine, 36*, 227–235.
Yin, R. R. (1978). *Changing urban bureaucracies: How new practices become routinized*. Santa Monica, CA: The Rand Corporation.
Yin, R. K. (1977). Production efficiency versus bureaucratic self-interest: Two innovative processes? *Policy Sciences, 8*, 381–389.
Zaltman, G., Duncan, R., & Holbek, J. (1973). *Innovations and organizations*. New York: Wiley.

PART IV

SOCIAL SYSTEMS

Community psychology is a substantive discipline linked by its values and modes of intervention, spanning a broad array of social issues. The preceding sections of this volume directly addressed conceptual maps, empirical foundations, and strategies and tactics for intervention—always with an eye toward our role relationships to others, and with an emphasis on mutuality and collaboration. It would be fair to note that these sections are divided somewhat arbitrarily, intended to provide alternative views of circumstances difficult to disentangle. Several of the chapters grouped in the empirical foundations section (Part II) could be here, organized around social systems, while some placed here might be appropriate for the section on concepts and frameworks (Part I). However, looking at the field with a map that locates social systems is yet another way to observe the field, one that emphasizes links among historical, bureaucratic, political, and structural realities largely determined by disciplinary traditions.

What holds the chapters in this section together are analyses bounded by organizational–bureaucratic constraints. Each of these considerations will, in any particular instance, be physically located in time and space, i.e., schools, medical settings, mental health centers, churches, courts, work settings, and so on. But each intervention, policy consideration, or research question must also be understood to reside within the context of particular social-system constraints that are created by, and therefore reflect, disciplinary cultures. While social systems do interact in complex ways (i.e., they are not completely bounded, closed systems), they each have their own dominant "ways," revealed in particular linguistic, attitudinal, behavioral, and communication conventions.

Although many different professionals can be found in each system, each will also tend to be dominated by the assumptions created by a particular group of professionals. Teachers and educational administrators who think in terms of curricula, school buildings, and classrooms, create a logic that is different from the logic of a system governed by lawyers, judges, and legislators, who think in terms of rights and obligations. Professionals trained in a religious vocation are going to use language differently, i.e., issues of hope, belief, and compassion may have greater salience as a way to frame issues than for those trained in medicine, where efficient delivery of expert treatment is the primary language. Medical settings where the physician, the nurse, and the social-service provider are confronted with third-party insurers and lawyers remain defined by assumptions about health and illness, but defining activity around citizen rights and health as opposed to disorder and disease will lead to different rules for behavior. Financing of services enters the picture in very different ways for each of these professionals. These differences have less to do with superficial notions such as "faith versus science" or who is more "moral," or least "self-serving," than with the deeper cultural assumptions of the various disciplines as they play themselves out in social-system contexts with their own peculiar organizational and ecological constraints. Sometimes disciplinary cultures will work well together, but sometimes they may be in conflict.

Despite their differences, mental health, medical, legal, educational, and religious professionals may be more similar to each other than to the people who participate in self- and mutual-help organizations. While every discipline likes to think of itself as client- or consumer-oriented, in most cases, regardless of the setting, there is a mix between the guild interests of professionals, maintenance interests of the settings, and genuine participation in goal-setting and decision-making by the supposed beneficiaries of the system.

A system defined by mental health professionals will be understood differently if it is defined by educators or lawyers, but neither one of these assures genuine participation on the part of children and families. Schools in which community members and other professionals have a voice will be different than those defined solely by the structural and linguistic conventions of any professional bureaucracy. Each profession will highlight different "rules of the game," but community members are not automatically well-represented in the rules of the game as written by any of the disciplines. Community psychologists, who are frequently called upon to span the boundaries of different systems and cultures, need to attend to more than the culture of our own discipline if we are to be effective "boundary spanners" (Kelly, 1992). Often community psychologists (who themselves also have guild and disciplinary interests) will need to advocate for (or with) those outsiders to professional power who the systems are supposed the serve. (For additional discussions on this topic see also Part I, especially the chapters on empowerment and on the ecological view; the Part II chapters on neighborhood and workplace participation; Part III on consultation, community organization, and the creation of settings; and Part V on ecological and qualitative research).

In the chapters that follow here, attention is centered on each of seven different systems (community mental health, community-based health interventions, the legal system, religious settings, the child and family welfare system, self-help groups and organizations, and school reform). There is also a chapter that addresses systems more generally, using a framework based in organizational psychology (and work settings). Obviously, systems are discussed here in terms of the issues they present to community psychology, and not every detail, every system, or all approaches to systems are represented, but those that are identified sample a spectrum of the issues and systems important to the concerns of community psychology.

We begin with Heller, Jenkins, Steffen, and Swindle's analysis of the community mental health system, a historical launching point for much of community psychology. They illustrate the power of current conceptual models (within both the disciplines and the popular culture) to mobilize change, pointing out some of the ways in which professionals may be a major impediment to (or catalyst for) change. Reading this chapter in light of Felner, Felner, and Silverman's conceptual arguments (see Part I) will provide a picture of both the possibilities and traps that await those who are willing to confront their own unexamined assumptions concerning mental health, including our most sacred ideas. Heller and his colleagues explore the possibilities of regional community mental health policies to foster collaboration among scientists and citizens. They emphasize new directions for state and local initiatives in training, planning, evaluation, and citizen participation.

Revenson and Schiaffino then discuss community-based health interventions, adopting the World Health Organization's definition of health as physical, mental, and social well-being, rather than as the absence of disease. They emphasize education to empower people through mediating structures, networks, and community institutions. They advocate multiple strategies for intervention consistent with many of the suggestions found in Part III of this volume. These authors argue for interventions that emphasize competence, a genuine knowledge of the culture of the people with whom one seeks to work, an emphasis on adoption of healthy lifestyles rather than risk factors, personal responsibility, and moral character. They describe interventions from the perspective of the problem, the setting, and the strategy, with detailed examples from the Minnesota Health Heart Project and AIDS prevention in the gay communities of New York and San Francisco, illustrating both a "top-down" and a "bottom-up" approach.

The third chapter in this section shifts our attention to systems organized around the various ways that religious settings contribute to individual and social concerns. This chapter is placed in this section on social systems because it presents religious organizations as mediating structures between individuals and communities. We may learn a great deal from work in religious contexts about the power of traditions, symbols, and organizational structures to generate continuity and shared individuality-in-community.

Pargament and Maton remind us that religious systems are not quasi-mental health institutions, and if we are to collaborate and learn from them we will need to approach religious settings on their own terms. They provide a rationale for why community psychologists may be interested in religion: It provides (1) a means to meet the primary human needs for meaning, belonging, and community, (2) a rationale and structure for working toward public good, and (3) a special access to marginal, disenfranchised, and minority groups.

Religious contexts are located in a system where community psychologists have many opportunities for collaboration. Examples here include peer counseling, drug abuse prevention, congregation development, economic sharing and barter programs, mentoring, and community-based development. But these authors also point us to sociological and anthropological analysis in order to supplement psychology's tendency to describe religious participation only in terms of individual dispositional orientations. Their conceptual framework, describing and distinguishing different institutions, is consistent with the type of consultation proposed by Trickett, Barone, and Watts (see Part III). Religious institutions can be analyzed at the local (organizational) level and as cultural institutions. Pargament and Maton provide a framework for distinguishing religious institutions in terms of theology, mission, and organization. Pathways of religious influence include social outreach as well as personal "inreach."

Like religion, legal institutions and assumptions are pervasive in any culture. The influence of law as the formal embodiment of social agreements is both direct and indirect, but, as the next chapter reminds us, the law is also practiced in contemporary social and political reality. Anyone with an interest in understanding a community will in some way confront the dynamics of its legal institutions. Here Melton highlights some of the ways in which the philosophy of legal realism has provided space for the input and involvement of social scientists. His discussion of policy formulations in a form accessible to actors in the legal system is reminiscent of the Phillips analysis of social policy (see Part III) as a venue for community psychology intervention.

Melton's analysis emphasizes the functions of law to cement collective identity and reify the myths and norms of a culture. Yet law also concretizes social structure in ways that may diminish the ability to change. Forms of legal intervention include direct regulation by threat or incentive, as well as indirect regulation by creating structures to facilitate certain kinds of behavior. One role for social scientists in the legal system is to match legal analysis with social reality and with the values and needs of communities. Practical assistance by community psychologists may involve the creation of new legal settings (see also the chapter by Cherniss and Deegan in Part III), collaboration with others to enable groups to make use of existing law, and raising awareness of legal entitlements.

Although child and family welfare could be addressed from within the mental health or community-based health care systems, or as central concerns in the context of both religious and legal systems, the fifth chapter of this section, by Knitzer, approaches child and family helping services as a system itself. In this chapter, children and families *per se* become the point of departure. Knitzer includes four core agencies and institutions in the family and child welfare system: child welfare agencies, mental health agencies, juvenile justice agencies, and schools. She takes the ecological approach into an analysis of the role of government and public responsibility. On the one hand Knitzer sees reason to be optimistic, as many efforts at reform hold promise for troubled children and families. For example, some of these reforms can be understood as deepening a commitment to families, rather than attempts to "rescue" children from them. Many seek to avoid removing children from their own communities, and to individualize (or to "familialize") treatments. Unfortunately, Knitzer points out, in order to access services, recent policies have emphasized that children and families must be experiencing serious and sustained crisis, and need to meet very specific categorical requirements. This leads, at the community level, to boundaries and structures that can prevent services from being smoothly delivered to people, many of whom do not fall into neatly ordered categories. It also tends to create gaps in services that no agency provides. In this context, Knitzer considers ways in which the boundaries of specific programs may become more permeable, i.e., through family-preservation programs, kinship foster-care, social support for parents and families, intensive case management, and cross-program collaboration at the local community level.

In the next chapter, taking a closer look at schooling itself as a system (including building, neighborhood, district, state, and federal structures), rather than viewing schools as one part of the child welfare system, Oxley considers issues in school reform with an emphasis on restructuring. Her aim is to develop a theory of school restructuring that underpins "communally organized" schools. She makes use of scholarship on effective schools and school-improvement programs, programs for social-emotional and intellectual goals, and interventions based on "house" systems and school–community collaboration.

Oxley argues that research and intervention in both psychology and education tend to obscure the social and organizational complexity of schools because of a preoccupation with individual- and classroom-level phenomena. Schools have an invisible culture, and restructuring of schools means restructuring at higher levels of organization. In this context, she suggests alternative schooling policies such as shared and collaborative decision-making, active learning, and mentoring, combined with organizational goals that include mastery of core subjects, critical-thinking skills, and non-traditional intelligences, social competence, and health. Oxley suggests that for community psychologists there must be a translation of the ideas of prevention, development, and social competence into the language of school-system regularities. In this regard, her thoughts on schools with respect to ideas about wellness, primary prevention, and ecological analysis, as addressed in Part I this volume, provide additional considerations for the conceptual frameworks of community psychologists, as does the suggestion that we involve ourselves in action research models for intervention and consultation (see Part III).

With Levy's chapter on self-help groups and organizations, the focus shifts from activities primarily developed within a professionalized disciplinary culture to those settings created by people who have elected, in many cases, to avoid the culture and control of the helping professions. Defining characteristics of such groups usually include commonality of an identified problem, members relating to each other as peers, and members playing dual roles as both providers and recipients of help. This makes such settings more easily responsive, accessible to members, and less costly than their professionalized counterparts. There is, to some extent, an ideological compatibility with community psychology. However, since the self-help system is necessarily less formalized than systems under professional control, it will also tend to be less accountable to professional scrutiny, and perhaps will be underresourced.

While self-help organizations may be thought of as communities of identity, similar to religious or ethnic organizations (see, for example, Humphreys & Rappaport, 1994) self-help group participants often seek supportive interpersonal assistance with problems in living, either separate from, or entirely outside of, professionalized helping systems. Self-help groups can therefore be viewed as interventions, social systems, or elements of social policy. In this chapter, Levy focuses on the particular set of issues involved in the methodology of conducting self-help research, especially around questions of outcomes.

Shinn and Perkins then turn our attention to what we can learn about social systems from the field of organizational psychology, particularly, but not exclusively, from the subfield of organizational development in the context of work settings. Community psychology and organizational development converge around many themes: the action research orientation originating with Levine, the processes and interventions of planned change, the tensions between research and practice, an ecological/systems orientation, advocacy of an extra-individual level of analysis, and the concern that within psychology organizational-level research is underdeveloped. Both fields are interested in work settings, especially the promotion of employee well-being, intersystem accommodation (i.e., work and family), and the structure of health and human-service organizations.

Shinn and Perkins review individual, group, intergroup, and organizational interventions in work settings, highlighting the use of survey feedback, job enrichment, and sociotechnical strategies. They attend to changes in overall organizational culture, including the beliefs, values, and assumptions held by organizational members, as well as the symbols and artifacts that reflect, sustain, and create them. While we have placed this chapter in the systems section of the volume, if read in conjunction with Part I it evokes an additional conceptual map, while in conjunction with Part II it presents empirical foundations, and in conjunction with Part III it suggests additional strategies and tactics for intervention.

REFERENCES

Humphreys, K., & Rappaport, J. (1994). Researching self-help/mutual aid groups and organizations: Many roads, one journey. *Applied and Preventive Psychology, 3*, 217–231.

Kelly, J. G. (1992). On teaching the practice of prevention: Integrating the concept of interdependence. In M. Kessler, S. E. Goldston, & J. M. Joffe (Eds.), *The present and future of prevention* (pp.251–264). Newbury Park: Sage.

Seidman, E. (1988). Back to the future, community psychology: Unfolding the theory of social intervention. *American Journal of Community Psychology, 16*, 3–24.

CHAPTER 19

Prospects for a Viable Community Mental Health System

Reconciling Ideology, Professional Traditions, and Political Reality

KENNETH HELLER, RICHARD A. JENKINS, ANN M. STEFFEN, AND RALPH W. SWINDLE JR.

The current community mental health system is undergoing severe retrenchment. With curtailment in federal funding, priorities are returning to what they were prior to 1950—private psychotherapy for the financially able and supportive care for chronic mental patients. Mental health centers are beginning to assume the functions of private psychiatric clinics and state mental hospitals—the systems of care they were intended to supplant. In the 1980s, the federal government began a steady and systematic withdrawal from community mental health centers, as well as from other health and human service programs. The responsibility for mental health care was returned to the states and to a growing private health care industry. This change produced a profound shift in service delivery, with the emphasis moving toward reimbursable services. Since inpatient services were being reimbursed at a higher rate than outpatient services, patients with a variety of disorders were more likely to be hospitalized than in the previous decade (Kiesler, 1980, 1982b). The noble experiment of the 1960s to empty the state hospitals had come full circle, with hospitalization now occurring more frequently in private, rather than public, facilities (Kiesler, 1982b; Kiesler & Simpkins, 1991). Since federal dollars for mental health care were being channeled to the states at continuously reduced levels, states that were unable to make up the shortfall increasingly were pressed to restrict their services to those clearly unable to care for themselves—the most severely disabled

KENNETH HELLER • Department of Psychology, Indiana University, Bloomington, Indiana 47405. RICHARD A. JENKINS • National Center for HIV, STD, and TB Prevention, Centers for Disease Control and Prevention, Atlanta, Georgia 30333. ANN M. STEFFEN • Department of Psychology, University of Missouri—St. Louis, St. Louis, Missouri 63121. RALPH W. SWINDLE JR. • Health Services Research and Development, VA Medical Center, Indianapolis, Indiana 46202.

Handbook of Community Psychology, edited by Julian Rappaport and Edward Seidman. Kluwer Academic/Plenum Publishers, New York, 2000.

clients. Similarly, community mental health centers, relying on state dollars, also began limiting their clientele to this same group, or to those with personal financial resources and private insurance (Jerrell & Larsen, 1986).

The original vision of community mental health included prevention programming, reaching underserved populations, fostering community awareness of social and environmental determinants of psychological dysfunction, and consultation to community caregivers to encourage the development of indigenous helping networks (Cowen, Gardner, & Zax, 1967). We think that, for the most part, these have remained interesting but untested ideas, and in those few instances in which demonstration projects have reported successful innovations, widespread diffusion and adoption has not occurred.

Our first goal of this chapter is to ask, "What happened?" Why is the vision of the community mental health movement still largely unfulfilled some 30 years after passage of the original legislation? Our second goal is to suggest some alternative directions that mental health services might take in the decades ahead. Much has been learned about prevention and treatment during this period, but this information will remain underutilized unless we understand why previous attempts at innovation could not be maintained.

The chapter will be organized as follows. First, we will present our views of the pressures and compromises that led to the passage of the community mental health centers legislation and its subsequent amendments. Our historical survey will be brief because the major issues have been reviewed elsewhere (Heller, Price, Reinharz, Riger, & Wandersman, 1984; Levine, 1981; Price & Smith, 1983). Next, we will discuss what we believe to be some of the weaknesses of the legislation and the reasons that community mental health centers have not lived up to their original promise. In so doing, we will pose some basic dilemmas about mental health care in the United States that continue to defy adequate planning and priority setting. Finally, we will describe the action we think should be taken to produce a viable community-oriented mental health system. Since retrospective analyses are by their very nature subjective, the reader is warned that what follows is not "fact," but our interpretation of events.

It has become fashionable to long for the "good old days" of the 1960s, and to blame the current malaise in the mental health system on the conservative federal climate and the withdrawal of federal funds. Although funding patterns clearly have a profound influence on programs, our own perspective suggests greater caution concerning what can be accomplished by federal initiatives alone. Serious impediments also can be found in public attitudes and in professional orientation and practices, and these will be highlighted in the current chapter.

THE COMMUNITY MENTAL HEALTH SYSTEM AS A CASE STUDY IN SOCIAL CHANGE

The community mental health "revolution" of the 1960s had both practical and ideological goals. At a practical level, CMH legislation was designed to overcome the deficiencies in mental health care that had become evident by the late 1950s, primarily by increasing the range, quality of, and access to, mental health services. At the time, public mental health care was the primary responsibility of state mental hospitals, a system that over the years had become overburdened through neglect. Services were designed for those requiring inpatient care, and hospitals often were placed at some distance from population centers. In addition, mental hospitals were not a high financial priority for many states, so services often were minimal and overcrowding was frequent. The net result was that patients who needed some form of mental health care often were required to become inpatients in a facility that removed them from work, family, and normal social interaction, but did little to encourage their recovery.

One solution to this problem was to provide money to the states to improve the quality of outpatient care. Beginning in 1948, this is exactly what happened. Section 314c of the Public Health Service Act allowed the National Institute of Mental Health (NIMH) to make block grants to states to support community mental health services and reduce the need for hospitalization (Buck, 1984). The purpose of these grants was to establish and expand outpatient psychiatric clinics. States could not use this money for inpatient care and were required to set up an administrative unit to oversee the clinics that was separate from the administration of the state hospitals (Buck, 1984). Thus, in the 1950s, the federal government was already encouraging the states to develop alternatives to their mental hospitals.

Not everyone agreed that alternatives to mental hospitals were needed. The Joint Commission on Mental Illness and Health, established by Congress in 1955 to develop a comprehensive plan for a national mental health program, called for a strengthening of the mental hospital system, not its abandonment. The emphasis in the Joint Commission report was on expanded treatment resources for severe mental illness, which included recommendations for training additional treatment personnel. Given the heavy representation of medical and psychiatric groups on the Commission, the emphasis on traditional treatment is not surprising (Snow & Newton, 1976).

In 1961, President Kennedy formed a special cabinet-level committee to analyze the Joint Commission report. This committee, which included top officials within the NIMH, was more reform-minded than the physician-dominated Joint Commission. Committee members were more interested in replacing the state system than in strengthening it. They also were aware of the minimal treatment most patients received in state institutions and generally agreed with the critics who felt that extended inpatient mental health care played a role in perpetuating symptomatic behavior. Their recommendation was to bypass the existing state system with a new network of federally funded centers.

The ideological underpinning of the 1963 CMH legislation was linked to the "New Frontier" agenda of the Kennedy administration, the goal of which was to reduce poverty and its psychological and social concomitants. The mandate of the community clinics to provide greater access to treatment was considered important, but insufficient. The Kennedy administration accepted the proposition that social conditions were causally linked to the development of mental disorder (Levine, 1981) and called for prevention programs to reduce its incidence.

The community mental health legislation that was approved by Congress in 1963 did not live up to this idealistic goal. Major changes were suggested by constituency groups opposed to the legislation (the American Medical Association, labor unions representing hospital workers, and communities in which mental hospitals were located as "captive" industries). The net result was that traditional clinical services were emphasized (e.g., inpatient, outpatient, partial hospitalization, and 24-hour emergency care). Prevention appeared almost as a footnote, as part of consultation and education services, and funds for training were not initially included. Although the legislation provided much less than they had wanted, the advocates of reform urged passage on the assumption that the act could be revised in future years.

Difficulties Encountered

Conceptual Ambiguity

Before 1960, federal programs were seen as helping state and local governments accomplish limited local objectives. Social welfare and mental health were considered to be local concerns. The "revolution" initiated by the Kennedy administration, and completed during the Johnson years, was to introduce the federal government as a primary actor in health and welfare issues. With the aid of a receptive social climate, health, education, social welfare, and mental health became part of a federal agenda (Price & Smith, 1983). Just as a foreign enemy had been vanquished in World War II, there was public optimism that domestic problems also could be overcome with a unified public resolve. The difficulty is that the confrontation of social problems is not the same as "wars" with external enemies against whom citizens can rally. Social and psychological problems involve entrenched attitudes and practices within the fabric of society, and there are no clear guidelines as to how to proceed. With regard to the mental health system, there was alarm over the warehousing of large numbers of people in custodial institutions, but most citizens, including federal planners, had no clear idea of what the alternatives should be (Hasenfeld, 1985). The solution proposed by the 1963 legislation mandated greater access to treatment, but suggested few changes in the model of service delivery. Prominent in the legislation were direct clinical services, similar to those already being provided by federally initiated community clinics as an expansion of state hospital services.

Bypassing State and Local Governments

What is remarkable about the 1963 legislation is that it ushered in a new partnership between professionals within NIMH and local mental health specialists that eventually bypassed state and local authorities. We believe that conservative state and county governments were seen as part of the problem, rather than a reflection of community sentiments. The "War on Poverty" and "Great Society" programs, of which the community mental health legislation was a part, sought a more direct link for dealing with social problems. If local and state programs were inadequate to address a multitude of human problems (as indeed they were), the solution proposed was not to upgrade these programs or to embark on changing community sentiments, but to bypass both. Change was to be legislated, and it was expected that deeply entrenched attitudes and practices would slowly "come around." The federal programs were to function as exemplars that would be readily adopted; hence, the willingness of federal officials to think of community mental health programs as demonstration projects whose federal contribution could be phased out after a few brief years. The result was that state governments became pass-through agencies, administering programs that they had no voice in shaping. State and local officials initially welcomed the influx of federal dollars; however, the lack of a local mandate became obvious when federal funds were withdrawn. The professional and community groups who were the beneficiaries of federal grants often represented narrow constituency groups with little skill or experience in developing local support for their programs.

The Disregard of Natural Communities

Hunter and Riger (1986) argue that "community" was a borrowed and inadequately understood concept in the formulation of the community mental health legislation. The concept of community was sufficiently nebulous that a variety of practices could be legitimized under its rubric. The term was attractive to citizens because it implied a "natural" process. At the same time, professionals could rally behind it because the decentralization provided by the proliferation of mental health centers meant an expansion of job opportunities in that field.

The manner in which natural communities were disregarded can be seen in the implementation of the "catchment area" concept, a major feature of the 1963 legislation. Each community mental health center was designed to serve a geographic area whose population was to be no less than 75,000 and no more than 200,000. The idea was to develop population-based services in manageable units. However, what often occurred in urban areas was that natural neighborhood boundaries were not observed because the criteria were numbers of people to be served and not areas defined by established social relationships (Hunter & Riger, 1986). As Heller et al. (1984) point out, the result was that

> Rather than serving an entire ethnic or racial neighborhood, for example, it was more likely that mental health catchment areas cut across different racial or ethnic neighborhoods. When this happened, it was difficult for any group to feel that the center was "theirs." the power of indigenous community groups to shape mental health programs to fit their needs was lessened while the control of center programs by professional groups was enhanced (p. 42).

Similar movement toward professional control occurred in rural areas where centers served heterogeneous socioeconomic and cultural groups with diverse traditions and little prior history of cooperation.

Ambiguities Concerning the Meaning of Citizen Involvement

Bypassing indigenous community groups represented a major point of vulnerability that threatened the long-term viability of community mental health centers. Although the centers provided greater access to mental health care, services were professionally defined and developed, and most citizens did not feel a sense of ownership in CMHC programs. When federal dollars were withdrawn in the 1980s, there was no groundswell of local support for the continuation of these programs with local tax dollars. Indeed, there was little sympathy for the once well-off mental health centers that were now competing with smaller local agencies also facing cuts in federal dollars.

The role of citizens in developing, controlling, and evaluating community mental health programs was left ambiguous in the legislation. While the drafters of the "Great Society" legislation had hoped to maximize citizen participation in community programs, it was never clear what "citizen participation" actually meant (Moynihan, 1969). Citizen participation in the development of mental health programs is generally conceded to have been a failure (Dowell & Ciarlo, 1983). Most mental health specialists did not receive group- or community-development training and did not know how to use community input. Community members of CMHC boards generally were not encouraged to provide leadership functions. Boards were usually dominated by a more informed technical staff and there generally were few incentives for board training. Furthermore, citizens were reluctant to get involved as long as the primary function of CMHCs was said to be patient care. After all, is not patient care a specialty endeavor?

But suppose the primary mandate of community mental health centers had been the enhancement of psychological and social functioning, rather than the treatment of disability. Most citizens would agree that they should have a say in shaping programs to enhance their own well-being; their active involvement in programs would have increased the likelihood of adoption and adherence. Here we see the power of conceptual models. Because treatment models defined the mental health field, both professionals and citizens alike assumed that the new mental health structures must serve treatment functions. This ideology was "built in" from the start and determined that the new centers would have a treatment, rather than a prevention, focus.

The action taken in developing the community mental health centers legislation reflected political expediency and the necessity of compromising with existing professional groups. Mental health officials at NIMH had a practical understanding of the political legislative process; they knew that they had to act while they had legislative momentum. They understood that a technology and commitment to community-oriented services was lacking, but felt that once centers were in place, targeted monies could then be made available to train and reorient staff. Since the public had become aware of the deficiencies of state mental hospitals, and reform of the mental health system had become part of the public agenda, it became important to get construction monies committed and mental health programs in place before public attention was diverted to another priority.

Problems Associated with Deinstitutionalization

The adequate treatment and care of chronic mental patients, historically, has been a major source of difficulty for the mental health professions. Deinstitutionalization, as a solution to this problem, has paradoxically increased public resistance to community mental health and is one factor in the suspicion of community-based programs.

The deinstitutionalization movement was fueled by a number of forces (Felton & Shinn, 1981). There was a strong belief that custodial mental institutions exacerbated psychotic symptomatology and social deficits. Another push came from cost-conscious legislators and bureaucrats who saw the benefits of antipsychotic medication as offering an opportunity to close expensive state hospitals. A third source of pressure for deinstitutionalization came from a series of judicial decisions affirming patients' right to treatment, which narrowed the grounds for involuntary commitment and treatment.

Unfortunately, while it was clear that many of the more dramatic symptoms of the major disorders could be managed by medication, little was understood at the time about the sort of support and supervision necessary to maintain patients in community and family settings. Local practitioners did not have an appropriate treatment technology for working with this patient population. Furthermore, many of the best-trained professionals had little interest in working with what was for them an unrewarding population.

By the mid-1970s, it was clear to officials within the NIMH that community mental health centers did not provide adequate care for chronic mental patients, and that new approaches to community treatment had to be advanced on a national scale. By this time, there were research findings concerning community approaches to treatment upon which new treatment technologies could be built (Fairweather, Sanders, Maynard, & Cressler, 1969; Paul & Lentz, 1977; Test & Stein, 1977). A major program of community-based care, the Community Support Program (CSP), was initiated, and was targeted specifically for that segment of the chronic population most susceptible to multiple hospitalizations and chronic role impairment (Love, 1984; Stroul, 1986). The new program was based on the maintenance of proper medication, social-skills training, and therapeutic and community support. Under this regimen, many patients could become significantly less symptomatic, were employable, and were more successful in resisting rehospitalization (Kiesler, 1982a; Pasamanick, Scarpitti, & Dinitz, 1967; Stein & Test, 1985). The new program also incorporated the recognition that some chronic patients could not live on their own and required a continuum of structured residential and therapeutic care in order to live in community settings. While staff-training inadequacies have persisted, the CSP program was accompanied by an aggressive training and education component that slowly penetrated CMHC standards of practice for this chronic population.

Unfortunately, the legacy of deinstitutionalization without treatment activated longstanding public fear of mental patients, and little was done initially to deal with these fears. It should come as no surprise that community members were angry and upset at what was generally perceived as the "dumping" of chronic mental patients into the community. Ironically, while we now have a much better idea of how such programs should be implemented (Anthony, 1989), the community mental health system was criticized in many quarters for failing its mandate, and insufficient funds were provided to mount effective community-support programs.

The cutback in community-support programs took place at the same time that various factors reduced economic opportunities for those with minimal job skills (e.g., increased automation, relocation of low-skill jobs to suburban locations, growth of technically sophisticated service-sector jobs). The result was, and continues to be, a rising tide of "homeless" families without the economic resources for self-care (Shinn & Weitzman, 1990). As is usually the case in a conservative climate, adverse social and economic conditions are minimized and individuals are "blamed" for their plight (Levine & Levine, 1970). The presence of chronic mental patients among the homeless, and the exaggeration of their numbers, strengthens the attribution of personal responsibility for poverty. As a result, the entire population of homeless individuals is denormalized and considered deviant and pathological. If one believes that the homeless are primarily mentally ill, then it is safe to conclude that what is needed is more restrictive care for these individuals, not greater economic opportunity.

There is a general perception that the community treatment of severe mental patients has been given a fair test and that it has failed. Given this perception, and the perceived link between community treatment and community mental health, the conclusion drawn in many circles is that community mental health also has failed a fair test. So, for many, the inevitable conclusion points once again to institutionalization.

Professional Resistance to Community Ideology and Practice

We believe that the resistance of mental health professionals to community mental health ideology and practice was severely underestimated. Most mental health specialists had no experience in public health medicine, nor did their models of treatment provide a place for public input. Treatment, which meant psychotherapy in the vast majority of cases, was considered a private and confidential exchange between patient and therapist. The unexpressed, but implicit, value stance of this enterprise was to free the patient from excessive conformity to the wishes of others. Whether phrased in terms of moderating the strength of superego influences or encouraging self-actualization, the basic idea was that the patient's problem was created by negative encounters with significant others. The therapist's job was to free the patient from "irrational beliefs" or influences that represented internalizations of the standards and wishes of others. From this conceptual stance, ties to others were most often seen as a source of stress, rather than support (Heller, 1979), and the involvement of others in treatment was generally seen as further increasing that stress. The one treatment modality that did engage family members—family therapy—shared the conceptual stance that families were a source of stress and misguided "paradoxical" communication that needed correction.

Not only did most treatment personnel have a conceptual bias against family and community members, but they also received little training in how to make constructive use of their input. So, while the intention of the community mental health centers legislation might have been to facilitate the involvement of the patient's network of family and friends in the helping process (Hunter & Riger, 1986), there was little likelihood that such a goal would be accomplished. The centers specialized in classical clinical treatment, the mode of operation that mental health professionals were prepared to offer.

DILEMMAS IN PLANNING COMMUNITY MENTAL HEALTH SERVICES

It is sobering to realize that proposals to revitalize the community mental health centers system with an infusion of new funds probably would meet with a similar fate as did the 1960s attempt at innovation. This is because many of the social and professional forces operating then are still with us today. Part of the problem is the way Americans conceptualize social problems, which often leads to counterproductive solutions.

Unexamined Societal Assumptions in Defining Problems and Proposing Solutions

Seidman and Rappaport (1986) provide a useful examination of the assumptions that undergird the social construction of reality in contemporary American society. They note that these unexamined, but implicit, premises "create simple, stereotyped problem definitions leading to similarly narrow and constrained solutions" (p. 5). Several assumptions that they outline are germane to our discussion of mental health policy and programs: (1) a tendency to require that all individuals be judged by a single standard; (2) generalizing from extreme examples; and (3) requiring uniform solutions to social problems. Thus, with regard to mental health policies, there is a common belief in a single standard of normality. We assume that people are either "normal" or "abnormal," with little attention to the true diversity in between. In generalizing from extreme examples, we expect mental patients to be unpredictable and dangerous, a characteristic of only an extreme few. Finally, we sponsor uniform solutions to the treatment of mental patients, and alternate between cycles of institutionalization and normalization of mental disorder, with neither solution adequate to the gradation of need that in fact represents reality.

A fourth unexamined assumption is a tendency toward pragmatism (Seidman & Rappaport, 1986), which influences us to see complex problems in simple terms. Thus, a common belief is that mental health policy represents the "public will" as transmitted to elected government representatives. What is usually ignored is the lobbying and influence displayed by professional interest groups that can overpower the public interest. Price and Smith (1983) present a convincing case that the amendments to the mental health legislation that occurred in the 1960s and 1970s benefited professional interest groups, but did very little to improve the welfare of disabled, poor clients. As Wildavsky (1979) points out, the problem with expecting simple solutions to work is that public policy problems do not have solutions that are applicable once and for all. It is our expectation of closure that is misleading, since problems are not so much solved as redefined, and superseded by the next policy crisis.

More than two decades ago, Campbell (1971) argued for an "experimenting society" in which there is a value commitment to social innovation and its evaluation. The commitment is to finding solutions, but not particular ones, to recurrent social problems. This distinction is important. Historically, in this country, we have been unwilling to work on complex social problems that are not amenable to quick solutions. In order to operate in this milieu, reformers have been forced to advocate specific solutions, exaggerating and overpromising what can be expected. If they are successful in receiving funds, they become identified with particular solutions, which they then have a vested interest in proving correct.

Campbell's point is that we should become oriented toward a process of problem definition and solution, rather than toward particular solutions, especially those that are funded on a massive scale but are inadequately evaluated. Using this criterion, the community mental health centers legislation represented problem definition and solution at its worst. The legislation was a highly compromised political response to social and economic pressures caused by the inadequate system of mental health care in the country at the time. It was amended over the years, not because research indicated that it was working either poorly or well, but because Congress found it expedient to respond to changing political problems by expanding the domain of mental health services to cover a wide array of social and psychological problems. Mental health agencies became responsible for drug abuse, rape, child abuse, and the problems of the elderly, and so on; these problems were defined as within the domain of mental health because treating them as such was an expeditious political solution.

Problems Created by Unexamined Professional Assumptions

The mental health professions are not immune to the social and ideological forces outlined above, and similar unexamined assumptions influence mental health theories and practices as well. Mental health practitioners accepted an expanded definition of their mission and readily embraced as mental health problems areas of functioning that would have been equally, if not more, responsive to economic, legal, or social solutions.

The press for simple problem definitions and explanations is reflected in the dominance of monoetiological theories (Bloom, 1985) and uniformity myths (Kiesler, 1966). While there is a general recognition that any given problem can have a number of causes, the theories that guide treatment have remained monoetiological. The field is marred by therapeutic "camps," in which practitioners apply the same solution to a wide assortment of problems with multiple causes. Despite calls for multifaceted etiological models (Price, 1974), little change can be expected as long as (1) the system is buffeted by political pressures that push for simplistic and universal solutions to complicated problems, (2) therapies are not evaluated, and (3) there are no incentives for clinicians to follow emerging research developments or to try new approaches that challenge their current methods (Cohen, 1985; O'Donohue, Curtis, & Fisher, 1985).

The Trap Created by an Exclusive Focus on Treatment and Rehabilitation

An axiom of community psychology and, more generally, public health practice, is that treatment does nothing to reduce the incidence of new cases. A likely scenario is that as the public becomes aware of treatment facilities, increasing numbers of individuals are referred and treatment resources soon become overtaxed. Service costs inevitably rise, and requests for funds for additional treatment personnel aggravate the perception that the problem is growing. As treatment budgets escalate, it does not take long for the public's patience and pocketbook to become exhausted. Critics then charge that the psychological approach was tried, and that it has failed. There are calls for other remedies, and these are likely to be more punitive solutions. Funds then move from treatment to incarceration. Unfortunately, this chronology becomes all too familiar when new problems are "discovered" to have psychological components, and are referred for solution to treatment-oriented mental health facilities.

This axiom also holds for the private mental health sector as new problems are "discovered" (e.g., addictions, stress, underachievement, chronic pain) leading to a proliferation of service programs with little empirical basis. The incidence of new "cases" increases as new problems are discovered, but the driving force behind this activity is the proliferation of treatment programs driven by the expanding supply of treatment professionals.

Solutions exclusively emphasizing treatment and rehabilitation place the mental health fields in a "no win" position for another reason. Treatment rhetoric fosters the illusion that problems are being solved. Yet, despite the statistics about the number of people who have been seen and "helped" by mental health services, it will be clear to most citizens that the incidence of disorder is not being reduced and, as a whole, society is not better off as a result of this activity. Not only will problems not have been solved, but society will have no better understanding of how such problems develop, nor will there be any structures in place that can be used by people for problem resolution.

Forces Maintaining the Status Quo

In the 1980s, federal dollars for mental health services were distributed to the states at continually reduced levels and, in many cases, states were unable to make up the shortfalls. This placed an increasing burden on mental health centers to generate more of their own revenues. Centers survived by trying to maximize revenues from insurance companies and other third-party sources, and increasing portions of center budgets have come from non-government revenues. As a result, services offered by community mental health centers became influenced by reimbursement standards set by the insurance industry. While market pressures forced centers to become more productive and efficient, services also reflected efforts at revenue generation, rather than being provided on the basis of need (Goplerud, Walfish, & Broskowski, 1985; Sorensen, 1985). Centers sought clients with the ability to pay for services, or with insurance and insurable conditions, while low-income clients without insurance were less likely to receive services.

When choice of treatment becomes determined by revenue considerations, incentives diminish for prevention, community-based treatment, or services for the indigent. For example, inpatient hospitalization for what were formerly considered outpatient disorders (eating disorders, stress reactions, problem drinking, moderate levels of depression, etc.) represents a new growth industry in both the public and private sectors. Companies can charge for psychiatric hospital days even though hospitalization is not needed, and in many cases is counterproductive to recovery and relapse prevention (Aviram, 1990; Marlatt & Gordon, 1985). For example, Miller and Hester (1986) report no compelling reason to recommend residential over nonresidential settings in the treatment of alcohol abuse.

The trend toward inpatient mental health care could be attenuated by the growth of health maintenance organizations (HMOs) and preferred provider organizations (PPOs), recent health care innovations that have gained momentum because of their appeal as cost-containment ventures. HMOs accept responsibility for furnishing mental health services to large organizations, and are paid on the basis of the number of persons covered by the contract, rather than the type or amount of service provided. PPOs are groups of health care providers who contract with organizations to provide services through negotiated fees for services. Both types of programs have incentives to reduce health care costs and, not surprisingly, emphasize outpatient, rather than inpatient, care and brief forms of therapy (Bloom, 1990). Unfortunately, cost containment has often led to questionable care decisions, particularly when HMOs and PPOs operate on a for-profit basis (Bloom, 1990; Kuttner, 1991). These approaches have also failed to stimulate prevention activities or innovative treatment, even though HMOs began with the intent of fostering preventive health activities (Flinn, McMahon, & Collins, 1987).

A second major source of factors that help to maintain the *status quo* involve traditions and practices within the mental health professions themselves. There are a number of reasons why innovative community models of service delivery are not likely to come from established professional groups. Practitioners have a vested interest in maintaining work settings that allow them to use the knowledge and skills acquired in professional training, and there are few financial incentives to upgrade these skills. Community intervention is taught in very few academic training programs, and there are not many opportunities to acquire new skills after graduate training. Outside of voluntary weekend workshops, formal opportunities for upgrading clinical and community skills do not exist. Most university psychology programs are not structured to provide postdoctoral training to mature practitioners, and the schism between academicians and practitioners is such that many in the latter group automatically dismiss such training as irrelevant to their needs. While one can hope that future generations of mental health practitioners will be more responsive to community approaches, the evidence seems to suggest that current students in the mental health professions are even more interested in private-practice models of service delivery than were their predecessors (Peterson, 1985). In addition, since the majority of current clinical practitioners are untrained in community approaches, few plans to restructure the mental health system are likely to succeed.

A third major impediment to mental health innovation is the tendency, described earlier, to search for unitary, uniform solutions to mental health problems (Seidman & Rappaport, 1986). For example, the idea of a single "comprehensive" mental health center comes from an era in which attending to psychological well-being automatically meant professional help (e.g., psychotherapy for "neurotic" disorders or supportive care for chronic mental patients). Consider the concept "continuity of care," which was used as a rationale for a single comprehensive mental health center. It was thought important to structure services for chronic mental patients so that they could retain the same treatment staff as they moved from hospital to community and back again. Consistent care would, of course, be less disruptive, so it was valuable for outpatient and inpatient services to be within the same administrative unit or facility. But a system of care that benefits chronic patients might not be suitable for others. Many citizens refuse to use a facility that is primarily identified with the care of chronic patients. Furthermore, "continuity of care" was meant to facilitate *professional* care. If one's goal is to facilitate *indigenous* care (network building, social support, community development projects, etc.) then housing such functions in a center primarily identified with treating mental illness does not make much sense. Naparstek, Biegel, and Spiro (1982) suggest that while organized neighborhoods might be effective in dealing with the environmental precipitants of disorder (e.g., reducing the effects of anomie or dislocation, or working toward improving the community's social and economic climate), they are less likely to be interested or effective in responding to entrenched psychological disorders.

NEW DIRECTIONS

A useful goal for a community-oriented service is to help citizens at local and regional levels understand vexing social and psychological problems, and to provide models for how such problems might be addressed. We believe that the focus should be on what can be accomplished for specific problems through collaborative planning between federal, state, and local governments, university training and research centers, and established professional and citizen groups. We will emphasize the role of state governments and local constituency groups because these units have been neglected in the past, and because they have a distinct role to play in future mental health planning.

Encouraging State and Local Initiatives

It is ironic that a *community* mental health system should be structured to provide so few opportunities for input from community members. This is because, as we have pointed out previously, community mental health legislation involved a liaison between the federal government and mental health professional groups that bypassed state and local governments. The latter were seen as entities that had for decades shunned their responsibilities for human welfare, resulting in overcrowded custodial hospitals and mental patient neglect. However, the unintended consequence of a liaison that excluded state and local groups was to further local denial and abdication of responsibility for mental health problems. Now that the federal government has withdrawn support from community mental health centers, state governments and local communities see little reason to assume a *new* burden, when funding is also being cut for programs that had been their traditional responsibility.

The federal program that was an active force in mandating standardized services ended in 1981 when the Mental Health Systems Act was revoked. With the exception of funds for the treatment of chronic mental disorders through Supplemental Security Income and Social Security Disability payments (Koyanagi & Goldman, 1991), there is no comprehensive federal community mental health program at the present time. A Block Grant program was established instead, which allowed states to use human services and mental health dollars as they wished. However, after years in which decisions were made at the federal level, many states did not have structures in place for informed policy decisions. Nevertheless, state governments became the arena for the shaping of mental health policy.

We believe that a key goal at the state level is to develop structures for establishing statewide public mental health priorities. State mental health administrators need to move beyond a focus on existing institutions and ask: What problems are we trying to solve with our mental health dollars? They then need to know the extent to which these problems are being solved, and what other solutions might be tried to accomplish these goals. Their commitment should be to finding solutions to vexing psychological and social problems, rather than being committed to particular solutions (e.g., mental hospitals or community mental health centers). While there will always be political lobbying by professional and patient advocacy groups to influence the mental health agenda, problems to be addressed also should be defined by needs assessment, rational planning, and priority setting (Morrell, 1979; Siegel, Attkisson, & Carson, 1978; Weiss, 1977; Weiss & Weiss, 1981). Problem solutions should be identified and supported based on research and evaluation. Thus, states need not be providers of direct services, nor do they need to maintain a heavy investment in institutions and the infrastructure needed to maintain them. They can instead use their funds to identify needs and to contract with service providers for programs to meet those needs, choosing from among providers on the basis of program fit and demonstrated program efficacy.

It must be recognized that suggestions such as those above fly in the face of mental health traditions. Historically, states have been providers of direct service, and the placement of state institutions has been a major source of patronage and political influence. States that attempt to close institutions or restructure funding patterns face opposition from groups that have a vested interest in the maintenance of institutional programs. Note how difficult it has been to close state hospitals despite the establishment of community mental health centers and the trend toward deinstitutionalization. A majority of states continue to maintain dual mental health systems. State hospitals and community mental health centers vie for financial support, with state hospitals receiving the bulk of mental health funds despite their much smaller patient population (Aviram, 1990; Carling, Miller, Daniels, & Randolph, 1987).

Some states have been able to break away from traditional, institution-based services. For example, one survey found that Wisconsin spent only 20% of its state mental health budget on state hospitals, while other states, such as New York, spent as much as 85% of their mental health budgets on such facilities (Aviram, 1990). Vermont transferred the functions of its lone state hospital to local CMHCs, with the goal of eliminating all but the forensic functions of the hospital (Carling, 1990; Carling et al., 1987). Other states developed plans to contract for services, rather than continuing to provide direct services themselves. These efforts have produced mixed results. For example, Illinois provided some funds to help establish local chapters of Grow, Inc., a mutual-help organization for chronic mental patients (Rappaport, Seidman, Toro, McFadden, Reischl, Roberts, Salem, Stein, & Zimmerman, 1985; Zimmerman, 1987). New Jersey funded a statewide self-help clearinghouse, helping expand an initially small program at a local community mental health center into a larger program offering information, referral, outreach, and training services for mutual aid groups and individuals interested in starting such programs (Madera, 1990). On the other hand, efforts to contract mental health services to private HMOs show considerable variability in the quality of care provided (Chang, Kiser, Bailey, Martins, Gibson, Schaberg, Mirvis, & Applegate, 1998; Johnsen, Morrissey, Landow, Starrett, Calloway, & Ullman, 1998; McFarland, Johnson, & Hornbrook, 1996). The financial incentives in for-profit HMOs is to offer minimal treatment and few specialist referrals. As a result, patients must be more aggressive in requesting treatment, a task that many socially impaired mental patients find difficult. Research indicates that the most effective treatments for chronic mental patients are either assertive community treatment (ACT) or intensive case management (Lehman, Dixon, Kernan, DeForge, & Postrado, 1997; Mueser, Bond, Drake, & Resnick, 1998; Mueser, Drake, & Bond, 1997). These models of service are rarely provided by HMOs, which typically do not look for clients. If anything, there are often bureaucratic barriers to treatment in for-profit HMOs that the severely mentally ill find difficult to surmount.

Since it seems that the current federal policy is to return the responsibility for initiatives in mental health to the states, it is important that structures be in place at the state level for informed policy decisions. At the present time, many states do not have planning or research and evaluation staff, so it is important to think of ways that such structures can be developed (Ridge, Pincus, Blalock, & Fine, 1989). Our suggestions will focus on an improved planning and evaluation capability at the state level, mechanisms for retraining current mental health personnel, and regional centers that can facilitate the implementation and evaluation of new prevention and treatment technologies.

Federal Support for Training, Planning, and Evaluation

A critical role for the federal government should be to support planning, research, and evaluation at the state level. Federal planners should resist the temptation to think that they "know what's best." Rather than imposing solutions, they could perform a more valuable service by upgrading the capacity of states to accomplish planning and evaluation. One way to realize this goal is for the federal government to provide training grants to states interested in upgrading their planning and evaluation capabilities (see, for example, Livingston & Srebnick, 1991).

A second federal function could be the provision of grants for training current mental health personnel. The original community mental health centers legislation did not include any funds for staff training, so there was no vehicle for existing staff to upgrade their skills. While universities did receive some monies earmarked for training in community mental health, their efforts were directed at training future generations of mental health workers, leaving existing mental health personnel essentially untouched. CMHC staff not only lacked training in community intervention, but also were essentially untrained in the newest methods of clinical treatment. For example, many center personnel are unaware of developments in the psychosocial rehabilitation of chronic mental patients (Leff & Vaughn, 1985; Paul & Lentz, 1977; Salem, Seidman, & Rappaport, 1988; Stein & Test, 1985; Test, 1981), and in many cases continue to flounder in the treatment of their most publicly visible clientele—deinstitutionalized mental patients. Only a small percentage of staff are aware of developments in conducting community-based prevention services, despite the growth of published material on the topic (Albee & Gullotta, 1997; Durlak & Wells, 1997; Heller, 1990; Price, Cowen, Lorion, & Ramos-McKay, 1988). Clearly, a mechanism is needed to provide mental health professionals with incentives and opportunities to upgrade their skills in emerging prevention and treatment technologies (Barlow, 1985; Edelstein & Michelson, 1986; Kelly, 1988; Marlatt & Gordon, 1985; Muniz, 1987; Price, Ketterer, Bader, & Monahan, 1980).

Training grants should be made available to universities and medical schools to upgrade the training of mental health personnel at all levels. One step in this direction is the NIMH Public-Academic Liaison program (PAL), which funds postdoctoral research fellowship training in state mental health agencies (Bevilacqua, 1991). This model of public agency and university cooperation could be adapted to other levels of professional training and other professional roles. Universities generally have played a minimal role in ongoing community education. With a downturn in enrollments in the late 1970s through the 1980s, a number of colleges and universities have found it profitable to develop vital adult education programs. Similar incentives could be provided to graduate programs in psychology to develop professional re-education programs, and to mental health personnel to upgrade their own conceptual and technical development. The inclusion of advanced training in mental health policy formation and in program development has the added advantage of providing a cadre of skilled personnel who could improve planning and evaluation at state and local levels.

While universities might be more willing to develop programs for mature professionals in this era of scarce training funds, what they would actually teach is, to some extent, a policy choice—state of the art treatment technologies and/or community intervention. The choice depends in part upon professional traditions, but also upon financial incentives. Prevention is more likely to receive prominence when there is a "market" for it. For example, Califano (1986) describes a prevention program adopted by the Johnson & Johnson company that provided a financial savings in terms of reduced absenteeism and lower health costs. The program had the following core elements: smoking cessation, weight control, nutrition, exercise, blood pressure control, stress management, and the advocacy of healthy life styles. Community mental health centers that have been able to maintain active prevention programs have done so by emphasizing income-generating projects that can then support programs with fewer resources (Godin, Carr-Kaffashan, & Hines, 1990; Schelkun, 1990).

Effective prevention or treatment programs are likely to be cost effective when they can be implemented with a minimum of professional personnel. An example is a prevention program developed by Olds (1988) for low SES pregnant teenagers about to have their first child, in which public-health nurses provided home visits oriented around health education and parenting skills, and encouraged links to supportive friends, family members, and human service agency staff (Olds, Henderson, Chamberlin, & Tatelbaum, 1986; Olds, Henderson, Tatelbaum, & Chamberlin, 1986). Other examples include consumer-run service programs funded by the Michigan Department of Mental Health to promote the community functioning of former mental patients (Mowbray, Chamberlain, Jennings, & Reed, 1988). Program elements involve support and life-skill training programs and a profit-making janitorial training and employment service. All are designed to reduce psychiatric hospitalization by providing support and promoting competence in community living, at a fraction of the cost of professionally administered programs.

Regional Centers for Innovation, Action Research, and Evaluation

Our recommendations for the development of policy research, enhanced professional training, and public participation clearly need to be implemented in a coordinated manner. We propose that the federal government redirect some of its allocations for research and training to a system of regional centers to promote better planning and greater innovation in service delivery. The purpose of such centers would be to serve as a resource for state and local communities to foster properly evaluated studies of attempts to solve pressing social problems. We envision a collaborative arrangement between scientists and citizens (Chavis, Stucky, & Wandersman, 1983) in identifying needs and in proposing and evaluating alternative attempts at problem resolution. The rationale for the regionalization of such centers is to maximize citizen involvement, as well as to respond to local conditions. This would facilitate the identification of stressors unique to particular subcultures, as well as the resources that particular localities possess. As Shinn has noted:

> Research that attempts to determine answers for all places and all time regarding the effects of programs that are implemented in vastly different ways with different populations in different locales with different needs may be doomed to failure. But studies in particular interventions, designed to answer questions framed in collaboration with local problem solvers, with provision for feedback to problem solvers in a time frame that permits action, may be very useful both to the problem solvers and to ... policy formulation (Shinn, 1987, p. 567–568).

Regional centers could provide incentives for university researchers to collaborate on program development and evaluation. Their knowledge of the literature could help local groups focus their efforts on manageable and achievable goals, avoiding some of the mistakes of the past. Early collaboration could insure the collection of usable evaluation data—a major problem when evaluation is considered only when a project has been in operation for a period of time. Researchers and their students would also benefit, and would gain an appreciation of real-life constraints as they attempt to put their ideas into practice in applied settings (Corbett & Levine, 1974).

Community control of these centers through citizen boards is important to insure that professionals do not dominate the center's agenda, and to address culturally appropriate definitions of needs and services (Cheung & Snowden, 1990). Final decisions about which problems to pursue and programs to fund should be determined by community groups and their representatives. Their decisions would be based on determining the most pressing problems in their area, as well as the resources available for problem resolution.

Community control of allocation decisions in the human service fields does not have a positive history of effectiveness or impartiality. Community boards for mental health centers are quite common, but they generally have not operated as effective, independent, decision-making bodies (Dowell & Ciarlo, 1983). Their decisions, to a large extent, have been shaped and influenced by their professional staff. Similarly, citizen boards of other human service organizations have been found to make allocation decisions that are often based on precedent and political influence, rather than on an assessment of community need or quality of service delivered (Steffen, 1987). Least successful are those community boards with a rotating membership of volunteers who serve with no particular mandate from defined constituency groups and who have little training or expertise. They are particularly vulnerable to influence by public and professional interest groups.

Our suggested remedy for this problem is to develop a system of election or appointment so that citizen members of regional center boards would be accountable to defined citizen constituency groups. This could be accomplished by special elections to fill board seats (similar to the way school boards are chosen in many communities) or by special appointment by local government officials (e.g., mayors, city or county councils). Either method has the advantage of increasing accountability since board members who consistently make unpopular decisions would fail to be re-elected or reappointed. Longer tenure, and the expertise that comes with tenure, also are more likely if members receive the acknowledgement and prestige associated with an areawide election or appointment.

We recognize that elections or appointments by local officials will tend to politicize the regional boards, but such a development is inevitable. After all, community control of allocation decisions really means political control. Of relevance here is the distinction between "social science" and "social system" solutions to social policy issues (Shadish, 1984). Social science solutions reflect the values and ideologies of the scientific community, which often are orthogonal to public values. On the other hand, "social system solutions ... reflect the pluralistic self interests of a policy shaping community" (Shadish, 1984, p. 728). As such, they are more likely to be implemented. Shadish uses the deinstitutionalization example to contrast the two. Whereas social scientists defined the problem as finding the best possible system of patient care, the problem for the "social system" was to determine where patients should live in communities that disliked having mental patients in their midst.

The tension we anticipate on the regional center boards will involve researchers advocating specific programs based on evaluation data, while community members decide which programs can be implemented given community values. Undoubtedly, bad decisions will sometimes be made. However, our expectation is that in the process both groups will be influenced by the ensuing dialogue and, over time, more effective programs will be chosen as communities become better educated concerning citizen needs and possible alternatives to meet these needs.

Regional centers should be supported by a number of sources (e.g., federal, state, local, and/or private funds) to insure greater financial stability. Federal funding is particularly vulnerable to shifts in the political climate. Conservative or liberal changes in the federal administration do not accurately reflect attitudinal shifts in the population at large. Presidential elections often are determined by differences of only a few percentage points in the popular vote, yet they have a profound ideological impact on federal responsiveness to social issues for years to come. State funds for mental health research and services are also reactive to political and budgetary vicissitudes (Elpers, 1989; Levin, Friedman, Nixon, & Zusman, 1989). Regional centers with multiple funding sources could be somewhat insulated from these political swings, particularly if they were successful in developing support among local constituency groups. The lack of consistent funding is a serious problem, and has been a major impediment in past efforts at program innovation. By the time a new program has been adequately developed and tested, a change in the political climate has often occurred and funds become unavailable for implementation.

Our proposal, then, involves federal funds as an initial catalyst for attracting state, local, and private support. Grant funds of this type also would be a stimulant for input and cooperation from governmental, academic, citizen, and service provider systems. Examples of university or medical school research collaboration with mental health agencies can be found in a number of states, in some cases funded by the Pew Foundation (Fine, Pincus, Ridge, James, Gregory, & Ennis, 1989; Talbott, 1991), but in only a few instances have these programs emphasized an explicit public health model (Neligh, Shore, Scully, Kort, Willett, Harding, & Kawamura, 1991).

There may be some classes of research for which regionalization possesses no particular benefit (e.g., research on the genetic determinants of schizophrenia or depression). On the other hand, the regional-centers concept would be useful in studying ecological factors in treatment, such as the community treatment of schizophrenics (Fairweather et al., 1969; Polak & Kirby, 1976) or the development of mutual aid organizations (Katz, 1981; Levine, 1988). Also, it is important to recognize that many of the practical problems associated with overcoming environmental risk factors in prevention and treatment research are not likely to be solved independent of concerted community efforts. For problems of this nature, scientists working alone lack the power to influence or implement change.

Community-based action projects to lower the incidence of coronary heart disease can serve as models for efforts that might be undertaken in the psychological sphere (e.g., Farquhar, Fortmann, Maccoby, Haskell, Williams, Flora, Taylor, Brown, Solomon, & Hulley, 1985; Leupker, Murray, Jacobs, Mittelmark, Bracht, Carlaw, Crow, Elmer, Finnegan, Folsom, Grimm, Hannan, Jeffrey, Lando, McGovern, Mullis, Perry, Pechacek, Pierie, Sprafta, Weisbrod, & Blackburn, 1994; McAlister, Puska, Koskela, Pallonen, & Maccoby, 1980; Puska, Nissenen, Tuomilehto, Salonen, Koskela, McAlister, Kottke, Maccoby, & Farquhar, 1985). Key elements of these projects involve:

- careful epidemiological research to demonstrate the existence of environmental and behavioral risks;
- community education efforts using the media to inform the public about risk factors and the action necessary to overcome them;
- follow-up community organization efforts with local community groups to enlist their cooperation in actively reaching their membership, emphasizing the importance of changes in norms, values, and practices; and, finally,
- formative evaluation occurring throughout the project so that feedback about what works can be used for improvements in the ongoing program.

Many of the practical problems concerning the implementation and evaluation of communitywide health projects have been already addressed (Altman, 1986; Farquhar, Fortmann, Wood, & Haskell, 1983) so that research centers would not have to start completely afresh in solving thorny implementation and evaluation issues. Examples of the manner in which regional centers can define and evaluate solutions to major health and social problems can be found in the work of the Stanford University Center for Disease Prevention, the Prevention Research Centers funded by NIMH, and the Veterans Administration Health Services Research and Development Field Programs (Goldschmidt, 1986). We believe that successful centers are those whose personnel understand the variety of roles and relationships needed to mount effective community programs (Chavis, Stucky, & Wandersman, 1983; Price, 1983).

Local Involvement in Community Mental Health

A major dilemma in planning mental health services for the 1990s and beyond is how to rekindle local concern and planning for psychological well-being—planning for all citizens, not just those in obvious psychological distress. In the years ahead, demographic changes in the population will introduce new constituency groups in need. Some examples are the aged, the under- and unemployed, and single-parent families living at or below the poverty line. Local communities with adequate funding sources are in the best position to deal with such problems.

An early example of active involvement of citizens and local officials in mental health prevention activities can be found in the Wellesley Program originally developed by Eric Lindemann in the late 1940s (Klein, 1968, 1987). Here was an instance in which mental health professionals encouraged citizens to become partners in programs that promoted optimal growth and development. The project was funded by the W. T. Grant Foundation and involved a multidisciplinary team from several schools and departments at Harvard University, in collaboration with local professional and lay groups. Their work extended from town planning to law enforcement, recreation, and education, and entailed a series of action programs based upon epidemiological risk data. For example, one major project involved a longitudinal study of kindergarten children and their families to predict later adaptation to school. Note that it was not expected that school and community problems would be permanently solved in Wellesley, but that a collaborative problem-solving structure would be set up by which these problems could be addressed.

There are several key ingredients in achieving community involvement. The first is that programs focus on everyday, recognizable problems, as defined by the people involved (Trotter, 1981). This step is necessary in order for the problem to be publicly "owned," that is, in order for people to take collective responsibility for the problem. A second important ingredient in developing community involvement is that people must feel competent in achieving some sort of problem resolution. People will not take action on problems that they do not believe are solvable. A third ingredient is the presence of structures that expedite group action. Projects may become part of the agenda of existing groups, or new problem-focused organizations may be developed.

These ingredients can be illustrated by the heart disease prevention programs described earlier. Risk factors for heart disease, e.g., smoking, fatty diet, and sedentary life styles, were identified and publicized so that people could understand those aspects of their own behavior that needed to be changed. People were shown how they could take action to overcome these risks, and there were follow-up contacts with organizations to work with group members in carrying out changes in health practices.

A major issue is whether environmental and behavioral risks can be identified for social and psychological problems in the same way as they have been identified for heart disease. Since we are not accustomed to thinking about social and psychological risk factors in this way, more research is clearly needed. Still there are some promising leads. For example, there is evidence that children who stay in school are better off socially and psychologically than those who drop out (Berrueta-Clement, Schweinhart, Barnett, & Weikart, 1987). When presented with the evidence and the social costs of inaction, we think that most people would support a campaign to improve schools and help children stay in school. With similar documentation, they also are likely to support programs for adequate nutrition, family stability, useful social roles for the elderly, full employment, and so on, all of which have been identified as factors contributing to the decreased likelihood of disorder (Blazer, 1982; Freeman, Klein, Kagan, & Yarbrough, 1977; Gelfand, Ficula, & Zabatany, 1986; Rosow, 1976; Seidman & Rapkin, 1983).

While most complex social and psychological problems are not easily solvable, through the decades there have been examples of how progress can be made when there is public ownership of problems and organized structures that encourage group action. Early examples are the Settlement Houses and adult-education classes that helped reduce disorder linked to poverty and ghetto life (Levine & Levine, 1970). Other examples are projects that focus on crime prevention, increasing educational opportunity and participation, creating a climate for better housing and jobs, forming community coalitions against substance abuse, or increasing the availability of medical services (Cook, Roehl, Oros, & Trudeau, 1994; Eugster, 1974; Lewis & Salem, 1981; Wagenaar, Murray, Wolfson, Forster, & Finnegan, 1994). As Stokols (1992) notes, we need not be deterred by the complexity of global environmental problems in order to take constructive action at local and regional levels.

The Extended Family Program operated by two religious organizations, the Little Sisters of the Assumption and the Dominican Sisters of the Sick Poor, provides an example of how interventions can be adapted to local community standards (Shinn, 1987; Shinn & Rosario, 1985). The goals of the program were to strengthen and stabilize at-risk families by improving family members' childrearing skills, and supporting the families in dealing with the various systems that impinged upon them. The primary agent in the program was a mature paraprofessional community member, a "grandmother," who worked with families in an "extended family" role. The grandmother was backed up at the agency by advocacy services and classes for parents, including experiential child-rearing classes for mothers in a playroom setting. Results of a pilot study showed improvements in mothers' parenting skills, family nutrition, and children's health during the period of family involvement in the program. The importance of the program is not in its positive results, since it has not yet been rigorously evaluated (Shinn, 1987); however, we see it as a model of how preventive mental health services might be delivered at the local level. Education and support are provided in a way that respects and builds on local norms and values. The indigenous grandmother received much more acceptance in the minority communities of New York City than would a more professionally trained middle-class worker. The service also was provided by an agency with an empowerment and advocacy ideology, and so probably received greater participant commitment than would an agency with a more "neutral" and distant professional stance.

We suspect that if citizens were asked how their mental health needs could be served, counseling and psychotherapy would be a low priority, chosen only under special circumstances. Higher priority is more likely to be given to projects that help overcome real-life stressors and provide a sense of competency and self-efficacy to participants. Viewed in this light, the options provided by the formal mental health system seem narrow indeed. Even during the years when federal support was readily available, no more than 2.5% of all CMHC staff hours were devoted to primary prevention activities (Swift, 1987).

Is a Viable Community-Based, Prevention-Oriented, Mental Health System Possible?

At this point, some readers may feel that we have taken leave of our senses. The 1980s saw the domination of a federal administration whose stance was to deny responsibility for social and psychological problems. The 1990s has produced little substantive change in terms of federal priorities and practices. Furthermore, the general record of most states and localities in attending to human services needs has not been particularly stellar. The mental health professions also have not distinguished themselves as advocates for the needy and underserved, nor have they rushed to adopt a preventive model—a point of view that has been disseminated in the literature for over two decades. Yet, the heart of our proposal involves proactive collaboration between all of these groups.

We believe that the current pessimism concerning the viability of community approaches reflects the political climate of the moment, and is as inaccurate a reading of what can be accomplished as was the unbridled optimism of the 1960s. Basic lifestyle attitudes and values, and the social institutions that they support, evolve slowly and are influenced more by demographic changes in the population and technological modification in the workplace than they are by current political events.

The stance of the Reagan and Bush administrations toward social and psychological problems involved a deliberate avoidance of responding to human needs until problems escalated to the point that behavioral disruptions become intolerable. Institutionalization was then advocated as the only alternative. A number of examples can be cited in which calls for institutionalization or incarceration reflect the consequence of earlier problem avoidance. For example, we spend more money building new prisons than in dealing with structural unemployment and inadequate educational opportunity, two major precipitants of crime. Unemployment among unskilled and semiskilled workers, as well as inadequate community support programs for marginally skilled workers and their families (as well as for deinstitutionalized mental patients), are factors in the rise of homeless populations in our cities (Shinn & Weitzman, 1990). Calls for institutionalizing these groups, for example, returning chronic mental patients to hospitals or jails (Belcher, 1988), while appealing to some in the short run, simply will not work as an exclusive national policy. Eventually the cost of warehousing large segments of our population will become excessively burdensome, as they did in the 1950s, and there will be mounting pressures for a change in policy. The point is rather simple: ignoring social inequities does not make problems associated with inequity disappear.

There is likely to be greatest community involvement when there is collective acceptance of responsibility for problems and community structures available to facilitate group action. These conditions are more likely for problems such as employment, education of children, health care, housing, public safety, transportation, and recreation. Entrenched psychological disorders (e.g., child and spouse abuse or chronic mental disorder) require more specialized treatment, but even here there is a supplementary role for indigenous help. It is important for mental patients to be treated with understanding and support, and not be deprived of normal social roles as family members or productive workers. The public can do a great deal to support and reinforce community functioning (e.g., Stein & Test, 1985). Patient self-help groups and mutual-help organizations also can be a boon to the management of dysfunctional behavior, and are important sources of indigenous treatment (Giarretto, 1981; Madara, 1990; Salem, Seidman, & Rappaport, 1988).

What can be expected in the years ahead from the mental health professions in terms of their engagement in collaborative public problem solving? As we have emphasized throughout this chapter, very few professionals have been trained with a public health/prevention or community development orientation. With the increasing growth of professional schools (Peterson, 1985), even fewer will adopt a community orientation in the years ahead. Freestanding professional schools are particularly oriented toward a traditional clinical, rather than a community or public health, treatment model. Since they graduate far more practitioners per program than university-based training programs, it is likely that future professional lobbying efforts will be increasingly devoted toward defense of professional guild prerogatives and less oriented toward public need. In many ways, we as a profession represent *the* major impediment to innovation within the mental health system. As swings once again occur in the political climate, there will be a renewed interest in domestic problems, and the public will turn to us for leadership. How will we respond? Without major changes in the training of mental health professionals, it is quite likely that our counsel will be the same as it was in the 1960s—increases in treatment facilities and treatment personnel.

CONCLUSION

We have attempted to provide an overview of the ideologies, fiscal contingencies, and political dynamics that have led to the current state of community mental health in the United States. We see these forces as contributing to the negation of public participation in policy making, the maintenance of traditional rehabilitation approaches, and the underdevelopment of public health and prevention strategies in the mental health arena. The result is a system that reflects professional ideologies and imperatives rather than community needs—a system that does not facilitate public ownership of mental health problems.

We have suggested that efforts to improve mental health practice should emphasize planning and evaluation at state and local levels, as well as increased collaboration between public and professional groups. In addition, we propose that universities be encouraged to participate in this process because they offer resources that can facilitate innovation and evaluation. Universities have contributed to the problems we have described by not being more connected to their home communities and by emphasizing individually oriented theories and solutions. Our proposal for regional centers leads naturally from the recognition that a publicly responsive mental health system must be accountable to local communities, and that research should play a major role in developing ecologically appropriate prevention and treatment programs (for examples see Livingston & Srebnick, 1991; Mechanic, 1991).

Our critique of the mental health system is not new (Aviram, 1990; Hasenfeld, 1985; Hunter & Riger, 1986; Levine, 1981; Price & Smith, 1983; Shadish, 1984; Snow & Newton, 1976); however, our suggestions for change are more radical than may be initially apparent. The coordination of academic, governmental, and practitioner groups represents not only structural reform, but also provides a vehicle for changing the ideology of community mental health practice toward a more ecologically based, community-oriented direction.

Many of those who have described the political and professional forces that have shaped the last 25 years of public mental health policy have generally come to the pessimistic conclusion that "the more things change, the more they stay the same" (Karr, 1849). The implication is that policy is driven by self-serving administrative and professional structures that, over the long run, subvert well-intentioned legislative initiatives. While we agree that these forces are important, our own views are less gloomy. We believe that the current configuration of mental health services will change because they are neither fiscally nor ideologically viable. In the decades ahead there will be public pressures for change, and our suggestions should improve public accountability and control through the development of more open problem-solving structures. But a key factor will be the stance taken by the mental health professions. Changes are needed in professional orientation and practice if we are to move toward a true community-oriented mental health system. While it is true that external political and financial pressures have shaped the current mental health system, to a much larger extent, current practice reflects our own conceptual models. It is for this reason that we believe that the building blocks for change reside much more in our own hands than many of us may realize.

ACKNOWLEDGMENTS. Preparation of this manuscript was facilitated by Grant #RO1MH41457 to KH. An earlier version of this manuscript benefited from the insightful comments of John W. Finney, Rudolph H. Moos, Julian Rappaport, and Edward Seidman.

REFERENCES

Albee, G. W., & Gullotta, T. P. (1997). *Primary prevention works.* Thousand Oaks, CA: Sage.

Altman, D. G. (1986). A framework for evaluating community-based heart disease prevention programs. *Social Science Medicine, 22,* 479–487.

Anthony, W. A. (1989). Research on community support services: What have we learned? Special issue: The community support system concept. *Psychosocial Rehabilitation Journal, 12,* 55–81.

Aviram, U. (1990). Community care of the seriously mentally ill: Continuing problems and current issues. *Community Mental Health Journal, 26,* 69–88.

Barlow, D. H. (1985). *Clinical handbook of psychological disorders.* New York: Guilford.

Belcher, J. R. (1988). Are jails replacing the mental health system for the homeless mentally ill? *Community Mental Health Journal, 24,* 185–195.

Berrueta-Clement, J. R., Schweinhart, L. J., Barnett, W. S., & Weikart, D. P. (1987). The effects of early educational intervention on crime and delinquency in adolescence and early adulthood. In J. D. Burchard & S. N. Burchard (Eds.), *Prevention of delinquent behavior: Primary prevention of psychopathology, Vol. 10* (pp. 220–240). Newbury Park, CA: Sage.

Bevilacqua, J. J. (1991). The NIMH public-academic liaison (PAL) research initiative: An update. *Hospital and Community Psychiatry, 42,* 71.

Blazer, D. G. (1982). Social support and mortality in an elderly community population. *American Journal of Epidemiology, 115,* 684–694.

Bloom, B. L. (1985). Focal issues in the prevention of mental disorder. In H. H. Goldman & S. E. Goldston (Eds.), *Preventing stress-related psychiatric disorders* (pp. 3–20). Washington, D.C.: U.S. Department of Health and Human Services. DHHS Publication No. (ADM) 85-1366.

Bloom, B. L. (1990). Managing mental health services: Some comments for the overdue debate in psychology. *Community Mental Health Journal, 26,* 107–124.

Buck, J. A. (1984). Block grants and federal promotion of community mental health services, 1946–65. *Community Mental Health Journal, 20,* 236–247.

Califano, J. A., Jr. (1986). *America's health care revolution.* New York: Random House.

Campbell, D. T. (1971). *Methods for the experimenting society.* Paper presented at the meetings of the Eastern Psychological Association, Washington, D.C., April.

Carling, P. J. (1990). Major mental illness, housing, and supports: The promise of community integration. *American Psychologist, 45,* 969–975.

Carling, P. J., Miller, S., Daniels, L. V., & Randolph, F. L. (1987). A state mental health system with no state hospital: the Vermont feasibility study. *Hospital and Community Psychiatry, 38,* 617–623.

Chang, C. F., Kiser, L. J., Bailey, J. E., Martins, M., Gibson, W. C., Schaberg, K. A., Mirvis, D. M., & Applegate, W. B. (1998). Tennessee's failed managed care program for mental health and substance abuse services, *JAMA, 279,* 864–869.

Chavis, D. M., Stucky, P. E., & Wandersman, A. (1983). Returning basic research to the community: A relationship between scientist and citizen. *American Psychologist, 38,* 424–434.

Cheung, F. K., & Snowden, L. R. (1990). Community mental health and ethnic minority populations. *Community Mental Health Journal, 26,* 277–291.

Cohen, L. H. (1985). Research utilization in community mental health: Some comments on O'Donohue, Curtis & Fisher (1985). *Professional Psychology: Research and Practice, 16,* 719–722.

Cook, R., Roehl, J., Oros, C., & Trudeau, J. (1994). Conceptual and methodological issues in the evaluation of community-based substance abuse prevention coalitions: Lessons learned from the national evaluation of the Community Partnership Program. *Journal of Community Psychology,* CSAP Special Issue, 155–169.

Corbett, F. J., & Levine, M. (1974). University involvement in the community. In H. E. Mitchell (Ed.), *The university and the urban crisis.* (pp. 137–162). New York: Behavioral Publications.

Cowen, E. L., Gardner, E. A., & Zax, M. (1967). *Emergent approaches to mental health problems.* New York: Appleton-Century-Crofts.

Dowell, D. A., & Ciarlo, J. A. (1983). Overview of the community mental health centers program from an evaluation perspective. *Community Mental Health Journal, 19*, 95–125.

Durlak, J. A., & Wells, A. M. (1997). Primary prevention mental health programs for children and adolescents: A meta-analytic review. *American Journal of Community Psychology, 25*, 115–152.

Edelstein, B. A., & Michelson, L. (1986). *Handbook of prevention*. New York: Plenum.

Elpers, J. R. (1989). Public mental health funding in California, 1959 to 1989. *Hospital and Community Psychiatry, 40*, 799–804.

Eugster, C. (1974). Field education in West Heights: Equipping a depressed community to help itself. In F. M. Cox, J. L. Erlich, J. Rothman, & J. E. Tropman (Eds.), *Strategies of community organization: A book of readings*, (pp. 291–303). 2nd ed. Itasca, IL: Peacock.

Fairweather, G. W., Sanders, D. H., Maynard, H., & Cressler, D. L. (1969). *Community life for the mentally ill: An alternative to institutional care*. Chicago: Aldine.

Farquhar, J. W., Fortmann, S. P., Maccoby, N., Haskell, W. L., Williams, P. T., Flora, J. A., Taylor, C. B., Brown, B. W. Jr., Solomon, D. S., & Hulley, S. B. (1985). The Stanford five-city project: Design and methods. *American Journal of Epidemiology, 122*, 323–334.

Farquhar, J. W., Fortmann, S. P., Wood, P. D., & Haskell, W. L. (1983). Community studies of cardiovascular disease prevention. In N. M. Kaplan & J. Stamler (Eds.), *Prevention of coronary heart disease: Practical management of the risk factors*. (pp. 170–181). Philadelphia: Saunders.

Felton, B. J., & Shinn, M. (1981). Ideology and practice of deinstitutionalization. *Journal of Social Issues, 37*, 158–172.

Fine, T., Pincus, H. A., Ridge, R., James, J. F., Gregory, D., & Ennis, J. (1989). Models of state funding for mental health research. *Hospital and Community Psychiatry, 40*, 383–387.

Flinn, D. E., McMahon, T. C., & Collins, M. F. (1987). Health maintenance organizations and their implications for psychiatry. *Hospital and Community Psychiatry, 38*, 255–263.

Freeman, H. E., Klein, R. E., Kagan, J., & Yarbrough, C. (1977). Relations between nutrition and cognition in rural Guatemala. *American Journal of Public Health, 67*, 233–239.

Gelfand, D. M., Ficula, T., & Zarbatany, L. (1986). Prevention of childhood behavior disorders. In B. A. Edelstein & L. Michelson (Eds.), *Handbook of Prevention*. (pp. 133– 152). New York: Plenum.

Giarretto, H. (1981). A comprehensive child sexual abuse treatment program. In P. B. Marzek & C. H. Kempe (Eds.), *Sexually abused children and their families* (pp. 179–198). New York: Pergamon.

Godin, S. W., Carr-Kaffashan, L. C., & Hines, P. M. (1990). The development and management of prevention services within a comprehensive, medical school-based, community mental health center. *Prevention in Human Services, 7*, 17–48.

Goldschmidt, P. G. (1986). Health services research and development: The Veterans Administration program. *Health Services Research, 20*, 789–824.

Goplerud, E. N., Walfish, S., & Broskowski, A. (1985). Weathering the cuts: A Delphi survey on surviving cutbacks in community mental health. *Community Mental Health Journal, 21*, 14–27.

Hasenfeld, Y. (1985). Community mental health centers as human service organizations. *American Behavioral Scientist, 28*, 655–668.

Heller, K. (1979). The effects of social support: Prevention and treatment implications. In A. P. Goldstein & F. H. Kanfer (Eds.), *Maximizing treatment gains: Transfer enhancement in psychotherapy*. (pp. 353–382). New York: Academic.

Heller, K. (1990). Social and community intervention. *Annual Review of Psychology, 41*, 141–168.

Heller, K., Price, R. H., Reinharz, S., Riger, S., & Wandersman, A. (1984). *Psychology and community change: Challenges of the future* (2nd ed.). Homewood, IL: Dorsey Press.

Hunter, A., & Riger, S. (1986). The meaning of community in community mental health. *Journal of Community Psychology, 14*, 55–71.

Jerrell, J. M., & Larsen, J. K. (1986). Community mental health services in transition: Who is benefiting? *American Journal of Orthopsychiatry, 56*, 78–88.

Johnsen, M. C., Morrissey, J. P., Landow, W. J., Starrett, B. E., Calloway, M. O., & Ullman, M. (1998). The impact of managed care on service systems for persons who are homeless and mentally ill. *Research in Community and Mental Health, 9*, 115–137.

Karr, A. (1849). In J. Bartlett (Ed.), *Familiar quotations*, Fifteenth edition, 1980. Boston: Little, Brown.

Katz, A. H. (1981). Self-help and mutual aid: An emerging social movement? *Annual Review of Sociology, 7*, 129–155.

Kelly, J. G. (1988). A guide to conducting prevention research in the community: First steps. *Prevention in Human Services, 6*, 1–174.

Kiesler, C. A. (1980). Mental health policy as a field of inquiry for psychology. *American Psychologist, 35*, 1066–1080.

Kiesler, C. A. (1982a). Mental hospitals and alternative care: Noninstitutionalization as potential public policy for mental patients. *American Psychologist, 37*, 349–360.

Kiesler, C. A. (1982b). Public and professional myths about mental hospitalization: An empirical reassessment of policy-related beliefs. *American Psychologist, 37*, 1323–1339.

Kiesler, C. A., & Simpkins, C. (1991). The *de facto* national system of psychiatric inpatient care: Piecing together the national puzzle. *American Psychologist, 46*, 579–584.

Kiesler, D. J. (1966). Some myths of psychotherapy research and the search for a paradigm. *Psychological Bulletin, 65*, 110–136.

Klein, D. C. (1968). *Community dynamics and mental health.* New York: Wiley.

Klein, D. C. (1987). The context and times at Swampscott: My/story. *American Journal of Community Psychology, 15*, 531–538.

Koyanagi, C., & Goldman, H. H. (1991). The quiet success of the national plan for the chronically mentally ill. *Hospital and Community Psychiatry, 42*, 899–905.

Kuttner, R. (1991). Sick joke. *The New Republic, 205*, 20–22.

Leff, J., & Vaughn, C. (1985). *Expressed emotion in families.* New York: Guilford.

Lehman, A. F., Dixon, L. B., Kernan, E., DeForge, B. R., & Postrado, L. T. (1997). A randomized trial of assertive community treatment for homeless persons with severe mental illness. *Archives of General Psychiatry, 54*, 1038–1043.

Leupker, R. V., Murray, D. M., Jacobs, D. R., Mittelmark, M. B., Bracht, N., Carlaw, R., Crowe, R., Elmer, P., Finnegan, J., Folsom, A., Grimm, R., Hannan, P. J., Jeffrey, R., Lando, H., McGovern, P., Mullis, R., Perry, C., Pechacek, T., Pierie, P., Sprafka, M., Weisbrod, R., & Blackburn, H. (1994). Community education for cardiovascular disease prevention: Risk factor changes in the Minnesota Heart Health Program. *American Journal of Public Health, 84*, 1383–1393.

Levin, B. L., Friedman, R. M., Nixon, D., & Zusman, J. (1989). A national study of state-supported psychiatric research institutes. *Hospital and Community Psychiatry, 40*, 388–392.

Levine, M. (1981). *The history and politics of community mental health.* New York: Oxford University Press.

Levine, M. (1988). An analysis of mutual assistance. *American Journal of Community Psychology, 16*, 167–183.

Levine, M., & Levine, A. (1970). *A social history of helping services: Clinic, court, school and community.* New York: Appleton-Century-Crofts.

Lewis, D. A., & Salem, G. (1981). Community crime prevention: An analysis of a developing strategy. *Crime and Delinquency, 27*, 405–421.

Livingston, J. A., & Srebnick, D. (1991). States' strategies for promoting supported housing for persons with psychiatric disabilities. *Hospital and Community Psychiatry, 42*, 1116–1119.

Love, R. E. (1984). The community support program: Strategy for reform? In J. A. Talbott (Ed.), *The chronic mental patient: Five years later.* (pp. 195–214). Orlando, FL: Grune & Stratton.

Madara, E. J. (1990). Maximizing the potential for community self-help through clearinghouse approaches. *Prevention in Human Services, 7*, 109–138.

Marlatt, G. A., & Gordon, J. R. (Eds.). (1985). *Relapse prevention: Maintenance strategies in the treatment of addictive behaviors.* New York: Guildford.

McAlister, A., Puska, P., Koskela, K., Pallonen, U., & Maccoby, N. (1980). Mass communication and community organization for public health education. *American Psychologist, 35*, 375–379.

McFarland, B. H., Johnson, R. E., & Hornbrook, M. C. (1996). Enrollment duration, service use, and costs of care for severely mentally ill members of a health maintenance organization. *Archives of General Psychiatry, 53*, 938–944.

Mechanic, D. (1991). Strategies for integrating public mental health services. *Hospital and Community Psychiatry, 42*, 797–801.

Miller, W. R., & Hester, R. K. (1986). Inpatient alcoholism treatment: Who benefits? *American Psychologist, 41*, 794–805.

Morell, J. A. (1979). *Program evaluation in social research.* New York: Pergamon.

Mowbray, C. T., Chamberlain, P., Jennings, M., & Reed, C. (1988). Consumer-run mental health services: Results from five demonstration projects. *Community Mental Health Journal, 24*, 151–156.

Moynihan, D. P. (1969). *Maximum feasible misunderstanding: Community action in the war on poverty.* New York: Free Press.

Mueser, K. T., Bond, G. R., Drake, R. E., & Resnick, S. G. (1998). Models of community care for severe mental illness: A review of research on case management. *Schizophrenia Bulletin, 24*, 37–74.

Mueser, K. T., Drake, R. E., & Bond, G. R. (1997). Recent advances in psychiatric rehabilitation for patients with severe mental illness. *Harvard Review of Psychiatry, 5*, 123–137.

Muñoz, R. F. (Ed.). (1987). *Depression prevention: Research directions.* Washington, D.C.: Hemisphere.

Naparstek, A. J., Biegel, D. E., & Spiro, H. R. (1982). *Neighborhood networks for humane mental health care.* New York: Plenum.

Neligh, G., Shore, J. H., Scully, J., Kort, H., Willett, B., Harding, C. M., & Kawamura, G. (1991). The program for public psychiatry: State-university collaboration in Colorado. *Hospital and Community Psychiatry, 42,* 44–48.

O'Donohue, W. T., Curtis, S. D., & Fisher, J. E. (1985). Use of research in the practice of community mental health: A case study. *Professional Psychology: Research and Practice, 16,* 710–718.

Olds, D. L. (1988). The prenatal/early infancy project. In R. H. Price, E. Cowen, R. Lorion & J. Ramos-McKay (Eds.), *Fourteen ounces of prevention: A casebook for practitioners.* (pp. 3–17). Washington, D.C.: American Psychological Association.

Olds, D. L., Henderson, C. R., Jr., Chamberlin, R., & Tatelbaum, R. (1986). Preventing child abuse and neglect: A randomized trial of nurse home visitation. *Pediatrics, 78,* 65–78.

Olds, D. L., Henderson, C. R., Jr., Tatelbaum, R., & Chamberlin, R. (1986). Improving the delivery of prenatal care and outcomes in pregnancy: A randomized trial of nurse home visitation. *Pediatrics, 77,* 16–28.

Pasamanick, B., Scarpitti, F. R., & Dinitz, S. (1967). *Schizophrenia in the community: Experimental studies in the prevention of hospitalization.* New York: Appleton-Century-Crofts.

Paul, G. L., & Lentz, R. J. (1977). *Psychosocial treatment of chronic mental patients.* Cambridge, MA: Harvard University Press.

Peterson, D. R. (1985). Twenty years of practitioner training in psychology. *American Psychologist, 40,* 441–451.

Polak, P. R., & Kirby, M. W. (1976). A model to replace psychiatric hospitals. *Journal of Nervous and Mental Disease, 162* 13–22.

Price, R. H. (1974). Etiology, the social environment, and the prevention of psychological dysfunction. In P. Insel & R.H. Moos (Eds.), *Health and the social environment.* (pp. 287–300). Lexington, MA: D.C. Heath.

Price, R. H. (1983). The education of a prevention psychologist. In R.D. Felner, L. A. Jason, J. N. Moritsugu, & S. S. Farber (Eds.), *Preventive psychology: Theory, research, and practice.* (pp. 290–296). New York: Pergamon.

Price, R. H., Cowen, E. L., Lorion, R. P., & Ramos-Mckay, J. (1988). *Fourteen ounces of prevention: A casebook for practitioners.* Washington, D.C.: American Psychological Association.

Price, R. H., Ketterer, R.F., Bader, B.C., & Monahan, J. (1980). *Prevention in mental health: Research, policy and practice.* Beverly Hills: Sage.

Price, R. H., & Smith, S. S. (1983). Two decades of reform in the mental health system (1963–1983). In E. Seidman (Ed.), *Handbook of social intervention.* (pp. 408–437). Beverly Hills: Sage.

Puska, P., Nissinen, A., Tuomilehto, J., Salonen, J. T., Koskela, K., McAlister, A., Kottke, T. E., Maccoby, N., & Farquhar, J. W. (1985). The community-based strategy to prevent heart disease: Conclusions from the ten years of the North Karelia project. *Annual Review of Public Health, 6,* 147–193.

Rappaport, J., Seidman, E., Toro, P. A., McFadden, L. S., Reischl, T. M., Roberts, L.J., Salem, D.A., Stein, C. H., & Zimmerman, M. A. (1985). Collaborative research with a mutual help organization. *Social Policy, 15,* 12–24.

Ridge, R., Pincus, H. A., Blalock, R., & Fine, T. (1989). Factors that influence state funding for mental health research. *Hospital and Community Psychiatry, 40,* 377–382.

Rosow, I. (1976). Status and role change through the life span. In R. H. Binstock & E. Shanas (Eds.), *Handbook of aging and the social sciences.* (pp. 457–482). New York: Van Nostrand Reinhold.

Salem, D. A., Seidman, E., & Rappaport, J. (1988). Community treatment of the mentally ill: The promise of mutual help organizations. *Social Work, 33,* 403–408.

Schelkun, R. F. (1990). Twenty years of primary prevention: Consultation, education and prevention at the Washtenaw County Community Mental Center. *Prevention in Human Services, 7,* 49–73.

Seidman, E., & Rapkin, B. (1983). Economics and psychosocial dysfunction: Toward a conceptual framework and prevention strategies. In R. D. Felner, L. A. Jason, J. N. Moritsugu, & S. S. Farber (Eds.), *Preventive Psychology: Theory, research and practice.* (pp. 175–198). New York: Pergamon.

Seidman, E., & Rappaport, J. (1986). *Redefining social problems.* New York: Plenum.

Shadish, W. R., Jr. (1984). Policy research: Lessons from the implementation of deinstitutionalization. *American Psychologist, 39,* 725–738.

Shinn, M. (1987). Expanding community psychology's domain. *American Journal of Community Psychology, 15,* 555–574.

Shinn, M., & Rosario, M. (1985). The extended family program: Final report to the Ford Foundation. Unpublished manuscript, New York University, New York.

Shinn, M., & Weitzman, B. C. (1990). Research on homelessness: An introduction. *Journal of Social Issues, 46,* 1–11.

Siegel, L. M., Attkisson, C. C., & Carson, L. G. (1978). Need identification and program planning in the community context. In C. C. Attkisson, W. A. Hargreaves, M. J. Horowitz, & J. E. Sorensen (Eds.), *Evaluation of human service programs.* (pp. 215–252). New York: Academic.

Snow, D. L., & Newton, P. M. (1976). Task, social structure, and social process in the community mental health center movement. *American Psychologist, 31*, 582–594.

Sorenson, J. E. (1985). Fiscal survival of community mental health in the 80's: Sharing demonstrated methods to increase revenues and decrease expenses. *Community Mental Health Journal, 21*, 223–227.

Steffen, A. M. (1987). *Decision making in human service organizations*. Unpublished manuscript, Indiana University, Bloomington, Indiana.

Stein, L. I., & Test, M. (Eds.). (1985). *The training in community living model: A decade of experience. New directions for mental health services, no. 26*. San Francisco: Jossey-Bass.

Stokols, D. (1992). Establishing and maintaining healthy environments: Toward a social ecology of health promotion. *American Psychologist, 47*, 6–22.

Stroul, B. A. (1986). *Models of community support services: Approaches to helping persons with long-term mental illness*. Boston: Center for Psychiatric Rehabilitation, Boston University.

Swift, C. (1987). Prevention planning in community mental health centers. In H. Jared & J. A. Morell (Eds.), *Prevention planning in mental health*. (pp. 75–110). Newbury Park, CA: Sage.

Talbott, J. A. (1991). The Pew project: A national effort to improve state–university collaborations. *Hospital and Community Psychiatry, 42*, 70.

Test, M. A. (1981). Effective community treatment of the chronically mentally ill: What is necessary? *Journal of Social Issues, 37*, 71–86.

Test, M. A., & Stein, L. I. (1977). A community approach to the chronically disabled patient. *Social Policy, 8*, 8–16.

Trotter, S. (1981). Neighborhoods, politics and mental health. In J. M. Joffe & G. W. Albee (Eds.), *Prevention through political action and social change*. (pp. 263–274). Hanover, NH: University Press of New England.

Wagenaar, A. C., Murray, D. M., Wolfson, M., Forster, J. L., & Finnegan, J. R. (1994). Communities mobilizing for change on alcohol: Design of a randomized community trial. *Journal of Community Psychology, SCAP Special Issue*, 79–101.

Weiss, C. H. (Ed.). (1977). *Using social research in public policy making*. Lexington, MA: Lexington Books.

Weiss, J .A., & Weiss, C. H. (1981). Social scientists and decision makers look at the usefulness of mental health research. *American Psychologist, 36*, 837–847.

Wildavsky, A. (1979). *Speaking truth to power: The art and craft of policy analysis*. Boston: Little, Brown.

Zimmerman, M. A. (1987). *Expansion strategies of a mutual help organization*. Paper presented at the Conference on Community Research and Action, Columbia, South Carolina.

CHAPTER 20

Community-Based Health Interventions

TRACEY A. REVENSON AND KATHLEEN M. SCHIAFFINO

An article published in the *New England Journal of Medicine* in early 1990 augured the current health care crisis when it concluded that a black man in Harlem was less likely to reach 65 years of age than a man in Bangladesh (McCord & Freeman, 1990). Americans spend more than 11% of the gross national product on health services—more than any other country. Health expenditures in the United States have risen from $26.9 billion in 1960 to $699.5 billion in 1990, and $1,035.1 billion in 1996 (U.S. Health Care Financing Administration, 1997). Paradoxically, these enormous health expenditures do not begin to assure better quality care or better health for all Americans. The differential gap in life expectancy for whites and blacks has been widening; a white female born in 1996 could expect to live about 79.7 years, a black female 74.2 years (Anderson, 1998; the comparable figures for males are 73.9 and 66.1). In 1997, an estimated 43.4 million Americans (15.3% of the population) were not covered by health insurance at any time during the year and the percentage nearly doubles (31.6%) for poor people.

It is time to face the reality of these appalling statistics, to develop new approaches to take preventive health services out of the sole province of hospitals, clinics, and emergency rooms, and to deliver them *in situ* to populations at highest risk. Community psychologists are uniquely prepared to join, if not lead, these efforts. Since its inception, community psychology has developed alternative paradigms for mental health and its treatment, exhibited a concern for underserved and disenfranchised populations, paid attention to social issues within ecological and empowerment frameworks, and developed a framework for a prevention science (Revenson & Seidman, in press; Yoshikawa & Shinn, in press). Community psychologists have expertise in broad-based mental health prevention strategies, and in reaching large numbers of people from different social strata, ages, and cultural backgrounds. Thus, the doors are wide open for community psychologists to extend and expand their paradigms, research designs, and intervention strategies to the realm of physical health.

TRACEY A. REVENSON • Department of Social-Personality and Health Psychology, CUNY Graduate Center, New York, New York 10016. KATHLEEN M. SCHIAFFINO • Department of Psychology, Fordham University, New York, New York 10458.

Handbook of Community Psychology, edited by Julian Rappaport and Edward Seidman. Kluwer Academic / Plenum Publishers, New York, 2000.

In this chapter, we provide a broad overview of community-based health interventions. First, we describe the sociopolitical context within which the focus on health promotion and disease prevention emerged. The defining features of community-based health interventions (CBHIs) are then presented, followed by descriptions of two exemplars, which contrast top-down and bottom-up approaches. The chapter concludes with a discussion of opportunities for community psychologists interested in intervention within the health system.[1]

Health is clearly more than the absence of the signs and symptoms of physical disease. The inclusive definition offered by the World Health Organization defines health as a state of complete physical, mental, and social well-being, and not as the mere absence of disease and infirmity (symptoms). We share that definition, and focus here on interventions designed to promote physical health. Of course, physical and mental health are inextricably intertwined.

THE CURRENT SOCIOPOLITICAL CONTEXT OF DISEASE PREVENTION AND HEALTH PROMOTION

With the exception of AIDS, the nature and patterns of disease over this century have changed from acute, infectious, and often fatal diseases to chronic disabling illnesses (Hinman, 1990). Heart disease, cancer, and stroke account for the greatest number of deaths in the United States and, with other chronic conditions, account for increased disability, hospitalization days, and lowered quality of life. Much of this illness and disability has been linked to behavioral or lifestyle factors (*Healthy People 2000*, 1990). The prime example is cigarette smoking, which has been implicated almost unequivocally in the development of lung cancer and coronary heart disease (Mattson, Pollack, & Cullen, 1987). The dramatic drop in mortality from infectious diseases such as tuberculosis, diphtheria, and polio over the past century was largely a result of advances in public health, accomplished by changes in the physical environment or through the use of preventive or therapeutic measures such as vaccines and antibiotics. No single-exposure preventive interventions comparable to vaccines can "remove" lifestyle risk factors.

Moreover, chronic diseases most often affect those people who have the least access to health care. Ethnic minority and elderly individuals, families living in poverty, and persons living in rural areas or inner cities are often in the poorest health, have multiple risk factors for serious illness, receive the poorest health care, have little or no insurance coverage, and are less likely to receive preventive care. For example, both among the poor and all persons alike, Latinos had the highest chance of lacking coverage: they account for 40.8% of poor persons and 31.6% of all persons, vs. 23.5% and 20.5% for blacks, and 31.3% and 14.2% for whites, respectively (U.S. Department of Commerce, 1994).

Psychology's contribution to the health system has revolved primarily around an individually oriented perspective, consistent with the foundations and history of the discipline (Yoshikawa & Shinn, in press). Similarly, most research and practice in behavioral medicine and health psychology has been directed toward individual differences in health status indicators, risk factors, and habits (Rodin & Salovey, 1990). While recognizing the importance of primary prevention, health psychologists concentrated their efforts on secondary prevention

[1]Guidelines for designing or implementing a community-based health intervention are beyond the scope of this chapter. For a more detailed discussion of specific intervention strategies, we recommend Altman & Goodman (in press); Stokols (1992); and Winett, King, and Altman (1989).

at the individual or small group level, to increase early detection of disease or encourage screening behavior (e.g., Aiken, Gerend, & Jackson, in press).

Not surprisingly, prevention efforts have not affected all segments of the American population equally. Despite medical progress in the past quarter century that has led to reductions in the major causes of death (cancer, heart disease, and stroke), many underserved and ethnic minority groups are lagging behind (Kingston & Smith, 1997; Liao & Cooper, 1995). For example, the age-adjusted mortality rate (for all causes) for blacks is approximately one and one half times that of whites (Macera, Armstead, & Anderson, in press). Approximately 31% of this excess mortality can be accounted for by six well-established risk factors related to behavior: smoking, alcohol intake, total serum cholesterol, blood pressure, obesity, and diabetes (Otten, Teutsch, Williamson, & Marks, 1990); an additional 38% can be accounted for by family income, despite the fact that these two classes of factors covary. Coronary heart disease as a cause of death among blacks far exceeds that of whites, with both physiological (e.g., hypertension, cardiovascular reactivity) and social environmental factors (e.g., racial stress, socioeconomic status) playing a role (Macera et al., in press). This suggests we look more closely at social-structural factors, including the economics of health care, that influence individual health practices.

Although recent emphases on disease prevention and health promotion among the medical and public health sectors provide a welcome contrast to the traditional medical model, disease prevention efforts have been defined and practiced by the medical community in ways that seriously limit their utility. Most behavioral and even community interventions focus on the individual as the target of change. Assumptions about the causes of illness in contemporary society and the causes of its "cure" underlie this focus. If the causes of illness are seen as the "fault" of the individual, through lifestyles characterized by stress, high-cholesterol diets, lack of exercise, smoking, alcohol and substance abuse, or failure to obtain routine medical care, then health interventions will be limited to persuading individuals to discontinue these behaviors, either through health education, fear appeals, or negative reinforcements. (Such was the basis of the infamous and ineffective slogan, "Just say no to drugs" by Nancy Reagan, and current MTV-style TV announcements about what drug use does to the brain.) In contrast, Stokols (1992), among others, urges us "to provide environmental resources and interventions that promote enhanced well-being among occupants of an area" (1992, p. 6).

FEATURES OF COMMUNITY-BASED HEALTH INTERVENTIONS

Community-based health interventions emphasize the use of education to empower people through mediating structures, networks, and community institutions (Altman & Goodman, in press; Winett, King, & Altman, 1989). Community-based approaches provide individuals with information and skills to initiate behavior change through naturally occurring structures and channels of influence, while developing and sustaining a supportive social environment that reinforces and sanctions the changes. *Achieving communitywide change requires an orchestrated effort aimed at the right target groups, with culturally appropriate messages, for a sustained period of time.*

Community-based health interventions can be distinguished from medical or behavioral health interventions in terms of their philosophy, values, and assumptions. First, CBHIs target not only individual behavior change, but a population, community, or setting as the *locus of intervention* (Seidman, 1990). For example, the Stanford Five-City Project (Farquhar, Maccoby, & Solomon, 1984) set a reduction in cardiovascular risk in the entire intervention community as one goal. To achieve this, a multifaceted educational campaign, including mass media, worksite, and school-based programs, was instituted with the participation of local health professionals and community settings (e.g., restaurants).

Second, the desired outcome or *locus of effects* (Seidman, 1990) is change on a community level, e.g., change in social norms, in conjunction with the aggregate-level behavior change that is used most often to measure program success. For example, an aggressive six-month campaign to change citizens' and local merchants' beliefs, actions, and policies regarding the sale of cigarettes to minors included communitywide media exposure, merchant education, and grassroots community organizing. The intervention lead to a reduction in the illegal sale of cigarettes to minors (from 74% pre-intervention to 39% postintervention; Altman, Foster, Rasenick-Douss, & Tye, 1989), an effect that was maintained six months after the intervention ended (Altman, Rasenick-Douss, Foster, & Tye, 1991). Achieving community-wide social change is much more difficult than changing an individual's behavior in a clinical or small group setting; at the same time, its impact is likely to be broader and long lasting (Winett et al., 1989).

Third, reflecting the core assumptions of community psychology, CBHIs draw on individual and community strengths, and emphasize adoption of healthy lifestyles as well as reduction of risk factors. This is accomplished by a two-pronged strategy of teaching individuals healthy behaviors within their natural environments and by creating environments that are conducive to health. For example, a worksite intervention not only would provide nutritional counseling and weight-loss programs for all employees, but also would build an on-site gymnasium, develop policies to allow employees to use it during work hours with no economic penalty, and provide healthy foods in cafeterias and snack machines. Other examples of healthy environments can be found in Stokols (1992).

Fourth, community-based programs emphasize the sociocultural context in understanding change processes. Unlike many behavioral interventions or wellness programs, CBHIs build these considerations into their programs. In order to reach underserved segments of the population, community-based programs must be tailored to the populations that will receive them, and should not rely on help-seeking efforts initiated by individuals. Several research studies illustrate the importance of placing health interventions within their cultural context. Patients who are poor, do not speak English well, or feel estranged from the unnecessarily complex health care system may avoid entering that system. Many Americans face cultural and language barriers when they *do* try to access care. For example, Latino patients may be more likely to construct and treat their symptoms according to culture-bound "folk medicine," including herbal remedies and spiritual healing (Landrine & Klonoff, in press), which is not understood or sanctioned by most medical practitioners. Thus, communication between patients and health care providers breaks down literally and figuratively.

The success of an intervention by Marin, Marin, Perez-Stable, Sabogal, and Otero-Sabogal (1990) demonstrates that a culturally anchored mass-media campaign can produce changes in a community's level of health information and awareness of available services (smoking-cessation programs). The educational awareness campaign reached the targeted population of less acculturated Spanish-speaking Hispanics, and effects were demonstrated, even though the intervention was brief. Similar success was found for an informational smoking-cessation intervention that included a mood-management component and was directed toward Spanish-speaking Latinos (Munoz, Marin, Posner, & Perez-Stable, 1997). Robbins, Allegrante, and Paget (1993) describe the process of modifying a structured education/mutual-help course designed for (white, middle-class) people with lupus for the Latino community.

Combining focus group techniques with individual interviews, and working to understand Latino patients' illness beliefs and group leaders' goals, the researchers were able to revise the course for cultural appropriateness and to make the course more appealing, accessible, and effective for the community.

Fifth, the developers of community-based intervention programs must be willing to "give them away" (Miller, 1969). Transferring ownership of programs and policies is essential to sustained change. When interventions cease, health behavior often reverts to pre-intervention risk levels, as demonstrated in the Multiple Risk Factor Intervention Trial (*MRFIT*; Hughes, Hymowitz, Ockene, Simon, & Vost, 1981). Most CBHIs are developed, implemented, and funded initially as action research (Argyris, Putnam, & Smith, 1985). The challenge is to insure that successful programs continue once research funding and researcher involvement is discontinued. The process of *community incorporation* (Winett et al., 1989) occurs when ownership is transferred to community leaders, so that the intervention continues in its original form, is modified to meet evolving community needs and resources, or incorporates new innovative components. The best strategy is to incorporate community ownership from the initial stages of program development. For example, the Stanford Five-City Project (Farquhar et al., 1984) built a gradual process of community incorporation into the research study, so that the full transfer would occur over a 12-year period, and community leaders were involved in decision-making and ownership from the outset.

Settings and Strategies for Intervention

The philosophy underlying CBHIs does not restrict their focus, methodology, or operation. In fact, it opens up a wide range of intervention possibilities. As a result, programs vary tremendously in scope, structure, content, and locus of effects, making it difficult to describe a modal CBHI or to compare program effectiveness. CBHIs can be described most easily in terms of their focus: the *problem*, such as reduction of cardiovascular risk factors; the *setting*, such as a school or worksite; or the intervention *strategy*, such as mass media. Many research-based interventions take a problem-centered approach, implementing a combination of strategies across multiple settings.

Medical Settings

Most health care still takes place within traditional medical settings; in 1995, $201.6 billion was spent for physician services for a medical complaint (U.S. Health Care Financing Administration, 1996). In one survey, 70% of smokers report that they would try to quit if asked by a physician (Ockene, 1987), a powerful indicator of the physician's referent power (Rodin & Janis, 1982). However, many patients do not undertake preventive health activities or comply with treatment, in part because of poor communication with physicians (Newman, Fitzpatrick, Revenson, Skevington, & Williams, 1996).

Physicians express little confidence in their ability to help patients change their health habits, and disagree on which health-promotion concepts are their responsibility to teach (Wechsler, Levine, Idelson, Rohman, & Taylor, 1983). This may be a result of the undervaluing of communication skills and health promotion within current medical education. For medical practice to be an effective setting for prevention, intervention efforts should shift from the current emphasis on individual behavior change needing personal motivation to setting and system-level changes among practitioners, medical educators, and insurers. For example, as the U.S. population ages, medical education for physicians, dentists, pharmacists, and other health professionals should include a basic understanding of the physiology and psychology of aging, and of the special problems and needs of the frail elderly. This could be accomplished best by teaching *in situ*, for example, through "teaching nursing homes" and routine visits to a geriatric medicine clinic. Similarly, fundamental changes in private and public insurance programs must address the fact that good health in late life involves a combination of medical, preventive, and social services.

Work Settings

Work settings are natural environments for the implementation of large-scale health promotion activities. Corporate executives are cognizant of the economic advantages of a healthy work force—reduced absenteeism and turnover, increased productivity and profits, and lower insurance premiums. Growth and interest in worksite health promotion continues at a remarkable rate. At least two-thirds of Fortune 500 companies (Hollander & Lengerman, 1988) and companies listed in Dun and Bradstreet (Fielding & Piserchia, 1989) reported at least one health-promotion program at their company. However, these programs were almost exclusively individually focused behavior-change programs, such as weight control, smoking cessation, blood pressure screening, stress management, and mental health counseling, particularly for drug or alcohol abuse. Attempts to modify the work environment have included "no smoking" areas, availability of nutritious foods in cafeterias and vending machines, and on-site exercise facilities (Terborg, 1988). Despite their existence, current worksite health promotion programs have not been very successful. Participation in programs is low because they require individual motivation to participate and because organizational support and commitment have been minimal. Thus, the worksite has not yet realized its potential as a health-promotion setting.

Schools

Schools are another natural community setting for health promotion, as they provide a day-to-day source of influence on youth. Most school-based clinics are organized by local health departments and school systems, with strong parental involvement (Dryfoos & Klerman, 1988). Public funding is provided at the state and local levels. Most clinics operate within a traditional medical model, providing physical examinations, screening for physical disorders (e.g., vision, hearing), and treating minor illnesses and accidents. Those adopting a more preventive model conduct gynecological examinations, and counsel and refer teenagers for family planning, sexually transmitted diseases, substance abuse, mental health problems, nutrition, and weight control; these clinics often go beyond the traditional role of "school nurse" in that many of the educational components are integrated into the classroom or other extracurricular activities (e.g., sports, health fairs). School-based clinics are most effective in reducing adolescent pregnancy rates and increasing condom use; the high use of services and student satisfaction are also used as indicators of success (Dryfoos & Klerman, 1988).

School-based programs are often reinforced in other microsystems (family, media, community organizations). For example, the school-based component of the Minnesota Heart Health Program (discussed in detail later in this chapter), developed the "Hearty Heart Home Team" to transfer cardiovascular prevention behaviors from school to home. Families of third-graders were mailed weekly packets of activities to be completed together, such as making grocery lists, preparing healthy meals, recognizing healthy snacks, and identifying foods high in salt and fat. (One such assignment was titled *Fruit, fruit, fruit for the home team!* Who says prevention can't be creative?) Points earned by completing these activities counted towards prizes, including a trip to Disney World.

Religious Institutions

Although data are only beginning to document the role of churches, synagogues, and religious fellowships in health-promotion efforts, they constitute a strong resource for the exchange of health information and a natural locale for the provision of services outside of medical settings. The role of the church as a social support system has been documented in several studies (Pargament & Maton, this volume), providing a sense of community and a means of resolving problems. The potential of this setting may be even greater in ethnic minority communities.

Mass Media

An early example of mass-media influence on health change was the partnership of the National Cancer Institute and the Kellogg company. A major advertising campaign informed the public of the connection between fiber consumption and cancer prevention. Individual actions were reinforced by printing the National Cancer Institute's toll-free cancer telephone hotline number on boxes of All-Bran Cereal and in television commercials. Sales of high-fiber cereals skyrocketed, and a large segment of the public was reached with information and resources concerning healthy diets and cancer prevention (Warner, 1987). This media strategy is now commonplace.

Most community-based interventions include a media component. Mass-media strategies are cost-effective; they reach a wide audience and rely on effective persuasion techniques, such as repetition and potent imagery. Moreover, they can be designed for particular audiences and reach low-income and ethnic minority families, who listen to radio and watch television more than affluent, majority culture families (McAlister, this volume).

Mass-media effects are greatest when combined with, and used to complement, other intervention strategies. For example, media interventions directed toward smoking cessation, in combination with self-help manuals, interpersonal support, and financial incentives, have been shown to boost smoking cessation rates among both middle-class and low-income populations and, when combined with a school-based curriculum, among African-American adolescents (Jason, 1998). A critical ingredient of effective mass-media health-promotion campaigns are those that work with local affiliates of the broadcast media and community-based businesses. This is both economically advantageous and assures community concern and ownership from the program's inception.

Community Organizing

In CBHIs, mediating structures such as families, churches and temples, schools, supermarkets, restaurants, and worksites are linked as agents in a communitywide effort to promote health. This serves a dual purpose. First, at the same time that health information is presented, social norms are developed that sanction healthy behaviors and make unhealthy behaviors less acceptable. Second, nesting programs within existing community organizations or developing new community structures (e.g., health councils) guarantees that structures will be left in place once researchers withdraw their participation. For example, in the successful North Karelia Cardiovascular Disease Prevention Project, project leaders travel throughout the country, establishing personal contacts with community leaders (local doctors, food industry representatives), local decision-making bodies, and the mass media, which would ensure that the intervention was carried out as designed and would continue (Puska, 1984).

A number of theorists and practitioners have proposed models of community organization that can be applied to health promotion efforts (Butterfoss, Wandersman, & Goodman, in press; Winett et al., 1989). Involvement of community groups in the design and implementation of interventions increases the likelihood that programs will reach their populations as originally designed, that both individual and societal change may occur, and that transfer of ownership of the interventions to community groups is smooth.

Environmental and Policy Change

The physical and social environment can be structured to support health promotion efforts through local initiatives, such as labeling heart healthy foods on restaurant menus (LeFebrevre, Peterson, McGraw, Lasater, Sennett, Kendall, & Carleton, 1986), and through state or national policy-level changes, such as forbidding the sale of cigarettes to minors (Altman et al., 1989). Health policies often involve what is called passive prevention (Williams, 1982), protecting individuals without action on their part (e.g., airbag laws) or with minimal individual action (e.g., laws requiring seatbelt use). A conceptual framework for creating health-promoting environments is presented in Stokols (1992).

EXEMPLARS OF COMMUNITY-BASED HEALTH INTERVENTIONS

To provide a more concrete picture of community-based health interventions, we now describe two community-based health interventions that contrast "top-down" vs. "bottom-up" approaches.[2] The first exemplar, the Minnesota Heart Health Program (MHHP), is a large-scale, multicomponent intervention that was initiated, funded, and implemented by the scientific community. Exemplifying action research within a community setting, it is navigated by an interdisciplinary team of scholars (physicians, psychologists, public health specialists, and health educators) and includes an extensive research component. The MHHP goes beyond a problem-centered approach (heart-disease prevention) to encompass setting- and population-based interventions within a developmental framework.

In the second exemplar, we describe the early efforts of the gay communities in New York and San Francisco to reduce the spread of human immunodeficiency virus (HIV) through communitywide behavior change. This exemplar is also problem-centered (AIDS prevention), but illustrates the potential power of citizen participation (Butterfoss et al., in press). Major changes in high-risk sexual practices among men who have sex with men and the resulting decline in the incidence of new AIDS cases can be attributed to concerted and persistent efforts from within the gay community, often in the absence of government concern.

In the first exemplar, scientists and health professionals create the conditions for commu-

[2]Many other excellent programs could have been described. We apologize to those colleagues who may feel slighted by our choice.

nity empowerment; in the second, the community empowers itself.[3] Nonetheless, the two exemplars share a number of elements: multiple strategies of change; intervention within naturally occurring, interconnected settings; culturally anchored messages for reaching the target population; a focus on facilitating social as well as individual change; reliance on multiple channels of communication, including mass media and mediating structures; and broad grass-roots participation.

The Minnesota Heart Health Program

The Minnesota Heart Health Program (MHHP) was a 10-year research and demonstration project to reduce morbidity and mortality from cardiovascular disease by modifying risk factors among the populations of three communities in Minnesota, North Dakota, and South Dakota, and maintaining these risk reductions over time (Mittlemark, Luepker, Jacobs, Bracht, Carlaw, Crow, Finnegan, Grimm, Jeffrey, Kline, Mullis, Murray, Pechacek, Perry, Pirie, & Blackburn, 1986). Using a sophisticated research design, the study involved six communities; each intervention community was paired with a comparison community and represents either a small town, a free-standing city, or a metropolitan area.

The project was designed to increase communitywide awareness of cardiovascular disease, generate participation in health education activities, and stimulate behavior changes that reduce risk. Risk-reduction programs targeted individuals, families, the school system, and health care professionals, and spanned both primary prevention efforts with the general population and secondary prevention efforts targeted toward high-risk groups. Both individual behavior and community change were targeted as loci of effects. Strategies included behavioral incentives, community organizing, direct educational efforts, and environmental support (Luepker & Perry, 1991).

The MHHP drew on social learning theory, persuasive communications, and diffusion-of-innovation models to involve community leaders and microsystems. Prior to intervention, community leaders were recruited to form an advisory board responsible for coordinating education activities, and together with project staff, formed a health council. Three citizen task forces were created to develop educational campaigns on smoking cessation, exercise, and dietary habits. This approach served to secure involvement by the community in later phases of the intervention and to maximize the likelihood of community incorporation. Another unique aspect of the MHHP was the involvement of community physicians both as recipients of educational interventions and as interventionists themselves (Mittlemark, Luepker, Grimm, Koettke, & Blackburn, 1988). Physicians were invited to join advisory boards, and educated to incorporate prevention into their medical practice.

Needs assessments were conducted prior to the implementation of specific educational campaigns. For example, 1203 students in two communities were surveyed regarding eating and exercise habits. Based on the findings, multicomponent educational programs were developed for three cardiovascular risk factors: smoking, blood pressure, and diet. The findings also suggested system-level environmental interventions within the school, such as, in the case of dietary change, reducing the fat and sodium levels of cafeteria offerings (a passive prevention strategy), labeling cafeteria food for nutritional content so that students could make

[3]No intervention can be purely top-down or bottom-up. The top-down effort we describe utilized existing community structures, and the bottom-up intervention tried to work with or change existing ones. We feel that this still provides an important contrast in the starting point and evolution of community-based health interventions.

healthier choices, and reinforcing those nutritional choices in health education classes. The programs also adopted a lifespan orientation, with programs targeting adults, adolescents, and younger children, and the interaction among age groups within the family.

Settings and Strategies

Media campaigns focused community interest on single risk factors for a defined period of time. Children and adolescents were involved in health education activities at screening centers in the community, and health education classes were conducted for adults in worksites, churches, and clubs. Other activities included community walks and advocacy activities directed toward changing food product labels. Sixty percent of age-eligible adults visited the screening centers (Mittlemark et al., 1986).

One particular program, the Quit and Win Contest, used behavioral incentives as a strategy for motivating communitywide behavior change. Prizes were awarded for maintenance of smoking cessation, with the grand prize being a week at Disney World. (A parallel campaign targeted at youths also utilized incentives; youths interviewed adults about their smoking habits, and the individual who interviewed the most adults won a 10-speed bicycle.) Each year of the intervention, individuals could enroll in the contest over a month-long period, scheduled to coincide with the Great American Smokeout. The contest generally recruited more than 5% of all adult smokers in the community and produced 30-day quit rates of about 40%, with abstinence rates of 20% at six-month and seven-month follow-ups. The contests recruited progressively fewer participants each year, with later contests yielding a participation rate of only 1%. When the enrollment period was extended to eight months, almost 7% of the entire smoking population of Bloomington, Minnesota pledged to quit, producing a 17% initial success rate and 11% abstinence at six months (Lando, Hellerstedt, Pirie, Fruetal, & Huttner, 1991). The history of the Quit and Win Contest illustrates the need to maintain vitality in ongoing programs, as well as the importance of community incorporation. Contest sponsorship was taken over from the MHHP by a local insurance company, which assured that the contest would continue; this commitment faltered during the period when community interest declined. The extended enrollment period employed in the Bloomington contest revitalized community interest and reestablished organizational support.

Because eating, exercise, and smoking habits appear to be learned in childhood and consolidated in adolescence, the MHHP included an emphasis on prevention with preadolescents. In addition to directly affecting children's behavior, it was believed that intervention with children might provide a vehicle for reaching their parents as well [an illustration of Kelly's (1971) notion of radiating effects].

"Hearty Heart and Friends" was a five-year nutrition education project whose major objective was the reduction of dietary fat and sodium consumption, and increased knowledge about healthy diets. Aimed at third and fourth graders, materials involved adventure books and filmstrips with cartoon characters who served as role models. In one book, Hearty Heart and several other residents of planet Strongheart journey to Earth. The Salt Sleuth's assignment is to teach Earth children to identify salt in food products and to provide tasty alternatives. Intervention components were school- and family-based, and materials were tailored to developmental level. The classroom component involved 15 sessions on food preparation, reading labels, monitoring heart rates, and aerobic activity; teachers were trained by MHHP staff. The program also included skills practice assignments to do at home with family members: Parents and children engaged in menu planning, preparing grocery lists, shopping, and meal preparation. The classroom component produced knowledge gain and attitude change, but had little impact on behavior, whereas the home-based component resulted in changes in shopping patterns and diet, specifically fat and carbohydrate intake (Luepker & Perry, 1991). The home-based component essentially reinforced the school-based component, demonstrating mesosystem change.

Another goal of the MHHP was to prevent the onset of smoking in early adolescence. Drawing on social psychological theories, educational programs emphasized the short-term dangers of smoking and built social skills to resist peer pressure through classroom presentations, small group discussion, and role-playing with peer and adult leaders (Perry, 1987). Although brief (six sessions over several weeks), the educational intervention had significant effects: Follow-up revealed that smoking rates had declined by the end of eighth grade, and were maintained through the end of ninth grade in the school that implemented a peer-led intervention. In contrast, smoking rates in schools that used adult leaders were similar to those in the schools that did not participate in the intervention. However, at the five- and six-year follow-ups, no significant differences were observed between the two types of interventions, and there was an increase in the number of adolescent smokers over time. However, this increase was smaller than that of the control schools, indicating that the intervention had been successful in delaying the onset of smoking (Luepker & Perry, 1991).

Community Incorporation

To assure that the interventions would be incorporated into the community after government funding ended and MHHP participation was withdrawn, particular care was given to systematic evaluation of each component. Evaluation included the identification of successful programs, as well as identification of components that had the greatest impact. Evaluation addressed four levels of change: the extent and growth of community resources and programs; feedback on the effectiveness of specific program components; monitoring program implementation, including community awareness and utilization rates; and evidence of individual, aggregate, and communitywide behavioral change.

Interventions were designed from the outset to be sensitive to community needs while maintaining the critical components of the intervention. One intended outcome of the school-based interventions was the incorporation of these programs into the school curricula; areas of need were identified by students and teachers, programs were phased in slowly with school board approval and faculty input, and evaluation results were shared with school staff.

Summary

The Minnesota Heart Health Project represents an ambitious effort to conduct theoretically driven research, thereby benefitting the community and expanding the scientific knowledge base. Given its sheer size and scope, the MHHP confronted a number of problems. One was the difficulty of maintaining the energy of innovation while fostering community ownership. Practical experience forced modifications of theoretically derived interventions (e.g., the Quit and Win Contest), and added to an understanding of persuasive communication and behavior change. The MHHP also struggled with its definition of success: What outcomes can be reasonably expected given the time frame and intensity of the interventions? (For example, should *delay* in the onset of adolescent smoking be considered a successful outcome or is *never smoking* the critical endpoint?) On a more positive note, the MHHP has contributed to an understanding of several issues that were not a central focus of the original research design. For example, the MHHP provided important information on gender differences in smoking onset among adolescents (Pirie, Murray, & Luepker, 1991). It also contributed to an appreciation of the relationship between smoking, body image, desire for thinness, and attitudes about sexuality among adolescent girls; these findings point to the need to conceptualize and study risk factors for eating disorders prior to program development (Leon, Perry, Mangelsdorf, & Tell, 1989).

AIDS Prevention within the Gay Community during the Early Years of the Epidemic

To illustrate how community-based health change can originate without research funding, scientific expertise, or professional support, we describe the efforts of the gay community to control HIV infection in two cities, San Francisco and New York, during the early years of the epidemic. These cities were the epicenters of the epidemic at that time, which necessitated urgent attempts at prevention. Given the gravity of the situation and the virtual absence of a government response, community-based voluntary organizations jumped in to fill a critical public health need (and two decades later, continue to expand and change to meet the changing face of the epidemic).

In 1984, almost 50% of the homosexual and bisexual men in San Francisco were infected with HIV, more than double that estimated only two years earlier (Winkelstein, Samuel, Padian, Wiley, Lang, Anderson, & Lewy, 1987). Epidemiological data from subsequent years charts a substantial decline in new HIV infections among homosexual and bisexual men. In San Francisco, the spread of infection declined from 18% for 1982 through 1984 to 4% in 1986 to 0.7% by mid-1987 (Winkelstein et al., 1987). More importantly, these declines could be attributed to reductions in unsafe sexual practices (Becker & Joseph, 1988; Schechter, Craib, Willoughby, Douglas, McLeod, Maynard, Constance, & O'Shaugnessy, 1988; Winkelstein, Wiley, Padian, Samuel, Shiboski, Ascher, & Loy, 1988), although neither changes in HIV status nor sexual practices could be attributed directly to any specific program. Educational materials prepared by community groups and the public health department were available, but study participants were not systematically exposed to specific health-promotion programs. Nevertheless, homosexual and bisexual men altered their sexual practices in a very short time period (Becker & Joseph, 1988).

The data for New York City present a similar epidemiological picture, with direct evidence linking behavior change with infection rates (Martin, Dean, Garcia, & Hall, 1989). Among a cohort of homosexual men, those who did not stop engaging in receptive anal intercourse as of 1985 were over three times as likely to be HIV positive as those who did. This protective effect of behavior change was even stronger among men who had the greatest number of sexual partners. Overall, sexual activity among gay men declined and safe sex practices were incorporated into sexual habits. For example, whereas half of the sample attended a bathhouse for sex at least once in 1981, only 8% had done so in 1987.

How was this community-level health change accomplished? To answer this question, we drew heavily on social histories of the AIDS epidemic, particularly Randy Shilts' comprehensive chronology, *And the Band Played On: Politics, People and the AIDS Epidemic* (1988). Other primary sources included the writings of Altman (1988), Arno (1988), Kramer (1989), Ouellette Kobasa (1990), and Perrow and Guillen (1990) on the history and politics surrounding the AIDS crisis and the response of voluntary organizations and the gay movement in the two cities. We chose to focus on the activities in San Francisco and New York as they had the highest proportion of gay men at the time. Although there are many similarities in the two cities' responses, we would like to emphasize that local government's response to the epidemic and the strength and identity of the gay communities was very different.

Mobilization of Community Resources

In both San Francisco and New York, community-based organizing among gay individuals became the nucleus of HIV-prevention activities. This was not wholly by choice: government and health care agencies that are expected to respond to public health crises failed to respond for a variety of reasons, including homophobia and discrimination, inability or refusal to understand the extent of the epidemic, and organizational failure (Perrow & Guillen, 1990).

The leaders of the San Francisco efforts were gay street organizers who knew little about public health principles, but a lot about community organizing. For example, finding that the San Francisco Department of Public Health was adopting a hands-off policy on AIDS education, a core of gay political activists mapped out their own education campaign:

> "Okay, we have to do an end run around these people," Bill [Krause] said to the group gathered at 79 Uranus Street. "We'll do it just like a political campaign. We'll get the message out about safe sex, and repeat it and repeat it until it sinks in. Target mailings. Brochures that speak to the audience. We've done it all before" (Shilts, 1988, p. 254).

The mobilization of the gay community proceeded in a somewhat different fashion in New York (Ouellette Kobasa, 1990; Perrow & Guillen, 1990). With early recognition that AIDS was disproportionately affecting homosexual men and that local government was paralyzed in its response, the gay community drew upon its resources—financial and professional—to create self-help voluntary organizations. The Gay Men's Health Crisis (GMHC) was founded in 1982 by a small group of well-educated, affluent professionals in business and the arts, who knew that a mysterious illness, first labelled as a "gay cancer," was striking many gay men, and that the medical profession was not responding.

Their actions underscored how badly the growing numbers of people with AIDS needed services. GMHC grew rapidly during its first months as the only organization to provide education, prevention, and counseling services to gay men in the city. Through volunteer efforts, GMHC wrote and distributed health recommendation brochures to a quarter million men, started a Buddy Program to provide tangible and emotional support, maintained a telephone crisis line, provided community outreach, organized weekly education forums, and developed financial and legal advising services. Today, GMHC is a very large non-profit voluntary organization with 260 paid staff members, with over 6600 active volunteers, that serves 8081 men, women, and children with AIDS, as well as 1076 family members and care partners annually, with an annual budget of $24.5 million (Gay Men's Health Crisis, 1998).

It is important to stress at this point a crucial difference between the development of AIDS services in the two cities. In San Francisco in 1984, the three largest programs received 62% of their funding from the city, whereas New York City was just beginning to provide funds. In San Francisco, the gay movement had gained legitimacy before the AIDS crisis, and was somewhat integrated into government structures. As Altman (1988) recounts, "San Francisco was prepared from early on in the course of the epidemic to devote resources to AIDS, and to develop a partnership between government and community-based organizations in the use of these resources" (p. 303). The Office of Lesbian and Gay Health within the San Francisco Department of Public Health was in place *before* the AIDS outbreak. One of Congressman Phil Burton's legislative assistants was assigned immediately to work full-time on AIDS issues. The San Francisco health department, allied with the gay community, organized a network of inpatient, outpatient, education, and support services. Thus, prevention efforts succeeded, in large part, because of *existing* channels for information and influence among the gay community.

In contrast, the gay men who founded GMHC or participated in its early fund-raising and service provision efforts were not already part of a well-defined or cohesive social movement. These early GMHC volunteers were not the gay activists of a prior decade; "they shared neither ideologies nor opinions about how organizations should be run" (Ouellette Kobasa, 1990, p. 284). Moreover, there was no integration or influence with city government. The New York City Office of the Mayor created an Office of Gay and Lesbian Health Concerns, but it appears to have done little in initiating programs or responding to voluntary organizations' requests. The potential strength of government to effect far-reaching and life-saving policies should not be overstated; in retrospect, city government did not respond in a responsible fashion.

Settings and Strategies

An aggressive public education campaign was instituted in San Francisco in 1984: a telephone hotline was created, signs were posted exhorting individuals to practice safe sex, and dramatic ads were placed in gay newspapers. These health messages originated from within the gay community and used frank language to deliver explicit safe-sex information materials that public agencies could not. Public service announcements were aired on radio and television. This media campaign quickly became a national model (Silverman, 1986).

Mass media were used whenever possible to provide information; this included both gay-oriented and more mainstream publications. Historical analyses show that there was minimal media coverage of AIDS. This lack of coverage can be attributed to a discomfort (some say repulsion) with what was assumed to be a disease of homosexuals, and the sexual language needed to describe its epidemiology. The federal government was no more forthcoming with information.

Gay newspapers, on the other hand, provided a consistent source of information. Some say that Larry Kramer's article, "1,112 and Counting," printed in the *New York Native* in March 1983 (cited in Kramer, 1989) irrevocably altered the context in which AIDS was discussed. Chastising federal and local government, the media, the medical establishment (including gay physicians), *and* gay community groups, Kramer used statistics forcefully to convince the gay community that they would need to change their sexual practices immediately and completely to avoid killing off the gay population. Although it aroused the wrath of many gay men, who branded Kramer an alarmist, "1,112 and Counting" mobilized the community to action.

Mere exposure to information does not lead directly to such pervasive behavior change. Messages need to motivate individuals to use the information and teach specific skills, which must then be reinforced for adoption and maintenance. It had become clear that educational campaigns were not achieving broad enough success, and that legal or policy-level interventions would be needed. Thus, support structures were put into place to reinforce the practice of safe sexual behaviors and changing social norms concerning anonymous sex. Community institutions that permitted unsafe behaviors (the bathhouses) became the next locus of intervention and the center of bloody political battles between gay activists and government officials, as well as among the activists themselves.

Early surveys of San Francisco gay men (McKusick, Wiley, Coates, Stall, Saika, Morin,

Charles, Hortsman, & Conant, 1985) had pointed to the bathhouses as a center of unsafe sexual activity. Even during the intensive media blitz on HIV transmission in the summer of 1983, bathhouse attendance increased. In some bathhouses, customers were encouraged to participate in safe-sex practices, such as mutual masturbation. However, men who attended the bathhouses remained far less likely to practice safe sex, even though they knew the risks.

As a result, a public health strategy of closing the bathhouses was proposed and was met with strong resistance. Bathhouse owners as well as gay organizations argued that such actions would constitute a denial of individual freedom and discrimination against gay establishments. The public position of the San Francisco Department of Public Health was that action should come from the gay community. In the end, bathhouse closing in San Francisco was accomplished in mid-1985 when undercover detectives established that patrons were ignoring the safe-sex alternatives available to them. (Similar events occurred in New York City, see Perrow & Guillen, 1990.)

Surprisingly, no significant educational efforts were made to target physicians who treated the gay population at sexually transmitted disease clinics; nor did these physicians initiate such efforts. Yet these settings provided a locus for finding the most concentrated sources of infection, and could have prevented thousands of new infections. By focusing efforts largely on education and individual behavior change, there were many missed opportunities in the early years of the epidemic.

Empowerment within the Gay Community

Looking back, the process of reducing AIDS in the gay community can be described as one of small wins (Weick, 1984). Health-policy modification was essentially a political process, won too slowly, at the expense of too many lives. Two problems in particular plagued these community-driven change efforts.

First, there was a profound tension involved in curtailing the epidemic while protecting individual civil liberties and avoiding renewed or increased discrimination. Public health concerns clashed with hard-won civil liberties. This tension was most strongly manifest *within* the gay community. Gay leaders advocating risk-reduction faced hostility and resistance from their peers. Gay community groups feared that the public focus on gay sexual practices might increase blaming the victim, inflame the new right's moralistic stance, and escalate homophobia. Even organizations such as GMHC maintained a passive position of informed choice: "You give people the information about how AIDS is transmitted and you let *them* make their own informed choice" (Shilts, 1988, p. 325, emphasis in original).

Second, the relationship between government and gay organizations was characterized more by distrust than cooperation. The efforts of the gay community were often met by an apathetic federal and local response to the epidemic, including failure or delay in notifying the public, providing research funds, and expanding health care facilities. Ironically, the success of the gay community in initiating education programs and providing numerous hours of volunteer service allowed city government to *remain* uninvolved, as it emphasized local control via community boards rather than supporting broader-based initiatives. In 1986–87 alone, GMHC provided direct client services estimated at an economic value of $2 million through its volunteer programs (Arno, 1988). A reliance on volunteer services also exposed the fragility of informal networks that were promoted as substitutes for publicly funded services. Many AIDS caregivers were themselves dying of the illness; who would care for them and for the people whose HIV infections would emerge over the next decade?

The AIDS epidemic has, in some ways, created or strengthened a psychological sense of community (Sarason, 1974). In San Francisco, warring gay political factions recognized the need to work together to effect large-scale change. In New York, the AIDS crisis brought many gay individuals together for the first time through the structure of the Gay Men's Health Crisis. Candlelight marches to lobby for federal support, annual Dance-a-Thons and AIDS Walks to raise funds, and demonstrations of remembrance, such as the Names project, serve to strengthen and reflect the community's solidarity.

The AIDS epidemic created a new generation of gay activists who, hopefully, will continue to fight the war of social injustices once this battle is won. "AIDS has changed the movement in ways [no one] could have anticipated in the headier days of the 1970s ... new people have come into the movement; many gay men who had hitherto regarded gay politics as irrelevant have become the front-line activists because of AIDS" (Altman, 1988, p. 310).

Although the gay community has won new legitimacy, it is not without new tensions and new battles (D'Augelli, this volume). For example, some have argued that GMHC's original goals have been co-opted, and that some activists have become the bureaucrats they originally despised. Internal struggles within the gay community in New York have led to the formation of more direct, confrontational, advocacy organizations, such as the AIDS Coalition to Unleash Power (ACT UP). Utilizing many of the rules for radicals delineated by Alinsky (1971), ACT UP has been successful in a number of arenas where GMHC has not, for example, challenging restrictive policies on experimental drugs.

A Need for Continued Prevention Efforts

The gay white men who created new settings and dealt with the AIDS epidemic in a directed manner were not completely powerless to begin with: They used their numbers, knowledge, and connections to disrupt the governmental *status quo* and to protect the health of their community. But that was then and this is now. The face of the AIDS epidemic has changed over the past decade and continues to change, including more people who are disempowered and without resources.

Although AIDS incidence remains highest among men who have sex with men (MSM), AIDS incidence increased in the 10-year span from 1986 to 1996 most dramatically among women, African-Americans, Hispanics, and people infected through heterosexual transmission or through injection drug use (Centers for Disease Control, 1998c). In the United States, African-Americans have been infected and affected disproportionately by HIV and AIDS. Of the total AIDS cases reported in 1997, 45% were reported among African-Americans (although they represent only 13% of the U.S. population), 33% among whites, and 21% among Hispanics. (The percentage of cases among Asians and American Indians remains less than 1%). Some of the increase among African-American and Hispanic populations has been attributed to intravenous drug use.

Clearly, HIV-prevention efforts must take into account socioeconomic and cultural issues, such as poverty, un- and underemployment, and poor access to health care. Current community-based efforts, sponsored by federal, state, and local agencies, include a wide range of programs, from individual-level behavior change for those who seek it (risk-reduction counseling, drug counseling) to street and community outreach services (needle exchange, HIV testing, helping at-risk individuals gain access to services). The Centers for Disease Control have instituted programs to assist national and community-based organizations serving the African-American community in building an infrastructure to provide HIV testing, counseling, and services; collaborations with religious institutions to encourage participation in HIV prevention efforts; and funding to assist minority organizations on the regional and national levels to provide HIV services within the community (Centers for Disease Control, 1998a).

The drop in new HIV infections among men since 1994 has been credited to earlier declines in HIV infections among white gay men, in part, as a result of targeted prevention efforts (Centers for Disease Control, 1998c). But the gay community cannot rest on its substantial laurels. Men who have sex with men (MSM) continue to account for the largest number of people reported with HIV/AIDS. In 1997, 21,260 AIDS cases were reported among MSM, compared with 14,698 among intravenous drug users and 8,112 among women and men who acquired HIV infection through heterosexual transmission (Centers for Disease Control, 1998b). There is a need for continuing HIV prevention among men who have sex with men, particularly young and minority MSM. Trends in the mid-1990s predicted a second wave of AIDS infection, particularly among gay and bisexual men younger than 25, as surveys indicated an increase in anal intercourse without condoms among this age group (Gross, 1993). Ongoing studies show that both HIV prevalence and risk behaviors remain high among young MSM, including those infected with HIV. In 1997, 47% of HIV diagnoses among adolescent males aged 13–19 and 53% of cases among men aged 20–24 were attributed to male-to-male sexual contact (Centers for Disease Control, 1998b). Moreover, among white MSM, AIDS incidence has been declining since 1994, reflecting in part the success of the prevention programs implemented in the 1980s. AIDS incidence among African-American and Latino MSM continued to increase until 1996, when the new combination drug therapies began to show an effect (Centers for Disease Control, 1998b). However, decline in AIDS attributed to the drug therapies is greater for white MSM than MSM of color, due perhaps to differential provision of these drugs.

Taken together, the recent data point to a strong need to design more effective, culturally anchored prevention efforts for younger gay and bisexual men. Community psychologists cannot make the assumption that the programs designed for an earlier generation of MSM will be equally effective with the current cohort. Younger gay and bisexual men are less concerned about becoming infected and more likely to take risks than their older peers. The explanations for this range from the personal to the political: a belief that AIDS is the plague of the older generation; fatalistic thinking that infection is unavoidable; HIV as a visible marker of a gay identity, creating an increased sense of belonging to the gay community and lives transformed by increased meaning; resistance to maintaining safe sex behaviors for one's entire lifetime; the hope of improved life expectancies for infected individuals raised by the successes of new highly active antiretroviral therapies; and lack of continued funding for prevention programs.

Moreover, cultural barriers to acknowledging homosexual activity within the African-American and Latino communities may hamper prevention efforts; for fear of being stigmatized, Latino men engaging in sexual relations with other men may not consider themselves homosexual and may discount educational messages targeted toward homosexuals (Marin, 1989). A 1997 scientific consensus conference sponsored by the National Institutes of Health reviewed existing data on the effectiveness of HIV behavioral interventions and concluded that "behavioral interventions to reduce risk for HIV/AIDS are effective and should be disseminated widely" (National Institutes of Health, 1997, p. 2); the report also concluded that comprehensive, community-based, culturally anchored programs work best.

Summary

This second exemplar described the ways a community conceptualized and responded to an acute health care crisis. These efforts account for most of the success in responding to the

AIDS epidemic and preventing HIV transmission. And through their actions, the gay community has been strengthened, even if it is not without tensions. For many individuals, participation in AIDS organizations offered an opportunity for empowerment.

A NOTE ON THE TREND TOWARD BLAMING THE VICTIM

The locus of effects of even the most exemplary community-based health interventions is centered on individual behavior change. This may reflect the resurgent interest in biobehavioral mechanisms underlying disease, the usual approach to "treatment" in psychology, or an outgrowth of a conservative political climate in which blaming the victim (Ryan, 1971) has become fashionable again. We would like to be able to conclude that community-based health interventions do not take a victim-blaming stance, but this is only partially true. As behavioral correlates of health are identified, they are regarded as the causes of disease and the means to better health. The health system is selling this idea, and we are buying. How often when reading obituaries do we consciously or unconsciously assign blame? A woman dies of lung cancer and we think "heavy smoker"; a young man dies of AIDS and we suppose unsafe sex. Health maintenance organizations are touted for their wellness programs, but these programs consist of standard behavioral programs, such as individual nutritional counseling or smoking-cessation programs.

This continued emphasis on individual responsibility for health has two consequences. First, it deflects attention from sociocultural influences on health practices (Landrine & Klonoff, in press). These may reflect different cultural models of illness and symptoms, as well as structural and economic barriers to the availability and utilization of health care. Second, it deflects attention away from more ingrained socioeconomic, environmental, and political forces that may, directly or indirectly, cause poor health—poverty, toxic wastes, urban crowding, or homelessness. These social conditions require far-reaching change, including legislative and economic reforms. These two perspectives—individual responsibility and social responsibility—are reflected in the dichotomy of active vs. passive modes of prevention (Williams, 1982).

The polarity between social and individual models of causation illustrates how the social construction of prevention will dictate the types of health interventions that are available. By sending the clear message that individuals are responsible for their own health, we have removed some of the pressure from institutions to engineer social change, e.g., to minimize environmental pollution and toxic waste. Community-based prevention efforts need to focus as strongly on societal and governmental responsibility as on individual behavior change. As Stokols suggests, "multifaceted interventions that incorporate complementary environmental and behavioral components and span multiple settings and levels of analysis are more likely to be effective in promoting personal *and* public health than those that are narrower in scope" (1992, p. 18, emphasis added).

A NEW SETTING FOR COMMUNITY PSYCHOLOGISTS

Community psychology and medicine have fundamental differences in their values, structures, incentives, and goals. Community psychology was born during the Great Society, when there was a keen interest in funding social programs. In some way, government funding priorities provided the impetus for preventive psychology, and continue to shape its evolution. Medicine is interested in preventive interventions largely in response to skyrocketing costs and an increasing need to care for a population that is living longer, with more chronic illnesses. Behavioral medicine initiatives have responded to the incentives of cost-cutting by offering a less expensive way to maintain a healthy nation. With that promise, however, psychologists must show not only that their interventions are effective but also *cost*-effective (Altman & Goodman, in press; Butterfoss et al., in press).

What can community psychology offer to the U.S. health care system? Foremost, we offer an ecological perspective to the social issues in which we engage (Revenson & Seidman, in press; Trickett, 1996). Community psychology has developed intervention theory relevant to large-scale change, and considers intervention paradigms that cut across psychobiological, social, and cultural levels (Revenson & Seidman, in press). Because most health problems do not have a single or simple cause, it is necessary to conduct primary prevention programs across multiple levels, enhancing the fit between people and their settings. We need to develop competent individuals and competent communities. The involvement of community psychologists in HIV prevention is one such road being taken (Peterson, 1998).

In an early call for community psychologists to become interested in physical health, Iscoe (1982) pointed out that mental health programs failed in part because of their lack of understanding of the daily lives, needs, and values of the communities in which they intervened. The same problems may befall many preventive health interventions, particularly those utilizing a one-size-fits-all strategy of behavior change. As we have emphasized throughout this chapter, community-based interventions must be culturally anchored within the target population. In addition, community psychologists need to be cognizant of the values, priorities, and constraints of another relevant culture—the U.S. health system. We know from past experience that system change will be thwarted if consultants repudiate the values of the system they are entering.

What can research and intervention in the health system offer community psychology? Community-based health interventions provide settings (some new, some not so new) in which community psychologists can *do* community psychology: clinics, hospitals, schools, work-sites. The research questions pose a fresh challenge to community psychologists, an opportunity to collaborate with interdisciplinary researchers and health care providers, and a potent opportunity to work on social problems of immediate and long-term relevance.

Let us also make a plea for more ecologically oriented research on *how*, *why*, *under what conditions*, *for how long*, and *for whom* community-based health interventions work. As with the design of interventions, the design of research needs to be attentive to the cultural diversity of its recipients (Hughes, Seidman, & Williams, 1993), as well as the influence of the social and political context on health and health behavior (Stokols, 1992). Such ecological considerations are critical in understanding the effects (or lack of effects) of particular program components, the choice of research sites, how the interventions and research components are implemented, and the role of community stakeholders.

We are reminded of the parable of the physician who stood on the banks of a river and pulled people floating downstream out as they swept by (McKinlay, 1979). The public health experts head upstream to determine who was pushing the people in; the outcome of their efforts is to refocus upstream and rescue the victims early. In this way, the parable serves as an illustration of secondary prevention. But in these dangerous waters lies the perfect opportunity for community psychologists: to engage in more upstream endeavors and keep people from falling into the river! Most current health interventions are neither mass-oriented nor directed toward healthy people or unhealthy environments. This is where the knowledge, values, and skills of community psychology can be of most value.

ACKNOWLEDGMENTS. The authors wish to thank Ed Seidman for his editorial expertise and decade of encouragement, David Koch for his excellent feedback on an earlier draft, and Eric Schrimshaw for providing updated statistics. David G. Altman served as the muse for this chapter, planting the seeds for ideas about the alliance between community psychology and health psychology.

REFERENCES

Aiken, L. S., Gerend, M. A., & Jackson, K. M. (in press). Subjective risk and health protective behavior: Cancer screening and cancer prevention. In A. Baum, T. A. Revenson, & J. E. Singer (Eds.), *Handbook of health psychology*. Mahwah, NJ: Erlbaum.

Alinsky, S. D. (1971). *Rules for radicals*. New York: Random House.

Altman, D. (1988). Legitimation through disaster: AIDS and the gay movement. In E. Fee & D. M. Fox (Eds.), *AIDS: The burdens of history* (pp. 301–315). Berkeley: University of California Press.

Altman, D. G., Foster, V., Rasenick-Douss, L., & Tye, J. B. (1989). Reducing the illegal sale of cigarettes to minors. *Journal of the American Medical Association, 261*, 80–83.

Altman, D. G., & Goodman, R. M. (in press). Community intervention. In A. Baum, T. A. Revenson, & J. E. Singer (Eds.), *Handbook of health psychology*. Mahwah, NJ: Erlbaum.

Altman, D. G., Rasenick-Douss, L., Foster, V., & Tye, J. B. (1991). Sustained effects of an educational program to reduce sales of cigarettes to minors. *American Journal of Public Health, 81*, 891–893.

Anderson, R. N. (1998). United States Abridged Life Tables, 1996. *National Vital Statistics Report, 47*(13). Hyattsville, MD: National Center for Health Statistics.

Argyris, C., Putnam, R., & Smith, D. M. (1985). *Action science: Concepts, methods and skills for research and intervention*. San Francisco: Jossey-Bass.

Arno, P. S. (1988). The future of voluntarism and the AIDS epidemic. In D. E. Rogers & E. Ginzburg (Eds.), *The AIDS patient: An action agenda* (pp. 56–70). Boulder, CO: Westview.

Becker, M. H., & Joseph, J. G. (1988). AIDS and behavioral change to reduce risk: A review. *American Journal of Public Health, 78*, 394–410.

Butterfoss, F. D., Wandersman, A., & Goodman, R. M. (in press). Citizen participation and health: Toward a psychology of improving health through individual, organizational and community involvement. In A. Baum, T. A. Revenson, & J. E. Singer (Eds.), *Handbook of health psychology*. Mahwah, NJ: Erlbaum.

Centers for Disease Control (1998a). Critical need to pay attention to HIV prevention for African-Americans. <http://www.cdcnpin.org/geneva98/issues/fafram.htm>; (accessed: 5 August 1998).

Centers for Disease Control (1998b). Need for sustained HIV prevention among men who have sex with men: Young and minority men at high risk. <http://www.cdcnpin.org/geneva98/issues/fmsmctx.htm> (accessed: 5 August 1998).

Centers for Disease Control (1998c). Trends in the HIV and AIDS epidemic. <http://www.cdcnpin.org/geneva98/trends/trends_3.htm> (accessed: 5 August 1998).

Dryfoos, J. G., & Klerman, L. V. (1988). School-based clinics: Their role in helping students meet the 1990 objectives. *Health Education Quarterly, 15*, 71–80.

Farquhar, J. W., Maccoby, N., & Solomon, D. S. (1984). Community applications of behavioral medicine. In W. D. Gentry (Ed.), *Handbook of behavioral medicine* (pp. 437–478). New York: Guilford.

Fielding, J. E., & Piserchia, P. V. (1989). Frequency of worksite health promotion activities. *American Journal of Public Health, 79*, 16–20.

Gay Men's Health Crisis (1998). Facts and statistics. <http://www.gmhc.org/glance/facts.html> (accessed: 5 August 1998).

Gross, J. (1993, December 11). Second wave of AIDS feared by officials in San Francisco. *The New York Times*, pp. A1, A10.

Healthy People 2000: National health promotion and disease prevention objectives. (1990). [DHHS Publication No. (PHS) 91-50212]. Washington, D. C.: U. S. Government Printing Office.

Hinman, A. R. (1990). 1889 to 1989: A century of health and disease. *Public Health Reports, 105*, 374–380.

Hollander, R. B., & Lengerman, J. J. (1988). Corporate characteristics and worksite health promotion programs: Survey findings from Fortune 500 companies. *Social Science & Medicine, 26*, 491–501.

Hughes, D., Seidman, E., & Williams, N. (1993). Cultural phenomena and the research enterprise: Toward a culturally-anchored methodology. *American Journal of Community Psychology, 21*, 687–703.

Hughes, G. H., Hymowitz, N., Ockene, J. K., Simon, N., & Vost, T. M. (1981). The multiple risk factor intervention trials (MRFIT). V. Intervention on smoking. *Preventive Medicine, 10*, 476–500.

Iscoe, I. (1982). Toward a viable community health psychology. *American Psychologist, 37*, 961–965.

Jason, L. A. (1998). Tobacco, drug and HIV prevention media interventions. *American Journal of Community Psychology, 26*, 151–188.

Kelly, J. G. (1971). The quest for valid preventive interventions. In G. Rosenbaum (Ed.), *Issues in community psychology and preventive mental health* (pp. 109–139). New York: Behavioral Publications.

Kingston, R. S., & Smith, J. P. (1997). Socioeconomic status and racial and ethnic differences in functional status associated with chronic diseases. *American Journal of Public Health, 87*, 805–810.

Kramer, L. (1989). *Reports from the holocaust: The making of an AIDS activist.* New York: St. Martin's.

Lando, H. A., Hellerstedt, W. L., Pirie, P. L., Fruetal, J., & Huttner, P. (1991). Results of a long-term community smoking cessation contest. *American Journal of Health Promotion, 5*, 420–425.

Landrine, H., & Klonoff, E. A. (in press). Cultural diversity and health psychology. In A. Baum, T. A. Revenson, & J. E. Singer (Eds.), *Handbook of health psychology.* Mahwah, NJ: Erlbaum.

LeFebvre, R. C., Peterson, G. S., McGraw, S. A., Lasater, T. M., Sennett, L., Kendall, L., & Carleton, R. A. (1986). Community intervention to lower blood cholesterol: The "know your cholesterol" campaign in Pawtucket, Rhode Island. *Health Education Quarterly, 13*, 117–129.

Leon, G. R., Perry, C. L., Mangelsdorf, C., & Tell, G. J. (1989). Adolescent nutritional and psychological patterns and risk for the development of an eating disorder. *Journal of Youth and Adolescence, 18*, 273–282.

Liao, Y., & Cooper, R. S. (1995). Continued adverse trends in coronary heart disease mortality among blacks, 1980–91. *Public Health Reports, 111*, 572–579.

Luepker, R. V., & Perry, C. L. (1991). The Minnesota Heart Health Program: Education for youth and parents. *Annals of New York Academy of Sciences, 623*, 314–321.

Macera, C. A., Armstead, C. A., & Anderson, N. B. (in press). In A. Baum, T. A. Revenson, & J. E. Singer (Eds.), *Handbook of health psychology.* Mahwah, NJ: Erlbaum.

Marin, G. (1989). AIDS prevention among Hispanics: Needs, risk behaviors, and cultural values. *Public Health Reports, 104*, 411–415.

Marin, G., Marin, B. V., Perez-Stable, E. J., Sabogal, F., & Otero-Sabogal, R. (1990). Changes in information as a function of a culturally appropriate smoking cessation community intervention for Hispanics. *American Journal of Community Psychology, 18*, 847–864.

Martin, J. L., Dean, L., Garcia, M., & Hall, W. (1989). The impact of AIDS on a gay community: changes in sexual behavior, substance use, and mental health. *American Journal of Community Psychology, 17*, 269–294.

Mattson, M. E., Pollack, E. S., & Cullen, J. W. (1987). What are the odds that smoking will kill you? *American Journal of Public Health, 77*, 425–431.

McCord, C., & Freeman, H. P. (1990). Excess mortality in Harlem. *New England Journal of Medicine, 322*, 173–177.

McKinlay, J. B. (1979). A case for refocussing upstream: The political economy of illness. In E. G. Jaco (Ed.), *Patients, physicians, and illness*, 3rd ed. (pp. 9–25). New York: Free Press.

McKusick, L., Wiley, J. A., Coates, T. J., Stall, R., Saika, G., Morin, S., Charles, K., Horstman, W., & Conant, M. (1985). Reported changes in the sexual behavior of men at risk for AIDS, San Francisco 1982–1984: The AIDS behavioral research project. *Public Health Reports, 100*, 622–628.

Miller, G. (1969). Psychology as a means of promoting human welfare. *American Psychologist, 24*, 1063–1075.

Mittlemark, M. B., Luepker, R. V., Grimm, R., Jr., Kottke, T. E., & Blackburn, H. (1988). The role of physicians in a community-wide program for prevention of cardiovascular disease: The Minnesota Heart Health Program. *Public Health Reports, 103*, 360–365.

Mittlemark, M. B., Luepker, R. V., Jacobs, D. R., Bracht, N. F., Carlaw, R. W., Crow, R. S., Finnegan, J., Grimm, R.H., Jeffery, R. W., Kline, F. G., Mullis, R. M., Murray, D. M., Pechacek, T. F., Perry, C. L., Pirie, P. L., & Blackburn, H. (1986). Community-wide prevention of cardiovascular disease: Education strategies of the Minnesota Heart Health Program. *Preventive Medicine, 15*, 1–17.

Munoz, R. F., Marin, B. V., Posner, S. F., & Perez-Stable, E. J. (1997). Mood management mail intervention increases abstinence rates for Spanish-speaking Latino smokers. *American Journal of Community Psychology, 25*, 325–344.

National Center for Health Statistics (1997). *Health, United States, 1995–96.* Hyattsville, MD: Public Health Service.

National Institutes of Health (1997, February). NIH consensus development statement: Interventions to prevent HIV risk behaviors. Washington, D.C.: U.S. Government Printing Office.

Newman, S., Fitzpatrick, R., Revenson, T. A., Skevington, S., & Williams, G (1996). *Understanding rheumatoid arthritis.* London: Routledge & Kegan Paul.

Ockene, J. K. (1987). Physician-delivered interventions for smoking cessation: Strategies for increasing effectiveness. *Prevention Medicine, 16,* 723–737.

Otten, M. W., Teutsch, S. M., Williamson, D. F., & Marks, J. S. (1990). The effect of known risk factors on the excess mortality of Black adults in the United States. *Journal of the American Medical Association, 263,* 845–850.

Ouellette Kobasa, S. C. (1990). AIDS and volunteer associations: Perspectives on social and individual change. *Milbank Quarterly, 68*(Supp. 2), 280–294.

Perrow, C., & Guillen, M. F. (1990). *The AIDS disaster: The failure of organizations in New York and the nation.* New Haven, CT: Yale University Press.

Perry, C. L. (1987). Results of prevention programs with adolescents. *Drug and Alcohol Dependence, 20,* 13–19.

Peterson, J. L. (1998). HIV/AIDS prevention through community psychology [Special issue]. *American Journal of Community Psychology, 26*(1).

Pirie, P. L., Murray, D. M., & Luepker, R. V. (1991). Gender differences in cigarette smoking and quitting in a cohort of young adults. *American Journal of Public Health, 81* 324–327.

Puska, P. (1984). Community-based prevention of cardiovascular disease: The North Karelia project. In J. D. Matarazzo, S. M. Weiss, J. A. Herd, N. E. Miller, & S. M. Weiss (Eds.), *Behavioral health: A handbook for health enhancement and disease prevention* (pp. 1140–1147). New York: Wiley.

Revenson, T. A., & Seidman, E. (in press). Looking back and moving forward: Reflections on a quarter century of community psychology. In T. A. Revenson, A. D'Augelli, S. E. French, D. Hughes, D. Livert, E. Seidman, M. Shinn, & H. Yoshikawa (Eds.), *Community psychology: A quarter century of theory, research, and action in social and historical context.* New York: Kluwer Academic/Plenum.

Robbins, L., Allegrante, J. P., & Paget, S. A. (1993). Adapting the systematic lupus erythematosus self-help (SLESH) course for Latino SLE patients. *Arthritis Care and Research, 6,* 97–103.

Rodin, J., & Janis, I. L. (1982). The social influence of physicians and other health care practitioners as agents of change. In H. S. Friedman & M. R. DiMatteo (Eds.), *Interpersonal issues in health care* (pp. 33–49). New York: Academic.

Rodin, J., & Salovey, P. (1990). Health psychology. *Annual Review of Psychology, 40,* 533–579.

Ryan, W. (1971). *Blaming the victim.* New York: Random House.

Sarason, S. B. (1974). *The psychological sense of community: Prospects for a community psychology.* San Francisco: Jossey-Bass.

Schechter, M. T., Craib, K. J. P., Willoughby, B., Douglas, B., McLeod, A., Maynard, M., Constance, P., & O'Shaugnessy, M. (1988). Patterns of sexual behavior and condom use in a cohort of homosexual men. *American Journal of Public Health, 78,* 1535–1538.

Seidman, E. S. (1990). Social regularities and prevention research: A transactional model. In P. Muehrer (Ed.), *Conceptual research models for preventing mental disorders* (pp. 145–164). [DHHS Publication No. (ADM) 90-1713]. Rockville, MD: National Institute of Mental Health.

Shilts, R. (1988). *And the band played on: Politics, people and the AIDS epidemic,* updated edition. New York: Penguin.

Silverman, M. (1986). The public health response. In V. Gong & N. Rudnick (Eds.), *AIDS: Facts and issues* (pp. 155–156). New Brunswick, NJ: Rutgers University Press.

Stokols, D. (1992). Establishing and maintaining healthy environments: Toward a social ecology of health promotion. *American Psychologist, 47,* 6–22.

Terborg, J. R. (1988). The organization as a context for health promotion. In S. Spacapan & S. Oskamp (Eds.), *The social psychology of health* (pp. 129–174). Newbury Park, CA: Sage.

Trickett, E. J. (1996). A future for community psychology: The contexts of diversity and the diversity of contexts. *American Journal of Community Psychology, 24,* 209–234.

U.S. Census Bureau (1998). Health Insurance Coverage—1997 <http://www.census.gov/hhes/hlthins/hlthins97/hig7t.html>: (accessed: 28 September 1997). [SB/94-28]. Washington, D.C.: U.S. Department of Commerce.

U.S. Health Care Financing Administration. (1996). National Health Expenditures by Type: 1980–1995. *Health Care Financing Review,* Fall. Washington, D.C.: U.S. Government Printing Office.

Warner, K. E. (1987). Television and health promotion: Stay tuned. *American Journal of Public Health, 77,* 140–142.

Wechsler, H., Levine, S., Idelson, R. K., Rohman, M., & Taylor, J. O. (1983). The physician's role in health promotion—A survey of primary care practitioners. *New England Journal of Medicine, 308,* 97–100.

Weick, K. (1984). Small wins: Redefining the scale of social problems. *American Psychologist, 39,* 40–49.

Williams, A. F. (1982). Passive and active measures for controlling disease and injury: The role of health psychologists. *Health Psychology, 1,* 399–410.

Winett, R. A., King, A. C., & Altman, D. G. (1989). *Health psychology and public health: An integrative approach.* New York: Pergamon.

Winkelstein, W., Samuel, M. Padian, N. S., Wiley, J. A., Lang, W., Anderson, R. E., & Levy, J. A. (1987). The San Francisco Men's Health Study: III. Reduction in human immunodeficiency virus transmission among homosexual/bisexual men, 1982–1986. *American Journal of Public Health, 77,* 685–689.

Winkelstein, W., Wiley, J. A., Padian, N. S., Samuel, M., Shiboski, S., Ascher, M. S., & Levy, J. A. (1988). The San Francisco Men's Health Study: Continued decline in HIV seroconversion rates among homosexual/bisexual men. *American Journal of Public Health, 78,* 1472–1474.

Yoshikawa, H., & Shinn, M. (in press). Facilitating change: Where and how should community psychology intervene? In T. A. Revenson, A. D'Augelli, S. E. French, D. Hughes, D. Livert, E. Seidman, M. Shinn, & H. Yoshikawa (Eds.), *Community psychology: A quarter century of theory, research and action in social and historical context.* New York: Kluwer Academic/Plenum.

CHAPTER 21

Religion in American Life

A Community Psychology Perspective

KENNETH I. PARGAMENT AND KENNETH I. MATON

Religion is woven tightly into the fabric of American life. In some ways, the essential "religiousness" of our culture is quite visible. The large number of congregations in any community, the key role of religious leaders and rituals during important transitions in life, the rapid expansion of ministry into television, and the prominence of religious traditions and holidays are clear signs of the salience of religion in the United States. Less visible, but perhaps more revealing, are some other indicators. For example, it is estimated that 94% of the American population believe in God; 88% believe God loves them; 81% believe we will be called before God on Judgment Day; 71% believe in life after death; more people have confidence in organized religion than in any other social institution; and religious figures such as Billy Graham, Mother Teresa, Pope John Paul II, and Archbishop Desmond Tutu are consistently named by Americans in their lists of most admired people (Gallup & Castelli, 1989).

What, if any, are the effects of religiousness in the United States? There is compelling evidence that religion is a potent force in society, shaping both individuals and institutions. Various dimensions of religiousness have been identified as significant predictors of a wide range of individual attributes and behaviors, such as racial prejudice, physical health and mortality, alcohol and drug abuse, nonmarital sexual activity, empowerment, mental health, psychosocial competence, and the outcomes of stressful experiences (e.g., Bergin, 1983; Hood, Spilka, Hunsberger, & Gorsuch, 1996; Koenig, 1994, 1997; Levin & Vanderpool, 1991; Maton & Wells, 1995; Pargament, 1997; Payne, Bergin, Bielema, & Jenkins, 1991; Schumaker, 1992). Religion has clear effects on social institutions as well. Benson and Williams (1982) demonstrated the strong relationship between the religious beliefs of members of the United States Congress and their voting behavior on eight significant issues. The 8.5 billion dollars in philanthropy provided by religious systems to other social institutions in 1985 was more than

KENNETH I. PARGAMENT • Department of Psychology, Bowling Green State University, Bowling Green, Ohio 43402. KENNETH I. MATON • Department of Psychology, University of Maryland Baltimore County, Catonsville, Maryland 21250.

Handbook of Community Psychology, edited by Julian Rappaport and Edward Seidman. Kluwer Academic / Plenum Publishers, New York, 2000.

twice as great as that provided by corporations and foundations (Jacquet, 1986). These resources were used to support refugee aid, emergency aid, shelter for the poor, advocacy, social justice, human rights, educational, food, and nutritional programs.

Despite its significance for individuals and institutions, religion has been neglected by psychologists and other mental health professionals for the greater part of this century (see Larson, Pattison, Blazer, Omran, & Kaplan, 1986; Weaver, Samford, Kline, Lucas, Larson, & Koenig, 1998). In more recent years, however, there have been signs of renewed interest in the study of religion. Given its concern with the individual-in-context and systemic change, the field of community psychology has a particularly important stake in the study of religious life.

In this chapter, we will examine religion in American life from a community psychology perspective. Traditional psychological approaches to religion, we will suggest, have often been individualistic, overly-simplified and overly-biased, and non-collaborative. Rather than focus on religion as an individual expression, we will examine religious institutions as they impact both individuals and communities. Our goal is to highlight the exciting opportunities for community psychology to learn about, learn from, and work with religious systems.

A BRIEF REVIEW OF PSYCHOLOGICAL APPROACHES TO RELIGION

It comes as a surprise to many psychologists that religion was a central topic of concern and study for the founders of psychology. Theoretical and empirical studies of religious education, worship, conversion, emotion, and experience by William James, G. S. Hall, J. H. Leuba, and E. D. Starbuck were regularly published by the *American Journal of Psychology* and, later, by the *Psychological Bulletin* in the late-19th and early-20th centuries. However, as psychology moved away from its philosophical roots, and as behavioral and psychoanalytic approaches became more prominent, interest in the psychological study of religion dropped sharply. The lack of religious study may have been influenced by the fact that, throughout the century, psychologists have been less religious as a group than the general population of the United States. Thus, they tend to underestimate the significance of religious phenomena (Beit-Hallahmi, 1974; Sarason, 1993; Shafranske & Malony, 1990).

The last 20 years have witnessed more of a rapprochement between psychology and religion sparked by an interest in pastoral counseling by religious communities, an interest in working with religious systems by community mental health professionals, and a greater appreciation of the importance of spirituality in both religious and professional communities. Developments in cognitive, social, and lifespan psychology have also led researchers to take a closer look at religion. This resurgence of interest in the psychology of religion is marked by what is becoming a significant body of theory and research (see Batson, Schoenrade, & Ventis, 1993; Hood et al., 1996; Wulff, 1997). Perhaps the most significant trend in this work is towards the conceptualization and measurement of religion as a multidimensional phenomenon, one which holds a variety of implications for the individual.

From a community psychology perspective, several issues of concern can be raised regarding the status of psychological approaches to religion. First, ever since James (1902) defined religion as "feelings, acts and experiences of individual men in their solitude" (p. 31), the psychological study of religion has been largely personological. A large portion of the research in the area has focused on identifying the different dispositional orientations of individuals to religion, and examining the implications of these orientations for various individual attitudes and behaviors (e.g., Donahue, 1985; Gorsuch, 1988). This has been a significant and fruitful research tradition. However, it leaves unanswered important questions about how religion is expressed by groups, families, and institutions; how religion is shaped by different events and contexts; and how religion, in turn, contributes to the lives of individuals and to society. Developments in the sociology and anthropology of religion that could help answer these questions have not been integrated into the psychological literature. Commenting on the individualism of religious research, Barton (1971) noted that:

> Researchers have proceeded to take people out of their actual social contexts and to limit their analysis to individual variables ... this is like a biologist putting his experimental animals through a meat grinder and taking every hundredth cell to examine under a microscope; almost all information about anatomy and physiology, about structure and function gets lost (p. 847).

A second concern from a community psychology perspective is the simplified and inflexible view many people (including psychologists) have of religion. Religious issues are often approached with either an undifferentiated positive or an undifferentiated negative stance. For example, in a study of indiscriminate proreligiousness, over 35% of a mixed sample of students and church members stated that "I always live by my religious beliefs"; approximately two-thirds of the sample stated that "This church has programs to meet the needs of all the members" (Pargament, Brannick, Adamakos, Ensing, Kelemen, Warren, Falgout, Cook, & Myers, 1987).

When it comes to religion, psychologists are no less prone to bias. Anti-religiousness is clear in the writings of several prominent psychologists who criticize religion on various grounds (e.g., Albee, 1982; Ellis, 1960; Freud, 1949). What these criticisms share is an exclusive focus on a particular type of religious expression. Other forms of religious expression go unmentioned and undistinguished from those seemingly dysfunctional approaches. Pro-religiousness among psychologists poses problems as well. More religiously sympathetic psychologists have focused on the question "What kind of religion is healthy or good?" The form of this question suggests that there is one type of religion good for everyone. It does not allow for the possibility that different forms of religion may offer different advantages and disadvantages depending on each individual's life experiences, personal preferences, and social context. In short, the anti-religious and pro-religious biases of psychologists lead to an oversimplification of religion in which the diversity of forms and effects of religious expression are neglected.

Finally, a community psychology perspective points to the relationship between psychological and religious communities as a source of concern. Psychologist, clergy, and congregation most often meet around mental health issues. Referrals of clinical cases by clergy are sought by mental health professionals. Psychologists are often involved in training clergy and congregation leaders as counselors. Mental health educational programs are offered to churches and synagogues. Certainly, many church/synagogue members have been helped through this process. However, the process is one-sided. Studies indicate that clergy refer far more cases to mental health professionals than they receive from mental health professionals (e.g., Carson, 1976; Koenig, Bearon, Hover, & Travis, 1991; Meylink & Gorsuch, 1986). Thus, while religious communities are drawing upon the unique resources of mental health professionals, mental health professionals are dealing with religious systems as if they were quasi-mental health institutions (Rappaport, 1981). Apparently overlooked in this process is the fact that religious systems are, simply put, religious; that is, they have missions, structures, theologies, and resources that distinguish them from other settings, including mental health centers (Pargament, Falgout, Ensing, Reilly, Silverman, Van Haitsma, Olsen, & Warren, 1991). When viewed as unique, multifaceted, and resourceful systems that may, at times, share the interests and concerns of psychologists, a broader set of opportunities for collaboration between psychological and religious communities emerges.

In recent years, community psychologists and others have begun to respond to these concerns. Community psychologists have applied their values, perspectives, and methods in an attempt to learn about, learn from, and work with religious systems (see Jason, 1997; Kloos, Horneffer, & Moore, 1995; Maton & Wells, 1995; Pargament, Maton, & Hess, 1992). While this work is yet in its infancy, a richer understanding of religion in American life is emerging.

RELIGION FROM A COMMUNITY PSYCHOLOGY PERSPECTIVE

Religion has been defined in a variety of ways. Common to these definitions, however, is a view of religion both as a social phenomenon, one involving a community of people who share a faith, and as an individual phenomenon, one involving a set of beliefs, practices, and feelings that place life experiences into a framework of Ultimate significance. Expressed individually or socially, religion has a dual character: It is involved in the construction and choice of pathways people take in their search for significance, and it is involved in the definition of significance itself (Pargament, 1992, 1997). What sets religion apart from other phenomena is the involvement of the sacred in this search for significance.

The religious institution is the primary system that bridges social and personal forms of religious phenomena. It is the gathering site for the fellowship of members. It provides opportunities for personal religious experiences. It is a central medium through which religious symbols, beliefs, rites, and traditions are transmitted to individuals. And it is a key channel through which religious ethics, values, and resources are transmitted to other institutions in society. In this sense, as Berger and Neuhaus (1977) note, religious institutions mediate between their members and a larger social matrix.

This chapter will focus on religious institution as the central phenomenon of interest, conceptualized at two levels of analysis. At the organizational level, local religious institutions, i.e., local churches, parishes, or congregations, will receive primary attention, as community psychologists have focused most of their attention on this level of analysis. Both the relationships of congregations to their members (inreach), as well as to individuals and organizations in the local community (outreach) will be examined. Much less work in community psychology has focused on other levels of analysis, such as the societal or cultural level, i.e., generalized cultural religious practices, beliefs, values, and norms. Reflecting the relative scarcity of community psychology work in this area, only a small portion of this chapter focuses on the societal level of analysis.

LEARNING ABOUT RELIGION

There are over 350,000 religious congregations in the United States, made up of approximately 148 million members and over 545,000 clergy, representing numerous denominations (Jacquet & Jones, 1991). These institutions vary in their functions, structure, values, goals, resources, members, leadership, traditions, activities, and context (Carroll, Dudley, & McKinney, 1986). They also vary dramatically in their impact on individuals and society. Consider the following examples: Only 8 of 29 ministers surveyed during the crisis over the admission of black students to Central High School in 1957 in Little Rock were active integrationists

(Campbell & Pettigrew, 1959). Over 100 million dollars was spent over a 15-year period by the church-based Campaign for Human Development to support over 2000 social justice programs (Evans, 1979). In 1978, several hundred members of the People's Temple in Jonestown were killed. Religious involvement has been associated with significantly lower rates of drug abuse and alcohol abuse (Benson, Wood, Johnson, Eklin, & Mills, 1983).

How do we make sense of this diversity in form and function of religious institutions? An ecological perspective provides a framework for understanding the varied intricate nature of religious life. From an ecological point of view, local religious institutions represent evolving organizational niches embedded in dynamic, changing environments. The nature of a specific religious institution is influenced by a multiplicity of factors, including member characteristics (e.g., SES, ethnicity), member needs, community locale (e.g., rural/suburban/urban; community composition and needs), the relationship to local community institutions and power structures, the cultural and religious tradition of both members and the larger denomination, and societal trends and forces. However, religious systems are not simply reactive. As they are being shaped by their broader milieu, they are also shaping it. Similarly, as they shape the lives of their members, they are, in turn, shaped by their members. Three key features help provide a framework for understanding the local ecology of religious systems and for distinguishing among religious institutions: theology, mission, and organization.

Theology

Religious systems throughout the world rest on a set of beliefs and values that prescribe a view of God or transcendent force in the Universe, a perspective on the nature of individuals and society, and a set of ideals regarding individual and social life. These beliefs and values offer a response to questions of ultimate meaning in life, such as how the world was created, why there is suffering in the world, the difference between good and evil, and what happens when we die. Of course the answers to these questions are very different among the religions of the world.

Even within western culture, there are marked differences in the theologies of religious institutions. Roberts (1990), for example, notes that theologies vary according to their source of doctrinal authority. He places theologies along a continuum ranging from Reversionism, in which the purity of original doctrines is stressed, to Orthodoxy, in which later historical revelations and interpretations are also authoritative, to Modernism, in which contemporary developments are accepted as authoritative and woven into the institution's theology. Theologies also differ in terms of the degree to which they focus on "this-worldly" or "other-worldly" concerns (Roozen, McKinney, & Carroll, 1984). This-worldy theologies emphasize the importance of establishing the Kingdom of God on *this* earth. Religious values and beliefs are expressed in concrete individual and social actions. Thus, there is no sharp distinction between the religious and the secular. Other-worldy theologies point to Heaven as the Kingdom of God. Here, emphasis is placed on the individual's relationship with God, and preparation for the world-to-come where the individual will receive his or her rewards or punishments for life experienced in this world.

Theologies may also be distinguished by the degree to which they challenge or comfort the individual and society (Berger, 1967; Glock, Ringer, & Babbie, 1967; Spilka & Bridges, 1991). Comforting theologies stress the soothing elements of faith as a means of bearing with the pain of life, and of keeping oneself and one's world together. Challenging theologies emphasize the transforming power of faith as bases for radical individual and social change.

Finally, theologies vary dramatically in their images of God and of the appropriate relationship between the individual and God. For example, grace-oriented theologies focus on God as a loving Deity, forgiving people for their sins, and embracing them in caring personal relationships. Sin-oriented theologies place greater emphasis on God as a stern powerful figure who punishes people for their transgressions.

Diverse contextual and personal forces shape religious world views. For example, Kelley (1977) has argued that rapid social change and the increasing complexities of modern life have led to the growth of religious institutions that adhere to strict religious thinking (reversionist) and provide a clear compelling sense of meaning in life. At the individual level, Benson and Spilka (1973) offer evidence that suggests that people with higher levels of self-esteem are more likely to adopt loving images of God.

Theologies also affect the response of the institution to the world and to its members. G. T. Marx (1967) notes that, historically, religion has served one of two diverse roles for blacks—either as an opiate or as a stimulus for radical social change. Surveying a group of black members of churches in the metropolitan United States, he found that the degree to which the members endorse a "this-worldly" versus "other-worldly" orientation was a crucial intervening variable. Members holding a this-worldy view were more likely to participate in social change efforts, while members holding an other-worldly view were more likely to "wait upon the Lord till (their) change comes."

Mission

As structures that mediate between the personal lives of the members and the larger social world, religious institutions develop both a public and a private character (Berger & Neuhaus, 1977). Underlying the stance the congregation takes both to the world and its members is a mission, a sense of purpose that guides the institution's actions and responses. There is, however, exceptional diversity in both the social and the personal missions of religious institutions.

Roozen et al. (1984), surveying over 400 leaders of Protestant, Jewish, Catholic, and non-denominational congregations, identified four types of public mission: (1) an activist orientation in which the congregation stresses social justice, a critical attitude about existing social structures, and systemic change; (2) a civic orientation in which the congregation supports existing social structures, seeks civil harmony, and avoids confrontation and conflict; (3) an evangelistic orientation in which non-members are encouraged to become new believers; and (4) a sanctuary orientation in which members are encouraged to withdraw from the stresses of society into the haven of the congregation. Maton and Pargament (1987) suggest two additional social orientations: (1) a social service orientation that focuses on assisting individuals inadequately served by the social system and (2) an avoidance orientation in which self-sufficient communities are established as a means of prohibiting contacts with the outside world.

Equally diverse are the personal missions of religious institutions. Strommen, Brekke, Underwager, and Johnson (1972) studied 316 congregations from the three major Lutheran bodies in the United States. They distinguished between two major orientations of the congregation to its members: a spiritual orientation that encourages the development of a transcendent meaning in life, a personal caring relationship with God, and a faith of emotional certainty, and a law orientation that stresses the importance of living by religiously based rules and traditions. Two further personal mission orientations may be distinguished: a growth orientation that challenges the individual to evaluate himself or herself critically and make personal improvements, and a maintenance orientation that supports the individual emotionally in his or her efforts to cope with the world (Pargament et al., 1991).

It is important to note that any given congregation may have multiple overlapping social and/or personal missions. For example, Roozen et al. (1984) report an association between activist and civic orientations, and between evangelical and sanctuary orientations. However, they also found that most congregations could be identified in terms of one or two dominant mission orientations.

Like the theology of an institution, missions are embedded in the context of a larger social milieu and the membership of the congregation. For example, as many urban congregations have moved to the suburbs, a number of the remaining religious institutions have shifted towards a more maintenance-oriented personal mission in response to the pressing needs of an increasingly impoverished membership (Maton & Pargament, 1987). In addition, many remaining mainline inner-city congregations have changed towards a more social activist or social-service public mission in response to deteriorating social conditions, such as homelessness (Cohen, Mobray, Gillette, & Thompson, 1991).

Organization

The theology and mission of religious institutions come to life through the organization of the congregation, and the organizations of religious institutions vary as dramatically as their theologies and missions. For example, religious institutions differ according to their degree of complexity and bureaucracy, with many institutions adopting complex hierarchical structures, while others develop more simplified communal organizations (Roberts, 1990). Religious institutions also evolve distinct processes for decision-making, communication, and generating and managing their resources. These processes are expressed through congregational climates diverse in their stability, flexibility, sense of community, social concern, emotional expressiveness, involvement in personal problems, and tolerance of individual differences (Pargament, Silverman, Johnson, Echemendia, & Snyder, 1983). Religious institutions also differ in their activities and practices. Some congregations emphasize regular religious practices (e.g., prayer, Bible study, services), and place special significance on life-transition rituals, such as baptisms, weddings, and funerals. Others place more of their energy into specialized helping approaches, such as pastoral counseling to members, group-based family-life enrichment programs, or self-help groups. And others emphasize activities that reach out to the larger community (Maton & Pargament, 1987). Finally, religious institutions may be distinguished in terms of their degree of embeddedness or active involvement in the diverse spheres of societal and individual life (Troeltsch, 1964).

The organization of the religious institution is shaped not only by its theology and mission, but also by its members and broader social context. In this vein, Pargament et al. (1983) found that congregations of different race, size, and denomination had distinctive climates. For instance, consistent with descriptions of the black church as a source of support and identity, small black Protestant congregations were characterized by a higher sense of community, stability, and social concern than white churches.

The organization of the religious institution can, in turn, shape its members and milieu. For example, Maton and Rappaport (1984) propose a number of relationships between religious organizational activities and behavioral change. They note that ongoing prayer groups, supportive relationships with fellow members, congregational norms focused on personal development, and high levels of commitment and involvement in the institution can help individuals deal with stressful life events, develop specific problem-solving skills, and enhance their psychological well-being.

The constructs of theology, mission, and organization provide a framework for understanding the religious institution as a complex multidimensional system, which can take many forms, and which is embedded in an individual–systems ecology. Clearly, however, these constructs are not independent of each other. Rather, the theology, mission, and organization of a religious institution are woven into richly intricate patterns. These patterns guide the institution along distinctive pathways that have significant and diverse implications for the member and for society.

Pathways of Religious Influence

Maton and Pargament (1987) describe and illustrate several pathways religious institutions take to influence society (outreach) and influence their members (inreach). They stress that it is important to avoid the temptation of evaluating these outreach and inreach pathways simplistically, that is, as either "all good" or "all bad." Rather, each of the pathways may be associated with psychosocial advantages and disadvantages. Finally, they note that, while these pathways reflect the dominant orientation of an institution, any institution may involve itself in more than one pathway. Using the constructs of theology, mission, organization, and psychosocial advantage and disadvantage as an organizing framework, several pathways of religious outreach and inreach can be articulated.

Social Outreach

The pathways of social outreach are described in Table 1. Rooted in a challenging, this-worldly theology of modernism, a number of religious institutions follow a *social action* pathway. This world view stresses the *corporate* (i.e., group-based or social-based) nature of sin. As a remedy, social action institutions adopt the mission of fundamental social systemic change. Towards this end, these institutions embed themselves deeply in social affairs through highly organized activities, including social protest, civil disobedience, community organization, political involvement, and participation in social policy formation. Social action institutions have the potential to reduce inequity and discrimination in other societal institutions, as well as to enhance the psychological well-being of involved individuals. Boyte (1984), for example, describes the beneficial political and psychological impact of (COPS), a parish-supported community-action organization for lower-income Mexican-Americans. Social action institutions may also encourage conflict and, in some cases, aggression to achieve social change (Gutierrez, 1973).

Other religious institutions follow a *social service* pathway. As seen in Table 1, these institutions also identify social problems in this world. However, they are more heavily influenced by a grace theology, and seek to improve the social system through work with underserved individuals, rather than through fundamental systemic change. Social service institutions involve themselves in a wide range of social support programs, including help for the elderly, homeless, poor, and deinstitutionalized; mentoring at-risk youth; social-skills training; and preparation for, and assistance through, life transitions (e.g., birth, marriage, parenting, divorce, retirement, death) (see Haugk, 1976; Pargament, 1982, for review). While rarely evaluated formally, descriptions of these programs suggest that they can contribute in a

Table 1. Social Outreach Pathways of Religious Institutions

Pathway	Theology	Mission	Organization	Advantages/ disadvantages
Social action	Challenge; this-world; modernism	Fundamental systemic change	Deeply embedded; social and political change	Institutional change/ conflict
Social service	This world; grace	Improve social system	Deeply embedded; social support programs	Social support/first-order change
Social conversion	Challenge; other-world; sin; revisionism	Evangelism	Moderately embedded; social control; evangelical	Member support/ intolerance; first-order change
Social conservatism	Comfort; this-world; orthodox	Support social system	Narrowly embedded; bureaucratic; traditional practices	Institutional protection/ maintenance of inequality
Social sanctuary	Comfort; other-world; grace	Protection from social system	Narrowly embedded; communal; pietistic and support activities	Member support/ maintenance of inequality
Social avoidance	Sin; reversion	Avoid social system	Narrowly embedded; social control; special practices	Alternative institution; member support/ dysfunctional member practices

significant way to the psychological, social, and material resources of many people facing serious problems. However, by responding to the individual needs of people experiencing social difficulties, social service institutions, like their mental health counterparts, have been criticized for "salving" rather than "solving" basic systemic problems (Berton, 1965).

Social conversion institutions also recognize problems in society. However, this pathway rests on a theology that views societal problems as a manifestation of individual sin; the solution lies in a focus on the other-worldly and a reversion to fundamental religious beliefs and practices. Thus, the mission of this institution is social change through evangelism. Social conversion institutions are often characterized by high levels of commitment among members, strict social controls, religious activities that stress the individual's personal relationship with God, and a variety of evangelism programs (e.g., hospital visits, religious literature, personal witnessing, religious media events). The social conversion pathway may offer a source of meaning, community, and structure to its members (McGaw, 1979). However, it may also be tied to a lack of tolerance for differences in beliefs and lifestyles. Furthermore, questions may be raised about the efficacy of individual religious development as the basis for social change.

Many religious institutions attempt to support and maintain existing social systems rather than radically change or reform them. This mission is a central element of the *social conservatism* pathway (see Table 1). Underlying this pathway is a more orthodox theology, which focuses on comfort rather than challenge in this world. Social conservatism institutions tend to adopt more complex, stable, bureaucratic structures, an emphasis on regular religious practices and traditions, and a relatively narrow scope limited to support for traditional institutions in society. While this support may play a key role in the protection of benevolent institutions, it may also perpetuate inequitable social conditions (e.g., Campbell & Pettigrew, 1959).

Other religious institutions view society more apprehensively, and try to protect their members from this world. Consistent with this mission, *social sanctuary* institutions stress spiritual comfort, an other-worldly view, and a grace orientation in their theology. The congregation also provides members with a supportive milieu through a more communal organization, a sense of community among the members, and religious activities that encourage a close relationship with God. In this pathway, members leave the "problems of the world" at the doorstep when they enter the congregation. As Kennell (1985) noted in a participant-observation study of an inner-city congregation, the social haven institution offers many members valuable support often missing in their environment. However, other theorists have suggested that this support occurs at the cost of more active social involvement (Block & Stark, 1965). In this sense, the social sanctuary congregation may also protect existing social institutions.

Yet another response to the view of evil in society is to actively avoid it. Table 1 indicates that the *social avoidance* pathway is based on a sin-oriented, reversionist theology. Members are challenged to avoid contact with existing social institutions. Alternative social structures are developed, often in isolation from the larger society. The organization of the social avoidance institution is typically characterized by charismatic leadership, high levels of control over members' behaviors, social solidarity, and special teachings and practices (Wilson, 1959). Social avoidance institutions tend to attract those who are less powerful and more alienated in society. While these institutions can generate potentially valuable alternative social structures, they can also encourage a loss of personal initiative and, at times, dysfunctional practices and norms (e.g., "Heaven's Gate").

Personal Inreach

Religious institutions also reach in to their members in a variety of ways. These pathways of personal inreach are presented in Table 2. Many congregations attempt to provide members with *personal structure* in their lives. Institutions that follow this pathway identify a law orientation as their key mission. Based on a sin-oriented, reversionist/orthodox theology, they offer their members a clear set of religiously based rules for living that define appropriate and inappropriate behaviors. The organization of these institutions stresses social control over members' actions, religious rituals and traditions, and a high degree of embeddedness in members' lives. Empirical evidence suggests that this type of system may provide members with a source of control over their impulses, a haven from a maladaptive subculture, and a system of personal and social support (Pargament, Echemendia, Johnson, Myers, Cook, Brannick, & McGath, 1987; Hood et al., 1996). However, there is also some evidence to indicate that more restrictive religious perspectives are tied to lower levels of personal competence and higher levels of interpersonal intolerance and prejudice (Benson & Spilka, 1973; Batson et al., 1993).

Other people turn to religious institutions for more limited purposes. As Table 2 shows, the institution may serve as a *personal defense* against feelings of weakness, anxiety, or loneliness, or as a *personal stress buffer* during crises or major life transitions. A number of studies have shown that people are more likely to become involved in religion during periods of stress, change, or personal distress (e.g., Lindenthal, Myers, Pepper, & Stein, 1970; Pargament, 1997; Pargament & Hahn, 1986). Maintenance of the individual in the world is the key personal mission of these institutions. Consistent with this mission is the comforting theology of the congregation, an active supportive clergy, and the use of religious rituals and congregation-based helping activities. However, since the scope of the institution in members' lives is narrow, these congregations often have difficulty generating sufficient resources to

TABLE 2. Personal Inreach Pathways of Religious Institutions

Pathway	Theology	Mission	Organization	Advantages/ disadvantages
Personal structure	Sin; reversionism; orthodox	Law	Deeply embedded; social control; traditional practices	Restraint; support/ intolerance; lower problem-solving skills
Personal defense/ stress buffer	Comfort	Maintenance	Narrowly embedded; active clergy; specialized helping; unstable	Support/dysfunctional beliefs and practices
Personal quest	Challenge; this-world; modernism	Growth	Deeply embedded; communal; autonomy	Competence; tolerance/ anxiety
Personal empowerment	Grace; comfort/ challenge	Spiritual/growth; maintenance	Deeply embedded; communal; pietistic activities	Interpersonal skills, well-being/instability
Personal identity	Orthodoxy; comfort	Maintenance; law	Moderately embedded; bureaucratic; traditional practices	Support/intolerance
Personal marginality	Varied	Varied	Varied	Competence/stress

maintain themselves. Personal defense and stress buffer institutions can provide their members with much needed support. Involvement in some religious groups has been found to moderate or deter the effects of negative life events (Ellison, 1993; Krause & Van Tran, 1989; Maton, 1989a, 1989b; Siegel & Kuykendall, 1990; Williams, Larson, Buckler, Heckman, & Pyle, 1989). For example, Maton found that both high levels of individual spiritual support (Maton, 1989a) and, at the organizational level of analysis, highly supportive congregations (Maton, 1989b) were related positively and in a stress-buffering fashion to individual well-being; apparently they protected individuals from the deleterious effects of varied and serious life stressors. Some institutionally related practices and beliefs, however, may interfere with the development of personal skills and the successful resolution of crises (e.g., Horton, Wilkins, & Wright, 1988; Pargament, Ensing, Falgout, Olsen, Reilly, Van Haitsma, & Warren, 1990).

Other religious institutions direct themselves towards the personal growth and development of their members. Institutions involved in the *personal quest* pathway espouse challenging, this-worldy, modernistic theologies that emphasize personal freedom and responsibility for human development. Communal-type organizations are developed that encourage individual autonomy, variety in religious expression, and personal search and change. Evidence indicates that members of this kind of institution have a greater sense of efficacy in life, are more willing to examine themselves critically, and are more tolerant and trusting of others (Pargament, Tyler, & Steele, 1979a). However, the lack of a simple definitive structure in the personal quest pathway may also result in higher levels of anxiety and insecurity among the members (Batson et al., 1993).

At the core of many religious institutions is the individual's personal relationship with God. The primary mission of the *personal empowerment* institution is spiritual—the development of an intimate relationship of members with a personal God (see Table 2). Underlying this pathway is a theology of a loving, caring, and powerful (i.e., impactful) Deity, actively influencing and transforming individuals and social environments—providing comfort and aid during times of personal need and providing challenge, in order to enable people to improve themselves and influence their social environments. Through its primary spiritual mission, the personal empowerment institution naturally incorporates missions focused on personal growth and maintenance as well. Specifically, this institution stresses activities that enhance the individual's relationship with God, such as prayer, fellowship groups, and Bible study, as well as being a communal supportive organization highly integrated in members' lives. In a number of studies, reports of a loving relationship with God have been associated with measures of mental health (Benson & Spilka, 1973; Batson et al., 1993). Maton and Rappaport, in their work with an empowering non-denominational fellowship, demonstrated the significant impact of this institution on the interpersonal skills and personal well-being of the members (Maton & Rappaport, 1984; Maton & Salem, 1995; Rappaport & Simkins, 1991). Yet, maintaining an empowerment pathway over time may be difficult, as it involves a continual balancing of challenging and comforting beliefs, and of spiritual and personal missions. Ultimately, the attempt to achieve and maintain this balance may prove draining and stressful, and/or may lead to an instability for individuals and congregations as one or the other form of belief or mission becomes predominant at a given point in time.

Religious institutions offer many people a source of identity in life. Congregations following a *personal identity* pathway provide a set of rituals, traditions, beliefs, images, and symbols that help their members define how they are both alike and different from others. They also adopt organizational structures that give members opportunities to define themselves and others in terms of particular roles. The theology of personal identity institutions is often orthodox, directed towards the mission of sustaining members in the world through adherence to religious traditions and laws. This pathway can play a significant role in the development and maintenance of the individual's sense of self and relation to the world, a function particularly crucial for minority and other marginal social groups (Herman, 1977). However, as Glock and Stark (1996) found in their study of anti-Semitism, intolerance and prejudice result when identity is based upon the *superiority* of particular teachings.

Finally, it is important to note that religious systems of all kinds can be reacted against as well as identified with. In this sense, any religious system may offer members the possibility of *personal marginality*. Marginality within religious systems may generate stress among members. Pargament, Tyler, and Steele (1979b) report that peripheral congregation status was associated with lower satisfaction than central status. However, marginality may also stimulate personal development (Rubin, 1982). Thus, Pargament and colleagues have also found marginal status to be associated with higher levels of personal competence, particularly within more restrictive religious institutions (Pargament, Johnson, Echemendia, & Silverman, 1985; Pargament et al., 1979b).

LEARNING FROM RELIGION

Religion has developed unique approaches to meeting people's needs and addressing social problems. Community psychology, in its attempt to prevent and alleviate individual and social problems, may benefit considerably from a careful examination of the strengths and weaknesses of the varied approaches adopted by religion. In this section, some of the dominant themes concerning religion and religious influence in American life, with direct relevance for community psychology, are reviewed. The implications of these themes for future research and action by community psychologists are discussed in the concluding section of this chapter.

Meeting Primary Human Needs for Meaning and Understanding

Central to diverse religious theologies is the provision of a world view that provides explanations and, in most cases, "ultimately hopeful" perspectives on life purpose and events, death, and history. The widespread presence of these themes across all religious world views points to a deep "need" in humans to find and create meaning, both in terms of universal issues and day-to-day events (Hood et al., 1996; Sarason, 1993). Empirical evidence suggests that in religious settings where theology, mission, and organization combine to uphold and/or challenge individuals, the influence of religion can be health promotive, stress buffering, and empowering (e.g., Maton & Pargament, 1987; Hood et al., 1996). The large number of Americans who continue to ascribe to a religious world view, in the context of a materialist and pragmatist dominant culture, underscores individuals' needs for understanding and meaning, and the capacity of religious systems to respond to these needs.

One important aspect of a religious world view is the extent and the conditions under which it influences individuals' psychological locus of control. The actual impact of religious world views on locus of control appears quite varied in nature. For instance, some theologies emphasize that God is in control of all events, and that ultimately all life stresses or situations will "work toward the good." The emphasis that God is in exclusive control of all situations, however, may lead to a passive approach to coping with personal life events and social injustices. On the other hand, the emphasis that God and the individual are partners working together, emphasized by some theologies, may enhance a sense of personal efficacy and efforts at social change (Hathaway & Pargament, 1990; McIntosh & Spilka, 1990; Pargament, Grevengoed, Kennell, Newman, Hathaway, & Jones, 1988; Schaefer & Gorsuch, 1991). Furthermore, the sense of control by a benevolent God may be particularly helpful in uncontrollable situations or crises where there are real limits to what an individual (Bickel, Sheers, Estadt, Powell, & Pargament, 1998; Jenkins & Pargament, 1988) or social group can accomplish. Thus, "letting go" of anxiety and personal control, and placing faith in God's ability to deal with uncontrollable personal or social events (Baugh, 1988; Cole & Pargament, 1999; Maton & Rappaport, 1984), may be a useful complement to psychology's traditional focus on enhancing personal control over events that are controllable. In short, some elements of external control, when integrated appropriately with an internal locus of control, may serve important functions, both on the individual and societal level (Pargament, Sullivan, Tyler, & Steele, 1982).

Meeting Primary Needs for Community and Belonging

In addition to providing meaning, religion as a social institution appears to provide a sense of community and belonging to millions of Americans. Religion contains distinctive assets in building interpersonal community. One asset is the potential for a holistic approach to the person—spiritual, psychological, interpersonal, and economic needs can all be legitimately addressed in religious settings (Anderson, Maton, & Ensor, 1991). A second distinctive asset is a rich heritage of tradition and symbols that facilitate the sense of continuity and shared history integral to community. A third distinctive asset is the voluntary, self-selected nature of religious involvement. Individuals apparently choose to join religious settings peopled by others who not only share religious backgrounds and beliefs, but who also share the same cultural, economic, and social statuses as themselves (Roberts, 1990).

In contemporary society, religious settings face many challenges in attempting to foster a sense of community (Roberts, 1991). The impersonalization and mobility of American communities, together with a prevailing materialistic and individualistic culture, may diminish cohesiveness within congregations. The fact that many of the traditional functions of religion have been taken over by other social institutions reduces the intrinsic capability of religion to establish viable community (c.f., Berger, 1967). Finally, the large size and traditional centralized organizational structure of many congregations also represent obstacles to community.

One apparently effective organizational response to these problems has been to base ongoing activities in small, decentralized units within the church. Ongoing small group prayer, bible study, and mission groups are increasingly frequent means of enhancing intimate sharing and interpersonal commitment among members of diverse congregations (Maton & Rappaport, 1984; McGaw, 1979; Wuthnow, 1994). Small group involvement likely contributes to an integrated, strengths view of participants, and provides the opportunity for balanced individual involvement in providing and giving (c.f., Maton, 1987). Finally, sustained small group involvement creates a more localized forum for involvement and control over decision-making, another factor apparently important for community (McMillan & Chavis, 1986).

A second organizational feature of many religious settings that likely facilitates belonging is the creation of participatory role opportunities for members. For instance, in an intensive study of a small Pentecostal congregation (less than 100 members) for disenfranchised, inner-city blacks, Williams (1974) found the presence of a large number of role positions: pastor, pastor's aide, choir president and members, church secretary, deacon board chairman and deacons, trustee board chairman and trustees, Sunday school superintendent and teachers, financial captains, local community "missionaries," and so on. Religious settings that effectively involve individuals in roles perceived as important likely contribute to both a sense of meaning and community among members (Maton, 1988).

A central task for religion in building community is to find a viable balance between individual "agency" (self-assertion) and "communion" (participation as part of a larger whole) (Bakan, 1966). Religion faces special dangers in this regard, as the special powers traditionally ascribed to religious leaders, and the fear of ostracism or sin, may promote a maladaptive suspension of individual judgment. Tragedies such as Jonestown and Heaven's Gate illustrate some of the conditions under which "agency" can be lost and "communion" can become destructive. Furthermore, the dangers of particularism are also paramount, especially when group boundaries become so firm that those who are different become labeled as "evil" or "ungodly," and negative consequences such as prejudice, discrimination, or violence may follow. On the other hand, in some settings the proper combination of individuality and community can prove extremely empowering, especially with leaders fully committed to the development of both individuals and community (e.g., Maton & Rappaport, 1984). Interestingly, in this regard some theoreticians have asserted that only religious settings are potentially capable of fully integrating individual freedom with lasting community, for instance, in the context of individuals fully committed to a community of fellow believers whose fundamental tenet is respect for each individual's unique search for meaning (Becker, 1968).

Beyond Narrow Individualism: Toward the Public Good

The classic structural-functional view of religion (Radcliffe-Brown, 1939) asserted that, as a social institution, religion exists not to meet the needs of individuals, but rather the needs or requirements of society as a whole. The shared values, beliefs, and norms of religion as an institution are viewed in this perspective as central to societal stability and social integration. Concern for others and prohibitions against greed and oppression are examples of contributions of religion viewed as necessary for the orderly development and maintenance of society.

Many of the original "religious" norms and values of Judaic-Christian religion are today interwoven into the civic culture of American society. However, while they are often pronounced, it appears that they are not always acted upon (Lasch, 1979). The narrow individualism of individual, family, and corporate life in America increasingly underscores the need for limits on individualism, and the need for a revival of institutions that generate more of a balance between individual needs and concern for the public good (Bellah, Madsen, Sullivan, Swidler, & Tipton, 1985; Sarason, 1986).

In contemporary society, religion continues to place limits on narrow individualism in a variety of ways. One way is through religious teachings on the importance of serving God and serving one's "neighbor." Thus, Judaism emphasizes the importance of *mitzvot*, or obligational commandments from God, including those focused on helping others in need. Different branches of Christianity focus on different applications of personal and/or social ethics (e.g., Carney, 1978; Hallie, 1979; Niebuhr, 1963), prayerful seeking of God's will rather than one's own desires, and on being a "servant" in one's everyday life. The latter term, "servant," emphasizes that the committed religious individual should focus on meeting the needs of others, especially those in greatest need, even at possible cost to oneself.

A related means by which religion can contribute to the public good is by generating overall conceptions, that is, "visions," of societal arrangements and practices consistent with the public good. The Judaic-Christian tradition, for instance in the Bible, offers visions of society in which sharing of material wealth, helping one's neighbor, and concern for the common good served to mediate between the individual and the collective. Modern social action congregations, such as the well-known Church of the Savior in Washington, D.C., articulate visions of a congregation knit together in a shared social justice ministry to the inner city and larger society. Martin Luther King shared a vision of a country in which "all God's children" were holding hands, together singing "free at last, free at last." New theologies, such as "liberation theology," have emerged to mobilize both the church and citizenry in Central America with visions of a new social order. Of course, the vision of the "public good" and the "good society" articulated by some popular leaders or theologians may represent values and class interests that contribute more to the maintenance of current social arrangements than to true social justice.

Special Access to the Marginal, Disenfranchised, and Minority Groups

One of the unique aspects of religion as a social institution is its special access to the poor and minorities. For instance, the church has historically stood at the center of community life and power in the black community, and apparently continues to be a significant influence today (Frazier, 1964; Hrabowski, Maton, & Greif, 1998; Maton, Hrabowski, & Greif, 1998; Maton, Teti, Corns, Vieira-Baker, Lavine, Gouze, & Keating, 1996; Moore, 1991). For many among the rapidly expanding Hispanic population in our country, Catholicism remains a way of life. When psychological needs arise, pastoral counseling and non-church-based religious healers of various kinds retain a central role for many minority and immigrant populations (e.g., Garrison, 1977; Wimberly, 1979). Finally, a significant amount of the services and social action for the disenfranchised comes directly from minority and mainline contributions of money and volunteer services. A community psychology interested in understanding and influencing the community dynamics, health care delivery, and individual needs of the disenfranchised in America needs to take seriously the central role of minority religion and institutional religion in America.

The special access and importance of religion for the disenfranchised appears to follow directly from the previous themes emphasized above: meeting needs for meaning, meeting needs for community, and extending beyond narrow individualism towards the public good. Thus, religion apparently helps those who are most negatively affected by uncontrollable external events and societal circumstances to develop a world view that provides meaning and understanding, as well as a source of optimism and hope for the future. Religious congregations can provide the disenfranchised with the interpersonal community, belonging, and meaningful roles most likely to be lacking in nonempowering social institutions (Kennell, 1985). Finally, for both the minority and mainline congregations, religious imagery and ethics provide a vision and a calling that allow people to reach beyond themselves to seek a greater public good, even in the midst of extremely stressful personal or community circumstances.

Of course, the role of religion in minority communities has the potential for negative as well as positive impacts. Specifically, it has been asserted that "otherworldly" religion is an "opiate" that diminishes social action efforts (G. T. Marx, 1967). In addition, it can be argued that social service outreach efforts distract attention and energy from the real preventive and systemic changes that would represent truly transforming and empowering change for disenfranchised minority communities.

WORKING WITH RELIGION AS A SYSTEM

The previous discussion has hinted of the potential benefits of collaborative work between community psychology and religion. Religious systems address many of the same individual and community concerns that community psychology addresses; these systems also have unique approaches, resources, and access that psychology lacks (Anderson, Maton, & Ensor, 1991). Both psychological and religious communities, then, appear to have much to gain from working together.

Unfortunately, as noted earlier, when psychologists have worked with the religious sector, the interactions have typically been one-sided. Ideally, collaboration with religion should be based on a "resource exchange" model (Kelly, 1986; Kloos, Horneffer, & Moore, 1995; Meylink & Gorsuch, 1986; Tyler, Pargament, & Gatz, 1983), encompassing a full recognition of, and respect for, the unique resources and limitations of religion and psychology.

Religious settings have not often been the focus of community psychology intervention efforts (e.g., Weaver et al., 1998). The existing examples, however, do portray a range of content areas and role relationships as a basis for collaborative efforts with religion, and illustrate the potential value in this work. Several that highlight the unique resources and dilemmas in working with religion will be presented below. Most of these interventions focus on efforts to enhance congregational inreach to its members. To date there are only a few published accounts of collaboration to influence congregational outreach to the community, or to launch efforts to influence cultural practices or basic social institutions in America (e.g., Eng & Hatch, 1991; Cohen et al., 1991; Maton & Seibert, 1991; Shifrin, 1991).

Peer Counseling: The Stephen Series

The Stephen Series is a system of one-to-one helping interactions with congregational members in need carried out by trained lay congregational helpers. The program was developed by Kenneth Haugk, an ordained minister and clinical psychologist (Haugk, 1985). The congregational members receiving help are often identified and referred by the minister; the Series estimates that after contact and encouragement by the minister, over 90% of members agree to accept help from the trained helpers. Those receiving help may be individuals undergoing specific life transitions or stresses, such as divorce, bereavement, and unemployment; or those suffering from physical or emotional problems. To date, over 30,000 congregational helpers have been trained, encompassing over 1100 congregations and over 40 denominations. While empirical evaluation research of the program has not been carried out, it is a program with a strong potential for widespread preventive and promotive influence.

Basic to the Stephen Series program are a series of training and supervision experiences. Initially, leaders from local congregations, often including the minister, receive two weeks of training provided by Stephen Series personnel. Those receiving the initial training then provide 50 hours of training to volunteer lay "Stephen ministers" in their congregation. The lay helpers are then ready to provide assistance to fellow members; however, they continue to receive supervision, education, and support bi-monthly.

The Christian concept of "the priesthood of all believers" serves as the underlying principle guiding the program (1 Peter 2:5–9). Concepts of Christian caring, along with psychological theory and methods, are presented in the training of the helpers. Included as training topics are listening skills, dealing with feelings, crisis intervention, assertiveness, the use of community resources, confidentiality, termination, the use of prayer in ministry, helping people with spiritual concerns, and other aspects of Christian caring.

The successful development of the Stephen Series by a psychologist-minister demonstrates the value of working with change agents who span the worlds of psychology and religion. Clearly, problems of legitimacy and of accurate knowledge of religious systems are likely to be greatly reduced in such efforts. Furthermore, it suggests that community psychologists have the potential to start in motion innovative change efforts in their own religious settings, which can then be disseminated to other settings.

Social Ecological Consultation: Multisite Drug Abuse Prevention Program

Roberts and Thorsheim (1987) used a social ecological consultation approach as part of a four-year drug abuse prevention field research project funded by the National Institute of Drug Abuse. The project focused on Lutheran congregations. Prior to initiation of any prevention programs, the investigators spent a full year consulting with various professionals, church leaders, and congregational members about possible approaches to drug abuse prevention. It was emphasized that each participating congregation would, with the consultation of the investigators, develop its own prevention program; thus the programs would be based on each congregation's unique strengths, resources, and problems. Ultimately, 50 congregations expressed interest in taking part in the program, and of these 24 were chosen—6 as chemical abuse information plus social support activities congregations, 6 as chemical abuse information only congregations, and 12 as control congregations.

Pastors in each of the 12 experimental congregations were asked to form 5-person teams and to identify a team leader. Workshops were held for all 12 of the teams in which the consultants presented information on chemical abuse and chemical abuse prevention. With the six information plus support congregations, the consultants worked closely with the pastors and teams to help plan congregational support activities, programs, meetings, and discussions unique to each congregation. As the authors state, a "partnership approach" was paramount throughout the consultation: "we assumed that we had much to learn from those with whom we were working ... we also hoped, through our own openness and honesty, to encourage trusting relationships and open expression of thoughts and feelings."

The authors report outcome data that indicated that consultation to experimental congregations was related to increased levels of congregational activity regarding abuse prevention, that increased levels of congregational activity was related to member "investment in community," and that increased levels of "investment in community" was inversely related to member alcohol consumption. Central to the "social ecology" consultation was the principle of tailoring each program to the specific needs and desires of the congregation. Furthermore, the locus of control for planning and initiating the prevention activities was clearly within congregational members, with the consultants serving primarily as emotional and technical resources.

Data-Based Change: The Congregation Development Program

Pargament and his colleagues (1991) have worked with over 50 churches and synagogues through the Congregation Development Program (CDP), a data-based assessment and feedback program designed to help congregations assess their strengths and weaknesses and plan for change. Through interviews, questionnaires, and visits, the CDP team gathers information about a variety of dimensions of congregation life: its structure; vision (e.g., personal and social mission) of what it should be about; psychosocial climate; priorities for change; satisfaction with programs, education, leaders, services, facilities, and clergy; and the role of religion in the individual lives of the members. The data are then interpreted jointly with the clergy and leaders of the congregation. Particular attention is paid to how the information can help the congregation move closer to its goals. A number of congregations have initiated significant changes in the congregation as a result of the CDP. These changes include new programming for the elderly, the development of small group projects to increase the sense of community in larger congregations, increased representativeness of church boards, and the development of five-year plans.

The CDP points to some unique challenges to working with religious systems: the need to address similarities and differences in values between psychologist and religious systems; the need to clarify differences between groups in methods for solving problems (i.e., faith and dogma versus data and empiricism); and the need to understand the unique nature of religious authority. However, the CDP also underscores the fact that religious systems are, in many ways, like other systems. For example, clergy and leaders respond to the data gathered by the CDP team with the same interest, hope, fears, resistance, and questions found in other systems.

Congregation-Based Economic Sharing: The Goods and Services Exchange

Maton helped to develop a congregation-based economic sharing and barter program as part of a four-year participant-inhabitant study of a non-denominational, religious fellowship (Maton, 1985). Nine members of the congregation participated as volunteer staff in the program. The staff members prepared position papers and spoke at congregational meetings, including Sunday services, about the biblical imperative for widespread sharing and exchanging of goods and services, both within and outside the churches. A congregational goods and services directory was then developed by distributing a checklist of 179 services and goods to all congregational members. Each person was asked to indicate those services and goods they were willing to provide, lend, or exchange. All information was computerized, allowing easy compilation and updating. A hard copy of the directory was printed for each staff member, categorized by type of service or good offered. Information was updated at six-month intervals.

The key component of the program was ongoing encouragement to church members to contact one of the nine staff members whenever they had an economic need. This person would then locate an individual in the directory with the appropriate resource. Either sharing or exchange could be arranged, depending on the desires of the two individuals involved. Examples of economic needs met were the repair of frozen house plumbing, lending a van for moving, painting an apartment, and giving away an old stove. An initial evaluation of program records indicated that many more people were willing to donate services or goods than to enter into exchange arrangements with a member in need. The idea of exchange apparently ran counter to the "freely giving" theology of the group, although project staff had tried to emphasize its importance in facilitating widespread adoption of economic sharing lifestyles.

This program demonstrated the possibility of mobilizing congregational members to donate time and energy for projects conceived as consistent with the theology and mission of the congregation. However, it also demonstrated that successful project components need to be carefully developed to fit the major beliefs and values of setting members.

Mentoring and Support for Inner-City Youth: Project RAISE

Project RAISE (Raising Ambition Instills Self Esteem) is a collaborative project involving Baltimore City schools, churches, and other community organizations (cf. Maton & Seibert, 1991). The project is aimed at providing inner-city youth with academic and social supports over a seven-year period in order to enable successful academic performance, high school graduation, viable career plans, and reduced psychosocial problems (i.e., teenage pregnancy, substance abuse, anti-social behavior). Thirteen community organizations, each committed to working with a single group of 60 students over the seven-year period, were recruited for the intervention. The 13 sponsoring organizations include six churches, three universities, two businesses, one government agency, and one fraternity. Each sponsor promises to recruit mentors for all students, to carry out regular after-school academic (e.g., tutoring) and cultural (e.g., museum visits) activities, and to contribute $10,000 in support of the students.

Two central RAISE program components are the mentors recruited by the sponsor and each sponsor's full-time program coordinator—in the case of the churches, both mentors and program coordinators are generally members of the sponsoring congregation. The mentor helps the student with academic subjects, serves as a model for personal success and responsibility, and provides attention, concern, and caring. The program coordinator organizes the mentoring and after-school activity components of the RAISE program, and also monitors and advocates for students in the schools on a daily basis.

The motivational and organizational bases of the religiously based RAISE mentors and program coordinators may provide distinct advantages when compared to their non-church-based counterparts (cf., Anderson et al., 1991). For instance, church-based mentors and coordinators may perceive a distinctive mission or calling from God to carry out this work, which may provide an especially deep and enduring commitment to the youth served. Also, religious congregations may be especially likely to provide mentors and program coordinators with the support needed to sustain their commitment and involvement over the seven-year project. In addition, parents and students may be more likely to trust and respond to outreach from church-based, rather than business or university-based, individuals, given the location of churches in the local community and the likelihood of common religious and/or cultural beliefs. Finally, the mentors and program coordinators who desire to make a more in-depth connection or special impact on the youth served (beyond periodic, one-on-one meetings) can naturally invite and involve students and parents in various congregational activities, while to do so in a business or university setting is much less feasible.

Indeed, research to date suggests distinctive impacts for the church-based sponsors. For instance, a survey focusing on those sponsoring organizations within three years of program involvement indicated that students served by the religious sponsors were more likely than those served by non-religious sponsors to currently have a mentor (75% vs. 35% of students, respectively); furthermore, among those students with a current mentor, the relationship with the mentor was of longer duration for those with church-based mentors (22.8 months vs. 8.3 months, respectively) (Maton, Seibert, & DeHaven, 1991). In addition, outcome analyses in which each group of RAISE students was contrasted with a non-RAISE comparison sample revealed more consistent academic gains (attendance, grades, promotions) among students served by congregational sponsors (Maton & Seibert, 1991; Maton et al., 1991). Research is currently planned to examine whether the positive effects of the church-based sponsors will continue over time.

Urban churches and other organizations (e.g., businesses) are increasingly involved in programs to help at-risk minority youth, including "adopt a school" programs, various outreach programs, and the provision of adult role models. In Project RAISE, religious organizations are central to an effort to provide mentoring and after-school support activities to disadvantaged youth, and may have a distinctive and positive impact on them.

Community-Based Development: A Partnership with Religious Institutions

Religious institutions have considerable clout when it comes to community development. Much of this clout is financial; churches and synagogues are among the chief providers of money for social and community action programs. But the clout goes beyond dollars. By their involvement in community development programs, religious institutions lend their prestige to the process of change; they enhance the legitimacy of social action to public officials and to the community itself (Maton & Wells, 1995; Speer, Hughey, Gensheimer, & Adams-Leavitt, 1995; Schorr, 1997).

Recognizing the unique resources of religious institutions, the Lilly Endowment developed a program of collaboration between local churches and other community organizations to revitalize communities (Scheie, Markham, Mayer, Slettom, & Williams, 1991). The program has four goals: (1) to stimulate greater religious institutional involvement in community revitalization, (2) to create new partnerships between religious and community organizations, (3) to strengthen community ministries, and (4) to attract new sources of funding for these activities (p. 5).

In 1989 28 grants were awarded nationally to various forms of religious-community partnership. Most of these partnerships have as their goal the rehabilitation and development of affordable housing for low- to moderate-income families. For example, several religious and community groups came together to form NOAH, the Neighborhood of Affordable Housing in East Boston. NOAH is currently rehabilitating and managing single-room housing units for the elderly, disabled, and working poor. It is also rehabilitating rental housing and converting a vacant church into a youth center.

Scheie et al. (1991) note that viable religious-community partnerships rest on an appreciation of the unique character of each system. They remind the community organization that religious institutions have a different mission—while bringing people to God may occur through community development, it is only one of many paths toward this end. And unlike the community organization, the church is not financially dependent on community revitalization for its survival. Further, religious systems are voluntary organizations that require the support of their members. Thus, they may work according to a longer timetable than the community organization. As Scheie et al. (1991) put it: "They [religious systems] have institutional memories that go back hundreds or thousands of years, and a future vision that stretches to eternity" (p. 75).

In spite of these differences, religious and community organizations have formed effective alliances in this program. As noteworthy as the program's success in community development is its success in obtaining an additional $45 million from sources other than the Lilly Endowment to sustain these partnerships and projects (Scheie et al., 1991). Moreover, the program appears to be increasing the sensitivity and commitment of these religious institutions to community needs, particularly the needs of the poorest. This program illustrates the powerful role the religious institution can play in community life when it looks beyond its own walls to the larger social world.

CHALLENGES, QUESTIONS, AND POSSIBILITIES FOR A COMMUNITY PSYCHOLOGY OF RELIGION

Clearly, religion is an integral part of American life. A very important implication for community psychology follows: *Without an understanding of religion in American life, an understanding of community in American life remains incomplete.* Thus, the processes of learning about, learning from, and working with religious systems are not only legitimate, but essential tasks, for community psychology. Progress has been made in each of these areas. And yet, not surprisingly, this work raises further challenges, questions, and possibilities for a community psychology of religion.

In moving from a person-centered, undifferentiated perspective to an ecological view that encompasses multiple levels of analysis, a richer, more complex picture of religion is beginning to emerge. Shaped by a myriad of personal and systemic forces, religion also affects individuals and society in a variety of ways. Yet the "whys, whens, and hows" of this transaction are far from clear. A key task for community psychology is to develop a deeper understanding of the processes through which religious institutions, both local and societal, take on their unique identity and, in turn, impact on their members and larger society. Many of the central concepts and methods of the discipline are well-suited to this task (Maton, 1993a). However, this research should encompass not only psychological perspectives, but sociological, anthropological, economic, and theological frameworks as well. In addition, this analysis requires a historical perspective and a diversity of research methods, including ethnographic and qualitative approaches (e.g., Maton, 1993b; Rappaport, 1995; Wuthnow, 1994).

Important implications for community research and action can be drawn from the unique responses of religion to concerns vital to our discipline: the need for meaning and understanding, the need for community and belonging, moving beyond a narrow individualism to a commitment to the public good, and responsivity to disenfranchised and marginal groups. For instance, concerning the need for meaning and understanding, intervention could be considered that enhance the world view, and the sense of historical and life "meaning" of individuals. These interventions could take place in collaboration with any of the primary social institutions, such as family, education, social services, business, or religion. In addition, religion's tradition of helping people come to terms with uncontrollable events points to the importance of careful evaluation of the conditions under which personal control, individualism, and empiricism diminish or enrich individual and social well-being.

The success of many religious systems at building community also underscores important targets for community research and action. Research programs should be geared to discovering the factors that build community in religious and other social settings as a foundation for consultation and intervention efforts. Particular attention should be paid to the idea of ongoing "small group base units," and of participatory role creation, to help restructure and enhance community in settings such as schools, neighborhoods, and places of work. Finally, focusing on our own discipline's needs for enhanced community, we might learn some valuable lessons from religious systems; in particular, the importance of explicit attempts to develop traditions, symbols, and organizational structures that generate continuity, contact, and shared individuality-in-community.

Insights from religious institutions also highlight the significance of research and interventions that help individuals and systems move beyond narrow individualism and to care, reflect, and take action about larger social issues. Particularly needed in our institutions are images and visions effective in empowering individuals and their systems to care for the well-being of themselves *and* each other, rather than at the expense of each other (Bakan, 1966; Sarason, 1987). Concepts, empirical methods, theoretical frameworks, and discourse languages that help generate these synergistic alternatives to narrow individualism are important priorities for our work (e.g., Bellah et al., 1985; Maton, 1987; Pargament & Myers, 1982).

The central role of religion and religious systems in the lives of the disenfranchised and marginal poses serious challenges for community psychology as a field. First and foremost, it raises questions about why so few linkages have been developed with religious systems, given the avowed interests of the discipline in aiding marginal and disenfranchised groups (see Kloos et al., 1995). Furthermore, it challenges researchers to undertake systematic study of the preventive and empowering potential of religious systems, both minority and mainline, which have access to disenfranchised and lower income groups (Maton & Wells, 1995). Finally, it underscores the need for intervention programs, at the individual and institutional levels, which bring together the complementary resources of religion and community psychology (Queen, 1997).

The increasing importance of spirituality in individual lives points to another potentially important area of focus for community psychology. Much of the current work on this topic has an individualistic, even anti-institutional, bias (Pargament, 1999; Zinnbauer, Pargament, & Scott, in press). Spirituality, however, cannot be understood outside of a larger social context. There are, in American society, a number of community settings, unaffiliated with religious institutions, that are explicitly designed to enhance spiritual development. For example, by the 1980s, it was estimated that 400 new spiritual organizations had been formed (Hood et al., 1996). Furthermore, many Americans meet regularly with others in some form of small group that builds upon, and/or contributes to, interests in spirituality (cf., Roof, 1993; Wuthnow, 1994). Included among these groups are a variety of settings that are not connected to institutionalized religion, such as self-help groups (e.g., Alcoholics Anonymous), women's spirituality groups, and certain men's self-development organizations (e.g., Mankind Project; Mankowski, Maton, Anderson, Burke, & Hoover, in press). Clearly, a community psychology of religion, broadly and meaningfully defined, needs to encompass the varied manifestations of spirituality in American culture, both within mainstream and non-mainstream religious traditions and across a diversity of settings that may or may not be allied with institutionalized religion. Taken together, they represent important sites to examine the confluence of the search for spirituality and community in American society, and the impact of this search on individual lives and the larger community.

As noted previously, most of the work in the community psychology of religion has taken place at the organizational, or local institutional, level of analysis. It is an important priority to continue research and interventions at this level. In addition, however, a central challenge for future research and action is to focus on religion at the cultural or social institutional level of analysis, as illustrated by the work of Bellah et al. (1985). Collaborative research with other social science disciplines may facilitate research at this level of analysis. Projects can also be implemented that attempt to support and develop denominational and ecumenical policies and theologies consistent with the cultural values of respect for diversity, the dignity and strength of the individual, and social justice. At the national level, this type of work would require close collaboration with major policymaking groups (e.g., the National Council of Churches; National Association of Black Churches; American Council of Bishops), and dialogue with theologians with a national influence. Alternatively, psychologists could aide in the creation of new religious settings (e.g., social action congregations) that may, in turn, influence mainline religion and culture.

In this chapter, we have stressed the importance of recognizing and respecting the unique resources and limitations of religion and of psychology. One final challenge, and a source of ongoing questioning, for a community psychology of religion concerns the most appropriate response to differences in values and world views between psychologist and religious institution. When there is substantial overlap in both the goals and chosen interventions of community psychologist and particular religious setting, value-related questions are less likely to come to the foreground. For example, both the psychologist and the religious community may feel comfortable in working towards a greater sense of community and competence within a congregation through active participative problem-solving methods. However, in other settings, differences in values may raise major dilemmas. For instance, what happens when the religious systems defines numerical growth as the *sine qua non* of well-being, while the psychologist believes that "bigger is not necessarily better"? Or, what happens when the psychologist and religious system differ in the value they place on certain religious problem solutions, such as deference to religious authority or passive forms of prayer?

There is no straightforward solution to the problem of differences in values and world views. Certainly, the psychologist must struggle with the tension between the need to promote his or her own values, and the need to affirm diverse ways of being human. The psychologist may then choose to work with more compatible systems, work within the system to create change, or work towards the creation of alternate settings. Regardless of the choice, value concerns should be an important topic of dialogue between psychological and religious communities as a prelude to work together. This dialogue may help prevent abuses of power, and promote greater trust and cooperation between groups.

In sum, as yet, our knowledge of religious systems is modest. What we do know highlights the important and challenging opportunities to learn about, learn from, and work with religious institutions. A community psychology perspective provides a significant framework for these basic and applied tasks. Further progress towards a community psychology of religion requires increased efforts on the part of our discipline to wrestle with the complexity, power, and diverse implications of religion in American life.

REFERENCES

Albee, G. W. (1982). Preventing psychopathology and promoting human potential. *American Psychologist, 9,* 1043–1050.

Anderson, R. W., Jr., Maton, K. I., & Ensor, B. E. (1991). Prevention theory and action from the religious perspective. *Prevention in Human Services, 10,* 9–28.

Bakan, D. (1966). *The duality of human experience: Isolation and communion in western man.* Boston: Beacon.

Barton, A. H. (1971). Selected problems in the study of religious development. In M. Strommen (Ed.), *Research on religious development* (pp. 836–855). New York: Hawthorn.

Batson, C., Schoenrade, P., & Ventis, W. (1993). *Religion and the individual: A social-psychological perspective.* New York: Oxford University Press.

Baugh, J. R. (1988). Gaining control by giving up control: Strategies for coping with powerlessness. In W. R. Miller and J. E. Martin (Eds.), *Behavior therapy and religion: Integrating spiritual and behavioral approaches to change* (pp. 125–138). Newbury Park: Sage.

Becker, E. (1968). *The structure of evil.* New York: G. Braziller.

Beit-Hallahmi, B. (1974). Psychology of religion 1880–1930: The rise and fall of a psychological movement. *Journal of the History of the Behavioral Sciences, 10,* 84–90.

Bellah, R. N., Madsen, R., Sullivan, W. M., Swidler, A., & Tipton, S. M. (1985). *Habits of the heart: Individualism and commitment in American life.* Berkeley: University of California Press.

Benson, P., & Spilka, B. (1973). God image as a function of self-esteem and locus of control. *Journal for the Scientific Study of Religion, 12,* 297–310.

Benson, P. L., & Williams, D. L. (1982). *Religion on capitol hill: Myths and realities.* New York: Harper & Row.

Benson, P. L., Woods, P. K., Johnson, A. L., Eklin, C. H., and Mills, J. E. (1983). *Report on 1983 Minnesota Survey on Drug Use and Drug-Related Attitude,* Minneapolis: Search Institute.

Berger, P. L. (1967). *The sacred canopy: Elements of a sociological theory of religion.* New York: Doubleday.

Berger, P. L., & Neuhaus, R. J. (1977). To empower people: The role of mediating structures in public policy. Washington, D.C.: American Enterprise Institute for Public Policy.

Bergin, A. (1983). Religiosity and mental health: A critical reevaluation and meta-analysis. *Professional Psychology, 14,* 170–184.

Berton, P. (1965). *The comfortable pew.* Toronto, Canada: McClelland and Stewart.

Bickel, C., Sheers, N. J., Estadt, B. K., Powell, D., & Pargament, K. I. (1998). Perceived stress, religious coping styles, and depressive affect. *Journal of Psychology and Christianity, 17,* 33–42.

Boyte, H. C. (1984). *Community is possible: Repairing America's roots.* New York: Harper and Row.

Campbell, E., & Pettigrew, T. (1959). Racial and moral crisis: The role of Little Rock ministers. *American Journal of Sociology, 64,* 509–516.

Carney, F. S. (1978). Ethics: Theological ethics. In W. T. R. Reich (Ed.), *Encyclopedia of Bioethics* (pp. 429–437). New York: Free Press.

Carroll, J., Dudley, C., & McKinney, W. (1986). *Handbook for congregational studies.* Nashville, TN: Abingdon.

Carson, R. J. (1976). *Mental health centers and local clergy: A source book of sample projects.* Washington, D.C.: Community Mental Health Institute.

Cohen, E., Mowbray, C. T., Gillette, V., & Thompson, E. (1991). Preventing homelessness: Religious organizations and housing development. *Prevention in Human Services, 10*, 169–186.

Cole, B., & Pargament, K. I. (1999). Spiritual surrender: A paradoxical path to control. In W. Miller (Ed.), *Integrating spirituality in treatment: Resources for practitioners* (pp. 179–198). Washington, D.C.: APA Books.

Donahue, M. J. (1985). Intrinsic and extrinsic religiousness: Review and meta-analysis. *Journal of Personality and Social Psychology, 48*, 400–419.

Ellis, A. (1960). There is no place for the concept of sin in psychotherapy. *Journal of Counseling Psychology, 7*, 188–192.

Ellison, C. G. (1993). Religious involvement and self-perception among Black Americans. *Social Forces, 71*, 1027–1055.

Eng, E., & Hatch, J. W. (1991). Networking between agencies and black churches: The lay health advisor model. *Prevention in Human Services, 10*, 123–146.

Evans, B. F. (1979). Campaign for human development: Church involvement in social change. *Review of Religious Research, 20*, 264–278.

Frazier, E. F. (1964). *The Negro church in America.* New York: Schocken.

Freud, S. (1949). *The future of an illusion.* New York: Liveright.

Gallup, G., Jr., & Castelli, J. (1989). *The people's religion: American faith in the 90's.* New York: MacMillan.

Garrison, V. (1977). Doctor, espiritista or psychiatrist?: Health-seeking behavior in a Puerto Rican neighborhood of New York City. *Medical Anthropology, (Spring)*, 66–191.

Glock, C. Y., Ringer, B. B., and Babbie, R. (1967). *To comfort and to challenge: A dilemma of the contemporary church.* Berkeley: University of California Press.

Glock, C., & Stark, R. (1966). *Christian beliefs and anti-Semitism.* New York: Harper.

Gorsuch, R. (1988). Psychology of religion. *Annual Review of Psychology, 39*, 201–221.

Gutierrez, G. (1988). *A theology of liberation.* London: SCM.

Hallie, P. (1979). *Lest innocent blood be shed.* New York: Harper and Row.

Hathaway, W. L., & Pargament, K. I. (1991). The religious dimension of coping: Implications for prevention and promotion. *Prevention in Human Services, 9*, 65–92.

Haugk, K. (1976). Unique contributions of churches and clergy to community mental health. *Community Mental Health Journal, 12*, 21–27.

Haugk, K. (1985). *Christian caregiving—a way of life.* Minneapolis, MN: Augsburg.

Herman, S. N. (1977). *Jewish identity: A social psychological perspective, Volume 48.* Beverly Hills: Sage.

Hood, R. W., Jr., Spilka, B., Hunsberger, B., & Gorsuch, R. (1996). *The psychology of religion: An empirical approach* (2nd ed.), New York: Guilford.

Horton, A. L., Wilkins, M. M., & Wright, W. (1988). Women who ended abuse: What religious leaders and religion did for these victims. In A. L. Horton and J. A. Williamson (Eds.). *Abuse and religion: When praying isn't enough* (pp. 235–246). Lexington, MA: Lexington Books.

Hrabowski, F. A. III, Maton, K. I., & Greif, G. (1998). *Beating the odds: Raising academically successful African American males.* New York: Oxford University Press.

Jacquet, C., Jr. (1986). *Yearbook of American and Canadian churches 1986.* Nashville: Abingdon.

Jacquet, C., Jr., & Jones, A. M. (1991). *Yearbook of American and Canadian churches 1991.* Nashville: Abingdon.

James, W. (1902). *The varieties of religious experience.* New York: Random House.

Jason, L. A. (1997). *Community building: Values for a sustainable future.* Westport, CT: Greenwood.

Jenkins, R., & Pargament, K. (1988). Cognitive appraisals in cancer patients. *Social Science and Medicine, 26*, 625–633.

Kelley, D. (1977). *Why conservative churches are growing.* New York: Harper & Row.

Kelly, J. (1986). Context and process: An ecological view of the interdependence of practice and research. *American Journal of Community Psychology, 14*, 581–599.

Kennell, J. (1985). *The role of a Nazarene church in the lives of its member: A test of three models.* Unpublished doctoral dissertation. Bowling Green State University, Bowling Green, OH.

Kloos, B., Horneffer, K., & Moore, T. (1995). Before the beginning; Religious leaders' perceptions of the possibility for mutual beneficial collaboration with psychologists. *Journal of Community Psychology, 23*, 275–291.

Koenig, H. G. (1994). *Aging and God.* New York: Haworth.

Koenig, H. G. (1997). *Is religion good for your health*? New York: Haworth.

Koenig, H. G., Bearon, L. B., Hover, M., & Travis, J. L. (1991). Religious perspectives of doctors, nurses, patients, and families. *Journal of Pastoral Care, 45*, 254–267.

Krause, N., & Van Tran, T. (1989). Stress and religious involvement among older blacks. *Journal of Gerontology and Social Sciences, 44*, S4–S13.

Larson, D. B., Pattison, E. M., Blazer, D. G., Omran, A. R., & Kaplan, B. H. (1986). Systematic analysis of research on religious variables in four major psychiatric journals, 1978–1982. *American Journal of Psychiatry, 143*, 329–334.

Lasch, C. (1979). *The culture of narcissism: American life in an age of diminishing expectations.* New York: Norton.

Levin, J. S., & Vanderpool, H. Y. (1991). Religious factors in physical health and the prevention of illness. *Prevention in Human Services, 9*, 41–64.

Lindenthal, J. J., Myers, J. K., Pepper, M. P., & Stein, M. S. (1970). Mental status and religious behavior. *Journal for the Scientific Study of Religion, 9*, 143–149.

Mankowski, E. S., Maton, K. I., Burke, C. K., Hoover, S. A., & Anderson, C. A. (in press). Collaborative research with a men's organization: Psychological impact, group functioning, and organizational growth. In E. Barton (Ed.), *Mythopoetic perspectives in men's healing work.* Westport, CT: Greenwood.

Marx, G. T. (1967). *Protest and prejudice.* New York: Harper & Row.

Maton, K. I. (1985). *Economic sharing among members of a religious setting: Patterns and psychological correlates.* Unpublished doctoral dissertation, University of Illinois at Urbana-Champaign.

Maton, K. I. (1987). *Towards an integrated, strengths model of the person in community research: The role of providing and receiving support to well-being.* Paper presented at the First Biennial Conference on Community Research and Action, Columbia, SC, May 20.

Maton, K. I. (1988, August). *A contributory, strengths, bidirectional perspective on congregational member well-being.* Paper presented at the 96th Annual Meeting of the American Psychological Association, Atlanta, GA.

Maton, K. I. (1989a). Community settings as buffers of life stress: Highly supportive churches, mutual help groups, and senior centers. *American Journal of Community Psychology, 17*, 203–232.

Maton, K. I. (1989b). The stress-buffering role of spiritual support: Cross-sectional and prospective investigations. *Journal for the Scientific Study of Religion, 28*, 310–323.

Maton, K. I. (1993a). A bridge between cultures: Linked ethnographic empirical methodology for culture-anchored research. *American Journal of Community Psychology, 21*, 701–727.

Maton, K. I. (1993b). Moving beyond the individual level of analysis in mutual help group research: An ecological paradigm. *Journal of Applied Behavioral Science, 29*, 272–286.

Maton, K. I., Hrabowski, F. A. III, & Greif, G. (1998). Preparing the way: A qualitative study of high achieving African American males and the role of the family. *American Journal of Community Psychology, 26*, 639–668.

Maton, K. I., & Pargament, K. I. (1987). The roles of religion in prevention and promotion. *Prevention in Human Services, 5*, 161–205.

Maton, K. I., & Rappaport, J. (1984). Empowerment in a religious setting: A multivariate investigation. *Prevention in Human Services, 3*, 37–72.

Maton, K. I., & Salem, D. (1995). Organizational characteristics of empowering community settings: A multiple case study approach. *American Journal of Community Psychology, 23*, 631–656.

Maton, K. I., & Seibert, M. (1991). *Third year evaluation of Project RAISE.* Unpublished evaluation report. University of Maryland Baltimore County, December.

Maton, K. I., Seibert, M., & DeHaven, G. (1991). *First year evaluation of Project RAISE II.* Unpublished evaluation report, University of Maryland Baltimore County, December.

Maton, K. I., Teti, D., Corns, K., Vieira-Baker, K., Lavine, J., Gouze, K. R., & Keating, D. (1996). Cultural specificity of social support sources, correlates and contexts: Three studies of African-American and Caucasian youth. *American Journal of Community Psychology, 24*, 551–587.

Maton, K. I., & Wells, B. (1995). Religion as a resource for well-being: Prevention, healing, and empowerment pathways. *Journal of Social Issues, 51*, 177–193.

McGaw, D. B. (1979). Commitment and religious community: A comparison of a charismatic and a mainline congregation. *Journal for the Scientific Study of Religion, 18*, 146–163.

McIntosh, D., & Spilka, B. (1990). Religion and physical health: The role of personal faith and control beliefs. In M. L. Lynn & D. O. Moberg (Eds.), *Research in the Social Scientific Study of Religion. Vol. 2* (pp. 167–194). Greenwich, CT: JAI Press.

McMillan, D. W., & Chavis, D. M. (1986). Sense of community: A definition and theory. *Journal of Community Psychology, 14*, 6–23.

Meylink, W. D., & Gorsuch, R. L. (1986). New perspectives for clergy–psychologist referrals. *Journal of Psychology and Christianity, 5*, 62–70.

Moore, T. (1991). The African-American church: A source of empowerment, mutual help, and social change. *Prevention in Human Services, 10*, 147–168.

Niebuhr, H. R. (1963). *The responsible self: An essay in Christian moral philosophy.* New York: Harper and Row.

Pargament, K. I. (1982). The interface among religion, religious support systems and mental health. In D. Biegel and A. Naperstak (Eds.), *Community support systems and mental health.* New York: Springer.

Pargament, K. I. (1992). Of means and ends: Religion and the search for significance. *International Journal for the Psychology of Religion, 2*, 201–229.

Pargament, K. I. (1997). *The psychology of religion and coping: Theory, research, practice.* New York: Guilford.

Pargament, K. I. (1999). The psychology of religion *and* spirituality? Yes and no. *International Journal for the Psychology of Religion, 9,* 3–16.

Pargament, K. I., Brannick, M., Adamakos, H., Ensing, D., Kelemen, M., Warren, R., Falgout, K., Cook, P., & Myers, J. (1987). Indiscriminate proreligiousness: Conceptualization and measurement. *Journal of the Scientific Study of Religion, 26,* 182–201.

Pargament, K., Echemendia, R., Johnson, S., Myers, J., Cook, P., Brannick, M., & McGath, C. (1987). The conservative church: Psychosocial advantages and disadvantages. *American Journal of Community Psychology, 15,* 269–286.

Pargament, K. I., Ensing, D. S., Falgout, K., Olsen, H., Reilly, B., Van Haitsma, K., & Warren, R. (1990). God help me (I): Religious coping efforts as predictors of the outcomes to significant negative life events. *American Journal of Community Psychology, 18,* 793–824.

Pargament, K. I., Falgout, K., Ensing, D. S., Reilly, B., Silverman, M., Van Haitsma, K., Olsen, H., & Warren, R. (1991). The congregation development program: Data-based consultation with churches and synagogues. *Professional Psychology, 22,* 303–404.

Pargament, K., Grevengoed, N., Kennell, J., Newman, J., Hathaway, W., & Jones, W. (1988). Religion and the problem solving process: Three styles of coping. *Journal for the Scientific Study of Religion, 27,* 90–104.

Pargament, K. I., & Hahn, J. (1986). God and the just world: Causal and coping attributions to God in health situations. *Journal for the Scientific Study of Religion, 25,* 193–207.

Pargament, K., Johnson, S., Echemendia, R., & Silverman, I. (1985). The limits of fit: Examining the implications of person-environment congruence in different religious settings. *Journal of Community Psychology, 13,* 20–30.

Pargament, K. I., Maton, K. I., & Hess, R. E. (Eds.). (1992). *Religion and prevention in mental health: Research, vision, and action.* Binghamton, NY: Haworth.

Pargament, K., & Myers, J. (1982). *The individual-system spiral: A foundation of value for action in community psychology.* Presented at American Psychological Association, Washington, D.C.

Pargament, K., Silverman, I., Johnson, S., Echemendia, R., & Snyder, S. (1983). The psychosocial climate of religious congregations. *American Journal of Community Psychology, 11,* 351–381.

Pargament, K., Sullivan, M., Tyler, F., & Steele, R. (1982). Patterns of attribution of control and individual psychosocial competence. *Psychological Reports, 51,* 1243–1252.

Pargament, K. I., Tyler, F., & Steele, R. (1979a). The church/synagogue and the psychosocial competence of the member: An initial inquiry into a neglected dimension. *American Journal of Community Psychology, 7,* 649–664.

Pargament, K., Tyler, F., & Steele, R. (1979b). Is fit It? The relationship between church/synagogue-member fit and the psychosocial competence of the member. *Journal of Community Psychology, 7,* 243–252.

Payne, I. R., Bergin, A. E., Bielema, K. A., & Jenkins, P. H. (1991). Review of religion and mental health: Prevention and the enhancement of psychosocial functioning. *Prevention in Human Services, 9,* 11–40.

Queen, E. L. II, (1997). Seeing ourselves in others: Changing civic roles for religious organizations. *Wingspread Journal, 19,* 10–12.

Radcliffe-Brown, A. R. (1939). *Taboo.* Cambridge, MA: Harvard University Press.

Rappaport, J. (1981). In praise of paradox: A social policy of empowerment over prevention. *American Journal of Community Psychology, 9,* 1–25.

Rappaport, J. (1995). Empowerment meets narrative: Listening to stories and creative settings. *American Journal of Community Psychology, 23,* 795–807.

Rappaport, J., & Simkins, R. (1991). Healing and empowerment through community narrative. *Prevention in Human Services, 10,* 29–50.

Roberts, B., & Thorsheim, H. (1987). A partnership approach to consultation: The process and results of a major primary prevention field experiment. In J. G. Kelly and R. Hess (Eds.), *The ecology of prevention: Illustrating mental health consultation.* Binghamton, NY: Haworth.

Roberts, K. A. (1990). *Religion in sociological perspective.* Belmont, CA: Wadsworth.

Roberts, K. A. (1991). A sociological overview: Mental health implications of religio-cultural megatrends in the United States. *Prevention in Human Services, 9,* 113–135.

Roof, W. C. (1993). *A generation of seekers: The spiritual journey of the baby-boomer generation.* San Francisco: HarperCollins.

Roozen, D., McKinney, W., & Carroll, J. (1984). *Varieties of religious presence.* New York: Pilgrim Press.

Rubin, J. Z. (1982). *Being a positively marginal Jew.* Paper presented at the American Psychological Association: Washington, D.C., August.

Sarason, S. B. (1986). And what is the public interest? *American Psychologist, 41,* 899–905.

Sarason, S. B. (1987). *Barometers of community change.* Invited address to the First Biennial Conference on Community Research and Action, Columbia, S.C., May 21.

Sarason, S. B. (1993). American psychology, and the needs for transcendence and community. *American Journal of Community Psychology, 21*, 185–202.

Schaefer, C. A., & Gorsuch, R. L. (1991). Psychological adjustment and religiousness: The multivariate belief-motivation theory of religiousness. *Journal for the Scientific Study of Religion, 30*, 448–461.

Scheie, D. M., Markham, J., Mayer, S. E., Slettom, J., & Williams, T. (1991). *Religious institutions as partners in community based program development: Findings from year one of the Lilly Endowment Program.* Minneapolis, MN: Rainbow Research.

Schorr, L. R. (1997). *Common purpose: Strengthening families and neighborhoods to rebuild America.* New York: Anchor.

Schumaker, J. F. (Ed.) (1992). *Religion and mental health.* New York: Oxford University Press.

Shafranske, E. P., & Malony, H. N. (1990). Clinical psychologists' religious and spiritual orientations and their practices of psychotherapy. *Psychotherapy, 27*, 72–78.

Shifrin, J. (1991). The religious community and mental illness: The problems—the possibilities. *Psychologists Interested in Religious Issues Newsletter, 16*, 1–15.

Siegel, J. M., & Kuykendall, D. H. (1990). Loss, widowhood, and psychological distress among the elderly. *Journal of Consulting and Clinical Psychology, 58*, 519–524.

Speer, P. W., Hughey, J., Gensheimer, L. K., & Adams-Leavitt, W. (1995). Organizing for power: A comparative case study. *Journal of Community Psychology, 23*, 57–73.

Spilka, B., & Bridges, R. A. (1991). Religious perspectives on prevention: The role of theology. *Prevention in Human Services, 9*, 93–112.

Strommen, M., Brekke, M., Underwager, R., & Johnson, A. (1972). *A study of generations.* Minneapolis, MN: Augsburg.

Troeltsch, E. (1931). *The social teachings of the Christian churches* (O. Wynn, trans.). New York: Macmillan.

Tyler, F., Pargament, K., & Gatz, M. (1983). The resource collaborator role: A model for interactions involving psychologists. *American Psychologist, 38*, 388–398.

Weaver, A. J., Samford, J., Kline, A. E., Lucas, L. A., Larson, D. B., & Koenig, H. G. (1998). What do psychologists know about working with clergy? An analysis of eight APA journals: 1991–1994. *Professional Psychology, 28*, 471–474.

Williams, D. R., Larson, D. B., Buckler, R. E., Heckman, R. C., & Pyle, C. M. (1989). *Religion and psychological distress in a community sample.* Paper presented at American Psychological Association, New Orleans, Louisiana.

Williams, M. D. (1974). *Community in a black Pentecostal church.* Pittsburgh, PA: University of Pittsburgh Press.

Wilson, B. R. (1959). An analysis of sect development. *American Sociological Review, 24*, 3–15.

Wimberly, E. P. (1979). *Pastoral care in the black church.* Nashville, TN: Abingdon.

Wulff, D. M. (1997). *Psychology of religion: Classic and contemporary* (2nd ed.). New York: Wiley.

Wuthnow, R. (1994). *Sharing the journey: Support groups and America's new quest for community.* New York: Free Press.

Zinnbauer, B. J., Pargament, K. I., & Scott, A. B. (in press). The emerging meanings of religiousness and spirituality: Problems and prospects. *Journal of Personality.*

CHAPTER 22

Community Change, Community Stasis, and the Law

GARY B. MELTON

A useful starting point for consideration of law and community psychology is to pose a literary existential question: why should a handbook on community psychology have a chapter on law? I suspect that the initial (and perhaps the only) answer that comes to the minds of most community psychologists is that the law represents a means of community change. One strategy that a community psychologist can stimulate when a class of people is mistreated is to "sue the bastards." Indeed, if the conventional wisdom is to be believed (and empirical data suggest that in this matter it should not; see Galanter, 1983; Trubek. 1984), the predominant American response to interpersonal and class conflict is to resort to litigation. In popular lore, Perry Mason; Judge Wapner (or his successor, mayor-turned-TV-judge Ed Koch); the litigators at McKenzie, Brackman; and most recently, a spate of dramatic prosecutors and public defenders are the referees in, and sometimes the initiators of, social conflict—the bearers of the "big stick" who will ensure that justice triumphs. Play in the political arena may be limited to those with numbers and bucks big enough to be noticed, but the power of the law (so the image goes) is there to be exercised by he who is right, not necessarily he who is privileged. The courts theoretically offer an even playing field in which all actors, regardless of their wealth or their power in other arenas, are empowered to defend and promote their interests.

This rather dramatic and awe-filled view of the law is not completely divorced from reality. However, few now would dispute the premise that the law is not simply a collection of autonomous neutral principles. Legal decision-making involves more than the judicial "slot machine" into which such principles, with nothing more, are dropped, and the logical answer emerges. The cliché that "we are all realists now" reflects the widespread recognition that judges *do* and, most legal scholars would argue, *should* make policy. The law includes abstract principles, but it also subsumes social and political reality.

Not only is the law less reliant on principles than many would claim, but often it is a nearly impotent or at least inefficient instrument in ensuring that those principles are fully

GARY B. MELTON • Institute on Family and Neighborhood Life, Clemson University, Clemson, South Carolina 29634.

Handbook of Community Psychology, edited by Julian Rappaport and Edward Seidman. Kluwer Academic / Plenum Publishers, New York, 2000.

applied. The law often is ineffectual in engineering social change, especially when authorities attempt to alter a particular behavior or relationship directly through application of sanctions for misconduct. Indeed, if it were otherwise in a democratic society, the law would be operating in a manner inconsistent with the principles on which it is grounded. Enacted, administered, and interpreted by elected representatives of the people (or individuals appointed by such officials), the law is presumed to *reflect*, not to change, the norms of the community.

In that regard, a better answer to the opening question may be the second response to be considered—that the law is the institution whose function most clearly is to reflect and promote the values of the community. Perhaps more than any other institution, the law serves, at its best, to cement a collective identity, to reify the myths and norms of the culture (see, e.g., Bellah, 1975; Geertz, 1980; Melton, 1987c). Indeed, if the law is successful in fulfilling its mission, development of a psychological sense of community may be nearly congruent with legal socialization (see Melton, 1992; Tapp & Levine, 1974). Therefore, the law as an institution should be a major focus of study for those who wish to understand the psychology of community life, and a major focus of intervention for those who wish to shape a shared sense of community.

Third, in a less positive sense, community psychologists might be interested in the law because the law may serve as an impediment to change. Not only does the law conserve the values of the culture and promote a sense of community, but it also concretizes social structures in ways that diminish their amenability to change. For example, reform of the social service and mental health systems frequently has been impeded by the corollary necessity of changing civil service and administrative structures (see, e.g., *New York State Association for Retarded Children, Inc., v. Carey*, 1978; Reppucci, 1977; Rothman & Rothman, 1984).

The law also may serve the interests of particular groups, apart from the interests of the community as a whole or even the principles on which the law is purported to rest. In that respect, as the scholars in the critical legal-studies movement have argued (see, e.g., Unger, 1983), legal doctrines often may be reconstructed to reach results consistent with the interests of privileged classes. For example, Rosen (1984) found decisions of the United States Supreme Court to be highly correlated with prevailing attitudes among affluent older Americans. Even if one moves outside an analysis of class conflict, it remains clear that, contrary to its role as moral guidepost, the law sometimes legitimizes and reifies the basest prejudices of the majority. The law long has catered to outrageous beliefs about people with mental disabilities (Melton & Garrison, 1987), and racial segregation and concomitant subjugation of blacks were sustained for nearly a century by an elaborate system of Jim Crow laws (Woodward, 1974). If community psychologists seek to promote social change, they must understand not only the ways that the law can be an avenue to empowerment of disenfranchised groups, but also the ways that the law stands in the way of change.

A fourth reason for considering the law in a handbook of community psychology is that the legal system is a forum in which policy is made or announced. A potential role of community psychology is to inform policymakers about human behavior and community life (Task Force on Psychology and Public Policy, 1986). In that sense, the primary purpose is not to change the principles that underlie the law, but instead to help the legal system to meet its own goals rationally and efficiently (see. e.g., Melton, 1987c, 1992). When an assumption about behavior is relevant to a legal analysis, community psychologists may inform legal decision-makers about scientific knowledge (or indeed may gather such information themselves) about the validity of the assumption. Such an approach, termed *social science in law* (Melton, Monahan, & Saks, 1987; Monahan & Walker, 1998), permits the law itself to set the agenda for community psychologists' work in the legal system. From that viewpoint, psychologists' success in the legal system is determined in large part by their ability to take an "inside" perspective and to frame their work so that it can be easily applied in legal analyses (Melton, 1987a, 1987b; Melton, Monahan, & Saks, 1987).

A final reason for community psychologists' attention to the law also may be conceptualized as *serving*, rather than changing, the law. At a micro level, the law is the institution that society has designated for resolution of conflict. Whether the matter at hand is the dissolution of a marriage, the compensation of an injured party, the determination of criminal blameworthiness, or the restraint of race-, gender-, or disability-based discrimination in education or employment, the courts are charged with expressing the conscience of the community and, in so doing, achieving just resolution of disputes. Armed with knowledge about factors affecting perceived justice (see, e.g., Lerner & Lerner, 1981; Lind & Tyler, 1988; Thibaut & Walker, 1978; Tyler, 1987, 1988), psychologists can assist in the development, implementation, and evaluation of legal procedures intended to match the law's own goals (see, e.g., Melton, Goodman, Kalichman, Levine, & Koocher, 1995; Melton & Limber, 1989).

To summarize, community psychology is potentially concerned with law in five ways: (1) a means of community change, (2) an expression of community identity, (3) an impediment to change, (4) a forum for policy development and implementation, and (5) the arbiter of micro-level conflict. Each of these functions will be considered in turn.

INSTRUMENTAL EFFECTS OF LAW: FORMS OF LEGAL INTERVENTION

Direct Regulation

Deterrence

To understand the effects of law, it is useful to consider the diverse ways in which its force can be applied. The most obvious means is through deterrence: fear of sanctions, whether criminal, civil (through the law of torts), or administrative. Few psychological researchers and theorists have studied deterrence (but see Carroll, 1978), despite the fact that it is an explicitly psychological concept. Instead, sociological and economic research ostensibly focused on deterrence in general has examined aggregate data, without the elimination of alternative explanations of law impact (or lack of it).

The most comprehensive and elegant conceptualization of deterrence was offered by Gibbs (1985), who noted the critical psychological elements of the concept: "Deterrence occurs when a potential offender refrains from or curtails criminal [or other illegal] activity because he or she *perceives* some threat of a legal punishment for contrary behavior and *fears* that punishment" (p. 87, emphasis added). In Gibbs's admittedly incomplete theory, a test of the deterrent effects of a law requires attention to 12 variables: (1) objective and (2) perceived certainty of an actual legal punishment; (3) presumptive and (4) perceived severity of a statutory or prescribed legal punishment; (5) objective and (6) perceived severity of an actual legal punishment; (7) objective and (8) perceived celerity of an actual legal punishment; (9) normative and (10) perceived normative scope of a statutory or prescribed legal punishment; (11) actual and (12) perceived actual scope of a statutory or prescribed legal punishment. Note that evaluation of deterrent effects requires knowledge of the law on the books, the law in practice, and citizens' perceptions of the law. No study yet has evaluated more than two of the 12 variables, and most of the variables have not been studied at all, especially in regard to specific deterrence (Gibbs, 1985).

Assessment of effects requires attention not only to multiple variables, but also to individual differences. Presumably, as Gibbs points out, most citizens comply with the law, regardless of fear of punishment. Combination of their perceptions with those of hard-core offenders renders the aggregate essentially meaningless. Researchers also generally have avoided the formidable task of studying *restrictive* (as opposed to *absolute*) deterrence. Even if a strategy of deterrence does not eliminate offensive behavior, it may reduce the frequency of misbehavior by offenders. Although little research has evaluated the tenets of deterrence theory, there is good reason to question the efficacy of deterrence in regard to the sorts of behavior most likely to be of concern to community psychologists. Notably, few remedies may be available for violations of institutionalized persons' civil rights by state officials. Hence, bureaucrats and politicians have little to fear as a result of violation of their constituents' civil rights, and there is little reason to believe that the perceived probability of punishment for such violations will be substantially greater than the actual probability.

Even the opportunities for obtaining access to the federal courts have narrowed significantly (Lampson, 1983; *Pennhurst State School & Hospital v. Halderman*, 1984). Even if politically and economically weak parties can formulate a given dispute with state officials in a justiciable manner (i.e., if they can frame a question for resolution in a court of law), they are apt to find themselves continually one-down. For example, a low-income criminal defendant is likely to have great difficulty in securing help in gathering evidence. On the other hand, the state has a fleet of investigators—the police. The defendant also is apt to have difficulty in exploring defenses without risking self-incrimination, although affluent defendants often can consult numerous experts without either providing the state with an additional means of exploring prosecutorial leads or divulging the opinions of any unfavorable experts (see Melton, Petrila, Poythress, & Slobogin, 1997, chap. 4). Similarly, parents involved in child protective cases often find that the state has control over the production of expert evidence that may be critical to dispositional decision-making, a point that the Supreme Court has acknowledged but given little weight in determining the requirements of due process (*Lassiter v. Department of Social Services*, 1981). Moreover, individuals in need of public support (e.g., through Social Security disability assistance) often find themselves subject to "bureaucratic justice" (Mashaw, 1983), in which administrative discretion can be applied in a seemingly arbitrary manner, and petitioners may lack the resources to pursue the matter. In that context as well, the petitioner commonly has little control over the development of the evidence.

Once access is gained, the plaintiffs in institutional litigation must meet a narrow standard for violation of civil rights, and no damages will accrue if the reason for such violation was a lack of funds (*Youngberg v. Romeo*, 1982). Courts also often have few practical remedies for noncompliance with injunctive relief. Because of the desire to avoid the appearance of judicial arrogance in a system of separation of powers, judges are not going to jail legislators for failure to appropriate sufficient funds or administrators for failure to initiate or implement policies to protect residents' rights. Indeed, state agencies are notorious for full compliance with court orders only when essentially no cost results from doing so. Otherwise, administrators typically will seek alternatives to compliance or will simply ignore the orders (Johnson, 1979).

Although courts may be more willing to intervene in matters involving private parties, disadvantaged classes often have difficulty in using the courts, even when they are not facing the state as adversary. In a classic article, Galanter (1974) pointed out the advantages of being a repeat player in the legal system, a position that is not limited to powerful persons or corporations, but that is certainly more common among them.

Repeat players understand the system and therefore are better able than inexperienced litigants to build a record to support their case. They enjoy economies of scale in the legal system and therefore are better able to purchase the services of specialists. They can adopt a strategy to maximize gains over the long term, including reform of the rules in litigation itself. Repeat players also are better able to determine the rules that matter (as opposed to those that are merely symbolic) and to calculate the odds of changing them. Equally important, they are able to establish informal relationships with the key players in the legal system. In short, repeat players, by virtue of experience, expertise, and resources, are ahead of one-shotters (the position occupied by most litigants from disadvantaged classes) even before the legal process begins. Even those legal institutions designed to provide access to the legal system (e.g., small claims courts) may be dominated by economically advantaged repeat players (but see Vidmar, 1984, 1987).

Thus, even if the courts are not completely powerless to deter institutional or corporate misbehavior, it must be recognized that the expected costs of violations of the law by powerful repeat players often are realistically low. In fact, the stick of the law may be most successfully applied in the relatively few instances in which powerful players are set against each other (e.g., large-scale antitrust litigation), with uncertain benefits to the general public.

Incentives

Although "sticks" may be associated more frequently with the law, "carrots" sometimes are available as well. Three forms of incentive systems apply. First, for government employees, the state may make merit pay and "perks" contingent on particular kinds of behavior or products. Second, the government may attach "strings" to government benefits, whether they are distributed to individuals, private programs, or other levels of government. Third, and most generally, the government may directly alter the marketplace, most commonly through use of the taxation power. When undesired behavior is relatively price-elastic, the government may decrease the frequency of the behavior by selective taxation. Conversely, other socially desirable behaviors (e.g., private investment in research and charitable organizations) may increase as a result of tax credits or deductions.

Research on such incentive systems indicates that they often are effective in changing individual or organizational behavior, a fact that should come as no surprise to readers who have sought government grants. Both individuals and organizations do "follow the money" in making choices. At an organizational level, for example, the availability of fiscal incentives may alter goals and behavior. Certainly the Education for All Handicapped Children Act (EAHCA [now known as the Individuals with Disabilities Education Act—IDEA], 1974), although never delivering the level of funding authorized, has resulted in substantial expansion and reorganization of school services for children with special educational needs. The promise of federal money has served as the carrot, inducing a variety of procedural, as well as substantive, changes in educational systems.

Analogously, the administrative threat of loss of federal funds probably was at least as effective in stimulating school desegregation as was the judicial threat of punishment for noncompliance with court orders to end discriminatory practices. The latter examples also illustrate the ambiguous psychological line between incentive systems and deterrence. Once government funds are expected, failure to obtain or retain such funds may appear punitive.

The potential efficacy of incentive systems is qualified by two matters that should be of interest to community psychologists. First, research suggests that marketplace regulation is most likely to be effective when is targeted to particular populations or situations. For example, tobacco use by adolescents (but not by adults) is reduced substantially by even a small increase in the price of cigarettes (Lewit, Coate, & Grossman, 1981). Given that addictive cigarette smoking typically begins in adolescence, an incentive system responsive to adolescents' behavioral patterns is likely to have substantial long-term effects on the frequency of smoking and, therefore, on public health (Arbogast, 1986; Garner, 1986; Warner, Ernster, Holbrook, Lewit, Pertschuk, Steinfeld, Tye, & Whelan, 1986).

Second, regulators must be sensitive to downstream effects (such as the link between adolescent and adult risk-taking behavior) and potential unintended effects. For example, in the late 1970s, the Consumer Product Safety Commission proposed regulations that would have required manufacturers of ladders to strengthen the three-step ladder commonly used for household tasks, such as changing light bulbs (see Orr, 1982). Although the proposed standards undoubtedly would have reduced injuries among users of stepladders, the substantial increase in cost that would have occurred might ultimately have resulted in greater injuries because more people would have avoided purchasing stepladders, instead relying on less stable means of reaching high objects.

Similarly, restrictive licensing laws may result in fewer services or more widespread use of low-quality services. Community psychologists may be sensitive to unintended diminution of innovative and nonprofessional services as a result of licensure of psychologists (Danish & Smyer, 1981). Other forms of social cost have been identified in other professions and trades. For example, licensure of electricians ironically increases the incidence of electrical injuries. The reason for such an effect, directly contrary to intended purposes, is probably that licensure decreases the pool of workers who can do electrical repairs, therefore increasing the cost of such services. As a result, more individuals probably try to do potentially dangerous home repairs that they are not competent to perform (Carroll & Gaston, 1981).

Of course, unintended positive side effects also can result from state regulation. For example, efforts in some states to decrease litter and waste of resources through a tax on non-returned soft-drink bottles have been shown also to result in a 60% reduction of emergency room visits for glass-related lacerations (Baker, Moore, & Wise, 1986).

Indirect Regulation

The effects that law does have on behavior may often result from the creation of social and political structures that facilitate a particular behavior more than direct regulation of the ultimately desired behavior. For example, the success of judicial orders for institutional change may be less the product of potential or actual penalties for noncompliance (i.e., deterrence), or of direct incentives for compliance, than the social-psychological sensitivity of the court in fashioning remedies designed to facilitate compliance. Although the appointment of a special master, a monitoring panel, a human rights committee, or even an entire agency to implement a decree, does not necessarily lead to compliance, it at least increases the salience of whatever contingencies for compliance exist and provides an ongoing establishment voice for powerless groups (see Herr, 1987; Melton, 1986; Mnookin, 1985; Rothman & Rothman, 1984). Moreover, specific elements of a decree (e.g., requirements for staff or the physical environment of an institution) may lead to conditions that prevent recurrence of intolerable conditions.

The legal structures that "demand" particular behavior need not be as overt as mechanisms established to facilitate judicial oversight. More generally, several areas of law are noteworthy for the ways in which they establish norms for community life and indirectly regulate behavior. Perhaps the most obvious example is land-use policy. Through zoning law, city councils and county boards of supervisors can undertake environmental-psychological interventions that shape not only the aesthetic qualities of the community, but also its social-class structure, its forms of recreation and "hangouts" for youth (see, e.g., *Aladdin's Castle v. City of Mesquite*, 1980), its range of employment opportunities, and numerous other dimensions of community life. For example, in Lincoln, Nebraska (a city in which I used to live), the city council has used its zoning authority to keep most movie theaters in the downtown area. Through direct regulation of theater owners, the city council has indirectly altered the behavior of the townspeople generally. Because the theaters are downtown, restaurants also have located downtown, and many people come downtown in the evenings for entertainment. The result is a livelier, more economically feasible, and more aesthetically pleasing downtown area, and probably (although such a hypothesis is difficult to validate) a greater sense of community.

Other indirect effects of law on social behavior are even more remote. Patent law, especially when combined with direct incentives (e.g., tax credits for research and development), effectively creates a society that devotes much of its resources to technological development. As the social and economic changes resulting from electricity, the automobile, and silicon chips illustrate, the law's role as social architect may be more potent, although perhaps less predictably so, than its function as direct allocator of rewards and punishments for particular behavior:

> Imagine a legislator at the turn of the century whose constituents ask how the law might help bring about the following changes: reduce the family to a kernel of its former self, reduce the control parents have of their children, increase premarital sexual activity, cause cities to bulge and flow outward, breaking into segments increasingly alienated from each other, and—while we're at it—send 54,000 people a year to cemeteries and another 2,000,000 to hospitals, pollute the air, and stimulate the growth of emergency medicine, insurance, and personal injury litigation and, in turn, the flowering of medical malpractice litigation.
>
> Assuming a turn-of-the-century legislator was persuaded to seek such changes, how might they be accomplished? The most effective way, apparently, would have been not by the usual method of trying to mandate such changes directly through law, but instead by using the law to promote the advent of the automobile. The law's greatest impact on behavior may be mediated through technology and through the social structures and contingencies that technology in turn creates (Melton & Saks, 1985, pp. 245–246).

In other instances, the law has profound, although still indirect, effects on community life by its structuring the boundaries of social institutions. For example, the most lasting effects of law on family life may emanate from sources other than family law (Melton, 1988). The definitions of *family* generally are found in other spheres of law. Consider the range in a partial list of legal issues in which the boundaries of a (legitimate) family are defined by the law on behalf of the community.[1]

[1]A Supreme Court decision (*Michael H. v. Gerald D.*, 1989) involving facts that the plurality hoped, perhaps naively, were extraordinary, illustrated the moral and practical significance of the law's definition of the boundaries of a family. In a highly fractionated decision (five opinions, with none of them signed in full by more than three justices), the Court rejected the claim to parental rights, including visitation, of a biological father who had related to his daughter as her father and who was prepared to provide economic support to a child who was conceived while the mother was married to another man. In an opinion written by Justice Scalia, a four-member plurality stated its belief that a challenge to a statutory presumption of paternity by the mother's husband would challenge "the historic respect—indeed, sanctity would not be too strong a term—traditionally accorded to the relationships that develop within the unitary family" (p. 123).

By contrast, in attacking the plurality's concept of the Constitution as a "stagnant, archaic, hidebound document steeped in the prejudices and superstitions of a time long past" (p. 141), Justice Brennan, joined by Justices Blackmun and Marshall, concluded:

> The atmosphere surrounding today's decision is one of make-believe. Beginning with the suggestion that the situation confronting us here does not repeat itself every day in every corner of the country ... moving on to the claim that it is tradition alone that supplies the details of the liberty that the

- Is a group of residents violating a zoning ordinance limiting a neighborhood to single-family residences?
- Is an individual eligible for compensation in tort for mental injuries incurred by witnessing the injury or death of a loved one, when the common law in the jurisdiction limits recovery by bystanders to family members?
- Is an individual's property immune from seizure for debts because it is a homestead?
- Is an individual a natural heir entitled to the benefits of a decedent's estate?
- When, if ever, does a parent cease to have financial responsibility for the care of an adult child? When, if ever, does the child become responsible for the health care and other necessities of life of the parent?
- Are the reciprocal economic responsibilities of cohabitants the same as those of spouses who have legally married?

In short, the law governs not only the structure of a family but its functions, and it often does so in circumstances in which there is no dispute within the family (or intimate group not legally recognized as a family). When an intrafamilial dispute does occur, the law can expand or contract the relationships at issue, with ultimate effects on the boundaries of the family, as demonstrated by the recent spate of legislation on grandparents' rights (Thompson, Tinsley, Scalora, & Parke, 1989).

Although the family is probably the most important example of such legal social architecture, it certainly is not unique. The law defines the nature and functions of corporations, partnerships, charitable voluntary associations, schools, and professions, as well as legal institutions themselves. By creating new structures or reifying customary relationships,[2] the law plays a largely invisible, but overarching, role in the everyday life of the community. Whenever one is a buyer or a seller, a borrower or a lender, a teacher or a student, a parent or a child, the law looms large in structuring the role and the relationship.

Government Speech

Thus far, I have considered ways that the power of the state is exerted to influence behavior. I turn now to overt, purposeful attempts to change behavior through law, but with minimal use of legal force. Even without imposition of punishments or rewards, or creation of new

---

> Constitution protects, and passing finally to the notion that the Court always has recognized a cramped vision of "the family," today's decision lets stand California's pronouncement that Michael—whom blood tests show to a 98 percent probability to be Victoria's father—is not Victoria's father. When and if the court awakes to reality, it will not find a world very different from the one it expects (p. 157).

In the conclusion to his dissent, one of the conservative members of the Court, Justice White, was less caustic but equally incredulous:

> I see no reason to debate the plurality's multilingual explorations into "spousal nonaccess" and ancient polity concerns behind bastardy laws. It may be true that a child conceived in an extra-marital relationship would be considered a "bastard" in the literal sense of the word, but whatever stigma remains in today's society is far less compelling in the context of a child of a married mother, especially when there is a father asserting paternity and seeking a relationship with his child. It is hardly rare in this world of divorce and remarriage for a child to live with the "father" to whom her mother is married, and still have a relationship with her biological father (pp. 161–162).

[2]Some entire areas of law are based on the institutionalization of social customs (e.g., contracts, commercial law, international law). Imposition of the force of law on such relationships reifies them and, in so doing, increases predictability of behavior and corollary diminution of risk. As noted later in this chapter, though, the cost is an inherent conservative influence that may retard desirable social change.

structures, the state still may affect behavior simply by "jawboning." The most notable examples of such a strategy probably have been the Public Health Service's long-term efforts to eliminate smoking and its recent public relations campaign to reduce the frequency of behavior that increases the risk of AIDS. At least in the former instance, the jawboning has consisted of both direct *government* speech and coercion of others to speak on behalf of the government (e.g., legal mandates for tobacco companies to put warning labels on packages of cigarettes).

Although government-sponsored media campaigns certainly are less intrusive than the use of the police power, they also present some problems about the limits of state authority. On the one hand, even the most ardent advocates of a *laissez-faire* approach to the marketplace generally favor means of ensuring that consumers have the information necessary for rational choice. Some might further argue that provision of such information so that the marketplace can regulate itself, in effect, is a particularly appropriate use of state resources in that it empowers consumers without requiring direct government intervention.

On the other hand, even commercial speech is protected by the first amendment (*Virginia Board of Pharmacy v. Virginia Citizens Consumer Council, Inc.*, 1976). Therefore, serious constitutional issues arise from strategies that rely on direct regulation of speech by corporate actors, whether through a requirement of some kinds of statements (e.g., the Surgeon General's warnings) or prohibition of others, especially when the intent is to *persuade* rather than merely *inform.* Indeed, such issues are present even when the method is relatively unintrusive, because the government itself is speaking, rather than requiring that unwilling parties provide (or refrain from providing) a particular message. Given the resources of the state, its credibility as a source, and its potential use of more forceful strategies, there is a danger that a vociferous government will drown out other voices.

The problem of deciding when injection of the government into public debates is justifiable or even necessary and when it is overly intrusive is not an easy one. Consider, for example, the dilemma faced by public-school officials when the school library contains books that espouse doctrines (e.g., racism) that most would find inconsistent with democratic ideals. On the one hand, if the school officials remain silent, they may inadvertently inculcate undesirable attitudes. On the other hand, if they remove the books from the shelves or even single the books out for negative commentary, they themselves practice (and symbolically teach) intolerance.

The difficulty of the problem is illustrated by the Supreme Court's response. In a 5–4 decision with seven opinions, the Court held that the first amendment prohibits removal of books from the library for political reasons, but the plurality also indicated that failure to purchase books for the same reason would be constitutional (*Board of Education v. Pico*, 1982).

Behavioral scientists may be able to contribute to resolution of policy debates through empirical study of *chilling effects* of government speech and action. Research might identify the situations in which official behavior can have the effect of suppressing free expression. The potential for such analysis was illustrated by Askin's (1972) brief to the U. S. Supreme Court alleging chilling effects of military surveillance of private citizens.

Beyond the constitutional issues raised by government speech, questions remain of the efficacy of large-scale media campaigns. Bonnie (1985) noted that, thus far, few effects of government-sponsored health-promotion campaigns have been observed:

> There is at present little evidence that discrete, time-limited media campaigns are effective in promoting healthy or safe behavior. While such campaigns may reinforce the attitudes and behaviors of

persons who are already inclined to behave safely, they appear to have little impact on the "high-risk" populations—in the context of driver safety, teenage and young-adult working-class drivers (p. 159).

Nonetheless, there is some evidence that failures of government media campaigns often have been the result of overly narrow messages and overly broad audiences. When the message is limited to raw information without attention to motivational factors, and when the medium is irrelevant to the group of most interest, there is little reason to expect even low-magnitude effects. Perhaps the clearest conclusion from research on the effects of government-sponsored media campaigns is that, to be effective, such campaigns must be targeted to particular audiences. For example, although public attention on the effects of smoking on fetal development has reduced the frequency of smoking by pregnant women, the reduction in smoking during pregnancy is highly correlated with the woman's level of education (Kleinman & Kopstein, 1987). Such a relationship is hardly surprising when prevention programs focus on dissemination of information through news programs and printed media.

It is likely that the Public Health Service's efforts and related government regulation of commercial speech (i.e., mandatory warnings on cigarette packs and proscription of televised advertising) were at least partially responsible for the sizeable drop in cigarette smoking by adults, especially men, that has occurred in the generation since the Surgeon General's report. However, as Bonnie (1985) has pointed out, other strategies might have been more effective, at least as supplements to the media campaigns. The government's stick could have been used to reach individuals indirectly. Tort liability could be imposed on physicians who fail to provide appropriate education and counseling for individuals in high-risk populations. Failure to warn about dangers of substance abuse during pregnancy, for example, could be a *per se* basis for a finding of negligence. Physicians would be likely to respond to such a threat of civil punishment, and they are especially credible sources on matters of personal health.

EFFICACY OF LEGAL INTERVENTION

Does Law Work?

As the discussion thus far illustrates, the question of whether law is effective in stimulating individual or community change is overly simple. At minimum, it is clear that enactment of law does not necessarily result in a change in behavior. The carrots and sticks available to the law often are limited, especially when corporate or institutional actors are involved. Even when parties are motivated to comply with the law, they may not know about changes in it. When the strategy is to use the courts to vindicate the rights of an individual or class, there may be problems in defining a justiciable dispute. To complicate matters further, as the case proceeds through the legal process and up the appellate ladder, the question at stake may vary substantially from the test issue originally posed (see Melton, 1986; Mnookin, 1985).

Even with such formidable obstacles, it also clearly is true that the law sometimes *does* create social change. As I already have noted, although the mechanism by which such change occurs often may be quite subtle and indirect, the change itself sometimes is far-reaching.

Indeed, sometimes the change not only may be profound but clearly intentional. Although the proper climate for desegregation may not have been present at the time of *Brown v. Board of Education* (1954), there also can be little doubt that the courts hastened the demise of racial segregation. Even though school desegregation did not have the effects on youth prejudice and self-esteem that were hypothesized (Stephan, 1978), implementation of court orders for desegregation commonly resulted in changes in community voting behavior and sociopolitical norms (e.g., election of African-American candidates, defeat of anti-busing candidates) within two to three years (Rossell, 1978).

When Does Law Work?

Given, then, that the law is neither omnipotent nor impotent, the question becomes one of identifying the circumstances in which law is likely to affect behavior. Answering that question is not easy. Changes in social and political climate often are coincident with changes in law. Indeed, there is little reason to expect a change in the law without a change in the prevailing mores and politics. Obviously, the legislature is presumed to follow shifts in popular sentiment. Changes in administrative decision-making, or enforcement of legislative or judicial decisions, also would be likely to reflect executive-branch officials' assessment of the preferences of the electorate. There is evidence that judges also are sensitive to prevailing attitudes and beliefs (Rosen, 1984).

Even relatively pristine quasi-experimental designs may not be able to distinguish the causes of changes in behavior toward conformity with new law. Moreover, to the extent that the law itself does result in altered behavior, the mechanism (e.g., whether a deterrent or a symbolic effect is at work) may remain unclear. Partly as a result, knowledge about the factors affecting compliance with the law still is fragmentary.

Zimring and Hawkins (1977) have presented perhaps the most cogent set of hypotheses about the instrumentality of law. Their analysis focuses on the degree of synchrony between law and social custom. Intuitively, the community unrest presented by use of deterrent threats to stimulate social change (as in the early days of court orders for school desegregation) is unlikely to be replicated when deterrent threats are employed to strengthen well-established social conventions. Indeed, in the latter context, social conflict might be induced by *failure* to exert the force of law to protect community norms.

Framing the phenomenon somewhat differently, if there is a substantial discrepancy between law and prevailing custom or between law and *important* custom, substantial force or threat of force will be necessary to obtain compliance. By important custom, I refer to behavior that reflects deeply held beliefs. For example, if illegal behavior is motivated by religious belief or political ideology, a substantial deterrent threat may be necessary to suppress the behavior. Similarly, if illegal behavior is economically rewarding or even essential to feasibility of the primary economic activity in a community, greater threats (or perhaps greater inducements) will be necessary to obtain compliance with the law. On the other hand, if law reflects the norms of the community, no carrots or sticks at all may be necessary. Simply providing cues through law about acceptable behavior may be enough.

Other factors that Zimring and Hawkins (1977) identified as probably affecting compliance are (1) the visibility of the custom at stake, (2) the reduction of social forces that have maintained the now-illegal behavior, and (3) the level of apparent need for reform. If the behavior is public, detection of noncompliance and, therefore, enforcement is likely to be relatively easy. In instances where individuals engage in now-illegal behavior reluctantly (for example, when restaurant owners maintained segregationist policies because of fear of alienating white customers), the change in law may give an excuse for behavior that conforms with their conscience. If a "clear and present danger" exists, law that upsets prevailing customs is more likely to be accepted.

Another influential conceptual framework was presented by Black (1976), whose approach is unique in his consideration of law as a quantitative variable—in essence, the degree of *force* of law. Although he has intended his series of theorems as purely descriptive statements of the variables affecting whether more or less law is present and applied, they effectively serve as explanations for the situations in which state power is or is not exerted. For example, Black has postulated that more law is present as social status rises (consider, e.g., the intricacies of corporate taxation and commercial law), but that the force of law is greater when it is applied downward in social status.

SYMBOLIC EFFECTS OF LAW

In general, I have considered the instrumentality of law, that is, the degree that the law accomplishes a particular behavioral objective. That emphasis reflects the way that psychologists and sociologists generally have approached law. Nonetheless, the more important effects of law (albeit even more difficult to study) probably are symbolic.

For example, psychologists have conducted hundreds of studies on jury behavior. Indeed, that topic is rivaled only by eyewitness testimony as a staple of psycholegal study (Saks, 1986). The fact that such topics are predominant itself reflects a sort of myopia, in that the choice of topics has emanated from the emphases of psychological research, rather than on the needs of the legal system. However, not just the choice of topic, but also its framework, reflects such a shortsightedness. Reflecting the instrumentalism of the social sciences, jury research almost universally has assessed the rationality of jury behavior: How good are jurors in comprehending and applying the law?

Although that question certainly is not trivial, it is not the only broad question about juries, and it may not be the most important one. Obviously, there are many possible mechanisms for decision-making, some of which may be more valid or rational than juries. The critical distinction, though, between juries and expert, or even mechanical, decision-makers is that juries are presumed to reflect the will of the community. Although the question has not been studied, we believe that judgment by a jury bears an inherent fairness; the litigants stand eyeball to eyeball with their peers who will judge them. Even if procedural reforms resulted in more accurate application of the law, such reforms might not be justified if they diminished the sense of justice experienced by the litigants or spectators. Moreover, juries' participation in legal decision-making may have important symbolic meaning for the jurors themselves and for the community as a whole.

More generally, law serves to provide cues to behavior that the community regards as laudable, permissible, or forbidden (see, generally, Melton & Saks, 1985). It *educates* the citizenry about the norms of the community and contributes to their internalization. Law also may serve to sensitize individuals to the harmful effects of prohibited conduct. In fact, when legal norms do comport with community norms, appeals to conscience generally have been shown to be at least as effective as, and sometimes more effective than, deterrent threats in preventing illegal behavior (see, e.g., Geller, Koltuniak, & Shilling, 1983; McNees, Egli, Marshall, Schnelle, & Risley, 1976; McNees, Kennon, Schnelle, Kirchner, & Thomas, 1980; Mecham, 1968; Schwartz & Orleans, 1967).

At the most abstract level, the law confirms the values of the community and contributes to development of a cultural identity. Anthropological research (e.g., Geertz, 1980; Pospisil, 1971; Nader & Todd, 1978) has shown the universality of law and the role of law in sustaining the body politic:

> [T]he state—and the law within it—functions as a parody of itself. The underlying theory of the state is imitated in its rituals. The law functions, then, as a symbolic representation of the ideals of the state, and it purports to teach the citizenry these principles, to serve as a model of natural social order (Melton & Saks, 1985, p. 252).

COMMUNITY PSYCHOLOGY IN LAW

Study of symbolic effects of law potentially will illuminate the ways that law may sustain the values of the community. Other activities that theoretically are system-preserving and appropriate for community psychologists are the development and diffusion of knowledge about behavioral assumptions in the law. Such tasks are conservative in that they provide information about the accuracy of assumptions that are critical to the development and implementation of legal policy consistent with the purported goals of the populace.

As a practical matter, though, such analyses often are reformist because they illuminate inaccuracies in prevailing assumptions in legal policy. My area of primary interest, children's rights, is illustrative. The law affecting the expression of liberty and privacy by adolescents has rested on assumptions about about their level of competence in decision-making, their vulnerability to psychological harm as a result of unwise decisions or decision-making itself, and the effects of decision-making by minors on family integrity (see generally *Bellotti v. Baird*, 1979; Koocher, 1987; Melton, Koocher, & Saks, 1983). Research has been virtually uniform in showing the assumptions of incompetence, vulnerability, and threats to family integrity to be erroneous, but the law has shown little recognition of such facts.

Despite the purported openness of juvenile and family law to behavioral science, the courts rarely have considered evidence that tests the assumptions that are fundamental to child and family policy (Melton, 1984). Failure by legal authorities to take developmental research into account in designing policy sometimes has appeared to reflect a willful desire to maintain myths that permit maintenance of paternalist policies and lip service to the liberty and privacy interests of minors (Melton, 1987c). Ironically, this approach has undermined efforts to build family-centered shared decision-making by parents and children (Melton, 1998a, 1998b).

However, capriciousness of legal authorities is probably not the full explanation of the failure to conform legal policy to knowledge about child development and family life. Specifically, psychologists probably share the blame in several ways. First, for too long, psychologists were, and too often still are, willing to offer opinions about youth welfare without any scientific foundation (Melton, 1984; Melton et al., 1997). Second, until relatively recently, psychologists avoided study of children and youth in real-life contexts and, therefore, failed to develop empirical data directly apposite to legal policy (cf. Bronfenbrenner, 1974). Third, even when relevant information was available, psychologists often failed through neglect or ignorance to diffuse research in a manner that it was likely to reach legal decision-makers. For example, despite the submission of numerous amicus briefs in the initial series of cases about adolescent abortion (perhaps the primary context in which constitutional doctrine about minors has been shaped), the amici generally ignored the relevant behavioral science research (Tremper, 1987). Fourth, few researchers have been sufficiently skilled in both empirical and legal analysis to frame research questions and resulting knowledge in ways that are likely to be persuasive to legal scholars and decision-makers.

At least on the topic of minors' competence, though, the state of both knowledge and diffusion of that knowledge has improved dramatically in recent years, in part because of the growth of a cadre of interdisciplinary scholars motivated to bring relevant knowledge to the legal system (see, e.g., Melton et al., 1987). Such scholars not only have increased relevant knowledge and framed it in a useful manner, but they systematically have examined the efficacy of various strategies for diffusing that knowledge (see generally Melton, 1987a, 1987b).

Such work on knowledge utilization is well within the tradition of community psychology. It entails study of the structural and personal factors that affect whether judges and other legal authorities learn of knowledge applicable to their decisions, whether they comprehend such information, and whether and how they use it. It further involves actual application of psychosocial research to increase the likelihood that judicial decision-making ultimately is consonant with the normative principles that underlie legal doctrines.

Active work to match legal analysis with social reality also comports with 20th-century jurisprudential theory (see Loh, 1984; Melton, Monahan, & Saks, 1987; Monahan & Walker, 1998). Since the legal realism movement of the New Deal era, legal scholarship has been unusually open to interdisciplinary approaches aimed ultimately at promotion of social welfare through law. Legal realism opened the door to consideration of what the law should be, not just what it is. This view has obtained even more credibility in legal scholarship with the growth of "law and ..." movements over the past two decades.

COMMUNITY PSYCHOLOGY IN A POST-REALIST LEGAL CONTEXT

The same trends are present in judicial decision-making, although judges have been slower than academicians to embrace the implications of legal realism. At least in part, this ambivalence has resulted from continuing doctrinal ambiguity about the proper role of social science within the law and the proper procedures for admitting such evidence into the judicial process (see, e.g., Bersoff, 1987; *Lockhart v. McCree*, 1986; *McKleskey v. Kemp*, 1987). Nonetheless, the legitimacy of some use of psychological research now is well settled, at least within the federal courts (Melton, 1987a, 1987b). Not only are psychological and sociological arguments now common in the Supreme Court, but conservative as well as liberal justices have criticized their colleagues for insufficient attention to social-scientific evidence on various issues. In a sense, this development indicates the degree of change that has occurred in the law. The furor that met footnote 11 (citing several social-science authorities) in *Brown v. Board of Education* (1954) now seems almost quaint.

At the same time, the reformist fervor that accompanied legal realism also may have abated. The social science in law perspective is relatively neutral politically. Although empirical evidence can be used to challenge the facial assumptions underlying the conventional order (see, e.g., *Hodgson v. Minnesota*, 1987), in principle, social science can be used as easily to sustain prevailing rules as to undermine them, depending on what the actual social reality is.

Indeed, some post-realist movements, although dependent on social-scientific methods and logic, are more in tune with the political right wing than social-welfare reformers. The law and economics movement is most clearly illustrative. Although the application of economic theory to the law need not have a conservative influence, law and economics as a scholarly movement has tended to glorify economic efficiency as a fundamental policy goal. Consequently, it has been welcomed by conservatives intent on preserving free-market approaches to public policy. The ideological compatibility is illustrated by the fact that two of the leading scholars of the movement, Richard Posner and Frank Easterbrook, were appointed by President Reagan to the Seventh Circuit Court of Appeals, and both were frequently mentioned as possible appointees to the Supreme Court when President Bush sought a conservative replacement for Justice Powell. Both are likely to resurface as potential Supreme Court appointees if a Republican succeeds President Clinton.

Indeed, psychology and law may be distinguished from some post-realist movements by its adoption, for the most part, of the values that underlay legal realism (Melton, 1990). Community psychology is challenged to explore ways of matching legal institutions to the needs of the community, and, in so doing, to assist in the creation of new legal settings that will facilitate the resolution of disputes and enhance perceived justice (see Melton, 1983).

At the same time, community psychology can help individuals and groups make use of existing law. For example, forensic psychology, when practiced in a community mental health center, offers the opportunity for psychologists to consult with attorneys about ways of dealing with clients with whom it may be difficult to communicate (Melton, Weithorn, & Slobogin, 1985). Psychologists also can assist legal authorities to educate litigants and witnesses about the means by which they can participate in the presentation of their cases (see Melton & Limber, 1989). Such efforts, when coupled with other sensible interventions (e.g., ongoing feedback about the process of the case), in effect empower the individuals involved in the legal process and increase their sense of being treated fairly (Lind & Tyler, 1988). Similarly, by using legal-socialization principles (see, e.g., Tapp & Levine, 1974) to teach individuals about their legal *entitlements* (see Tapp & Melton, 1983), community psychologists can induce beliefs that citizens are indeed law-creators, and that the law does not stop at the courthouse door. Such strategies are highly consistent with the values embedded in both the legal system and community psychology.

To summarize, although the legal system sometimes is the problem more than the solution, the fact remains that fundamental legal values (e.g., those embedded in the Bill of Rights) are largely compatible with the prevailing values in community psychology. Although the law sometimes serves as an impediment to change, it also serves to reify and sustain the core values of the community. In the end, psychologists might view the legal system as a series of opportunities for empowerment of individuals and groups, with psychologists best able to assist the legal system in meeting its goals and matching legal settings and procedures with the knowledge and expectations of citizens.

REFERENCES

Aladdin's Castle v. City of Mesquite, 630 F.2d 1029 (5th Cir. 1980), *rev'd in part and remanded*, 455 U.S. 283 (1982).

Arbogast, R. (1986). A proposal to regulate the manner of tobacco advertising. *Journal of Health Politics, Policy, and Law*, *11*, 393–422.

Askin, F. (1972). Chilling effect: A view from the social sciences. *Columbia Human Rights Law Review*, *4*, 59–88.

Baker, M. D., Moore, S. E., & Wise, P. H. (1986). The impact of "bottle bill" legislation on the incidence of lacerations in childhood. *American Journal of Public Health*, *76*, 1243–1244.

Bellah, R. N. (1975). *The broken covenant: American civil religion in time of trial.* New York: Seabury.

Bellotti v. Baird, 443 U.S. 622 (1979).

Bersoff, D. N. (1987). Social science data and the Supreme Court: *Lockhart* as a case in point. *American Psychologist*, *42*, 52–58.

Black, D. (1976). *The behavior of law*. New York: Academic.

Board of Education v. Pico, 457 U.S. 853 (1982).

Bonnie, R. J. (1985). The efficacy of law as a paternalistic instrument. In G. B. Melton (Ed.), *Nebraska Symposium on Motivation: The law as a behavioral instrument*, (Vol. 33, pp. 131–211). Lincoln: University of Nebraska Press.

Bronfenbrenner, U. (1974) Developmental research, public policy, and the ecology of childhood. *Child Development, 45,* 1–5.

Brown v. Board of Education, 347 U.S. 483 (1954).

Carroll, J. M. (1978). Psychological approach to deterrence. *Journal of Personality and Social Psychology, 36,* 1512–1520.

Carroll, S. L., & Gaston, R. J. (1981). Occupational restrictions and the quality of services received: Some evidence. *Southern Economic Journal, 47,* 959–976.

Danish, S. J., & Smyer, M. A. (1981). Unintended consequences of requiring a license to help. *American Psychologist, 36,* 13–21.

Galanter, M. (1974). Why the "haves" come out ahead: Speculations on the limits of legal change. *Law and Society Review, 9,* 95–160.

Galanter, M. (1983). Reading the landscape of disputes: What we know and don't know (and think we know) about our allegedly contentious and litigious society. *UCLA Law Review, 31,* 4–71.

Garner, D. W. (1986). Tobacco sampling, public policy and the law. *Journal of Health Politics, Policy, and Law, 11,* 423–439.

Geertz, C. (1980). *Negara: The theatre state in nineteenth-century Bali.* Princeton, NJ: Princeton University Press.

Geller, E. S., Koltuniak, T. A., & Shilling, J. S. (1983). Response avoidance prompting: A cost-effective strategy for theft deterrence. *Behavioral Counseling and Community Interventions, 3,* 28–42.

Gibbs, J. P. (1985). Deterrence theory and research. In G. B. Melton (Ed.), *Nebraska Symposium on Motivation: Vol. 33. The law as a behavioral instrument* (pp. 87–130). Lincoln: University of Nebraska Press.

Herr, S. S. (1987). The future of advocacy for persons with mental disabilities. *Rutgers Law Review, 39,* 443–486.

Hodgson v. Minnesota, 827 F.2d 1191 (8th Cir. 1987) (reh'g granted and opinion vacated and withdrawn), 497 U.S. 417 (1990).

Johnson, C. A. (1979). Judicial decisions and organization change: Some theoretical and empirical notes on state court decisions and state administrative agencies. *Law and Society Review, 14,* 27–56.

Kleinman, J. C., & Kopstein, A. (1987). Smoking during pregnancy, 1967–80. *American Journal of Public Health, 77,* 823–825.

Koocher, G. P. (1987). Children under law: The paradigm of consent. In G. B. Melton (Ed.), *Reforming the law: Impact of child development research* (pp. 3–26). New York: Guilford.

Lampson, M. (1983). Senate subcommittee reviews Justice Department's enforcement of Section 504 and CRIPA. *Mental Disability Law Reporter, 7,* 492–493.

Lassiter v. Department of Social Services, 452 U.S. 18 (1981).

Lerner, M. J., & Lerner, S. C. (Eds.). (1981). *The justice motive in social behavior: Adapting to times of scarcity and change.* New York: Plenum.

Lewit, E. M., Coate, D., & Grossman, M. (1981). The effects of government regulation on teenage smoking. *Journal of Law and Economics, 24,* 545–569.

Lind, E. A., & Tyler, T. R. (1988). *The social psychology of procedural justice.* New York: Plenum.

Lockhart v. McCree, 476 U.S. 162 (1986).

Loh, W. D. (1984). *Social research in the judicial process: Cases, readings, and text.* New York: Russell Sage Foundation.

Mashaw, J. L. (1983). *Bureaucratic justice: Managing social security disability claims.* New Haven, Connecticut: Yale University Press.

McCleskey v. Kemp, 481 U.S. 279 (1987).

McNees, M. P., Egli, D. S., Marshall, R. S., Schnelle, J. F., & Risley, T. R. (1976). Shoplifting prevention: Providing information through signs. *Journal of Applied Behavior Analysis, 9,* 399–405.

McNees, M. P., Kennon, M., Schnelle, J. F., Kirchner, R. E., & Thomas, M. M. (1980). An experimental analysis of a program to reduce retail theft. *American Journal of Community Psychology, 8,* 379–385.

Mecham, G. D. (1968). Proceed with caution: Which penalties slow down the juvenile traffic offender? *Crime and Delinquency, 14,* 142–150.

Melton, G. B. (1983). Community psychology and rural legal systems. In A. W. Childs & G. B. Melton (Eds.), *Rural psychology* (pp. 359–380). New York: Plenum.

Melton, G. B. (1984). Developmental psychology and the law: The state of the art. *Journal of Family Law, 22,* 445–482.

Melton, G. B. (1986). Litigation *In the interest of children*: Does anybody win? *Law and Human Behavior, 10,* 337–353.

Melton, G. B. (1987a). Bringing psychology to the legal system: Opportunities, obstacles, and efficacy. *American Psychologist, 42,* 488–495.

Melton, G. B. (Ed.). (1987b). *Reforming the law: Impact of child development research.* New York: Guilford.

Melton, G. B. (1987c). The clashing of symbols: Prelude to child and family policy. *American Psychologist, 42*, 345–354.

Melton, G. B. (1988). The significance of law in the everyday life of children and families. *Georgia Law Review, 22*, 851–895.

Melton, G. B. (1990). Law, science, and humanity: The normative foundation of social science in law. *Law and Human Behavior, 14*, 315–332.

Melton, G. B. (1992). The law is a good thing (psychology is, too): Human rights in psychological jurisprudence. *Law and Human Behavior, 16*, 381–398.

Melton, G. B. (1998a). Parents *and* children. *Family Futures, 2*, 10–14.

Melton, G. B. (1998b). *Facilitating children's participation: A framework for legal reform*. Report to the Israeli Ministry of Justice.

Melton, G. B., & Garrison, E. G. (1987). Fear, prejudice, and neglect: Discrimination against mentally disabled persons. *American Psychologist, 42*, 1007–1026.

Melton, G. B., Goodman, G. S., Kalichman, S. C., Levine, M., & Koocher, G. P. (1995). Empirical research on child maltreatment and the law. (Report of the American Psychological Association Working Group on Legal Issues Related to Child Abuse and Neglect). *Journal of Clinical Child Psychology, 24*(Suppl.), 47–77.

Melton, G. B., Koocher, G. P., & Saks, M. J. (Eds.). (1983). *Children's competence to consent*. New York: Plenum.

Melton, G. B., & Limber, S. (1989). Psychologists' involvement in cases of child maltreatment: Limits of role and expertise. *American Psychologist, 44*, 1225–1233.

Melton, G. B., Monahan, J., & Saks, M. J. (1987). Psychologists as law professors. *American Psychologist, 42*, 502–509.

Melton, G. B., Petrila, J., Poythress, N. G., Jr., & Slobogin, C. (1997). *Psychological evaluations for the courts: A handbook for mental health professionals and lawyers* (2nd ed.) New York: Guilford.

Melton, G. B., & Saks, M. J. (1985). The law as an instrument of socialization and social structure. In G. B. Melton (Ed.), *The law as a behavioral instrument* (pp. 235–277). Lincoln: University of Nebraska Press.

Melton, G. B., Weithorn, L. A., & Slobogin, C. (1985). *Community mental health centers and the courts: An evaluation of community-based forensic services*. Lincoln: University of Nebraska Press.

Michael H. v. Gerald D., 491 U.S. 110 (1989).

Mnookin, R. H. (Ed.) (1985). *In the interest of children: Advocacy, law reform, and public policy*. New York: W. H. Freeman.

Monahan, J., & Walker, L. (1998). *Social science in law: Cases and materials* (4th ed.). Westbury, NY: Foundation Press.

Nader, L., & Todd, H. (Eds.). (1978). *The disputing process: Law in ten societies*. New York: Columbia University Press.

New York State Association for Retarded Children, Inc., v. Carly. 393 F. Suppl. 715 (E.D.N.Y. 1978).

Orr, L. D. (1982). Goals, risks, and choices. *Risk Analysis, 2*, 239–242.

Pennhurst State School & Hospital v. Halderman, 465 U.S. 89 (1984).

Pospisil, L. (1971). *Anthropology of law: A comparative theory*. New York: Harper & Row.

Repucci, N. D. (1977). Implementation issues for the behavior modifier as institutional change agent. *Behavior Therapy, 8*, 594–605.

Rosen, D. (1984). Democracy and demographics: The inevitability of a class-based interpretation. *University of Dayton Law Review, 10*, 37–96.

Rossell, C. H. (1978). School desegregation and community social change. *Law and Contemporary Problems, 42*, 133–183.

Rothman, D. J., & Rothman, S. M. (1984). *The Willowbrook wars*. New York: Harper & Row.

Saks, M. J. (1986). The law does not live by eyewitness testimony alone. *Law and Human Behavior, 10*, 279–280.

Schwartz, R. D., & Orleans, S. (1967). On legal sanctions. *University of Chicago Law Review, 34*, 274–300.

Stephan, W. G. (1978). School desegregation: An evaluation of predictions made in *Brown v. Board of Education*. *Psychological Bulletin, 85*, 217–238.

Tapp, J. L., & Levine, F. J. (1974). Legal socialization: Strategies for an ethical legality. *Stanford Law Review, 27*, 1–72.

Tapp, J. L., & Melton, G. B. (1983). Preparing children for decision making: Implications of legal socialization research. In G. B. Melton (Ed.), *Children's competence to consent*, (pp. 215–233). New York: Plenum.

Task Force on Psychology and Public Policy. (1986). *American Psychologist, 41*, 914–921.

Thibaut, J., & Walker, L. (1978). A theory of procedure. *California Law Review, 66*, 541–566.

Thompson, R. A., Tinsley, B. R., Scalora, M. J., & Parke, R. D. (1989). Grandparents' visitation rights: Legalizing the ties that bind. *American Psychologist, 44*, 1217–1222.

Tremper, C. R. (1987). The high road to the bench: Presenting research findings in appellate briefs. In G. B. Melton (Ed.), *Reforming the law: Impact of child development research* (pp. 199–231). New York: Guilford.

Trubek, D. (1984). Turning away from law. *Michigan Law Review, 82*, 824–835.

Tyler, T. R. (1987). The psychology of disputant concerns in mediation. *Negotiation Journal, 3*, 367–374.

Tyler, T. R. (1988). What is procedural justice? *Law and Society Review, 22*, 301–355.

Virginia Board of Pharmacy v. Virginia Consumers Council, Inc., 425 U.S. 748 (1976).

Unger, R. M. (1983). The critical legal studies movement. *Harvard Law Review, 96*, 561–676.

Vidmar, N. (1984). The small claims court: A reconceptualization of disputes and an empirical investigation. *Law and Society Review, 18*, 515–550.

Vidmar, N. (1987). Assessing the effects of case characteristics and settlement forum on dispute outcomes and compliance. *Law and Society Review, 21*, 155–164.

Warner, K. E., Ernster, V. L., Holbrook, J. H., Lewit, E. M., Pertschuk, M., Steinfeld, J. L., Tye, J. B., & Whelan, E. M. (1986). Promotion of tobacco products: Issues and policy options. *Journal of Health Politics, Policy, and Law, 11*, 367–392.

Woodward, C. V. (1974). *The strange career of Jim Crow*. New York: Oxford University Press.

Youngberg v. Romeo, 457 U.S. 309 (1982).

Zimring, F., & Hawkins, G. (1977). The legal threat as an instrument of social change. In J. L. Tapp & F. J. Levine (Eds.), *Law, justice, and the individual in society: Psychological and legal issues* (pp. 60–68). New York: Holt, Rinehart and Winston.

CHAPTER 23

Helping Troubled Children and Families

A Paradigm of Public Responsibility

JANE KNITZER

As America enters the 21st century, there is growing debate about the extent to which the schools, a central socializing institution, are structured to produce the kind of workforce that America needs (National Education Goals Panel, 1995; Toch, 1991). On a much less public level, another debate about structure is also taking place—the structure of the social service system that seeks to improve outcomes for a large and vulnerable group of children at risk of school and life failure. Broadly writ, the helping systems for such children and families typically include at least four core public agencies and institutions that, sequentially or concurrently, but typically without regard for one another, serve the children and families: these are the departments of social service, including child welfare agencies; mental health agencies; juvenile justice agencies; and schools (often special education programs, but sometimes regular education).

In recent decades, pressures on these social service systems grew: There was an escalation of multineed families facing not only poverty, but often additional burdens such as homelessness; substance abuse; high levels of community violence; exposure to physical, sexual, or emotional abuse; or any other multiple risk factors that place families and the children within them at risk of diminished opportunities and outcomes (National Commission on Children, 1991; Children's Defense Fund, 1991; Danziger, 1990). During the 1980s and the early 1990s, there was considerable experimentation and calls for reform across these social service systems, notwithstanding, or perhaps partially propelled by, the shrinking dollars available for families with special needs. This led to considerable innovation and even the development of new research paradigms. By the late 1990s, however, a competing framework emerged—managed care. Although originally conceived in relation to health care issues, the

JANE KNITZER • National Center for Children in Poverty, School of Public Health, Columbia University, New York, New York 10032.

Handbook of Community Psychology, edited by Julian Rappaport and Edward Seidman. Kluwer Academic/Plenum Publishers, New York, 2000.

concept of managed care, rather than cross-system collaboration, represents an alternative paradigm of public, and indeed private, responsibility. How this paradigm clash will play out remains unknown at the time of this writing.

This chapter focuses primarily on the developments related to the paradigm that predated managed-care initiatives. This is primarily because a central aim is to provide a perspective on service delivery issues, and to relate them to an emerging base of social science knowledge and theory. This is in contrast to the managed care phenomenon, which has emerged largely as a cost-efficiency strategy and, at least for troubled children and families, is not grounded within the practice experience of developmental and community knowledge. Given this, the purpose of this chapter is to examine the forces behind the reform momentum, as well as to highlight the barriers to broad-scale change in the delivery of helping services to troubled children and families. To that end, the chapter has three goals: to highlight the role of the federal government in both facilitating and inhibiting a shift in the prevailing paradigm; to examine service developments that carry the seeds of a new paradigm further; and to speculate on the implications of new policy and practice developments for community psychologists, for our understanding of the change processes at various levels of government and, ultimately, for long-term change in the definition of public responsibility to multineed children and families.

THE ANALYTIC FRAMEWORK

Because our analysis examines intersecting factors at various levels of government and across systems, it is appropriate to apply an ecological perspective to the discussion. Such a perspective provides a framework though which to view the dominant, traditional paradigm that is the object of change strategies, as well as a lens through which to examine the structural and value shifts that are gaining limited, but significant, legitimacy. In so doing, it draws heavily on the work of both Hobbs and Bronfenbrenner. As early as 1978, Hobbs first called attention to the power of an ecological perspective to heighten our understanding of helping interventions (Hobbs, 1978). Shortly thereafter, Bronfenbrenner (1979) articulated his theory of ecology, in this instance focusing not on interventions, but on the mechanisms and processes of human development. Envisioning what amounts to a "nested" theory of human development, he described four sets of relationships/conditions that influence a child's development: the child in relation to his own immediate environment (i.e., his family, his school); the family in relationship to other systems that directly affect the child (i.e., the schools); the factors that indirectly affect the child through the family (i.e., the family's employment patterns), and the larger political and social factors (i.e., public policy or larger ideologies) that affect both the child and the family indirectly.

However, although recognizing the power of institutional forms beyond the community (i.e., public policy as shaped through the courts and legislation), Bronfenbrenner, a developmental psychologist, focused most of his analysis on the child in the context of family and immediate community (Bronfenbrenner, 1980, 1986). Further, his emphasis was on normal development. But spurred by the power of an ecological metaphor that, by definition, emphasizes and stimulates analyses of both positive and negative reciprocal relationships among and between professionals and clients, individuals and families, and agencies and institutions, the concept has now taken hold across a broad range of human service domains. So, for example, the literature reveals the use of an ecological framework in analyses of the fields of child mental health, social work, and child welfare, as well as healthcare (Apter & Propper, 1988; Combrinck-Graham, 1990; Gerhardt, 1989; Kemp, Whittaker, & Tracey, 1997; Munger, 1991).

Most of these analyses share a common approach, articulating the way specific informal networks and social support systems, as well as more formal agencies and institutions, impinge upon the functioning of one family. The locus of attention in these analyses is the family/child unit and the services and institutions with which the family comes into direct contact. The analyses are relatively silent, however, about the ways in which public, and specifically national, policies affect the shape of the social service delivery system at the state and local levels. Yet, national policies are often an invisible determinant of the degrees of freedom that individual agencies and professionals have in responding to family needs. Further, in placing the family system at the center of the analysis, they also tend to ignore the significance of one other important determinant of outcome, the relationships *across* different service systems at both the state and (especially) local levels (i.e., child welfare, juvenile justice, child mental health, education), for these too shape outcomes for the often shared families that the systems serve. This analysis seeks to shift the figure ground balance; placing not the families, but the larger ecological factors that so significantly determine the degrees of freedom an individual service provider has in working with children and families.

THE CHANGING MANDATES OF PUBLIC RESPONSIBILITY

As a context for examining the efforts to move toward a new paradigm for the delivery of publicly supported social services, this section provides an overview of the evolution of public responsibility, with an emphasis on the legacy of the legislative directions of the past.

The history of social services for children and adolescents in this country, particularly those who are poor, is a long one (Bremner, 1970). Originally, public responsibility for these children was seen almost entirely as a local function. Reflecting an early manifestation of "blaming the victim," treatment for poor, orphaned, or abandoned children was often harsh, and marked by placement in institutions once known as "poor houses." As reports of abuse of these children surfaced during the late 19th century, states began to take a more active role, often creating boards of overseers to visit these institutions and report publicly on the conditions they found (Bremner, 1970).

The turn of the century brought significant changes as the settlement-house movement challenged the institutional model and sought to integrate new immigrant families into the fabric of the community (Bremner, 1970; Costin, 1983, 1985). Social work emerged as a profession, and the array of organizations seeking to respond to needy children and families expanded. Gradually, child welfare functions, focused on neglected, abandoned, and dependent (i.e., poor) youth, became more differentiated and new institutions were created. Foremost among these were the juvenile courts. Initially started in Chicago, these spread rapidly as an effort to respond to the "deviant" behavior of the many immigrant children flooding some of the large cities. Seen by some as a reasonable response to a social threat, and by others as a clear manifestation of an effort to stamp out ethnic differences, the courts soon became central in the lives of poor and troubled families. Indeed, it was the judges who, out of frustration, called for the development of child-guidance clinics, which could offer more help than they could from the bench. Thus, during the 1930s these too, largely capitalizing on new child-development and mental-health concepts, were added to the network of services and functions (Levine & Levine, 1992).

As services and courts grew, so did the web of public policies affecting dependent, neglected, and abandoned children, as well as children brought before the courts as delinquent, and eventually as status offenders (a status offense is an act that would not be considered a problem were it not committed by a minor). At first, the activity was largely confined to the state level, reflected in the passage of statutes defining the conditions under which state authority could be used to intervene in family life and to place children either in foster homes or in state institutions for the delinquent (Bremner, 1970). Gradually, however, the federal role became increasingly significant.

The Growing Federal Role

Pre-1960

Congress enacted specific legislation related to the social welfare of children and families as early as 1819, setting aside land for schools for deaf children. But not until the latter half of the 20th century did the federal government assume an increasingly active role in influencing the shape of the social service system, both at the state and community levels (Bremner, 1970; Knitzer, 1987). The first substantive legislation pertaining to social services for children and families was enacted in 1934 as part of the Social Security Act. It encouraged states to create public child-welfare agencies in all jurisdictions of the state, and provided funds for foster care.

The 1960s and 1970s

Federal activity with respect to social services for children and families between the New Deal and the Great Society was limited, although Congress did enact the School Lunch Program, largely to provide a market outlet for farmers (Steiner, 1976). However, this all changed during the 1960s and early 1970s (Knitzer, 1987; Levitan, 1969; Steiner, 1976). In response to the heightened commitment of that time to deal with poverty, other federal legislation was (and continues to be) enacted that had a major bearing on the support services available to poor, often minority, and troubled children and their families.

Juvenile Justice. With respect to troubled children and families, the initial focus of attention, spurred by an interest by President Kennedy, was juvenile delinquency. This culminated in 1974 in the passage of the Juvenile Justice and Delinquency Prevention Act (JJDP), which provided funds for a range of community-based services. (Until that time, federal attention to juvenile delinquency had been confined to juveniles charged with federal offenses).

The JJDP legislation was, in many ways, groundbreaking. As was the case with Head Start (Zigler & Valentine, 1979), Congress used social-science theory (that delinquency was environmentally determined and that changing the environment would change behavior) to justify the enactment of a new federal approach (Levitan, 1969). Growing from the theory, the legislation was not simply focused on youth in crisis. Rather, the goal was more ambitious—to use federal dollars to prevent delinquency; to prevent, in other words, an undesirable social and personal outcome. As a result, in its early years, JJDP was a catalyst for the development of a broad range of programs that went far beyond traditional (and limited) notions of social services, narrowly viewed as face-to-face casework and counseling. Instead, they revisited some of the more comprehensive strategies and approaches of the old settlement-house movement of the 19th century reformers. Although this broad, preventive approach was not sustained during the Reagan–Bush years, the early funds spawned a range of innovative youth initiatives, and strengthened a commitment to develop specialized services for adolescents.

During those "heady" days of the 1960s and early 1970s, when there was a widespread belief that poverty could be if not conquered, then at least reduced, there was also a more targeted effort to strengthen social services. To this end, in 1974 Congress created Title XX of the Social Security Act, called the Social Services Title. In rhetoric characteristic of a frontier mentality, that legislation took as its goal enhancing not family, nor child and family functioning, but "self-sufficiency," in particular economic self-sufficiency. Not surprisingly, the funds for the program were initially used largely to support childcare for parents in job-training programs.

Special Education. A federal commitment related to social services was reflected in the provisions of the 1974 landmark Education for All Handicapped Children Act (EHA), now known as the Individuals with Disabilities Education Act (IDEA). Reflecting the *zeitgeist* of the 1960s and 1970s that included a focus on the rights of the disenfranchised, the law set forth a series of rights and protections for children, including the development of a written *individualized* education plan and periodic reviews of progress. It also guaranteed parents a voice in school-related decision-making, laying the groundwork for strong family advocacy on behalf of children with special educational needs. Most significantly, from a social-service perspective, the legislation required schools not only to educate such children, but to provide them with related support services, including counseling, therapy, and social services if these were necessary to enable the children to learn.

In fact, implementation of this aspect of the law has been particularly problematic, especially for troubled children with emotional or behavioral problems (Knitzer, Steinberg, & Fleisch, 1990). But as a matter of policy, this country is now on record defining a role for social services within or limited to the schools for children with special needs. Moreover, as concern with educational issues escalates on the policy agenda, there is new interest in revisiting the role of social services within a school context for all children, and particularly for children at risk of school failure (Levy & Copple, 1989; Center for the Future of Children, 1992).

Child Abuse. Finally, from the perspective of social services, federal activity of the 1970s is notable because it marked the first Congressional response to child abuse, a reality garnering increased visibility due to both the availability of x-ray technology and the recognition of the battered child syndrome (Levine, 1992). Thus, again in 1974 (a banner year for children and social services), Congress enacted the Child Abuse Treatment and Prevention Act. The law required that in order to access federal funds for abused children, each state had to establish a system to report and investigate allegations of abuse. Congress mandated, in other words, the creation of what has become the child-protection system. Although funds through this legislation were (and continue to be) very limited, its impact on the social-service system has been enormous (Kamerman & Kahn, 1991).

The 1980s

During the 1980s there were two federal legislative developments that have had major implications for rethinking the ways in which social services to children and families are delivered. Both were in response to documentation of serious problems in the ways in which public dollars were expended on behalf of troubled children and families, particularly those involved with the child-welfare system, the mental health system, or both.

Child Welfare. During the 1970s, concern about child-welfare practices escalated, as analyses by advocates and others both nationally and within individual states found troubling patterns (Knitzer, Allen, & McGowan, 1978; National Commission of Children in Need of Parents, 1978). Close to half a million children were being removed from their homes and placed in foster care, with virtually no efforts to provide services to enable the families to keep their children. Yet, in a distortion of a social contract, once in placement, the children were virtually abandoned, with little effort to reunite them with their own families or to place them, as an alternative, in adoptive homes. Moreover, analyses of the limited statistical data available suggested that life for children in foster care was quite different from the idealized image; many children experienced frequent moves and frequent changes of caseworkers. For minority children, disproportionately represented in child welfare, the burden was even greater—more time in care and even less stability. The most striking finding, however, was that the problem was exacerbated by federal policies. The legislation of the 1930s that had once marked a positive reform effort was getting in the way of providing services to children in their own families. Virtually 80% of the available funds could only be used for out-of-home placement, a small percentage for family-based services, and nothing to encourage adoption.

Congress deemed this an unacceptable situation, and in the waning days of the Carter administration, dramatically revamped the federal role (Jacobs & Davies, 1992). This increased the funds that could be used to provide "preventative services," that is, services to families as alternatives to out-of-home placement; provided new funds to encourage the adoption of children who could not return to their biological families; and established a system of protections for children in foster care centering around periodic administrative and court reviews to prevent children from becoming lost in the system. The law, known as P.L. 96-272, the Adoption Assistance and Child Welfare Act, also sought to protect the rights of parents of children in placement by ensuring them a voice in these periodic procedures (Allen & Knitzer, 1983).

Predictably, this new legislation was not embraced by the Reagan administration, which, despite its vocal proclamations of commitment to family, sought aggressively to undermine the law, first by failing to write regulations (which must be in place for a law to take effect) and then by failing to monitor the implementation of the regulations. Nonetheless, as discussed in the next section, the family-focused ideology of the law has served as a spur to the development of new approaches to child-welfare services.

Children's Mental Health. In contrast to the federal role in child welfare, the federal role in children's mental health has been inconsistent and very limited. The first flurry of attention to children's mental health was in 1972 (Meyers, 1985). At that point, as an afterthought to the Community Mental Health Centers Act, and as a response to a Congressionally appointed Joint Commission on the Mental Health of Children, Congress permitted both community mental health centers and free-standing child-guidance centers to develop special programs for children (and presumably their families, although this was never made explicit). In crafting the legislation, Congress authorized awards for up to seven years. But while those agencies receiving grants were protected, Congress itself had a change of heart, and the legislation was repealed two years later.

Not until 12 years later did Congress again examine the question of public responsibility to children and adolescents in need of mental health services, partially in response to a national report by the Children's Defense Fund. That report examined the response of the mental health system to emotionally disturbed children who were the responsibility of mental health agencies or other child-serving systems. It found such children to be virtually "unclaimed" by any public system (Knitzer, 1982). Fewer than one-half of the state departments of mental health even had a person assigned to such children, and the state role was limited either to providing in-patient care alone or, in some states, in-patient and some out-patient care, primarily through mental health centers. Families were largely ignored or treated as if they caused the problem. Most significantly, the report highlighted the reality that the vast majority of children in need of mental health services were not the direct responsibility of mental health agencies. Rather they were in the care and often the custody of child welfare, juvenile justice, and special education.

Two years later, with very little fanfare, Congress authorized the National Institute of Mental Health (NIMH) to allocate $1.5 million to create the Child and Adolescent Service System Program (CASSP). In contrast to the detailed child-welfare reform legislation, in this instance there was no authorizing legislation, but instead merely budgetary authority for a small new program. However, although CASSP was, by federal standards, a very small program, it has been an important one. In particular, in contrast to the child-welfare reform strategy, CASSP has focused attention on the need for a systems approach to reform (Stroul, 1996). It provides no money for direct services, but instead served as a catalyst to the states, challenging them to strengthen state leadership on behalf of the children within state departments of mental health, and to insist that state mental health actively link with other child-caring agencies, particularly child welfare and special education.

But CASSP also sought to transform the traditional children's mental health paradigm in three other significant ways (Knitzer, 1987). First, CASSP encouraged states to strengthen the array of community-based services to meet the needs of troubled children who needed a more intensive response than out-patient care as an alternative to out-of-home placement (Stroul & Friedman, 1986). To this end, CASSP encouraged demonstrations in communities to implement the concept of a community-level system of care, encompassing both non-residential services (i.e., crisis intervention, day treatment, respite care for families) and residential services, including professional/therapeutic foster home families. Second, CASSP encouraged the emergence of a strengthened parental voice, seeding family-support groups across the country, along with technical assistance and even a new national organization. Third, CASSP raised the consciousness of child and family mental health professionals about the importance of attention to the ethnic and cultural context in which mental health services are delivered (Cross, Barzon, Dennis, & Isaacs, 1989; Isaacs & Benjamin, 1991).

Policy Mandates and Messages of the 1980s and Early 1990s

Taken together, changes in federal laws governing the allocation of public dollars for troubled and high-risk children and families reflect, to varying degrees, several themes that carried with them the seeds of a new approach to service delivery. First, they reflect a deepening commitment to families usually written off as "dysfunctional" and/or blamed for a child's problem. This is enormously significant. If parents, even parents with multiple and complex needs, are viewed as having strengths that can be mobilized on behalf of their children, professionals must build a service-delivery system in a new image—one charged to help parents parent more effectively, whatever obstacles they face, as long as a child's safety can be assured.

Behind this radical shift in orientation lay a dramatic questioning of the *status quo*. However haltingly, the notion that children can be "rescued" from their families, class, and culture, which propelled many of the early social-service initiatives, has been tested and found wanting on many different levels. To that end, public-policy mandates in child welfare, mental health, and special education begin to call upon social-service delivery systems to focus new attention on how to work with, rather than abandon, families beset by difficulties that may limit their parenting capacity. For example, the amendments to child-welfare legislation sought to stimulate the field to develop new technologies for working with families that include substance abusers, a disturbingly widespread problem, particularly in communities with a high concentration of low-income families.

The second theme, closely intertwined with the first, is a deepening policy commitment to avoid the unnecessary out-of-home placement of children. Thus, in different ways, each of the systems is charged, to the extent possible, to keep children with their own families and in their own communities. According to the child-welfare laws, placement must be "in the least restrictive setting," and "reasonable efforts" must be made to prevent placement. The special-education laws call for placement in the most normal setting; CASSP, in its emphasis on developing a range of services to supplement traditional in- and out-patient care, seeks to operationalize a way to prevent placement by ensuring that a range of sufficiently intensive alternatives are available within the community. In part, as noted above, this thrust represents a growing questioning of the merits of removing children from their own homes and families; in part it reflects attention to economics. Out-of-home residential care is getting prohibitively expensive, and foster parents, the backbone of the placement system, harder to recruit (Citizens for Missouri's Children, 1989; Knitzer & Cole, 1989a, 1989b).

The third theme, especially visible in legislation crafted during the 1970s, is the emphasis placed on protecting the rights of children (and to a lesser extent, families) to *individualized services*, those that are tailored to a particular set of needs and strengths. This is most evident in special-education legislation, which requires an individualized education plan and, further, establishes a series of due-process procedures that theoretically were intended to ensure a parental voice in school decision-making. Similarly, the child-welfare legislation of the 1980s set forth a series of checks and balances largely centering around reviews of children in placement, in order to hold public systems accountable for the fates of individual children.

These protections have, in fact, spawned a great deal of both individual and class-action litigation over the years. Yet there is a widespread sense that, however important, the procedural approach to protections has had mixed outcomes, involving families and systems in adversarial battles, diverting energies from the quality of services for parents to ensure their voice in the decision-making, and, in effect, creating the illusion of accountability (Kamerman & Kahn, 1989; Knitzer, Steinberg, & Fleisch, 1990). A response to this was visible at two levels. The first could be seen in the ever-changing federal legislative framework, particularly the special-education laws. To that end, when a right to appropriate services was extended to infants and toddles with development delays, families, not just children, were encouraged to explore non-adversarial dispute-resolution mechanisms, such as mediation.

Perhaps more significantly, however, and a testament to the effort to focus on substantive, rather than merely procedural, compliance with the spirit of the laws, service providers and policymakers alike began to explore ways to make the service system more responsive to the individualized (perhaps "familized" would be a better word) mandate. This is important because of the potential impact on real children and families (as discussed later). But it is also important because it represents an interesting example of the dynamic interplay between concepts embedded in public policy, and the ways in which one decade's innovative concepts can stretch a field in not necessarily predictable ways. Policymakers speak of the unanticipated consequences of particular policies. In that instance the consequence appears to be a catalyst for new practice strategies.

Focusing on the family, on avoidance of unnecessary out-of-home care, and on individualizing services are all concepts given special credibility in the policy context in recent years. But, however important these themes are, they get "played out," indeed, integrated into the earlier structure of federal legislation that is governed by two salient principles; first, that in order to access federally supported social services, a child and family must be experiencing a serious or sustained crisis and, second, access to services are categorical, reimbursed through a funding stream generated by a particular legislation, related to a particular service system, and bound by particular eligibility criteria and limits. Stated differently, even if analysis reveals that there are common themes across individual pieces of legislation; in practice, it remains very difficult to manipulate the legislation to develop, at the community level, a seamless service-delivery system where system boundaries and structure do not get in the way of service.

THE VIEW FROM THE FIELD: THE PREVAILING PARADIGM

Viewed from a state and community perspective, there are essentially four public systems that to varying degrees are either legally mandated or expected to provide help to children in their care—child welfare, juvenile justice, mental health, and special education. Each of these is represented typically by a single agency or unit. (The names and functions vary somewhat from state to state and community to community). At the direct service level, social services to children and families are typically provided by either private, mostly non-profit agencies (e.g., family service agencies, battered women and children's aid societies) or by public agencies such as community mental health centers and local child welfare offices. (As noted, a recent phenomenon of for-profit managed care has also emerged). Typically, these local agencies are paid with public funds through contracts, third-party reimbursements, or direct budget lines from any or all of the public systems charged with responsibility for the children and adolescents. Before exploring the new developments that are visible within the field, first consider the prevailing paradigm for social services for children and their families.

Despite calls for more respect for families, cross-system collaboration at the community level, and efforts to direct dollars to family and community-based services and away from unnecessary out-of-home care, widespread change within these systems is still illusory. Instead, the three defining aspects of the prevailing paradigm at the state and local level reflect tradition and historical legacies. First, overall, the social-service delivery system remains a vertical one. Individual service delivery systems, even if serving the same children and families, typically have few formal mechanisms for working together on behalf of a specific child or family. Second, even within specific service delivery systems, categorical programs are administered in ways that narrow service options, so, for example, except in unusual circumstances, funds for out-of-home placements cannot be diverted to support home and community-based services. Third, individuals, rather than families, continue to be defined as the "client."

The end result is that, structurally, the service delivery system at both the state and local levels remains much as it has been traditionally—separate systems with limited mandates. At the state level, an ecological map would show a picture of vertical columns representing the different service agencies, typically with narrow, if any, passageways from one to the other. Instead, each system is responsible for a distinct, rather narrowly defined population of children and, only to varying degrees, the child's family. Child welfare, originally mandated to provide a range of social services to a range of children, today focuses largely on abused and neglected children (Kamerman & Kahn, 1991). Juvenile justice services children who come before the courts as delinquents or status offenders, offering largely probation or institutionalization. Mental health agencies serve "mentally ill," seriously emotionally disturbed children or behaviorally disordered children (whatever label is chosen), largely determined by whether they have a psychiatric diagnosis; notwithstanding CASSP, mental health agencies still deal with them largely in traditional, office-based out-patient therapy, residential treatment, or hospitals.

At the local level, the system-by-system approach feeds into other sets of problems. For example, there are often gaps in particular types of services that no agency provides (for example, day-treatment programs or therapeutic preschool programs). Sometimes each agency provides similar services with multiple administrative structures, and sometimes one system provides a needed service but is inaccessible to clients of another system. Private providers, especially those running large agencies, often try to structure a coherent array of services even with these constraints. So, in an effort to meet the needs of the families and children who come before them, they become adept at getting categorical funds from a broad range of funding sources. In New York City, for example, a study of 35 settlement houses found each received funding from 21 different programs, many serving the same types of families (United Neighborhood Houses of New York, 1991). Even so, arbitrary restrictions and funding limits defeat the intent to enhance families and community services. A program for children at risk of dropping out can serve only target children, but not their siblings. (United Neighborhood Houses of New York, 1990). Or, programs targeted to substance abusers aged 15 and up cannot work with 13-year-old abusers. Similarly, programs designed for children with serious behavioral and emotional problems cannot provide any support to other family members, again, particularly siblings. In other instances, families with young children and adolescents may end up with (to paraphrase Mother Goose) "so many case workers they don't know what to do." Clearly, from many perspectives, the prevailing social-services paradigm is increasingly cumbersome to both public- and private-sector providers, particularly to those who work with families with a wide variety of complex needs, often in low-income communities.

Research data from the 1980s provide a slightly different rationale for making the multiple systems dealing with troubled children and families more permeable. This evidence suggests that many of the troubled and at-risk children and adolescents often exhibit the same kinds of behaviors, and need many of the same kinds of services, regardless of whether they are the responsibility of mental health, child welfare, juvenile justice, or even special education (Knitzer, 1982; Rutter, 1979). For example, child welfare officials all over the country are reporting that higher proportions of the children, adolescents, and families they serve have more serious emotional and behavioral problems than in the past (Virginia Department of Social Services, 1986). Overall estimates suggest that anywhere from one third to one half of the children in the child welfare system need mental health and other specialized family-support services (Knitzer, 1989). One study (Trupin, Low, Forsyth-Stephens, Tarico, & Cox, 1988) found an even higher rate. Mental health officials report that children who come before out-patient mental health agencies increasingly look like the same children who come before child welfare agencies. In Congressional testimony, mental health center directors from all regions of the country reported that the children being referred to clinics are more violent, more substance abusing, and more disturbed than previously (United States House of Representatives, Select Committee on Children, Youth, and Families, 1987).

For children in placement, the patterns of overlapping need are even more dramatic. Studies of children in residential treatment facilities show little variation in either diagnoses or past histories whether they are placed by mental health or child welfare agencies (Citizens for Missouri's Children, 1989). A multistate study of the placement of children in out-of-home care found that when a child is placed through a child welfare agency, it is largely a function of whether problems were identified by school or not, rather than of the severity of the problems (Friedman, Silver, Duchnowski, Kutash, Eisen, Brandenburg, & Prange, 1988). Youth in detention through the juvenile justice system show similarly high levels of emotional disturbance, with many of the same kinds of family patterns that are reflected in the mental health caseload already described. Moreover, we also know that many of the troubled children and adolescents who need services are served by multiple systems, either sequentially or concurrently. A New York State study, capturing the pattern others have also noted, found that 41% of the children in mental health facilities were veterans of the department of social services, as were 40% of those in juvenile-justice facilities (Cocozza & Ingalls, 1984).

But beyond research, there was one other force acting as a spur to a paradigm shift—the increasing stress on the systems. Homelessness, violence, and drugs, all conditions damaging to the mental health of children and families, are ever more visible, and account for a sharp rise in foster-care placement rates following a decline in the early 1980s. Those who seek to improve outcomes for the most troubled children and families are feeling overwhelmed and increasingly concerned about maximizing the impact of the services that they can provide. This coupled with the mandates embedded in public policies have set the stage for new attention to the generation of reform strategies designed to change both service interventions and the ecology of service system interactions, particularly at the community level.

TOWARD A NEW VISION: RESTRUCTURING THE SOCIAL SERVICE SYSTEM

Effective change in the area of social service, as indeed is the case with change in virtually any area that involves the family, public institutions, and public policies, is dependent upon three components. First, it is necessary that there be some models of programmatic approaches that embody the appropriate principles and practices. Second, if there is to be large- (or even moderate-) scale implementation, there must also be responses from policy-makers either at the state or federal level or both. They are faced with the task of providing incentives and a supportive context for institutionalizing the new directions. Third, and this is typically the most difficult, the fiscal, professional, and other barriers that may get in the way of implementing new practice and policy directions must be addressed. Consider next efforts to create alternative approaches to programs and policies, and to confront the barriers that lock the social services system into traditional paradigms.

New Service Assumptions and Strategies

Thinking Families

The rhetoric of social services have always included lip service to the family—placement is the last resort, according to child welfare, for example. Instead, too often families have been disrespected and discounted.

For this reason, it is significant that the most visible and widespread service development for troubled children and families has been the growth of family-focused services that seek, in very concrete and direct ways, to empower highly stressed, and typically very poor, families. Particularly relevant for the purposes of this chapter are the family-focused approaches to end the inappropriate removal of children from their families. For both the mental health and the social service community, these approaches have largely centered on the emergence of strategies to serve the children and families *in their own homes*, with intensive, short-term interventions called family preservation services (Allen & Larson, 1998; Knitzer & Cole, 1989a, 1989b, Whittaker, Kinney, Tracy, & Booth, 1988). The roots of family preservation services go back to the days when settlement-house workers went into homes routinely and helped families with concrete needs. But family preservation services are also deeply linked to new therapeutic strategies, particularly family systems therapy and behavioral interventions, that are, in turn, grounded in solid theoretical frameworks; crisis intervention, social learning, and family systems theories, with different programs emphasizing one over the other (Barth, 1988). Most importantly, they are also linked to a value orientation that seeks to empower families, even families facing the most desperate odds by helping them define, prioritize, and solve problems.

The most well-known and the most replicated of these intensive, short-term program models is the Homebuilders program, begun in 1974 by several psychologists working in a child welfare agency (Whittaker et al., 1988). The Homebuilders program is interesting in several respects: it is not only home-based, that is workers go into the homes to see the families, but it is also very short term, limited to four to six weeks. However, it is an exceptionally intensive service, with families receiving as much as 20 hours a week of face-to-face therapy during the intervention. (Other family preservation programs, typically less intensive, last for up to three months). The intensity of the intervention, in fact, turns the traditional therapeutic timetable on its head, so that in the course of a short-term intervention, families are likely to receive almost as much therapy as they would in a year of traditional outpatient visits. Moreover, family-preservation services also extend the notion of traditional limits of therapy to include a concrete commitment to helping a family meet its basic needs. Thus, in the Homebuilders program, the therapist engages families and wins their trust, often by helping them get food, housing, or benefits.

There are still many unanswered questions about this service approach. Skeptics argue to date that the data are equivocal as to whether family-preservation services avoid, or merely postpone, placement, and call for more sensitive measures of impact on individual and family functioning (Wells & Beigel, 1992). Others focus on exploring how to strengthen the approach. What kinds of follow-up do families need when they are in these programs? Can the impact of the service be strengthened if closer links are made with the early childhood and the school community (Knitzer, 1996). In a New York City program, for example, families themselves expressed more concern about the school-related problems of their children than any other problems (Mitchell, Tovar, & Knitzer, 1989). But there can be no question of the significance of family preservation as a powerful catalyst for challenging the comfortable out-of-home paradigm that particularly pervades child welfare and mental health.

Family-preservation services, however, are not the only manifestation of a new service stance toward families. The growth of kinship foster care, in which children who cannot be with their own mothers and fathers are placed with relatives (who are reimbursed), also marks a recognition that family ties matter, and matter a great deal to children. In New York City, for example, one half of the children in the foster care system are in relatives' homes (Legal Aid Society, 1992). At one level, this calls for a rethinking of the mandates of the federal child welfare legislation, which require that children either be returned to their own parents or adopted. (A significant proportion of relatives do not wish to adopt, but are willing to provide care to children for long periods of time). At another level, it marks a dramatic extension of efforts to build a social-service system that is supportive of families.

In addition, and also of great potential significance in improving the delivery of direct services, are the efforts, largely spurred by the children's mental health community, to redefine the relationship between parents and professionals so that parents are treated as allies and advocates, rather than as merely victims or problems. In exploring this development, Friesen and Koroloff (1990) highlight the evolution of service approaches from a system in which parents were seen as the cause of a child's problem and the target of change efforts, to a system where professional tried to provide supportive psychotherapy and groups, to an effort to supplement these professionally driven services with parent-organized and/or parent-led support groups. While the road to this new view of parents is rocky, and traces of earlier and stigmatizing approaches are still all too present, alternative philosophies, emphasizing teaching and helping parents to cope, empowering them, and respecting their strengths, are expanding.

There is one other significant manifestation of the growing centrality of a family perspective; that is, the emergence of what has been called the "family support movement" (Zigler & Weiss, 1985). Its roots lie in the efforts within the child development community to strengthen families' capacity to provide nurture and positive early childhood experiences to young children. To that end, many communities are developing family resource centers, places where parents, particularly those stressed by the unremitting burdens of poverty, can have respite from the demands of child care, learn better techniques of interacting with their children, and have a chance to build their own self-esteem through a broad range of activities. In some instances, family resource programs are targeted to a specific subset of families, such as teen mothers, who are especially likely to benefit from a program that enhances their understanding of how children develop, that provides concrete help, and that enables them to connect with both mentors and other parents in similar situations. So, for example, the state of Maryland has set up a network of such programs. Elsewhere, the programs are linked to early childhood programs. No rigorous or long-term evaluations of such efforts have yet been undertaken, but the effort to rebuild a sense of family, community, and support marks a new use of public dollars, and a new professional paradigm (Dunst, Trivette, & Deal, 1988; Knitzer & Page, 1996; Zigler & Weiss, 1985).

Related to this effort, it should also be noted that there is growing interest not only in using the school as a hub for the delivery of social services to children, but as a hub for family support services as well. To that end, for example, San Diego County developed a comprehensive support program in an elementary school serving a very poor community. Armed with documentation that the school population consumed 10% of the county social-service budget, and that one third of the school's families were involved with multiple county social-service agencies, the county stationed workers from the different agencies at the school site, empowered them to intervene earlier, and tracked the experiment to see its impact. Drawing on much the same impulses, the state of Kentucky embarked on an ambitious project to create family resource centers linked to elementary schools throughout the state. The importance of careful research to document the impact of these efforts cannot be overstated, nor can the challenge such multidimensional service system research poses to the field.

Individualizing Services

As noted earlier in this chapter, in 1974 Congress called for individual education plans. Mental health agencies have long called for individualized treatment plans. But, for the most part, efforts to individualize services have been spotty. Spurred largely by the CASSP momentum, a new trend is emerging—a commitment to tailor a mix of services to the unique needs of a particular child and family. Sometimes known as individualized services, and sometimes as "wrap-around services," the approach is rooted in the assumption that funds and services should be reallocated and used creatively for children in their own homes and communities. So, for example, mental health dollars in one community were used to pay for a behavioral coach to help a child learn to ride a bike and thus foster success with peers. On a systemwide basis, the concept was first used in North Carolina (Behar, 1985). Subsequently, the strategy was refined by the Alaska CASSP program, which developed innovative and carefully individualized treatment plans to return children to Alaska who were in out-of-home placement in the "lower 48." Efforts to test out the limits of the concept are escalating (Boyd, Reditt, & Clark, 1992). This, in turn, is spurring additional reform efforts, focused on creating pools of "flexible human service dollars" to enable workers to purchase the services that cannot otherwise be provided. In a corollary effort to build unified approaches to families, many communities are also creating cross-system teams to do treatment/service planning and assessment (as well as monitoring). Such teams, with respect to wrap-around services, become particularly important as a protection against arbitrary determinations. The goal is to set guidelines and accountability mechanisms that will give providers flexibility to use service funds creatively, but at the same time, responsibly.

Fostering Cross-System Collaboration

Calls for coordination and collaboration across agencies working with the same family are as routine as rhetoric in a political season about children being this nation's greatest resource. And yet, here too, efforts to operationalize the rhetoric are generating new intervention approaches. This is reflected in two ways; first, in the efforts to develop strategies to "glue" a package of services from different providers together and, second, in the efforts to create forum and processes for service providers, and sometimes parents, public officials, and the business community as well to come together at a community level to find new ways of making decisions about individual children and families, about how to allocate dollars for community services, and about how to build in meaningful accountability checks.

The emergence of intensive case management across different human service fields is the inevitable consequence of a human service system trying to meet the complex needs of families who require the involvement of multiple service agencies. To this end, across all human service fields, interest in what is generically a form of intensive case management is emerging, although increasingly, and in response to objections from parents who do not like the implication that they or their children are a "case" to be "managed," other terms (i.e., family specialist, family advocate, care coordinator) are gaining wider usage. Whatever the name, the essential task is to "glue" a package of services together for a specific child and family (Knitzer, 1982). Informally, the job description is to "do whatever it takes" to provide the appropriate mix of services and supports. More formally, the job typically entails working with a treatment team in the development of service plans, monitoring the service plans, troubleshooting, providing a caring ear for children and families, and navigating the bureaucracies to make sure that what is supposed to happen, happens. While there have been such efforts in the past (Apter, Apter, Trief, Cohen, Wooklock, & Harootunian, 1978; Knitzer, 1982), current efforts seem more likely to be institutionalized, in part because it is now possible to use Medicaid funding for them. Further, although the strategy to date has touched only a small number of children, and the training implications have not been well articulated, the approach echoes a theme of the family preservation initiatives (Burchard & Clarke, 1990). Rebuilding families is labor-intensive; and intensive involvement, even if on a time limited basis, may be more effective for families, and more cost efficient for the public coffers, than the usual once-a-week, or once-a-month, encounters.

The second approach to attacking the fragmentation of services that is bemoaned in virtually any community in this country involves creating (either by state option or local initiative) mechanisms that deliberately require or foster cross-system collaboration. In effect, this is the community-level counterpart of case management, service coordination, and individualized services. Central to the effort to implement cross-system collaborations is the notion that, taken together, the range of social services within a specific geographic area form a *de facto* system of care. Mechanisms are emerging to make explicit this *de facto* system of care, to identify gaps in services, and to generate strategies to reallocate funds (and to the extent possible, in a constraining fiscal climate, to expand them). In effect, by inventing, if not reinventing, a communitywide network view of typically discrete social services, local-level providers and policymakers are focusing an ecological lens at the community level. Stimulated by the work of Stroul and Friedman (1986), as they have evolved, community-based cross-system collaborations have three components: ensuring that each community has a range of non-residential, as well as residential, support services; providing a mechanism to permit the community, through its public officials, advocates, and business representatives and providers to make consensual decisions about what programs are needed to fill in the gaps and how resources should be allocated; and identifying case-management capacity to permit active planning and monitoring of individual cases.

Changing State Policies

Not surprisingly, emerging state-level policy initiatives to improve social services to children and families bear a very direct relationship to the service developments just described. Paralleling the service developments, state-level policy strategies largely involve efforts to stimulate the delivery of intensive in-home and school-based services, as well as efforts to foster cross-system collaboration and to expand systems of care.

Family Preservation in Statute

Nurtured by the active encouragement of the Edna McConnell Clark Foundation and the development, with extensive foundation support, of national training, technical assistance, and support capacity, states are increasingly enacting legislation to ensure a statewide distribution of family preservation services. Thus, in a true example of what Elmore (1983) calls "social policy making as strategic intervention," 31 states developed major initiatives designed to ensure the spread of the services throughout the state (Edna McConnell Clark Foundation, 1990). Federal legislation in the early 1990s was, in fact, called the Family Preservation, Family Support, and Adoption Assistance Act. In 1997, however, this was superseded by the Safe Families and Adoption Assistance Act.

The development of strong family support services are proving attractive to policymakers for three major reasons. First, they can serve as a powerful test of the need for placement, thus meeting the policy mandate of both the child welfare and mental health systems to avoid unnecessary out-of-home placement. Second, in a cost-containment era, intensive, short-term services are demonstrably fiscally effective, costing substantially less than even the least expensive out-of-home placement. Third, such services are particularly attractive to policymakers because they seem effective for a broad spectrum of clients. Data show success in working with abused and neglected children, emotionally disturbed children, children facing hospitalization, and court-involved children. Moreover, since the focal point is the family, there are likely to be spin-off impacts for siblings as well as the target child at imminent risk of placement.

Policy Incentives for Cross-System Collaboration

The second major theme in social service policy initiatives at the state level is not as developed, but nonetheless potentially very significant. It involves the deliberate effort to foster cross-system collaborations using policy carrots and sticks. In Pennsylvania, for example, using the CASSP model and pooled moneys from mental health and education, the state supported a statewide network of CASSP coordinators, charged to facilitate the development of cross-system approached to serving troubled children and families. In Virginia, the state has moved steadily from an early effort to pool funds on behalf of specific children bouncing from system to system, to an effort to use pooled funds to seed services to broaden the availability of community-based day treatment, in-home services, and therapeutic fostercare, to supporting a demonstration effort in selected communities to create a system of care that goes beyond just those children identified as seriously emotionally disturbed.

The concept of reforming social services by strengthening the capacity within the community to link services across systems, and to do collaborative case planning, interventions, and monitoring is seen, in fact, as so compelling a change strategy that several foundations have created major initiatives to provide incentives to communities to revisit the customary way of doing business. But they have also sought to leverage change from the states, inviting them to participate in the initiative and insisting that the states agree to certain additional reforms, such as fiscal innovation. The Robert Wood Johnson Foundation, for example, supported a seven-site project focused on improving services to seriously emotionally disturbed children and adolescents using a community-collaboration approach (Beachler, 1990). Similarly, the Anne E. Casey Foundation mounted several community-driven initiatives focused specifically on improving outcomes for children and families in poor, urban communities. The role of foundations in fostering cross-system initiatives at the state and community level is particularly interesting because this is not a theme that has been sounded in federal legislation (although at the administrative level there is interest in service coordination).

Facing the Dilemmas and Barriers

This chapter is premised on two assumptions; first, the recent past has yielded important new insights about how to improve the ways in which we, as a society, respond to the needs of multineed children and families and, second, the social service system for children and families does not work as effectively as it could (even given limited resources). Taking the analysis further, there appear to be five major reasons for the difficulty and complexity of implementing new directions.

Pro-residential Bias

Since the early days of the "child-savers" and the "orphan trains," providing services to poor and troubled children has meant taking them from their homes. Today, this pro-residential bias continues to be pervasive not only among the mental health and the child welfare professionals, but also among legislators, even though evidence suggests an out-of-home placement strategy is not necessarily more effective and, indeed, often has negative consequences for the children (Lewis, 1980). The notion that it is possible to provide services of comparable intensity to the best of residential treatment to children and families in their own homes is simply not yet widely accepted, although the kinds of home-based services highlighted earlier are beginning to challenge the still-too-common paradigm that "intensive" must equal "out-of-home."

Anti-parent Bias

Closely related to the bias in favor of out-of-home placement is the bias against families, particularly poor families. Notwithstanding efforts to empower such families through both services and statutory protections, both workers and public officials continue to doubt the extent to which these families can be helped. In fact, in some ways, as substance abuse becomes one of the most common reasons that children are at risk, this belief may be escalating. The task, in response, is to increase the capacity to differentiate between those families who can be helped and those families where it is impossible to make gains—not to write off families in general. This is a challenge that the social service field has not yet mastered, notwithstanding the proliferation of risk-assessment scales.

Cross-System Suspicion

The third attitudinal barrier with which those seeking to strengthen cross-system collaboration must contend is essentially a cross-cultural barrier. Notwithstanding the likelihood that similar impulses motivate those who become psychologists or social workers, once they become part of a particular system, within-system socialization is powerful. Indeed, very often, although the children and adolescents move across systems, workers and public officials do not. This means there is often also a high level of ignorance or misinformation about the mandates and *modus operandi* of other systems. So, for example, there is often great skepticism on the part of child welfare agencies about whether mental health can really come through for them. Mental health personnel typically understand very little about child welfare laws. Educators often know little about how child welfare functions. Clearly then, in moving forward on a collaborative cross-system social-service agenda, either implicitly or explicitly, there must be opportunities for both policymakers and workers to talk to each other, to build a common language, and to own together the new service ideas. They must, in short, master different cultures.

Fiscal Barriers

The fourth barrier is fiscal. At one level, the problem has to do with the level of resources. As the problems of families escalate with rising substance abuse, homelessness, and poverty, the intervention task becomes more complex, even as the funding shrinks. At another level, there is also an issue about whether the existing resources are allocated in the most effective way and, indeed, whether potential resources are used, particularly to pay for the range of services families may need. This is largely a political problem, rooted in both attitudes to the poor and in the ways legislative committees are structured. They, too, often exist in isolation, with mental health committees, for example, having no connection with child welfare committees. At the state level, the signs are encouraging, as state legislatures are creating their own version of a cross-system policy change—special children's committees—charged to look at child and families policy through a coherent lens. At the federal level, recent changes toward the devolution of responsibility to the state and community may be helpful. At issue, however, is the Congressional Committee structure that promotes categorical programs.

The Town/Gown Gap

It takes enormous energy and effort to implement both program-level and policy-level innovations. Typically, the strategies emerge at the level of direct service, and are then used to justify reshaping public policies (although in the legislative process, or during subsequent implementation, sometimes the spirit of the innovation is lost). Typically, the academic community is not involved. This in turn creates new problems. The feedback loop between program providers, advocates, and policymakers is often better than the loop between activists within the human service system and the academic communities that frame research questions and, most significantly, train the next generation of human-service providers. Thus, it is of increasing concern that clinicians continue to be trained only in office-based interventions, rather than home, school, and community-based strategies (a focus lost from the early days of community psychology), and that, across disciplines, there is little effort to train human-service providers who can function comfortably in a cross-disciplinary, cross-system context. This creates a strange dilemma. Providers wonder where they will recruit staff to work in new ways with children and families, even as policymakers seek to expand mandates to implement these models.

LESSONS AND IMPLICATIONS

Thus far, this discussion has provided an overview of some of the themes that have undergirded efforts to improve both access to, and the quality of, social services afforded to troubled children and families, (Stroul & Friedman, 1996). Old dilemmas and problems remain, but at the same time, the new directions highlighted here are gaining visibility and to some extent, stability, although they are also being challenged by the managed-care paradigm. While there is little systematic research from which to draw formal lessons about the evolving social services paradigm, it does appear to have four sets of implications. First consider the implications for community psychologists.

Viewed from the perspective of community psychologists, at least three points are particularly interesting about these new developments. In the first place, the reform directions are consistent with at least two of the most important principles of community psychology: attention to ecological realities and attention to the goodness of fit between a person and his or her environment (Munger, 1991). The growing respect for viewing troubled families through an ecological lens is reflected at the direct-service level in the way that intensive in-home services are being shaped. (In a number of programs, for example, therapists and families even develop eco-maps as a way of both engaging them and identifying potential sources of untapped informal support). Similarly, respect for the ecology of service systems is reflected in the new attention to the potential of case management for multineed and multiservice user families. These are a direct response to a long overdue recognition that service systems within a community and at the state level are, like it or not, welded together in an ecological system, and that pressure on one part inevitably results in a reaction in another part.

The concern with the "person–environment fit" theme is, in some ways, more tentative but, ultimately, more promising, reflecting a policy commitment to better individualize interventions to meet the needs of children and families, regardless of the door through which they enter the service system. In this respect, federal policies have been a catalyst, propelling the field first to attend to procedural due-process issues and, more recently, to the meaning of substantive process. Toward this end, the new service developments highlighted in this chapter are particularly promising, reaching toward flexibility of dollars and individualized service interventions and real (as opposed to paper) cross-system and cross-professional linkages.

The third theme described in this chapter that resonates within community psychology is the renewed attention to the concept of community evident particularly in the efforts to foster cross-system perspectives at both the state and community levels. These new directions affirm the potential role of community in supporting troubled children and families. At the same time, a caveat is in order. It should be noted that the community settings targeted, for the most part, do not reach deeply into the urban areas most beset by poverty areas of the kind most recently described by Wilson (1987) as home to the "underclass," those stuck in poverty with few routes of escape and few models of alternatives.

Finally, and of a different nature, the emphasis on communitywide service system issues poses a real challenge for both the academic community and, particularly, the research community to test out methodologies that are sensitive enough to respond to the complex evaluation challenges the new service paradigm poses.

Viewed from still a broader perspective, the events of the last two decades with respect to the helping systems, as well as the ways in which public responsibility to poor and/or vulnerable children and families is being redefined, have also highlighted several lessons about social change in general. First, during the 1960s and 1970s, the catalyst for social change was clearly the federal government. During the 1980s and into the 1990s, foundations have become major players in seeking to shape social change processes, largely by holding out incentives to the states and communities to serve as a laboratory for new approaches in much the same way the federal government held out incentives earlier. During the late 1990s, the pendulum may be shifting again as "devolution," the transfer of responsibility for a range of governmental functions, shifts from the federal level to the state and local levels. Whether the changes will be institutionalized, and what foundation strategies will be needed facilitate this if outcomes are positive remains to be seen.

Second, based on the experience in implementing reform efforts, it is also clear that technical assistance, training, and a kind of cheerleading support function make a big difference, no matter what the investment of money. This is particularly true in terms of the impact of a CASSP-type framework throughout the policy community and of the spread of the concept of family-preservation services. What is interesting, however, is that much of the technical assistance and support has been generated at the national level. There is very little experience with states fostering such networks and support, yet ultimately, if the kind of changes envisioned by the proponents of a paradigm shift are to prevail, perhaps a next-generation task will be for states to provide similar support, technical assistance, and "cheerleading."

Third, although public policies for the population of children and families are often derided as ineffective and unresponsive, the evidence of service providers reaching to implement the spirit of the laws, for example, through the concept of "wrap-around services" is promising. It suggests an elasticity in public policy that may be important given the fact that legislative changes are made very incrementally, with add-ons to old paradigms more typical than total restructuring. (Even for the Individuals with Disabilities Education Act, which was once landmark, radical legislation is now being reframed and conceptualized in light of changing definitions of responsive service).

It is too early to proclaim that we are in the midst of a paradigm shift in the way we conceptualize social services for multineed, high-risk children and families in this country, or that the directions highlighted in this paper bespeak lasting change (Illback, Cobb, & Joseph, 1997; Knitzer, 1997). But it is clear that, building on the framework of due-process protections established through the reforms of the 1960s and 1970s, new attention is being turned to issues of quality as well as a sharpened concern with concrete outcomes. Even more significantly, we are also beginning to elaborate on and enhance the range of home and community-based service models and slowly to recognize the significance of service intensity. This, along with a meaningful interagency focus at all levels of the service-delivery system, may be the route toward what is, in fact, a new view of the ecology of the social service system for children and families. The implementation challenge is enormous and fraught with many difficulties, but the vision of a more responsive system appears to be becoming a reality in concept and, in some scattered places, in practice as well.

But there are also important limits. The new directions described in this chapter, however innovative, largely reach the circle of children who will cost the public money no matter what—in placement, in jails, or in special education. To access most of the interventions described here, a child must have been abused, court-involved, or even at the point of out-of-home placement. The challenge of early intervention, particularly for those children in what has been called "double jeopardy," exposed to the risks of poverty along with specific biological or environmental assaults (Kaplan-Sanoff, Parker & Zuckerman, 1991), still garners only limited policy support. It is true that there are some efforts to create a network of family support services for less at-risk parents and children (Weiss & Jacobs, 1988; Zigler & Weiss, 1985), but stable funding for these efforts are woefully limited. Fundamentally, across all levels of government, the short-term cost-containment mentality prevails. This has been dramatic in the last few years as managed care becomes the new "buzzword." This is neither to disparage the significance of the efforts described here, nor the enormity of the tasks of instituting these on a systemwide, rather than a demonstration, basis. But at the same time, the future agenda must also address the issues of early intervention, and indeed, the broader issues of poverty that breed so many of the problems with which the social service institutions are now confronted.

REFERENCES

Allen, M.L., & Larson, J. (1998). *Healing the whole family: A look at family care programs.* Washington, D.C.: Children's Defense Fund.

Allen, M. L., & Knitzer, J. (1983). Child welfare: Examining the policy framework. In B. McGowan & W. Meezan (Eds.), *Child welfare: Current dilemmas: future directions* (pp. 93–141). Itasca, IL: Peacock.

Apter, S., Apter, D., Trief, P., Cohen, N., Wooklock, D., & Harootunian, B. (1978). *The BRIDGE program: Comprehensive psychoeducational services for troubled children and families.* Washington, D.C.: National Institute of Mental Health.

Apter, S., & Propper, C. (1988). Ecological perspectives on youth violence. In S. Apter & A. Goldstein (Eds.), *Youth violence: Programs and prospects* (pp. 140–159). New York: Pergamon.

Barth, R. P. (1988). Theories guiding home-based intensive family preservation services. In J. Whittaker, J. Kinney, E. Tracey, & C. Booth (Eds.), *Improving practice technology for work with high risk families: Lessons from the Homebuilders Social Work Education Project* (pp. 91–114). Seattle: Washington Center for Social Workers Research, University of Washington.

Beachler, M. (1990). The mental health services program for youth. *Journal of Mental Health Administration, 17,* 115–121.

Behar, L. (1985). Changing patterns of state responsibility: A case study of North Carolina. *Journal of Clinical Child Psychology, 14,* 185–195.

Boyd, L. A., Reditt, C. A., & Clark, H. B. (1992). *Fostering individualized services: A wrap around study.* Tampa: Florida Mental Health Institute. Draft.

Bremner, R. H. (1970). *Children and youth in America.* Vols. I, II, & III. Cambridge, MA: Harvard University Press.

Bronfenbrenner, U. (1979). *The ecology of human development: Experiments by nature and design*. Cambridge, MA: Harvard University Press.

Bronfenbrenner, U. (1980). The ecology of childhood. *School Psychology Review*, *9*, 294–297.

Bronfenbrenner, U. (1986). The ecology of the family as a context for human development. *Developmental Psychology*, *22*, 723–742.

Burchard, J. D., & Clarke, R. T. (1990). The role of individualized care in a service delivery system for children and adolescents with severely maladjusted behavior. *The Journal of Mental Health Administration*, *17*, 148–160.

Center for the Future of Children. (1992). *School linked services: The future of children*, *2*. Available from the David and Lucille Packard Foundation, Los Altos: CA.

Children's Defense Fund. (1991). *The state of America's children*. Washington, D.C.: Author.

Citizens for Missouri's Children. (1989). *Where's my home? A study of Missouri's out of home placement*. Washington, D.C.: Author.

Cocozza, J., & Ingalls, R. (1984). *Characteristics of children out of home*. Albany: New York State Council on Children and Families.

Combrinck-Graham, L. (1990). *Giant steps: Therapeutic interventions in mental health*. New York: Basic Books.

Costin, L. B. (1985). The historical context of child welfare. In J. Laird & A. Hartman (Eds.), *A handbook of child welfare: Context, knowledge and practice* (pp. 34–60). New York: Free Press.

Costin, L. B. (1983). *Two sisters for social justice: A biography of Grace and Edith Abott*. Chicago: The University of Illinois Press.

Cross, T., Barzon, B., Dennis, K., & Isaacs, M. (1989). *Toward a culturally competent system of care*. Washington, D.C.: Georgetown University Child Development Center.

Danziger, S. M. (1990). Anti-poverty policies and child poverty. *Social Work Research Abstracts*, *26*, 17–24.

Dunst, C., Trivette, C., & Deal, A. (1988). *Enabling and empowering families: Principles and guidelines for practice*. Cambridge, MA: Brookline Books.

Edna McConnell Clark Foundation. (1990). *Keeping families together: Facts about family preservation*. New York: Author.

Elmore, R. (1983). Social policy making as strategic intervention. In E. Seidman (Ed.), *Handbook of social intervention* (pp. 212–236). Beverly Hills, CA: Sage.

Friedman, R., Silver, S., Duchnowski, A., Kutash, K., Eisen, M., Brandenburg, N., & Prange, M. (1988). *Characteristics of children with serious mental disturbances identified by public systems as requiring services*. Unpublished manuscript. Tampa: University of South Florida, Florida Mental Health Institute.

Friesen, B., & Koroloff, N. (1990). Family-centered services: Implications for mental health administration and research. *Journal of Mental Health Administration*, *17*, 26–47.

Gerhardt, U. (1989). *Ideas about illness: An intellectual and political history of medical sociology*. New York: New York University Press.

Hobbs, N. (1978). Families, schools and communities: An ecosystem for children. *Teacher's College Record*, *79*, 756–766.

Illback, R.J., Cobb, C..T., & Joseph, H.M. (Eds.). (1997). *Integrated services for children and families: Opportunities for psychological practice*. Washington, D.C.: American Psychological Association.

Isaacs, M., & Benjamin, M. (1991). *Towards a culturally competent system of care: Vol. II*. Washington, D.C.: Georgetown University Child Development Center.

Jacobs, F., & Davies, M. (1991). Rhetoric or reality? Child and family policy in the United States. *Social Policy Report*, *5*, 1–25.

Kamerman, S., & Kahn, A. (1989). *Social services for children, youth and families in the United States*. Greenwich, CT: Annie E. Case Foundation (reprinted, 1990, in *Children and Youth Services Review*, *12*, 1–184.

Kamerman, S., & Kahn, A. (1991). Is child protection driving child welfare? Where do we go from here? *Public Welfare*, *48*, 9–13.

Kaplan-Sanoff, M., Parker, S., & Zuckerman, B. (1991). Poverty and early childhood: What do we know and what should we do? *Infants and Young Children*, *4*, 58–76.

Kemp, S.P., Whittaker, J.K., & Tracey, E.M. (1997). *Person–environment practice: The social ecology of interpersonal helping*. Hawthorne, NY: Aldine DeGruyter.

Knitzer, J. (1982). *Unclaimed children: The failure of public responsibility to children and adolescents in need of mental health services*. Washington, D.C.: Children's Defense Fund.

Knitzer, J. (1987). *Federal policies and the well-being of children. A report to the W.T. Grant Foundation*. New York: Bank Street College of Education.

Knitzer, J. (1989). *Emerging collaborations between child welfare and mental health*. New York: Bank Street College of Education.

Knitzer, J. (1996). Meeting the mental health needs of young children and their families. In B. Stoul (Ed.), *Children's mental health: Creating systems of care in a changing society*. Baltimore: Paul H. Brookes.

Knitzer, J. (1997). Services integration for children and families: Lessons and questions. In R.J. Illback, C.T. Cobb, & H.M. Joseph, Jr. (Eds.), *Integrated services for children and families: Opportunities for psychological practice*. Washington, D.C.: American Psychological Association.

Knitzer, J., & Cole, E. (1989a). *Family preservation services: The program challenge for child welfare and child mental health systems*. New York: Bank Street College of Education.

Knitzer, J., & Cole, E. (1989b). *Family preservation services: The policy challenge to state child welfare and mental health systems*. New York: Bank Street College of Education.

Knitzer, J., & Page, S. (1996). *Map and track: State initiatives for young children and families*. New York: National Center for Children in Poverty, Columbia University School of Public Health.

Knitzer, J., Steinberg, Z., & Fleisch, B. (1990). *At the schoolhouse door: An examination of programs and policies for children with behavioral and emotional problems*. New York: Bank Street College of Education.

Legal Aid Society, Juvenile Rights Division. (1992). *Kinship Foster Care: A policy paper prepared for Symposium on Kinship Foster Care convened by the Association of the Bar of the City of New York*.

Levine, M. (1992). Child protection legislation: Origins and evolution. *The Child Youth and Family Quarterly, 15*, 2–3. Division 37. Washington, D.C.: American Psychological Association.

Levine, M., & Levine, A. (1992). *Helping children: A social history*. New York: Oxford University Press.

Levitan, S. (1969). *The great society's poor law*. Baltimore: Johns Hopkins Press.

Levy, J., & Copple, C. (1989). *Joining forces: A report from the first year*. Alexandria, VA: National Association of State Boards of Education.

Lewis, M. (1980). The undoing of residential treatment: A follow-up study of 51 adolescents. *Journal of the American Academy of Child Psychiatry, 19*, 160–171.

Meyers, J. (1985). Federal efforts to improve mental health services for children: Breaking a cycle of failure. *Journal of Clinical Child Psychiatry, 14*, 182–187.

Mitchell, C., Tovar, P., & Knitzer, J. (1989). *The Bronx Homebuilders Program: An evaluation of the first 45 families*. New York: Bank Street College of Education.

Munger, R. (1991). *Child mental health from the ecological perspective*. Lanham, MD: University Press of America.

National Commission on Children. (1991). *Beyond rhetoric: A new American agenda for children and families*. Washington, D.C.: U.S. Government Printing Office.

National Commission on Children in Need of Parents. (1978). *Who knows? Who cares? Forgotten children in foster care*. New York: Institute for Public Affairs.

National Education Goals Panel. (1995). *The national education goals report*. Washington, D.C.: U.S. Government Printing Office.

Rutter, M. (1979). Protective factors in children's responses to stress and disadvantage. In M.W. Kent & J.E. Rolf (Eds.), *Competency in children* (pp. 45–74). Hanover, NH: University of New Hampshire Press.

Steiner, G. (1976). *The children's cause*. Washington, D.C.: The Brookings Institution.

Stroul, B., & Friedman, R. (1986). *A system of care for severely emotionally disturbed children and youth*. Tampa: Florida Mental Health Institute, University of South Florida.

Toch, T. (1991). *In the name of excellence: The struggle to reform the nation's public schools. Why it's failing and what should be done*. New York: Oxford University Press.

Trupin, E., Low, B., Forsyth-Stephens, A., Tarico, V., & Cox, G. (1988). *State children's mental health system analysis*. Seattle: Department of Community Psychiatry, University of Washington.

United Neighborhood Houses of New York, Inc. (1991). *Increasing the effectivness and replicability of the settlement house*. New York: Ford Foundation.

United States House of Representatives, Select Committee on Children, Youth and Families. (1987). *Children's mental health: Promising responses to neglected problems*. Washington, D.C.: U.S. Government Printing Office.

United States House of Representatives, Select Committee on Children, Youth and Families. (1989). *No place to call home. Discarded children in America*. Washington, D.C.: U.S. Government Printing Office.

Virginia Department of Social Services (1986). *Report of a task force on the status of older children in foster care*. Richmond, VA: Virginia Department of Social Services.

Wells, K., & Biegel, D. (1992). Intensive family preservation services research. Current status and future agenda. *Social Work Research & Abstracts, 28*, 21–25.

Weiss, H., & Jacobs, F. (1988). *Evaluating family programs*. New York: Aldine De Gruyter.

Whittaker, J., Kinney, J., Tracy, E., & Booth, C. (Eds.). (1988). *Improving practice technology for work with high risk families: Lessons from the Homebuilders Social Work Education Project*. Seattle: Washington Center for Social Welfare Research, University of Washington.

Wilson, W. J. (1987). *The truly disadvantaged: The inner city, the underclass, and public policy*. Chicago: The University of Chicago Press.

Zigler, E., & Weiss, H. (1985). Family supported system: An ecological approach to child development. In R. Rappoport (Ed.), *Children, youth and families: The action-research relationship*. New York: Cambridge University Press.

Zigler, E., & Valentine, J. (Eds.). (1979). *Project Head Start: A legacy of the war on poverty*. New York: Free Press.

CHAPTER 24

The School Reform Movement

Opportunities for Community Psychology

DIANA OXLEY

The 1983 publication of "A Nation at Risk," commissioned by then Secretary of Education Terrel Bell, was the watershed event for efforts to improve the performance of the nation's public schools. A first wave of reforms aimed at strengthening and augmenting flagging educational standards was soon overtaken by a second wave of efforts to completely restructure the entire system of education. Elements of both standards-raising and restructuring have persisted, although the former enjoys greater political support and conviction (Weinstein, 1996).

The reform movement does not emanate from idealist visions like those of the 1960s alternative school movement. They arise from an urgent, pragmatic desire to maintain the economic competitiveness of the U.S. Indeed, the impetus for reforms recalls the 1950s launching of the U.S.S.R. space shuttle Sputnik. In the wake of Sputnik, the U.S. took steps to strengthen math and science instruction in order to regain its technological lead. The resemblance between the two reform eras ends there, however. First, current interest in educational improvement attends an era of decreased trust in public institutions and willingness to finance them. Second, there is the sense that the 21st century, the information age, and the rapid pace of change, make more profound demands on the population as a whole than previous technological expansion. National educational policy, while restricted to goal-setting and very much concerned with raising math and science competencies, nevertheless has a wider-ranging focus which includes developmental readiness, school safety, and universal literacy (U.S. Department of Education, 1991; National Education Goals Panel, 1995).

The educational problems we face today have been much more broadly defined than those of the 1950s. How do we achieve higher levels of academic mastery and equity in educational outcomes, yet with static or shrinking educational budgets? Diverse answers abound, which rest on quite different conceptualizations of underlying problems. Conservative views have predominated at the national level and in many states: "what works" in terms

---

DIANA OXLEY • Department of Special Education and Community Resources, University of Oregon, Eugene, Oregon 97403.

Handbook of Community Psychology, edited by Julian Rappaport and Edward Seidman. Kluwer Academic / Plenum Publishers, New York, 2000.

of educational practice is known (U.S. Department of Education, 1986, 1987); the problem is to overcome resistance to change. In other words, the problem has been cast in terms of human motivation. On the other hand, a spate of educational proposals by national advocacy organizations (Carnegie Council on Adolescent Development, 1989; Children's Defense Fund, 1988) and others (Noddings, 1992) points to a different set of more radical problems and solutions: The needs of children and especially adolescents, at the end of this century are very different than in the past, and call for quite different educational arrangements, public commitments, and community collaboration.

Community psychologists are well positioned to contribute to educational reform given their ecological, preventive, and social interventionist perspectives. Their eschewal of purely person-centered, unilevel, and positivist scientific approaches to problems, and their fundamental preoccupation with social-psychological phenomena coincide with warnings against single-level studies and narrowly framed interventions in the educational arena (National Academy of Education, 1991). The success of school reform, in fact, may rest on the ability of reformers to adopt this more broad-based, larger-vision perspective.

The aim of this chapter is to provide a framework with which to pursue school reform. I first delineate some important, ecological parameters of schooling to which research and intervention should be oriented. Then, I develop the case for school restructuring as opposed to school improvement, contrast individual-level and school-level reforms and educational and social psychological approaches, and offer a conceptual framework and underlying theory for school restructuring (Oxley, 1994a). I conclude with suggestions for the conduct of future research on educational issues.

SCHOOL AS A COMPLEX SOCIAL SYSTEM

The ecology of schools encompasses children and adults in various roles, social groups, and settings not limited to classrooms; a complex organizational structure; cultural norms and values; temporal patterns; and physical structures. Classrooms, clubs, student council, halls, cafeterias, faculty lounge, and meetings are all settings where teaching and learning are shaped (Barker & Associates, 1978; Kelly, 1979). Units of school organization, such as grade levels, academic tracks and departments, programs, and administrative units constitute additional important mediators of what students learn. Schools combine contradictory elements of a bureaucratic hierarchy and a loosely coupled system to create a workplace culture that makes straightforward predictions about individual behavior impossible (Boyd, 1991). The length of the class period, school day, and school year dictate activity in a largely taken-for-granted manner.

Yet, research and intervention in both psychology and education often ignore and obscure the social and organizational complexity of schools because of their preoccupation with individual-level phenomena. Researchers continue to examine relationships between factors that are used to characterize the school as a whole (for example, size, student and faculty composition, *per capita* spending) and educational outcomes as if none of these variables intervene in a significant way. Student- and classroom-based reforms remain just that, and too infrequently consider the invisible cultural and structural aspects of school (Sarason, 1982; Sarason & Klaber, 1985).

School settings, organizational units, and the school as a whole constitute appropriate units of analysis because they are the naturally occurring, ecological units of school activity. But, schools, in turn, are constrained by ever more inclusive units of organization (Bronfenbrenner, 1979; Seidman, 1988), and sources of school problems are often found in the relationships between these units. Thus, it is important to locate schools simultaneously within the larger context of the community, for example, neighborhood and school district, and beyond, for example, state and federal bureaucracies.

Interventions that attempt to address these diverse elements of schooling and their interrelationships stand a much better chance of producing results with broad and stable psychological meaning than change efforts that are focused only on individuals, whether students or teachers. However, such interventions are also difficult to mount given their challenging conceptual requirements, their indirect connection to policy goals, and the very fact of their wide range of intended effects.

THE CASE FOR SCHOOL RESTRUCTURING

In the 1980s the public's perception of the need for school improvement fueled a flurry of state and local reforms that augmented teacher salaries and introduced teacher competence testing; student performance standards were raised, and school accountability for meeting these standards was increased through closer monitoring of test results. In general, states' spending for education increased, often in relation to the establishment of categorical programs for needy student populations (for example, dropout prevention programs). Legal challenges to wide disparities in funding across school districts were made in several states.

The evidence suggests, however, that these measures had little or no impact on academic achievement. For example, national high school completion rates improved little (National Center for Education Statistics, 1991), and international comparisons of student achievement data continued to show U.S. students ranking well below their counterparts in other industrialized countries (Lapointe, Meade, & Phillips, 1989). Indeed, a sizable body of research casts doubt on whether enhanced resources alone can have positive effects on student performance (Coleman, Campbell, Hobson, McPartland, Mood, Weinfield, & York, 1966; Walberg & Fowler, 1987). Further, it is clear that heightened scholastic standards are meaningless unless institutionalized means of meeting these standards are found.

Analysts argued that these reform policies were too narrowly targeted at inputs and outputs, while leaving the fundamental structure of schools untouched (Carnegie Task Force on Teaching as a Profession, 1986; National Governors' Association, 1986). A several-decade-long history of failed reforms, mostly classroom based, also points to the unchanged structure of schools as a barrier to well-conceived, yet circumscribed, reform efforts (Cuban, 1986). A spate of analyses of schools, particularly secondary schools, shows that the problems of education are deeply rooted in the structure of the curriculum, teaching profession, and school management (Boyer, 1983; Goodlad, 1984; Powell, Farrar, & Cohen, 1985; Sizer, 1984).

Further, the performance of inner-city schools has convinced many that nothing short of a complete overhaul of the school system will render them functional. It is in the inner city that the bureaucratic structure of schools, its scale and remote administration, along with other traditional structures such as age-grading and academic tracks, have assumed their most dysfunctional forms (Carnegie Foundation for the Advancement of Teaching, 1988; Committee for Economic Development, 1987; National Coalition of Advocates for Students, 1985).

These arguments for school restructuring overtook earlier improvement efforts. The goal of restructuring was nothing less than to develop a new organizational form (or forms) of schooling, which included new authority structures, new staff roles, reorganized curriculum and instruction, and new systems of accountability (David, Purkey, & White, 1989). There was the explicit recognition that restructuring at the school level must be accompanied by restructuring at higher levels of the educational system as well (Cohen, 1988; Elmore, 1988; Linney & Seidman, 1989).

Many school districts pursued diverse reforms under the rubric of restructuring, for example, site-based management and shared decision-making among administrators, teachers, and parents; house systems and other school-within-a-school plans; and community collaborations. Inner-city school districts made the strongest response to calls for reform, commensurate with the dire need to improve their performance in relation to culturally diverse, underachieving student populations. Many of the individual reforms that these schools implemented had clear potential; they had a theoretical and/or empirical base. However, it is unclear whether individual reforms add up to an effectively restructured school.

Critics also charged that the restructuring concept had not been defined sufficiently to permit distinctions between reforms that constitute restructuring and those that did not (Olson, 1988). Some researchers avoided defining restructuring by using a continuum that ordered schools according to how far they departed from traditional practices (Newmann & Associates, 1996). Further, the link between these reforms and desired educational goals is often difficult to demonstrate (Finn, 1990). Finally, and not surprisingly, some districts' approaches to restructuring were found to be "desperate remedies for desperate times," based on little more than faith (Cuban, 1991).

In order to pursue restructuring in a meaningful way, schools require unifying conceptual and theoretical frameworks that identify the key components of a comprehensive approach to school reform and show how the different strategies are linked to each other and to desired educational goals. There need not be one best approach to restructuring. The existence of competing theories may not only provide schools with options better suited to individual circumstances, but also serve to inform each one's continued development.

The conceptual framework I offer here has several aims. First, the framework integrates areas of consensus across extant works as well as complementary aspects of different approaches to school reform. Second, the framework addresses the peculiar educational needs of inner-city youth, but within the larger context of the requirement to rely upon state-of-the-art, empirically sound educational strategies that are highly recommended for all children. Third, the framework speaks to the ecological complexity of educational systems, that is, the multiple, interdependent dimensions and levels on which schooling is organized.

In the following sections, I detail the knowledge bases on which the conceptual framework for school restructuring rests. Works in the areas of effective schools, school-improvement programs, house systems, and school–community collaborations are reviewed. They are offered as underpinnings for an approach to school improvement that links students' intellectual development to their social, emotional, and physical growth, as well as linking teacher empowerment to student achievement. These bodies of work are contrasted with at-risk student programs, a concurrent and widely pursued solution to the problem of academic failure defined in terms of students' developmental deficits as opposed to system shortcomings.

PROGRAMS FOR AT-RISK STUDENTS

The problem of student attrition has generated a good deal of research, as well as programmatic responses at city, state, and federal levels of government. The shortage of skilled labor, combined with high dropout rates among our largest and rapidly growing population subgroups, Hispanics and African Americans, made dropout prevention a priority among policy makers, especially in those states and urban centers where these minorities are concentrated (Institute for Educational Leadership, 1986; U.S. Department of Education, 1987).

Academic research has tended to focus on the question of why students drop out from the standpoint of student characteristics. That is, variation across individuals, as opposed to schools or communities, is identified as a source of explanation of student attrition. Studies examined variables such as race, poverty, parental level of education, history of educational achievement, and self-reported reasons for dropping out, (for example, pregnancy, need to provide family support, and dislike of school), in relation to school completion (Ekstrom, Goertz, Pollack, & Rock, 1986; Rumberger, 1983; Steinberg, Blinde, & Chan, 1984). Only a few analyses sought to delineate sociocultural arguments for dropping out (Fine, 1986; Fine & Rosenberg, 1983) and to explore systematically the contribution of school characteristics (Wehlage & Rutter, 1996). At best, the research helped clarify the relative importance of diverse student attributes in dropping out; at worst, it obscured institutional contributions. For example, poverty was shown to be more directly linked to student attrition than race, yet less widely understood is that the concentration of poverty in schools explains student attrition better than does student poverty (New York State Education Department, 1987a).

Not surprisingly, both educators and researchers have responded to the dropout problem with victim-blaming interventions. Dropout prevention is operationalized as a program, often classroom-centered, delivering augmented services to students who are segregated from others on the basis of documented risk criteria (Orr, 1987; Wehlage, 1983). Virtually no discussion of the appropriateness of different interventions for schools of different descriptions has appeared, since that presumes a school-level analysis of the problem. A special program for targeted students presumes that the school is suitable for the majority of students. Yet, by the criteria used, many schools in inner cities are composed of majorities of at-risk students (Oxley, 1988). Targeted services in this context seem arbitrary. Only where a small minority of students drop out does it seem defensible for dropout prevention to take the shape of an exclusively student-focused intervention as opposed to school and/or system change. Even this logic fails if we consider that at-risk students may merely be the most sensitive indicators of problems to which larger numbers of students respond in less obvious ways.

Ecology of Inner-City Schools

The ecology of schools located in poor, inner-city neighborhoods quickly dilutes the positive effects that a circumscribed dropout prevention program might have on students. Evaluations of dropout prevention programs in New York City showed that while programs had limited success in bringing students back into school, they did not alter significantly students' long-term attendance, academic achievement, and chances of graduating (Grannis, Riehl, & Pallas, 1989; New York City Board of Education, 1989). Yet, New York City programs incorporated most of the features considered to be essential components of dropout prevention, for example, health services, counseling, job placement, and a small school-within-a-school environment.

Inner-city schools share several attributes in common. The following list does not exhaust these attributes, but points out conditions both within the school and in the school's relationship to the larger educational system that distinguish these schools and have implications for dropout prevention (Hess & Greer, 1986; Council of the Great City Schools, 1987; Foley & Oxley, 1986; Oxley, 1988):

1. They are often large and overcrowded; have high proportions of poor, language-minority, African American and Hispanic youth; and experience high student mobility.

2. They have difficulty attracting and retaining high-quality teachers who are otherwise able to compete successfully for positions in schools serving high-achieving students.
3. They are underfunded relative to schools serving better students within the community and outside it. Urban schools are often more expensive to operate given the higher overhead costs (building maintenance, teacher salaries) as well as the extra resources needed for disadvantaged students.
4. The existence of unzoned magnet and other special schools with higher admission standards draws the best students away from poor neighborhoods, producing higher proportions of marginal students and reputations of being "last resorts" for the schools that must serve students in these areas.
5. Federal and state categorical programs make additional funds available to schools serving students with special needs, but restrict staff's freedom to spend the money as they see fit. Separate funding streams require the creation of multiple, separately administered programs that create competition for students, staff, space, and materials; place additional burdens on school management; cause discontinuities in students' course of study and treatment; and detract from a schoolwide sense of mission and community.
6. They are managed by large, remote bureaucracies that are often more sensitive to community political pressures than school needs; policy formulation is a slow, complicated process of negotiation among different interest groups, including the most powerful constituents, city and state government divisions, advocacy groups, and labor; and the politicized environment of the district office creates high turnover of district leaders and discontinuities in school policy, which, in turn, cause cynicism among school staff.

It should be clear how many new programs for at-risk youth fall far short of addressing the conditions that are likely to influence the holding power of schools located in the inner city. But these programs also have unforeseen negative side effects in inner-city schools because they fail to take into consideration the ecological environment: Students, who are already likely to feel inferior by virtue of the school they attend, feel they are labeled negatively by their peers for participating in a dropout prevention program; returning truants intensify space demands in already overcrowded schools, creating disincentives for retrieval; administrators reallocate resources to accommodate dropout prevention programs, creating additional turf conflicts; school staff feel their school is further stigmatized by a state- or city-imposed dropout prevention program; and local school autonomy and flexibility are further eroded by overly prescriptive state and city programs (Oxley, 1988).

EDUCATIONAL MODELS OF SCHOOL-LEVEL INTERVENTIONS

Schoolwide reform on a national basis was spurred by the effective schools movement (Edmonds, 1979, 1981) and school improvement programs (SIP) (Purkey, Rutter, & Newmann, 1985). Staff who adopted the effective schools model of reform sought to install a set of features associated with high-functioning schools, while participants in SIP set out to establish a school improvement planning process involving shared decision-making. Taken together, the effective schools and school improvement programs loosely describe a school restructuring model that incorporates both process and goal. The goal, an effective school as defined by characteristics that have been empirically linked to school success, addresses to some extent the criticism that restructuring is unconnected to student outcomes. Effective schools and SIP are discussed in the following section, before turning to social-psychological approaches to school-level reform that are needed to flesh out a school restructuring model.

Effective Schools

The literature on effective schools provides support for the view of the school as a meaningful unit of analysis and level of intervention—over and above the classroom where most academic interest has been focused. The research spans a large number of studies that demonstrate relationships between school characteristics and positive student outcomes (see Purkey & Smith, 1983, and Rowan, Bossert, & Dwyer, 1983, for reviews of this literature). Although there is overlap among the effective features that have been identified, different schools have pursued different effective schools models. One of the most popular of these lists strong administrative leadership, high expectations for children's achievement, an orderly atmosphere conducive to learning, an emphasis on basic-skill acquisition, and frequent monitoring of pupil progress as the critical ingredients of school success (Edmonds, 1979).

In an attempt to generate a more theoretically defensible, as well as empirically based, set of effective school features, Purkey and Smith (1983) drew from the literature on school organizational theory and implementation research as well as from effective schools. Their list of effective school characteristics includes: school-site management, instructional leadership, curriculum articulation, parental involvement, staff development, staff stability, recognition of student success, maximized learning time, and district support. In addition, they include a group of variables they view as instrumental to creating a productive social climate: collaborative planning and staff collegiality, sense of community, clear goals and high expectations commonly shared, and order and discipline.

The research is not unassailable. Besides the inherent difficulty in documenting causal relationships between complex, school-level attributes and outcomes, a serious limitation of these studies is their overreliance on a restricted range of academic performance measures, often standardized achievement tests. Clearly, such tests do not tap the range of intellectual skills that are currently deemed important, for example, critical thinking, computer, and writing skills (Good & Weinstein, 1986), nor do they recognize the full range of human capabilities, such as musical, spacial, and bodily aptitudes (Gardner, 1983), whose development may be crucial to many individuals' growth and self-esteem.

Further, schools are about much more than academic proficiency; they are major agents of socialization, the so-called hidden curriculum of schools (Hamilton, 1983). Effective schools therefore should be defined in terms of the acquisition of both intellectual and social skills because of their interdependencies (DeVries, 1997) and because the public expects schools to exert a positive influence in both areas. A few of the effective schools studies examined outcomes that included student self-reliance (Brookover, Beady, Flood, Schweitzer, & Wisenbaker, 1979) and delinquency (Rutter, Maughan, Mortimore, Ouston, & Smith, 1979). Clearly, however, additional research is needed to document relationships between school features and student outcomes in the areas of social, moral, and emotional development. This research needs to examine the many non-classroom behavior settings where important social learning occurs and, in so doing, may provide additional evidence and specification for features such as collaborative planning and sense of community to which the effective schools research has tended to be insensitive.

Despite such shortcomings, some argued that the effective schools research identified unquestionably important features of schooling and was strong enough to permit interventions (Purkey & Smith, 1985). However, the weak record of effective schools programs suggests that intervention based on such formulations is not straightforward. Indeed, effective school characteristics subsume a large set of unexplicated social and organizational processes. The labels attached to these features belie the complexity of the social relationships and distributions of time, space, power, and human resources they represent. In addition, effective schools programs specified neither the structures needed to support these processes nor the structural barriers that complicate their implementation.

School Improvement Programs

SIPs complemented effective schools models to the extent that they dealt primarily with a process of planning and implementing school reform, and only secondarily with goals. The assumptions that SIPs hold in common are that school-level consensus-building among a broad group of staff is needed to drive any successful school improvement effort, and that school improvement plans will vary from school to school, reflecting the unique conditions found in each (Purkey, Rutter, & Newmann, 1985).

The impetus for the widespread adoption of SIPs around the country was the increasing recognition among policymakers of the decisive role played by local school staff in implementing policies formulated by outside agents, whether they are district, state, or federal educational policymaking bodies (Bremen & McLaughlin, 1977). If school staff have the power to thwart or channel policy in unexpected directions, then giving them greater input into shaping policy is less likely to result in policies that insult staff's sense of professional independence or disregard important local exigencies.

While many SIPs revolved around the implementation of effective schools features (Miles & Kaufman, 1985), others pursued more open-ended strategies. For example, the New York State Education Department (1987) mandated a school improvement planning process involving: (1) the establishment of a committee composed of the principal, teachers' union representative, members of the staff and student body, and parents, (2) the identification of significant problem areas often concerned with, but not limited to, areas of substandard school performance, and (3) the establishment of goals and short-term objectives that must first be achieved to reach these goals.

Ironically, district- or state-mandated school improvement programs fashioned after this bottom-up approach often created staff resistance because, in the final analysis, they still left school staff without the resources to follow through with implementing the program. At a minimum, staff require time to plan that, in turn, may require relief from some classes or compensation for participation in extended workshops. Second, staff require knowledge about how to conduct a collaborative planning process and about school improvement models such as effective schools. Districts and states sometimes made such resources available to schools, however, in large school districts, like New York City, these resources were spread far too thinly to be effective (Educational Priorities Panel, 1988).

Even more difficult to obtain are the necessary adjustments in the authority structure of the school system to enable school staff to engage in true shared decision-making with the principal and his or her cabinet and with district and state officials. A national survey of school improvement programs showed that in the majority of cases where principals indicated they had a program, less than 50% of staff surveyed were aware it existed, and in urban school districts, where district support is viewed as a problematic feature of schooling, district officials typically did not participate in school planning committees (Purkey, Rutter, & Newmann 1985).

Clark and McCarthy (1983) analyzed schools' participation in a district-initiated SIP over the adoption, implementation, and institutionalization phases of its evolution. They concluded that the balance of power shared among the teachers, principal, and district officials in each participating school was crucial to maintaining long-term pursuit of school improvement. The district directed schools to establish a planning committee. The schools that managed to sustain school improvement planning longest maximized their ownership and initiative by allowing a teacher to serve as the chairperson in charge of carrying out committee work, and by employing the district representative as a facilitator and the principal as supervisor. In this way, successful schools may have managed to create a collaboration among equals corresponding appropriately to their complementary, yet, in practical terms, equivalent knowledge and responsibilities.

SOCIAL PSYCHOLOGICAL MODELS OF SCHOOL-LEVEL INTERVENTIONS

Effective schools and school improvement programs give us a "leg up" to the task of school restructuring because they provide a rationale and a rudimentary framework for school-level reform. As pointed out earlier, however, most effective schools models are based on a narrow conception of schooling as an intellectual process, a limitation that Purkey and Smith (1983, 1985) and school improvement programs begin to address. Two approaches to school-level reform that directly address social–psychological and sociocultural failings of schools are now presented.

One of these, the house system or school-within-a-school (SWS) plan, offers an alternative organizational model of schooling whose primary objective is to enhance student and staff relationships. While its central focus is organizational structure, the literature on house systems also identifies the kinds of organizational processes that they are intended to support. The second, a school–community collaboration, describes a process of enhancing these same social relationships and, secondarily, structures that support these processes. Research has documented the benefits of both in broad developmental terms. As such, these school reform models delineate relevant school structures and processes that the foregoing educational approaches inadequately detailed or overlooked altogether.

House Systems and SWS Plans

Houses and SWSs comprise a strategy for organizing a school into smaller units for the purpose of creating a more stable and cohesive social context for learning. Small groups of staff and students are assigned to a house or subschool on a permanent basis, and all aspects of schooling, including instruction, support services, administration, and extracurricular activities, are replicated within each subschool. Ideally, subschools are further broken down into interdisciplinary teacher teams who share a group of students in common (Oxley, 1990; Plath, 1965; Ratzki, 1988). Students take most, if not all, their courses from the team, obtain counseling from subschool staff, and have an opportunity to participate in their own subschool extracurriculars. SWS staff have the authority to make and carry out decisions affecting the education of their students (Plath, 1965; Oxley, 1990). Some functions are also maintained centrally. Usually, a schoolwide administrator supervises the subschools and building operations. Some courses and activities may be offered on a schoolwide basis to permit students to pursue a wider variety of interests than their subschool staff can support.

Houses and SWSs are hardly a new concept in school organization. They enjoyed popularity in the 1960s and 1970s as a means of reducing the human costs of increased high school size. Few SWS plans survived to the present. The well-entrenched hierarchical system of school governance and continued trend toward curriculum diversification eroded the small school approach. SWSs again rose to the top of national school reform agendas in the 1980s (Goodlad, 1984; National Coalition of Advocates for Students, 1985; Carnegie Foundation for the Advancement of Teaching, 1988). Strategies for organizing schools into smaller units were made a matter of policy in a number of school districts where large school size and student alienation predominate. These strategies hold more promise than they had previously because they coincide with other policies that encourage wider participation in decision-making and strengthening the basic curriculum.

Theories of organization (Kimberly, 1976), setting size (Barker & Associates, 1978), and student alienation (Newmann, 1981) suggest that small schools or small units within large schools promote social processes needed to sustain effective organizational functioning. These processes include extensive interaction and familiarity among students and staff, vertical and horizontal communication among staff, and student involvement in school activities. Research on school size provides support for these theoretical assertions (Crain & Strauss, 1986; Gottfredson, 1985; Lee & Smith, 1995; Lindsay, 1982; Pittman & Haughwout, 1987).

Research on SWSs, although less plentiful, is consistent with the studies of school size. My study of the implementation of house systems in New York City high schools documented more positive social relationships among students and between students and their teachers, greater student participation in extracurricular activities, a stronger sense of community, and a higher rate of passing courses among students in better-implemented houses (Oxley, 1990). Similarly, in a study of a subschool within a larger unrestructured school, subschool students perceived more social cohesion and teacher guidance and passed more courses than students at large, and subschool teachers collaborated more with colleagues and had broader contact with students than did teachers at large (Oxley, 1997b). At the middle-school level, Felner and colleagues' research (1997) on organizing teachers and students into small learning communities showed that high-functioning teacher teams working with no more than 120 students (the same ratio as in the high school subschool) obtained higher student achievement behavior and well-being than more fragmented arrangements.

Qualitative analysis of staff's efforts to implement SWSs revealed that academic departments, tracks, and special programs posed significant obstacles to restructuring (Oxley, 1990, 1997c). These specialized structures are made possible by large organizational size and are difficult to maintain alongside SWSs. Each subschool does not have a sufficient number of students to permit their being sorted into homogeneous classes designed for particular ability levels and other characteristics, a questionable practice in any event (Oakes, 1985). Schools in which SWSs were better implemented eliminated some tracks and programs and resolved the tension between subschools and academic departments by integrating the two to some extent. For example, department heads were made coordinators of subschools with curricular emphases that corresponded to their subject area. Similarly, student support services that are normally organized as separate, specialized activities were also integrated to some extent. In one school where each grade-level cohort constituted a house, grade-level advisors were made house coordinators. In all schools, however, SWSs uneasily coexisted with the traditional school structure.

The research on SWSs provides further support for effective schools features, such as curriculum articulation and those related to a favorable school climate, since they overlap with SWSs attributes shown to have positive social psychological as well as academic consequences for students. Most important, SWSs link rather abstract effective schools features to the kinds of concrete school structures needed to support them.

School–Community Collaboration

The school–community approach developed by Comer (1976, 1985, 1987) over the past 20 years is based on the notion that schools do not serve students well because they are disjunctive with their surrounding communities, particularly those located in the inner city. School staff and students often do not share the same culture due to differences in race, class, and life experience and, as a result, lack mutual understanding and trust. The economic and social forces that bring diverse groups together in the same community make these communities generally less cohesive and supportive. Schools have not changed to compensate for these societal changes since they have not been organized, historically, to respond directly to their communities.

In order to create a more supportive school culture, school–community collaborations seek to involve parents more integrally in the operation of the school, to broaden the base of input into formulating school policy, and to support students through less punitive behavioral interventions and restructured school programs. Comer defines the collaboration as a process or set of activities that university change agents help school staff establish. Nevertheless, given the interrelatedness of structure and process, Comer's (1987) description of his program specifies some structural as well as programmatic elements:

1. A representative governance/management body composed of principal, parent, teachers, and support staff directs the overall process of school improvement consisting of needs assessment and program development.
2. A parent participation group composed of paid part-time aides assists teachers and collaborates in the development of workshops for other parents.
3. A mental health team provides direct services to children and development assistance to parents in creating workshops.

University change agents and their trainees help school staff develop adult and child empowerment processes out of which evolve concrete curricula, programs, and interventions that vary from school to school. The practices of keeping teachers with their students for two years, retaining slow learners in regular classrooms, and using a social-skills curriculum have been developed, but are not offered as prescriptive features of the school–community approach. The open-endedness of Comer's model may be a function, to some extent, of the simpler and more flexible organization of elementary schools where these programs were initiated. One might argue that school–community collaborations in secondary schools have to include a SWSs strategy that, in effect, organizes the school along elementary school lines, for example, smaller-scale, and a more coherent curriculum, to give staff the same order of flexibility to develop additional programs.

Studies indicate that one long-standing school–community program sharply increased academic performance and the school's relative standing in terms of student attendance, incidence of serious behavior problems, and staff attendance and turnover. A sample of students drawn from the program school three years after they left it demonstrated higher achievement and perceived school competence relative to a control group (Cauce, Comer, & Schwartz, 1987).

A CONCEPTUAL FRAMEWORK OF SCHOOL RESTRUCTURING

The different routes taken to school improvement are instructive in that together they address a complementary set of issues that serve to describe a multidimensional framework for school restructuring. Restructuring depends on the specification of a mutually reinforcing group of processes, structures, and goals because of the ecological interdependence of such key dimensions of schooling (Eisner, 1985). Some may argue that one or another of these is primary, for example, that performance goals (Finn, 1990; Wiggins, 1991) should be used to dictate the rest. However, the simultaneous focus on process, structure, and goal helps compensate for the limitations associated with each. A concentration on goals or processes does not necessarily lead to the deep structural changes needed to support them. Purely structural formulae do not inform the educational processes that directly affect learning.

The framework used to guide school restructuring must also apply to different levels of the educational system. A several-decade-long history of failed educational reforms, mostly classroom-based, points to the need to address aspects of the classroom and school simultaneously (Cuban, 1986), as well as higher levels of the system such as the school district (Elmore, 1988). In the next sections I specify the structural, processual, and goal parameters of the school restructuring framework and depict the changed contours of schooling at multiple levels. I also briefly describe traditional school structure and functioning to highlight the differences between the two approaches.

Traditional School Structure

Schools appear to be a combination of bureaucratic and loosely coupled structures (Purkey & Smith, 1983; Boyd, 1991). They conform to a bureaucratic model of organization in that management is centralized and staff roles are highly differentiated. School policy is formulated by individuals at the top of the administrative hierarchy and communicated to line staff who are expected to act in accordance with the policy. School functioning is organized as narrowly defined activities performed by individuals who specialize in these activities. Thus, administration, student support, and instruction are sharply bounded functions, each of which is further divided into discrete tasks carried out by different people. Schools, like bureaucracies in general, tend to be organized on a large scale. Large size is required to support specialized personnel and, in theory, affords an economy of scale since a centralized management system does not need to grow as fast as the organization as a whole. For example, both small and large schools have only one principal.

Schools diverge from the bureaucratic model in that administrative and instructional functions are much less tightly coupled than one would expect to find in a bureaucracy. The independence of teachers afforded to a large extent by the isolation of the classroom appears to diffuse the effect of school directives. Moreover, the qualitative nature of measures of teacher performance as well as the difficulty in interpreting measures of student performance limit administrators' ability to use such feedback directly in managing the organization.

Alternative School Structures

Current critiques of schooling and school improvement models converge to a great extent on the kinds of generic attributes of organizational structure that are needed to create a supportive context for teaching and learning. They include, but are not limited to, the following six interdependent features:

1. Small organizational scale: downsized district offices, smaller schools, house systems, instructional clusters (Boyer, 1983; Bryk, Lee, & Smith, 1990; Carnegie Council on Adolescent Development, 1989; Carnegie Foundation for the Advancement of Teaching, 1988; Children's Defense Fund, 1988; Committee for Economic Development, 1987; Goodlad, 1984; National Coalition of Advocates for Students, 1985).
2. Decentralized management: local community school boards, school-based management, house systems (Carnegie Council on Adolescent Development, 1989; Committee for Economic Development, 1987; David, Purkey & White, 1989; Oxley, 1990, 1997b; Purkey & Smith, 1983, 1985).
3. Broad-based decision-making bodies: school-governance councils composed of administrators, teachers, parents, and students (Boyer, 1983; Carnegie Council on Adolescent Development, 1989; Comer, 1985; Committee for Economic Development, 1987; Goodlad, 1984; National Coalition of Advocates for Students, 1985; Purkey & Smith, 1985; Sizer, 1984).
4. Cross-role/discipline collaborative groups: school-community partnerships, integrated social services, interdisciplinary teacher teams (Carnegie Council on Adolescent Development, 1989; Children's Defense Fund, 1988; Comer, 1985; David, Purkey & White, 1989; Purkey & Smith, 1985; Sizer, 1984).
5. Bridges across temporal gaps in schooling: school transition programs, cross-year teacher-student groups (Children's Defense Fund, 1988; Comer, 1985; Ratzki, 1988).
6. Heterogeneous instructional groups: mainstreaming programs, elimination of academic tracks and pull-out programs (Carnegie Council on Adolescent Development, 1989; Goodlad, 1984; National Coalition of Advocates for Students, 1985; Oakes, 1985; Oxley, 1994b; Wang, Walberg, & Reynolds, 1988).

These structures describe an organization composed of small, relatively autonomous, interdisciplinary groups of staff and students who work together over extended periods of time guided and supported by parents and supervisors situated at both middle and high levels of the organization. Because management responsibilities are shared among a wider group of individuals, administrators are able to devote some of their time to other functions, such as instruction and student support, thereby closing the gaps between these functions. Staff–student groups are small enough that informal as well as formal structures can be used to convey opinions and information so that the groups remain flexible and responsive. Collaborations among school staff with varying kinds and levels of expertise help reduce gaps in service delivery and redundancy.

Cross-role collaborations between school staff and outside agents such as universities, parents, health and social services, and businesses are also key to school restructuring. Of special importance is the establishment of linkages between school districts and universities and colleges that allow for an ongoing interchange between university trainers and researchers and school practitioners. Permanent partnerships with universities are needed to eliminate the cultural discontinuity that exists between schools and universities to the point of creating not only knowledge gaps, but outright hostility.

Finally, a basic building block of a restructured school are instructional groups based on a heterogeneous mix of individuals with respect to entry-level abilities, gender, and ethnicity. Contrary to the long-standing, pervasive, but discredited (Oakes, 1985) practice of grouping students with like abilities, heterogeneously grouped students force teachers to deal with the unique needs of each student rather than their presumed shared characteristics (Wang, 1992). Students' varied strengths are recognized and shared with others. Moreover, the social and cultural differences of group members are made an integral part of the curriculum, and learning how to consider issues from different perspectives becomes a means of furthering cognitive development (New York State Social Studies Review and Development Committee, 1991). In the same way, more experienced teachers are grouped with newer and weaker teachers so that the former can mentor the latter.

Traditional Educational Practices

Haberman (1991) has identified a typical urban style of teaching that he labels the pedagogy of poverty. It consists of a one-way form of communication between teachers and students wherein the teacher issues information, directions, assignments, tests, homework, and grades and attempts to gain student compliance through close monitoring of student behavior and punishment, if necessary. In response to this directive, controlling pedagogy, students spend a great deal of instructional time trying to manipulate and reduce the power of teachers (Haberman, 1991; Oxley, 1990). Beyond classroom instruction, again, one-way communication predominates: teachers inform parents and police student behavior throughout the school, while administrators instruct teachers and maintain records on students.

Alternative School Processes

The alternative structural elements listed previously are required to support a set of interdependent management, teaching, and learning activities that have been advanced in the recent school advocacy and research literatures:

1. *Shared decision-making*: teachers, parents, and students help formulate policy (Boyer, 1983; Comer, 1985; Committee for Economic Development, 1987; Goodlad, 1984; National Coalition of Advocates for Students, 1985; Purkey & Smith, 1985; Purkey, Rutter, & Newmann, 1985; Sizer, 1984)
2. *Collaborative work*: students engage in cooperative learning; teachers develop programs and skills in consultation with other teachers, support staff, and parents (Children's Defense Fund, 1988; Comer, 1985; Council of Chief State School Officers, 1990; David, Purkey & White, 1989; Newmann & Thompson, 1987; Purkey & Smith, 1985; Purkey, Rutter, & Newmann, 1985; Wang, 1992)
3. *Active learning/inquiry*: students initiate learning; teachers formulate and evaluate new techniques (Children's Defense Fund, 1988; McCombs, 1991; Sizer, 1984; Wang & Palincsar, 1989)
4. *Mentoring/guidance*: Students mentor their peers; teachers mentor students and each other (Children's Defense Fund, 1988; Committee for Economic Development, 1987; Ratzki, 1988)

Shared decision-making and collaborative planning drive the work of the organization. Importantly, these activities are consistent with the predominantly verbal mode in which teachers operate. Teachers also function as inquirers on an ongoing basis, continuing to extend their knowledge and mirroring the learning process for students. Students function as "workers" (Sizer, 1984), discover answers, produce knowledge, and help one another in the process. Students learn how to work together with other students, teachers, and their parents to achieve their educational objectives (Ratzki, 1988). They have opportunities to participate in school government and rule-making and social activities as part of the school's explicit social and moral curriculum (Power, Higgins, & Kohlberg, 1989). Finally, school staff guide and counsel students, helping them to understand themselves and their world.

Traditional Educational Goals

The body of research on effective schools already discussed reflects a much more restricted range of educational goals than that for which schools are actually held accountable. U.S. public education has a long-standing commitment to well-rounded student development. This commitment, however, has been expressed in terms of the provision of "extras," such as health and physical education, sports programs, student government, and fine arts, participation in which is completely disconnected to mastery of "serious courses."

Alternative Goals

The alternative school processes already listed are geared to achieving a wider range of formal social, emotional, moral, physical, and intellectual developmental goals than is presently the case:

1. Mastery of core subjects, including English, math, social studies, and science (Carnegie Foundation for the Advancement of Teaching, 1988; Powell, Farrar, & Cohen, 1985; Sizer, 1984)
2. Higher-order intellectual functioning, including problem-solving and critical thinking (Carnegie Council on Adolescent Development, 1989; Children's Defense Fund, 1988; Good & Weinstein, 1986; Newmann & Associates, 1996; Segal, Chipman, & Glaser, 1985; Sizer, 1984)
3. Development of nontraditional intelligences, including kinesthetic, spatial, musical, and intrapersonal (Children's Defense Fund, 1988; Eisner, 1988; Gardner, 1983)
4. Social and moral capabilities (Carnegie Council on Adolescent Development, 1989; Children's Defense Fund, 1988; Comer, 1985; Committee for Economic Development, 1987; Power, Higgins, & Kohlberg, 1989; Weissberg, 1987)
5. Good health (Carnegie Council on Adolescent Development, 1989)

These educational goals are based on the explicit recognition that intellectual, social, moral, and physical development are interdependent and on the philosophy that schools should be devoted to helping students realize their full human potential, rather than serving only the narrower aims of the society, for example, employability. The widespread conviction that educators have pursued a too broad and shallow curriculum and should emphasize core academic subjects need not deter educators from providing opportunities for students to develop artistic, musical, mechanical, and other talents. Reading and writing instruction, for example, can be pursued in the context of teaching fine arts and shop and vice versa. Cross-disciplinary teacher teams make such integration and reinforcement of skills across subjects feasible. In addition, teachers can direct students to use the concepts, facts, and skills taught in core courses as tools for increasing their understanding of themselves and the conditions in which they live. In other words, increased mastery of math, English, and so on need not mean more and harder courses by these names but, instead, instruction that links so-called academic subjects to the cultivation of a broad array of non-traditional abilities, such as personal and social intelligence (Gardner, 1983).

Indicators of the progress that students make toward these goals can be created to provide both students and teachers with feedback about how well they are doing. Such indicators could include measures of improvement as well as absolute level of mastery. Demonstrations of student competence in different areas should be integrated as much as possible to be meaningful (Sizer, 1984). Student portfolios that contain work products requiring collaboration with peers and teachers, initiative and persistence in carrying out long-term projects, as well as mastery of particular academic skills and facts would help to offset constrictive standardized tests.

Summary

Successful school restructuring requires the application of a generic and causally related set of structures, processes, and goals at multiple levels of the educational system. The structures that have been delineated here define a context that supports educational processes that are considered to be instrumental to attaining the broad goals of child development. Certainly, additional specifications and dimensions of school restructuring could be and have been identified, even causally related (Conley, 1991) and ecology-minded ones (Eisner, 1988). The goal here is to organize complementary approaches to school reform into a framework that provides both conceptual coherence and a measure of ecological validity.

Many of the individual reforms described here, if not necessarily the unified framework, have proven politically feasible. The Chicago School District implemented a radically restructured governance system that gives authority over schools to local community boards. Likewise, New York City reduced the scale of central bureaucracies by shifting personnel to intermediate-level jurisdictions and schools, and limited the size of schools that could be built. The Los Angeles, Columbus, Philadelphia, New York, and Boston school districts adopted house/charter systems at high and/or middle school levels. Nationally, school-based management and shared decision-making became the watchwords of reform after the lead of the Dade County School District (Committee for Economic Development, 1987). Many districts, including those in New York (New York State Education Department, 1987) and Philadelphia, pursued policies geared to making schools into "child development centers that would be a central point of contact for children's services," (*Philadelphia Inquirer*, May 6, 1990), in effect, collapsing the public agencies of health, recreation, juvenile justice, and libraries into one in schools and requiring schools to operate on a longer day, year-round schedule consistent with their broader mandate. More recently, the Philadelphia School District organized schools into K–12 clusters to increase continuity of practice and support for students (Newberg, 1995). State departments of education have established learning objectives that replace graduation requirements that stipulate the number of credit hours needed in different subjects, thus paving the way for curriculum integration.

Toward a Theory of School Restructuring

The theory that underpins the above framework can best be described as a theory of a communally organized school that both requires and responds constructively to diverse characteristics of students and their families. Communal organization refers to a social group that is bound by personal as well as utilitarian ties (Bryk, Lee, & Smith, 1990). Members of a community care about one another on the basis of shared values and experiences and, in addition, perform practical functions for each other. Communities bestow feelings of belonging and identity. In the context of a school community, teachers' roles are not limited to instruction and professional interchange. Teachers also function as friends, supporters, and advisors to students and colleagues, alike.

Research on communal relations in school is consistent with other framework specifications. Small schools and the organization of large schools into small units are more conducive to students' sense of belonging and involvement in school activities and staff collegiality than are large schools (Bryk & Driscoll, 1988; Lindsay, 1982; Oxley, 1990, 1997b; Pittman & Haughwout, 1987). Shared learning experiences, as measured by limited differentiation of courses and academic tracks, are integral to communal schooling, while racial and socioeconomic similarities are not (Bryk & Driscoll, 1988).

"Treatments" for racial and cultural diversity are a nearly ubiquitous feature of school reform agendas. The "all children can learn" maxim promulgated by school districts, parent outreach, bilingual programs, and linkages with social service agencies give an idea of the range of such treatments. However, approaches to school restructuring seldom stipulate diversity as a necessary ingredient. On the contrary, efforts in several large cities to establish schools that serve and are staffed by African-American males rest on the view that the intellectual development of African-American males is best pursued within a homogeneous social context.

The report of the New York State Social Studies Review and Development Committee (1991) helps to turn common notions of diversity on their heads. The committee's controversial conclusions were that social studies instruction should cover a broad range of cultures, examine social problems from differing cultural perspectives, and draw upon students' own backgrounds and experiences. On that basis, schools with heterogeneous populations of students can offer a learning context that is intellectually rich, while schools with homogeneous student bodies must rely on less compelling means of bringing differing perspectives and experiences into the curriculum. Indeed, the availability of diverse cultures and language skills remains a unique, though still untapped, resource of the inner city.

Communal school organization has special relevance to inner cities and to the changing conditions in which adolescents and their families live. School communities offer a means of enculturating diverse social and cultural groups to the extent that they lead individuals to identify with the values and goals of the school as a whole. At the same time, school communities have a greater than ordinary capacity to recognize individual and group differences and to employ these differences as pedagogical tools. The school community curriculum represents less a fixed and independent entity than a dynamic transaction between existing knowledge bases and particular community contexts over time. What students learn is not divorced from how they live.

I offer this theory as one formulation of a restructured school. It is consistent with a growing literature on school communities (Bryk & Driscoll, 1988; Carnegie Council on Adolescent Development, 1989; Fine, 1992; Gregory & Smith, 1987; Newmann, 1993; Sergiovanni, 1994) that seeks to advance a personally supportive and socially cohesive form of schooling that is also flexible and dynamic (Louis & Miles, 1990), as distinct from the traditional bureaucratic structure of schools (Bryk, Lee, & Smith, 1990).

Other theories of school restructuring are possible. Implicit in the various approaches that are being taken to education reform are alternative formulations of what schooling requires to serve children effectively. As noted above, the communal theory of schooling delineated here diverges quite clearly from the idea of organizing schools around shared characteristics of students, as male African-American and special-needs schools do. It also can be distinguished from school choice (Chubb & Moe, 1988) and school charter (Shanker, 1988) models, both of which alter the authority structure to spur open-ended processes for school change. The latter approaches appear to empower stakeholders and to serve the interests of student diversity but, in fact, invoke marketplace forces while begging the question, altogether, of what constitutes democratic schooling.

Articulation of the theories that underpin these approaches is important because it clarifies the line of reasoning and empirical support on which reform programs rest and, thus, enables school districts to evaluate their options more rigorously. Moreover, the application of strong, competing theories of school restructuring serves to inform each other's ongoing development and allows comparative theory testing. Ultimately, empirical tests of the interrelationships among the elements of the theory delineated here and comparisons with other theories on student outcomes will determine the relative merit of a communal theory of school restructuring.

FUTURE RESEARCH

The theory testing described above only hints at the nature and scope of research that community psychologists need to conduct to further the development of schooling as an instrument of children's as well as adults' intellectual and socioemotional growth. The school reform debate not only raises numerous questions about education *per se*, but also taps into basic belief systems, political views, and social consciousness that may well determine the course of the reform movement. The examination of such complex questions challenges even our most vaunted theoretical notions, research paradigms, and tools.

Ecological versus Psychological Constructions of School Interventions

If community psychologists are to address schooling on its own terms, they must translate constructs such as primary prevention, adolescent development, and social competence into the language of school system processes and regularities. In other words, we must translate those terms that define our field and bring us to the point of doing research and intervention in schools into school-context-defined issues. Otherwise we will continue to contribute to the unhealthy discontinuity that exists between the concerns of educators and psychologists. For example, teachers defend their exclusive role as classroom instructors and refer out "discipline problems," while guidance counselors and school psychologists address student behavior problems but, traditionally, have little input on educational practice. Social-competence building occurs in special classes and infrequently in relation to socially supportive schoolwide structures and processes.

The precepts of primary prevention lead community psychologists to study features of schools in relation to psychological processes in order to design therapeutic interventions in them. Inherent in this task is the limiting notion of psychological wellness as the level and phenomenon of interest. Its starting point is a set of constructs defined independently of ecological context. Even though interest in primary prevention leads us to a consideration of context, it necessitates conceptualizing the environment in individual-level terms that relate to health and well-being. The researcher must abstract from the environment elements that can be viewed as direct inputs to individual functioning, for example, perceived social support. Thus, primary prevention research in schools tends to focus on children's functioning in relation to teacher and classroom variables and treats school-level attributes as if they were directly accessible to children and not mediated by intermediate-school structures and functions.

Felner and colleagues (Felner, Ginter, & Primavera, 1982; Felner & Adan, 1988) address these shortcomings to some extent. Their primary prevention project aims to increase beginning students' adjustment to high school by augmenting the social support available to them. It can achieve this by manipulating key school-structure and process variables that affect social support provision: Project teachers handle their students' administrative and counseling needs, rather than the several staff members who ordinarily carry out these functions, and students have classes with a subset of the entering ninth-grade class in a demarcated area of the school building in order to create a smaller and more stable social context for peer interaction.

On the other hand, the intervention fails to locate these variables in the broader context of school functioning and, therefore, does not identify the range of variables that influence, if indirectly, the effectiveness and long-term sustainability of the intervention. For example, the reorganization of the project teachers' role is not linked to changes in the school's administrative hierarchy, which limits classroom teachers' capacity to act decisively as a student advisor/advocate. Further, the assignment of students to classes does not consider educational programming rules that determine which students can be grouped together for instruction. The result of even relatively broad-based primary prevention interventions like this one is that they put the burden of change on line staff, while leaving the system mostly unchanged. An unintended negative side effect of these low-level interventions is teachers' reluctance to participate or their eventual burnout.

In place of approaching the school as a conjunction of child and school factors, researchers can engage school-defined problems, activities, reactions to interventions, and other ecological phenomena as beginning, if not end, points. Unique syntheses of people, activities, places, and times define the character of schools. These behavior settings (Barker & Associates, 1978), transactional units (Oxley, Haggard, Werner, & Altman, 1986), and social regularities (Seidman, 1988) shape individual expression. Efforts to identify regularities, such as fragmented learning, teacher isolation (Eisner, 1986), uniform treatment of students, organizational self-protection (Miles, 1981), student disruption/teacher attempts at control (Oxley, 1990), and student resilience (Oxley, 1990) have helped to illuminate the nature of schooling and particular types of schools. However, researchers need to expand our knowledge of how these patterns of functioning are related to organizational structure and goals, characteristics of different stakeholder groups, temporal patterns, physical attributes, and student outcomes. These recommendations echo Seidman's (1990) reconceptualization of prevention as the development of programs, settings, and policies in a context-sensitive manner.

Research that has identified school ecology issues relevant to school reform as well as primary prevention includes studies of school governance processes (Gruber & Trickett, 1987), school administrators' acquisition of information relevant to school change (Saunders & Repucci, 1977), educational philosophy and climate (Trickett, McConahay, Phillips, & Ginter, 1985), and school structure as it relates to the efficacy of consultation efforts (Goldman

& Cowan, 1976). Lenrow and Cowden's (1980) analysis of human delivery systems links the preference for bureaucratic management of schools and other public agencies to its perceived association with science and rational modes of problem solving. These authors suggest that reform of these institutions cannot proceed without addressing these basic cultural underpinnings. The impermanence of school reforms made over the last several decades sadly bears out this point (Bloom, 1988; Cuban, 1986, 1997; Oxley, 1997a).

Finally, community psychologists need to direct much more of their research to examining school problems and change efforts within their larger political and economic contexts. Sarason (1990) points out more starkly than most that the success of school reform depends on the alteration of existing power relationships among administrators, teachers, and students, a linkage that a growing number of policymakers at local and state levels of government accept. Fine (1990) links the politics of urban schools, that is, the unequal allocation of state funds and related school-level disincentives to the abandonment of failing students. At the heart of urban, as well as rural, school problems is the unresolved question of the political and economic worth of poor students. The abiding need for community psychologists to join with professionals in other fields, such as education, economics, and political science, is still largely unmet.

Action Research as *Modus Operandi*

Action research seems most able to accommodate the ecological complexity of schools. Researchers have not only the school reform agenda to consider, but also the ecological impact of conducting research itself. In particular, researchers who join with practitioners in change efforts justify their presence in a setting where serious problems exist, as do tensions between practitioners and researchers that spring from the researchers' discrepant goals and language (Billington, Washington, & Trickett, 1981; Weinstein, Soule, Collins, Cone, Mehlhorn, & Simontacchi, 1991). Second, action research provides the opportunity to observe the social system's dynamic operation. Researchers' examination of the schools' response to their presence and reaction and long-term adaptation to the intervention may provide greater insights into school ecology than its routine functioning (Lewin, 1951). Moreover, the relative long-term basis on which action research must be conducted is consistent with the complexity of the phenomena under study.

Under this model of research, the researcher becomes part of what is studied. His or her objectivity ceases to be a rigid requirement; indeed, the impossibility of pure objectivity is recognized, but not treated as a deficiency. Truth is viewed less as an unchanging reality than as something that constantly shapes and reshapes itself in accordance with the forces present (Capra, 1975). The researcher is not present to record the impact of a program passively, but to help the program realize its potential. This *modus operandi* is consistent with a transactional world view that seems to be emerging in community psychology (Altman & Rogoff, 1987).

Two studies illustrate many of the above points extremely well. Eisner (1986) shadowed students and teachers across their days to arrive at descriptions of the school experience. In order to produce meaningful interpretations of these descriptions, Eisner used both university-based researchers with teaching experience and teachers in the schools they studied to produce a set of accounts or "educational criticisms," which were developed through a structured process of description, interpretation, evaluation, and identification of themes. Eisner's methodology not only rejects the myth of objective observation, but depends upon the observers' access to the phenomenon through their subjective knowledge of education and upon extensive immersion in the school experience, itself, in the style of anthropology. Although the goal of Eisner's research was not change per se, his use of teachers as researchers empowered them to act as problem solvers in their own right.

Weinstein et al.'s (1991) efforts to heighten teachers' expectations for at-risk students through systemic intervention also relied on an active partnership among researchers and teachers. Weinstein et al. sought to replace classroom- and school-level instructional regularities characterized by low expectations for students with high expectancy practices. The university–school collaboration, of necessity, involved mutual accommodation: researchers dropped research jargon and negotiated the design of reforms with educators; teachers studied research materials and jointly authored a research article. Their analysis of the collaboration and findings of limited program impact contribute much more to an understanding of school ecology than conventional, static descriptions of interventions yielding more positive effects. Felner et al.'s (1991) observation that Weinstein's intervention might have had greater success had it drawn more widely on the school reorganization literature points out once again the ecological complexity of schools and the narrowness of even multilevel interventions that do not target sufficient aspects of the organization to permit successful implementation of the program.

CONCLUSIONS

Community psychologists have an important opportunity to contribute to current preoccupations with school reform, particularly school and educational system restructuring. Our commitment to ecological formulations of problems and expertise in a broad spectrum of behavior position us well to help carry out meaningful educational change. The discussion of contemporary approaches to enhancing academic achievement presented earlier serves to point out the limitations of different models and the need for synthesizing complementary aspects of them. The conceptual framework of a restructured school that I offer is intended to accomplish some of this synthesis and, thereby, to help sustain the current momentum for systems change.

The future of school restructuring depends on the interdependent activities of empirical evaluation of school change efforts and continued development of conceptual and theoretical formulations of alternative forms of schooling. In order to pursue ecologically valid and, ultimately, effective interventions, community psychologists must consider objective patterns of behavior, how behavior is organized with respect to units of people, space, and time; key dimensions of school organization such as goals and structure; and relationships to settings at higher levels of school system and community organization. Research may necessitate longer investments of time and the performance of useful roles in the setting that legitimate the researcher's prolonged presence, as well as serve to acquaint the researcher more intimately with the setting.

Since community psychology research itself is influenced by an ecology of scholarly activity nested in academic departments and universities, changes in these contexts are needed to support changes in the conduct of research. For example, community psychology staff and students may need to locate themselves in community settings on a semipermanent basis; they may find it advantageous to assume community roles, such as advocate, that academicians tend to view as inconsistent with a positivist brand of science; and a wider variety of publication routes may need to be developed to document their activity more fully and continuously.

Our research and intervention in schools should not represent the opportunistic examination of community-psychology-defined constructs, but rather, attempts to resolve urgent school issues, that is, ecologically valid problems. Our efforts in schools will do more to further the development of theories of empowerment (Rappaport, 1987) and social intervention (Seidman, 1988) on which our field uniquely depends than do activities that remain "closer to home."

REFERENCES

Altman, I., & Rogoff, B. (1987). World views in psychology: Trait, interactional, organismic, and transactional perspectives. In D. Stokols, & I. Altman, (Eds.) *Handbook of environmental psychology*, 7–40. New York: Wiley.

Barker, R., & Associates. (1978). *Habitats, environments, and human behavior.* San Francisco: Jossey-Bass.

Berman, P., & McLaughlin, M. (1977). *Federal programs supporting educational change: Factors affecting implementation and continuation. Vol. 7.* Santa Monica, CA: Rand.

Billington, R., Washington, L., & Trickett, E. (1981). The research relationship in community research: An inside view from public school principals. *American Journal of Community Psychology, 9*, 461–479.

Bloom, S. (1988). Structure and ideology in medical education: An analysis of resistance to change. *Journal of Health and Social Behavior, 29*, 294–306.

Boyd, W. (1991). What makes ghetto schools succeed or fail? *Teachers College Record, 92*, 331–362.

Boyer, E. (1983). *High school: A report on secondary education in America.* New York: Harper & Row.

Bronfenbrenner, U. (1979). *The ecology of human development.* Cambridge, MA: Harvard University Press.

Brookover, W., Beady, C., Flood, P., Schweitzer, J., & Wisenbaker, J. (1979). *School social systems and student achievement: Schools can make a difference.* New York: Praeger.

Bryk, A., & Driscoll, M. (1988). *The school as community: Theoretical foundation, contextual influences, and consequences for students and teachers.* Madison: National Center on Effective Secondary Schools, University of Wisconsin.

Capra, F. (1975). *The tao of physics.* Toronto: Bantam.

Carnegie Council on Adolescent Development. (1989). *Turning points: Preparing American youth for the 21st century.* Washington, D.C.: Carnegie Council on Adolescent Development, Carnegie Corporation of New York.

Carnegie Foundation for the Advancement of Teaching. (1988). *An imperiled generation: Saving urban schools.* Princeton, NJ: Carnegie Foundation for the Advancement of Teaching.

Carnegie Task Force on Teaching as a Profession. (1986). *A nation prepared: Teachers for the 21st century.* New York: Carnegie Forum on Education and the Economy.

Cauce, A., Comer, J., & Schwartz, B. (1987). Long term effects of a systems-oriented school prevention program. *American Journal of Orthopsychiatry, 57*(1), 127–131.

Children's Defense Fund. (1988). *Making the middle grades work.* Washington, D.C.: Children's Defense Fund.

Chubb, J., & Moe, T. (1988). Politics, markets, and the organization of schools. *American Political Science Review, 82*, 1065–1087.

Clark, T., & McCarthy, D. (1983). School improvement in New York City: The evolution of a project. *Educational Researcher, 12*(4), 17–24.

Cohen, M. (1988). *Restructuring the education system: Agenda for the 1990s.* Washington, D.C.: National Governors' Association.

Coleman, J., Campbell, E., C., McPartland, J., Mood, A., Weinfeld, F., & York, R. (1966). *Equality of educational opportunity report.* Washington, D.C.: U.S. Government Printing Office.

Comer, J. (1976). Improving the quality and continuity of relationships in two inner-city schools. *Journal of the American Academy of Child Psychiatry, 15*, 535–545.

Comer, J. (1985). The Yale-New Haven primary prevention project: A follow-up study. *Journal of the American Academy of Child Psychiatry, 24*, 154–160.

Comer, J. (1987). New Haven's school-community connection. *Educational Leadership*, 13–16.

Committee for Economic Development. (1987). *Children in need: Investment strategies for the educationally disadvantaged.* Washington, D.C.: Committee for Economic Development.

Conley, D. (1991). *Restructuring schools: Educators adapt to a changing world.* Eugene, OR: ERIC Clearinghouse on Educational Management.

Council of Chief State School Officers. (1990). *Voices from successful schools: Elements of improved schools serving at-risk students and how state education agencies can support more local school improvement.* Washington, D.C.: Author.

Council of the Great City Schools. (1987). *Results in the making.* Washington, D.C.: Council of the Great City Schools.

Crain, R. & Strauss, J. (1986). *Are smaller high schools more or less effective?* Baltimore, MD: Center for Social Organization of Schools, Johns Hopkins University.

Cuban, L. (September, 1986). Persistent instruction: Another look at constancy in the classroom. *Phi Delta Kappan,* 7–11.

Cuban, L. (November 20, 1991). All-male African-American public schools: Desperate remedies for desperate times. *Education Week, 11*(12), 36.

Cuban, L. (1997). Change without reform: The case of Stanford University School of Medicine, 1908–1990. *American Educational Research Journal, 34,* 83–122.

David, J., Purkey, S., & White, P. (1989). *Restructuring in progress: Lessons from pioneering districts.* Washington, D.C.: National Governors' Association.

DeVries, R. (1997). Piaget's social theory. *Educational Researcher, 26,* 4–17.

Edmonds, R. R. (1979). Effective schools for the urban poor. *Educational Leadership, 37,* 15–27.

Edmonds, R. R. (1981). Making public schools effective. *Social Policy, 12,* 56–60.

Educational Priorities Panel. (1988). *Evaluation of the New York City Comprehensive School Improvement Process.* New York: Educational Priorities Panel.

Eisner, E. (1986). *What high schools are like: Views from the inside.* Stanford, CA: Stanford University.

Eisner, E. (1988). The ecology of school improvement. *Educational Leadership,* 24–29.

Ekstrom, R., Goertz, M., Pollack, J., & Rock, D. (1986). *Who drops out of high school and why? Findings from a national study. Teachers College Record, 87,* 356–373.

Elmore, R. (1988). *Early experience in restructuring schools: Voices from the field.* Washington, D.C.: National Governors' Association.

Felner, R., & Adan, A. (1988). The school transitional environment project: An ecological intervention and evaluation. In R. Price, E. Cowen, R. Lorion, & J. Ramos-McKay, (Eds.), *Fourteen ounces of prevention: A casebook for practitioners,* (pp. 111–122). Washington, D.C.: American Psychological Association.

Felner, R., Ginter, M., & Primavera, J. (1982). Primary prevention during school transitions: Social Support and environmental structure. *American Journal of Community Psychology, 10,* 277–290.

Felner, R., Jackson, A., Karak, D., Mulhall, P., Brand, J., & Flowers, N. (March, 1997). The impact of school reform for the middle years. *Phi Delta Kappan,* 528–532, 541–550.

Felner, R., Phillips, R., DuBois, D., & Lease, M. (1991). Ecological interventions and the process of change for prevention: Wedding theory and research to implementation in real world settings. *American Journal of Community Psychology, 19,* 379–387.

Fine, M. (1986). Why urban adolescents drop into and out of public high school. *Teachers College Record, 87*(3), 393–409.

Fine, M. (1990). *Framing dropouts: Notes on the politics of an urban high school.* Albany, NY: SUNY Press.

Fine, M. (1992). *Chart(er)ing urban school reform: Philadelphia style.* Philadelphia, PA: Philadelphia Schools Collaborative.

Fine, M., & Rosenberg, P. (1983). Dropping out of high school: The ideology of school and work. *Journal of Education, 165,* 257–272.

Finn, C. (1990). The biggest reform of all. *Phi Delta Kappan, 71,* 584–592.

Foley, E., & Oxley, D. (1986). *Effective dropout prevention: An analysis of the 1985–86 program in New York City.* New York: The Public Education Association.

Gardner, H. (1983). *Frames of mind: The theory of multiple intelligences.* New York: Basic Books.

Goldman, R., & Cowan, P. (1976). Teacher cognitive characteristics, social system variables, and the use of consultation. *American Journal of Community Psychology, 4,* 85–98.

Good, T., & Weinstein, R. (1986). Schools make a difference: Evidence, criticisms, and new directions. *American Psychologist, 41,* 1090–1097.

Goodlad, J. (1984). *A place called school: Prospects for the future.* New York: McGraw-Hill.

Gottfredson, D. (1985). *School size and school disorder.* Baltimore, MD: Center for Social Organization of Schools, Johns Hopkins University.

Grannis, J., Riehl, C., & Pallas, A. (1988). *Evaluation of the New York City Dropout Prevention Initiative.* New York: Teachers College, Columbia University.

Gregory, T., & Smith, G. (1987). *High schools as communities: The small school reconsidered.* Bloomington, IN: Phi Delta Kappa Educational Foundation.

Gruber, J., & Trickett, E. (1987). Can we empower others? The paradox of empowerment in the governing of an alternative public school. *American Journal of Community Psychology,, 15*, 353–371.

Haberman, M. (1991). The pedagogy of poverty versus good teaching. *Phi Delta Kappan, 73*, 290–294.

Hamilton, S. (1983). The social side of schooling: Ecological studies of classrooms and schools. *The Elementary School Journal, 83*, 313–334.

Hess, G., & Greer, J. (April, 1986). *Educational triage and dropout rates.* Paper presented at the American Educational Research Association Annual Convention, San Francisco, CA.

Institute for Educational Leadership. (1986). *School dropouts: Everybody's problem.* Washington, D.C.: Institute for Educational Leadership.

Kelly, J. (Ed.). (1979). *Adolescent boys in high school: A psychological study of coping and adaptation.* New York: Wiley.

Kimberly, J. (1976). Organizational size and the structuralist perspective: A review, critique, and proposal. *Administrative Science Quarterly, 21*, 571–597.

Lapointe, A., Mead, N., & Phillips, G. (1989). *A world of differences: An international assessment of mathematics and science.* Princeton, NJ: Educational Testing Service.

Lee, V., & Smith, J. (1995). Effects of high school restructuring and size on gains in achievement and engagement for early secondary school students. *Sociology of Education, 68*, 241–270.

Lenrow, P., & Cowden, P. (1980). Human services, professionals, and the paradox of institutional reform. *American Journal of Community Psychology, 8*, 463–484.

Lewin, K. (1951). Frontiers in group dynamics. In D. Cartwright, (Ed.), *Field theory and social science: Selected theoretical papers by Kurt Lewin.* Chicago: University of Chicago Press.

Lindsay, P. (1982). The effect of high school size on student participation, satisfaction, and attendance. *Educational Evaluation and Policy Analysis, 4*, 57–65.

Linney, J., & Seidman, E. (1989). The future of schooling. *American Psychologist, 44*, 336–340.

Louis, K., & Miles, M. (1990). *Improving the urban high school: What works and why.* New York: Teachers College Press.

McCombs, B. (1991). Motivation and lifelong learning. *Educational Psychologist, 26*, 117–127.

Meier, D. (1987). Central Park East: An alternative story. *Phi Delta Kappan, 68*, 753–757.

Miles, M. (1981). Mapping the common properties of schools. In R. Lehming, & M. Kane, (Eds.), *Improving schools: Using what we know.* Beverly Hills, CA: Sage.

Miles, M., & Kaufman, T. (1985). Directory of effective schools programs. In R. J. Kyle (Ed.), *Sourcebook on effective schools.* Washington, D.C.: National Institute of Education.

National Academy of Education. (1991). *Research and renewal in education.* Stanford, CA: Stanford University, School of Education.

National Center for Education Statistics. (1991). *Dropout rates in the United States: 1990.* Washington, D.C.: U.S. Government Printing Office.

National Coalition of Advocates for Students. (1985). *Barriers to excellence: Our children at risk.* Boston: Author.

National Commission on Excellence in Education. (1983). *A nation at risk: The imperative for educational reform.* Washington, D.C.: Superintendent of Documents, U.S. Government Printing Office.

National Education Goals Panel. (1995). *The national education goals report.* Washington, D.C.: Superintendent of Documents, U.S. Government Printing Office.

National Governors' Association. (1986). *Time for results: The governors' 1991 report on education.* Washington, D.C.: National Governors' Association.

New York City Board of Education. (1989). *High School Attendance Improvement Dropout Prevention Program 1987–1988.* New York: New York City Board of Education.

New York State Education Department. (February, 1987a). Concentration of poverty in schools linked to dropout rates above the statewide average. *Learning in New York, 8.*

New York State Education Department (1987b). *Increasing high school completion rates: A framework for state and local action.* Albany: New York State Education Department.

New York State Social Studies Review and Development Committee. (1991). *One nation, many people: A declaration of cultural interdependence.* Albany: New York State Education Department.

Newberg, N. (May, 1995). Clusters: Organizational patterns for caring. *Phi Delta Kappan*, 713–717.

Newmann, F. (1981). Reducing alienation in high schools: Implications of theory. *Harvard Educational Review, 51*, 546–564.

Newmann, F. (1993). Beyond common sense in educational restructuring: The issues of content and linkage. *Educational Researcher, 22*, 4–13, 22.

Newmann, F., & Associates. (1996). *Authentic achievement: Restructuring schools for intellectual quality.* San Francisco, CA: Jossey-Bass.

Newmann, F., & Thompson, J. (1987). *Effects of cooperative learning on achievement in secondary schools: A summary of research*. Madison: National Center on Effective Secondary Schools, University of Wisconsin-Madison.

Noddings, N. (1992). *The challenge to care in schools*. New York: Teachers College Press.

Oakes, J. (1985). *Keeping track: How schools structure inequality*. New Haven, CT: Yale University Press.

Olson, L. (1988). The restructuring puzzle. *Education Week*, 7–8, 11.

Orr, M. (1987). *What to do about youth dropouts*? New York: SEEDCO.

Oxley, D. (1988). *Effective dropout prevention: The case for schoolwide reform*. New York: The Public Education Association.

Oxley, D. (1990). *An analysis of house systems in New York City neighborhood high schools*. Philadelphia, PA: Temple University.

Oxley, D. (1994a). Organizing for responsiveness: The heterogeneous school community. In M. Wang & E. Gordon (Eds.), *Educational resilience in inner-city America: Challenges and prospects*, (pp. 179–190). Hillsdale, NJ: Erlbaum.

Oxley, D. (1994b). Organizing schools into small units: Alternatives to homogeneous grouping. *Phi Delta Kappan*, *7*, 521–526.

Oxley, D. (1997a). *Organizing schools into small units: Implications for a cultural change process*. Presented at the American Education Research Association, Chicago, IL.

Oxley, D. (1997b). Theory and practice of school communities. *Educational Administration Quarterly*, *33*, 624–643.

Oxley, D. (1997c). Making community in an inner city high school. In D. Sage (Ed.), *Inclusion in secondary schools*. Port Chester, NY: National Professional Resources.

Oxley, D., Werner, C., Altman, I., & Haggard, L. (1986). Transactional qualities of neighborhood social networks: A case study of "Christmas Street." *Environment and Behavior*, *18*, 640–677.

Philadelphia Inquirer. (May 6, 1990). Funding problems place city schools at crossroad.

Pittman, R., & Haughwout, P. (1987). Influence of high school size on dropout rate. *Educational Evaluation and Policy Analysis*, *9*, 337, 343.

Plath, K. (1965). *Schools within schools: A study of high school organization*. New York: Teachers College, Columbia University.

Powell, A., Farrar, E., & Cohen, D. (1985). *The shopping mall high school*. Boston: Houghton-Mifflin.

Power, F., Higgins, A., & Kohlberg, L. (1989). *Lawrence Kohlberg's approach to moral education*. New York: Columbia University Press.

Purkey, S., Rutter, R., & Newmann, F. (1985). *U.S. high school improvement programs: A profile form the High School and Beyond Supplemental Survey*. Madison: Wisconsin Center for Education Research.

Purkey, S., & Smith, M. (1983). Effective schools: A review. *The Elementary School Journal*, *83*, 427–452.

Purkey, S., & Smith, M. (1985). School reform: The district policy implications of the effective schools literature. *The Elementary School Journal*, *85*, 353–389.

Rappaport, J. (1987). Terms of empowerment/exemplars of prevention: Toward a theory for community psychology. *American Journal of Community Psychology*, *15*, 121–148.

Ratzki, A. (1988). Creating a school community: One model of how it can be done. *American Educator*, *12*(1), 10–17, 38–43.

Rowan, B., Bossert, S., & Dwyer, D. (1983). Research on effective schools: A cautionary note. *Educational Researcher*, *12*(4), 24–31.

Rumberger, R. (1983). Dropping out of high school: The influences of race, sex, and family background. *American Educational Research Journal*, *20*, 199–220.

Rutter, M., Maughan, D., Mortimore, P., Ouston, J., & Smith, A. (1979). *Fifteen thousand hours: Secondary schools and their effects on children*. Cambridge, MA: Harvard University Press.

Sarason, S. (1982). *The culture of the school and the problem of change*. Boston: Allyn and Bacon.

Sarason, S. (1990). *The predictable failure of school reform*. San Francisco: Jossey-Bass.

Sarason, S., & Klaber, M. (1985). The school as a social situation. *Annual Review of Psychology*, *36*, 115–140.

Saunders, J., & Reppucci, D. (1977). Learning networks among administrators of human service institutions. *American Journal of Community Psychology*, *5*, 269–276.

Segal, J. W., Chipman, S. G., & Glaser, R. (Eds.). (1985). *Thinking and learning skills: Vol. I Relating instruction to research*. Hillsdale, NJ: Erlbaum.

Seidman, E. (1988). Back to the future, Community Psychology: Unfolding a theory of social intervention. *American Journal of Community Psychology*, *16*, 3–24.

Seidman, E. (1990). Social regularities and prevention research: A transactional model. In Muehrer, P. (Ed.) *Conceptual research models for preventing mental disorders*. Rockville, MD: National Institute of Mental Health.

Sergiovanni, T. (1994). *Building community in schools*. San Francisco, CA: Jossey-Bass.

Shanker, A. (1988). A charter for change. *New York Times*, July 10, p. E7.

Sizer, T. (1984). *Horace's compromise: The dilemma of the American high school*. Boston: Houghton-Mifflin.

Steinberg, L., Blinde, P., & Chan, K. (1984). Dropping out among language minority youth. *Review of Educational Research, 54*, 113–132.

Trickett, E., McConahay, J., Phillips, D., & Ginter, M. (1985). Natural experiments and the educational context: The environment and effects of an alternative inner-city public school on adolescents. *American Journal of Community Psychology, 13*, 617–643.

U.S. Department of Education. (1983). *A nation at risk: The imperative for educational reform*. Washington, D.C.: U.S. Department of Education.

U.S. Department of Education. (1986). *What works: Research about teaching and learning*. Washington, D.C.: U.S. Government Printing Office.

U.S. Department of Education. (1987). *Schools that work: Educating disadvantaged children*. Washington, D.C.: U.S. Government Printing Office.

U.S. Department of Education. (1991). *America 2000: An education strategy*. Washington, D.C.: U.S. Department of Education.

Walberg, H., & Fowler, W. (1987). Expenditure and size efficiencies of public school districts. *Educational Researcher, 16*(7), 5–15.

Wang, M. (1992). *Adaptive education strategies: Building on diversity*. Baltimore: Paul H. Brookes.

Wang, M., & Palincsar, A. (1989). Teaching students to assume an active role in their learning. In M. Reynolds, (Ed.), *Knowledge base for the beginning teacher* (pp. 71–84). Oxford: Pergamon.

Wang, M., Walberg, H., & Reynolds, M. (1988). A scenario for better-not separate-special education. *Educational Leadership, 50*(2), 35–38.

Wehlage, G. (1983). *Effective programs for the marginal high school student*. Bloomington, IN: Phi Delta Kappa.

Wehlage, G., & Rutter, R. (1986). Dropping out: How much do schools contribute to the problem? *Teachers College Record, 87*, 374–392.

Weinstein, R. (1996). High standards in a tracked system of schooling: For which students and with what educational supports? *Educational Researcher, 25*(8), 16–19.

Weinstein, R., Soule, C., Collins, F., Cone, J., Mehlhorn, M., & Simontacchi, K. (1991). Expectations and high school change: Teacher-researcher collaboration to prevent school failure. *American Journal of Community Psychology, 19*, 333–363.

Weissberg, R. (1987). Teacher ratings of children's problem and competence behaviors: Normative and Parametric characteristics. *American Journal of Community Psychology, 15*, 387–401.

Wiggins, G. (1991). Standards, not standardization: Evoking quality student work. *Educational Leadership, 48*(5), 18–25.

CHAPTER 25

Self-Help Groups

LEON H. LEVY

Among the various mental and physical health intervention modalities, none are likely to be as compatible with the values, goals, and ideology of community psychology as self-help groups (SHGs). Ecologically, while they are part of the community's health care delivery system, their roots are in the community, rather than in the various professional disciplines that staff the other components of that system. Furthermore, they are the only component of the delivery system whose sanction for existence comes from its immediate beneficiaries, rather than from the sociopolitical structure. While SHGs were initially born out of dissatisfaction with the established health care system (Katz & Bender, 1976), their surge in growth and their prevalence today can largely be explained by the changes in the social and cultural climate of America following the social and political eruption of the 1960s, which left in its wake, among other things, counterculturalism, the consumer movement, and a devaluation of the respect and privileges traditionally accorded professionals and others in authority. Thus, SHGs are the component of the health care system most likely to be identified with, and accessible, to the community served by the system.

At the level of public policy, SHGs hold the promise of increasing the community's health care resources at minimal cost to its citizens. And at the individual level, because SHGs are for the most part under the control of their members themselves, participation in these groups should enhance their members' sense of empowerment, which may itself have positive mental health consequences (Rappaport, 1987).

Despite their ideological compatibility, however, before community psychology as an empirically based discipline can give SHGs their full endorsement, much remains to be known about their effectiveness. Put more positively, there is much about SHGs that commends them to community psychology as an appropriate and important arena of research. Indeed, given their proliferation and popularity—estimates of the one-year prevalence of participation in SHGs range from 7.5 million in 1992 (Lieberman & Snowden, 1994) to over 10 million in 1999 (Jacobs & Goodman, 1989)—it would not be hyperbole to say that the need for research on their effectiveness is urgent.

Systematic research and scholarship concerned with SHGs are of quite recent vintage, beginning in 1976. That year saw the publication of both *Support Systems and Mutual Help*

LEON H. LEVY • Department of Psychology, Virginia Commonwealth University, Richmond, Virginia 23229.
Handbook of Community Psychology, edited by Julian Rappaport and Edward Seidman. Kluwer Academic / Plenum Publishers, New York, 2000.

(Caplan & Killilea, 1976), *The Strength in Us* (Katz & Bender, 1976), and a special issue of *The Journal of Applied Behavioral Science* (*12*, 1976) devoted to SHGs. Together, these three publications summarized the state of conceptualization and research on SHGs up to that time and did much to set the direction for future work on this topic. Readers are referred to these publications for a historical perspective on the current research scene.

This chapter will selectively review the research literature on SHGs since 1976 from three different perspectives: From a mental health perspective, it will be concerned with their effectiveness and with the processes and mechanisms that subserve their role as clinical interventions; from an organizational perspective, its focus will be on their growth and functioning as social systems; and from the perspective of public policy, it will consider the implications of our current knowledge of SHGs for public support of SHGs, and for their role as an integral component of the organized health care delivery system. It will be helpful, however, to begin with a brief discussion of the defining characteristics of SHGs and with a consideration of the particular methodological problems associated with research on them.

DEFINING CHARACTERISTICS OF SELF-HELP GROUPS

In his pioneering articulation of the concept of support systems, Caplan (1974) clearly captured many of the essential characteristics of SHGs. He defined support systems as "continuing social aggregates that provide individuals with opportunities for feedback about themselves and for validations of their expectations about others, which may offset deficiencies in these communications within the larger community context" (pp. 4–5). He went on to note that within these social aggregates,

> The person is dealt with as a unique individual. The other people are interested in him in a personalized way. They speak his language. They tell him what is expected of him and guide him in what to do. They watch what he does and they judge his performance. They let him know how well he has done. They reward him for success and punish or support him if he fails. Above all, they are sensitive to his personal needs, which they deem worthy of respect and satisfaction (pp. 5–6).

Caplan considered SHGs to be support systems, referring to them as "mutual-help groups of 'people in the same boat' " (p. 23). Thus, they have also been characterized as "ready-made social support systems in specific domains of problems" (Shumaker & Brownell, 1984). However, while it is true that SHGs are formed around particular problems or afflictions shared by all their members, there are other, more specific characteristics that should also be noted that distinguish them from other support systems and from the other components of the health care system.

Unlike other social support systems, such as family and friends, because all the members of SHGs share the same problem, they relate to each other as peers within the context of their group, each acting as both a provider and a recipient of help, focused on their common problem or condition. These three characteristics of SHGs, commonality of problem, members relating to each other as peers, and members playing dual roles as both providers and recipients of help, are often cited as keys to understanding the unique effectiveness of SHGs (Gartner & Riessman, 1977; Levine & Perkins, 1987). This is not to say that there are no hierarchies of roles within SHGs but, in contrast to professional care systems, the roles are functionally defined and open to any member qualified and willing to perform them.

SHGs also differ from naturally occurring social support systems in that they are intentional, and their activities are guided, in varying degrees, by particular ideologies concerning the nature of their members' affliction and how it can be effectively dealt with (Levine & Perkins, 1987). These ideologies vary in their elaborateness and in how clearly they are articulated, but they usually provide members with a new way of viewing their problem, or with a new world view (Humphreys, 1996; Kennedy, Humphreys, & Borkman, 1994), infusing them with a sense of purpose and direction, much as the theories of health professionals do for them. How these ideologies figure in the effectiveness of SHGs, however, is a question awaiting empirical study, although there has been some interesting speculation (Antze, 1976).

The final defining characteristic of SHGs is that their origin, sanction for existence, and the control over their mode of operation rest with the members of the group themselves; they are autonomous. Although some groups that are nationally organized, such as Alcoholics Anonymous (AA), clearly prescribe how individual chapters are to operate, and others, such as Parents Anonymous, have professional sponsors, the sense of autonomy is very much a part of all SHGs. And this sense is certainly justified when they are compared with the professional components of the health care system.

This autonomy has a number of consequences for SHGs, not all of which are necessarily salutary. It frees them from the dogma under which "establishment" health care professions labor, thus allowing them to take a more pragmatic approach to dealing with their members' problems. It places greater responsibility upon the shoulders of members for both the successes and the failures of their groups, which can be therapeutically beneficial. But it also deprives them of access to the sources of financial and technical support usually available to other human services agencies. And, not being a part of the "establishment," SHGs are not subject to its demands of accountability. As a consequence, SHGs may be expected to (and have been found to) exhibit considerable variability in their performance (Roberts, Luke, Rappaport, Seidman, Toro, & Reischl, 1991) and in their effectiveness. This latter consequence, of course, has important implications for the design of research on SHGs and for the generalizability of research findings. It also complicates the advocacy and development of public policies concerned with SHGs.

As elements in the definition of SHGs, these characteristics distinguish between those groups, such as Recovery, Inc, and Overeaters Anonymous, which I consider to qualify as SHGs; and groups such as Weight Watchers, a proprietary group; and Mothers Against Drunk Driving, an advocacy group. It must be recognized, however, that it remains an empirical question which of these characteristics, either singly or in combination, are essential to the unique effectiveness of SHGs.

SELF-HELP GROUPS AS CLINICAL INTERVENTIONS

Problems Associated with Research on Self-Help Groups

The extent and quality of empirical research on SHGs is surprisingly limited given their prominence on the contemporary human services scene and the encouragement of such research by The President's Commission on Mental Health (1978). But the reasons for this become readily apparent once we consider the methodological problems encountered in conducting this research.

Although none of the design and analysis problems are unique to SHGs, many become more intractable and acute in the case of SHGs for reasons that are largely intrinsic to these groups. Because membership in SHGs is largely self-defined, problems in sampling and in the definition of the population being sampled are virtually insoluble. It is difficult to assure the validity of characterizations of the specific modes of operation of particular SHGs because of the high variability found in the practices of SHGs, even among those affiliated with the same national self-help organization. Further, it is impossible to utilize any kind of research design involving randomized assignments either to alternative treatments or to control groups without doing violence to the essential nature of SHGs, even if they were willing to sanction such a study.

Apart from these obvious design problems, the quality of data in SHGs research is a serious problem because they generally prohibit the use of any on-site, within-meeting recording devices and because they do not maintain any archival records. Thus, although most SHGs will cooperate with investigators, they do so under conditions that, while understandable in terms of their own concerns and values, make the acquisition of high quality, reliable data quite difficult, at best.

This means that any kind of process research (e.g., Levy, 1976; Lieberman, 1983; Rappaport, Seidman, Toro, McFadden, Reischle, Roberts, Selam, Stein, & Zimmerman, 1985; Wollert, Levy, & Knight, 1982) must depend upon on-site observers using complex coding schemes to record interactions as they occur, intensive post-meeting interviews with members, or survey questionnaires completed by members. Since the first two approaches are extremely labor intensive and costly, questionnaires have become the most common source of data on the processes and activities found in SHGs. But, as with all self-report measures, the quality of the data thus obtained is entirely dependent upon the accuracy of member's responses, which is difficult to assess. Moreover, since SHG members are neither trained observers nor psychologically trained, it also limits the subtlety and complexity of the processes that can be studied.

Most of these problems are common to field studies in the behavioral sciences. They are threats to internal validity, construct validity, and external validity, as defined by Cook and Campbell (1979). Since most of these threats are well known to those familiar with the psychotherapy research literature, and a more extended discussion of them as they present themselves in the case of SHGs may be found elsewhere (Levy, 1984), I would like to focus here on a particular dilemma that may be unique to the problem of outcome research with SHGs and that has not heretofore been described. This dilemma involves what might be termed the *intrinsic positive bias effect* in SHG outcome research. It is present in field studies whenever SHGs are compared with other interventions or with matched control groups, and is due to the following unique combination of factors:

1. *Differential mortality in membership.* As compared with a matched comparison or control group, at any given point in time, or over any specified time period, SHGs will contain more individuals who are benefitting from their membership than who are not, since those who are not benefitting are more likely to have dropped out due to the relative ease of doing so.

2. *Differential competence and adjustment.* Participation in a SHGs requires a certain level of social competence and interest in social relationships. Lieberman and Videka-Sherman (1985), for example, found that members of a widowed persons SHG were more likely than nonmembers to be active in social organizations and clubs. Thus, as compared with any matched group of comparably distressed individuals, SHG members are likely to have higher levels of interest and competence in social relationships, and to the extent that these are factors in personal adjustment and in the ability to benefit from interpersonally mediated therapeutic interventions, SHG members, on the average, should be better able than nonmembers to benefit from SHG participation.

3. *Differential utilization of ancillary sources of help.* Consistent with point 2, it is

reasonable to expect that SHG members, as compared to nonmembers, will tend to make more use of other sources of support and help, particularly from their social networks (Lieberman, 1979). These ancillary sources of help, either by themselves or in interaction with the SHGs, thus confer a special advantage on SHG members *vis-à-vis* nonmember controls.

4. *Differential motivation.* In joining a SHG, members make a commitment, at some level, to changing and to taking an active role in changing, which may not be present, or as strong, in nonmembers. Thus, as compared with any matched group of comparably distressed individuals, SHGs are likely to be composed of members with higher levels of motivation to work on their problems.

While any one of these factors may also apply to other forms of therapy, their convergence in SHGs provides them with an intrinsic advantage in any outcome study in which they are compared with matched nonmember control groups. This would seem to make an obvious case for denying credibility to the results of any outcome study that did not make use of a randomized treatment design. But to eliminate the confounding, were it possible through some cleverly contrived means of randomly assigning individuals to SHGs and to alternative forms of intervention, would pose equally serious interpretive problems.

And herein lies the dilemma: *In contrast to any other intervention, a SHG does not exist as an intervention apart from its members who are both the instrumentality and the objects of the intervention; change the characteristics of its membership and the intervention is changed as well.* The very fact that individuals are members of SHGs long enough to contribute data to any evaluation of their effectiveness suggests that they find this mode of intervention a congenial (and possibly an effective) one, and that it probably represents a good match with their beliefs, attitudes, and personalities. This cannot be said of any other mode of intervention, since in no other mode are individuals so free to become engaged and disengaged.

Thus, random assignment of individuals to SHGs and to other forms of intervention would result in a fundamental distortion of the natural ecology of these groups—some people would be in SHGs who normally would not be and vice versa. The *composition* of the SHGs' membership would be different in some indeterminate, but probably nontrivial, way from that of naturally formed SHGs. And to the extent that the effective functioning of any group is dependent upon its particular mix of interactants, such randomly formed SHGs would not be representative of naturally forming SHGs in either their membership or their functioning. Thus, while randomization might eliminate the intrinsic positive bias effect, it would do so at the cost of introducing a negative bias relative to naturally formed SHGs, and the knowledge so obtained would have little applicability to the question that motivated the research in the first place.

Is there any solution to this dilemma? There may be if we are willing to drop the null hypothesis approach to testing for treatment effects as Meehl (1978) has cogently proposed. Meehl has argued that for most research in psychology, especially in the "softer" areas such as clinical psychology, the null hypothesis, taken literally, is always false, and that its falsification, even in the predicted direction, provides weak support for the substantive theory in question. There are just too many subtle, extraneous, uncontrolled factors that could have interacted in some complex fashion with the independent variable to produce the effect.

The alternative that Meehl proposes is testing for consistency with predicted experimental outcomes; in the present context, this would consist of testing for consistency with explicitly stated treatment outcomes expected of particular SHGs along particularly defined dimensions. The research designs required to produce such data already exist, ranging from simple pre-post designs to interrupted time-series analyses. A particularly useful approach for SHGs would be the goal-attainment scaling procedure advocated by Kiresuk and Lund (1978) for the assessment of programs and interventions. Essentially this requires defining the course and/or outcome for particular targets of intervention by particular SHGs that would be taken as evidence for their effectiveness.

This would solve the intrinsic positive bias dilemma and would have two other salutary consequences as well: It would force researchers to seriously confront the criterion problem in the course of stating the treatment outcomes that they would count as successful and, having specified these, it would lay the groundwork for a cost-effectiveness assessment. Too often, outcome studies, and not only those involving SHGs, rely upon catch-as-catch-can findings of significant differences among the many dependent variables included in the design without any consideration of either their order of importance or the actual levels of gain achieved. The result, while possibly having some theoretical value, is certainly nothing that would aid either a clinician in deciding whether to make a referral to a SHG or a policymaker deciding whether to foster their further growth.

Of course, outcome research, or summative evaluations, represent only one genre of SHG research. Considerably less problematic from a design standpoint are process research and formative evaluation research—research concerned with how SHGs function as intervention modalities, since these involve essentially within-group designs. Perhaps in part because this kind of research is less methodologically problematic and is intrinsically interesting, it is currently where most SHG research, as well as the most creative and innovative thinking, is found (Powell, 1994). At the same time, however, while this research is process focused, its findings can ultimately provide the foundation for the enhanced effectiveness of SHGs.

Research on the Effectiveness of Self-Help Groups

Although SHGs are most often thought of as functioning in a secondary prevention role, they have also been proposed as primary preventive interventions (Borman, 1982; Hermalin, 1979; Silverman, 1972). Since there have been no studies of SHGs' effectiveness in this latter role, we will be concerned only with findings concerning their effectiveness as agents of secondary prevention. As might be expected from the preceding discussion, the amount of research that passes muster by the most liberal interpretation of quasi-experimental design is quite small. For this reason, and because of the limited number of studies involved, I believe that it will be more instructive to generalize about the characteristics of the data on SHGs than about what is said concerning the effectiveness of SHGs. Therefore, this discussion will be structured so as to highlight the two most salient characteristics of these findings, rather than in terms of individual studies.

The first characteristic of these data is the prevalence of what we might term *perspectival discrepancies*. These discrepancies occur between data representing SHG members' perspectives, that is, their reports of the benefits that they have derived and their assertions of the personal value of the group to them, and data reflecting researchers' perspectives, represented by formal and informal measures of SHG member levels of symptomatology, adjustment, or improvement.

The second characteristic of SHG outcome data is their *nonuniformity*. This is found in individual differences in particular measures of benefits derived by members within a particular SHG (which may be expected), in differences among the various measures of benefit found within a particular study (which must be troubling since such differences are rarely predicted), in measures of the effectiveness of different SHGs affiliated with the same self-help organization, and in the outcomes of groups dealing with different conditions (which, again, may not be surprising, but which must be dealt with).

Perspectival Discrepancies

Most investigators have followed Strupp and Hadley's (1977) proposed model for the evaluation of psychotherapy outcomes in adopting outcome criteria of SHG effectiveness. These represent three different perspectives (Hinrichsen, Revenson, & Shinn, 1985; Lieberman & Bond, 1979; Levy, 1984): the members', the group's, and the researchers'. This recognizes that the goals of individual SHG members may not coincide with those of the group itself, and that these both, in turn, may be different from those sought by the investigator who represents the interests of the professional community and, ultimately, society at large. Thus, for example, an individual may join Alcoholics Anonymous to save his job and regain his self-respect, and will consider the group effective if he has achieved these goals, even if he has not become abstinent. AA, on the other hand, will only count the achievement of abstinence as success, while a researcher may use moderate drinking, as well as abstinence and several measures of psychosocial adjustment, to gauge the group's effectiveness.

Although the expectation of discrepancies is implicit in the notion of representing different perspectives in the evaluation of intervention outcomes, because there is no consensus on how to deal with such discrepancies, finding them can pose a potentially serious problem for SHGs. This is because while the popularity and growth of SHGs derive largely from their members' views of their value, their legitimacy as interventions from society's standpoint rests largely on the assessments of their effectiveness by researchers' criteria. Although similar discrepancies are frequently found in psychotherapy research, and its efficacy is subject to constant challenge, psychotherapy's legitimacy has never been questioned because it is practiced by professionals. SHGs do not enjoy such immunity.

In a survey study of the impact of Mended Hearts, a SHG established to help heart surgery patients and spouses adapt to their surgery, Videka (1979) compared heart surgery patients who were members of Mended Hearts with a demographically comparable group of nonmember heart surgery patients on a variety of measures of psychosocial adaptation (e.g., depression, anxiety, self-esteem, and use of psychotropic medication). With the exception of retired members, she found essentially no differences between members and nonmembers on these measures, even when she controlled for members' involvement in the organization.

Yet, when members were asked to rate Mended Hearts on the dimensions of relevance to their needs, enjoyableness, helpfulness, and informativeness, 60% rated their group as relevant to their needs, 70% as enjoyable, 68% as helpful, and 71% as informative. And when asked to rate their satisfaction with the chapters, 50% rated them as "very satisfactory" or "could not be better" and another 36% rated them as "satisfactory;" only 14% rated their chapter as "very unsatisfactory." Thus, although the researcher's measures suggested that Mended Heart members derived little benefit from their membership, the members apparently felt otherwise.

Similarly, in a study of Compassionate Friends, a SHG for bereaved parents, Videka-Sherman and Lieberman (1985) found no evidence that the group had any impact on members' psychosocial adjustment with respect to such dimensions as depression, anxiety, somatization, and self-esteem. Nevertheless, group members reported that they had become more self-confident (65), more in control of their situations (72%), happier (61%), less depressed (60%), less anxious (60%), less guilty (44%), less angry (44%), less isolated (50%), and freer to express feelings (77%). Although it is true that the dimensions on which members were asked to rate themselves were not identical to those that failed to reveal any treatment effect, the divergence in perspectives is nevertheless striking.

This divergence was also found in a study of the Scoliosis Association, Inc., an organization of peer support groups for people with scoliosis and their families (Hinrichsen, Revenson, & Shinn, 1985). Although members reported high levels of satisfaction with their chapters, they fared no better than a nonmember comparison group on measures of psychosocial adjustment. However, the failure to find a treatment effect in this otherwise well-designed and well-analyzed study may be due in part to how SHG membership was defined, and we shall digress briefly because this brings up two important methodological problems in this area.

Hinrichsen et al. (1985) defined a member as anyone who had attended at least one scoliosis club meeting, thus (reasonably) excluding individuals who might pay dues to the Scoliosis Association but not attend any meetings. The nonmember comparison group in the study was composed of individuals who had written to the Scoliosis Association in response to a magazine article, thus indicating some interest in the group, but had not joined or attended a meeting.

This method of defining membership points to the fact that there is no consensus on the definition of membership among researchers. The extent of this problem is exemplified by the fact that attendance at only one group meeting counted as membership in Hinrichsen et al.'s (1985) study, while Lieberman and Videka-Sherman (1986) required attendance at three meetings in their study. This lack of consistency among investigators on so fundamental a question as the definition of membership can only contribute to inconsistencies in outcome findings from one study to another.

Actually, there are two problems here: the definition of SHG membership and the measurement of attendance as an index of the "dosage" received of whatever the group provides that is supposed to be beneficial. Membership and dosage are not identical, nor are attendance and dose. SHG members' attendance at meetings is frequently irregular, and many consider themselves members of a group although they rarely attend its meetings, or do so only on an as-needed basis. Thus the question of what "membership" itself, irrespective of attendance, may contribute to the effects of SHGs is worthy of study. This may vary with the type of group, and my guess is that it may involve the extent to which membership itself contributes to the members identities.

SHG attendance is viewed, either implicitly or explicitly, as a measure of exposure to the hypothesized influence of a group and as having a dose–response relationship with outcomes. This is reasonable at first glance, but vexing at second. Valid attendance data are virtually impossible to obtain because SHGs do not keep attendance records and would be averse to researchers doing so for a variety of reasons, including protecting the privacy of members. Although Yeaton (1994) has demonstrated a way in which valid attendance records could be obtained that would protect member privacy, its complexity of implementation and logistical demands place it beyond the reach of all but the most generously funded researchers (if any exist).

But even were it possible to obtain valid records of meeting attendance, using them as a measure of dosage or exposure to the impact of SHG on members is problematic for another reason: doing so requires the assumption that the dose delivered at each SHG meeting is uniform for each member and for every meeting of the group, which is obviously untenable.

Videka (1979) appears to have attempted to address this problem by assessing members' amount of involvement in Mended Hearts. A measure of involvement was also used by Lieberman and Videka-Sherman (1986) in a study of a widowed persons' group. However, although degree of involvement may be an important variable in its own right, it is no more satisfactory as a substitute for dosage in evaluating SHGs than it would be acceptable as an alternative to number of sessions in the evaluation of psychotherapy. Thus, the problem of controlling for level of exposure or dosage in assessing effectiveness remains on the table.

While addressing these and other methodological problems may reduce the extent of perspectival discrepancies in SHG outcome research, it is unlikely to eliminate them. Therefore, for the reasons noted at the beginning of this section, investigators need also to give their attention to the theoretical question of how to construe these discrepancies when they occur. The obvious answer that they reflect differences in criteria only begs the question.

Nonuniformity of SHG Outcome Data

Although the doctrine of the uniformity of nature may be of doubtful validity (Cohen & Nagle, 1934), such is our yearning for order and certainty that we implicitly assume its truth and tend to be disconcerted when we encounter phenomena that are not in conformity with it. As a consequence, there is a tendency to devalue or distrust phenomena that fail to pass the test of uniformity. If separate studies of five different SHGs were to find that members of three of these appeared to benefit from their membership, while members of the remaining two did not, we are likely to doubt the effectiveness of all five SHGs rather than just of the two that failed; the evidence for the effectiveness of the SHGs acquires the stigma of inconsistency. For this reason, it is important to confront the lack of uniformity or consistency found in SHG outcome data, consider its sources, and determine how it can be reduced, where appropriate.

One obvious source of nonuniformity of findings across studies may be their use of differing methodologies or research designs. This is illustrated in the case of the differing conclusions drawn by Stunkard at two points in time about the effectiveness of TOPS (Take Off Pounds Sensibly) as a weight-control intervention. Based upon a cross-sectional analysis of the weight-loss records of 22 TOPS chapters, he first reported that the average TOPS member loses about 15 pounds, and described TOPS as "a uniquely successful self-help approach to obesity" (Stunkard, 1972, p. 143). Following a two-year longitudinal study of TOPS, however, in which he followed individual members and also kept track of drop-outs, his conclusion was quite different: "Although a small percentage of persons joining TOPS are able to lose substantial amounts of weight and to maintain weight loss, for the vast majority of members, TOPS is a relatively ineffective method of weight control" (Levitz & Stunkard, 1974, p. 426).

There is no way of estimating the extent to which differing (and in some cases faulty) methodologies have contributed to the nonuniformity of SHG outcome data, but it is likely to be considerable. While the solution may not necessarily lie in standardizing research designs in outcome studies, the area would benefit if investigators and journal editors could arrive at a consensus as to the minimum requirements for an adequate design and methodology in this area. This has occurred to a good extent in connection with psychotherapy research, and it should be possible here as well.

A second source of nonuniformity in outcome findings is the lack of precision in the definition and use of the "self-help group" label by professionals (Gartner & Reissman, 1977; Katz & Bender, 1976; Powell, 1987), as well as the general population. This leads to considerable heterogeneity in the nature of the groups included under the SHG rubric. The consequences are strikingly illustrated in the contrast between Stunkard's (Levitz & Stunkard, 1974) pessimistic appraisal of TOPS' effectiveness as a SHG weight-control agent, cited above, and Lieberman's (1986) optimistic report of the findings of "a large scale prospective study of over 10,000 members of Norwegian self-help groups" (p. 97) in which the average weight loss for those completing an eight-week course in these groups was 15.2 pounds, and that after four years between 30% and 35% had maintained or increased their weight loss, while only 15% had regained all they had lost or increased their weight (Grimsmo, Helgesen, & Borchgrevink, 1981).

The findings for the Norwegian groups are clearly at variance with those for TOPS. However, it appears that, in addition to this study's design and methodology differing markedly from Stunkard's, the groups involved were also quite different from TOPS, and from SHGs in general. At best, they might be described as following a self-help format. The first clue to this effect is in the Grimsmo et al.'s neutral reference to the groups only as "lay groups," and their further statement that they were built upon self-help principles. Although the Norwegian "slim clubs," as they were called, were led by hostesses who had themselves been club members, club membership involved participation in an eight-week course, for which there was a required fee and in which members were given a low-calorie diet, encouraged to do physical exercise, and avoid alcohol—all departures, in varying degrees, from practices found in conventionally defined self-help groups (e.g., Katz & Bender, 1976; Levy, 1976; Powell, 1987).

How many, or which, of these differences might have contributed to the differences in outcomes found by Levitz and Stunkard (1974) and by Grimsmo et al. (1981) is, of course, an open question. There may also have been other factors—cultural, genetic, historic, and sampling—that contributed to the differences in outcomes. But the point remains that until there is greater precision in the use of the designation "self-help group" by researchers and authors doing SHG outcome studies and authors of articles describing results of these studies, readers of secondary sources may be pardoned if they conclude that the evidence for the effectiveness of SHGs is intrinsically unreliable. This could be detrimental to the pursuit of further research on this question, as well as to the welfare of SHGs and their prospective members.

This source of apparent unreliability in outcome findings, unlike others, is one that could be significantly reduced if researchers and writers on SHGs could agree to adopt labeling conventions that would reduce the heterogeneity in the structure and operation of the groups now found under the SHG rubric. Clearly distinguishing between "classical" SHGs, hybrid SHGs (Powell, 1987), SHG format groups (such as Grimsmo et al.'s "slim clubs"), and support groups of various kinds, in both the research and secondary literature, would benefit the general public's understanding of the differences between these kinds of groups and what they have to offer, as well as SHGs' future place in the health care and human services arenas.

A final source of apparent nonuniformity in outcome findings is the almost exclusive focus on main effects in SHG effectiveness research and the failure to recognize that orderliness or uniformity in the effects of so complex a process as SHG interventions is unlikely to be found at so gross a level of analysis. If orderliness is to be found across different outcome studies, it is much more likely to be found at the level of interactions between the characteristics of the groups, their focal problem, and their members. Moreover, besides explaining the presence or absence of main effects, significant interactions can contribute to our understanding of SHGs and provide the basis for the enhancement of their effectiveness.

It would be unfortunate if this focus on perspectival discrepancies and nonuniformity of outcome data were to lead to the impression that there is little or no credible evidence of SHG effectiveness. This is not true. Although subject to a variety of methodological caveats, the balance of outcome studies that involve any kind of comparison group is in the positive direction. Lacking, however, is the particularized knowledge as to which SHGs are effective interventions, for whom, and for what conditions. But it is, in principle, an obtainable and worthy pursuit. In the meantime, scientists, clinicians, policymakers, and the public are faced with having to make decisions about SHGs under conditions of uncertainty. Thus, the question is: what stance should be taken toward this uncertainty? For scientists, the answer is easy: uncertainty equals challenge and opportunity. For policymakers, the answer is different and more complex. Thus, we will consider this question further when we discuss the policy implications of SHG research findings in the final section of this chapter.

Self-Help Group Mechanisms and Processes

There is a fairly substantial body of writings on how self-help groups function, much of it antedating systematic research on their effectiveness and largely speculative and anecdotal (Dean, 1971; Gartner & Riessman, 1977; Hansell, 1974, 1976; Katz, 1970; Robinson & Henry, 1977; Trice & Roman, 1970; Wechsler, 1960). Systematic empirical research on this question is of more recent vintage and considerably less extensive (Levy, 1979; Wollert, Levy, & Knight, 1982; Lieberman, 1979, 1983; Rappaport & Seidman, 1987), but growing in quantity and diversity (Powell, 1994). Even in the absence of clear evidence of the effectiveness of SHGs, such research can be of value. It can further our knowledge of the nature of SHGs, and it can identify the processes and mechanisms that might be responsible for whatever effectiveness they are found to possess. Moreover, in bootstrapping fashion, to the extent that certain of these mechanisms and processes are found to be associated with the effectiveness of particular groups, this knowledge can lead to the further improvement of SHGs' effectiveness.

The approach taken by Levy and his colleagues (Levy, 1979; Wollert, Levy, & Knight, 1982) drew upon a review of the extant literature on SHGs and close observations of meetings of a diverse array of 16 SHGs. Based upon these observations, Levy and his research team inferred the operation of 11 processes that functioned as mechanisms of support and change in the groups. Four of these were behavioral in their focus, and seven were cognitive. It was expected that the importance of each of these processes would vary as a function of the nature of each group's focal problem and the approach taken in dealing with it.

In addition to these processes, Levy and his colleagues (1979) also identified 28 help-giving activities that they had observed occurring in these groups. These were to be used in describing the operation of SHGs and in process-analytic studies concerned with questions of effectiveness and group differences. Some of these activities are also found in individual psychotherapy or behavior therapy; others have been found more commonly in various other kinds of groups.

In a subsequent study (Wollert, Levy, & Knight, 1982), nontechnical, behavioral descriptions of these activities were incorporated in questionnaires that were distributed to group members who were asked to rate their frequency of occurrence in their group meetings. The groups represented were chapters of Alcoholics Anonymous, Overeaters Anonymous, Parents Anonymous, and Take Off Pounds Sensibly, all representing what Levy and his colleagues termed *behavior control groups*, and Emotions Anonymous, Make Today Count, and Parents Without Partners, which represented *stress coping groups*. Correlations between mean group ratings of the frequency of occurrence of each of the 28 activities for all possible pairs of groups ranged between .38 ($p > .05$, between PA and one of the two TOPS chapters) and .88 ($p < .01$, between EA and PWP), with all but three correlations above .53 ($p < .01$), indicating considerable similarity among these groups, regardless of type, in the relative frequency with which they engaged in the various help-giving activities.

Additionally, differences were found between behavior control and stress coping groups.

Mann–Whitney *U* tests between the mean group-rated frequencies of the various help-giving activities by members of the two types of groups revealed that members of behavior control groups reported significantly more frequent use of personal goal setting and positive reinforcement than members of stress coping groups. Behavior control groups also had higher mean ratings for 9 of the 10 other behaviorally focused activities, while mean ratings for the remaining 16 activities were not consistently higher for either of the two types of groups. Although these findings certainly require further investigation, particularly through the use of directly observed frequencies of group activities, they do make intuitive sense since they suggest that behavior control groups actually do rely more heavily on behavioral techniques than do stress coping groups.

Members of both types of groups reported the frequent use of supportive (empathy, instillation of hope, mutual affirmation, justification, normalization), expressive (catharsis, sharing, self-disclosure), and insight-oriented (explanations, functional analysis, discrimination training) activities. They were also consistent in reporting infrequent use of confrontive interpersonal behaviors (confrontation, seeking feedback, offering feedback) and certain types of behaviorally oriented activities (modeling, extinction, punishment, behavioral rehearsal). These findings suggest that both types of groups take a relatively broad-spectrum approach to helping their members, not only in dealing with their members' identified personal problems, but also in attempting to meet their needs for empathic understanding, a sense of meaning, and an opportunity to express their feelings and share their experiences with one another.

Lieberman (1979, 1983) has also been interested in change mechanisms in SHGs and their perceived helpfulness. Using a survey approach, and utilizing large samples of several thousand, involving several different SHGs, he focused on change mechanisms that were derived from the psychotherapy and group process literature (Lieberman, Yalom, & Miles, 1973; Yalom, 1975), supplemented by additional mechanisms particularly identified with SHGs. A number of these mechanisms, such as normalization and feedback, are either similar or identical to those studied by Levy and his colleagues. His findings cannot be compared with Levy's, however, because his respondents were asked to rate each item or experience for its helpfulness to them, rather than its frequency of occurrence. But Lieberman's data can provide some insight into which experiences or mechanisms SHG members judge to be most helpful and least helpful. It is uncertain, however, how these judgments relate either to the prevalence of the mechanisms or to their actual effectiveness as agents of change.

In several studies involving a number of different SHGs, Lieberman (1979, 1983) has found both similarities and differences between groups in the mechanisms their members find most helpful. Two mechanisms, however, were found to rank high among almost all groups: normalization (or universalization) and support. Beyond these, Lieberman found considerable variation among the groups in the mechanisms that they judged to be helpful; this was true even when he narrowed his focus to SHGs that dealt with bereavement following loss of a spouse or a child. This led Lieberman (1983) to conclude that "we are unable to provide reasonable generalizations regarding the linkage between change mechanisms and a specific type of change" (p. 250).

While this conclusion well summed-up Lieberman's findings, its generalization beyond them must be subject to the caveat that it rests on participants' self-reports (Nisbitt & Wilson, 1977). Unfortunately, this is true of much of SHG research (including my own). At the same time, however, self-reports are also behaviors and should not, and can not, be cavalierly dismissed.

In a project that is likely to remain unmatched for its comprehensiveness and complexity, Rappaport and Seidman and their associates (Rappaport et al., 1985) have managed to go well beyond self-report data. Through a unique circumstance, they were able to conduct an intensive longitudinal study of a single self-help organization over an extended period of time. The group is GROW, a SHG intended for persons with a history of severe psychopathology. It began in Australia and expanded to the United States in 1978 at the invitation of O. H. Mowrer. In 1981, with about a dozen groups established in central Illinois, the founder of GROW, Father Keogh, approached Rappaport and Seidman offering them an opportunity to evaluate GROW's effectiveness. After due deliberation about such a study's feasibility and about their ability to maintain the study's scientific integrity, they developed a comprehensive plan of study of GROW as both a social organization and a clinical intervention. Supported by the National Institute of Mental Health, the study has yielded such a prodigious amount of quantitative and qualitative data that it can be only briefly described here.

The project makes use of a continuous, comment-by-comment coding system, in which all comments during a group meeting are assigned to one of the following mutually exclusive categories: *support*, *interpretations*, *direct guidance*, *requests for feedback*, *personal questions*, *impersonal questions*, *self-disclosures*, *information-giving*, *group process*, *agreement*, *negative*, and *small talk*. Observers using the system were trained to a high degree of reliability, equal to or exceeding a kappa of .70, and were tested periodically to assure that they maintained this level. Observations were made over a 28-month period of 529 different meetings of the 15 Grow groups, which encompassed 822 different members.

For an average GROW meeting, it was found that support, interpretations, and direct guidance, combined, accounted for 24% of all comments, and that personal questions and its counterpart self-disclosures together accounted for another 9%. Thus, a substantial portion of GROW meetings appears to be devoted to providing help within a personalized informational context. Also found was a relatively high frequency of support (7%), defined as comments that are encouraging, approving, or offer tangible assistance, which, together with the similarly high frequency of agreement comments (8%) and low frequency of comments coded as negative (2%), conveys a positive, supportive image of GROW, similar to that which emerged from both Lieberman's and Levy's findings.

In an example of process research, Toro (1987) examined changes in group behavior over time in a subsample of 83 newcomers who had attended five or more meetings. Repeated measures ANOVAs for each of the 12 comment categories and for total comments revealed significant increases in their comments in the categories of support, interpretations, group process, and negative, and in their total comments. These changes seem to reflect the newcomers' increasing comfort in their new role as GROW members and their socialization into this role. Ultimately, it should be possible to determine whether these changes represent the modal pattern of entry into the GROW way of life and how this, and other patterns, relate to the different membership careers of GROW members. More generally, the behavioral recording system used in this study allows for detailed studies of sequential relationships between behaviors within meetings, differences between groups in interaction patterns, and, most importantly, the relationship of all of these with the adjustment outcomes of GROW members.

While it may seem unfortunate at first glance that the generalizability of the findings of this undertaking may be limited to a single SHG organization serving a geographically limited population, it is likely the case that it will only be through intensive studies such as this that we will ever gain the finely detailed knowledge of how SHGs work and what accounts for their effectiveness. The study also brings up the enormous investment in time, money, and talent that obtaining this knowledge will require, and raises the important policy question of whether society is ready to meet this need.

SELF-HELP GROUPS AS SOCIAL SYSTEMS

Fully understanding SHGs requires taking a broader view of them as social systems, in terms of their dynamics and their relation to other systems—an ecological view, as recently proposed by Maton (1994). In a particularly interesting study of how *systemic organizational supports* are related to the prevalence and survival of SHGs, Leventhal, Maton, and Madara (1988) identified three major types of systemic organizational support structures: national self-help organizations (NSHOs), such as Alcoholics Anonymous and Recovery, Inc., which provide support to their local chapters through their well-developed ideologies and methods for dealing with their members' problems, and their knowledge and experience in the organization and conduct of groups; self-help clearinghouses (SHCs) which provide support to a broad diversity of groups through referral of new members to the groups and by providing technical assistance in the formation of groups as well in their operation; and local health/social service agencies, which may sponsor or provide assistance to specific types of groups.

Drawing upon the statewide files of the New Jersey Self-Help Clearinghouse (NJSHC) for 1983 and 1984, Leventhal et al. (1988) tested two hypotheses concerning NSHOs and SHGs' prevalence and survival. The first, the affiliation-superiority hypothesis, predicted that SHGs affiliated with an NSHO will enjoy an advantage over nonaffiliated groups, such that they will have greater net growth rates and be more numerous than unaffiliated groups. This hypothesis was only partially supported. In support of the hypothesis, the proportion of affiliated groups for 1983 and 1984 was 89.8% and 87.1%, respectively, in both cases significantly greater than what would be expected were affiliated and unaffiliated groups equal in number. (This significant inequality held even when AA, Al-Anon, and Alateen were excluded from the analysis, although the percentage of total groups is much less.)

Contrary to the hypothesis, however, affiliated groups showed only a 1.3% growth rate over the year, which was significantly lower than the 25.9% growth rate of unaffiliated groups. When both the birth and death rates of the groups were analyzed, however, it was found that this difference in net growth was due to the significantly higher birth rate for unaffiliated groups (40.0% vs. 14.3% for affiliated groups), and the similar mortality rates for affiliated and unaffiliated groups: 13.0% and 14.1%, respectively. Thus, were these rates to continue indefinitely, the time would come when the affiliation-superiority hypothesis would be completely falsified.

Parenthetically, the overall birth rate during the 1983–1984 period for all SHGs in the NJSHC files was 16.2%, while their death rate was 8.1%, yielding a net growth rate of 8.1%. A subsequent study (Maton, Leventhal, Madara, & Julien, 1989) using these same files for the period from 1984–1986 revealed an annual growth rate of 9.0%. Should these growth rates be anywhere near representative of the national growth rate for SHGs, this would further emphasize the importance of SHGs as objects of study.

The second hypothesis tested by Leventhal et al. (1988) was that there would be differential rates of change in rates of birth, mortality, and net growth between SHGs affiliated with different NSHOs. This was based on their assumption that there would be differences in how effectively the different NSHOs worked with their respective affiliates, as well as in the affiliated groups' membership and focal problems. When the NSHOs were effective, it was reasoned, their affiliated groups should have higher birth rates and lower death rates. To test this hypothesis, they compared these rates for the 11 NSHOs that had the largest number of in-state affiliated groups.

Clear support for this hypothesis was found in the highly significant difference between the 10.8% growth rate for AA groups as compared with the .8% growth rate for all other affiliated groups combined. This difference was due to the AA groups' very low 2.1% mortality rate as compared with the combined affiliated groups' 13.5% mortality rate, and the essential absence of a difference in their birth rates.

Also of interest were different discernable patterns of growth and decline among the different affiliated groups. Leventhal et al. believe that these patterns are the product of a complex interaction between the current state of the community, with its values, problems, and resources, contemporary society at large, the needs addressed by these various groups, their effectiveness in meeting these needs, and their effectiveness as self-maintaining systems within their current environment.

Building upon this study, but using the NJSHC files from 1984–1986, Maton et al. (1989) analyzed the effects on SHGs' birth and death rates of national affiliation, professional involvement, and member focal problem (life stress, medical condition, and behavior control) in a sample of 3,152 different groups. Using log linear logit analyses, they found that professional involvement among unaffiliated groups was associated with lower group mortality, but that it was associated with higher mortality among affiliated groups. They also found that unaffiliated behavior control groups had higher odds for both mortality and birth than either unaffiliated life stress or medical groups. Thus, it appears that the possible benefits of professional involvement in SHGs and of affiliation with a NSHO may be contingent upon both group and member characteristics. In addition to the scientific implications of these findings, Maton et al. also discuss a number of their practical implications for professionals working with SHGs.

There have been various attempts over the years to investigate the structural and organizational characteristics of SHGs, but these have been largely descriptive (e.g., Katz & Bender, 1976; Traunstein & Steinman, 1973; Todres, 1980). As early as 1957, Katz had proposed a stage sequence in the development SHGs, identified as origin, informal organization, emergence of leadership, formal organization, and professionalization. Were certain consequences for a group's viability or functioning to follow from its location at one or another of these stages, or from the rate at which it reached each stage, such a schema would be of considerable value. Although there has been speculation along these lines, to date there has been no empirical evidence that this is the case, or that all groups necessarily follow this sequence (Katz, 1981).

A recent empirical study by Maton (1988) focused upon three internal structural characteristics of SHGs that might be expected to affect their functioning. Using a specially constructed questionnaire, Maton investigated the relationship between perceived *group order and organization, role differentiation*, and *leadership* in SHGs and their members' well-being, represented by measures of *depression* and *self-esteem*, respectively. He also obtained members' appraisals of the extent to which they felt that they had benefitted from their membership in their group, measured by a *group benefits* scale, and of their satisfaction with the way their group operated, measured by a *group satisfaction* scale.

The study involved 144 members of 15 SHGs, five each from three SHG organizations—Compassionate Friends, Multiple Sclerosis, and Overeaters Anonymous—chosen deliberately to represent three distinctly different group types. Maton found that the three organizations differed significantly on each of the organizational characteristics. Although members of the three types of groups did not differ significantly on either depression or self-esteem, they did differ significantly on both group benefits and group satisfaction. Hierarchical multiple regression analyses, controlling for group type, revealed that role differentiation was negatively related to depression and positively related to self-esteem; order and organization was positively related to group benefits; and leadership was positively related to group satisfaction. There were no significant group type by organizational characteristic interactions, indicating that the patterns of relationship were consistent across the three types of SHGs.

Although they are correlational and based upon self-reports, these findings break new ground in SHG research in demonstrating the potential importance of organizational variables as determinants of both member well-being and appraisal of their groups. Longitudinal studies and the use of other measurement approaches should now follow. But the findings, as they stand, are consistent with the self-help philosophy of the value of members sharing of responsibilities (role differentiation), and they suggest areas of attention—organizational development and leadership training—that may be important for both SHGs and the professionals working with them in enhancing their viability and effectiveness.

The development of self-help clearinghouses that serve as information and referral agencies for individuals in search of SHGs is an interesting phenomenon in its own right. Beginning as small shoe-string operations, some of them, such as the New Jersey Self-Help Clearinghouse, have become sophisticated, state-aided operations. In addition to maintaining computerized databases on SHGs in their areas, they often provide consultation to SHGs and agencies wishing to establish SHGs and sponsor workshops, conferences, and SHG fairs. There are now well over 40 clearinghouses in North America (Powell, 1987), and they continue to grow in number and have now formed their own network (Miller and Wollert, 1986). Evidence of their potential as systemic organizational supports (Leventhal et al., 1988) for SHGs may be found in Madara's (1986) report that during a period of three and a half years the consultation provided by the New Jersey Self-Help Clearinghouse led to the development of 207 new SHGs in the state, many of types not previously available.

Organizationally, self-help clearinghouses and SHGs are almost symbiotically linked, since clearinghouses could not exist without SHGs, and SHGs have much to gain from the existence of clearinghouses. Yet, neither clearinghouses nor their linkage with SHGs have yet to garner very much research attention (Meissen & Warren, 1994; Wollert & The Self-Help Research Team, 1987). Since clearinghouses are likely to be organizationally stable structures, frequently associated with community social agencies, they could serve as bridges between SHGs and both the community and its health care system. For the same reason, they could also serve as vehicles for the allocation of funds to SHGs, where these are needed. Before these possibilities can be realized, however, much more will have to be known about clearinghouses, regarding both their organization and function.

SELF-HELP GROUPS AND PUBLIC POLICY

Although many might agree that SHGs would benefit from a public policy that fosters research aimed at enhancing their effectiveness and their optimal utilization within the health care delivery system, and some might also agree that such a policy should also include direct aid to SHGs, there is also good reason to be concerned about possible unintended consequences of such a policy: Would it lead to government intrusiveness in SHGs' operations? Would it alter some intrinsic quality of SHGs that might reduce their effectiveness? Would it result in a reduction in the quality of health care as individuals are shunted to SHGs in the interests of cost containment when they actually require professional care? These questions require more extended consideration than they can be given in the brief space available here, but I raise them in order to indicate some of the issues that public policy advocates must confront.

More fundamentally, however, I believe that there are also two problems that SHG advocates should be aware of as they contemplate entering the public policy arena. The first is that they enter it from a position of weakness rather than strength with respect to empirical evidence of SHGs' effectiveness. The form and severity of this problem are most likely to vary with whether advocacy is at the national, state, or local level, but it will be present and must be dealt with. I suggest one way in the next section, which proposes reconstruing SHGs more broadly, as social institutions.

The second problem, related to the first, is how, given the current state of knowledge and research concerning SHGs' effectiveness, we as scientists can responsibly advocate public support for SHGs as a health care resource. I believe there may be three grounds upon which this can be done. The first is a that they are already being used as such by growing numbers of people and may soon rival psychotherapy in the number of persons turning to them for help (Jacobs & Goodman, 1989), with the possibility that SHGs they may eventually replace psychotherapy as the major modality for mental health care delivery (Prochaska & Norcross, 1982; Tyler, 1980). Whether that possibility is realized or not, prevalence of SHG usage argues strongly for funding for research that will increase our understanding of them and enhance their effectiveness.

The second ground, related to the first, is that just as increasing numbers of people are turning to SHGs on their own, the private and nonprofit sectors of the health care system—HMOs and managed behavioral health care companies—are also including them in their continuum of care. To assure the quality of care provided by them, governmental regulation requires more and better knowledge about SHGs, their effectiveness, and how they can be utilized.

Finally, I believe that a cogent case can be made that, for many causes of human suffering, such as chronic mental illness, drug abuse, and membership in socially victimized groups, SHGs may be uniquely qualified to complement the services rendered by professionals (Salem, Seidman, & Rappaport, 1988).

With respect to public, as well as private and nonprofit-sector, policy advocacy, the ultimate question that must be addressed is SHGs' effectiveness—it is their bottom line. This is the obvious and necessary policy question with respect to their utilization, while at the same time it is the SHG research community's task to show how their research is the obvious and necessary path to its answer.

Self-Help Groups as Social Institutions

Without sacrificing our integrity as scientists, I believe that on the basis of what is already know about SHGs, an argument can be made for public support for SHGs. This rests upon the view that public support for SHGs should not rest only on their effectiveness as clinical interventions, as they are more than clinical interventions. Instead, SHGs may be seen more broadly as only the most recent manifestation of an evolving social institution (Jacobs & Goodman, 1989) built around a shared ideology of the value of cooperation, shared experience, personal responsibility, and mutual help in the achievement of a common end. As such, this institution dates back to the beginning of civilization (Katz and Bender, 1976; Kropotkin, 1972) and certainly played a major role in the history of the development of our country. Thus, SHGs are institutions that are consistent with some of our society's most fundamental values, both in their aims and in their means of achieving these aims. This may be why they have proven so popular.

If this view of SHGs is accepted, then just as public support is provided for other social institutions, such as the family, universal education, and our economic system, despite the absence of conclusive evidence of their efficacy and, in fact, sometimes in spite of documented instances of their failures, support should also be provided for SHGs. The question thus becomes not whether to advocate support for SHGs, but the purposes for which to recommend support and the forms that this might take.

Forms and Purposes of Support for Self-Help Groups

Support for individual SHGs and for SHG organizations might include direct financial and technical support, and indirect support in the form of public endorsements of their value and utility, public service announcements, and educational programs aimed at giving the public a better understanding of what SHGs do and how to shop for one. Many individual, local SHGs receive support within their communities in the form of meeting rooms, referrals, consultations, and occasional financial contributions. However, there are no formally established structures through which federal and state financial support could be directly provided to these groups. And it would probably be difficult to develop such structures because of the loosely organized nature of the groups. Such support could be provided, however, through regional self-help group clearinghouses (Wollert et al. 1987) since they have (or could develop) the organizational stability and professional core necessary to assure accountability in the use and distribution of this support.

The amount of money SHGs usually need is not very large and is usually for mundane purposes such as telephones and postage, but it could be crucial in some instances. For example, a local chapter of the Chronic Pain Association, Inc. that had experienced remarkable growth was forced to abandon a publicity plan that could have led to further growth because it lacked the funds for the postage necessary to reply to all the inquiries anticipated (C. Lidz, personal communication, 1987). It is also likely that if SHGs knew funds were available for their use, they might come up with less mundane uses for it, such as sending members to leadership workshops and developing educational forums.

Providing federal or state funding and other forms of support to SHGs through regional clearinghouses, rather than directly to either individual chapters or their national organizations, would help reduce threats to their autonomy that might result were they to receive it directly from the public coffers. It would also put these clearinghouses in a good position to serve as brokers (noncoercively, of course) between researchers and individual SHGs. Better yet, where these clearinghouses are affiliated with universities or other research organizations, they could themselves become self-help group research and development centers (Meissen & Warren, 1994).

A PROPOSED RESEARCH AGENDA

Within recent years there has been a rapid growth of alternative approaches to the conceptualization and study of SHGs (Powell, 1994), many which promise to enrich our understanding of their operation by bringing different levels of analysis to bear and by broadening the horizon of meaning in addressing questions about outcomes and effectiveness (Humphreys & Noke, 1997; Kennedy, Humphreys, & Borkman, 1994; Luke, Roberts, & Rappaport, 1994; Rappaport, 1994; Schubert & Borkman, 1994). Viewed from a public policy standpoint, I believe that the focus of these and future studies should be on two broad objectives: the assessment and enhancement of SHGs' effectiveness, and how SHGs can be most effectively integrated within a comprehensive approach to health care delivery, which will increasingly come under the constraints of managed care.

To achieve the first objective, programmatic research is needed to identify the processes that operate within SHGs and how they relate to outcomes. Achieving the second will require identifying the functions that SHGs are most uniquely qualified to perform, most cost-effectively, in relation to the other components of the health care system in dealing with particular health and mental health problems. This question has yet to be addressed by SHG researchers. It is a systems-level question that will require a multidisciplinary approach, including the policy sciences and the behavioral and social sciences.

Our current knowledge of the processes that operate in SHGs and how these and other factors relate to outcomes is best described as embryonic. Useful leads are provided by the early work of Lieberman and Levy, and by more recent research using ecological narrative and other new paradigms (Humphreys & Noke, 1997; Kennedy, Humphreys, & Borkman, 1994; Luke, Roberts, & Rappaport, 1994; Maton, 1994; Rappaport, 1994; Schubert & Borkman, 1994). Following these leads and enlarging upon them, research must ultimately make it possible to specify how particular actions within a SHG interact with each other in relation to particular outcomes, both proximal, in terms of members' responses and subsequent group functioning, and distal, in terms of member's levels of psychosocial functioning and physical health. Only knowledge of this degree of specificity (or approximating it) can serve as a basis for the assessment and enhancement of SHGs' effectiveness.

Research on the integration of SHGs within the total health delivery system is badly needed and should be given high priority. It would serve the interests of SHGs by legitimizing their role within the system, and it would serve the interests of both the system and the community by increasing the resources and efficiency of the system in meeting the community's health care needs. Such research need not pose a threat to SHGs of being co-opted or of putting their autonomy in jeopardy, since it would recognize their autonomy as one of their intrinsic characteristics. It is also possible, however, that out of this research a place might also be found for new kinds of "hybrid" SHGs (Jacobs & Goodman, 1989; Powell, 1985), which include professionals in supportive or ancillary roles.

In this research, as well as in research on processes and outcomes, it will be important to take into account two variables that have thus far not been very salient in research on SHGs. The first is the condition or problem dealt with by the SHG, and the second is a developmental variable, the point where members are in the course of dealing with their problem when they enter a SHG. With regard to the first dimension, it may be expected that SHGs serve different functions for persons with different problems. For the deinstitutionalized, chronically mentally ill, for example, SHGs may supplement the episodically available services of mental health professionals, in part by providing them with a niche in which they can restructure their lives (Salem, Seidman, Rappaport, 1988). Although SHGs may generally function as a niche for their members, regardless of their problem (Levine & Perkins, 1987), how it serves this function may vary depending upon the condition or problem being dealt with by its members. For substance abusers, for example, SHGs may best serve as an adjuvant to other forms of individual treatment through the reinforcement provided for maintenance of behaviors that act to control their abuse behavior. For the bereaved, they would obviously serve a very different function (Levy, Derby, & Martinkowski, 1993). Research identifying the range of these different SHG functions vis-à-vis their problem focus should thus be given high priority, since this knowledge is essential in determining the SHGs' place within the health care system's response to each patient's needs.

From a developmental perspective, it seems reasonable to expect that whether a person's problem is alcoholism, having been a victim of physical violence, or bereavement, where they are in the trajectory of their response to their problem, may make them differentially responsive to what SHGs may have to offer them. Research on this question would thus also contribute to our knowledge of the optimal mix and timing of professional and SHG intervention.

Factors affecting access to SHGs or their utilization is a cross-cutting issue that must also be addressed by SHG researchers. There is substantial evidence that SHGs are underutilized by the poor minorities (Snowden & Lieberman, 1954; Humphreys & Woods, 1994), but this may be true for other individuals with respect to particular SHGs as well. The reasons for this are likely to be many and diverse, including the image held of SHGs and of those who decline to join them (Levy & Derby, 1992), lack of knowledge about them, and cultural factors. Clearly, SHGs may not be for everyone or for every condition, but it would serve the public interest to be able to chart the parameters that determine their fit in each case.

Finally, research is needed on the role of professionals in the growth and functioning of SHGs. Professionals could and, in some cases, have contributed significantly to their establishment and to enhancing their effectiveness. Research by Maton (1989) cited earlier suggests that the benefits of professional involvement may vary as a function of the type of group. While the potential contributions that professionals might make to SHGs have long been recognized (Caplan, 1974; Powell, 1987), there has not been any systematic research concerning how they have worked with SHGs and with what effect.

In addressing the research agenda I have just proposed, as well as in dealing with the numerous methodological and epistemological problems encountered in self-help group research, I should also like to recommend that we begin to broaden our conceptions of acceptable approaches to research. Specifically, I believe that there is much to be gained by exploring the contributions to useful knowledge in this area that can be made through qualitative as well as quantitative research. An excellent case has been made recently for venturing beyond the familiar horizon of logical positivism by contributors to Powell (1994) and by Tebes and Kraemer (1991). Tebes and Kraemer clearly show how the knowledge gained in doing so in the study of self-help groups may complement and elucidate the knowledge gained through more established, quantitative means.

CONCLUSIONS

As an emerging social institution, as well as a therapeutic modality likely to become a major participant in the provision of health and mental health care in the future, SHGs should have a significant claim on the attention of community psychologists. For these reasons also, SHGs have a legitimate claim to the support, economic and otherwise, of society. Public policy concerning the provision of such support, however, has yet to be formulated. The thrust of this policy is likely to be influenced in no small degree by the findings of research on the effectiveness of SHGs and their role within the health care delivery system. While community psychologists may take the lead in this research, if it is to serve the needs of policy development as well as science, it will require the participation of the policy sciences, as well as the behavioral and social sciences. As this chapter has made clear, SHGs pose a daunting challenge to researchers who venture into this area. Yet, to those who are undaunted by the challenge, the rewards can be many. These include the experience of working with SHG members themselves, learning from their struggles, courage, and wisdom, and the experience of finding solutions to problems and answers to questions that may have a direct effect on the future shape of health care delivery and on the general welfare of society.

REFERENCES

Antze, P. (1976). The role of ideologies in peer psychotherapy organizations: Some theoretical considerations and three case studies. *Journal of Applied Behavioral Science, 12*, 323–346.

Borman, L. D. (1982). Helping people to help themselves—self-help and prevention: Introduction. *Prevention in Human Services, 1*, 3–15.

California Department of Mental Health. (1984). *A survey of California adults regarding their health practices and interest in health promotion plans.* Sacramento, CA.

Caplan, G. (1974). *Support systems and community mental health.* New York: Behavioral Publications.

Caplan, B., & Killilea, M. (Eds.). (1976). *Support systems and mutual help: Multidisciplinary explorations.* New York: Grune & Stratton.

Cohen, M. R., & Nagel, E. (1934). *An introduction to logic and the scientific method.* New York: Harcourt, Brace.

Cook, T. D., & Campbell, D. T. (1979). *Quasi-experimentation: Design and analysis issues for field settings.* Chicago: Rand McNally.

Dean, S. R. (1971). Self-help group psychotherapy: Mental patients rediscover willpower. *International Journal of Social Psychiatry, 17*, 72–78.

Gartner, A., & Riessman, F. (1977). *Self-help in the human services.* San Francisco: Jossey-Bass.

Grimsmo, A., Helgesen, G., & Borchgrevink, C. (1981). Short-term and long-term effects of lay groups on weight reduction. *British Medical Journal, 283*, 1093–1095.

Hansell, N. (1976). *The person-in-distress: On the biosocial dynamics of adaptation.* New York: Human Sciences.

Hermalin, J. (1979). Enhancing primary prevention: The marriage of self-help groups and formal health care delivery systems. *Journal of Clinical Child Psychology, 8*, 125–129.

Hinrichsen, G. A., Revenson, T. A., & Shinn, M. (1995). Does self-help help? An empirical investigation of scoliosis peer support groups. *Journal of Social Issues, 41*, 65–87.

Humphreys, K. (1996). World view change in Adult Children of Alcoholics/Al-Anon self-help groups: Reconstructing the alcoholic family. *International Journal of Groups Psychotherapy, 46*, 255–263.

Humphreys, K., & Noke, J. M. (1997). The influence of posttreatment mutual help group participation on the friendship networks of substance abuse patients. *American Journal of Community Psychology, 25*, 1–16.

Humphreys, K., & Woods, M. D. (1994). Researching mutual-help groups participation. In T. Powell (Ed.), *Understanding the self-help organization: Frameworks and findings* (pp. 62–87). Thousand Oaks, CA: Sage.

Jacobs, M. K., & Goodman, G. (1989). Psychology and self-help groups: Predictions on a partnership. *American Psychologist, 44*, 536–545.

Katz, A. H. (1970). Self-help organizations and volunteer participation in social welfare. *Social Work, 15*, 51–60.

Katz, A. H. (1981). Self-help and mutual aid: An emerging social movement? *Annual Review of Sociology, 7*, 129–155.

Katz, A. H., & Bender, E. I. (Eds.). (1976). *The strength in us: Self-help groups in the modern world.* New York: New Viewpoints.

Kennedy, M., Humphreys, K., & Borkman, T. (1994). The naturalistic paradigm as an approach to research with mutual-help groups. In T. Powell (Ed.), *Understanding the self-help organization: Frameworks and findings* (pp. 172–189). Thousand Oaks, CA: Sage.

Kiresuk, W. A., & Lund, S. H. (1978). Goal attainment scaling. In C. C. Attkisson, W. A. Hargreaves, M. J. Horowitz, & J. S. Sorenson (Eds.), *Evaluation of human service programs* (pp. 341–370). New York: Academic.

Kropotkin, P. (1972). *Mutual aid. A factor of evolution.* New York: New York University Press (originally published in 1902).

Leventhal, G. S., Maton, K. E., & Madara, E. J. (1988). Systemic organizational support for self-help groups. *American Journal of Orthopsychiatry, 31*, 75–87.

Levine, M., & Perkins, D. V. (1987). *Principles of community psychology: Perspectives and applications.* New York: Oxford University Press.

Levitz, L. L., & Stunkard, A. J. (1974). A therapeutic coalition for obesity: Behavior modification and patient self-help. *American Journal of Psychiatry, 131*, 423–427.

Levy, L. H. (1976). Self-help groups: Types and psychological processes. *Journal of Applied Behavioral Science, 12*, 310–322.

Levy, L. H. (1979). Processes and activities in groups. In M. A. Lieberman & L. D. Borman (Eds.), *Self-help groups for coping with crisis: Origins, members, processes, and impact* (pp. 234–271). San Francisco: Jossey-Bass.

Levy, L. H. (1984). Issues in research and evaluation. In A. Gartner & F. Riessman (Eds.), *The self-help revolution* (pp. 155–172). New York: Human Sciences.

Levy, L. H., & Derby, J. F. (1992). Bereavement support groups: Who joins; who does not; and why. *American Journal of Community Psychology, 20*, 649–662.

Levy, L. H., Derby, J. F., & Martinkowski, K. S. (1993). Effects of membership in bereavement support groups on adaptation to conjugal bereavement. *American Journal of Community Psychology, 21,* 361–381.

Lieberman, M. A. (1979). Help seeking and self-help groups. In M. A. Lieberman & L. D. Borman (Eds.), *Self-help groups for coping with crisis: Origins, members, processes, and impact* (pp. 116–149). San Francisco: Jossey-Bass.

Lieberman, M. A. (1983). Comparative analysis of change mechanisms in groups. In H. H. Blumberg, A. P. Hare, V. Kent, & M. Davies (Eds.), *Small groups and social interaction, Vol. 2* (pp. 239–252). London: Wiley.

Lieberman, M. (1986). Self-help groups and psychiatry. *American Psychiatric Association Annual Review, 5,* 744–760.

Lieberman, M. A., & Bond, G. G. (1979). Women's consciousness raising as an alternative to psychotherapy. In M. A. Lieberman & L. D. Borman (Eds.), *Self-help groups for coping with crisis: Origins, members, processes, and impact* (pp. 150–163). San Francisco: Jossey-Bass.

Lieberman, M. A., & Borman, L. (1979). *Self-help groups for coping with crises.* San Francisco: Jossey-Bass.

Lieberman, L. A., & Videka-Sherman, L. (1986). The impact of self-help groups on the mental health of widows and widowers. *American Journal of Orthopsychiatry, 56,* 435–449.

Lieberman, M. A., & Snowden, L. R. (1994). Problems in assessing prevalence and membership characteristics of self-help group participants. In T. J. Powell (Ed.), *Understanding the self-help organization: Frameworks and findings* (pp. 32–49). Thousand Oaks, CA: Sage.

Lieberman, M. A., Yalom, I. D., & Miles, M. B. (1973). *Encounter groups: First facts.* New York: Basic Books.

Luke, D. A., Roberts, R., & Rappaport, J. (1994). Individual, group context, and individual-group fit predictors of self-help group attendance. In T. Powell (Ed.), *Understanding the Self-Help organization: Frameworks and findings* (pp. 88–114). Thousand Oaks, CA: Sage.

Madara, E. J. (1986). A comprehensive systems approach to promoting mutual aid self-help groups: The New Jersey Self-Help Clearinghouse Model. *Journal of Voluntary Action Research, 15,* 57–63.

Maton, K. I. (1988). Social support, organizational characteristics, psychological well-being and group appraisal in three self-help populations. *American Journal of Community Psychology, 16,* 53–77.

Maton, K. I. (1994). Moving beyond the individual level of analysis in mutual-help group: research: An ecological paradigm. In T. Powell (Ed.), *Understanding the self-help organization: Frameworks and findings* (pp. 136–153). Thousand Oaks, CA: Sage.

Maton, K. I., Leventhal, G. S., Madara, E. J., & Julien, M. A. (1989). Factors affecting the birth and death of mutual help groups: The role of national affiliation, professional involvement, and member focal problem. *American Journal of Community Psychology, 17,* 643–671.

Meehl, P. E. (1978). Theoretical risks and tabular asterisks: Sir Karl, Sir Ronald, and the slow progress of soft psychology. *Journal of Consulting and Clinical Psychology, 46,* 806–834.

Meissen, G. J., & Warren, M. L. (1994). The self-help clearinghouse: A new development. In T. C Powell (Ed.), *Understanding the self-help organization: Frameworks and findings* (pp. 190–211). Thousand Oaks, CA: Sage.

Miller, S., & Wollert, R. (1986). *Report on the Dallas self-help clearinghouse conference.* Ottawa: Secretary of State.

Nisbett, R. E., & Wilson, T. C. (1977). Telling more than we can know: Verbal reports on mental processes. *Psychological Review, 84,* 231–259.

Powell, T. J. (1985). Improving the effectiveness of self-help. *Social Policy, 16,* 22–29.

Powell, T. J. (1987). *Self-help organizations and professional practice.* Silver Spring, MD: National Association of Social Workers.

Powell, T. J. (1994). *Understanding the self-help organization: Frameworks and findings.* Thousand Oaks, CA: Sage.

President's Commission on Mental Health (1978). Task Panel on Community Support Systems. *Report to the President,* Vol. 2 (Appendix). Washington, D.C.: U.S. Government Printing Office.

Prochaska, J. D., & Norcross, J. C. (1982). The future of psychotherapy: A Delphi poll. *Professional Psychology, 13,* 620–627.

Rappaport, J. (1987). Terms of empowerment/exemplars of prevention: Toward a theory of community psychology. *American Journal of Community Psychology, 15,* 117–148.

Rappaport, J. (1994). Narrative studies, personal stories, and identity transformation in the mutual-help context. In T. Powell (Ed.), *Understanding the self-help organization: Frameworks and findings.* (pp. 115–135). Thousand Oaks, CA: Sage.

Rappaport, J., & Seidman, E. (1987). Overview of the Grow research project. Paper presented at the First Biennial Conference on Community Research and Action, Columbia, SC.

Rappaport, J., Seidman, E., Toro, P. A., McFadden, L. S., Reischle, T. M., Roberts, L. J., Selam, D. A., Stein, C. H., & Zimmerman, M. A. (1985). Finishing the unfinished business: Collaborative research with a mutual help organization. *Social Policy, 15,* 12–25.

Roberts, L. J., Luke, D. A., Rappaport, J., Seidman, E., Toro, P. A., & Reischl, T. M. (1991). Charting uncharted terrain:

A behavioral observation system for mutual help groups. *American Journal of Community Psychology, 19,* 751–737.
Robinson, D., & Henry, S. (1977). *Self-help and health: Mutual aid for modern problems.* London: Robertson.
Salem, D. A., Seidman, E., & Rappaport, J. (1988). Community treatment of the mentally ill: The promise of mutual-help organizations. *Social Work, 33,* 403–408.
Schubert, M. A., & Borkman, T. (1994). Identifying the experiential knowledge developed within a self-help group. In T. Powell (Ed.), *Understanding the self-help organization: Frameworks and findings* (pp. 227–246). Thousand Oaks, CA: Sage.
Shumaker, S. A., & Brownell, A. (1984). Toward a theory of social support: Closing the conceptual gaps. *Journal of Social Issues, 40,* 11–36.
Silverman, P. R. (1972). Widowhood and primary prevention. *The Family Coordinator, 21,* 95–102.
Snowden, L. R., & Lieberman, M. A. (1994). African-American participation in self-help groups. In T. Powell (Ed.), *Understanding the self-help organization: Frameworks and findings* (pp. 50–61). Thousand Oaks, CA: Sage.
Strupp, H. H., & Hadley, S. W. (1977). A tripartite model of mental health and therapeutic outcomes. *American Psychologist, 30,* 187–197.
Stunkard, A. J. (1972). The success of TOPS, a self-help group. *Postgraduate Medicine, 18,* 143–147.
Tebes, J. K., & Kraemer, D. T. (1991). Quantitative and qualitative knowing in mutual support research: Some lessons from the recent history of scientific psychology. *American Journal of Community Psychology, 19,* 739–756.
Todres, R. (1980). *Self-help groups: Analysis of organizational characteristics.* Presented at Annual Meeting of American Orthopsychiatric Association, Toronto, Canada.
Toro, P. A. (1987). Behavioral changes among members of a mutual aid organization. Paper presented at the First Biennial Conference on Community Research and Action, Columbia, SC.
Traunstein, D., & Steinman, R. (1973). Voluntary self-help organizations: An exploratory study. *Journal of Voluntary Action Research, 2,* 230–239.
Trice, H. M., & Roman, P. M. (1970). Delabeling, relabeling, and Alcoholics Anonymous. *Social Problems, 17,* 538–546.
Tyler, L. E. (1980). The next twenty years. *Counseling Psychologist, 8,* 19–21.
Videka, L. M. (1979). Psychosocial adaptation in a medical self-help group. In M. A. Lieberman & L. D. Borman (Eds.), *Self-help groups for coping with crisis: Origins, members, processes, and impact* (pp. 362–386). San Francisco: Jossey-Bass.
Videka-Sherman, L., & Lieberman, M. A. (1985). The effects of self-help and psychotherapeutic intervention on child loss: The limits of recovery. *American Journal of Orthopsychiatry, 55,* 70–81.
Wechsler, H. (1960). The self-help organization in the mental health field: Recovery, Inc., a case study. *Journal of Nervous and Mental Disease, 130,* 297–314.
Wollert, R. W., Levy, L. H., & Knight, B. G. (1982). Help-giving in behavior control and stress coping self-help groups. *Small Group Behavior, 13,* 204–218.
Wollert, R., and the Self-Help Research Team (1987). The self-help clearinghouse concept: An evaluation of one program and its implications for policy and practice. *American Journal of Community Psychology, 15,* 491–508.
Yalom, I. D. (1975). *The theory and practice of group psychotherapy,* 2nd ed. New York: Basic Books.
Yeaton, W. H. (1994). The development and assessment of valid measures of service delivery to enhance inference in outcome-based research: Measuring attendance at self-help group meetings. *Journal of Consulting and Clinical Psychology, 62,* 686–694.

CHAPTER 26

Contributions from Organizational Psychology

MARYBETH SHINN AND DENNIS N. T. PERKINS

This chapter is concerned with what community psychologists can learn from organizational psychology about changing organizations to promote individual empowerment and well-being. As such, it focuses largely, but not exclusively, on that part of organizational psychology known as organizational development. We begin by discussing convergences and divergences between organizational and community psychology. We then selectively survey interventions undertaken by organizational psychologists at the individual, group, intergroup, and organizational levels, as well as at the boundaries between individuals and organizations, and speculate about which types of interventions are most useful to community psychology. Next, we examine limitations on the transfer of knowledge from organizational psychology to the types of organizations with which community psychologists typically deal. Finally, we discuss how value differences between organizational and community psychology may promote, rather than hinder, learning.

CONVERGENCES AND DIVERGENCES

Community psychology might think of organizational psychology as an older sibling, from whom there is much to learn. The family resemblance is strong. Both organizational and community psychology claim the action research of Kurt Lewin as a parent, are concerned with processes of intervention and planned change, experience the tension between research and practice, have an ecological or systems orientation, and advocate extra-individual levels of analysis. Yet both complain that theory and research at the organiational level are underdeveloped (Keys & Frank, 1987; Pfeffer, 1985). Works on organizational psychology and organizational change are frequently structured around individual, group, and organizational

MARYBETH SHINN • New York University, Center for Community Research and Action, Department of Psychology, New York University, New York, New York 10003. DENNIS N. T. PERKINS • The Syncretics Group, Branford, Connecticut 06505.

Handbook of Community Psychology, edited by Julian Rappaport and Edward Seidman. Kluwer Academic / Plenum Publishers, New York, 2000.

levels of analysis (e.g., Huse & Cummings, 1985; Katz & Kahn, 1978; Pfeffer, 1985; Porras & Robertson, 1992; Schneider, 1985).

Organizational psychology is more advanced than community psychology in analyzing relations across levels of analysis (e.g., Mowday & Sutton, 1993; Roberts, Hulin, & Rousseau, 1978; Rousseau, 1985), although organizational theorists bemoan the paucity of empirical research (e.g., Wilpert, 1995). An intuitive example concerns the correspondence or "goodness of fit" between individual jobs, the design of a work group, an organization's structure and strategy, and its external environment. Lack of correspondence between structures at different levels, like poor fit between individuals and environments, can have adverse consequences for organizations and for the people in them.

To illustrate, Huse and Cummings (1985, p. 55) describe an attempt to enrich jobs in a plant producing surgical sutures by adding variety, autonomy, and opportunities for the employees to participate in decision-making about how to go about the work. The attempt failed because the structure of the organization, the work, and the external environment left little to decide: the market for sutures was stable, production runs were long and closely scheduled, the technology for producing the sutures was highly certain, and the jobs required only minimal interaction. Efforts to make jobs less routine, in this case, simply disrupted performance; hiring employees who expected to participate in decision-making led to dissatisfaction, absenteeism, and turnover. Although theories of organization–environmental relations (e.g., Davis & Powell, 1992) are beyond the scope of this chapter, we discuss fit between organizational characteristics and organizational interventions in the following.

If organizational and community psychology are siblings, however, they are not identical twins. One obvious difference is in the settings where they choose to work, while another, perhaps more central, distinction involves values. The bottom line for organizational psychologists is typically the productivity, efficiency, and profitability of the organization; for community psychologists it is more often empowerment of the disenfranchised and the well-being of individuals in their social contexts. However, the two types of goals are often compatible or even synergistic, a point to which we will return. Organizational development frequently involves increasing the autonomy of those at the bottom of the organizational hierarchy or creating opportunities for them to exert influence. There is some evidence that people-oriented management policies and corporate profits are correlated (Pfeffer, 1998a; Schuster, 1986).

Organizational productivity and individual well-being cannot always be made to converge, however, despite the efforts of humanistic practitioners of organizational development (Alderfer, 1977b; Friedlander & Brown, 1974; Walton & Warwick, 1973). Organizational psychologists, who are typically invited in by management, are most likely to work at higher organizational levels. If they do work at other levels, it may still be in the service of those at the top, or in one cynical view, "making some people happier at the job of making others richer" (Ross, 1971, p. 583). Community psychologists, whether invited by management or unions, or when suggesting interventions on their own initiative or at the behest of advocacy groups, should have special concern for more disadvantaged or exploited workers. They might bring the powerful technology of organizational psychology to social movement organizations, human service agencies, and other groups concerned with social welfare.

Despite these different emphases, several areas of organizational theory and practice seem especially relevant to community psychology. One, the special provenance of many theorists and practitioners of organizational development, is the promotion of employees' well-being in all work organizations. The workplace plays a parallel role in the lives of many adults to the role school plays for children. Just as schools have served as a locus for prevention activities with children, so the workplace may serve for adults.

Organizational efforts to promote both individual and organizational health by increasing worker autonomy, involving workers in decisions that affect them, and giving workers both psychological and fiscal ownership of their organizations are easily cast in community psychology's language of empowerment (Klein, this volume). Organizational psychology may provide the most systematic body of research extant on efforts to empower people and on planned change. Community psychology's concerns that prevention efforts not subvert individual rights in the name of meeting needs (Rappaport, 1981), and that empowerment efforts involve the substance as well as the trappings of empowerment (Serrano-Garcia, 1983/84), are echoed, or more accurately, foreshadowed, by concerns of many organizational theorists that their techniques not subvert individual freedom or the equalization of power in society (Alderfer, 1977b; Friedlander & Brown, 1974; Ross, 1971; Walton & Warwick, 1973).

A second point of convergence is at the boundaries of organizational life, or in the realm Murrell (1973) called intersystem accommodation. Transitions into or out of organizations, as in hiring, retirement, or layoffs, are likely to be stressful for individuals, as are daily efforts to combine multiple roles, for example, as worker and parent. Katz and Kahn (1978, p. 46) called on Allport's (1933) concept of partial inclusion to understand that organizational roles represent only a "psychological slice" of their incumbents, although organizations sometimes demand more. Both organizational and community psychologists have interests in helping organizations to ease role transitions for individuals and to accommodate their members' other roles.

A third area of convergence concerns commonweal organizations, such as government or the police; mutual benefit organizations, such as labor unions, self-help groups, or political advocacy organizations; and human service organizations (Blau & Scott, 1962, p. 43 ff.). Here, the bottom lines of organizational effectiveness and empowerment or well-being of individuals often converge. Although organizational psychologists have long studied non-profit and public-sector organizations, community psychologists, with some notable exceptions (e.g., Keys & Frank, 1987), have too often remained ignorant of their efforts.

A final area of convergence concerns efforts to accommodate and benefit from diversity. Driven by the increasing demographic diversity of both workers and consumers in the United States, the rise of multinational corporations in which people from different cultural backgrounds are brought together, as well as legal mandates to avoid discrimination, organizational psychologists have theorized about and developed programs to help workplaces accommodate employees with different backgrounds and to promote effective interactions among diverse workers (Jackson & Associates, 1992; Triandis, Kurowski, & Gelfand, 1994).

ORGANIZATIONAL INTERVENTIONS AT INDIVIDUAL, GROUP, AND INTERGROUP LEVELS

What Changes Stem from Individual-Level Interventions in Organizations?

We believe that individual-level interventions within organizational contexts are often misguided, whether the target is organizational or individual change. Katz and Kahn (1978, p. 658) dubbed the effort to change organizations by changing individuals the "psychological fallacy" because organizational outcomes depend on processes at higher levels of analysis (see also Beer, 1976). Organizations may also be relatively poor loci for individual-level efforts to change individuals, because of ways that organizational conditions constrain individual behavior and coping efforts (Kanter, 1977). Efforts to change individual behavior in organizations may require change in these conditions. In an empirical review of 131 field studies, Macy and Izumi (1993) concluded that individual-level interventions produced low improvements on financial, behavioral, and attitudinal measures.

Attempts to change individuals in organizational contexts also raise concerns for individual rights. Consider the example of employee assistance programs, an increasingly common form of secondary prevention directed at early identification and treatment of substance abuse and mental health problems that manifest themselves at work (e.g., Hartwell, Tyler, Steele, French, Potter, Rodman, & Zarkin, 1996; Steele, 1988; Trice & Roman, 1972). Advocates point to the "leverage" the workplace has in inducing workers to confront problems and seek treatment, but leverage may quickly become coercion. Organizational and community psychologists might instead redirect some employee assistance efforts from case finding and treatment at the individual level to primary prevention at the organizational level, e.g., by promoting health for all employees, reducing job stressors, and changing organizational norms that foster use of substances to cope with stress (Allen & Linde, 1981). Sonnenstuhl (1988) describes the potential of these approaches for reducing substance abuse, and offers an extended case study (1996) of how sandhogs (who work underground building tunnels and other systems) transformed an occupational culture of drinking into one of sobriety.

What Changes Stem from Group-Level Interventions in Organizations?

A number of organizational interventions make use of the power of groups to motivate change (Cartwright, 1951; Hackman, 1992; Lewin, 1951). Do group-level interventions lead to individual or to organizational change? The answers are complicated by historical developments in the interventions themselves.

Laboratory training, sensitivity training, or simply T- (for training) groups represent an early form of organizational intervention (e.g., Benne, Bradford, Gibb, & Lippitt, 1975; Schein & Bennis, 1965). T-groups were designed to provide members with insight into their own behavior and its impact on others, sensitivity to others' behavior, and an understanding of group dynamics via experiential learning and feedback (e.g., Campbell & Dunnette, 1968). They were also intended to change organizations by changing managers (French & Bell, 1983).

Initially, T-groups were composed of strangers who met in unstructured, face-to-face groups with a trainer. The "here and now" of members' behavior within the group formed the grist for self-examination and group feedback. There is considerable evidence that such T-groups changed members' self-perceptions and their behavior as viewed by others, at least initially, but participants often found it difficult to apply and maintain their skills in the "back-home" situation, especially if organizational norms did not support the changes (Argyris, 1979; Beer, 1976; Campbell & Dunnette, 1968; Smith, 1975). Studies rarely examined whether improvements extended to task or organizational performance.

Over time, changes in groups' composition and structure made organizational change more plausible (French & Bell, 1983). First, stranger groups were replaced by "cousin groups" of employees from the same organization who did not work together, or by intact "family" work groups, in order to promote transfer of learning to the back-home environment (Beer, 1976). The "there and then" of ordinary group functioning supplemented the "here and now" of stranger T-groups as a subject for examination (Beer, 1976; Woodman & Sherwood, 1980). According to Blake, a prime mover in these developments, it was "learning to *reject* T-group, stranger-type labs that permitted [organizational development] to come into focus" (letter quoted by French & Bell, 1983, p. 16; emphasis in original). Second, the types of group-level interventions became more varied. External consultants focused on task performance ("team building") or process analysis, and elaborate, multistage interventions, such as the managerial grid (Blake, Mouton, Barnes, & Greiner, 1964) were developed.

Group-level approaches to organizational development have spawned an enormous research literature and even a healthy number of reviews and meta-analyses covering as many as 574 studies (Golembiewski, Proehl, & Sink, 1982). Overall, the reviews indicate positive effects of group-level interventions on employees' attitudes and group process (e.g., Neuman, Edwards, & Raju, 1989; Porras & Berg, 1978; Sundstrom, De Meuse, & Futrell, 1990; Woodman & Sherwood, 1980), job behaviors such as absenteeism (e.g., Guzzo, Jette, & Katzell, 1985; Nicholas, 1982), organizational productivity or performance (e.g., Guzzo et al., 1985; Nicholas, 1982; Porras & Berg, 1978), or any other outcomes that were measured (Golembiewski et al., 1982). Macy & Izumi (1993) found that group-level interventions (contrasted with individual and system-wide interventions) produced the highest improvements in behavioral outcomes such as absenteeism, turnover, and complaints, and Guzzo and Dickson (1996) concluded that, irrespective of interventions, organizational structures based on work teams appeared to be more effective on a variety of dimensions than more traditional bureaucratic structures.

It is difficult to draw clear conclusions about the relative merits of different types of interventions; reviews differ in the types of interventions found most effective or find few differences among types (e.g., Golembiewski et al., 1982; Porras, 1979). The reviews classify particular interventions inconsistently[1]; indeed, there are few pure types. Many studies incorporated elements of several intervention strategies simultaneously or sequentially (Kaplan, 1979; Porras & Berg, 1978). The strategies themselves continued to evolve. The methodological difficulties of proving causality in field studies of organizations also lead to different conclusions, with some authors accepting only experimental studies with artificial groups as sufficiently rigorous for inclusion, and others rejecting these entirely on grounds of external validity. These difficulties and others have led some organizational theorists, like many community theorists (e.g., Tolan, Keys, Chertok, & Jason, 1990), to call for research methods that involve group members in the research, have longer time frames, and include rich descriptions of context and dynamics (Beer & Walton, 1987).

Overall, the evidence of effectiveness of group-level interventions is sufficiently positive that community psychologists should consider employing them in the settings where they work. We speculate that, as a class, group-level interventions may be especially important in small community-based organizations where the organization is essentially a group (e.g., self-help groups, small alternative organizations). They may also be of particular value in community organizations of any size where different racial, cultural, or professional backgrounds or constituencies of group members interfere with group process. In schools and other organizations where professionals operate relatively independently of one another (Cherniss, 1980, p. 72 ff; Weick, 1976), group interventions may be less relevant to task performance, but may be important to counteract teachers' frequent experience of loneliness and isolation (Keys & Bartunek, 1979).

What Can Organizational Research Tell Us about Social Support?

Social support is not an organizational intervention, but it is an interpersonal or group activity relevant to individual well-being in organizational contexts. It should come as no

[1]For example, the study mentioned most often in the various reviews (Blake et al., 1964) was classified as a T-group experience by Campbell and Dunnette (1968), as team-building by Nicholas (1982), as process consultation with other non-group-level activities by Kaplan (1979), and, we infer, as a "managerial grid" intervention by Porras and Berg (1978), the only authors to have such a category.

surprise to community psychologists well-versed in the study of social support that researchers have found beneficial effects of support from co-workers and supervisors in the workplace in general (House, 1981; House & Wells, 1978; Kobasa & Puccetti, 1983; LaRocco, House, & French, 1980; LaRocco & Jones, 1978), and in human service organizations (Jayaratne & Chess, 1984; Shinn, Mørch, Robinson, & Neuner 1993; Shinn, Rosario, Mørch, & Chestnut, 1984). A particular contribution from organizational theory is the analysis of ways organizational structures may foster or constrain social support (see House, 1981). For example, House and Wells (1978) attributed the minimal impact of social support from co-workers in a manufacturing plant to a technology that did not permit individual interaction. Similarly, Shinn, Wong, Simko, and Ortiz-Torres (1989) found weak effects of co-worker support in white-collar organizations where co-workers were not allowed to help or, in some cases, even to talk to, one another. Cherniss (1980, p. 93) argued that interventions to promote support must address organizational conditions that constrain social interaction. Incentive plans may be one such strategy, with unit-wide or company-wide bonuses for performance more likely to nurture cooperation and support than pay plans based on individual performance (Lawler, 1977).

What Changes Stem from Intergroup Interventions?

Intergroup interventions are intended to reduce dysfunctional conflict between groups. Where groups in conflict operate independently, interventions can be aimed at keeping the groups separate or limiting the circumstances under which they can interact (Huse & Cummings, 1985, p. 141). When groups are interdependent or when structural or contextual factors promoting conflict cannot be addressed, other solutions may be tried (Beer, 1976). One is rotation or exchange of personnel, so that members of each group learn more about the other's activities and perspectives. Another is direct negotiation, with or without the help of third-party consultants (Huse & Cummings, 1985, p. 142).

Third-party consultants can extract constructive outcomes from organizational conflict (e.g., Walton, 1969) by sustaining the mutual motivation of participants to engage in conflict resolution or using process skills to provide support, encourage openness, and maintain optimum tension levels between protagonists. This role requires considerable skill, since the interventionist must turn antagonism into problem-solving (Filley, 1975, p. 5) by creating a climate of trust and acceptance.

Yet another solution to conflict between groups is intergroup problem-solving. Blake, Shepard, and Mouton (1964, p. 114–195) described a process in which each group met separately with a consultant to develop "images" of itself and the other group. The groups then met together to exchange images and to clarify them in discussion. The next steps depended on the type of groups. In the case of a union-management conflict, the two sides worked separately with consultants to develop evidence for the other side's images. In the case of conflict between headquarters and a field unit, functional groups from the two units met together to discuss functional problems. In each case, all participants reconvened to share observations, compile a consolidated list of key issues and sources of friction, and plan next steps. Long-term follow-up was deemed essential. Blake, Shepard, et al. (1964, p. 122) even used a modified design with one party when the other party in the conflict declined to participate.

Unfortunately, most evaluations of intergroup interventions are anecdotal (Beer, 1976). Beer suggested that although such interventions are most likely to work when the groups in conflict have superordinate goals, these goals do not always exist. Golembiewski et al. (1982, p. 91) found that, overall, intergroup interventions have higher rates of both positive and negative effects than many other interventions. An implication is that conflicts, once they surface, must be dealt with skillfully, or they may escalate.

A potential cause of intergroup conflict of special interest to community psychologists is inequality in power, status, or competence as, for example, between staff and clients of a service system. Here, third-party consultants can serve as a counterweight to equalize situational power imbalances. Or, by working to increase the power and competence of the lower-status group, they may help to redress the imbalance and lay the groundwork for better relations (Beer, 1976). Another such cause is race or ethnicity. The evolution of racial and ethnic conflicts may depend on whether divisions parallel hierarchical levels in an organization or members of minority groups are embedded in a hierarchy dominated by majority members. Pushed by legislation regarding employment discrimination and pulled by desires to draw on the best talents of an increasingly diverse labor force, many work organizations bring people from different ethnic groups together to a greater extent than do other social institutions, and some organizational psychologists have given attention to resolving conflicts (Alderfer & Thomas, 1988).

We believe that intergroup interventions may be especially useful in community organizations. In human service or public-sector organizations, staff and clients, different groups of staff, or different constituencies may vary on ethnic, racial, gender, socioeconomic, or professional dimensions that impede understanding and cooperation. Conflict in voluntary or social movement organizations may arise from differing roles (e.g., paid staff *vs.* volunteer), or ideology and goals (Riger, 1983/84). Golembiewski et al. (1982) found intergroup interventions to be more common in the public sector than in the private sector.

ORGANIZATIONAL INTERVENTIONS AT THE LEVEL OF THE ORGANIZATION

Klein (this volume) describes organizational interventions, such as quality of work-life programs and employee ownership, that may empower workers. Here we discuss three other forms of intervention at the organizational level that may be valuable for community psychologists: survey feedback, job enrichment, and design of socio-technical systems, especially the creation of autonomous work groups. We briefly introduce the ideas of organizational culture and cultural change.

What Is the Value of Survey Feedback?

French and Bell (1983) gave survey feedback, or survey-guided development, equal standing with laboratory training in the origins of organizational development. This intervention technique is based on the systematic collection of attitudinal data from, and subsequent feedback to, all members of the organization, starting at the top and working down in functional teams. All members are involved in analysis, interpretation, and the design of corrective action steps (French & Bell, 1990, p. 169). Data are usually gathered with questionnaires, but interview data and company records may be used. Some authors (e.g., Beer, 1976) argued that the scientific quality of the data is less important than client ownership of them. Unless the survey focuses on areas of respondents' concerns, and the values implicit in it are congruent with the respondents' own, clients may reject the data as invalid or irrelevant (Mohrman, Mohrman, Cooke, & Duncan, 1977).

In large organizations, data feedback typically begins with the top manager or executive team. Frequently consultants conduct "cascades" of data feedback for family groups reporting to managers at successively lower organizational levels. At each stage, group members discuss the data gathered from their own group, diagnose problems, plan action steps, and prepare for data feedback to the next lower organizational level (Huse & Cummings, 1985, p. 131). Some observers (Nadler, 1980; Shaskin & Cooke, 1976, as quoted in Huse & Cummings, 1985, pp. 133–134) have suggested that feedback to intact work groups is most appropriate where work groups are relatively independent or when within-group issues are key. If groups are interdependent or systems-level problems exist, problem-solving should instead occur in cross-linked groups or special task forces.

Practitioners of survey feedback differ in emphasizing its importance for group process, including development of problem-solving norms of openness, trust, and collaboration (e.g., Miles, Hornstein, Calder, Callahan, & Schiavo, 1971), or for correcting problems in organizational functioning that have been pinpointed in the survey data and in subsequent discussions (e.g., Hausser, Pecorella, & Wissler, 1975). The first use of survey-feedback is a group-level intervention; the second is an organizational-level intervention.

The organizational psychology model of survey feedback, sometimes in conjunction with other techniques, has been used in schools (e.g., Brown, 1972; Coughlan & Cooke, 1974; Miles, Hornstein, Callahan, Calder, & Schiavo, 1969; Mohrman et al., 1977) and psychiatric hospital wards (Ellsworth, 1973), among others. Moos and his colleagues (Moos, 1973; Pierce, Trickett, & Moos, 1972) independently developed a parallel technique based on feedback of discrepancies between real and ideal social climates in an in-patient ward and in a community setting. Shinn, Perkins, and Cherniss (1980) then combined the two approaches in a study of group homes for youths. These studies showed positive changes in participants' attitudes and convergence of real and ideal social climates where the action planning phases were well-developed, but several studies found detrimental changes for control groups not involved in problem-solving (Brown, 1972; Coughlan & Cooke, 1974; Ellsworth, 1973). Where groups were led by peers rather than supervisors or external change agents, the perceived legitimacy of the groups and the legitimacy, skill, and support accorded their leaders were critical to success (Mohrman et al., 1977).

Nadler (1977, p. 78) suggested that feedback of data showing poor performance leads to frustration unless the recipients have mechanisms to solve their problems, and Pasmore (1976) also warned against raising expectations without fulfilling them. Friedlander and Brown (1974) and Beer (1976) agreed that changes were unlikely without follow-up after the feedback meeting. In Golembiewski et al.'s review (1982), diagnostic activities were more likely than most other classes of organizational development to have negative effects, although it is not clear whether the interventions so classified went beyond diagnosis to action.

Bowers (1973) provides further evidence for the importance of fully implementing problem-solving processes. In a comparative study of four organizational development activities in 23 organizations, he found survey feedback led to the most positive changes in both managers' and employees' perceptions of a range of organizational variables. The two control conditions involved some return of survey data but no problem-solving meetings: When data were returned to supervisors at all levels, there were mixed changes. When data were returned only to the top manager, both managers' and employees' perceptions grew more negative.

In his review, Nicholas (1982) also distinguished between degrees of involvement in group activity after feedback of survey data. He found survey feedback alone to be the least successful of four types of human-process interventions in affecting job behavior and performance, although survey feedback with team building had an average rate of success. Neuman et al. (1989) and Porras and Berg (1978), who did not make the distinction, found survey feedback comparable to other interventions in affecting attitudes and productivity.

In human-service organizations, survey feedback involving clients as well as staff can provide one mechanism for integrating client opinions into development efforts. Where this has been tried, staff and client perceptions were often closer than either group had expected (Shinn et al., 1980), and this fact facilitated problem-solving. Problem-solving with regard to the work climate, as it affects staff, as well as to the social climate, as it affects clients, might be an important tool to alleviate staff burnout. On the other hand, survey feedback is not a quick fix. Keys (1986) noted the process can be cumbersome. Survey design, data collection, feedback, and problem-solving require a sustained commitment from a relatively stable group of participants. Where staff or client turnover is high, survey feedback is unlikely to be successful (Shinn et al., 1980).

What Is the Value of Job Enrichment?

Survey-guided development can lead to a plethora of organizational changes, depending on the problems uncovered in the diagnostic data and the solutions generated in response. Job enrichment involves a prescribed set of changes appropriate under more limited circumstances: when jobs themselves are insufficiently motivating, and when various organizational systems (described below) will support change (Hackman & Oldham, 1980; Oldham & Hackman, 1980). Organizational theorists reason that routine and unmotivating jobs may have costs (in lost productivity, absenteeism, or sabotage) that exceed the benefits of efficient division of labor (Beer, 1976). For community psychologists, making work more interesting might be an end in itself.

Organizational psychologists have traditionally distinguished between job enlargement, or increasing the variety of tasks in a job by incorporating functions from a horizontal slice of the organization, and job enrichment, which incorporates tasks from higher vertical levels (e.g., Beer, 1976). Hackman and Oldham (1980, p. 77) suggested that the key dimensions of motivating jobs are variety in the skills needed, significance of the work for other people, the extent to which the worker completes a whole or identifiable piece of work rather than just a fraction of one (task identity), autonomy or discretion in how the work is carried out, and feedback about the effectiveness of one's performance. These dimensions are not empirically independent (Nystrom, 1981), and all can be targets for enrichment.

If a careful diagnosis indicates that job enrichment is in order, possible steps include combining tasks, especially so that they form meaningful whole units, giving the individual worker some of the responsibility and authority previously vested in supervisors, allowing workers to establish direct, unmediated relationships with the system's clients, and giving workers feedback on how they are doing, often by making them responsible for quality control or giving them access to performance records (Hackman & Oldham, 1980, p. 135). For example, a case-management system in which each caseworker coordinates all services for a small group of clients offers more enriched jobs than a system in which workers specialize in particular services and a supervisor allocates services to clients. In the case-management system, the worker is responsible for the whole client, engages in a greater variety of activities, has more discretion, along with the client, in determining what services are most appropriate, and gets feedback from the client as to the success of the mix of services chosen.

Cummings and Molloy (1977, p. 86) reviewed 28 studies of job restructuring. The variables most commonly manipulated (the "action levers") were, in decreasing order of frequency, autonomy or discretion, variety, information or feedback, and training; most studies manipulated several variables. Results were overwhelmingly positive, with improvements in the quality of products found in all 17 studies that measured this variable, and improvements in costs, productivity, attitudes, and job withdrawal behaviors (absenteeism and turnover) also found in the vast majority of studies where these were measured. Nicholas (1982) divided an overlapping set of 24 studies into job enlargement, job enrichment, and job enrichment with worker participation in the redesign. The first two were associated with improvements in job behaviors and productivity just under half the time; the small set of enrichment studies involving worker participation had positive effects on 70% of the variables studied. Guzzo et al. (1985) found that productivity improved an average of 0.42 standard deviation units in studies of work redesign, although Neuman et al. (1989) found smaller and more variable effects on satisfaction and other attitudes. Golembiewski et al. (1982) found at least a balance of positive over negative effects in over 90% of 84 private-sector "technostructural" interventions, including job enlargement.

Oldham and Hackman (1980) caution that several organizational systems can constrain job-enrichment programs. Some technologies, for example an assembly line, do not permit workers enough discretion so that meaningful amounts of autonomy, variety, or feedback can be built into jobs. Rigid personnel systems with narrow job descriptions or financial and quality control systems may not provide enough room to maneuver. Personnel systems may be governed by union–management negotiations; control systems are often bound by legal or contractual arrangements with customers. Unless these constraining systems are loosened, changes in jobs may not be meaningful. Similarly, training, career development, compensation, and supervision practices can undo changes once implemented. Before undertaking enrichment programs, careful diagnosis is necessary to determine not only whether jobs are unmotivating, but also whether organizational systems will permit and sustain change.

One reason that other organizational systems are so conservative with respect to changing jobs is that changes have ripple effects. As Nystrom (1981, p. 282) put it, "overtly redesigning one job covertly redesigns adjacent jobs." The supervisor's job in particular may be impoverished as workers' jobs are enriched, requiring compensating changes in the supervisory role (Nystrom, 1981; Oldham & Hackman, 1980; Walton & Schlesinger, 1979).

Hackman and Oldham (1980, p. 82; Oldham & Hackman, 1980) also considered whether enriched jobs fit with individual employees' needs for challenge and growth. Jobs that might motivate one employee might "stretch" another too far. Organizations with a mission may be especially likely to overextend workers, without regard for individual needs or compensating support. In a set of group homes with which the authors consulted, child-care workers were on duty from the time the children awoke until they went to bed, and remained on call for problems throughout the night. Their responsibility for the whole child was supposed to match that of real parents, who never go off duty. Not surprisingly, the child-care workers turned over at the rate of 200% per year. Excessive zeal to enrich jobs or demands for high levels of commitment in social movement or human service organizations may be one cause of burnout and turnover (e.g., Riger, 1983/84).

What Is the Value of Socio-technical Intervention?

Another intervention focused on the nature of work itself is the socio-technical systems approach. This approach focuses on the technological demands of the task, the social organization of workers performing it, and the fit between the two. The socio-technical systems interventions initiated by the British Tavistock group are among the most impressive success stories in organizational development (see review by Katz & Kahn, 1978, p. 701 ff.). Although the settings—British coal mines (Trist & Bamforth, 1951), Indian textile mills (Rice, 1958), and a variety of Scandinavian manufacturing plants (Norstedt & Aguren, 1973; Thorsrud, Sorensen, & Gustavsen, 1976)—may seem exotic to community psychologists, the approach itself is relevant to many community organizations.

In principle, socio-technical interventions give equal consideration to social and technological changes but, in practice, the most common changes are in group design, along lines that seem independent of technology. Concomitant changes in technology, skill development, or reward systems may accommodate the group work (Cummings, 1981; Pasmore, Francis, & Haldeman, 1982). The approach typically involves creating semi-autonomous work groups that together perform a variety of tasks previously broken up into individual jobs. Individual work roles are enlarged to create greater variety in tasks, identification with the product as a whole rather than with some small aspect of it, and say in the way work is organized. Work groups are strengthened by increasing their authority, autonomy, and opportunity for interaction, and pay structures are frequently altered to reward group, rather than individual, productivity.

Socio-technical systems interventions do for work groups what job enrichment does for individuals. Cummings (1978) noted that, in job enrichment, designers manipulate work variables to increase individual motivation; in socio-technical systems the same variables are deemed necessary for cooperation and self-regulation in groups. For example, skill variety and autonomy may be motivating to workers; in groups they also provide flexibility to adjust to changing environmental and task conditions, such as the changing challenges of a seam of coal in the coal mine or the demands posed by different types of thread in the textile mill. When there is uncertainty over the environment ("boundary transactions") or the task itself ("conversion activities"), external supervisors may be less equipped to regulate the activities of a work group than are the employees who are closer to the uncertainty (Cummings, 1978).

Since the creation of self-regulating work groups is parallel to job enrichment, the earlier caveats about organizational support apply here as well. Hackman and Oldham (1980, p. 224) advocated the simpler tack of designing jobs for individuals unless there is a compelling argument favoring group-level design. Cummings (1978) offered several criteria: First, the group task should be a self-completing whole composed of interdependent parts. Without interdependence, there is little reason to engage in group work. Second, the group should control its own boundaries. It needs a well-defined physical territory, control over rates of inputs and outputs, sufficient skills to free it from reliance on external resources, and responsibility for boundary decisions, such as quality control, to free it from dependence on external regulators. Third, the group should control its task, including work methods, production goals, and knowledge of results.

Results of socio-technical interventions in the literature are overwhelmingly positive. In a review of 134 studies, Pasmore et al. (1982) found positive results over 80% of the time for productivity, costs, absenteeism, attitudes, safety, grievances, and quality when these variables were measured. Cummings and Molloy (1977, p. 40) and Nicholas (1982) found similar improvements in smaller reviews. In meta-analyses, Guzzo et al. (1985) estimated the improvement in productivity to be 0.62 standard deviation units; Beekun (1989) found productivity increases averaging 0.49 standard deviation units and reductions in escape behaviors (absenteeism, turnover) of 0.30 standard deviation units.

Creation of autonomous work groups might be considered by many human service, mutual benefit, and social movement organizations. Indeed, the groups have much in common with the "team approach" used by many human service agencies, the "lodge" program developed by Fairweather, Sanders, Maynard, and Cressler (1969) to help psychiatric patients live and work in the community, and the collective work and decision-making structures often used by feminist organizations (Riger, 1983/84). Certainly tasks are uncertain in many social movement, mutual benefit, and human service organizations, and political, regulatory, and funding environments may fluctuate. The argument that those who are closest to the uncertainty should make decisions about how to adapt is a reasonable one.

Socio-technical interventions into technology, in addition to group organization, would seem especially appropriate for high-tech service organizations such as hospitals (Chisholm & Ziegenfuss, 1986), although Pasmore, Petee, and Bastian (1986) suggested that the traditional authority of the physician, and the association of specialization with occupational status in health care settings, are cultural barriers to the creation of autonomous work groups. Several authors (Chisholm & Ziegenfuss, 1986; Hackman & Oldham, 1980, p. 65) have complained about the theory's vagueness regarding what changes should be made under what circumstances, and about its lack of attention to individual differences. Still, the potential value of socio-technical approaches to community organizations seems great.

Two relatively recent reviews categorized interventions rather differently than we do here. Macy and Izumi (1993) did not include survey feedback as an intervention (presumably preferring to classify the changes that arose out of such interventions). They included the formation of autonomous or semi-autonomous teams, along with changes in feedback and reward systems, flexible schedules, and many other changes that involved power and control among their "structural action-levers," whereas job enrichment and less autonomous group approaches (among many others) were seen as "human-resource action-levers." In language more familiar to community psychologists, structural action-levers would be those that changed social regularities (Seidman, 1988, 1990), and human-resource action-levers would work within existing regularities. "Technical action-levers," of which those most relevant to human service organizations might be introduction of new computer hardware or software systems, were a third category. (The authors posited, but could not find studies of, a fourth category of "total-quality management action-levers.") In their review of 131 field studies, they found the largest effects for the small number of interventions that involved all three types of action-levers, but all groupings of interventions that included structural changes were more successful than those that confined themselves to changes in human resources. Improvements in attitudinal outcomes (e.g., satisfaction, commitment) were harder to produce than improvements in either financial outcomes (e.g., quantity and quality of production, costs) or behavioral outcomes (e.g., absenteeism, turnover). Interventions that encompassed systemwide change produced the largest financial improvements, and group-level interventions led to the highest behavioral improvements.

Porras and Robertson (1992) also adopted a rather different categorization of interventions as involving organizing arrangements, social factors, technology, or physical settings, with all but the last taking place at multiple levels, from the individual to the organization. Overall, they found fewer than half of the outcome variables assessed to show positive changes, although there were relatively few negative changes. Technological interventions were least likely to produce positive change.

Can Changes in Organizational Culture be Managed?

Recent literature on organizational change has begun to focus on organizational culture (Beer & Walton, 1987; Schein, 1990) and vision (Porras & Silvers, 1991). Culture includes the beliefs, values, and assumptions held by organizational members, the symbols or artifacts that reflect them (Schein, 1990), along with norms for behavior (Kotter & Heskett, 1992). Vision includes these and adds organizational purpose and mission (Porras & Silvers, 1991). Cultures may evolve naturally or cultural changes may be forced by environmental circumstances or by mergers or acquisitions.

Although there are descriptions of ways that organizational leaders can mold cultures (e.g., Kotter & Haskett, 1992; Pfeffer, 1998b; Schein, 1990) and, in the case of the sandhogs who transformed an occupational culture (Sonnenstuhl, 1996), evidence for transformations from the bottom of the hierarchy, there is as yet little empirical evidence for effects of planned interventions into organizational culture. Change efforts that are not compatible with an organization's culture are unlikely to be successful (Porras & Robertson, 1992).

Kotter and Haskett (1992) defined adaptive cultures as those able to satisfy three major groups of stakeholders (customers, employees, and stockholders), and found that companies who did so were more successful, by standards of expansion in sales, income, workforce size, and value of stock, than companies that did not. Community psychologists might pay attention to the evolving literature in this area, especially since many of the organizations we deal with are guided by a strong sense of mission, and must satisfy multiple stakeholders.

Who Receives and Benefits from What Interventions?

Friedlander and Brown (1974), p. 334) pointed out that most human-process interventions (including group and intergroup methods) have been undertaken with management groups, whereas socio-technical interventions typically focus on blue-collar or lower-level white-collar employees. Nicholas (1982), for example, found 13 human-process interventions among white-collar workers, 2 for both collar colors, and none for just blue-collar workers. By way of contrast, 15 technostructural interventions were directed at white-collar workers and 20 at blue-collar workers. Similarly, in Bowers' (1973) study, training interventions were confined to top management, whereas survey feedback involved workers at all organizational levels. From this distributional evidence, Nicholas (1982, p. 539) concluded that human-process interventions "were most successful when aimed only at salaried workers." Other observers might infer a class bias in researchers' views about who can benefit from interventions aimed at insight and problem-solving or interpersonal skills. Community psychologists might have different biases here as well. Guzzo et al. (1985) found that improvements in productivity as a result of organizational interventions were larger for managerial/professional and sales workers than for blue-collar and clerical workers, but suggested that this may have been due to the relatively high success rates of the training interventions that were typically confined to the former groups.

Can Organizational and Community Change Facilitate Each Other?

Pfeffer (1998b) reviewed studies suggesting that organizations model their structure and practices on others with which they share directors or with which they interact. Nevertheless, Trist (1986) observed that diffusion of successful innovations among organizations is slow. He contended that diffusion could be accelerated if organizational innovations were linked to a wider process of community change. As an example, he described how an area-wide labor-management committee, with advisors from the community and stimulus from a university, facilitated quality-of-work-life projects in numerous organizations over a 14-year period, and contributed to the economic revitalization of a declining industrial area. Similarly, Clamp (1987a, 1987b) described how the Mondragon system of federated cooperatives revitalized another declining industrial area in the Basque region of Spain by promoting the development of new cooperatives and support structures. The cooperatives, whose managers were responsible to democratically elected boards, weathered a later economic downturn with much less dislocation of workers than in other Spanish industries. Although the conditions that fostered the success of these interventions may be rare, the models suggest avenues that community psychologists might follow in promoting community and organizational change.

INTERVENTIONS AT THE BOUNDARIES BETWEEN INDIVIDUALS AND ORGANIZATIONS

We have described multiple levels of intervention to promote organizational change. Next we consider interventions to ease changes in relationships between individuals and organizations. These include major life transitions at the beginning and end of employment, and daily shifts between work and other aspects of life. Transitions are often stressful, and interventions to ease them may promote individual well-being.

What Helps Individuals Joining Organizations?

Just as community psychologists have intervened to ease students' transition to school (Bloom, 1971; Felner, Ginter, & Primavera, 1982), organizational psychologists have worked on strategies for selection and socialization of workers. Typical unstructured interviews are not terribly valid as a selection device, and more valid tests take time and effort to develop (Guion & Gibson, 1988; Schmitt & Robertson, 1990). Hackman and Oldham (1980, p. 25) argued that selection and training are not very helpful in the common case where people are overqualified for jobs. Recruitment procedures that lure prospective applicants with exaggerated glowing descriptions of jobs can lead to anger when new recruits begin to experience organizational reality, and raise ethical issues as well (Porter, Lawler, & Hackman, 1975).

To counter such problems, Wanous (1975, 1977) proposed the simple yet radical solution of providing job applicants with a "realistic job preview," and letting them decide for themselves whether to join the organization described. This strategy replaces the typical panoply of unrealistic promises with a balanced presentation of accurate, detailed information about the work environment as it really exists. The medium for presenting information—brochures, films, visits—is less important than the frank tone.

It might at first appear that such candor would make it difficult, if not impossible, to recruit new employees. In the majority of studies in which realistic previews were tested, however, no adverse effects were found. Also, it seems likely that those who selected themselves out because of accurate advance information eventually would have left anyway, often after expensive training or, in human service settings, establishing soon-to-be-severed relationships with clients. In the "realistic preview" cases cited by Wanous (1977), the survival rate for the control group, which received the usual orientation, was lower than for those whose jobs were portrayed truthfully. The meta-analysis by Guzzo et al. (1985), however, found essentially no effect of job previews on job withdrawal behaviors. Neuman et al.'s (1989) meta-analysis observed weak, but consistent, positive effects on job attitudes.

Other researchers have focused on socialization of new recruits. In a classic experiment, to which we will return in our conclusion, Gomersall and Myers (1966) studied the socialization process of a manufacturing plant experiencing production problems. Workers assembled complex electronic products under conditions of rapid and continuous technological change, a process that required considerable skill. Although it is not unusual for workers to experience tension when starting a job, the anxiety level in this organization was exceptionally high. New employees were subjected to "initiation"—actually, hazing—by veterans. They also faced an overwhelmingly complicated training program, conducted by busy supervisors so familiar with the technology that they had lost touch with the psychological state of new employees. Perhaps most harmful, new operators were fearful of discussing their problems with supervisors, and thus kept concerns to themselves. Predictably, these conditions affected job performance, turnover, and, ultimately, productivity.

In response, the researchers instituted an experimental socialization program. Before the newcomers could be frightened by the veteran employees, they were given time to become acquainted with the organization, to ask questions, and to relax. New employees were told to expect success, based on data that 99.6% of those hired eventually learned the necessary skills. They were told to disregard rumors and, as in a realistic job preview, presented with good and bad facts about the job. They were encouraged to ask questions, and assured that lack of understanding was to be expected in the beginning. And they were given accurate characterizations of their individual supervisors. "The absolute truth was the rule." (At a minimum, it is impressive that the researchers were able to establish absolute truth.) The program was a success. Relative to a comparison group socialized in the ordinary manner, training time, costs, absenteeism and tardiness, and waste in the manufacturing process and rejects were all cut by half or more. Similar socialization processes might be useful in schools, or any other organizations that routinely absorb new members.

What Helps Workers Leaving Organizations?

Janis and Mann (1977, pp. 155 ff., 367 ff.) suggested that anticipating possible negative consequences of decisions, as made possible by both realistic job previews and orientations to good and bad points of a job, aids in reaching good decisions and serves to inoculate people against potential setbacks. Realistic previews might thus be valuable to workers who are retiring, being laid off, or changing jobs. Layoffs and plant closings may be especially stressful (Jahoda, 1979; Kasl, Gore, & Cobb, 1975; Liem & Rayman, 1982) because of the involuntary nature of the change, the stress of unemployment itself, and the difficulty workers are likely to have finding alternative employment in a tight labor market.

Caplan, Vinokur, Price, and van Ryn (1989; Vinokur, van Ryn, Gramlich, & Price, 1991; Vinokur, Price, & Schul, 1995) designed an intervention involving training in job seeking, inoculation against setbacks, and social support for workers who had recently lost jobs. In a large field experiment, those offered the intervention were less likely to become depressed and more likely to become reemployed than the control group. They also had higher earnings and more job satisfaction. Among people who had not yet found adequate new jobs, those in the experimental group had more motivation to continue the search and a higher sense of self-efficacy in seeking employment. People who were at greatest risk for depression tended to self-select themselves into the intervention.

Taber, Walsh, and Cooke (1979) described a community effort to ease the impact of a plant closing with coordinated proactive services for unemployed workers and those anticipating unemployment. Organizational psychologists helped to set up an impressive community council involving company and union representatives, as well as social service agencies, financial institutions, colleges, hospitals, and so on. The case study shows the value of organizational theory to coordinating an ad hoc interorganizational group—a task in which community psychologists often participate.

How Can Organizations Help Workers Manage Daily Transitions?

Hiring and layoffs or retirements mark one form of temporal transition to and from work. Another form takes place daily as workers move between work and other facets of their lives. Motivated in part by strategic responses to the changing demographics of the labor force, and by changing institutional beliefs about appropriate roles for employers, (e.g., Friedman, 1987; Goodstein, 1994; Offermann & Gowing, 1990; Rousseau, 1997), many organizations have made a variety of efforts to accommodate the workplace to family life. Zedeck and Mosier (1990) surveyed a number of these, including maternity and paternity leave (still abysmal by European standards), various forms of assistance with child and dependent care, part-time work and job sharing, home-based work, and relocation assistance. Unfortunately, there is still little evidence that such programs help employees to balance work and family demands. Kirchmeyer (1995) surveyed managers across a variety of firms about their companies' practices with respect to non-work obligations, and the managers' own organizational commitment. She found that organizational practices such as flexibility in hours, work arrangements, and other accommodations that allowed employees to meet their own non-work responsibilities, were more highly associated with organizational commitment than efforts to meet employees' non-work needs directly, e.g., by provision of recreational facilities, counseling, or on-site day care. An organizational perspective that work and other aspects of life are separate domains, so that organizations should make no efforts to accommodate workers' outside needs, was associated with lower commitment.

Flexible work hours or "flexitime" programs are one common attempt to ease these daily transitions. Although originally developed as a solution to traffic congestion, flexitime was later conceptualized as an intervention in worker autonomy (Cummings & Molloy, 1977). Flexitime permits workers some discretion in scheduling work hours to fit with their family, personal, or even physiological needs. A number of reviews have found salutary effects of flexitime in such areas as job attitudes, absenteeism, tardiness, productivity, ease of child care, and usage of personal time (Cummings & Molloy, 1977; Golembiewski, 1985; Golembiewski & Proehl, 1978; Neuman et al., 1989; Nollen, 1982; Ronen, 1981; Silverstein & Srb, 1979), although Neuman et al. (1989) found no effect on job satisfaction. Guzzo et al. (1985) found an average productivity gain of 0.30 standard deviation units.

Kanter (1977) suggested that flexitime should be especially helpful to working parents. Winett and Neale (1980), in a small-sample study, found that working parents who took advantage of flexitime spent almost an hour more with their families each day. Staines and Pleck (1985) did not measure flexitime *per se*, but found that perceived control over the hours or days one worked moderated the adverse effects of non-standard schedules (e.g., night-shift work) on family life in a nationally representative sample of workers who were married or parents. Two studies, however, cast doubt on the value of flexitime for parents. Shinn et al. (1989) found that whereas perceived flexibility in job hours had mild benefits for parents in eight organizations, the availability of flexitime programs had no effects on well-being. Two-fifths of the parents said that their child-care arrangements constrained their use of flexitime.

Bohen and Viveros-Long (1981) found flexitime to be associated with positive outcomes for single people and childless couples, but not for parents in their public-sector sample. As flexitime programs become more prevalent at work, community psychologists might work to make other institutions such as child care more flexible as well, so that those whose lives are bounded by multiple institutions may reap the benefits of flexibility.

MATCHING INTERVENTIONS TO SETTINGS

The failure of flexitime programs to aid the group they were expected to help most in two studies is just one illustration of how efforts at organizational change may go awry. Although interventions may fail because they are ill-conceived or poorly implemented, or because of local events, a more interesting reason for failure may be a mismatch between the intervention and the setting. Efforts to promote organizational change must fit the culture of the organization (Beer & Walton, 1987) and the nation (Faucheux, Amado, & Laurent, 1982). Keys (1986) proposed diagnosing organizational problems to determine where to begin: Any serious conflict must be dealt with first, or the consultation abandoned, because unresolved conflict can undermine other efforts. If skills are deficient, then competencies should be improved. Finally, if skills are adequate, one can use them to improve organizational processes such as goal-setting, meeting procedures, and assessment of change.

In addition to characteristics of particular organizations that may constrain change, certain classes of settings have enough features in common to suggest cautions, if not guidelines, for prospective change agents. We briefly consider three broad and overlapping classes of settings with which community psychologists often deal: public sector organizations, human service organizations, and new settings.

In discussing the limits of popular techniques for organizations of concern to community psychologists, we do not mean to encourage pessimism. Golembiewski et al. (1982) found similar success rates for 270 public-sector and 304 private-sector interventions. Guzzo et al. (1985) found identical positive effect sizes for interventions in for-profit and non-profit organizations, and even larger effects for interventions in government. Macy and Izumi (1993) reported slightly larger overall effect sizes for interventions with "non-manufacturing, non-profit" organizations than for manufacturing and non-manufacturing, profit-making organizations. Sensitivity to differences between types of organizations should allow even better results.

What Features Constrain Change in Public-Sector Organizations?

Golembiewski (1985) described a number of features of public organizations that could constrain change (p. 13 ff.) and then cited an unpublished thesis by Proehl evaluating the extent to which these features actually hindered 270 organizational development efforts in government and other public organizations (p. 45 ff.). The most frequent single constraint was procedural rigidity imposed by law or civil service rules. Rules may proscribe new authority and reward structures, such as group pay plans. Similar constraints on redesigning work or developing autonomous work groups in the private sector (mentioned above) may not be as formidable. McConkie (1985) detailed how the basic assumptions and values of the bureaucratic model guiding most public-sector organizations are foreign to organizational development.

A set of constraints that were collectively even more pervasive than procedural rigidity in

Golembiewski's (1985) review arose from the diverse interests, values, and incentives of different players. In a federal agency, for example, these players include both houses of Congress, congressional committees, political appointees, the protected (civil) service, and other federal agencies with competing objectives. The media and interest groups external to the government provide close scrutiny. Numerous groups may have veto power over changes that threaten their interests.

The interface between different branches of government or between political appointees and career civil servants may be especially volatile. (In the private sector, the dividing line between management and workers is far lower in the administrative hierarchy, and middle- or lower-level managers who do not promote policies decided at the top can be replaced more easily.) The relatively rapid turnover of political appointees also makes linkages with career civil servants weak. To keep control, superiors may avoid delegation to subordinates or consciously promote fragmentation rather than integration.

Golembiewski (1985, p. 291 ff.) posited guidelines for working "at the interface" of conflicting interests in public organizations: The intervenor should work for the development of the system as a whole, rather than for a particular client (who may have initiated the intervention). He or she must take an interstitial role, be comfortable with marginality, maintain access to and from multiple groups, create balance between competing groups, and manage tensions between those with higher and lower levels of power. The intervenor should strive to "mobilize commonalities," but should realize that these may not always exist; clarifying points of disagreement may also be valuable.

Interventions should aim at changes in policy and structure, not just in patterns of interaction. The latter may fail because the system inhibits change or because differences are irreconcilable; the former has more potential for prevention, not just temporary amelioration. The intervenor must be prepared for mercurial changes in conditions; he or she should pick strategic spots and times to create success and be prepared for the uneven, "hurry up, then wait," pace of change.

Because of the "special texture of the arena," the intervenor may have to take on roles ordinarily eschewed in the private sector. He or she must be willing to take risks, to be "the point person" for change. The intervenor may become a go-between or mediator, but must avoid entering into power competitions. Perhaps most important, the intervenor must keep conscious of potential conflicts in values with system members. Value congruence is not always necessary, but sensitivity to conflicts is.

What Features Constrain Change in Human Service Organizations?

Human service organizations overlap somewhat with the public-sector organizations Golembiewski analyzed, but also possess a distinct set of characteristics. As Cooke (1985) noted of schools, human service organizations are often engaged in the complex and uncertain task of changing people. Their methods are ambiguous, particularly with respect to effectiveness, and there are few competitive pressures that might motivate change. Human service organizations operate in turbulent environments on which they are dependent for clients and funding. Like public-sector organizations, they are targets of multiple competing influences. They may be buffeted by community crises and subjected to public scrutiny. All these factors may lead administrators of human service organizations to adopt a defensive, reactive stance inhospitable to organizational development (Cooke, 1985).

Administrators in the human services frequently lack, or believe they lack, the fiscal resources for organizational development. A sense of the seriousness of their mission may prevent them from diverting staff time from service provision to organizational change or professional growth, particularly if an off-site intervention might be perceived as a boondoggle, or even as fun. They may subordinate staff welfare to the welfare of clients, despite evidence that staff burnout impedes performance (e.g., Lazaro, Shinn, & Robinson, 1984).

The task of human service organizations is complicated by what Kouzes and Mico (1979, p. 457) described as three distinct "domains" or spheres of influence with contrasting principles, measures of success, structural arrangements, and work modes. The "policy domain" is where governing policies are formulated. For human service organizations, this domain is often occupied by a board of directors, where representatives of the local community may serve. The guiding principle is legitimacy by the consent of the governed; success is measured by just, impartial, and fair decisions; the structure usually involves representation; and work modes involve negotiating, bargaining, and voting.

The "management domain," by contrast, operates on principles of hierarchical control and coordination. Cost efficiency and effectiveness are its measures of success, and bureaucracy its structure. Its work mode is linear control. These two domains mirror those of government organizations, with the "policy domain" perhaps less complex. In the private sector, the "management domain" usually dominates.

The third, the "professional domain," however, is unique to the human services. It is occupied by professionals who provide services and operates according to principles of self-regulation and autonomy. Its measures of success are quality of care and adherence to professional standards; its structure is collegial; and its mode of work is individualized, client-specific problem-solving.

Although each of the three domains is organized in ways that promote its primary task, the discordance in principles, success measures, structures, and work modes between domains serves to separate them. Occupants of different domains develop different and sometimes incompatible identities, visions of reality, norms of behavior, and rhythms of change, and they frequently struggle with one another for power and control.

Kouzes and Mico's (1979) view of the role of change agents in human service organizations is quite similar to Golembiewski's vision for public-sector organizations more generally: no matter how they are brought in, they must take the system as a client, and avoid alliances with any one part, although they must acknowledge that the goals of the policy domain have priority. Techniques for dealing with intergroup conflict are especially important. Informal collateral organizations, with members drawn from each of the conflicting groups, can sometimes solve problems outside of the usual administrative structure (Alderfer, 1977a; Zand, 1974). Intergroup problem-solving and imaging techniques (Blake et al., 1964), or training of managers in negotiation skills and integrating roles may also be useful.

Human service organizations may also share many characteristics of what Alderfer and Berg (1977) called "underbounded systems," namely unclear authority structure, uncertain role definitions, and confused communication patterns. For example, Alderfer (1980) describes an elementary school with two warring parents' groups, who were reluctant to even appear in meetings with each other, and a third parent–teacher steering committee formed by the principal in response to an externally funded citywide project to promote improved leadership in schools. Teachers and unaffiliated parents worried about getting caught up in the battle, and the principal's authority was undermined. Teachers also lacked a common agreement about their roles towards each other and the "learning centers," which were intended to promote cooperation across grade levels. A community environment of population and economic decline, and community demands on school space also impinged on the school. The key managerial task in such settings is to move the organization away from this underbounded condition; intervention activities should facilitate this process. For example, the consultant attempted to clarify the roles of the competing parents' groups to each other and to the steering committee, and worked internally with teachers and the principal on the principal's leadership role and style.

Unfortunately, many popular interventions strategies were developed to reduce boundaries, substitute participatory decision-making for autocratic control, and open up communications in organizations that can be characterized as "overbounded." A common cause of failure of organizational development may be the application of interventions designed for overbounded systems to underbounded problems (Alderfer, 1980, p. 271).

Other authors make comparable observations about what they call "organized anarchies" (Cohen, March, & Olsen, 1972), "loosely-coupled systems" (Weick, 1976), and "underorganized systems" (Brown, 1980). Brown (1980) contended that change efforts in underorganized systems should tighten, rather than loosen, organization by enhancing leadership; expanding the role of informal cultural mechanisms reflected in myths, norms, language, and values; elaborating or clarifying organizational structure; and clarifying, rationalizing, automating, or professionalizing technology. Similarly, Tichy (1985) argued (with respect to hospitals that lack professional management) that it behooves organizational development specialists to focus on basic issues such as managerial competence, the organization's capacity to carry out strategic planning, and the fit between strategy and organizational design. Leitko and Szczerbacki (1987) advocated increased oversight of human service agencies, clearer policies and rules, and formal management training for administrators to counter diffusion of authority. Strong leadership, networking, and strategic vision can serve to integrate power centers of professional groups and administrators.

Brown (1980) maintained that not only the goals of organizational development but also the process, the role of the change agent, and the ethical dilemmas differ for overorganized and underorganized systems. Typical change efforts developed for overorganized systems, "assume the existence of an identifiable system that must be penetrated ('entry') to gain concealed information ('diagnosis') as a prelude to opening up the system ('intervention')" (p. 190). Change in an underorganized system, on the other hand, starts with identification of the relevant entities. The task is not so much one of penetration as of inclusion. The relatively independent subsystems must then be convened and organized.

The role of the change agent, according to Brown (1980), should mirror the degree of organization ultimately desired in the system. In an underorganized system, the role may be relatively well-defined and authoritative, and the structure of the relationship should be clearly specified. But attempts to increase organization in underorganized systems involve questions of changing or preserving the distribution of power. Violations of members' autonomy may be a greater risk than violations of privacy. An authoritative consultant role leads to pressures to take sides on polarized issues. The value dilemmas may be greater, or at least more salient, than for a consultant in an overorganized system who does not come to grips with issues of power. Hence, Brown (1980) argued, the consultant to underorganized systems needs the political competence to understand the systems' dynamics and to manage his or her own role and values.

What Features Constrain Change in New Settings?

Interventions designed for overbounded systems may be especially inappropriate for settings undergoing the throes of organizational creation (Cherniss, this volume; Kimberly,

Miles, & Associates, 1980; Perkins, 1981; Perkins, Nieva, & Lawler, 1983; Sarason, 1972). Perkins et al. (1983) described severe problems created by the introduction of participatory management in a new plant with a sophisticated technology. A mandate to engage in collaborative decision-making was broadly interpreted to mean that almost any form of managerial control was inappropriate. An egalitarian structure was applied to all problems, even when technical expertise was unequally distributed, or when time pressures rendered group-centered decisions unworkable. In a new organization with ill-defined authority relationships and managers afraid to set limits, this "one person, one vote" decision-making structure had the effect of exaggerating the lack of internal boundaries.

The essential managerial task in a new organization is to create a set of system characteristics—authority relations, role definition, and so forth—that are congruent with each stage of the organizational life cycle. At the inception of a new organization, this means creating boundaries where none previously existed. As the organization matures, however, these structures will evolve and system characteristics must be continually adjusted to maintain an optimal degree of "boundedness."

Of course, new organizations are founded in the for-profit as well as the non-profit sector; community agencies may be bureaucratic and overbounded rather than underbounded and chaotic. Matching of interventions to settings requires a diagnosis of the actual client organization, not simply an assumption of characteristics or constraints based on labels or stated goals.

CONCLUSIONS

We began this chapter by citing conceptual similarities between community and organizational psychology siblings, but with a central difference in "bottom line" values. Put starkly, one sibling focuses on empowerment and well-being, the other on productivity and profitability. This distinction is exaggerated, but the siblings do wear different conceptual lenses, and differences in perspective affect both research and intervention. Yet, paradoxically, it may be that the organizational psychologist's concern for productivity can provide a basis for changes that would be dismissed were they to be justified solely on the basis of humanitarian values.

Take our earlier description of Gomersall and Myers' (1966) experiment in organizational socialization as an example. In their firm, a community psychologist might have chosen new workers' anxiety as the dependent variable, searching for independent factors that could be used to alleviate stress and strain. But the research team, consisting of an industrial psychologist and a plant manager, saw job performance as a key dependent variable that was, in turn, affected by anxiety. They then turned to the socialization process as the likely point of intervention in a causal chain ending in job competence.

The socialization program was a significant success when viewed through the lens of organizational effectiveness. But the program also helped individual employees, who experienced a more humane introduction to the organization. Because productivity had been an explicit part of their research design, there were data to support the introduction of such a program in settings where an appeal based on humanitarian values might not prevail. This research might even be useful in promoting more thoughtful socialization processes for other organizations (for example, universities) with less easily measured "bottom lines."

This study is no aberration. Katzell and Guzzo (1983) found improvements in satisfaction and other job attitudes in about three-quarters of 67 experiments that were designed to increase worker productivity, although Macy and Izumi (1993) and Porras and Robertson (1992) found attitudinal changes to be more rare. Pfeffer (1998a, p. 64) reviewed research showing that the financial success and longevity of companies were associated with a variety of management strategies that also produce high levels of commitment from workers: employment security, selective hiring of new workers, decentralized decision-making and self-managed teams, relatively high compensation contingent on organizational performance, extensive training, reductions in status distinctions among levels in the organizational hierarchy, and extensive sharing of financial and performance information.

In the final analysis, we believe that both organizational and community siblings are searching for ways of helping individuals and collectivities to benefit by mutual association. Whether these collectivities are private corporations, block associations, hospitals, or *kibbutzim*, they must ultimately be concerned with providing products or services. A pragmatic awareness of the importance of the bottom line, viewed through the lens of an organizational psychologist, can thus provide guidance for community psychologists who place well-being or empowerment first in their lexicon of values. At the same time, since organizations can achieve their objectives only with the sustained commitment of people, organizational psychologists can learn a great deal from those whose attention is focused on the welfare of the individual.

This is a challenging idea. It implies that we need to listen to those whose values may be quite different from our own. But it may also be the best way to help organizations, and the people who live in them, thrive.

ACKNOWLEDGMENT. We thank Scott Santos of the Delta Consulting Group for his assistance with the literature search for this chapter.

REFERENCES

Alderfer, C. P. (1977a). Improving organizational communication through long-term intergroup intervention. *The Journal of Applied Behavioral Science, 13*, 193–210.

Alderfer, C. P. (1977b). Organization development. *Annual Review of Psychology, 28*, 197–223.

Alderfer, C. P. (1980). Consulting to underbounded systems. In C. P. Alderfer & C. L. Cooper (Eds.), *Advances in experiential social processes, Vol. 2*, (pp. 267–295). New York: Wiley.

Alderfer, C. P., & Berg, D. N. (1977). Organizational development: The profession and the practitioner. In P. H. Mirvis & D. N. Berg (Eds.), *Failures in organization development and change: Cases and essays for learning* (pp. 89–110). New York: Wiley.

Alderfer, C. P., & Thomas, D. A. (1988). The significance of race and ethnicity for understanding organizational behavior. In C. L. Cooper & I. T. Robertson (Eds.), *International review of industrial and organizational psychology, Vol. 2* (pp. 1–41). New York: Wiley.

Allen, R. F., & Linde, S. (1981). *Lifegain*. Englewood Cliffs, NJ: Appleton.

Allport, F. H. (1933). *Institutional behavior*. Chapel Hill: University of North Carolina Press.

Argyris, C. (1979). Reflecting on laboratory education from a theory of action perspective. *The Journal of Applied Behavioral Science, 15*, 296–310.

Beekun, R. I. (1989). Assessing the effectiveness of sociotechnical interventions: Antidote or fad? *Human Relations, 42*, 877–897.

Beer, M. (1976). The technology of organization development. In M. D. Dunnette (Ed.), *Handbook of industrial and organizational psychology* (pp. 937–993). Chicago: Rand McNally.

Beer, M., & Walton, A. E. (1987). Organization change and development. *Annual Review of Psychology, 38*, 339–367.

Benne, K. D., Bradford, L. P., Gibb, J. R., & Lippitt, R. O. (Eds.). (1975). *The laboratory method of changing and learning*. Palo Alto, CA: Science and Behavior Books.

Blake, R. R., Mouton, J. S., Barnes, L. B., & Greiner, L. E. (1964). Breakthrough in organization development. *Harvard Business Review, 42*(6), 133–155.

Blake, R. R., Shepard, H. A., & Mouton, J. S. (1964). *Managing intergroup conflict in industry*. Houston: Gulf Publishing.

Blau, P. M., & Scott, W. R. (1962). *Formal organizations: A comparative approach.* San Francisco: Chandler.

Bloom, B. L. (1971). A university freshman preventive intervention program: Report of a pilot project. *Journal of Consulting and Clinical Psychology, 37,* 235–242.

Bohen, H. H., & Viveros-Long, A. (1981). *Balancing jobs and family life.* Philadelphia, PA: Temple University Press.

Bowers, D. G. (1973). OD techniques and their results in 23 organizations: The Michigan ICL study. *The Journal of Applied Behavioral Science, 9,* 21–43.

Brown, L. D. (1972). Research action: Organizational feedback, understanding, and change. *The Journal of Applied Behavioral Science, 9,* 21–43.

Brown, L. D. (1980). Planned change in underorganized systems. In T. G. Cummings (Ed.), *Systems theory for organization development* (pp. 181–203). Chichester, England: Wiley.

Campbell, J. P., & Dunnette, M. D. (1968). Effectiveness of T-group experiences in managerial training and development. *Psychological Bulletin, 70,* 73–104.

Caplan, R. D., Vinokur, A. D., Price, R. H., & van Ryn, M. (1989). Job seeking, reemployment, and mental health: A randomized field experiment in coping with job loss. *Journal of Applied Psychology, 74,* 759–769.

Cartwright, D. (1951). Achieving change in people: Some applications of group dynamics theory. *Human Relations, 4,* 381–392.

Cherniss, C. (1980). *Professional burnout in human service organizations.* New York: Praeger.

Chisholm, R. F., & Ziegenfuss, J. T. (1986). A review of applications of the sociotechnical systems approach to health care organizations. *The Journal of Applied Behavioral Science, 22,* 315–327.

Clamp, C. (1987a). History and structure of the Mondragon system of worker cooperatives. In E. M. Bennett (Ed.), *Social intervention: Theory and practice* (pp. 349–370). Lewiston, NY: Edwin Mellen.

Clamp, C. (1987b). Managing cooperation at Mondragon: Persistence and change. In E. M. Bennett (Ed.), *Social intervention: Theory and practice* (pp. 371–392). Lewiston, NY: Edwin Mellen.

Cohen, E. M., March, J. G., & Olsen, J. D. (1972). A garbage can model of organizational choice. *Administrative Science Quarterly, 17,* 1–25.

Cooke, R. A. (1985). Organizational development in school systems. In E. F. Huse & T. G. Cummings, *Organization development and change* (3rd ed., pp. 410–418). St. Paul, MN: West.

Coughlan, R. J., & Cooke, R. A. (1974). *The structural development of educational organizations.* Unpublished manuscript, University of Michigan.

Cummings, T. G. (1978). Self-regulating work groups: A socio-technical synthesis. *Academy of Management Review, 3,* 625–634.

Cummings, T. G. (1981). Designing effective work groups. In P. C. Nystrom & W. H. Starbuck (Eds.), *Handbook of organizational design, Volume 2: Remodeling organizations and their environments* (pp. 250–271). New York: Oxford University Press.

Cummings, T. G., & Molloy, E. S. (1977). *Improving productivity and the quality of work life.* New York: Praeger.

Davis, G. F., & Powell, W. W. (1992). Organizational–environment relations. In M. D. Dunnette & L. M. Hough (Eds.), *Handbook of industrial and organizational psychology, Vol. 3,* (2nd ed., pp. 269–313). Palo Alto, CA: Consulting Psychologists Press.

Ellsworth, R. B. (1973). Feedback: Asset or liability in improving treatment effectiveness? *Journal of Consulting and Clinical Psychology, 40,* 383–393.

Fairweather, G. W., Sanders, D. H., Maynard, H., & Cressler, D. L. (1969). *Community life for the mentally ill: An alternative to institutional care.* Chicago: Aldine.

Faucheux, C., Amado, G., & Laurent, A. (1982). Organizational development and change. *Annual Review of Psychology, 33,* 343–370.

Felner, R. D., Ginter, M., & Primavera, J. (1982). Primary prevention during school transitions: Social support and environmental structure. *American Journal of Community Psychology, 10,* 277–290.

Filley, A. C. (1975). *Interpersonal conflict resolution.* Glenview, IL: Scott, Foresman.

French, W. L., & Bell, C. H., Jr. (1983). A brief history of organization development. In W. L. French, C. H. Bell, Jr., & R. A. Zawacki (Eds.), *Organization development: Theory, practice, and research* (pp. 15–19). Plano, TX: Business Publications.

French, W. L., & Bell, C. H., Jr. (1990). *Organization development: Behavioral science interventions for organization improvement* (4th ed.). Englewood Cliffs, NJ: Prentice-Hall.

Friedlander, F., & Brown, L. D. (1974). Organization development. *Annual Review of Psychology, 25,* 313–341.

Friedman, D. E. (1987). Work vs. family: War of the worlds. *Personnel Administrator, 32*(8), 36–39.

Golembiewski, R. T. (1985). *Humanizing public organizations.* Mt. Airy, MD: Lomond.

Golembiewski, R. T., & Proehl, C. W., Jr. (1978). A survey of the empirical literature on flexible work hours: Character and consequence of a major innovation. *Academy of Management Review, 3,* 837–852.

Golembiewski, R. T., Proehl, C. W., Jr., & Sink, D. (1982). Estimating the success of OD applications. *Training and Development Journal, 36(4)*, 86–95.

Gomersall, E. R., & Myers, M. S. (1966). Breakthrough in on-the-job training. *Harvard Business Review, 44*(4), 62–72.

Goodstein, J. D. (1994). Institutional pressures and strategic responsiveness: Employer involvement in work-family issues. *Academy of Management Journal, 37*, 350–382.

Guion, R. M., & Gibson, W. M. (1988). Personnel selection and placement. *Annual Review of Psychology, 39*, 349–374.

Guzzo, R. A., & Dickson, M. W. (1996). Teams in organizations: Recent research on performance and effectiveness. *Annual Review of Psychology, 47*, 307–338.

Guzzo, R. A., Jette, R. D., & Katzell, R. A. (1985). The effects of psychologically based intervention programs on worker productivity: A meta-analysis. *Personnel Psychology, 38*, 275–291.

Hackman, J. R. (1992). Group influences on individuals in organizations. In M. D. Dunnette & L. M. Hough (Eds.), *Handbook of industrial and organizational psychology, Vol. 3*, (2nd ed., pp. 199–267). Palo Alto, CA: Consulting Psychologists Press.

Hackman, J. R., & Oldham, G. R. (1980). *Work redesign*. Reading, MA: Addison-Wesley.

Hartwell, T. D., Steele, P., French, M. T., Potter, F. J., Rodman, N. F., & Zarkin, G. A. (1996). Aiding troubled employees: The prevalence, cost, and characteristics of employee assistance programs in the United States. *American Journal of Public Health, 86*, 804–808.

Hausser, D. L., Pecorella, P. A., & Wissler, A. L. (1975). *Survey-guided development: A manual for consultants*. Ann Arbor, MI: Institute for Social Research.

House, J. S. (1981). *Work stress and social support*. Reading, MA: Addison-Wesley.

House, J. S., & Wells, J. A. (1978). Occupational stress, social support, and health. In A. McLean, G. Black, & M. Colligan (Eds.), *Reducing occupational stress* (pp. 8–29). DHEW (NIOSH) Publication No. 78-140. Washington, D.C.: U. S. Department of Health, Education, and Welfare.

Huse, E. F., & Cummings, T. G. (1985). *Organization development and change* (3rd ed.). St. Paul, MN: West.

Jackson, S. E., & Associates (1992). *Diversity in the workplace: Human resource initiatives*. New York: Guilford.

Jahoda, M. (1979). The impact of unemployment in the 1930's and 1970's. *Bulletin of the British Psychological Society, 32*, 309–314.

Janis, I., & Mann, D. (1977). *Decision making: A psychological analysis of conflict, choice, and commitment*. New York: Free Press.

Jayaratne, S., & Chess, W. A. (1984). The effects of emotional support on perceived job stress and strain. *The Journal of Applied Behavioral Science, 20*, 141–153.

Kaner, R. M. (1977). *Work and family in the United States: A critical review and agenda for policy*. New York: Russell Sage.

Kaplan, R. E. (1979). The conspicuous absence of evidence that process consultation enhances task performance. *The Journal of Applied Behavioral Science, 15*, 346–360.

Kasl, S., Gore, S., & Cobb, S. (1975). The experience of losing a job: Reported changes in health, symptoms, and illness behavior. *Psychosomatic Medicine, 37*, 106–122.

Katz, D., & Kahn, R. L. (1978). *The social psychology of organizations* (2nd ed.) New York: Wiley.

Katzell, R. A., & Guzzo, R. A. (1983). Psychological approaches to productivity improvement. *American Psychologist, 38*, 468–472.

Keys, C. B. (1986). Organization development: An approach to mental health consultation. In F. V. Mannino, E. J. Trickett, M. F. Shore, M. G. Kidder, & G. Levin (Eds.), *Handbook of mental health consultation* (pp. 81–112). U.S. Department of Health and Human Services, National Institute of Mental Health. Washington, D.C.: U.S. Government Printing Office, DHHS Publication No. (ADM)86-14460.

Keys, C. B., & Bartunek, J. M. (1979). Organization development in schools: Goal agreement, process skills, and diffusion of change. *The Journal of Applied Behavioral Science, 15*, 61–78.

Keys, C. B., & Frank, S. (1987). Community psychology and the study of organizations: A reciprocal relationship. *American Journal of Community Psychology, 15*, 239–251.

Kimberly, J. R., Miles, R. H., and Associates. (1980). *The organizational life cycle: Issues in the creation, transformation, and decline of organizations*. San Francisco: Jossey-Bass.

Kirchmeyer, C. (1995). Managing the work-nonwork boundary: An assessment of organizational responses. *Human Relations, 48*, 515–536.

Kobasa, S. C. O., & Puccetti, M. C. (1983). Personality processes and individual differences in resistance to stress. *Journal of Personality and Social Psychology, 45*, 839–850.

Kotter, J. P., & Haskett, J. L. (1992). *Corporate culture and performance*. New York: Free Press.

Kouzes, J. M., & Mico, P. R. (1979). Domain theory: An introduction to organizational behavior in human service organizations. *The Journal of Applied Behavioral Sciences, 15*, 449–469.

LaRocco, J. M., House, J. S., & French, J. R. P., Jr. (1980). Social support, occupational stress, and health. *Journal of Health and Social Behavior, 21*, 202–218.

LaRocco, J. M., & Jones, A. P. (1978). Co-worker and leader support as moderators of stress-strain relationships in work situations. *Journal of Applied Psychology, 63*, 629–634.

Lawler, E. E., III. (1977). Reward systems. In J. R. Hackman & J. L. Suttle (Eds.), *Improving life at work: Behavioral science approaches to organizational change* (pp. 163–225). Santa Monica, CA: Goodyear.

Lazaro, C., Shinn, M., & Robinson, P. E. (1984). Burnout, job performance, and job withdrawal behaviors. *Journal of Health and Human Resources Administration, 7*, 213–234.

Leitko, T. A., & Szczerbacki, D. (1987). Why traditional OD strategies fail in professional bureaucracies. *Organizational Dynamics, 15*(3), 52–65.

Lewin, K. (1951). *Field theory in social science.* (pp. 229–236). New York: Harper & Row.

Liem, R., & Rayman, P. (1982). Health and social costs of unemployment. *American Psychologist, 37*, 1116–1123.

Macy, B. A., & Izumi, H. (1993). Organizational change, design, and work innovation: A meta-analysis of 131 North American Field Studies—1961–1991. In R. W. Woodman & W. A. Pasmore (Eds.), *Research in organizational change and development, Vol. 7* (pp. 235–313). Greenwich, CT: JAI.

McConkie, M. L. (1985). Organization development in the public sector. In E. F. Huse & T. G. Cummings, *Organization development and change* (3rd ed., pp. 418–426). St. Paul, MN: West.

Miles, M. B., Hornstein, H. A., Callahan, D. M., Calder, P. H., & Schiavo, R. S. (1969). The consequences of survey feedback: Theory and evaluation. In W. Bennis, K. Benne, & R. Chin (Eds.), *The planning of change* (pp. 457–468). New York: Holt, Rinehart & Winston.

Miles, M. B., Hornstein, H. A., Calder, P. H., Callahan, D. M., & Schiavo, R. S. (1971). Data feedback: A rationale. In H. A. Hornstein, B. B. Bunker, W. W. Burke, M. Gindes, & R. J. Lewicki (Eds.), *Social intervention: A behavioral science approach* (pp. 310–315). New York: Free Press.

Mohrman, S., Mohrman, A., Cooke, R., & Duncan, R. (1977). A survey feedback and problem-solving intervention in a school district: "We'll take the survey but you can keep the feedback." In P. H. Mirvis & D. N. Berg (Eds.), *Failures in organization development and change: Cases and essays for learning* (pp. 149–189). New York: Wiley.

Moos, R. H. (1973). Changing the social milieus of psychiatric treatment settings. *The Journal of Applied Behavioral Science, 9*, 575–593.

Mowday, R. T., & Sutton, R. I. (1993). Organizational behavior: Linking individuals and groups to organizational contexts. *Annual Review of Psychology, 44*, 195–229.

Murrell, S. A. (1973). *Community psychology and social systems: A conceptual framework and intervention guide.* New York: Behavioral Publications.

Nadler, D. A. (1977). *Feedback and organization development: Using data-based methods.* Reading, MA: Addison-Wesley.

Nadler, D. A. (1980). Using organizational assessment data for planned organizational change. In E. E. Lawler III, D. A. Nadler, & C. Cammann (Eds.), *Organizational assessment: Perspectives on the measurement of organizational behavior and the quality of work life* (pp. 72–90). New York: Wiley.

Neuman, G. A., Edwards, J. E., & Raju, N. S. (1989). Organizational development interventions: A meta-analysis of their effects on satisfaction and other attitudes. *Personnel Psychology, 42*, 461–489.

Nicholas, J. M. (1982). The comparative impact of organizational development interventions on hard criteria measures. *Academy of Management Review, 7*, 531–542.

Nollen, S. D. (1982). *New work schedules in practice: Managing time in a changing society.* New York: Van Nostrand Reinhold.

Norstedt, J. P., & Aguren, S. (1973). *The Saab-Scania report.* Stockholm: Swedish Employers Confederation.

Nystrom, P. C. (1981). Designing jobs and assigning employees. In P. C. Nystrom & W. H. Starbuck (Eds.), *Handbook of organizational design, Volume 2: Remodeling organizations and their environments* (pp. 272–301). New York: Oxford University Press.

Offermann, L. R., & Gowing, M. K. (1990). Organizations of the future: Changes and challenges. *American Psychologist, 45*, 95–108.

Oldham, G. R., & Hackman, J. R. (1980). Work design in the organizational context. In B. M. Staw & L. L. Cummings (Eds.), *Research in organizational behavior, Vol. 2* (pp. 247–278). Greenwich, CT: JAI.

Pasmore, W. A. (1976). The Michigan ICL study revisited: An alternative explanation of the results. *The Journal of Applied Behavioral Science, 12*, 245–251.

Pasmore, W., Francis, C., & Haldeman, J. (1982). Sociotechnical systems: A North American reflection on empirical studies of the seventies. *Human Relations, 12*, 1179–1204.

Pasmore, W., Petee, J., & Bastian, R. (1986). Sociotechnical systems in health care: A field experiment. *The Journal of Applied Behavioral Science, 22*, 329–339.

Perkins, D. N. T. (1981). *Toward a theory of intervention in new organizations*. Unpublished manuscript, Yale University, New Haven, CT.

Perkins, D. N. T., Nieva, V. F., & Lawler, E. E., III. (1983). *Managing creation: The challenge of building a new organization*. New York: Wiley.

Pfeffer, J. (1985). Organizations and organization theory. In G. Lindzey & E. Aronson (Eds.) *Handbook of social psychology Vol. 1* (3rd ed., pp. 379–440). New York: Random House.

Pfeffer, J. (1998a). *The human equation: Building profits by putting people first*. Boston: Harvard Business School Press.

Pfeffer, J. (1998b). Understanding organizations: Concepts and controversies. In D. T. Gilbert, S. T. Fiske, & G. Lindzey (Eds.), *Handbook of Social Psychology Vol. 2* (4th ed., pp. 733–777). New York: Oxford University Press (McGraw-Hill).

Pierce, W., Trickett, E., & Moos, R. (1972). Changing ward atmosphere through staff discussion of the perceived ward environment. *Archives of General Psychiatry, 26*, 35–41.

Porras, J. I. (1979). The comparative impact of different OD techniques and intervention intensities. *The Journal of Applied Behavioral Science, 15*, 156–178.

Porras, J. I., & Berg, P. O. (1978). The impact of organization development. *Academy of Management Review, 3*, 249–266.

Porras, J. I., & Robertson, P. J. (1992). Organizational development: Theory, practice, and research. In M. D. Dunnette & L. M. Hough (Eds.), *Handbook of industrial and organizational psychology Vol. 3* (2nd ed., pp. 269–313). Palo Alto, CA: Consulting Psychologists Press.

Porras, J. I., & Silvers, R. C. (1991). Organization development and transformation. *Annual Review of Psychology, 42*, 51–78.

Porter, L. W., Lawler, E. E., & Hackman, J. R. (1975). *Behavior in organizations*. New York: McGraw-Hill.

Rappaport, J. (1981). In praise of paradox: A social policy of empowerment over prevention. *American Journal of Community Psychology, 9*, 1–25.

Rice, A. K. (1958). *Productivity and social organization: the Ahmedabad experiment*. London: Tavistock.

Riger, S. (1983/84). Vehicles for empowerment: The case of feminist movement organizations. *Prevention in Human Services, 3*(2/3), 99–117.

Roberts, K. H., Hulin, C. L., & Rousseau, D. M. (1978). *Developing an interdisciplinary science of organizations*. San Francisco: Jossey-Bass.

Ronen, S. (1981). *Flexible working hours: An innovation in the quality of work life*. New York: McGraw-Hill.

Ross, R. (1971). OD for whom? *The Journal of Applied Behavioral Science, 7*, 580–585.

Rousseau, D. M. (1985). Issues of level in organizational research: Multi-level and cross-level perspectives. In L. L. Cummings & B. M. Staw (Eds.), *Research in organizational behavior, Vol. 7* (pp. 1–37). Greenwich, CT: JAI.

Rousseau, D. M. (1997). Organizational behavior in the new organizational era. *Annual Review of Psychology, 48*, 515–546.

Sarason, S. B. (1972). *The creation of settings and the future societies*. San Francisco: Jossey-Bass.

Schein, E. H. (1990). Organizational culture. *American Psychologist, 45*, 109–119.

Schein, E. H., & Bennis, W. G. (1965). *Personal and organizational changes through group methods: The laboratory approach*. New York: Wiley.

Schmitt, N., & Robertson, I. (1990). Personnel selection. *Annual Review of Psychology, 41*, 289–319.

Schneider, B. (1985). Organizational behavior. *Annual Review of Psychology, 36*, 573–611.

Schuster, F. E. (1986). *The Schuster report: The proven connection between people and profits*. New York: Wiley.

Seidman, E. (1988). Back to the future, community psychology: Unfolding a theory of social intervention. *American Journal of Community Psychology, 16*, 3–24.

Seidman, E. (1990). Pursuing the meaning and utility of social regularities for community psychology. In P. Tolan, C. Keys, F. Chertok, & L. Jason (Eds.), *Researching community psychology: Issues of theory and methods* (pp. 91–100). Washington, D.C.: American Psychological Association.

Serrano-Garcia, I. (1983/84). The illusion of empowerment: Community development within a colonial context. *Prevention in Human Services, 3*(2/3), 173–200.

Shinn, M., Mørch, H., Robinson, P. E., & Neuner, R. A. (1993). Individual, group, and agency strategies for coping with job stressors in residential child care programmes. *Journal of Community and Applied Social Psychology, 3*, 313–324.

Shinn, M., Perkins, D. N. T., & Cherniss, C. (1980). Using survey-guided development to improve program climates: An experimental evaluation in group homes for youths. In R. Stough & A. Wandersman (Eds.), *Optimizing environments: Research, practice, and policy* (pp. 124–135). Washington, D.C.: EDRA.

Shinn, M., Rosario, M., Mørch, H., & Chestnut, D. E. (1984). Coping with job stress and burnout in the human services. *Journal of Personality and Social Psychology, 46*, 864–876.

Shinn, M., Wong, N. W., Simko, P. A., & Ortiz-Torres, B. (1989). Promoting the well-being of working parents: Coping, social support, and flexible job schedules. *American Journal of Community Psychology*, *17*, 31–55.

Silverstein, P., & Srb, J. H. (1979). *Flextime: Where, when, and how?* Key issues series, No. 24, Ithaca, NY: Cornell University.

Smith, P. B. (1975). Controlled studies of the outcome of sensitivity training. *Psychological Bulletin*, *82*, 597–622.

Sonnenstuhl, W. J. (1988). Contrasting employee assistance, health promotion, and quality of work life programs and their effects on alcohol abuse and dependence. *The Journal of Applied Behavioral Science*, *24*, 347–363.

Sonnenstuhl, W. J. (1996). *Working sober: The transformation of an occupational drinking culture*. Ithaca, NY: ILR Press/Cornell.

Staines, G. L., & Pleck, J. H. (1985, August). *Work schedules, flexibility, and family life*. Paper presented at the meetings of the American Psychological Association, Los Angeles.

Steele, P. D. (Ed.) (1988). Substance abuse and the workplace: Special attention to employee assistance programs. Special Issue, *The Journal of Applied Behavioral Science*, *24*(4), 315–469.

Sundstrom, E., De Meuse, K. P., & Futrell, D. (1990). Work teams: Applications and effectiveness. *American Psychologist*, *45*, 120–133.

Taber, T. D., Walsh, J. T., & Cooke, R. A. (1979). Developing a community-based program for reducing the impact of a plant closing. *The Journal of Applied Behavioral Science*, *15*, 133–155.

Thorsrud, E., Sorensen, B. S., & Gustavsen, B. (1976). Sociotechnical approach to industrial democracy in Norway. In R. Dubin (Ed.), *Handbook of work, organization, and society* (pp. 421–464). Chicago: Rand McNally.

Tichy, N. M. (1985). Organizational development in health care. In E. F. Huse & T. G. Cummings, *Organization development and change* (3rd ed., pp. 432–437). St. Paul, MN: West.

Tolan, P., Keys, C., Chertok, F., & Jason, L. (Eds.) (1990) *Researching community psychology: Issues of theory and methods*. Washington, D.C.: American Psychological Association.

Triandis, H. C., Kurowski, L. L., & Gelfand, M. J. (1994). Workplace diversity. In H. C. Triandis, M. D. Dunnette & L. M. Hough (Eds.), *Handbook of industrial and organizational psychology Vol. 4*, (2nd ed., pp. 769–827). Palo Alto, CA: Consulting Psychologists Press.

Trice, H. M., & Roman, P. M. (1972). *Spirits and demons at work: Alcohol and other drugs on the job*. Ithaca, NY: New York State School of Industrial and Labor Relations, Cornell University.

Trist, E. (1986). Quality of working life and community development: Some reflections on the Jamestown experience. *The Journal of Applied Behavioral Science*, *22*, 223–237.

Trist, E. L., & Bamforth, K. W. (1951). Some social and psychological consequences of the long-wall method of coal getting. *Human Relations*, *4*, 3–38.

Vinokur, A. D., Price, R. H., & Schul, Y. (1995). Impact of the jobs intervention on unemployed workers varying in risk for depression. *American Journal of Community Psychology*, *23*, 39–74.

Vinokur, A. D., van Ryn, M., Gramlich, E. M., & Price, R. H. (1991). Long-term follow-up and benefit-cost analysis of the Jobs Project: A preventive intervention for the unemployed. *Journal of Applied Psychology*, *76*, 213–219.

Walton, R. E. (1969). *Interpersonal peacemaking: Confrontations and third party consultation*. Reading, MA: Addison-Wesley.

Walton, R. E., & Schlesinger, L. A. (1979). Do supervisors thrive in participatory work systems? *Organizational Dynamics*, *7*(3), 25–38.

Walton, R. E., & Warwick, D. P. (1973). The ethics of organizational development. *The Journal of Applied Behavioral Science*, *9*, 681–698.

Wanous, J. P. (1975). A job preview makes recruiting more effective. *Harvard Business Review*, *53*, 166–168.

Wanous, J. P. (1977). Organizational entry: The individual's viewpoint. In J. R. Hackman, E. E. Lawler, & L. W. Porter (Eds.), *Perspectives on behavior in organizations* (pp. 126–135). New York: McGraw-Hill.

Weick, K. E. (1976). Educational organizations as loosely coupled systems. *Administrative Science Quarterly*, *21*, 1–19.

Wilpert, B. (1995). Organizational behavior. *Annual Review of Psychology*, *46*, 59–90.

Winett, R. A., & Neale, M. S. (1980). Results of an experimental study on flextime and family life. *Monthly Labor Review*, *103*(11), 29–32.

Woodman, R. W., & Sherwood, J. J. (1980). The role of team development in organizational effectiveness: A critical review. *Psychological Bulletin*, *88*, 166–186.

Zand, D. E. (1974). Collateral organization: A new change strategy. *The Journal of Applied Behavioral Science*, *10*, 63–89.

Zedeck, S., & Mosier, K. L. (1990). Work in the family and employing organization. *American Psychologist*, *45*, 240–251.

PART V

DESIGN, ASSESSMENT, AND ANALYTIC METHODS

A complete compendium of measurement and methodological issues in community psychology would require its own handbook. No such goal is intended here. However, the four chapters in this section, read in conjunction with one another, highlight many of the most interesting problems of design, assessment, and analysis for our field. Collectively, these chapters present an approach that emphasizes contextual awareness and ecological validity, either directly or by reference to further reading. Individually, each chapter offers a somewhat different perspective on the issues of assessment.

Much of psychological research has been based on measures of individuals, social climates, observational inventories, physical environment indices, demographics, social indicators, and geographic information systems—each assessed as if frozen in time, culturally bound, and laden with theoretical assumptions. We begin this section with Linney's chapter on contextual assessment, a central issue for community psychologists, most of whom hold a systems, ecological point of view in theory and practice. How can we approach empirical research with that same sensitivity?

Linney describes conceptions of context as shared perceptions, material surroundings, and social regularities. In this chapter, demographic measures are discussed as "proxy" variables, while social regularities are seen to involve ratios and temporal patterns (Seidman, 1988). Linney asserts a conceptualization of context that views physical and social material as opportunities for, and constraints on, action. She proposes multimodal and transactional models to assess multidimensional, dynamic relationships. The behavior setting or standing pattern of behavior is highlighted as a unit of analysis. Linney suggests strategic sampling of contexts, multimethods and analysis of linkages among levels of analysis, and qualitative and descriptive methods, as well as assessment of stability and change over time.

In the next chapter, Shinn and Rapkin address the complexities of cross-level research, wherein one is interested in relationships among two or more variables at different levels of analysis, a central conceptual, methodological, and analytic problem for the community psychologist. Their chapter addresses problems that arise with a "mismatch" between conceptualization and measurement. Shinn and Rapkin specifically propose the use of hierarchical linear statistical models. Five types of cross-level relationships, varying by nature and direction of effect between levels, are discussed, including effects of variables at one level on variables at another level, deviations from a group standard, controlling for multiple-level relationships by decomposition of aggregate correlations, moderating effects of variables at one level on another, and effects of person–environment fit. At the heart of their chapter is a conceptual map that articulates an essential theme of community psychology: Our concepts require both individual and systems variables, and our analyses (conceptual as well as analytic) must address this fact, if we are to have a genuine community psychology.

Programs for change benefit from a conscious consideration of the criteria: How will we know if we have seen change? How will we know if our interventions are worth dissemination? There are many ways to analyze data—a topic that is beyond the scope of this volume. However, considerations of the nature of change and its conceptualization are of some importance to community psychology. The chapter by Tanaka concerns statistical models for change using a "construct-focused approach." We include it in this section because the desire to stimulate, facilitate, or encourage change is so central to why we engage in the strategies and tactics of community intervention in the first place.

In this context, we view statistical measurement of change as yet another strategy for gaining both understanding and support for our work. As noted in our earlier remarks concerning the other sections of this volume, it is not that we think policy decisions and social changes are simply rational decisions made on the basis of who has the most appropriate statistical analysis; but rather, such analysis can contribute to the activity of the community psychologist as much as the craft of community collaboration. Awareness of, if not expert status in, a range of competencies for thinking about change are a part of the community psychologist's repertoire.

Tanaka reminds us that methods for analysis are tools; they are only as good as our projects and our constructs. If the project is ill-conceived or our constructs are not meaningful over time, methods for analysis will not save us. This chapter repeatedly highlights the interconnections of method and theory in a sophisticated way, using examples relevant to community work. It highlights some of the problems associated with assessment of change, including its conceptualization in terms of multiple processes, dimensions, and units. Statistical methods appropriate to different conceptualizations of change are offered. Structural equation models with latent variables are suggested as well suited to correlational data in longitudinal designs. Changes in means and variances and covariances are discussed in terms of growth curve or autoregressive models. Time series and survival models are introduced. Tanaka reminds us of the problems of "lagged effects," and of the possibility that we may not be measuring the same construct over time. Among the other important reminders for those of us who seek to evaluate change in community work is the importance of both multiple measures and within-group analysis to understand why an intervention works for some, but not for others.

The final chapter in this section, by Stewart, tells yet another story about how to conduct research while doing community work. He reminds us that the roots of qualitative approaches to research are both longstanding and contemporary in the social sciences. In university psychology departments, qualitative methods have been, until quite recently, marginalized. There is little formal training available without going to other disciplines. But Stewart points us to a variety of sources where we can find exemplars. He explicitly rejects the juxtaposition of quantitative and qualitative as either/or propositions for our field, and instead proposes an educational information-sharing approach to increasing our methodological options.

Community psychology, with its emphasis on diversity of voice, cultural understanding, and local context is ideally positioned in terms of its values and goals to make good use of qualitative methods, ranging from interview to participant observation, from ethnography to interpretative and critical analysis. These are methods suitable to amplify the voices of those who have been silenced, to foreground the expertise of the oppressed, and to honestly portray ourselves as a part of that process, even as we try to represent "others." We can use as many tools as we can find in the business of understanding and fostering individual, social, and community change, and Stewart makes the case that qualitative research belongs in the armamentarium of the community psychologist.

In addition to pointing the reader toward the philosophical and practical underpinnings of qualitative work, Stewart's chapter raises a variety of ethical questions that pose important dilemmas for our field, whatever one's choice of method. It may be that all community work is what Stewart calls, "an ethically tricky proposition." While advocating for a plurality of methods, Stewart also asks us to be critical analysts of our own assumptions, practices, and procedures. In this sense his chapter, like much of the field of community psychology, is sympathetic to the notion of a critical psychology (see Fox & Prilleltensky, 1997, for an overview of that related field).

REFERENCES

Fox, D., & Prilleltensky, I. (Eds.). (1997). *Critical psychology: An introduction.* Thousand Oaks, CA: Sage.

Seidman, E. (1988). Back to the future, community psychology: Unfolding the theory of social intervention. *American Journal of Community Psychology, 16*, 3–24.

CHAPTER 27

Assessing Ecological Constructs and Community Context

JEAN ANN LINNEY

From its earliest beginnings, "the reciprocal relationships between individuals and the social systems with which they interact" (Bennett, Anderson, Cooper, Hassol, Klein, & Rosenblum, 1966, p. 7)—the study of persons in ecological context—has been a central theme for community psychology. Much of the thinking in this field has been predicated on the assumption that the behavior of individuals can be better understood when contextual factors are considered, a proposition well explicated by Lewin (1935) and Bronfenbrenner (1979, 1995), but translated into research and action in only limited ways. For at least 75 years ecological context has been silently recognized as an essential dimension for understanding human behavior, but most research in psychology has followed a strategy of studying individual variation with context held constant.

Recently there has been a resurgence in attention to the role of context stimulated both by limitations in studying only individuals and by new developments in several research areas. Ease of access to multivariate statistical techniques has enabled researchers to examine relational patterns between indices of context and measures of individual behavior, and to statistically model their separate and joint contributions (Bryk & Raudenbush, 1992; Kenny, 1996; Kenny & Judd, 1996). New research in behavior genetics has focused attention on the role of the environment in understanding how genes may be expressed and modified (Plomin & Neiderhiser, 1992; Neiderhiser, Reiss, & Hetherington, 1996; Reiss, 1997). Developmental research has increasingly incorporated family, peer group, and school variables in predictive models (Coie, Watt, West, Hawkins, Asarnow, Markman, Ramey, Shure, & Long, 1993). Greater awareness of cross-cultural variation in social, personality, and cognitive phenomena have further highlighted ecological contributions. Both community psychologists and preventionists have called for greater attention to assessment of context to enhance adoption and implementation of interventions (Blakely, Mayer, Gottschalk, Schmitt, Davidson, Roitman, & Emshoff, 1987; Kelly, 1990, 1991).

JEAN ANN LINNEY • Department of Psychology, Barnwell College, University of South Carolina, Columbia, South Carolina 29208.

Handbook of Community Psychology, edited by Julian Rappaport and Edward Seidman. Kluwer Academic / Plenum Publishers, New York, 2000.

CONCEPTIONS OF ECOLOGICAL CONTEXT

What is meant by ecological context and how has context been studied? Like theories of individual behavior, context has been conceptualized in several quite different ways and studied with different methodologies. Despite considerable discussion about the importance of contextual influences and person–situation psychology, there is not consensus with respect to a conceptual framework to guide research, nor a common set of constructs, variables, instruments, or methodologies.

Conceptualizations of context have developed from personality research on person–situation interactions. Context has been defined as the shared perceptions of members of the setting, patterns of interpersonal relationships, and the effect of variation in a quantifiable contextual stimulus such as resource availability (cf. Walsh, Craik, & Price, 1992). Much of this work has had the goal of understanding individual response to contextual variation, with context viewed as a factor moderating individual behavior.

Others theorists have suggested that context should be studied as a construct separate and distinct from the specific persons involved in the setting, as a set of "rules" or operations that characterize the setting, set the agenda, and prescribe limits for behavior of individuals in the setting (Seidman, 1988; Trickett, Kelly, & Todd, 1972). One example of this approach, the social ecology model, draws concepts from biological ecology and general systems theory positing important ecological processes separate and distinct from the individual inhabitants of any particular context. Consistent with the premise that context is distinct from the perceptions and behavior of the setting inhabitants, physical environmental features of settings and social indicator data have also been studied as "person-free" indices of context.

A third perspective on context is based on the transactional supposition that individual behavior and situations must be considered simultaneously, rather than in some separate or sequential causal relationship (e.g., Barker, 1968, 1987; Altman & Rogoff, 1987); that behavior and context are inextricably intertwined. Transactional perspectives, more than other views, have stressed the importance of studying development and change over time in persons and settings. As presently articulated, transactional conceptions of context tend to rely on qualitative, naturalistic research methods.

Community and developmental psychologists have suggested that ecological context should be conceptualized at multiple levels (Bronfenbrenner, 1979; Rappaport, 1977; Seidman, 1987). While several schematic frameworks have been proposed using different terminology (e.g., micro, meso, exo, macro, or individual, small group, organization, community), they share the assumption that there are multiple layers of context that mutually influence one another. Analysis at each level of context enhances understanding of behavior or functional patterns at another level. For example, studies of classroom student–teacher interaction patterns may be better understood and explained by considering the overarching goals of the school as an institution and its role in the community. Successful implementation of cooperative learning in school classrooms, for example, may be limited by the competing institutional agenda of sorting, rank ordering, and selecting functions that the education system serves for other community systems (Tyack & Cuban, 1995; Wagner, 1990).

Most conceptions of ecological context posit some model of mutual reciprocity in which persons affect context and context affects persons. There is considerable debate, however, about the nature of these patterns of influence, and the appropriate methods for determining the mediating and moderating effects. Context as an entity for study is more likely a moving, changing target, rather than a fixed stage upon which behavior unfolds (Linney, 1991). As developmental processes have become more prominent in theories of individuals, so too it has also become increasingly important to focus on dynamic models of ecological context. Pairing the notion of changing individuals with changing contexts greatly increases the complexity of these models, however, and presents a formidable challenge for measurement and modeling.

Before describing specific approaches to assessing context, it is important to recognize that the particular model or conceptual framework of ecological context and the strategy chosen for studying it is dependent on the nature of the questions guiding a particular project. For the developmental or clinical researcher, context is typically a less salient focus than the individual and, thus, indices of context most prevalent within this arena are likely to address the immediate context (e.g., small groups, family, peer networks) and be most obviously connected to individuals. Analysts of public policy, organizational behavior, and service-system design are more likely to focus on the system of settings, with less attention paid to the specific individuals occupying those settings. Increasingly, these perspectives are overlapping, but it is important to recognize that differences in frameworks and assumptions have resulted in alternative conceptual models and assessment strategies.

In the following sections, assessment strategies and specific instruments derived from different conceptual models of context are described. The intention here is to provide the reader with perspective on the scope of methods potentially available and some consideration of the advantages, limitations, and applications of these multiple approaches.

Context as Participant Perceptions of the Environment

The most widely used assessments of settings and environments are instruments based on Murray's (1938) theory of person–environment interaction, which posits that individuals respond to environments in both idiosyncratic and normative ways. Murray suggested that environments convey normative expectations for behavior, what he called environmental press. Shared perceptions of persons in any given setting are considered evidence of environmental press, and thus have been conceptualized to be characteristics of the setting, or its environmental demands. Based on this conceptual framework, Moos and colleagues developed the social climate scales to assess the shared perceptions of the members of a setting (Moos, 1994).

The social climate scales define three primary dimensions characterizing a setting: (1) a relationship dimension with components such as supportiveness, involvement, and cohesion; (2) a personal development dimension including autonomy and self-enhancement; and (3) a system maintenance and change dimension comprised of components like order, clarity, and control in the setting. Persons in the settings report their perception of that setting and their perception of the ideal for the setting on a set of true–false items pertaining to each of the three primary dimensions. Each social climate measure yields a profile of scores based on the aggregated responses of the members of the setting for the primary dimensions and associated subscales. Social climate scales are available for several small group and organizational settings, including work and family environments, university residence halls, psychiatric inpatient settings, correctional settings, community treatment settings, supported community-living facilities, and classroom environments.

The social-climate scales are probably the most commonly used quantitative measures of context at the small-group and organizational levels of analysis. They yield easily acquired, face-valid assessments of a specific setting. Subscale scores have been statistically related to measures of individual well-being, such as job satisfaction and psychological adjustment (Repetti & Cosmas, 1991), individual-involvement indices like school attendance (Moos,

1979; Moos & Moos, 1978), and outcomes of treatment, like recidivism among juvenile offenders (Moos, 1975). The scales have been used to describe variation within a class of settings, e.g., sheltered-care environments (Timko & Moos, 1991), and in consultation and intervention programs (Bliss, Moos, & Bromet, 1976).

This model of ecological assessment has not been without criticism. Factor analytic studies of the social climate scales failed to confirm the theoretically specified subscale structure of the instruments (e.g., Alden, 1978; Boake & Salmon, 1983). Some have suggested that the measures are not more than assessments of overall satisfaction by the members of the setting (Brady, Kinnard, & Friedrich, 1980; Wilkinson, 1973), rather than a measure of qualities of the environment that are separate and distinct from the responding individuals (Hall & Pill, 1975). Shared-method variance between the social climate scales and other self-report measures has also been suggested to account for the statistically significant correlations typically reported.

Trickett, Trickett, Castro, and Schaffner (1982) have reported low correlations between scores on the classroom environment scale derived from students and those of independent observers, even after extended observations in the same classrooms. Raviv, Raviv, and Reisel (1990) report differences in social climate measurements between teachers and students in the same classroom. These findings suggest that the measures are tapping perceptions of members that appear to be dependent not only on membership in the setting, but also on one's role in the setting. The weak correspondence between observers and setting members suggests that the scales may not assess characteristics of the environment separate and distinct from the experience of membership.

Despite conceptual and psychometric criticism, the social climate scales are widely used and have demonstrated significant relationships with behavioral outcomes that have practical importance, such as recidivism among juvenile offenders and grades in school. It may be that the social climate measures do a better job at identifying individuals who are likely to succeed than other individual-level assessments, or that the measures can identify combinations of organizational practice and individual affect related to successful outcomes.

Repetti and colleagues (Repetti, 1987; Repetti & Cosmas, 1991) compared individual perceptions and aggregated perceptions of the workplace as predictors of individual outcomes. They report that aggregated ratings were more predictive of individual job satisfaction than the individual's own ratings, but individual ratings were more closely associated with measures of depression and anxiety than aggregated perceptions. This pattern of findings suggests that setting characteristics may be important correlates of setting specific behavior and attitudes, for example, job satisfaction, but less relevant to broader indices of adjustment, consistent with theoretical models hypothesizing the interdependence of person and setting.

Extensive research with the social climate scales leaves a number of unanswered questions with respect to what they are measuring, and further suggests that ecological context can be associated with individual behavior in several differing ways, yet to be studied in depth. Processes accounting for the predictive relationships that have been reported are not only of theoretical importance, but also of practical significance. Articulation of these linkages can be useful in prescribing characteristics of settings that might guide change efforts, thus leading to desirable outcomes for the setting participants.

Whether the social climate measures assess a unique construct reflecting the integration of personal variables and the social setting, or are simply assessments of the individual's personal construal of their environment is not clear. Nevertheless, this assessment strategy appears to have descriptive validity, although its prescriptive utility is yet to be been convincingly demonstrated. Work with the social climate scales and this conceptualization of context supports the value of examining both subjective and objective dimensions of environments.

Study of the same individuals across different settings and the degree to which experience in one setting affects another may be fruitful directions for future research. This method may provide a means for studying similarity in perceptions of identification of common ecological dimensions across situations, the differential predictive power of individual perceptions, and the role of collective perceptions in the behavioral patterns of different types of settings. Longitudinal analyses of members entry into and departure from different settings are needed to better understand the person–setting relationship and the role of setting perception for understanding individual behavior.

Context as Objective and Observable Dimensions

Observation Inventories

A few ecological constructs and specific setting types have been assessed following a traditional psychometric approach to measurement development in which a contextual construct is hypothesized, items thought to reflect the construct are rationally generated, and a subset of items empirically are selected using data from large samples and criterion groups to establish discriminant validity. The PASS (Program Analysis of Service Systems; Wolfensberger & Glenn, 1975) is an example of this approach.

The PASS is a comprehensive rating of the degree to which a treatment setting reflects the construct of normalization (Wolfensberger, 1972). The measure includes 48 ratings theoretically defined as indicators of the normalization construct, for example, physical integration of the facility with the community; proximity to community resources; socially integrative programs and images; projection of deviant images through the physical environment; programming and staffing; age-appropriate facilities and programming; resident autonomy and rights as reflected in activities, programs, and routines; quality and comfort in the setting; and overall model coherency and administration consistent with the normalization ideology. Each item of the measure is rated after two to three days of observation in the setting by each of the members of a team of four to six observers. Each observer completes the ratings independently, with disagreements resolved by discussion and consensus. The individual-item ratings are combined to form a total PASS score for the agency or program, and a subscale score reflecting the quality of the physical facilities. The authors intended the instrument to be used in the evaluation and certification of residential settings for the mentally retarded, particularly for the purposes of stimulating change toward more normalizing settings. Following standard procedures for measurement development, Flynn and Heal (1980) examined internal consistency and item intercorrelations. The instrument has been modified for use in the assessment of residential facilities for other groups (Linney, 1982b; Mulvey, Linney, & Rosenberg, 1987).

The PASS is an example of measurement development for a construct defined in terms of contextual indicators. It focuses exclusively on the setting, policies, and organizational procedures that theoretically should reflect the concept of normalization. Use of the measure does not rely on the reports or perceptions of the members of the setting. Rather, indices are directly observed or available from the archives and records of the setting (e.g., staff development, evaluation procedures). The measure incorporates physical and social facets of the setting, as well as administrative policy and staffing.

Normalization as a construct, like some other constructs in community psychology, has most commonly been measured by assessing the degree to which members of the setting change. That method of assessment does not directly assess the environment, but rather the effectiveness of the setting in modifying the performance and behavior of the individuals present. In contrast, the PASS measures the construct directly at the setting level, following a traditional model of instrument development applied to an ecologically defined construct. While it does not assess the transactional aspects of a normalizing setting (i.e., how the setting interfaces with its members), the instrument can be useful in developing taxonomies of settings based on the normalization construct, and data from the PASS could be related to patterns of individual resident outcomes, thus providing important descriptive information.

A number of other observation instruments for assessment of specific environments have been developed following this psychometric procedure, e.g., the Hospice Environmental Survey (Taylor & Perrill, 1987), which assesses the extent to which hospice settings provide a "homelike atmosphere," the Environmental Assessment Index (Poresky, 1987), for rural home environments, and the School Environment Inventory (Linney, Forman, & Levy, 1988), assessing observable indicators of student and teacher morale, rigidity, and responsiveness to student behavior. The Assessment Profile for Early Childhood Programs (Abbott-Shim & Sibley, 1987) and the Home Observation for Measurement of the Environment (HOME) (Caldwell & Bradley, 1994) combine measurement of physical environmental indices with observer ratings of interaction patterns, norms, and policies. The items included in these instruments were derived from a theoretically specified model of ideal environmental influences for each setting.

Observation inventories like these are based on the construct-validation approach to measurement development, which is well established in psychology. Measures of this type might be developed for other prominent constructs in the field (e.g., empowerment, sense of community) at the small-group, organizational, and community levels of analysis. Instruments developed within this methodological and conceptual framework could include assessment of the physical features of the environment, global interaction patterns, and norms and policies regarding adaptation and resource exchanges. They are, however, generally "snapshot" measures describing the setting, and not measures of process or transaction. While items are grounded in observable actions, the calibration of response options may limit their sensitivity in detecting change. Another caution with this type of measure is cross-cultural applicability. In operationalizing an ecological construct, it is likely that the indicator items may reflect a particular cultural perspective. The HOME, for example, values a child-centered, visually and physically stimulating environment with substantial parent–child interaction. The measure may have limited validity in communities in which sibling relationships and peer teaching are more prominent.

Physical Environment Indices of Context

Context can be conceptualized as the physical characteristics of a setting—a conceptual definition that separates the person from the setting. In traditional laboratory research, physical characteristics of the experimental situation are frequently held constant on the assumption that these may have an effect on the identified variables being studied. So also outside of the laboratory, physical features of environments have been related to social behavior, development, and satisfaction for the persons in the setting. For example, space and furniture arrangement can significantly affect the social behavior of patients in hospital settings (Zimring, Carpman, & Michelson, 1987). Seating arrangements in the elementary school classroom have been associated with levels of social interaction and on-task behavior (cf. Gump, 1987). The availability of toys and manipulable objects in the home has been associated with developmental competence (cf. Wohlhill & Heft, 1987).

Craik and Feimer (1987) use the term "technical environmental assessments" to describe a class of physical environmental measurements that are based on the use of standard metrics (e.g., decibel level, units per specified area) and typically involve observable, tangible environmental qualities such as space, color, furniture arrangement, or lighting. There is a large body of research in environmental psychology that involves these physical environmental indicators and the effect of differing environmental conditions on the behavior of the individuals in those environments (cf. Stokols & Altman, 1987; Sundstrom, Bell, Busby, & Asmus, 1996).

The range of physical characteristics that might be measured is unlimited. Variables representing multiple levels of analysis can be formed from counts, ratios, or ratings done by an observer. At the small-group level of family or classroom, for example, such indices might include the number of books available, arrangement of furniture, distribution of space by function, or distribution of personal space per person. An evaluative and qualitative dimension can be incorporated within assessments of the physical environment by training observers to rate the quality of the setting and its objects, e.g., the amount of wear and tear on furniture, cleanliness of the facility, or litter in the yard. At the organizational level, physical environmental measures might include the size of the student body in a school, the number of classrooms in the building, or student/teacher ratios. Communities might be assessed in terms of the percentage of space devoted to parks, outdoor lighting levels, or the ratio of different types of housing units.

Naturalistic observation of behavior in settings that systematically vary on selected physical dimensions can inform both understanding of the limit-setting capacity of a context as well as patterns of behavioral adaptation. The ways in which inhabitants modify the physical setting may provide important insight into ideal person/environment matches, a relational construct important to a community psychology perspective. In providing limits or parameters for behavior, physical environment features both trigger and inhibit specific patterns of social behavior, cognitions, and learning. For example, research on furniture arrangements in residential psychiatric treatment settings contributed to hypotheses about the need for privacy and personal space as conditions for social behavior. Likewise, physical environments can be arranged to better match the psychological needs of setting inhabitants, as demonstrated in Lawton's research on physical characteristics of living units for elderly or disabled persons (cf. Lawton, 1990), for example. Both observation and experimentation with changeable features of the physical environment are useful strategies for enhancing understanding of person/situation transactions and incorporating context into theories of individual behavior.

In contrast to the social climate scales, technical environmental assessments of the environment are based on a unidimensional conception of the environment, i.e., in terms of its physical characteristics. Certain ubiquitous environmental features may be unrelated to the perceptions and behavior of the people living and working in the settings. For example, indices of pollution may be imperceptible to the inhabitants of the setting, although in the long term they are likely to have a significant impact on the behavior and well-being of the inhabitants. Conversely, for a number of physical environmental characteristics, it is the perception of the inhabitants that may be more predictive of the impact of the environment on persons than the objective level of those physical variables. Research on crowding provides an illustration. While there is some disagreement as to the specific measure that best defines crowding, it can be defined in objective terms, and the same objective level of crowding can be experienced by individuals in a variety of places. Depending on the place and the expectations of the individuals, however, a given level of crowding will be experienced with more or less discomfort and will have a differential impact on behavior (Baum & Paulus, 1987). Likewise, Wandersman and Hallman (1993) have shown that the presence of a toxic-waste site can affect citizen perceptions of well-being and reports of health problems, regardless of the actual threat to health.

The physical environment sets limits for living environments, and as such is an important contextual dimension to assess. Measures of the physical environment have been predictive of patterns of behavior for groups of setting participants. Predictions of behavior and adjustment for a single individual seem to be enhanced by the inclusion of subjective perceptions in addition to technical environmental measures. Research with a physical environmental conceptualization of context can be extremely useful in the design of settings (e.g., neighborhoods, workplaces, residential facilities) and in the study of behavior patterns over time, as these change the physical environment and are changed by the environment.

Demographic and Social Indicator Measures of Context

A common way to operationalize context is the use of a demographic variable to represent some condition outside the person. For example, "family context" might be operationalized as the number of parents in the home or household size. "Neighborhood context" could be indicated by the percentage of owner-occupied homes in a specified area, and "community context" as the modal socioeconomic status derived from census tract data. These single demographic indicators can hardly be called conceptually derived variables, yet they represent indicators of ecological dimensions and provide easily obtained and quantifiable indices appropriate for use in statistical modeling. Many of these so-called contextual indices have been significantly correlated with individual behavior, for example, the single-parent family, high neighborhood crime rates, and high rates of public assistance in the community have been associated with rates of illegal drug and alcohol use by adolescents. Unfortunately, these demographic indices can be misleading and need to be interpreted primarily as proxy variables or covariates of other contextual processes.

Given the complexity of conducting contextual assessments and the very limited attention by researchers to contexts outside of the family, continued use of demographic variables may be one easy way to insure inclusion of some contextual information in future research. If examined in light of their status as proxy variables, social indicators have the potential to heighten awareness and move researchers into more detailed and conceptually sophisticated assessments of contextual processes.

Another useful approach to contextual assessment is analysis of social indicator data. Social indicators are a class of measures usually available in public archives and databanks, which can be conceptualized as indices of community health or well-being (Heller et al., 1984). Social indicators are readily available on a range of population variables like growth and mobility rates, crime, economic status (e.g., employment rates, business development, retail sales), mental health (e.g., suicide rates, hospital admissions), physical health (e.g., infant mortality, hospital admissions, emergency medical calls, medical prescriptions filled), and education (e.g., per student expenditures, drop-out rates, college and technical school enrollments).

Rather than measures of a particular conceptual model of environmental context, social indicators are more accurately viewed as the correlates and outcomes of social and environmental processes occurring in a community of interest. They might also be considered proxy variables representing other community quality-of-life dimensions. Indices like rates of enrollment in higher education, sales tax receipts for purchase of alcohol, and *per capita* rates of video poker machines tell us something about community values, attitudes, and activity patterns. A single indicator may reflect multiple facets of community life, e.g., higher-education enrollment rates may be indicative of community attitudes toward education, the quality of the schools, economic resource levels, and the availability of higher-education institutions.

Recent research has sought to examine the mechanisms by which social-indicator indices affect the adjustment and well-being of those in the settings. For example, Simons, Johnson, Beaman, Conger, and Whitbeck (1996) examined the mediators of community context on adolescent conduct problems and psychological distress. Community disadvantage was operationalized as a composite of three social indicators: the proportion of adult males unemployed or working only part time, the proportion of citizens receiving government financial assistance, and the proportion of adults with less than a high school education. Structural-equation models showed that community disadvantage boosted the probability of conduct problems among adolescent boys by disrupting effective parenting. The models show direct effects of community disadvantage on adolescent male behavioral outcomes, but these effects are better understood by examining the social indicator data as part of a multilevel ecological model. Similarly, Wilson (1995) has provided an intriguing analysis of unemployment as an index of community context. His research on hyperpoor neighborhoods has shown that high levels of unemployment result in the breakdown of important organizing dimensions within a community. He argues that regular employment contributes to the maintenance of time as an organizing factor in community life, which has implications for school attendance, predictable routines in family life, and neighborhood interactions.

Social indicator data provide a useful strategy for assessment at the community level of analysis, which is infrequently assessed. Contextual assessment at this level has been elusive in part because of problems with the definition and boundaries of a community, the diversity within any single community, and the ready identification of organizations and smaller units comprising the community. Social indicator data accommodate many of these problems because the data can be aggregated to match different definitional boundaries of community or locality, as well as varying time segments. Time-series analysis, in combination with epidemiological methods, can be used to describe community patterns or lead to hypotheses about interdependencies and causal relationships (Kellam, 1991; Kellam & Rebok, 1992). Dooley and Catalano (1988), for example, examined relationships between economic conditions and mental health status. Using available social indicator data on employment and psychiatric admissions in several locales, they simulated a quasi-experiment with differing economic conditions, leading to the conclusion that changes in economic conditions have a causal relationship with rates of psychiatric hospital admission.

As archival data, social indicators are always subject to instrumentation threats to validity (i.e., changes in the recording procedures) and do not have demonstrated construct validity. Like assessment at the individual level, however, the use of multiple items or indicators is desirable. A single social indicator is the parallel of a single item at the individual level of assessment. Some single items can be robust and predictive, but generally a set of related items is preferable for measuring the manifestations of a process or construct. As with social indicator data, multiple indices considered together provide a more reliable analysis of the phenomenon in question. For example, the community context relevant to alcohol and other drug use might be assessed with social indicators such as alcohol sales, DUI arrests, and traffic accidents involving alcohol. These data could be disaggregated for smaller reporting areas such as precincts, municipalities, or counties, or by source of purchase (e.g., restaurants and bars versus liquor stores) to identify variations within a community and to assess effects of an intervention at the community level. Any one of these indicators considered in isolation may lead to inaccurate or incorrect conclusions, while the set of indicators provides possible replication of effects.

The technology of Geographic Information Systems (GIS) offers exciting possibilities for the quantitative study of social indicator data to examine social ecological processes and change at the community level. GIS mapping techniques construct three-dimensional maps of community resources (i.e., any of a number of social indicator variables) and can be examined for patterns of change over time or contingencies in developmental patterns among different indicators. Geographers have used the technique to study associations between demography and cultural practices, patterns of community growth and development, and relationships among natural resource availability, economic development, and housing development (Cowen, 1992). The technology is already being used in human services planning and management with existing databases maintained by federal and state governments (Warnecke, 1993). Application of this technology with community and neighborhood data can be useful in identifying demographic regularities and patterns of interrelationships, which lead to hypotheses about ecological and community processes. It offers a potentially important comparative analytic tool for the study of social ecology principles (Trickett, Kelly, & Todd, 1972) at the community level, allowing for examination of interdependence among community subsystems, as well as analysis of the patterns of resource cycling.

Context as Social Regularities

Seidman (1988) proposed the study of social regularities as a contextual construct for community psychology. He defined social regularities as the regular or routine patterns of interchange among the elements of a setting, the connections and linkages that define relationships within and between levels of analysis. Seidman identified *differences* and *ratios* as indicators of social relations, and *temporal patterns* among those ratios and differences as the foci for examination of social regularities. As illustration of this conceptual frame he cites Linney's (1986) study of the impact of school desegregation policies, in which change in the ratios of black and white children placed in special education classes over time was examined. It was hypothesized that, to the extent that the school system was based on a pattern of social regularities in which black children were systematically sorted into lower academic groups, desegregation of the school buildings might disrupt typical sorting patterns. Maintenance of this characteristic social regularity might be manifest in a change in rates of placement in special education (another sorting mechanism within the school), such that the desegregation intervention would result in a shift in the site of the sorting regularity. Linney's analysis showed a slight increase in the percentage of children placed in special education and a substantial change in the racial composition of the classes—evidence of change in social regularities at the school-building level following the desegregation.

Mulvey and Hicks' (1982) examination of the adaptation of the juvenile justice system to policy change affecting the definitions of delinquency provides another example of analysis of social regularities using archival data. Their time-series analysis of juvenile-offense record data demonstrated that the juvenile justice system continued to process youth at the same rate and in much the same manner despite what appeared to be dramatic change in policy. Following the policy change prohibiting court processing of status offenses, Mulvey and

Hicks found no change in the total numbers of youth processed through the system as compared to the time period before the policy change, but found substantial changes in the types of charges being prosecuted (i.e., a substantial decline in status offenses and a corresponding increase in misdemeanors). Mulvey and Hicks' use of archival data in time-series analysis shed light on the effect of a policy-level intervention and the system adaptations occurring as a response.

Conceptualization of context as its characteristic social regularities implies setting-specific operationalization, e.g., patterns of student placement in the school and patterns of processing youth in the juvenile justice system, but the derivation of ratios and temporal patterns as the specific metric allows study of these patterns across time and settings. This makes the social regularities contextual frame particularly useful for study of interlevel interdependencies (e.g., small group to organizational) and examination of cross-level effects.

Choice of the relevant indicators and patterns for analysis within this conceptual framework is not always obvious. A fairly rich understanding of the setting and consideration of setting assumptions is necessary to identify relevant processes and associated indicators. Case study and ethnographic work will be important sources of insight into community processes to be examined. For example, Orvik (1991) has suggested study of the community context for persons with mental illness in terms of community absorption rates, a construct that might be defined with social indicator data, such as employment rates for persons with serious mental illness or residential patterns including apartment living. Analysis of regularities longitudinally and across sites is likely to generate hypotheses about how identified patterns serve the setting and what other adaptations may occur simultaneously with change.

Theoretically informed research with social indicator data and indices of rates and change offer new directions for description of community process and change over time. Multivariable, longitudinal research across neighborhoods and communities can be greatly facilitated with use of data routinely collected by others. Archival data allows for analysis of longer time series, including time periods preceding an intervention, policy change, or other community event possibly triggering change, and the construction of quasi-experimental designs with larger sample sizes. This type of analysis can be extremely useful in the generation of hypotheses about context and community processes, which can subsequently be studied in greater depth with other methodologies.

Multimodal Environmental Assessment

Measurement of psychological constructs has been significantly influenced by Campbell and Fiske's (1959) model of multitrait, multimethod approaches to construct validation. Assessments that incorporate multiple methods, informants, and constructs are valued across most of the social sciences. Consistent with this approach, Moos and Lemke (1996) developed a multimodal assessment procedure for living environments that includes four domains and measures reflecting three conceptual definitions of context. The Multiphasic Environmental Assessment Procedure (MEAP) is an illustration of a comprehensive, conceptually based environmental-assessment procedure developed initially for assessment of nursing homes and other sheltered-care living facilities. The specific items on the MEAP reflect the environmental features of those settings, e.g., wheelchair accessibility and the presence of handrails in the bathrooms, but the instrument has been modified successfully for use in other types of community residential settings (Arns, 1990; Linney, 1982a).

The MEAP includes four instruments. The Physical and Architectural Features Checklist assesses recreational resources, safety features, space availability, community accessibility, physical amenities, and so on, primarily the physical environmental features of the setting. The Policy and Program Information Form assesses aspects of program regularities and stated policies guiding activity in the setting such as selectivity in admission, expectations for resident functioning, resident control, provisions for privacy, and tolerance for deviance. The Resident and Staff Information Form taps information about the socio-demographic characteristics of residents and staff, residents' current level of functioning *vis à vis* independence, leisure activities, and participation in activities outside the facility. The fourth instrument is a social climate scale assessing resident perceptions of interpersonal relationships, opportunities for personal growth, and mechanisms of system maintenance in the facility.

The MEAP reflects a multidimensional model of context hypothesizing that the physical environment, organizational features, social regularities, and perceptions of the individuals in the setting jointly constitute the social environment. Moos and colleagues have shown that MEAP profiles differentiate types of facilities, providing evidence for the validity of the instrument (Lemke & Moos, 1986; Timko & Moos, 1991, Moos & Lemke, 1996). Like the social climate research, the dimensions are also related to selected resident outcomes (e.g., Lemke & Moos, 1986; Timko & Moos, 1989).

The MEAP has been used most extensively in descriptive research on residential facilities for the elderly. Like the PASS, it can be useful in establishing and maintaining quality standards in these facilities. Additional research is needed, however, to establish predictive validity and sensitivity to change in organizations. The instrument provides a comprehensive descriptive picture of a setting, incorporating different models of context; however, surprisingly little work has been done examining the relationships among different conceptual definitions of context included within this assessment procedure. For example, how do physical environmental variables relate to participant perceptions of the setting? To what extent are the different conceptualizations of context redundant? How does change in one area translate into change in other domains? By including multiple definitions of context in a single measure, use of the MEAP affords an opportunity to examine the multiple dimensions of context.

Toward Transactional Models of Context

The contextual models discussed thus far could be criticized for their failure to (1) address the complexity of contextual variation, (2) adequately recognize the multifaceted nature of context, (3) assess change over time, and (4) assess the interdependence of persons and context. However operationalized, context is most often depicted as the backdrop against which the behavior of individuals unfolds. Like individuals, however, contexts change with time and are both influenced by, and exert influence on, the individuals who participate in the setting.

Transactional theorists have articulated the importance of studying the dynamic relationship between persons and contexts (Altman & Rogoff, 1987; Kellam & Rebok, 1992; Sameroff, 1990). Developmentalists in the transactional perspective suggest that different contextual domains may be more or less salient for accomplishment of developmental tasks at different points in the individual's lifespan, and in light of the personal resources available to individuals (Sameroff, Seifer, & Bartko, 1997). For example, an infant with physical disabilities may need enhanced stimulation from the maternal context and additional supports from the physical context in order to accomplish normative developmental tasks. Another infant possessing enhanced cognitive and physical resources may accomplish the same developmental tasks with reduced stimulation from the ecological context. Throughout the lifespan, any one contextual domain will be variably salient.

A transactional framework enhances previous contextual models by consciously recognizing both the multifaceted nature of context and the need to incorporate a temporal dimension into any model of person–setting relationships. The more dynamic and multidimensional model of transactions better approximates the reciprocity and interaction hypothesized in the person–environment fit construct of community psychology.

Embodied in the notion of transactional person–environment concepts are constructs that characterize matches or relationships as the unit of study, rather than simply as combinations of persons and good or bad elements of an environment. Unfortunately, operationalization of these relational, interdependent constructs remains elusive. Our closest approximations may best be captured in contemporary notions of behavior setting theory and qualitative efforts at description of context.

Behavior Setting Analysis

Three decades ago, Barker (1965, 1968) proposed the study of behavior settings as the primary unit of analysis for understanding behavior. By definition, the behavior setting encompasses both physical and behavioral dimensions, and considers persons and situations as inseparable. A behavior setting is distinguished by time and space boundaries and "a standing pattern of behavior." Barker posited that neither the physical characteristics of the environment nor the individual behavior patterns of the persons in the setting alone can account for the streams of activity observed in any place. Rather, he suggested that the synomorphic relationship between the physical environment and behavior patterns, what he called the behavior setting, should be the unit of analysis. Classic behavior setting theory stipulates that the persons in a setting are largely interchangeable, with the same patterns of behavior occurring irrespective of the specific individuals, and that behavior settings have an operating system for preservation of the standing patterns of behavior, including deviance-control operations.

An illustration of the significance of this conceptual framework can be found in understanding a baseball game. One can learn very little about the game of baseball (a standing pattern of behavior) by studying the baseball field before the players come out of the locker room. This would be analogous to studying the physical environment alone. Similarly, we would not be able to determine the rules of the game or the contingencies determining the behavior of the individual players by focusing on each player in isolation (the common, individual-level focus of psychological research), or by studying their perceptions of the game, the ballpark, or teammates. Imagine, for example, two hours of observation of the first-base player alone, without the context of the field, other players, and sequences of action surrounding the player. Very little could be learned about what this player is doing and why, and it would be quite difficult to predict or change the behavior of the player with only observational data available. Barker suggests that it is the combination of the physical field and the distribution of players on the field that allows us to learn about the standing patterns of behavior constituting the baseball game, i.e., the regular patterns of movement and the rules governing and predicting that motion.

Behavior setting analysis as an assessment procedure involves, first, the identification of behavior settings in the system of interest. This is accomplished by observation and rational delineation of behavior settings, judging each setting with time, boundary, and synomorphy criteria (Barker, 1968; Schoggen, 1989; Wicker, 1979). Each behavior setting meeting these criteria is then described quantitatively and/or qualitatively on dimensions such as duration, number and type of participants, primary functions (e.g., education, religion, hygiene, sustenance), types of behavior (e.g., thinking, talking, expressing emotion), pressure for participation, and participatory roles (leader, active functionary, onlooker, or audience). This procedure yields a descriptive record of behavior settings in a given system, allowing for comparison among behavior settings and across systems.

Behavior setting surveys, as initially described by Barker, can be an exceedingly lengthy process. Barker and colleagues spent over a year in an exhaustive description of the behavior settings in a single community (Barker & Wright, 1955). The behavior setting methodology has been applied in schools (Barker & Gump, 1964; Schoggen & Schoggen, 1988), churches (Wicker, 1969), health care settings (Willems, 1976), courtrooms (Ross, 1982), residential treatment facilities (Linney, Webb, & Rosenberg, 1985), and work settings (Oxley & Barrera, 1984). These applications have involved smaller systems (e.g., a group home) or specific types of behavior settings (e.g., court hearings), and thus make assessments more feasible by requiring substantially less time. Wicker (1979) has suggested both time and event sampling to streamline the assessment procedure.

The validity of the behavior setting construct and the assessment strategy have been evidenced in the derivation of "manning" theory (Barker, 1968; Wicker, McGrath, & Armstrong, 1972). Wicker (1987) reviewed the use of behavior setting theory and methodology for documenting community life, assessing the social impact of organizations and institutions within a community, diagnosing community needs, analyzing organizational structure, analyzing health service delivery systems, and consulting on organizational problems. He has elaborated new directions for behavior setting methodology to include analysis of their generation and development. Drawing on case study and ethnographic methods, Wicker has illustrated the importance of a developmental temporal analysis of settings, and the need for greater attention to the ways in which they are shaped by actor's intentions.

Behavior setting methods have not been widely used, perhaps in part because they appear quite cumbersome. Cluster analysis and factor analysis of behavior setting data (Luke, Rappaport, & Seidman, 1991; Price & Blashfield, 1975) has indicated more comprehensive clusterings of behavior setting characteristics representing functional components.

Behavior setting technology provides a method that is quite consistent with the assessment needs of community psychology research. The physical environment and participant behavior are integrated. Quantitative indices not specific to one type of setting can be generated, e.g., time and space parameters, number and type of participants, and functions. Indices representing role and power relationships, the kinds of transactional and relational constructs postulated by community psychologists, can be examined. The technology has applicability to culturally diverse settings, although, as an observational technique, it is not clear to what extent the observer's own perceptions influence the use of the behavior setting technology.

Behavior setting methodology can be applied to multiple levels of analysis. It provides a strategy for examining role relationships among the members of small group settings and the types of behavior patterns in which they engage. At the organizational or community level, systems can be described in terms of the relative frequency of specific types of behavior settings. For example, Linney, Webb, and Rosenberg (1985) described community group homes in terms of the percentage of behavior settings characterized by residents functioning as leaders or joint functionaries. This quantitative index allowed comparison across settings and the analysis of relationships between behavior setting characteristics and selected outcomes or products of the setting. Luke, Rappaport, and Seidman (1991) demonstrated associations between behavior setting "phenotypes" in a mutual help organization and change among its members. Second-order indices, like ratios or empirically derived phenotypes, increase the utility of behavior setting data for theory development and model testing.

Most of the work with behavior setting methodology has considered behavior settings as discrete units. There have been few analyses of the links between and among behavior settings. Wicker's (1988) descriptive work on the creation of small businesses began to qualitatively examine the relationships among behavior settings linked by common people and objectives. Unfortunately, only a very small number of scientists appear to be working within this framework. Little work has focused on the deviance control processes hypothesized as part of each behavior setting, nor on the factors influencing change in behavior settings. Wicker's (1982, 1992) writing on the life cycle of behavior settings and temporal factors affecting change are important directions for understanding change and stability at the organization and community levels.

DIRECTIONS FOR FUTURE WORK

Several quite different conceptualizations of ecological context (both objective and subjective, quantitative and qualitative) available for study of community processes and person–environment transactions have been described. Despite a substantial increase in the appearance of the terms "environmental," "ecological," and "contextual" in the published literature, there has been very limited work on systematic measurement of social and community context in the past decade. There is neither a "gold standard" for contextual assessment, nor even a common set of constructs generally examined by researchers. Understanding of the reciprocal relationships between individuals and environments might be advanced with the expectation that research and action initiatives will at least systematically sample and describe contexts at multiple levels, pay greater attention to multitrait–multimethod models of measurement development and to longitudinal study, and pay attention not only to change, but to mechanisms contributing to stability in contexts.

Strategic Sampling of Contexts

Moving from the individual to other levels of analysis raises unit-of-analysis issues, as well as questions about appropriate sample size for adequate statistical conclusion validity. These issues are basic to our current research methodologies; however, they may be premature considerations given the level of theoretical and operational specification currently characterizing the field of contextually grounded research and action. Concerted attention needs to be directed toward systematic sampling of environmental domains to improve the statistical probabilities of identifying significant relationships. Without measures of contextual variables and sufficient variation on those constructs, quantitative analysis cannot identify a significant role for context.

Strategic sampling of settings (whether organizations, neighborhoods, or communities), combined with theory-guided ecological assessment, can begin to provide the missing data on diversity in ecological domains and identify the preliminary structure of relationships among multiple contextual levels. Barker and Gump's (1964) study of school size is a good illustration of this approach. Their research involved only 13 schools; however, they varied strategically on an organizational dimension of theoretical importance to behavior setting theory, i.e., size.

Multitrait–Multimethod Analysis

Traditional measurement development and construct validation models involve examination of intercorrelations among instruments hypothesized to be related (and unrelated). In ecological assessment there has been little analysis of interrelationships among the several assessment techniques currently available. Several of the techniques share conceptual overlap and involve assessment of the same or similar domains, yet we know almost nothing about the convergence of these procedures, nor in what ways they account for the unique variance in the settings or have differential predictive utility. Linney (1982a) found high correlations between scores on a modified MEAP and a modified PASS in the assessment of residential facilities for juvenile offenders. Unfortunately, the sample was not large enough for the statistical procedures necessary to estimate the proportions of unique variance contributed by each procedure. More of this kind of multimeasure construct validation research is needed. Use of multiple methods, like behavior setting analysis and social climate assessments, in one study may enhance our understanding of the processes contributing to the unique ecologies of settings.

Articulation of Linkages among Levels of Analysis

The levels-of-analysis contextual schema postulates interdependence and mutual influence among the several levels, including processes similar to Kelly's (1971) notion of radiating impact. Strategies for assessing cross-level transactions and relationships are needed to elaborate our understanding of context. Theoretical and practical questions, such as how school policies on special services (organization level) influence the individuals in that organization, or how change in role relationships like cooperative/joint tasks among individuals in a workplace (small group), affect organizational policies on promotion and remuneration need to be examined. These examples of cross-level interdependence require both a theoretical framework within which to conceptualize relationships, and a measurement strategy that assesses or characterizes the pathways of influence.

In intervention efforts it is not uncommon for the target of intervention and the locus of effect to be at different levels. There are numerous examples of policy or organizational restructuring that has the intention of affecting change at the individual or small-group level (e.g., the creation of Head Start centers, neonatal rooming-in hospital policies, use of quality circles in the workplace). With cross-level effect as the desired outcome, measurements at each of the levels of effect and intervention are minimally necessary to evaluate the presence or absence of change, and to elucidate patterns of reciprocity and effect among identifiable levels of context. To identify mechanisms of cross-level change and the transactions contributing to observed change, assessment of interlevel junctions and processes are necessary.

The significance of cross-level relationships has been demonstrated in patterns of covariation between indices at two or more levels of analysis, for example, cooperative learning classrooms and individual self-esteem (Slavin, 1983), and change in school procedures for student grouping and subsequent drop-out rates (Felner & Adan, 1988; Felner et al., 1997). Progress is needed toward identifying the processes that link the several levels of analysis and the mechanisms that affect change among them.

Stability and Change

Community psychology is concerned with understanding stability and change in social systems and effects on individuals. Concepts such as second-order change (Watzlawick, Weakland, & Fisch, 1974), social regularities (Seidman, 1988), and patterns of resource exchange and social ecology (Trickett, Kelly, & Todd, 1972) imply both stability and change in the functioning of social systems. These concepts also reflect transactional, dynamic, systemic qualities. Transaction and interaction are processes difficult to capture in traditional measurement instruments. Many, if not most, of the measurements used in psychology are best described as static snapshots of unidimensional constructs. The snapshot or measurement reflects "how much" of the construct is present at that time, and we assess change by looking for a difference in that level at a later time. The transactional nature of the phenomena of interest to community psychology requires more than monodimensional, linear conceptions of either stability or change. With the development of multivariate statistical techniques, we can move beyond the unidimensional limitation; however, linear causal models and reductionism continue to dominate our thinking and hence our measurement and analysis.

Stability and change as primary phenomena of interest make it essential that measurements be sensitive and precise in order to detect and characterize patterns of change. These patterns may be subtle, may result in qualitatively different states, and, for cross-level change, may involve distinctly different sets of variables. Further complicating this picture is the unknown temporal dimension of change, both in terms of when the effect of an intervention may be detected and how systems change over time (Lorion, 1990).

Examining change from a multilevel perspective requires that we think of constructs in multiple forms. Developmental researchers have postulated constructs that may manifest in different forms across the age span. Poor attachment, for example, may be evidenced in the "strange situation" in infancy, as disruptions in peer relations in childhood, and as failures in intimacy during adulthood (Allen, Aber, & Leadbetter, 1990; Main, Kaplan, & Cassidy, 1985). For the community psychologist, parallel conceptions of contextual constructs must be hypothesized. These parallel manifestations may be evident across the lifespan of the individual or setting, across settings, or from one level of analysis to another. For example, racism might be evident in individual attitudes and behavior, specific hiring and firing policies at the department or small-group level, and purchasing policies governing selection of vendors at the organizational level. Research on school desegregation provides an illustration of the need to examine multiple indicators of the same construct at several levels. While many schools achieved racial balance relative to other schools (a common operational definition of desegregation), within each school, change in policies on student placement resulted in resegregation at the small-group or classroom level. In this illustration, racial balance at the organizational level is not consistent with the same indicator at the small-group level because of an organizational policy specifying how the small groups form.

Efficient Use of Qualitative and Descriptive Methods of Study

Anthropological methods and constructs focusing on patterns of exchange, networks, and rules governing relationships provide fruitful directions for research at the non-individual level. For example, anthropologists have compared cultures on the basis of kinship networks derived from biological relationships, functional relationships, and relative importance to some reference individual. The focus is less on comparison to a standard, and more on a descriptive understanding of patterns of relationship and the rules that determine those relationships.

Other disciplines may provide community psychology researchers with potential measurement strategies. Morgan (1983) has compiled an interesting set of papers discussing methodologies from a variety of disciplines that can inform community psychology. Anthropological techniques for identifying kinship patterns and social organizational structures should be explored. Sociological analysis of social networks appears to have useful implications for description of community processes and change. Analysis of social support via social network analysis is well known to community psychologists; however, our focus has tended to be on the outcomes for individuals and our networks anchored by a target subject. Sociologists analyze networks as patterns of resource exchange, social interaction, and racial integration at the community level. Use of the technique for analysis of community-level processes may offer some important new directions for study of person–environment fit constructs.

Many of the key concepts in community psychology remain to be operationalized outside of the individual level. For the most part, we continue to focus on easily acquired indices of the environment, such as socioeconomic status, family structure, and the individual's perception of the environment. Given the rhetoric about the importance of context, use of "quick and dirty" assessments is unfortunate. At best these indices are proxies for other ecological processes, and usually share enough method variance with other individual self-report data that they appear as weak correlates, readily discarded in a multivariate analysis. Greater attention must be directed toward inclusion of meaningful contextual assessments, both qualitative and quantitative, both for focused analysis of person–setting transactions as well as for enhanced understanding of processes at the individual level. Future work in this area will benefit from strategic and systematic sampling of contexts and focused attention toward measurement and characterization of important contextual dimensions.

REFERENCES

Abbott-Shim, M. & Sibley, A. (1987). *Assessment Profile for Early Childhood Programs.* Atlanta, GA: Quality Assist.

Alden, L. (1978). Factor analysis of the Ward Atmosphere Scale. *Journal of Consulting and Clinical Psychology, 46,* 175–176.

Allen, J. P., Aber, J. L., & Leadbetter, B. J. (1990). Adolescent problem behavior: The influence of attachment and autonomy. *Psychiatric Clinics of North America, 13,* 455–467.

Altman, I. & Rogoff, B. (1987). World views in psychology: Trait, interactional, organismic, and transactional perspectives. In D. Stokols & I. Altman (Eds.), *Handbook of environmental psychology,* Vol. 1 (pp. 7–40). New York, Wiley.

Arns, P. G. (1990, August). *The ideal community residential care facility: Can the experts agree?* Paper presented at the 98th annual meeting of the American Psychological Association, Boston.

Barker, R. G. (1965). Explorations in ecological psychology. *American Psychologist, 20,* 1–14.

Barker, R. G. (1968). *Ecological psychology: Concepts and methods for studying the environment of human behavior.* Stanford, CA: Stanford University Press.

Barker, R. G. (1987). Prospecting in environmental psychology: Oskaloosa revisited. In D. Stokols & I. Altman (Eds.), *Handbook of environmental psychology,* Vol. 2 (pp. 1413–1432). New York, Wiley.

Barker, R. G. & Gump, P. V. (1964). *Big school, small school.* Stanford, CA: Stanford University Press.

Barker, R. G., & Wright, H. F. (1955). *Midwest and its children: The psychological ecology of an American town.* New York: Harper & Row.

Baum, A., & Paulus, P. (1987). Crowding. In D. Stokols & I. Altman (Eds.), *Handbook of environmental psychology,* Vol. 1 (pp. 533–570). New York, Wiley.

Bennett, C. C., Anderson, L. S., Cooper, S., Hassol, L., Klein, D. C., & Rosenblum, G. (Eds.) (1966). *Community psychology: A report of the Boston conference on the education of psychologists for community mental health.* Boston: Boston University Press.

Blakely, C. H., Mayer, J. P., Gottschalk, R. G., Schmitt, N. M., Davidson, W. S., Roitman, D. B., & Emshoff, J. G. (1987). The fidelity-adaptation debate: Implications for the implementation of public sector social programs. *American Journal of Community Psychology, 15*, 253–268.

Bliss, F. H., Moos, R. H., & Bromet, E. J. (1976). Monitoring change in community-oriented treatment programs. *Journal of Community Psychology, 4*, 315–326.

Boake, C., & Salmon, P. G. (1983). Demographic correlates and factor structure of the Family Environment Scale. *Journal of Clinical Psychology, 39*, 95–100.

Brady, C. A., Kinnard, K. L. & Friedrich, W. N. (1980). Job satisfaction and perception of social climate in a mental health facility. *Perceptual and motor skills, 51*, 559–564.

Bronfenbrenner, U. (1979). *The ecology of human development*. Cambridge, MA: Harvard University Press.

Bronfenbrenner, U. (1995). Developmental ecology through space and time: A future perspective. In P. Moen & G. Elder (Eds.), *Examining lives in context: Perspectives on the ecology of human development* (pp. 619–647). Washington, D.C.: American Psychological Association.

Bryk, A., & Raudenbush, S. (1992). *Hierarchical linear models*. Newbury Park, CA: Sage.

Caldwell, B. M., & Bradley, R. H. (1994). Environmental issues in developmental follow-up research. In S. L. Friedman (Ed.), *Developmental follow-up: Concepts, domains and methods* (pp. 235–256). San Diego: Academic.

Campbell, D. T., & Fiske, D. W. (1959). Convergent and discriminant validation by the multitrait-multimethod matrix. *Psychological Bulletin, 56*, 81–105.

Coie, J. D., Watt, N., West, S. G., Hawkins, D., Asarnow, J., Markman, H., Ramey, S., Shure, M., & Long, B. (1933). The science of prevention: A conceptual framework for and some directions for a national research program. *American Psychologist, 48*, 1013–1022.

Cowen, D. J. (1992). *Proceedings: 5th International Symposium on Spatial Data Handling (Charleston, SC)*. Columbia: University of South Carolina.

Craik, K., & Feimer, N. (1987). Environmental assessment. In D. Stokols & I. Altman (Eds.), *Handbook of environmental psychology*, Vol. 2 (pp. 891–918). New York: Wiley.

Dooley, D., & Catalano, R. (1988). Psychological effects of unemployment. *Journal of Social Issues, 44*.

Felner, R. D. & Adan, A. (1988). The school transitional environment project: An ecological intervention and evaluation. In R. Price et al. (Eds.), *Fourteen Ounces of prevention* (pp. 111–122). Washington, D.C.: American Psychological Association.

Felner, R., Jackson, A. W., Kasak, D., Mulhall, P., Brand, S. & Flowers, N. (1997). The impact of school reform for the middle grades: A longitudinal study of a network engaged in Turning Points-based comprehensive school transformation. In R. Takanishi (Ed.), *Preparing adolescents for the twenty-first century: Challenges facing Europe and the United States* (pp 38–69). New York: Cambridge University Press.

Flynn, R. J. & Heal, L. W. (1980). *A short form of PASS-3 for assessing normalization: Structure, interrater reliability and validity*. Unpublished manuscript, Purdue University School of Science at Indianapolis, Indianapolis, IN.

Gump, P. (1987). School and classroom environments. In D. Stokols & I. Altman (Eds.), *Handbook of environmental psychology*, Vol. 1 (pp. 691–732). New York: Wiley.

Hall, D. & Pill, R. (1975). Social climate and ward atmosphere. *Social Science and Medicine, 9*, 529–534.

Heller, K., Price, R., Reinharz, S., Riger, S., Wandersman, A. & D'Aunno, T. (1984). *Psychology and community change: Challenges for the future*. Homewood, IL: Dorsey.

Kellam, S. G. (1991). Developmental epidemiological framework for family research on depression and aggression. In G. R. Patterson (Ed.), *Depression and aggression in family interaction*. Englewood Cliffs, NJ: Erlbaum.

Kellam, S. G., & Rebok, G. (1992). Building developmental and etiological theory through epidemiologically-based preventive intervention trials. In J. McCord & R. Tremblay (Eds.), *Preventing antisocial behavior: Intervention from birth through adolescence* (pp. 162–195). New York: Guilford.

Kelly, J. G. (1971). The quest for valid preventive interventions. In G. Rosenblum (Ed.), *Issues in community psychology and community mental health* (pp. 109–140). New York: Behavioral Publications.

Kelly, J. G. (1988). *Designing prevention research as a collaborative relationship between citizens and social scientists*. Office of Substance Abuse Prevention Monograph-3, Prevention Research Findings (pp. 148–154). Rockville, MD: U.S. Department of Health and Human Services.

Kelly, J. G. (1990). Changing contexts and the field of community psychology. *American Journal of Community Psychology, 18*, 769–792.

Kelly, J. G. (1991). *Context, communities and prevention*. Paper prepared for the Second National Prevention Research Conference, Washington, D.C., June.

Kenny, D. A. (1996). The design and analysis of social-interaction research. *Annual Review of Psychology, 47*, 59–86.

Lawton, M. P. (1990). Residential environment and self-directedness among older people. *American Psychologist, 45*, 638–640.

Lemke, S. & Moos, R. H. (1986). Quality of residential settings of elderly adults. *Journal of Gerontology, 41*, 268–276.

Lewin, K. (1935). *A dynamic theory of personality*. New York: McGraw-Hill.

Linney, J. A. (1982a). "Alternative" facilities for youth in trouble: Descriptive analysis of a strategically selected sample. In J. Handler & J. Zatz (Eds.), *Neither angels nor thieves: Studies in deinstitutionalization of status offenders* (pp. 127–175). Washington, D.C.: National Academy Press.

Linney, J. A. (1982b). Multicomponent Assessment of Residential Services for Youth (MARSY). In J. Handler & J. Zatz (Eds.), *Neither angels nor thieves: Studies in deinstitutionalization of status offenders* (pp. 740–779). Washington, D.C.: National Academy Press.

Linney, J. A. (1986). Court-ordered school desegregation: Shuffling the deck or playing a different game. In E. Seidman & J. Rappaport (Eds.), *Redefining social problems* (pp. 259–274). New York: Plenum.

Linney, J. A. (1991). *Community context in prevention science*. Task Force Report for the Second National Prevention Science Conference, National Institute of Mental Health, Washington, D.C.

Linney, J. A., Forman, S. G., & Levy, M. (1988). *Multisource, observational assessment of school environments*. Project SCCOPE Technical Report, University of South Carolina, Psychology Department.

Linney, J. A., Webb, D., & Rosenberg, M. (1985). *A time sampling procedure for behavior setting analysis in treatment facilities for juvenile offenders*. Poster presentation at the annual meeting of the Southeastern Psychological Association, Atlanta, GA.

Lorion, R. P. (1990). Developmental analyses of community phenomena. In P. Tolan, C. Keys, F. Chertok, & L. Jason (Eds.), *Researching Community Psychology: Issues of theory and methods* (pp. 32–41). Washington, D.C.: American Psychological Association.

Luke, D. A., Rappaport, J., & Seidman, E. (1991). Setting phenotypes in a mutual help organization: Expanding behavior setting theory. *American Journal of Community Psychology, 19*, 147–167.

Main, M., Kaplan, N., & Cassidy, J. (1985). Security in infancy, childhood and adulthood: A move to the level of representation. *Monographs of the Society for Research in Child Development, 50*(1–2), 66–104.

Moos, R. H. (1975). *Evaluating correctional and community settings*. New York: Wiley.

Moos, R. H. (1979). *Evaluating educational environments: Procedures, measures, findings and policy implications*. San Francisco: Jossey-Bass.

Moos, R. H. (1994). *The Social Climate Scales: A user's guide (2nd Ed.)*. Palo Alto, CA: Consulting Psychologists Press.

Moos, R. H., & Lemke, S. (1996). *Evaluating residential facilities: The Multiphasic Environmental Assessment Procedure*. Thousand Oaks, CA: Sage.

Moos, R. H. & Moos, B. S. (1978). Classroom social climate and student absences and grades. *Journal of Educational Psychology, 70*, 263–269.

Morgan, G. (Ed.) (1983). *Beyond Method: Strategies for social research*. Beverly Hills, CA: Sage.

Mulvey, E. P., & Hicks, A. (1982). The paradoxical effect of a juvenile code change in Virginia. *American Journal of Community Psychology, 10*, 705–721.

Mulvey, E. P., Linney, J. A., & Rosenberg, M. (1987). Organizational control and treatment program design as dimensions of institutionalization in settings of juvenile offenders. *American Journal of Community Psychology, 16*, 525–546.

Murray, H. A. (1938). *Explorations in personality*. New York: Oxford University Press.

Neiderhiser, J. M., Reiss, D., & Hetherington, E. M. (1996). Genetically informative designs for distinguishing developmental pathways during adolescence: Responsible and antisocial behavior. *Development and Psychopathology, 8*, 779–791.

Orvik, J. M. (1991). The dropped out: Redescribing chronic mental illness as a question about communities. In M. Roberts & R. Bergner (Eds.), *Advances in Descriptive Psychology*, Vol. 6 (pp. 271–297). Greenwich, CT: JAI.

Oxley, D., & Barrera, M. (1984). Undermanning theory and the workplace: Implications of setting size for job satisfaction and social support. *Environment and Behavior, 16*, 211–234.

Plomin, R., & Neiderhiser, J. M. (1992). Genetics and experience. *Current Directions in Psychological Science, 1*, 160–163.

Poresky, R. H. (1987). Environmental Assessment Index: Reliability, stability and validity of the long and short forms. *Educational and Psychological Measurement, 47*, 969–975.

Price, R. H. & Blashfield, R. K. (1975). Explorations in the taxonomy of behavior settings: Analysis of dimensions and classifications of settings. *American Journal of Community Psychology, 3*, 335–351.

Rappaport, J. (1977). *Community psychology: Values, research and action*. New York: Holt Rinehart & Winston.

Raviv, A., Raviv, A., & Reisel, E. (1990). Teachers and students: Two different perspectives?—Measuring social climate in the classroom. *American Educational Research Journal, 27*, 141–157.

Reiss, D. (1997). Mechanisms linking genetic and social influences in adolescent development: Building a collabortive search. *Current Directions in Psychological Science, 6*, 100–105.

Repetti, E. L. (1987). Individual and common components of the social environment at work and psychological well-being. *Journal of Personality and Social Psychology, 52,* 710–720.

Repetti, R. L., & Cosmas, K. A. (1991). The quality of the social environment at work and job satisfaction. *Journal of Applied Social Psychology, 21,* 840–854.

Ross, J. S. (1982). *A behavior setting analysis of policy change in juvenile court proceedings.* Unpublished master's thesis, University of Virginia, Charlottesville.

Sameroff, A. J. (1990). *Prevention of Developmental Psychopathology Using the Transactional Model: Perspectives on Host, Risk Agent, and Environment Interactions.* Paper prepared for the National Conference on Prevention Research, National Institute on Mental Health, Washington, D.C.

Sameroff, A. J., Seifer, R., & Bartko, W. T. (1997). Environmental perspectives on adaptation during childhood and adolescence. In S. S. Luthar (Ed.), *Developmental psychopathology: Perspectives on adjustment, risk and disorder* (pp. 507–526). New York: Cambridge University Press.

Schoggen, P. (1989). *Behavior settings: A revision and extension of Roger G. Barker's "Ecological psychology".* Stanford, CA: Stanford University Press.

Schoggen, P., & Schoggen, M. (1988). Student voluntary participation and high school size. *Journal of Educational Research, 81,* 288–293.

Seidman, E. (1987). Toward a framework for primary prevention research. In J. A. Steinberg & M. M. Silverman (Eds.), *Preventing mental disorders: A research perspective* (pp. 2–19). Washington, D.C.: US Government Printing Office.

Seidman, E. (1988). Back to the future, community psychology: Unfolding a theory of social intervention. *American Journal of Community Psychology, 16,* 3–24.

Simons, R. L., Johnson, C., Beaman, J., Conger, R. D., & Whitbeck, L. B. (1996). Parents and peer group mediators of the effect of community structure on adolescent problem behavior. *American Journal of Community Psychology, 24,* 145–172.

Slavin, R. (1983). *Cooperative learning.* New York: Longman.

Stokols, D., & Altman, I. (Eds.) (1987). *Handbook of environmental psychology.* New York: Wiley.

Sundstrom, E., Bell, P. A., Busby, P. L., & Asmus, C. (1996). Environmental psychology. *Annual Review of Psychology, 47,* 482–512.

Taylor, J. H., & Perrill, N. K. (1987). The Hospice Environment Survey: Pilot test of a new measurement instrument. *Omega Journal of Death and Dying, 18,* 237–250.

Timko, C., & Moos, R. H. (1989). Choice, control and adaptation among elderly residents of sheltered care settings. *Journal of Applied Social Psychology, 19,* 636–655.

Timko, C., & Moos, R. H. (1991). A typology of social climates in group residential facilities for older people. *Journal of Gerontology, 46,* 160–169.

Trickett, E. J., Kelly, J. G., & Todd, D. M. (1972). The social environment of the high school: Guidelines for individual change and organizational development. In S. G. Golann & C. Eisdorfer (Eds.), *Handbook of community mental health* (pp. 331–406). New York: Appleton-Century-Crofts.

Trickett, E. J., Trickett, P. J., Castro, J. J., & Schaffner, P. (1982). The independent school experience: Aspects of the normative environments of single sex and coed secondary schools. *Journal of Educational Psychology, 74,* 374–381.

Tyack, D. & Cuban, L. (1995). *Tinkering toward utopia: A century of public school reform.* Cambridge, MA: Harvard University Press.

Walsh, E. B., Craik, K. H., & Price, R. H. (Eds.) (1992). *Person-environment psychology: Models and perspectives.* Hillsdale, NJ: Erlbaum.

Wagner, L. (1990). Social and historical perspectives on peer teaching in education. In H. C. Foot, M. J. Morgan, & R. H. Shute (Eds.), *Children helping children* (pp. 21–42). Chichester, UK: Wiley.

Wandersman, A. H., & Hallman, W. K. (1993). Are people acting irrationally? Understanding public concerns about environmental threats. *American Psychologist, 48,* 681–686.

Warnecke, L. (1993). Geographic information systems in human services. *Government Imaging, 2,* 15–16.

Watzlawick, P., Weakland, J. H., & Fisch, R. (1974). *Change: Principles of problem formation and problem resolution.* New York: Norton.

Wicker, A. W. (1969). Size of church membership and members' support of church behavior settings. *Journal of Personality and Social Psychology, 13,* 278–288.

Wicker, A. W. (1979). *An introduction to ecological psychology.* Monterey, CA: Brooks-Cole.

Wicker, A. W. (1987). Behavior settings reconsidered: Temporal stages, resources, internal dynamics, and context. In D. Stokols & I. Altman (Eds.), *Handbook of environmental psychology,* Vol. 1 (pp. 613–653). New York: Wiley.

Wicker, A. W. (1988). Life cycles of behavior settings. In J. E. McGrath (Ed.), *The social psychology of time: New perspectives* (pp. 182–200). Beverly Hills, CA: Sage.

Wicker, A. W. (1992). Making sense of environments. In E. B. Walsh, K. H. Craik, & R. H. Price, (Eds.) *Person-environment psychology: Models and perspectives* (pp 157–192). Hillsdale, NJ: Erlbaum.

Wicker, A. W., McGrath, J. E. & Armstrong, G. E. (1972). Organizational size and behavior setting capacity as determinants of member participation. *Behavioral Science, 17*, 499–513.

Wilkinson, L. (1973). As assessment of the dimensionality of Moos' social climate scale. *American Journal of Community Psychology, 1*, 342–350.

Willems, E. P. (1972). The interface of the hospital environment and patient behavior. *Archives of Physical Medicine and Rehabilitation, 53*, 115–122.

Willems, E. P. (1976). Behavioral ecology, health status, and health care: Applications to the rehabilitation setting. In I. Altman & J. F. Wohlhill (Eds.), *Human behavior and environment: Advances in theory and research*, Vol. 1 (pp. 211–263). New York: Plenum.

Wilson, W. J. (1995). Jobless ghettos and the social outcomes of youngsters. In P. Moen & G. Elder (Eds.), *Examining lives in context: Perspectives on the ecology of human development* (pp. 527–543). Washington, D.C.: American Psychological Association.

Wohlhill, J. F., & Heft, H. (1987). The physical environment and the development of the child. In D. Stokols & I. Altman (Eds.), *Handbook of environmental psychology*, Vol. 1 (pp 281–328). New York: Wiley.

Wolfensberger, W. (1972). *The principle of normalization in human services*. Toronto: National Institute on Mental Retardation.

Wolfensberger, W. & Glenn, L. (1975). *PASS-3, A method for the quantitative evaluation of human services*. Toronto: National Institute on Mental Retardation.

Zimring, C., Carpman, J. R., & Michelson, W. (1987). Design for special populations: Mentally retarded persons, children, hospital visitors. In D. Stokols & I. Altman (Eds.), *Handbook of environmental psychology*, Vol. 2 (pp. 919–950). New York: Wiley.

CHAPTER 28

Cross-Level Research without Cross-Ups in Community Psychology

MARYBETH SHINN AND BRUCE D. RAPKIN

A central tenet of community psychology is that human behavior must be understood in context. Community and other ecologically oriented psychologists have proposed typologies of contexts for behavior (Altman & Rogoff, 1987; Barker, 1968; Bronfenbrenner, 1979, 1986; Murrell, 1973; Rappaport, 1977; Seidman, 1988), with the twin goals of understanding the interplay of people and contexts, and of exhorting psychologists to include ever-broader contexts of behavior in their theory, research, and intervention practices. Typically, the typologies are organized from narrower to broader contexts or from lower to higher levels of analysis.

Higher levels of analysis may be distinguished from lower ones in that they may involve: (1) multiple individuals, (2) units with internal structure and social organization, and (3) patterns of interactions or reciprocal relations between individuals, groups, and social systems. In the extreme, represented by the world view Altman and Rogoff call transactional, the entities disappear into "a *confluence* of inseparable factors that depend on one another for their very definition and meaning" (1987, p. 24; emphasis in original), and relationships become paramount. Some authors require that units at different levels of analysis have a hierarchical relationship to one another (e.g., Rousseau, 1985). Several approaches explicitly or implicitly consider the physical, social, or temporal environment of behavior as an extra-individual unit of analysis.

This chapter focuses on cross-level research, which involves relationships among vari-

Note: Portions of this chapter represent a revision and expansion of an earlier publication by Shinn (1990). Mixing and matching: Levels of conceptualization, measurement, and statistical analysis in community research. In P. Tolan, C. Keys, F. Chertok, & L. Jason (Eds.), *Researching community psychology: Issues of theory and methods* (pp. 111–126). Washington, D.C.: American Psychological Association.

MARYBETH SHINN • Center for Community Research and Action, Department of Psychology, New York University, New York, New York 10003. BRUCE D. RAPKIN • Memorial Sloan-Kettering Cancer Hospital, New York, New York 10021.

Handbook of Community Psychology, edited by Julian Rappaport and Edward Seidman. Kluwer Academic / Plenum Publishers, New York, 2000.

ables at more than one level of analysis. We use the word "group" as a shorthand for groups, settings, organizations, and social systems with recognizable boundaries. We assume that there are multiple individuals in each group, typically not selected at random. Further, we assume that observations of individuals are not independent; indeed, group members are linked by virtue of occupying a common setting and interacting with one another. When multiple groups are involved, they are comparable in structure and function and membership is mutually exclusive. Thus, our discussion pertains to a wide spectrum of social systems, including families, work places, classrooms, mutual help groups, churches, neighborhoods, residential facilities, and graduate programs. Some of the methods we discuss may generalize to less-bounded groups (e.g., an individual's social network, informal groups, transient gatherings). It may also be quite fruitful to apply these methods to studies of groups nested within higher levels of organization (e.g., classrooms in school districts, families in neighborhoods). However, we draw most of our examples from situations where individuals are members of settings with relatively distinct boundaries.

This chapter begins by distinguishing cross-level research from within-level and multi-level research. We offer a typology of cross-level relationships, including direct influences and contextual effects. Psychologists are accustomed to measuring variables at the individual level. To do cross-level research, we need better methods for assessing variables at extra-individual levels of analysis. Thus, we discuss ways of assessing group-level variables directly and methods for describing groups in terms of their members, particularly in ways that highlight the diversity of individual experiences and perspectives. We close with a discussion of cross-level processes or dynamic relationships among groups or environments and the individuals within them.

DEFINING RESEARCH IN TERMS OF LEVELS OF ANALYSIS

Within-Level and Multi-Level Research

Cross-level research may be contrasted with within-level and multi-level research. Within-level research involves research at a single-level of analysis, in psychology usually at the individual level. Much existing research in community psychology is of this type. Within-level research may deal with populations, ignoring social structure, as in many studies of prevention, and with an individual's patterns of relationships with other people, as in many studies of social support. It may examine the effects of a particular environmental condition or manipulation, but typically does not attempt to understand social structures and patterns of reciprocal relations involving units at more than one level.

More rarely, within-level research involves a single extra-individual level of analysis. For example, Tausig (1987) studied relationships among human service agencies and identified patterns of relationships that might indicate "cracks" in the mental health service system. These included the absence of relationships among agencies where they might be expected, unsatisfactory relationships, and haphazard rather than consistent patterns of contact between pairs of agencies with similar functional relationships.

Multi-level research (Rousseau, 1985) concerns relationships between independent and dependent variables at a given level that *replicate or generalize* across two or more levels. As an example, Rousseau cites a review by Staw, Sandelands, and Dutton (1981), which suggests that individuals, groups, and organizations respond similarly to threat, defined as an environmental event with impending negative or harmful consequences for the entity. At each level, threat leads to restriction in information and constriction in control, and consequently to well-learned, dominant, or rigid responses. Staw et al. (1981) hypothesized that such responses are adaptive when environmental changes are small, but are potentially maladaptive under conditions of great turbulence or radical change.

Multi-level research may have considerable power to generate hypotheses about the applicability of understanding garnered at one level to constructs and processes at another level. For example, hypotheses about the differential effectiveness of problem-focused and emotion-focused coping at the individual level might be extended to activities undertaken by work groups or organizations to assist members (Shinn & Mørch, 1983; Shinn, Mørch, Robinson, & Neuner, 1993). But multi-level theories are as likely to obscure as they are to clarify if they are only anthropomorphic metaphors (e.g., Rousseau, 1985). To exploit multi-level models requires a *composition theory* that specifies the relationships between variables at different levels presumed to be functionally similar (Roberts, Hulin, & Rousseau, 1978, p. 84; Rousseau, 1985). The notion of environmental threat, for example, is more similar across individuals, groups, and organizations than is the notion of constriction of control.

Barker (1968) and Wicker (1990) suggest that multi-level theories, in which relationships are replicated across levels of analysis, are rarely useful. They argue that systems at different levels of analysis are incommensurate, that is, they follow different laws. An engineer and an economist explain the movement of a train carrying wheat across the plains of Kansas according to completely different principles, both true, both relevant, but as incompatible "as the price of wheat in Chicago and the horsepower of the engine" (Barker, 1968, p. 12). Indeed, the boundaries between systems are defined by the points at which different principles are required to explain their behavior (Wicker, 1990). Wicker argued that each system should be analyzed in terms appropriate to it, and not solely in terms of concepts borrowed from another level.

When higher-level units are assessed by aggregating information gathered about lower-level units, different relationships may be found in analyses at different levels of aggregation. Attempts to generalize from one level to another have been dubbed the ecological fallacy. Robinson (1950) first demonstrated this problem. Using census data, he showed, for example, that although foreign birth and illiteracy displayed a mild positive correlation at the individual level, the percentage of foreign-born persons in a state was negatively correlated with the percentage of illiterate persons, because foreign-born people tended to settle in states with high literacy rates. Disparate processes accounted for the correlation at the two levels.

In the ecological fallacy, one typically has data on aggregates and wishes to make inferences about individuals. The reverse is also possible. Glick and Roberts (1984) point out that one cannot infer the effects of participatory decision-making on organizational performance from data about individual performance. Participatory decision-making may enhance organizational effectiveness via organizational innovation or improved work procedures that reflect the inherent interdependence of workers in organizations. Measures of short-term individual performance that fail to model the interdependence may miss this phenomenon.

Cross-Level Research

Cross-level research (also called mixed-level, e.g., Glick, 1980) involves relationships among two or more variables at different levels of analysis. Expanding on a typology offered by Rousseau (1985, p. 16), we identify five types of cross-level relationships:

1. Direct effects of variables at one level on variables at another level
2. Frog-pond effects, or effects of deviations from a group standard
3. Study of relationships at multiple levels, each controlling for the other via the decomposition of aggregate correlations
4. Moderating effects of a variable at one level on a relationship at another level, or person by environment interaction
5. Effects of person-environment fit

We will provide examples of these five relationships and address theoretical and methodological issues for each. Generally, statistical approaches for each type of cross-level research have developed independently of the others, although all are adapted from regression and ANOVA models. One important exception to this trend is represented by Bryk and Raudenbush's (1992) work on hierarchical linear models. They offer an integrated analytic approach to the evaluation of a large variety of cross-level relationships. Although the same analytic results can be obtained in other ways, we find Bryk and Raudenbush's approach to have considerable heuristic value for thinking about cross-level relationships in general. Thus, before discussing approaches to the study of different cross-level relationships, it is useful to introduce the basic elements of their model.

Hierarchical Linear Models in Cross-Level Research

Hierarchical linear models (HLM) can be used to analyze different types of data in which lower-level observations are nested within a higher-level unit, including multiple observations of a given entity (repeated measures), as well as cases within groups. HLM is a direct extension of multiple regression. It attempts to account for the variance in some dependent variable measured at the lowest level, using independent variables measured at that level and at higher levels. Although HLM can accommodate any number of levels, we consider the two-level case, applied to individuals nested within groups.

In HLM, the "level 1" model describes a regression equation predicting the dependent variable from independent measures at the individual level. This model is estimated for each group. That is, HLM generates estimates of regression coefficients (intercept and slopes) for each group. In the next step of HLM, within-group regression coefficients serve as dependent measures in "level 2" equations. Group differences in intercept and slope are predicted by independent variables measured at the group level. There is a level 2 model for each level 1 regression coefficient. Coefficients estimated in these level 2 models indicate how much each level 1 regression coefficient can be accounted for by group membership, or by variables measured at the group level. Residual variance in the level 2 equations indicates the portion of the level 1 effect that cannot be explained by differences among groups. Results of level 2 equations are substituted back into the level 1 equation to provide an overall model, decomposing each level 1 regression coefficient into effects related to group differences and effects that are specific to each group.

By including or excluding various terms in the level 1 and level 2 equations, HLM can reproduce various familiar analyses. For example, if the only term in the model is the estimate of how group membership accounts for differences in within-group intercepts, HLM is equivalent to a one-way between-groups ANOVA with random effects (that is, how much does the intercept or group mean account for variance in the dependent variable). Adding a single independent variable at the individual level is equivalent to ANCOVA. As we discuss in the following sections, HLM can be used to estimate the various types of cross-level relationships identified above.

Bryk and Raudenbush (1992) discuss the advantages of HLM over other approaches to cross-level analysis. Maximum likelihood methods used in HLM provide independent and unbiased estimates of group and individual-level effects. Compared to HLM, other techniques (e.g., aggregate correlations, individual-level regressions with group-level variables distributed over cases) tend to underestimate the effects of group influences on individual-level outcomes. As might be expected, HLM is most applicable to situations where there are fairly large numbers of observations at each level of analysis (Laren, 1991). This makes sense if we consider that HLM's estimation of within-group parameters depends on the stability of regression coefficients within each group. Even so, as Bryk and Raudenbush (1992) discuss, HLM can take into account the measurement precision of each parameter by adjusting unreliable within-group effects for aggregate effects.

Bryk and Raudenbush warn that the validity of HLM depends on proper specification of effects at each level. For example, an apparent group-level difference may be due to the omission of an individual difference variable associated with group membership. HLM requires careful attention to potential influences within and across levels. Theoretical considerations must guide applications of HLM. We develop our discussion of HLM further, in considering the five types of cross-level relationships discussed in the following.

Effects of Variables at One Level on Variables at Another Level. Direct relationships between contextual (group or environmental) factors and individual variables are the type of cross-level relationship most commonly studied in community psychology. For example, Felner, Ginter, and Primavera (1982) described an intervention that promoted ninth graders' attendance, grades, and self-esteem by restructuring the role of homeroom teachers to increase students' sense of support and accountability, and by reorganizing class assignments so that students had a more consistent peer group.

Cross-level models of this type typically involve a downward flow of influence from higher to lower levels of analysis: the asylum coerces the behavior of both inmates and staff (Goffman, 1961); degree of urbanicity affects the structure of social networks (Fischer, 1977); individuals adopt the "standing pattern of behavior" in settings they enter (Barker, 1968). Indeed, Bryk and Raudenbush's (1992) HLM specifically assumes that higher-level factors influence lower-level phenomena. In HLM, group-level variables explain variance among within-group intercepts (that is, mean differences among groups).

Although often assumed, a downward flow is not inherent in the concept of cross-level analysis (Rousseau, 1985). Community psychologists who study social action are particularly interested in the influence of "change agents," who attempt to catalyze change in settings (e.g., Seidman, 1983). Activists may also create new settings that accord with their values and goals (Cherniss, this volume; Sarason, 1972). These settings may later serve as models to influence others, or may simply exist as alternative structures for those who participate in them. Individuals may also have profound effects on the membership and activities of settings. For example, faculty (and often students in graduate programs) select new students and faculty and determine the curriculum. People in positions of authority usually have the most influence, but settings vary in the extent to which they allow influence and participation in decision-making from people at lower levels.

Bidirectional models, in which the agents of change are influenced, absorbed, or co-opted by the larger units they are creating or changing, are also possible and are often the most accurate representation of interdependence across levels. Children are influenced by their family systems, but also participate in molding them. Mutual-aid groups influence the behavior of their members, but people also create mutual-help groups, and the groups frequently attempt to influence social and political regularities affecting their members and others who are similarly situated (Rappaport, Seidman, Toro, McFadden, Reischl, Roberts, Salem, Stein, & Zimmerman, 1985). Goldenberg (1971) provides a fascinating description of bidirectional influence in the creation of a setting.

Frog-Pond Effects. A second type of cross-level relationship is the effect of individual differences from a group standard or a "frog-pond effect" (Firebaugh, 1980). For example, Seidman and Rapkin (1983) found that relative poverty (distance from a group standard) was more potent than absolute level of resources in explaining crime rates. Wechsler and Pugh (1967) showed that rates of first admissions to mental hospitals in Massachusetts among people with specific demographic characteristics (age, marital status, birthplace, profession) were higher in communities where those characteristics were relatively rare than in communities where they were common. Brown (1968) demonstrated that college students randomly assigned to live on floors of a residence hall where few others shared their academic interests became less certain of their career goals and were more likely to change their majors than students in the majority, regardless of initial interests. Sometimes, as in these examples, discrepancies from group norms in either direction may put individuals at risk. In other cases, only deficits, such as relative poverty, are problematic. There might also be benefits for esteem and accomplishment of positive discrepancies (being a "big frog").

Again, influence may be bidirectional. Individuals who are outliers from their groups may be at risk and, over time, we might expect them to conform to group influences or to leave. On the other hand, outliers may begin to affect group perceptions or patterns of interaction. For example, research on the "risky shift" in group decision-making suggests that an individual who possesses a cogent argument that is not widely shared is likely to move the group towards his or her point of view (Vinokur & Burnstein, 1974). Outliers may be viewed as deviants, opinion leaders, troublemakers, revolutionaries, rate busters, or role models. Indeed, individuals who deviate from their groups in ways that are deemed positive are often chosen as leaders in order to influence the group.

Frog-pond effects are relatively simple to analyze by partialing out or subtracting the group mean from each individual's score. The difference scores reflect the deviation of each individual from his or her own particular "frog-pond." When mean differences among groups or settings are appreciable, deviation scores may provide a very different picture than raw scores. Note that a frog-pond effect involves a correlation in the full (that is, ungrouped) sample. Bryk and Raudenbush (1992) discuss frog-pond effects in terms of "centering" variables in the level 1 model around group means (level 2 models need not be invoked). Either or both independent and dependent variables may be centered, depending on questions of interest. For example, students having high achievement relative to classmates may report higher relative or absolute levels of self-esteem.

Decomposition of Aggregate Correlations. An extension of the study of individual deviations from group means involves the decomposition of overall correlations into group and individual components. The basic question here is whether the observed correlation between two variables in the full sample can be explained by the fact that individuals are in groups. For example, in a study of the relationship between school performance and perceived support from classmates, one may ask whether the effect occurred at the group level (the best performers tend to come from the most supportive classes), the individual level (students who perceive that there is more support tend to perform better, regardless of their class), or some combination. Statistical techniques can help determine whether aggregate data can be interpreted as reflecting group-level phenomena, individual-level phenomena, or both (Dansereau,

Alutto, Markham, & Dumas, 1982; Dansereau, Alutto, & Yammarino, 1984; Dansereau & Markham, 1987; Glick & Roberts, 1984; Kenny, 1985; Kenny & La Voie, 1985; see Hall, 1988, for a review).

All of these methods involve decomposing a full-sample correlation into individual and group-level components. The individual component is based on deviation scores of individuals from their group means, identical to the frog-pond effect but with deviation scores computed for both variables in the correlation. Correlations based on deviation scores are termed pooled within-group correlation coefficients. The group-level component reflects the covariance remaining after pooled within-group effects are removed from total covariance.

HLM provides a flexible approach to decomposing within- and between-group correlations (Bryk and Raudenbush, 1992). As discussed earlier, HLM is concerned with accounting for the distribution of within-group regression coefficients. In order to decompose the correlation between X and Y, HLM would use the group mean of X to predict the intercepts of within-group (level 1) equations predicting Y from X. In other words, the model estimates the effect of mean differences in X on mean Y, as well as the average within-group relationship between X and Y. As we discuss below, HLM allows much more sophisticated analysis of group-level influences on correlations.

Most authors concerned with decomposition of correlations into between and within components simply treat the raw, group-level correlation as the group-level effect. By way of contrast, Kenny and La Voie (1985) argue that decomposition of the full-sample correlation into group- and individual-level terms does not control for the fact that correlations at the group level are not independent from within-group correlations. They illustrate the point with a thought experiment using the individual-level variables of height and weight. Of course, in a full, ungrouped sample, height and weight should be correlated due to their individual-level connection. If a large enough number of individuals are randomly assigned to pseudogroups, group means should be equal, and the individual-level correlation (that is, the correlations of the deviations of height and weight scores around their group means) should equal the ungrouped correlation. In other words, we would expect no group-level effect. However, if groups are small, so that random assignment does not equate them, there would still be a correlation at the group level due to the fact that the group with the heaviest individuals on average would also have the tallest. This correlation of group means can be thought of as the group-level correlation that would be expected due to the individual make-up of the group, since there is no group-level process linking height and weight. Kenny and La Voie (1985) suggest adjusting the raw group-level correlation for the corresponding within-group term. In essence, this yields an estimate of the group-level correlation above and beyond that which would be expected given the distribution of individuals into groups. These authors further suggest disattenuating the group-level correlation for the "unreliability" suggested by within-group variance—that is, lack of agreement within groups. (HLM also corrects for this sort of unreliability in parameter estimates.) Although there is no appropriate test for the significance of the estimated and disattenuated group-level correlation, this statistic provides a sense of the strength of the group effect after individual-level confounds are removed. The estimated effect can be contrasted with the raw group-level correlation to determine the effect of the statistical adjustments.

Interpretation of the within- and between-group correlations depends on their magnitude and (for unadjusted effects) significance. If only the pooled within-group correlation is large, then the relationship between variables is localized at the individual level. Similarly, if the group component is large, the setting-level interpretation would be applied. When correlations at both levels are large, some interesting possibilities arise. The case where strong group- and individual-level effects are in the same direction suggests that individual and group factors act in concert to produce the full-sample effect. For example, if performance and perceived support are positively correlated at both the individual and the classroom levels, the findings would suggest that children who perceive more support than their classmates also perform better, and that supportive classrooms are associated with good overall performance, above and beyond this individual effect. Correlations at different levels can also be in *opposite* directions. Using the classroom example, a positive group effect coupled with a negative individual effect may suggest a within-class triggering process, with students who perform poorly pulling for relatively more support from their classmates. Alternatively, a negative group-level correlation, together with a positive individual-level correlation, suggests that peer support is diminished (or perhaps, competition is greater) in high-performing classrooms, although children still benefit from relatively more support from peers. Note that large group and individual effects in opposite directions may yield full-sample correlations near zero.

Methods for separating group and individual-level effects may bring important new insights out of existing data. Florin, Giamartino, Kenny, and Wandersman (1988) used Kenny and La Voie's (1985) method to reanalyze data on the social climates of 17 block associations. The data were originally analyzed at the level of the block association only, since analyses of variance showed group effects for eight of ten climate measures (Giamartino & Wandersman, 1983). Perhaps the largest differences in results of the two analyses were in the area of time involvement. Whereas Giamartino and Wandersman (1983) reported that no social-climate variables were related to the time members spent working in their organizations, upon reanalysis, four dimensions appeared important. Members spent more time in organizations that were more cohesive, tolerant of expressions of negative feelings, open to sharing of personal feelings, and intolerant of uncoordinated, independent action. A number of individual-level effects, independent of group effects, also emerged. Methodological cautions in applying this technique are that there is no significance test for the corrected group-level correlation and that the consequences of violating the formal requirement that individuals be randomly assigned to groups are unclear.

Person by Environment Interactions

It is important to note that methods to decompose the correlation between variables into within- and between-group components tacitly assume that the individual-level correlation can be described meaningfully by a pooled correlation based on all groups. This assumption may not be warranted in many cases. For example, support and performance may be positively correlated in one classroom, negatively correlated in another, and uncorrelated in a third. Pooled within-group correlations may obscure these important between-group differences in the correlation of two variables. One global test for comparability of within-group correlations is provided by Box's (1948) M statistic, which assesses the similarity of variance–covariance matrices for two or more groups. If M is significant, it suggests that groups are not comparable, and that pooled correlations may be misleading.

Clearly, mere identification of the presence of group differences in correlations is not sufficient. Rousseau (1985) complained that, all too frequently, a moderating effect of group membership is asserted when a main effect is found in one setting and not in another, without any effort to understand why this occurs. It is important to determine what it is about groups that moderates the individual-level effect.

HLM is specifically geared to identifying and explaining within-group differences in correlations (Bryk & Raudenbush, 1992). In HLM, within-group regression slopes generated at the individual level are treated as outcomes in equations at the group level. This makes it possible to identify variables at the group level associated with systematic differences in the correlations among individual-level variables. This sort of effect can be interpreted as an interaction between a group-level variable and an individual-level variable in predicting the individual outcome. To take a hypothetical example, the individual-level correlation between time spent talking and satisfaction may be negative in newly formed mutual-help groups (where members are still getting to know one another, and are happy not to be put "on the spot"), but positive in older groups (where members who are more engaged may talk more than those who are bored or alienated). This interaction effect can be tested by using longevity as a group-level predictor in HLM, and observing whether this accounts for within-group regressions of satisfaction on talking.

HLM is not the only approach available for describing person by environment interactions. Maton's (1989) evidence for the stress-buffering effect of social support at the setting level provides an important example of identifying a group moderator. Using hierarchical multiple regression, Maton assessed the supportiveness of settings by averaging the perceptions of setting members and showed that, under some circumstances, the relationship between perceived stressors and experienced distress (both assessed at the individual level) was reduced in more supportive settings.

Identifying group-level moderators of individual-level relationships depends more on theoretical than methodological considerations. However, statistically testing such relationships requires sufficient setting variance in the group characteristic of interest, and enough settings to rule out spurious explanations. Even when it is not possible to identify specific group-level characteristics that explain group moderator effects, it may be useful to treat the within-group correlation as a group-level variable, in the same way we treat "proportion of women" or "average satisfaction" as descriptions of groups.

Person–Environment Fit

Person–environment fit (P–E fit) or congruence models may be thought of as special cases of setting interactions with individual variables: setting characteristics are presumed to moderate the relationship between some person characteristic and adjustment (French, Rodgers, & Cobb, 1974). Carp and Carp (1984) provide an excellent review and synthesis of these models, especially as they pertain to the assessment of older adults. We will briefly outline some of the main considerations of P–E fit models as a major branch of cross-level research.

Conceptually, it is useful to distinguish three aspects of P–E fit. Most basic is the similarity or difference of the individual from other people in the setting—essentially, the relationship captured in the frog-pond effect. Overall measures of similarity might be constructed by summing the deviation of individuals from group means across relevant measures, or by constructing a profile of scores. It is important to note that different dimensions of similarity may have very different functions in a setting. For example, in a study of nursing-home residents, Ruggiero and Rapkin (1991) found that perceived support was enhanced by similarity in neighborhood background between residents and others on their ward, but diminished by similarity in age.

A second dimension of P–E fit involves the ability of an individual to meet environmental "press" for different kinds of performance, and for the environment to supply the resources an individual needs to adapt (Carp & Carp, 1984; French et al., 1974). This model of P–E fit was well articulated by Lawton and Nahemow (1973), who describe fit in terms of Helson's

(1964) notion of adaptation level. People at or near an optimal fit are in a homeostatic relationship with their environments, but imbalances may arise from changes in either the individual's needs and abilities, or in the environment's resources and demands. Individuals can adapt to relatively minor imbalances. Indeed, Lawton and Nahemow (1973) suggest that facing demands slightly greater than one's adaptation level can enhance adjustment, and that individuals with higher levels of competence can adapt to a wider range of demands and resources. However, too great a shift away from the optimal level in either direction can produce maladjustment. This model of person–environment congruence is broadly applicable to any personal competencies and environmental demands that impinge on one another. For example, to understand or enhance self-disclosure in a mutual-help group, one might consider supports and group norms specific for this behavior. A different set of environmental features might be examined with respect to members' provision of tangible support to one another.

A third aspect of P–E fit is the congruence between environmental features and personal preferences or the closeness of the environment to some personal ideal. A number of authors (Kahana, 1975; Moos, 1974) have used perceived environment or "real" social-climate dimensions that parallel measures of preference or "ideal" social climate: for example, how much privacy is there, and how much privacy do you prefer? With parallel or commensurate scales such as these, one can design a range of congruence coefficients to represent degree of fit, taking into account level of preference and direction of deviation (Kahana, Liang, & Felton, 1980). However, Kahana (1975) points out that perceptual ratings may be confounded by preference ratings—individuals who do and do not value privacy may use different criteria to rate a setting as "very private." Indeed, measures of P–E fit based solely on individual perceptions are probably best conceptualized as single-level, rather than cross-level, measures. If the environment is assessed directly, via key informants, or via aggregate perceptions of people within it, one avoids the confound and obtains a cross-level measure. Carp and Carp (1984) take a further step away from commensurate scales. They propose an integrated, theory-driven approach to assessing P–E fit, by describing person and environment characteristics on their own terms, and identifying interaction effects that predict outcomes.

Cross-Level Research in Community Psychology

These five types of cross-level relationships open up exciting avenues for community research. Indeed, we contend that cross-level research should be at the core of community psychology. This goal is reflected in the oxymoronic nature of the field's name. "Community" refers to extra-individual contexts; "psychology" refers to individual experience (cf. Hobfoll, 1990; Keys & Frank, 1987a). Constructs such as empowerment or P–E fit are exciting when they embody a cross-level relationship between the individual and the social system. When they are defined in terms of individual psychological variables, such as locus of control for empowerment or satisfaction with the environment for P–E fit, they lose their community flavor. Were we to lose this ultimate connection to the individual, we would cease to be psychologists, but when we confine ourselves to the individual level, we lose our community identity.

Of course, community psychologists may be concerned with relationships between settings or with effective functioning of groups or organizations as targets of research or intervention, but we study these higher levels of analysis not just for their own sake, but also for their impact on individual well-being. Such research is relevant to community psychology when characteristics of the extra-individual units have clear theoretical implications for individual outcomes. For example, Tausig (1987) studied patterns of relationships among agencies providing social services in order to identify structural barriers to referrals of individuals from one service to another and, by extension, lack of easy access by individuals to relevant services.

Although we advocate cross-level studies, it is not our goal to prescribe a narrow set of research questions or methodologies. As our discussion may suggest, cross-level research encompasses a wide variety of designs. The diversity of approaches may at first seem disconcerting. There is no prescription for determining the proper way to analyze cross-level data. As researchers who have approached this class of problems have learned, methods must often be "home grown." It should be self-evident that cross-level methods must follow from cross-level questions. Multiple methodologies may yield multiple insights into the behavior of people in context.

In order to do cross-level research, we need strategies for assessing extra-individual variables in ways that capture their significance for individual outcomes and behavior. The next two sections describe methods for assessing extra-individual units directly and by using information about their constituent parts.

MEASURING EXTRA-INDIVIDUAL UNITS DIRECTLY

This section describes measures of groups and other extra-individual units that are not constructed from information about individuals, that is, group-level measures that match group-level conceptualizations. McGrath and Altman's (1966) review of research on small groups showed that studies of relationships between variables at different levels were relatively rare, and that cross-level relationships reached significance only about two-thirds as often as relationships among measures within a single level. Wicker (1990) took this as evidence that different levels are incommensurate. It may also be evidence that both cross-level theory and assessment methods need further development.

It is relatively easy to devise measures of groups or environments at the group level: for example, size, location in space or in an organization's structure, function or mission, policies, longevity. It is harder to think about extra-individual variables that are proximally related to individual behavior. To develop such measures, we need theory to guide us to constructs of potential functional significance.

Seidman's (1988, 1990) notion of social regularities may be especially fertile ground for cultivating the necessary theory. Social regularities are patterns of constancy in relationships between individuals and social systems, often indexed by differences or ratios. For example, it was the genius of Barker and colleagues (Barker, 1987; Barker & Gump, 1964; Wicker, McGrath, & Armstrong, 1972) to translate the distal variable of organizational size into the more proximal social regularity of manning or staffing, or the ratio of the number of setting inhabitants to the number of social roles available. The conceptualization in terms of social regularities rather than physical entities made it easier to see differences in tolerance for diversity and in mechanisms for regulating behavior in under- and overstaffed settings. Similarly, in daycare centers, group size is less important than staff–child ratio in predicting children's engagement and cognitive development (Whitebook, Howes, & Phillips, 1990), because staff–child ratio is, in turn, associated with the attention that children receive. Staff education and training levels are also important, presumably because they enable teachers to relate to children more effectively and in age-appropriate ways.

In evaluating physical environments, the most fruitful variables are again those that have functional significance or that convey symbolic messages to inhabitants. For example, Proshansky, Ittelson, and Rivlin (1970) showed that adding drapes and more comfortable furnishings to an uncomfortable solarium on a psychiatric ward led patients to use the room more frequently and actively. The refurnished room was more functional and conveyed new expectations for behavior. Theories of defensible space (Newman, 1972; Perkins, Florin, Rich, Wandersman, & Chavis, 1990) suggest that areas that can be readily observed and that have symbolic markers of ownership, such as fences or block-watch signs, are less likely to be robbed or vandalized.

Symbolic meanings may be especially important to vulnerable or devalued groups. Wolfensberger (1972) judged the extent of normalization in facilities for mentally retarded people, that is, the degree to which they created culturally normative environments so as to promote normative behavior. Both institutional furnishings and childlike decorations, such as pictures of clowns, convey the message to residents that they are not normal adults who could expect to live in homes. Rapkin (1987) identified characteristics of the procedures and policies in agencies employing elder community volunteers that either reflected or refuted a negative social construction of old age. For example, an agency that regularly tries to find a temporary replacement when a volunteer is absent conveys the message that the volunteer's role is important for the agency's operation. This runs counter to the stereotype that old age equals obsolescence. Similarly, Shinn, Knickman, Ward, Petrovic, and Muth (1990) suggested that shelter conditions such as lack of privacy, bolted down furniture, admonishing posters, unnecessary regimentation, and filth symbolically undermined the dignity of homeless residents.

An important criterion for selecting setting-level characteristics is their ability to facilitate or inhibit individual adaptation. Consider, for example, the case of elders seeking long-term care services at home. Barriers to access exist at a variety of levels in the social system. First, at the policy level, individuals may face a range of eligibility criteria based on income, degree of impairment, available resources at home, citizenship, and place of residence, to name a few. Second, public information and media may not offer the information elders need to find or compare the services they desire. Third, at the community or neighborhood level, the organization of services and relationships among agencies may affect accessibility of services. Fourth, agencies may effectively bar clients through lack of transportation, inadequate hours of operation, or insensitivity to cultural and language factors. Fifth, individuals may encounter norms against using services in their families, churches, or other primary groups.

As this example demonstrates, group and setting-level constructs that affect individuals' behavior abound (for other examples, see Keys & Frank, 1987b; Moos, 1973; Moos & Lemke, 1984; Stokols, 1981). Once such constructs are conceptualized and assessed using methods appropriate for the particular phenomenon of interest, and at a particular level, they can be used in cross-level analyses. For example, it might be meaningful to compare individual-level outcomes of elder home-care recipients in communities with different configurations of services or different norms about care at home.

MEASURING GROUPS WITH INFORMATION ABOUT INDIVIDUALS

So far we have used the word "level" to mean what Katz and Kahn called "level of conceptualization" (1978, p. 13), that is, the level of theory or understanding, the level at which conclusions are drawn and generalizations made. In the preceding section, we emphasized measures of groups that are framed at the group level. However, the level of conceptualization sometimes differs from both the level of measurement and the level to which data are assigned for statistical analysis (Rousseau, 1985). A central question for cross-level research concerns the consequences of a mismatch between level of conceptualization and level of measurement.

Lewin (1952) argued that, whereas it is possible to objectively and reliably measure units of any size with methods fitted to the unit, any "attempt to determine reliably large macroscopic units by observing microscopic units ... is bound to fail" (p. 244). Katz and Kahn (1978, p. 13), on the other hand, held that researchers must distinguish between levels of conceptualization and levels of measurement, but that the two need not match. Although levels of conceptualization and measurement co-vary in the natural sciences (so that, for example, the psychological experiences of color vision cannot be fully understood by measuring the physiological processes), in the social sciences, higher-level (emergent) phenomenon may be observed in the interrelated actions of individuals. In studying organizations, they argue, one should take the social-system level as the conceptual starting point, but one typically constructs measures using information from or about individuals. Systems-level concepts direct the selection of individual-level data and dictate their use.

Katz and Kahn (1978, p. 13) offer the example of the introduction of a new piece-rate payment plan in an industrial enterprise. A researcher could study resulting phenomena at the individual level, focusing, for example, on the worker's needs for economic gains. Or one could examine group-level norms that limit or legitimate production rates. In both cases, one would ask questions of or observe the behavior of individuals, but the data would be used to draw different inferences.

Let us pursue Katz and Kahn's assertion that one can assess extra-individual units of conceptualization by asking individuals, using the example of economic needs and group norms. It is not hard to imagine assessing workers' needs for economic gains by asking individuals. If need is defined by an individual's subjective state, there may be no better approach. However, if norms are considered not simply cognitive expectations, but also social standards that regulate attitude and behavior (Sherif, 1936, e.g., p. 85), it is less clear that individual perceptions are a good way to measure them. How should one proceed? Should one ask individuals directly about the existence or strength of norms or the extent to which they are shared and then *average* the responses? Or should one ask each individual what the presumed norms are and then look at the *variability* of responses? Does disagreement among group members indicate lack of norms, lack of reliability in measuring them, or perhaps the existence of subgroups for whom norms operate in very different ways? To answer these questions, we need more insight into both problems in measuring extra-individual phenomena by collecting data from individuals, and, as Katz and Kahn (1978) put it, how data from individuals should be used to shed light on higher levels of conceptualization.

Describing Groups in Terms of the Average Member

The typical way of using individual-level data to describe groups is to take the mean of members' scores. The group mean necessarily transcends the perspective of any one individual. However, the use of the mean to describe a setting implies that the attribute being measured is expected to be the same for all group members. Individual deviation from the mean is treated as measurement error. This kind of understanding of "persons-in-settings" closely parallels the logic of analysis of variance (ANOVA), where the group is presumed to exert a uniform main effect on individual members, and where differences are treated as error variance. Methods like the intraclass correlation for testing the agreement among ratings of group members are all based on ANOVA.

When is it appropriate to use the mean as a measure of the setting? Many authors suggest first calculating an intraclass correlation or other coefficient of consistency or interrater reliability among group members (Dansereau et al., 1984; Kenny & La Voie, 1985). James (1982) placed great weight on measures of interrater agreement, and Guion (1973) suggested that perceptions be accepted as measures of organizational attributes only if they are virtually unanimous. Glick (1985) eschewed agreement among individuals as a criterion for reliability of an organizational attribute and instead emphasized the extent to which organizations can be reliably differentiated from one another. Of course, group differentiation is useful only when (1) multiple groups are measured and (2) groups are expected to vary. At the least, the differentiation criterion imposes certain requirements for sampling settings. Joyce and Slocum (1984) adopted both these criteria for construct validity and added a third: predictable relationships between aggregate measures and other variables at organizational or individual levels.

One construct that has become particularly identified with the strategy of aggregation across individuals to describe settings is social climate (e.g., James & Sells, 1981; Moos, 1974, 1984). Social climates based on aggregated perceptions within intact groups have had impressive successes, according to Joyce and Slocum's third criterion of predicting other group or organizational phenomena. In one example of criteria that share no perceptual method bias with climate, classroom climates that are task-oriented and set specific academic goals, while maintaining both supportive relations and structure, are associated with gains on standardized achievement tests. In another, treatment climates that lack peer or staff support, that are disorganized, and have unclear rules and procedures have high drop-out rates (Moos, 1984). Below, we discuss how agreement among group members emerges. At this point, we consider ways to describe groups in terms of individuals that go beyond mean scores.

The Whole is More Than the Mean of the Parts: Describing the Group in Terms of the Diversity of Members

When average individual measures do not demonstrate high interrater agreement, discriminate among settings, or display interpretable relationships with external criteria, it seems reasonable to conclude that the mean is more a statistical artifact than an intrinsically meaningful property of the setting. Under such conditions, some authors conclude that it is necessary to reject the group level of analysis in favor of treating cases as disaggregated individuals (e.g., Dansereau et al., 1984). Although we agree that it is difficult to interpret the mean (or other measure of central tendency, such as a median) as a valid group characteristic under such circumstances, it also seems unreasonable to proceed as if individuals are no longer in groups. Even if group members' scores do not converge, they are still linked by virtue of membership. The mean is by no means the only meaningful information that may be derived about the aggregate characteristics of individuals in a group.

This section addresses issues that arise in deriving and analyzing alternative group-level measures that describe the diversity of group members. It begins with the relatively straightforward identification of subgroups within a larger group, considers the continuous variables that indicate position within a group, and then examines the univariate and multivariate distributions of variables. Subsequent subsections describe groups in terms of members' relationships and regularities in members' social behavior.

Identification of Subgroups

One potential cause of within-group heterogeneity is the existence of subgroups that are internally homogenous but distinct from one another. The distinctions may arise from individual attributes or from the different experiences the environment affords to different individuals. A community psychology that values cultural relativity must recognize that subgroups often view extra-individual phenomena through distinctive lenses; settings that foster the growth of one subgroup may do so at the expense of another. Opportunities, for example, vary systematically for individuals by age, race, gender, sexual orientation, social class, or place in an organization's structure. If a teacher calls on boys more than girls and listens more patiently to their responses, boys and girls may perceive the classroom environment very differently. Differential experiences may also be haphazard: The tourist whose pocket is picked has a lower impression of the city than one whose visit is more benign.

Recognition of the fact that a single environment may exert different pressures or provide different opportunities for different subgroups led Chein (1954) to propose a middle ground between the objective or physical environment (in Gestalt psychologists' terms, the geographical environment) and the perceived or social environment (in Gestalt terms, behavioral). He labeled this middle ground the geo-behavioral or objective-behavioral environment, that is, the environment looked at objectively from the point of view of understanding behavior. Recognition of multiple subenvironments allows one to examine their effects, Chein contended, without abandoning the geo-behavioral environment for a psychological analysis of individuals.

Morris, Shinn, and Dumont (1999), for example, examined barriers to the integration of women and ethnic minority officers in a police department. They theorized that precincts would differ in the extent to which they supported or excluded women and minorities, and that these differences could be measured via officers' perceptions. However, both main effects of demographic subgroup (white male, minority male, female), as well as interactions between the precinct and the subgroup in predicting views of the commanding officer's support and fairness, suggested that the precinct environments differed systematically for different demographic subgroups. Relationships among variables also differed, to some extent, for different subgroups. For example, for women and minority men, the commanding officer's sensitivity to diversity (as assessed by the average view of group members within the precinct) was positively related to job satisfaction; for white men, the relationship was reversed.

Differences Related to Within-Group Roles and Positions

Not only demographic differences, but also roles or positions, may influence people's perceptions and experiences in a group. Positions may be defined formally or informally based on achieved or ascribed characteristics within the group (seniority, rank, job title), or in society at large (age, social class, gender). The association between position and other variables is an important property of groups. For example, do long-term residents in a community differ in income (or in neighborhood satisfaction) from newcomers? Do people who, in Barker's (1968, p. 51) terms, penetrate more deeply into behavior settings experience different pressures to participate than others who are less involved?

The number and variety of positions evident in a setting constitute group-level variables, necessarily measured at the group level of analysis. Alternatively, the association of position with other variables assessed at the individual level is an important way to describe groups. For example, at the classroom level, do students in an accelerated reading group view competition differently than do their classmates? Choice of measures of the association between position and other variables depends on the level of measurement of each. For instance, in a study of differences in attitudes toward patients among doctors, nurses, orderlies, and volunteers at a hospital, eta-square ratios could be computed to provide information about the proportion of variance in attitudes due to staff roles.

Distributions of Variables

Describing group members according to their status on some positional variable, or examining the association of position with other variables, can be generalized to consideration of univariate and multivariate distributions of group members on any variables of interest. Measures of distribution provide richer descriptions of groups than is provided by measures of central tendency. Measures of variability, such as the standard deviation or inter-quartile range are always interesting. Fuller descriptions are particularly useful where data are multimodal or skewed, where distributions are truncated, where outliers or the tails of distributions are of special interest, and where outliers heavily influence means. For example, communities are better described by the number of residents at various income levels than by mean income and standard deviation, in part because we are likely to be interested in the very rich and the very poor. Joint distributions of several variables, such as income, family structure, age, gender, and ethnicity, are also important descriptors of groups. There are certainly differences between communities (or companies or nations) in which income distributions are narrow or broad, in which income is (or is not associated) with ethnicity or gender, and in which level of income is positively or negatively associated with change in income over time.

Theoretical questions may motivate examination of particular characteristics of a distribution. Consider how the distribution of production rates can be used as a group-level measure in our earlier example of norms for production. When workers are paid on a piece-work basis, that is, according to the number of units of output they produce, they typically worry that if production goes too high, management will pay less for each unit produced. Thus, norms arise that set an informal ceiling on individual production, with negative sanctions for rate-busters. If all group members are sufficiently capable and motivated to achieve, then all should perform at or near the ceiling, and the overall distribution should be narrow. If workers are not equally motivated or capable, the distribution should be skewed with a long tail at lower rates of production, a mode at the norm, and an immediate drop to near zero frequency above the norm. In self-report measures, those whose production was far below the norm might not be aware of its existence; those performing at or near the norm, especially those with a strong economic need to go beyond it, might be acutely aware. Hence, lack of agreement on norms might reflect differential places in the distribution rather than lack of norms.

The distributions of production rates is, of course, an aggregate of individual rates, but with a difference. If the production rates are seen as individual measures, each individual datum has the same status as any other. But if production rates are seen as part of a distribution, then each datum has meaning only as it relates to the overall pattern. That pattern is a group-level indicator of the norm under investigation (cf. McGrath & Altman, 1966, p. 19). As these examples suggest, there are several ways that the distribution of a single variable across members of a setting can be represented, just as there are multiple measures of central tendency. Choice of a distributional statistic depends upon the aspects of heterogeneity and group composition to be highlighted, including variance, range, skewness, kurtosis, or the difference between the median and the mean. Groups could also be characterized in terms of their fit to a normal distribution or some other theoretically relevant ideal. Factors that guide selection of the proper statistic include whether deviations from central tendency are meaningful, whether the distribution comprises various identifiable groups, and whether differences between extreme members are of interest. Other guiding considerations include group size, the number and reliability of distributional properties of interest, and the desire to compare different groups in terms of their distributions.

When there is more than one variable of interest, describing the diversity of groups takes on added complexity. One approach to dealing with multiple measures is to describe the univariate distribution of each. Thus, in a given classroom, perceived peer support may be bimodal, achievement level may be distributed uniformly, and attendance may show virtually no variability. The multivariate situation also provides the opportunity to examine relationships among measures within subgroups. Two other flexible alternatives to the empirical description of multivariate distributional properties of a group include correlational methods and cluster analysis. Depending upon questions of interest to the researcher, correlation matrices may be used to derive within-group correlations, regressions, or factor structures, which may, in turn, be compared across groups. Thus, it is possible to distinguish classrooms where grades are predictable from student's ethnicity and social class from classrooms where these variables are orthogonal. Cluster analytic methods can be used to identify subgroups of setting members with similar profiles of scores. For example, if members of a setting have a common perception of social climate, all members' profiles of ratings on relevant climate scales would converge. However, if some members perceive more order and rule clarity, and others experience more support, group members may display different patterns of scores. These profiles could be identified by cluster analyses of members within each setting. Settings could be compared regarding the number of clusters, the presence of similar profiles of scores, and the proportion of members associated with each profile.

As mentioned previously, tests of the appropriateness of group means as a measure include interrater reliability, group differences, and convergence with other measures. Although there is no direct analogue to inter-rater reliability, some similar criteria might be applied to the evaluation of the appropriateness of distributional measures. One might determine whether two measures of a given construct display similar degrees of heterogeneity. A group that is highly variable on one measure of supportive exchange should be similarly variable on an alternate measure. The shape of the distribution of scores in different groups can be compared using non-parametric tests, such as the Komolgorov–Smirnov tests (see Siegel, 1956). Correlations with independent criteria might be especially helpful for establishing confidence in measures of distributional features. For example, co-workers identified as having similar patterns of perceptions using cluster analysis might be expected to work in proximity to one another, to have similar roles, or to share some other feature that might account for their common point of view. Ability to detect such within-group relationships depends on sample size.

Describing the Group in Terms of Members' Relationships

Up to this point, the methods that we have discussed treat measures of individuals as independent observations. Central tendency, distributional, and positional statistics combine or contrast scores, but they do not take into account ways in which group members' scores may be directly and causally related to one another. For example, co-workers' perceptions of their jobs may be based upon a common social construction of reality that emerges from daily interactions. Although such interdependencies in the behavior of members of the same setting are commonplace, our roots in individual psychology often lead us to ignore them, and to treat members as independent units of analysis. An additional problem arises if a group contains important subgroups or positional variables that we do not recognize. In this case, systematic variance that could be linked to group or position is lumped with individual variance.

To understand the dependencies among individuals' scores, or to identify subgroups of people whose attitudes or behaviors are linked, we may want to assess members' connections and interpersonal ties inside (and outside) the group. More or less familiar techniques from sociometry or social-network analysis can be used to describe who is connected to whom, or who is involved in specific kinds of exchanges. For example, to determine whether members influence one another's ratings of social climate in a setting, sociometric measures or behavioral observations might be used to discern how frequently different members interact. A matrix of scores could be formed, with elements indicating the degree of contact between every possible pair of individuals. Thus, in a setting with 20 participants, this matrix would have 190 unique elements, representing the degree of contact between every possible dyad. A second matrix of similar dimensions could be formed, indicating the profile distance between each pair of members' social climate ratings. Entries in this matrix will be smaller for dyads who share a similar view of the setting. Comparison of these matrices would determine the association of members' perceptions and interaction frequencies. A simple negative correlation between the corresponding elements of the two matrices would suggest that more interaction produces less distance in perception. The robustness of this correlation might be studied by using different variables and methods to compute profile distance between group members (Rapkin & Luke, 1993), by using different measures of contact between members, and/or by computing correlations that omit dyads involving certain people, chosen at random. Methods might depend on whether influence is presumed to be unidirectional or bidirectional.

Regularities in Members' Social Behavior in Groups

Frequencies, types, and directions of contact among members of a social group, particularly if modeled over time, are themselves important measures of group characteristics. For example, Sarason (1982, p. 105) described the behavioral regularity in American schools that teachers, not students, ask almost all of the questions. Patterns of interaction can be related to the achieved and ascribed characteristic of group members, distinguishing, for example, between classrooms where girls and boys do and do not interact, and between organizations where communication across hierarchical levels is unidirectional or bidirectional.

A more fine-grained approach to the assessment of regularities in group behavior can be adopted from methods developed for the study of dyadic interaction by Gottman (1979). These methods begin with the behavioral observation of individuals involved in an ongoing exchange or dialogue. The stream of behavior is divided into units demarcated by changes of speaker, and coded according to the content and/or affect the actor conveys. These procedures are common to many behavioral observation systems. What is unique about Gottman's approach is the way data are treated after being coded. Rather than simply counting how frequently each actor engages in each behavior, Gottman preserves the sequential order in which units occur. This makes it possible to assess the probability that a particular actor will emit a target behavior, given the preceding behavior of others in the group.

Roberts (personal communication, 1991) discussed the possibility of using methods of sequential analysis to study interactions in mutual-help groups. Consider the following hypothetical example: If we are interested in assessing group regularities around self-disclosure, we may observe that self-disclosure by some group member occurs in 15% of all observational units. However, members' disclosures may occur in 65% of the units immediately following the leader's self-disclosure. This conditional probability (of members' disclosure given leader's disclosure) can be tested to see if it is significantly different from the base rate of disclosure. If so, it would indicate that there is a lag 1 relationship between leader disclosure and member disclosure in this group. Lag 1 means that the target behavior immediately follows the antecedent condition. Longer lags may also be examined. Note that a relationship in one group is established using data derived exclusively from that group. In other groups, the same conditional probability may be equal to the base rate of disclosure, indicating no contingent relationship, or it may be significantly less than the baseline, indicating that leader self-disclosure inhibits, rather than encourages, member self-disclosure.

The use of sequential analysis to establish social regularities in interactions holds much potential for cross-level research. Groups may be compared in terms of the strength of various antecedents and consequences of target behaviors. This analytic approach can be extended to take account of group members' positions and relationships. Different contingencies may hold for women and men, blacks and whites, newer and older members, or members who do and do not have relationships outside the group.

Sequential methods are not easy to apply. Even in studies of dyads, with behavior coded in a relatively small number of categories, the number of possible antecedent and consequent relationships is large. In groups with multiple actors, the problem is compounded by the number of possible focal individuals. This situation is simplified somewhat if individual differences can be subsumed under role or status characteristics of members, as suggested above. However, in approaching analyses such as these, *a priori* specification of theoretically interesting relationships may be necessary to help keep one's bearings in a sea of data analytic options.

UNDERSTANDING THE CROSS-LEVEL PROCESSES BEHIND GROUP DIFFERENCES

The previous two sections have outlined a variety of methods for assessing extra-individual units of analysis. Simply establishing group differences does not, of course, explain them. In this final section, we describe cross-level processes that, over time, may lead to group differences, aid in the formation of group norms, or create fit between persons and environments. These processes may be studied in their own right or as potential confounds for other processes in which the researcher is more interested.

Schneider and Reichers (1983) described three mechanisms that lead to common perceptions of an environment: (1) grouping of individuals who share common perspectives (or characteristics) via selection, attraction, and attrition; (2) common experiences of the objective environment (which we include in a broader category of socialization described below); and (3) social interaction leading to a shared social construction of reality. Agreement among members in describing a group or organization, although an extra-individual phenomenon, thus may reflect more than just the objective environment. Similar issues arise in understanding group-level effects that do not depend on perception. Wicker (1972) described processes leading to what he called "behavior–environment congruence," or the conformity of behavior to the different programs of different environments. Most of his processes involve individual learning or shaping of behavior by the setting (socialization), or the choices of the individual to enter and remain in the setting and of the setting to welcome or exclude the individual (selection, attraction, and attrition).

Distinguishing among these cross-level processes is critical to developing interventions to promote change. Similarly, in evaluating "environmental treatments," one must distinguish group-level effects that reflect what goes on in the group from effects arising from selection, attraction, and attrition of group members and, in the case of perceptual measures, from changes in perceptual anchors as a result of social interaction. For example, do graduates of a drug treatment program stay free of drugs more successfully than a sample of addicts on the street because of the graduates' experience in the program (socialization), because they were motivated to get off drugs (attraction), or because they were dropped from the program if they failed to stay clean (attrition)? Do they agree that the program's rules are fair rather than arbitrary because they all experience the same environment (socialization), because of group discussion (social construction of reality), or because those with different perspectives have left (attrition)? Techniques for demonstrating differences and apportioning variance are not sufficient to answer these questions, particularly when data are collected at a single point in time.

One critique of many of the methods we have described for assessing groups is that they suggest a static relationship between stable person and environment features. To understand the emergence and maintenance of behavior–environment congruence requires putting this relationship into a dynamic context. In the next sections, we describe selection, attraction, and attrition; social construction of reality; and socialization as means of developing group consensus and between-group differences in perceptions and behavior. We also discuss some ways we might recognize these processes in action.

Selection, Attraction, and Attrition

Selection, attraction, and attrition are clearly bidirectional processes. Settings select and reject or eject members, just as members choose setting (Barker, 1968, p. 171; Wicker, 1972). Wicker (1972) suggested that both individuals and settings make decisions about each other according to a social exchange model. Each accepts the other when the rewards for doing so exceed the comparison level for alternatives. Often this is an ongoing process. Students are attracted to, and decide to apply to, certain graduate psychology departments in light of alternatives such as other psychology programs, law school, or a job, on the basis of the short- and long-term rewards they expect from each setting. The psychology departments each select a subset of the applicants for admission, in comparison with the other applicants in their pool. Then the students who have been selected by each department choose whether to attend in light of the (often smaller) comparison set now available to them. After entering, students who cease to find a program rewarding may leave; if they fail to meet program standards, they may be asked to leave. Wicker (1972) noted that there is a certain asymmetry between people and settings. Settings can often accommodate a variable number of inhabitants, so in admitting a particular member, the comparison set includes admitting no one. Individuals, on the other hand, have to choose some setting, although it need not be a graduate program in psychology. Both individuals and settings may work actively to increase their comparison set: Programs send out recruitment materials to increase their applicant pools and students apply to multiple programs to increase their options.

The combined effects of selection, attraction, and attrition are to create groups that are relatively homogenous in some dimensions. Psychology graduate students, for example, are likely to have more impressive undergraduate records than a random sample of college graduates, but probably know less chemistry than a random sample of medical students. If students in the more prestigious graduate programs have more impressive records than those in less prestigious programs, and also go on to publish more articles, one might ask whether the differential publication rates are due to the training (socialization) students receive in the more prestigious programs, or simply to control over group membership via selection, attraction, and attrition.

It is not always easy to determine whether group differences are due to control of group membership rather than to socialization, even with longitudinal data. In principle, within-group similarity and between-group differences due to selection and attraction should be manifest at the outset, whereas effects due to socialization should develop over time; however, this criterion is not helpful if the outcome (e.g., publication rates) cannot be assessed until some time has passed. If within-group similarity is due to attrition, outliers should be more likely to leave than those who fall closer to the central tendency of the group.

Effects of selection and socialization can be modeled with a regression-discontinuity design (Cook and Campbell, 1979, p. 137) if selection is based entirely on some measured criterion, so that individuals are selected for the socialization experience (the treatment) if, and only if, they exceed some cutoff score, and if outcome data are available for those who are and are not selected. When posttest scores are regressed on pretest scores, socialization effects show up as differences in intercept or slope of the regression line at the cutoff point. Selection effects are estimated by the slope itself. Alternately, if a substantial group of people are essentially equal on the selection criterion, one can conduct an experiment within this group, randomly selecting some to be exposed and others to be denied exposure to the socializing treatment. Of course, psychologists who cheerfully advocate random assignment to other people's programs may be reluctant to conduct a randomized experiment in their own graduate school admissions. To study the effects of attrition, one can examine differences between those who leave and those who stay and, if possible, include those who left in any follow-up studies.

When one cannot control selection and obtain information on those not selected, one may still model the selection process. For example, in a study of alternative models for sheltering homeless families, an important question was whether nonprofit shelters placed families in housing more quickly than did city-run shelters or welfare hotels because the nonprofit shelters "creamed" the best clients. Shinn et al. (1990) found consensus among directors of the nonprofit sites, the city official in charge of assigning families to shelters, the operators of the computer-matching system, and the families themselves that neither shelters nor families could circumvent the city's assignment of families to shelters. However, some nonprofit sites did control resident composition with limits on family size or prohibited older children or men. Non-profit shelters also had the right to institute eviction proceedings against residents. Although eviction was rarely used, the possibility probably influenced residents' behavior.

Social Construction of Reality: Development of Shared Perspectives

Typically, selection and attraction affect group homogeneity at the outset, whereas socialization and the social construction of reality both reduce variance over time. Often, development of shared perspectives is seen as an artifact to be controlled in assessing "real" change. Golembiewski, Billingsley, and Yeager (1976) offer an intriguing example: They assessed members' perceptions of the authority structure of their organization before and after an intervention designed to increase levels of participation in decision-making. Although respondents agreed at posttest that the environment was more participatory than before, direct comparison of pretest and posttest scores indicated a shift in the opposite direction. Golembiewski et al. (1976) suggested that the intervention did change the organization in the direction of greater participation, but that it changed respondents' visions of participatory processes even more, so that the discrepancy between vision and reality increased. The shared perspective of the organization as less participatory than before was, in this analysis, an artifact, created by stretching of the perpetual yardstick. One may attempt to eliminate such stretching of rubber yardsticks, (e.g., by anchoring rating scales), or one may study changes in perceptual frames as a phenomenon of interest, but one ignores them at one's peril.

In addition to complicating the assessment of other cross-level effects, the development of shared perspectives (or the failure to develop them) are cross-level phenomena worthy of research in their own right. Social psychologists examine development of consensus and polarization in laboratory groups and in juries (Moscovici, 1985; Rodin, 1985). Community psychologists might study how neighborhood groups identify problems and set priorities for solving them. In all these cases, influence is likely to be bidirectional. That is, individuals may influence the group, and the group influences individuals within it. People or events outside the group may also have profound effects. For example, a widely publicized incident of police brutality in one community may lead to polarization in perspective between police officers and citizens in another community.

Finally, one might study the relationship between the development of consensus and other variables. For example, Cherniss and Krantz (1983) drew on case studies of two human service organizations where staff had high levels of ideological or religious commitment in order to suggest that the development of ideological community may avert staff burnout. Riger (1983/84) similarly used qualitative data to consider the relative costs and benefits of collective decision-making structures based on consensus in feminist-movement organizations. Although development of shared perspectives may sometimes be seen as a nuisance variable that complicates the measurement of socialization processes, in these examples it seems to be a part of those processes.

Socialization

By socialization, we mean the cross-level processes by which settings influence individuals' characteristics, behavior, and attitudes, and the parallel processes by which individuals influence settings. Hackman (1992) distinguishes two kinds of group influence on members: ambient stimuli, comprising information that is available to setting inhabitants as part of the structure and regular procedures of a setting (desks in a classroom where the students all sit facing a standing teacher who speaks); and discretionary stimuli, which are supplied to particular members (the teacher tells a noisy student to "pipe down"). In the language of systems theory, both kinds of group influences are forms of feedback to members. Discretionary feedback may include rewards or sanctions, access to or denial of opportunities, or informal support and rejection in social interaction. Ambient feedback may be contained in the physical and social structure of the setting, procedural regularities, written rules and policies, and even the observable discretionary feedback directed at others.

Wicker (1972) similarly distinguishes between operant learning, in which the individual receives direct positive or negative reinforcement for an act, and observational or instructional learning, in which signs and symbols (such as "shallow water: do not dive") shape behavior without the need for direct reinforcement. Wicker invokes behavior-setting theory (Barker, 1968) to suggest when such discretionary stimuli are likely to be forthcoming. People in a setting monitor the environment for events, e.g., a noisy student or a broken light fixture, that may disrupt their goals and the program of the setting. When disruptions occur, they seek to correct them with either deviation-countering mechanisms (e.g., telling the student to "pipe down") or vetoing mechanisms that remove the problem from the setting (e.g., sending the student to the principal).

Correcting disruptions is one way that individuals may influence their settings. Not all people are equally sensitive to disruptions; those with greater authority and responsibility are more likely to both notice and correct them. Specialization in functions may also occur, so that a janitor may be responsible for fixing (or replacing) a broken light fixture, whereas a teacher is responsible for admonishing (or ejecting) an unruly student (Wicker, 1972).

The choice between deviation-countering and vetoing mechanisms depends on the relative costs of each, and these costs may, in turn, depend on whether the setting has enough members to carry out its behavioral program. Settings that are understaffed (undermanned, Barker & Gump, 1964) are more likely to tolerate marginal performances and to use deviation-countering mechanisms to bring behavior into line. Settings that are overstaffed are less tolerant, and are more likely to use vetoing mechanisms. Thus, a group of four 9-year-olds attempting to play baseball may tolerate a 4-year-old or even a mother on the team. A group of thirty 9-year-olds is likely to relegate all such misfits, and even some marginal 9-year-olds, to the sidelines (Barker, 1968, p. 181).

Settings can be compared in terms of the range of diversity they tolerate, the specific issues that pull for feedback, and the rate at which individual members are socialized to some criterion. The type and degree of socializing influences exerted in a setting probably depend on both individual values (for example, the value setting members place on conformity versus diversity) and on setting characteristics, in addition to staffing levels. For example, the payment system in a factory might determine both the distribution of production rates and the specific group members and behaviors subject to feedback. In a piece-work system, sanctions would be reserved for those whose production was too great; in a group-reward system, sanctions or assistance would be offered to those whose production was too low. Newcomers might be ignored in the first system until they became a threat; in the second, they might be singled out for help to bring them up to par.

Study of the process of socialization must often involve direct observation of the ambient and discretionary stimuli in an environment. In the case of discretionary feedback, it is important to understand its nature, who exerts it, and its targets. How is feedback distributed among people in different subgroups, in different organizational positions, or at different points in a distribution? Study of newcomers to the group will often be fruitful, because oldtimers may have long ago reached some equilibrium position. Careful choice of variables may sometimes illuminate the processes at work. In our ongoing example of norms that limit production rates, we might examine the shape of learning curves over time. If a production ceiling results from natural limits on skill or technology, workers' learning curves might approach it with gradual deceleration, and will never exceed the top (subject to minor fluctuations of course). If the ceiling results from social norms, the deceleration might be abrupt, and individuals might exceed the ceiling, only to be brought back into line by the disapprobation of peers.

Simple observation of changes over time in a single group's attitudes or behaviors is usually insufficient to identify socialization processes. Changes in attitudes may be due to stretching of perceptual yardsticks, as noted above; changes in both attitudes and behavior could also result from maturation, or from external trends that have nothing to do with the group. Some rival explanations can be ruled out when comparison groups subject to the same maturational and external influences or comparison measures that are immune to perceptual biases are available for study.

Because both ambient and discretionary stimuli may convey different meanings to people in different subgroups, it may be useful to interview carefully sampled group members about the stimuli they observe and the pressures they experience. For example, a waiting room with magazines full of white faces and with pictures of white people on the walls may seem unexceptional to whites, but may provide a clear message that they are not welcome to people of color. A pin-up of a scantily dressed woman in an office may inform other women that they will not be taken seriously there, and gays will feel that their sexual orientations are devalued. An intellectual argument that faculty members experience as stimulating and fun may be perceived as threatening by a first-year graduate student. Once again, we must recognize diversity within a single social environment.

CONCLUSIONS

In this chapter, we have tried to sketch a conceptual and methodological road map that covers some (but by no means all) of the terrain involved in cross-level research. Cross-level methods often seem to demand trade-offs: rigor versus practicality, diversity versus parsimony, scientific convention versus untried innovation. Given the complexity of social systems, we believe that these trade-offs come with the territory. The reward, we believe, is a rich understanding of people in context. Cross-level research methods and assessment tools can incorporate a variety of both qualitative and quantitative approaches. By challenging assumptions that environments are the same for all participants and that all individuals are well-represented by group means, cross-level tools can also help us to understand the diversity of people's experiences. As we have said repeatedly, cross-level methods must be guided by cross-level questions. Because theory and methods develop in tandem, we hope that this survey of cross-level research questions, assessment methods, and processes will stimulate community psychologists' efforts to conceptualize as well as to study phenomena involving multiple levels of analyses.

REFERENCES

Altman, I., & Rogoff, B. (1987). World views in psychology: Trait, interactional, organismic, and transactional perspectives. In D. Stokols & I. Altman (Eds.), *Handbook of environmental psychology* (pp. 7–40). New York: Wiley.

Barker, R. G. (1968). *Ecological psychology: Concepts and methods for studying the environment of human behavior*. Stanford, CA: Stanford University Press.

Barker, R. G. (1987). Prospecting in environmental psychology: Oskaloosa revisited. In D. Stokols & I. Altman (Eds.), *Handbook of environmental psychology* (pp. 1413–1432). New York: Wiley.

Barker, R. G., & Gump, P. V. (1964). *Big school, small school: High school size and student behavior*. Stanford, CA: Stanford University Press.

Box, G. E. P. (1949). A general distribution theory for a class of likelihood criteria. *Biometrika, 36*, 362–389.

Bronfenbrenner, U. (1979). *The ecology of human development*. Cambridge, MA: Harvard University Press.

Bronfenbrenner, U. (1986). Ecology of the family as a context for human development: Research perspectives. *Developmental Psychology, 22*, 723–742.

Brown, R. D. (1968). Manipulation of the environmental press in a college residence hall. *Personnel and Guidance Journal, 46*, 555–560.

Bryk, A. S., & Raudenbush, S. W. (1992). *Hierarchical linear models: Applications and data analysis methods*. Newbury Park, CA: Sage.

Carp, F. M., & Carp, A. (1984). A complementary/congruence model of well-being or mental health for the community elderly. In I. Altman, M. P. Lawton, & J. F. Wohlwill, *Elderly people and the environment* (pp. 279–336). New York: Plenum.

Chein, I. (1954). The environment as a determinant of behavior. *Journal of Social Psychology, 39,* 115–127.

Cherniss, C., & Krantz, D. L. (1983). The ideological community as an antidote to burnout in the human services. In B. A. Farber (Ed.), *Stress and burnout in the human service professions* (pp. 198–212). New York: Pergamon.

Cook, T. D., & Campbell, D. T. (1979). *Quasi-experimentation: Design and analysis for field settings.* Boston: Houghton-Mifflin.

Dansereau, F., Jr., Alutto, J. A., Markham, S. E., & Dumas, M. (1982). Multiplexed supervision and leadership: An application of within and between analysis. In J. G. Hunt, U. Sekaran, & C. A. Schriesheim (Eds.), *Leadership: Beyond establishment views* (pp. 81–103). Carbondale, IL: Southern Illinois University Press.

Dansereau, F., Alutto, J. A., & Yammarino, F. J. (1984). *Theory testing in organizational behavior: The varient approach.* Englewood Cliffs, NJ: Prentice-Hall.

Dansereau, F., & Markham, S. E. (1987). Levels of analysis in personnel and human resources management. *Personnel and Human Resources Management, 5,* 1–50.

Felner, R. D., Ginter, G., & Primavera, J. (1982). Primary prevention during school transitions: Social support and environmental structure. *American Journal of Community Psychology, 10,* 277–290.

Firebaugh, G. (1980). Groups as contexts and frog ponds. In K. H. Roberts & L. Burstein (Eds.), *Issues in aggregation, New Directions for Methodology of Social and Behavioral Science, Vol. 6* (pp. 43–52). San Francisco: Jossey-Bass.

Fischer, C. S. (1977). *Networks and places: Social relations in the urban setting.* New York: Free Press.

Florin, P., Giamartino, G. A., Kenny, D. A., & Wandersman, A. (1988). *Uncovering climate and group influence by separating individual and group effects.* Unpublished manuscript, University of Rhode Island.

French, J. R. P., Jr., Rodgers, W., & Cobb, S. (1974). Adjustment as person–environment fit. In G. V. Coelho, D. A. Hamburg, & J. E. Adams (Eds.), *Coping and adaptation* (pp. 316–333). New York: Basic Books.

Giamartino, G. A., & Wandersman, A. (1983). Organizational climate correlates of viable urban block organizations. *American Journal of Community Psychology, 11,* 529–641.

Glick, W. (1980). Problems in cross-level inferences. In K. H. Roberts & L. Burstein (Eds.), *Issues in aggregation, New Directions for Methodology of Social and Behavioral Science, Vol. 6* (pp. 17–30). San Francisco: Jossey-Bass.

Glick, W. H. (1985). Conceptualizing and measuring organizational and psychological climate: Pitfalls in multilevel research. *Academy of Management Review, 10,* 601–616.

Glick, W. H., & Roberts, K. H. (1984). Hypothesized interdependence, assumed independence. *Academy of Management Review, 9,* 722–735.

Goffman, E. (1961). *Asylums: Essays on the social situation of mental patients and other inmates.* New York: Anchor.

Goldenberg, I. I. (1971). *Build me a mountain: Youth, poverty, and the creation of new settings.* Cambridge, MA: MIT Press.

Golembiewski, R. T., Billingsley, K., & Yeager, J. (1976). Measuring change and persistence in human affairs: Types of change generated by OD designs. *Journal of Applied Behavioral Science, 12,* 133–157.

Gottman, J. (1979). *Marital Interaction.* New York: Academic.

Guion, R. M. (1973). Note on organizational climate. *Organizational Behavior and Human Performance, 9,* 120–125.

Hackman, J. R. (1992). Group influences on individuals in organizations. In M. D. Dunnette & L. M. Hough (Eds.), *Handbook of Industrial and Organizational Psychology, Vol. 3* (2nd ed., pp. 199–267). Palo Alto, CA: Consulting Psychologists Press.

Hall, R. J. (1988). *A level of analysis approach to construct validity and relationship issues in perceived climate and job satisfaction measures.* Unpublished doctoral dissertation, University of Maryland.

Helson, H. (1964). *Adaptation level theory.* New York: Harper & Row.

Hobfoll, S. E. (1990). Person–environment interaction: The question of conceptual validity. In P. Tolan, C. Keys, F. Chertok, & L. Jason (Eds.) *Researching community psychology: Issues of theory and methods* (pp. 164–167). Washington, D.C.: American Psychological Association.

James, L. R. (1982). Aggregation bias in estimates of perceptual agreement. *Journal of Applied Psychology, 67,* 219–229.

James, L. R., & Sells, S. B. (1981). Psychological climate: Theoretical perspectives and empirical research. In D. Magnusson (Ed.). *Toward a psychology of situations: An interactional approach* (pp. 275–295). Hillsdale, NJ: Erlbaum.

Joyce, W. F., & Slocum, J. W., Jr. (1984). Collective climate: Agreement as a basis for defining climates in organizations. *Academy of Management Journal, 27,* 721–742.

Kahana, E. (1975). A congruence model of person–environment interaction. In P. G. Windley, T. Byerts, & E. G. Ernst (Eds.), *Theoretical developments in environments for aging.* (pp. 181–214). Washington, D.C.: Gerontological Society.

Kahana, E., Liang, J., & Felton, B. J. (1980). Alternative models of person–environment fit. *Journal of Gerontology, 35*, 584–595.

Katz, D., & Kahn, R. L. (1978). *The social psychology of organizations* (2nd ed.). New York: Wiley.

Kenny, D. A. (1985). The generalized group effect model. In J. R. Nesselroade & A. von Eye (Eds.), *Individual development and social change: Exploratory analysis* (pp. 343–357). Orlando, FL: Academic.

Kenny, D. A., & La Voie, L. (1985). Separating individual and group effects. *Journal of Personality and Social Psychology, 48*, 339–348.

Keys, C. B., & Frank, S. (1987a). Community psychology and the study of organizations: A reciprocal relationship. *American Journal of Community Psychology, 15*, 239–251.

Keys, C. B., & Frank, S. (Eds.) (1987b). Organizational perspectives in community psychology [Special issue]. *American Journal of Community Psychology, 15*(3).

Laren, D. (1991). *The use of hierarchical linear modeling with data from the panel study of income dynamics.* Unpublished manuscript. University of Michigan, Institute for Social Research.

Lawton, M. P., and Nahemow, L. (1973). Ecology and the aging process. In C. Eisdorfer and M. P. Lawton (Eds.), *Psychology of adult development and aging* (pp. 619–674). Washington, D.C.: American Psychological Association.

Lewin, K. (1952). Behavior and development as a function of the total situation. In D. Cartwright (Ed.), *Field theory in social science: Selected theoretical papers by Kurt Lewin* (pp. 238–303). London: Tavistock. (Original work published in 1946.)

Maton, K. I. (1989). Community settings as buffers of life stress? Highly supportive churches, mutual help groups, and senior centers. *American Journal of Community Psychology, 17*, 203–232.

McGrath, J. E., & Altman, I. (1966). *Small group research: A synthesis and critique of the field.* New York: Holt, Rinehart & Winston.

Moos, R. H. (1973). Conceptualizations of human environments. *American Psychologist, 28*, 652–665.

Moos, R. H. (1974). *Evaluating treatment environments: A social ecological approach.* New York: Wiley.

Moos, R. H. (1984). Context and coping: Toward a unifying conceptual framework. *American Journal of Community Psychology, 12*, 5–25.

Moos, R. H., & Lemke, S. (1984). Supportive residential settings for older people. In I. Altman, M. P. Lawton, & J. F. Wohlwill (Eds.), *Elderly people and the environment* (pp. 159–190). New York: Plenum.

Morris, A., Shinn, M., & Dumont, K. (1999). Contextual factors affecting the organizational commitment of diverse police officers: A levels of analysis perspective. *American Journal of Community Psychology, 27*, 75–105.

Moscovici, S. (1985). Social influence and conformity. In G. Lindzey & E. Aronson (Eds.), *Handbook of social psychology, Vol. II* (3rd ed., pp. 347–412). New York: Random House.

Murrell, S. A. (1973). *Community psychology and social systems: A conceptual framework and intervention guide.* New York: Behavioral Publications.

Newman, O. (1972). *Defensible space: Crime prevention through urban design.* New York: MacMillan.

Perkins, D. D., Florin, P., Rich, R. C., Wandersman, A., & Chavis, D. M. (1990). Participation and the social and physical environment of residential blocks: Crime and community context. *American Journal of Community Psychology, 18*, 83–115.

Proshansky, H. M., Ittelson, W. H., & Rivlin, L. G. (1970). The influence of the physical environment on behavior: Some basic assumptions. In H. M. Proshansky, W. H. Ittelson, & L. G. Rivlin (Eds.), *Environmental psychology: Man and his physical setting* (pp. 27–37). New York: Holt, Rinehart, & Winston.

Rapkin, B. D. (1987). *The personal goals of elder community volunteers.* Unpublished doctoral dissertation. University of Illinois at Urbana–Champaign.

Rapkin, B. D., & Luke, D. (1993). Cluster analysis in community research: Epistemology and practice. *American Journal of Community Psychology, 21*, 247–277.

Rappaport, J. (1977). *Community psychology: Values, research, and action.* New York: Holt, Rinehart & Winston.

Rappaport, J., Seidman, E., Toro, P. A., McFadden, L. S., Reischl, T. M., Roberts, L. J., Salem, D. A., Stein, C. H., & Zimmerman, M. A. (1985). Collaborative research with a mutual help organization. *Social Policy, Winter, 15*, 12–24.

Riger, S. (1983/84). Vehicles for empowerment: The case of feminist movement organizations. *Prevention in Human Services, 3*(2/3), 99–117.

Roberts, K. H., Hulin, C. L., & Rousseau, D. M. (1978). *Developing an interdisciplinary science of organizations*, San Francisco: Jossey-Bass.

Robinson, W. S. (1950). Ecological correlations and the behavior of individuals. *American Sociological Review, 15*, 351–357.

Rodin, J. (1985) The application of social psychology. In G. Lindzey & E. Aronson (Eds.), *Handbook of Social Psychology, Vol. II* (3rd ed., pp. 805–881). New York: Random House.

Rousseau, D. M. (1985). Issues of level in organizational research: Multi-level and cross-level perspectives. In L. L. Cummings & B. M. Staw (Eds.), *Research in organizational behavior, Vol. 7* (pp. 1–37). Greenwich, CT: JAI.
Ruggiero, J., & Rapkin, B. D. (1991). *Similarity of institutionalized elders to their support networks: Effects on well-being*. Unpublished manuscript, New York University.
Sarason, S. B. (1972). *The creation of settings and the future societies*. San Francisco: Jossey-Bass.
Sarason, S. B. (1982). *The culture of school and the problem of change*. Boston: Allyn and Bacon.
Schneider, B., & Reichers, A. E. (1983). On the etiology of climates. *Personnel Psychology, 36*, 19–39.
Seidman, E. (Ed.) (1983). *Handbook of social intervention*. Beverly Hills: Sage.
Seidman, E. (1988). Back to the future, community psychology: Unfolding a theory of social intervention. *American Journal of Community Psychology, 16*, 3–24.
Seidman, E. (1990). Pursuing the meaning and utility of social regularities for community psychology. In P. Tolan, C. Keys, F. Chertok, & L. Jason (Eds.) *Researching community psychology: Issues of theory and methods* (pp. 91–100). Washington, D.C.: American Psychological Association.
Seidman, E., & Rapkin, B. (1983). Economics and psychosocial dysfunction: Toward a conceptual framework and prevention strategies. In R. D. Felner, L. A. Jason, J. N. Moritsugu, & S. S. Farber (Eds.), *Preventive psychology: Theory, research, and practice* (pp. 175–198). New York: Pergamon.
Sherif, M. (1936). *The psychology of social norms*. New York: Harper.
Shinn, M., Knickman, J. R., Ward, D., Petrovic, N. L., & Muth, B. J. (1990). Alternative models for sheltering homeless families. *Journal of Social Issues, 46*(4), 175–190.
Shinn, M., & Mørch, H. (1983). A tripartite model of coping with burnout. In B. Farber (Ed.), *Stress and burnout in the human service professions* (pp. 227–240). New York: Pergamon.
Shinn, M., Mørch, H., Robinson, P. E., & Neuner, R. A. (1993). Individual, group, and agency strategies for coping with job stressors in residential child care programmes. *Journal of Community and Applied Social Psychology, 3*, 313–324.
Siegel, S. (1956). *Non-parametric statistics*. New York: McGraw-Hill.
Staw, B. M., Sandelands, L. E., & Dutton, J. E. (1981). Threat rigidity effects in organizational behavior: A multilevel analysis. *Administrative Science Quarterly, 26*, 501–524.
Stokols, D. (1981). Group X place transactions: Some neglected issues in psychological research on settings. In D. Magnusson (Ed.), *Toward a psychology of situations: An interactional perspective* (pp. 393–416). Hillsdale, NJ: Erlbaum.
Tausig, M. (1987). Detecting "cracks" in mental health service systems: Application of network analytic techniques. *American Journal of Community Psychology, 15*, 337–351.
Vinokur, A., & Burnstein, E. (1974). the effects of partially shared persuasive arguments on group-induced shifts: A group problem-solving approach. *Journal of Personality and Social Psychology, 29*, 305–315.
Wechsler, H., & Pugh, T. F. (1967). Fit of individual and community characteristics and rates of psychiatric hospitalization. *American Journal of Sociology, 73*, 331–338.
Whitebook, M., Howes, C., & Phillips, D. (1990). *Who cares? Child care teachers and the quality of care in America* (Final report of the National Child Care Staffing Study). Oakland, CA: Child Care Employee Project.
Wicker, A. W. (1972). Processes which mediate behavior-environment congruence. *Behavioral Science, 17*, 265–277.
Wicker, A. W. (1990). Levels of analysis as an ecological issue in the relational psychologies. In P. Tolan, C. Keys, F. Chertok, & L. Jason (Eds.), *Researching community psychology: Issues of theory and methods* (pp. 127–131). Washington, D.C.: American Psychological Association.
Wicker, A. W., McGrath, J. E., & Armstrong, G. E. (1972). Organization size and behavior setting capacity as determinants of member participation. *Behavioral Science, 17*, 499–513.
Wolfensberger, W. (1972). *Normalization: The principle of normalization in human service*. Toronto, Canada: National Institute on Mental Retardation.

CHAPTER 29

Statistical Models for Change

J. S. Tanaka

Themes involving "change" recur in psychological research with great frequency. For example, the efficacy of social interventions and policy decisions is often measured in terms of whether change can be observed in whatever units are being assessed (e.g., people, classrooms, organizations; cf., Judd & Kenny, 1981). Lifespan developmental studies are often concerned with the "natural" or "historical" changes that occur either within or across individuals (e.g., Nesselroade, 1988). Finally, under some research circumstances, investigators are interested in differentiating change that occurs as a function of development from change that occurs as the result of some social intervention (e.g., research in developmental epidemiology; Kellam, 1990).

Despite the centrality of research questions involving change, there have been numerous methodological problems associated with trying to interpret the nature of change. Different (and often not explicit) assumptions about how change occurs can dramatically alter conclusions reached from the same data. This was seen, for example, in the multiple analyses of the Head Start educational intervention effect (e.g., Bentler & Woodward, 1978; Campbell & Erlebacher, 1975; Magidson, 1977; Tanaka, 1982). Difficulty in assessing change has been a longstanding concern in the methodological literature (e.g., Bereiter, 1963; Cronbach & Furby, 1970; Goldstein, 1979; Harris, 1963; Kenny & Campbell, 1989; Nesselroade, 1988; Nesselroade & Baltes, 1979; Rogosa, 1980; Rogosa & Willett, 1985b; Willett, 1988), and continues to occupy the efforts of methodologists, as can be attested to by the appearance of edited volumes by Collins and Horn (1991) and von Eye (1991) on this topic.

Many of these problems and the substantive (mis)interpretations they engender are rooted in a common conceptualization of change as a single process. It will be argued here that change can reflect a myriad of different phenomena, of which only a subset may be relevant in a particular study. Researchers can be misled by temptations to map into fixed statistical templates for analyzing change. These issues are further clouded by confusing methods for studying changes in interunit variability with methods for studying changes in intraunit variability. In this chapter, these different definitions of change and their substantive implications will be described. Change will be conceptualized as occurring along many different

J. S. Tanaka • Late of the Departments of Educational Psychology and Psychology, University of Illinois at Urbana–Champaign, Champaign, Illinois 61820.

Handbook of Community Psychology, edited by Julian Rappaport and Edward Seidman. Kluwer Academic / Plenum Publishers, New York, 2000.

dimensions, each with its own meaning. Emphasis will be placed on *a priori* determinations of the type of change of interest within a particular research question, and the subsequent adoption of statistical tools that will allow the appropriate conclusions to be drawn. It is hoped that sufficient guidance can be provided to allow researchers to recognize how particular questions about change can be articulated in statistical models.

Discussion of change assessments have typically centered around issues of examining data from longitudinal studies. The possibility of change occurring in cross-sectional studies is often ignored. However, as has been noted (e.g., Panter, Tanaka, & Wellens, 1992), change processes might be effectively modeled for durations as short as interitem response intervals. While current discussion of these issues concerns the respondent as an "information processor," similar concerns have been noted classically in the context of measurement reactivity (e.g., Nunnally, 1975). Microanalytic methods (e.g., Gottman, 1981; Gottman & Roy, 1990) explicitly model data obtained over short time epochs. For the most part, these time-series models will not be considered here. West and Hepworth (1991) provide a good introduction to this area.

The methods to be discussed here follow the usual description as it occurs in longitudinal research, where the units of time are typically days, months, or years, and the units of assessments are individuals. However, it should be recognized that these methods can also be employed when the units of time may be appreciably shorter (e.g., minutes, seconds, and milliseconds) with different levels for the units of assessment (e.g., individuals, organizations, school districts). To avoid the typical presentation of these statistical models of change as being applicable only at the level of individuals, the term "unit" will refer generally to the entity in which change is being studied (Seidman, 1988).

The organization of this chapter is as follows. First, different ways of conceptualizing the change process at a descriptive level are presented. Next, statistical methods are proposed to deal with these different conceptualizations of change. Structural equation models with latent variables (e.g., Loehlin, 1987; Tanaka, Panter, Winborne, & Huba, 1990) are used as the organizing framework to discuss these statistical developments. These models are particularly well-suited to the correlational data typically encountered in longitudinal models, but are not limited to non-experimental designs (cf., Tanaka et al., 1990). Hypotheses regarding both changes in means (location) and in variances/covariances (scale) are discussed, as they are typically represented in terms of either growth curve or autoregressive models. Strictly intraunit-level or "time series" (cf., Kenny & Campbell, 1989) models are reviewed briefly. A brief discussion of event history or survival models follows. The chapter concludes with the theoretical and conceptual limitations of the proposed framework.

ASSESSING CHANGE: A CONSTRUCT-FOCUSED APPROACH

The discussion of change presented here is couched in terms of *constructs* rather than their specific operationalizations (i.e., particular measures). The idea of focusing on constructs rather than measures is consistent with the representation of psychological theory operating at the level of constructs (e.g., Cronbach & Meehl, 1955; Loevinger, 1957). Some have equated this perspective with issues of construct validity from the domain of psychometrics (e.g., Bentler, 1978); however, it should be noted that a somewhat broader definition of construct validity is used here than might be typically found in texts on psychometric theory.

To illustrate the concepts underlying this treatment of construct validity, it can be noted, for example, that psychologists are generally interested in inferred attitudinal structures rather than in particular attitude measures. Observed measures are imperfect vehicles for attempting to understand unobservable psychological processes. In other words, when we set out to measure psychological constructs of interest, we know that we will not be able to measure a particular observed manifestation of the construct with perfect reliability. This is equally true of both "behavioral" and "self-report" data.

The focus on constructs allows us to clearly differentiate problems in measurement from problems of theory. This perspective illustrates that psychological theories are not bound to any one specific measurement operationalization. This was systematically addressed in a conceptual (although not statistical) way in Campbell and Fiske's (1959) delineation of the multitrait, multimethod matrix. In this formulation, different assessment strategies could be employed to triangulate on a psychological construct of interest (see also Patterson & Bank, 1986). While the importance of multiple assessments has long been recognized in psychological research, the majority of psychological studies only employ a single way of operationalizing a construct of interest *within* a given study. In this single-indicator approach, implicit equivalencies are made between the psychological construct of interest and a particular measurement of that construct. Hence, the success or failure of a theory necessarily becomes bounded to a measurement perspective, a problematic endpoint to a process that did not initially depend so closely on measurement.

As noted by Campbell and Fiske (1959) and later reiterated by others (e.g., Bentler, 1978; Cook & Campbell, 1979; Houts, Cook, & Shadish, 1986; Patterson & Bank, 1986), it is generally preferable to have multiple indicators of the same construct, ideally from multiple assessor perspectives. In employing such multimethod and multiagent assessments, we can then disaggregate common, construct-level effects from effects that are attributable to a particular operationalization of the construct or factors that are unrelated to the construct (e.g., method variance).

While this approach shares some conceptual ideas with psychometric methods, a broader implication of such a focus can be easily expanded to encompass all types of behaviors. In fact, it can be argued that psychological research grounded in the principles of reliability and validity (i.e., the "non-experimental" or "correlational" paradigms in psychology) have always been concerned with multiple assessments (through examination of multiple items) and their interrelatedness (through examination of how well those multiple items can be aggregated), and thus, from the perspective adopted here, have reflected a greater sensitivity to theoretical and empirical concerns for ruling out threats to the invalidity of a study.

This construct-oriented approach also allows us to discuss statistical models for change that have constructs rather than measures as their primary focus. In other words, latent variable structural-equation modeling will provide a frame for this discussion (e.g., Tanaka et al., 1990). While it is not necessarily the case that all of the statistical models that are presented are strictly latent variable models, all of the models presented will be concerned with measurement error in an effort to address the "glop" often present in data (Bank, Dishion, Skinner, & Patterson, 1990).

Specifications of Types of Change

There are three major classes of statistical models that can be considered when answering questions related to change. Schematically, an organizational structure for these models is presented in Figure 1.

Time as a Predictor

Population-averaged models
  Questions: Can change be detected across units of analysis across time?
  Does a construct demonstrate stability across units of analysis over time?
  Examples: Repeated measures analysis of variance
  Autoregressive models

Subject-specific models
  Question: How much variability in change exists across units?
  Examples: Growth curve models
  Intensive single unit designs

Times as an Outcome

Survival/Event history mdoels
  Question: What are predictors of the time it takes for a particular event to occur?
  Examples: Survival analysis/Event history analysis

FIGURE 1. A schematic organization for understanding change.

The first major conceptual dimension along which longitudinal models can be evaluated is whether time is treated as a predictor variable or as an outcome variable. Appropriate research questions when time is treated as a predictor include issues of the stability of a construct over time or the longitudinal trajectory of a construct over time. When time is treated as an outcome variable, questions such as the length of time it takes for some outcome to occur or remit are relevant.

In regard to time in predictor models, there are two types of questions that can be distinguished. In psychometric work, these have been referred to as questions involving intraindividual versus interindividual change (e.g., Buss, 1979; Nesselroade, 1990). In a biometric context, Zeger, Liang, and Albert (1988) refer to these as "subject-specific" and "population-averaged" models. Fundamentally, this distinction refers to the extent to which heterogeneity among the units of analysis is incorporated into the specification of a model. Intraindividual or subject-specific modeling approaches include information about subject heterogeneity, while interindividual or population-averaged modeling does not. While it has been typically the case that issues of change have historically focused on the latter, later work in longitudinal modeling has emphasized the complementarity of both approaches (e.g., McArdle & Epstein, 1987; Nesselroade, 1988; Rogosa, 1988).

An organizing principle in looking at both types of change is provided by Cattell's description of the "data box" (e.g., Buss, 1979; Cattell, 1966, 1988). Other authors have extended these ideas into explicitly stated statistical-mathematical models of change, couched in terms of interindividual change invoking concepts such as stability (e.g., Gollob & Reichardt, 1987; Hertzog & Nesselroade, 1987; Nesselroade, 1988; Rogosa, 1979; Rogosa & Willett, 1985b; Tanaka & Huba, 1987), intraindividual change invoking concepts such as growth (e.g., Labouvie, 1981; McArdle, 1986, 1988; McArdle, & Epstein, 1987; Rogosa, Brandt, & Zimowski, 1982; Rogosa & Willett, 1985a; Willett, Ayoub, & Robinson, 1991), and intraindividual change looking explicitly at change as it occurs in an intensively observed unit of analysis (e.g., Kenny & Campbell, 1989; Nesselroade & Ford, 1985).

The "data box," which organizes measurement facets, provides a useful point of departure for this discussion. While the original development of "data box" ideas took place in the context of factor analytic work, they represent a general way to think about different "slices" of data. The ideas are particularly well-suited for studying change, since these designs necessarily include data collection over multiple modes or facets. For example, a longitudinal design might involve measurements on a number of respondents on multiple variables at several time points. Here, three different measurement facets are involved: respondents, variables, and time. However, it is typically the case that only two of these three facets are considered in analyses. Further, selection of the two facets to be used in analysis can be thought to imply interest in either interunit (measurements and respondents) or intraunit (measurements and time) change. Figure 2 presents a schematic of the data matrix.

Time As a Predictor

Assessment of interunit change represents the dominant theme in psychologists' understanding of the meaning of change. From this perspective, change is defined over units. This would represent R-type analysis using the Cattellian description. The particular aspect of the data box that is examined involves the crossing of respondents and variables, with time serving as a replication factor.

At the other end of the change continuum using time as a predictor, intraunit approaches take another perspective on the data array, involving measurements on a single respondent over multiple time points. Of particular interest in this type of analysis are the correlations among occasions that index the degree of intraunit consistency. To quote Comrey (1973, p. 221), P-techniques have the "greatest potential in (clinical) research involving variables that exhibit substantial real fluctuations in the individual over time." Nesselroade (1988) elaborated this point and suggested that conditions exist where multiple observations on a single unit would yield information similar to assessing many individuals in a single cross-section.

Intermediate to these perspectives are models where a sample of units is assessed

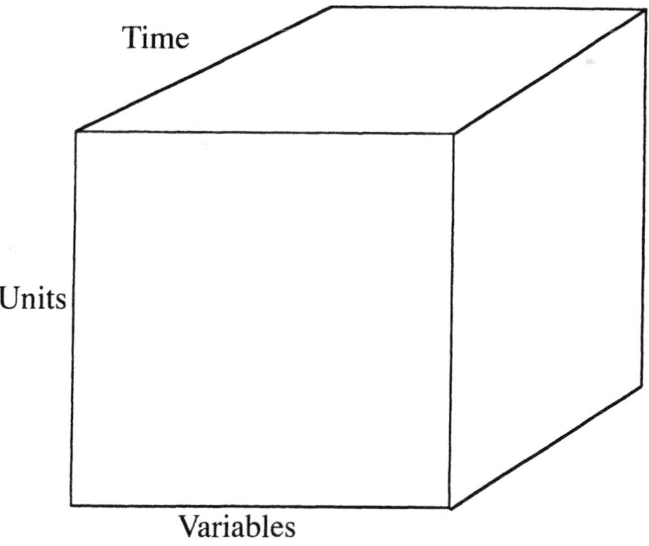

FIGURE 2. A "data box" (following Cattell, 1966) representing the measurement of N units measured on p variables at t occasions.

repeatedly over time. Rather than hypothesizing that units' prior assessments will affect their subsequent status, as in the autoregressive or psychometric models of change, all assessments on a given unit are hypothesized to be a direct function of time. Cattell (1966, 1988) characterized such models as T-type analyses, later discussed as growth curve models (e.g., Burchinal & Appelbaum, 1991; McArdle & Epstein, 1987; Willett et al., 1991).

Research questions of interest often involve the assessment of patterns of within-unit change. However, this conceptualization of change is clearly different from the standard psychometric perspective of looking at average change aggregated over individuals. The difference between these models can be summarized in terms of what is being measured in assessing change. In R-type models, one is interested in average change where aggregation is over a sample of units expected to demonstrate uniform, homogeneous change over time (i.e., all units are changing at the same rate). In contrast, T-type models consider within-unit change allowing for possible differences in the rate or variability of change patterns across the sample of units. Thus, some units may change at an accelerated rate, some may change more slowly, and others may not change at all. Finally, intensive, within-unit approaches to change, as characterized by P-type analyses, attempt to understand the change process as it occurs for a single unit of analysis.

The strengths and weaknesses of the different approaches can be demonstrated concretely in an example. Consider a data taken from ten subjects at two time points representing assessments pre- and posttreatment. Hypothetical data for these ten subjects are presented in Table 1, and are graphically displayed as a function of time in Figure 3.

Looking at any single respondent, we see that differences are exhibited from pretest to posttest, with some respondents demonstrating increases, while others exhibit decreases. However, if one were to conduct the within-subjects *t*-test for these data, a *t*-value of 0 would be obtained. The conclusions drawn from this nonsignificant finding would be correct: On the average, there is no difference between pretest and posttest scores. However, this statistical summary does not adequately characterize the change observed in any individual among these ten subjects.

TABLE 1. Hypothetical Change Data for Ten Subjects

Subject	Time 1 (T1)	Time 2 (T2)	δ(T2 − T1)
1	15.0	18.0	+3.0
2	20.0	20.0	0.0
3	17.0	16.0	−1.0
4	15.0	13.0	−2.0
5	21.0	25.0	+4.0
6	18.0	23.0	+5.0
7	17.0	16.0	−1.0
8	25.0	22.0	−3.0
9	24.0	19.0	−5.0
10	15.0	15.0	0.0
Mean	18.7	18.7	0.0
Standard deviation	3.7	3.8	3.2

Note: δ denotes the difference function applied to the variables within the parentheses.

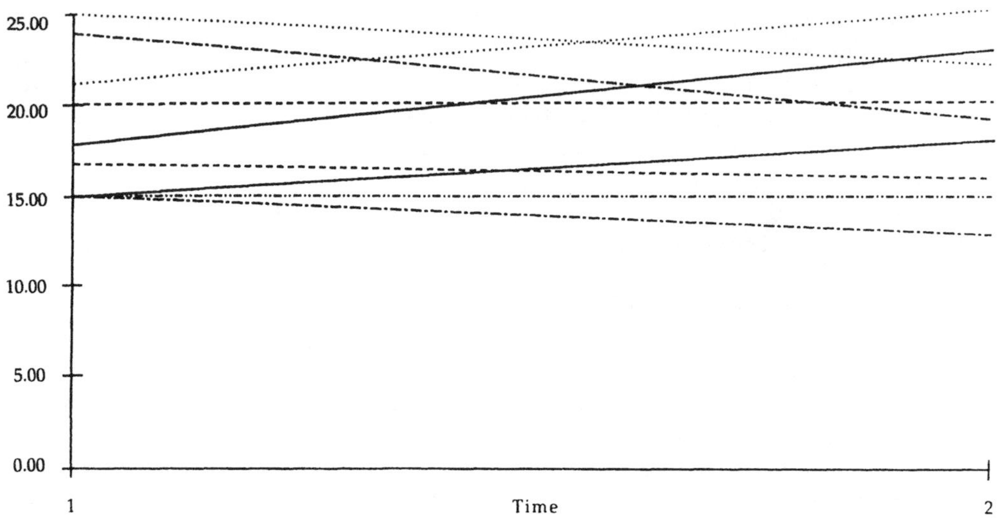

FIGURE 3. Table 1 data graphed as a function of time.

Time As an Outcome

In addition to research questions that are framed in terms of the longitudinal course of psychological constructs, we can also ask questions where time is considered to be an outcome. For example, we might be interested in whether an intervention designed to provide more socially supportive environments to elderly persons in the community reduces their rate of entry into formal nursing-home care. As another example, we might be interested in the effects of an intervention focusing on structured adolescent peer-group activities in decreasing the rates of high school dropout. The conceptual link between these two examples lies in their common interest in modeling the time until a particular event occurs.

As is the case for statistical models where time is a predictor, different literatures have referred to these models in different ways. For example, in biometrics, this class of models is often called hazard modeling or survival analysis (e.g., Agresti, 1990). In the sociological literature, these models are referred to as event-history models (e.g., Allison, 1984). While these models have been typically underutilized in the psychological literature, a paper by Rogosa and Ghandour (1991) demonstrates the applicability of these ideas to behavioral data.

Given a conceptual framework in which time can be seen as either a predictor or an outcome, we can next go on to discuss how questions about change in longitudinal designs might be articulated.

Asking Questions about Change

By recognizing the interdependencies between a psychological construct of interest and its particular operationalizations, questions about change over time can be framed in a number of different ways. However, an initial question might involve whether it is *meaningful* to study change given the constructs we have measured. Hertzog and Nesselroade (1987) discuss an example where asking questions about change simply is not meaningful when, for example, a construct might be expected to be highly consistent within time, but highly unstable across time. Thus, an initial question which might be asked is: *Are concepts regarding change relevant for the given constructs being studied?* Implicit in this question are issues that are often taken for granted or unquestioningly accepted as being "good" demonstrations of assessment reliability. For example, it is possible that we might not expect a particular time-limited assessment to have strong test–retest reliability if the construct in question changes over time. A particular construct might be sensitive to a number of factors (e.g., weather, time of day, an argument with a spouse) that would not be expected to have predictable stability across time. One can, of course, ask about the influence of these exogenous factors on the construct over time; however, questions about the time-to-time stability of the construct without considering these exogenous influences may be meaningless.

While this issue might seem obvious, it sometimes appears in more subtle forms. For example, consider a quasi-experimental design looking at the effects of a new type of classroom instruction on the mathematics abilities of school-aged children from second to fourth grade. If mathematics abilities are measured at the beginning of the second grade and at the end of fourth grade, it is unclear whether identical types of mathematics performance are being assessed, particularly if different assessments are used at the two time points. While examining individual change in mathematics abilities in light of the intervention is a reasonable hypothesis, the precise definition of what "mathematics abilities" are must be clearly understood to illustrate its potential for change. Lord (1958) made a related point about measurement comparability over time.

Given this latter perspective, it is reasonable to ask whether, for specific research questions, a hypothesis involves change in the same construct across an observational period (e.g., quantitative changes in distributional orderings or level across time), or shifts to a qualitatively different construct (e.g., the nature of what is being assessed changes across time). Such questions obviously transcend issues of construct labelling and instead reflect the particular assumptions made by investigators in examining longitudinal phenomena. Viewed from this perspective, a question regarding the relevance of examining psychological change is an initial precondition for examining change. In this chapter, it will be assumed that the longitudinal invariance of constructs can be evaluated empirically, since complexities arise for these constructs in the analysis of longitudinal data. If it is meaningful to assess change in a definitionally invariant psychological construct, one might next ask how construct stability can be assessed. It is also relevant to ask where this change might be observed: within an analysis unit or across analysis units.

Latent Variable Modeling: A Statistical Overview

Rather than provide a review of latent-variable structural-equation modeling in general, this chapter will focus specifically on those aspects of this statistical methodology that are applicable to the study of change. Interested readers interested in the basic introductions to latent variable modeling can refer to the treatment of this topic in texts by Loehlin (1987) and Bollen (1989). Such comprehensive references will be useful to the extent that topics such as data non-normality (e.g., Bentler, 1983; Browne, 1982, 1984; Huba & Harlow, 1986, 1987), sample size (e.g., Tanaka, 1987), model fit (e.g., Tanaka, 1993), and model misspecification (e.g., Kaplan, 1988; MacCallum, 1986) cannot be addressed here.

However, there is a statistical view presented in this chapter that, in other work (LaDu &

Tanaka, 1995), has been forwarded as an important way in which to think about the incremental utility of fitted models. Rather than focusing on the overall fit of any single model, this chapter will emphasize the comparative fit of competing *substantive* models for a given set of observations. While such a view is not inconsistent with early writings in this area, nor with similar thinking in the context of general linear models [see, for example, the discussion of increments in squared multiple correlation values that form the heart of the Cohen and Cohen (1983) presentation of multiple regression], it has been generally overlooked in the latent variable modeling literature. From perspective of improving social science theory, Meehl (1990) and others (e.g., Humphreys, 1990) have argued about the utility of such incremental thinking.

THE STUDY OF INTERUNIT CHANGE

As has been pointed out by a number of authors, any examination of change critically depends on the time lag associated with when hypothesized changes are thought to occur. A two-wave experiment looking at change over a six-month interval will not yield results if the phenomenon under investigation has a two-year developmental trajectory. Thus, it is important to ascertain the time lags over which change is hypothesized to occur. Gollob and Reichardt (1987) have discussed the importance of failing to account for lagged effects, even in the context of only having cross-sectional data. A more fundamental consideration of this problem is the issue of whether the construct being measured remains the same across time.

Assessing Construct Stability: The Role of Construct Definition

In many psychological studies, the same measure is employed across time to assess change. This promotes a nominalistic fallacy of equating a particular measure with a theoretical construct of interest. Even if a fixed measure is employed across multiple measurement occasions, it is possible that construct definition is altered across time. This has been pointed out in work by Knowles (1988) and others (e.g., Panter et al., 1992), who argue that multiple administrations of a particular measure may change the meaning of such measures for respondents.

Operationally, we can define different ways in which to construe possible changes in meaning. A fundamental change that is central to many longitudinal investigations is the notion that level differences will be observed in the construct of interest over time. Thus, for example, we may want a particular intervention to lower rates of delinquency or the experience of psychological distress, or to raise performance on a mathematics aptitude test in a treatment group relative to a control group.

However, as is the case in general linear models statistical methods [e.g., univariate or multivariate analysis of variance models (ANOVA, MANOVA)], the evaluation of such level hypotheses depends critically on assumptions about variable scaling across time. In its familiar form, such assumptions are presented in terms of homogeneity of variance (homoscedasticity) or covariance matrix assumptions for the ANOVA and MANOVA models, respectively. These assumptions simply reflect the idea that variables must be expressed in comparable scaling units in order to test the level hypotheses of interest.

Finally, an issue that is tied to the concern of Knowles (1988) and others (Panter et al., 1992) is that of whether the construct being assessed remains invariant across time. When a construct is only represented by a single measured assessment, it is not a testable hypothesis; it must be assumed that the single measure is not altered in terms of its meaning for a respondent. However, evaluation of such an assumption is critical if one is to talk about change in a single construct as opposed to a nomological net containing multiple constructs.

The strength of a latent-variable modeling approach is that each of these hypotheses is testable. In addition to being able to test hypotheses related to potential shifts in level and scale, the multiple-measure approach emphasized in latent-variable modeling allows for evaluation of hypotheses related to the invariance of construct definition.

The three levels of questions within the study of interunit change can be viewed hierarchically in the reverse order in which they have been presented here. In other words, an initial question that must be evaluated by an investigator is the extent to which the same construct is being assessed over time, so that it is meaningful to ask questions about change. If this precondition has been met, then one can go on to ask questions about scale invariance, addressing the analog of the homoscedasticity assumption of latent variable models. Finally, if both of these preconditions are met, then one can go on to ask the substantively interesting question of interest: Are level changes observed in the target construct? Not only are these questions organized hierarchically, but the to-be-tested hypotheses involve explicit model comparisons within this hierarchy. We will develop this presentation by working through the exact latent variable models to be tested at each stage of this hierarchy.

Do the Constructs of Interest Maintain Definitional Invariance Across Time, i.e., Is a Definitionally Identical Construct Being Measured at All Time Points?

Figure 4 is a diagram of a two-wave longitudinal latent-variable model. Following one standard for the presentation of these models, circles depict latent variables, while squares denote their measured variable indicators. In this case, each latent variable has the same four measured-variable indicators at each of the two time points. A necessary condition to demonstrate the definitional consistency of the latent variable across the two times points is the invariance of measured variable—latent-variable relations. That is, each measured variable has identically the same relation in magnitude and sign to what is assumed to be the same latent variable across time.

Conceptually, this across-time invariance demonstrates that the latent variable does not change in terms of its definition relative to the particular measured variable indicators that were employed. If such invariance cannot be demonstrated, then there are other (in this case, unmeasured) influences on the latent variable that are serving to change its definition over time. Substantive interpretation of such changes might include the kinds of cognitive reinterpretations of the operationalizations of a construct over time suggested by Knowles (1988) and Panter et al. (1992). Within a hypothesis-testing framework provided by latent-variable structural-equation models, examining this hypothesis involves tests of the "measurement model," the interrelations between measured and latent variables over time. Hence, a null hypothesis of invariant factor structure requires that these factor loadings be equal over time (e.g., Meredith, 1964a, 1964b).

Across-Time Construct Invariance

An initial hypothesis to be tested is that of construct invariance. One cannot meaningfully discuss change in a statistical sense unless the construct being assessed maintains the same

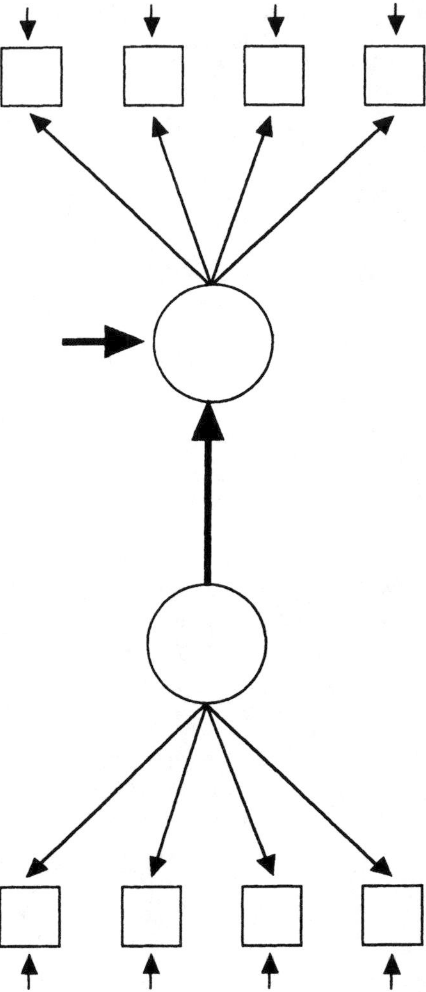

FIGURE 4. A two-wave longitudinal model with identical measured variables at each time point.

definition across the assessment period. The evaluation of construct invariance involves the comparison of two models. These models are "nested," referring to the fact that one model being tested can be thought of as a simplification of the other model. In this strategy, one model serves as a baseline for a comparison model of interest. A model with unconstrained across-time factor loadings (i.e., with no equality constraints across time) is tested first and serves as the baseline.

Let us assume the Figure 4 model is a diagrammatic representation of data obtained from 250 subjects at two points in time.[1] While, as is pointed out by Rogosa (1988), more than two time points are desirable in longitudinal assessment, this simple example will adequately demonstrate issues in construct invariance. The covariance matrix and means for these eight variables are presented in Table 2.

[1]In fact, these data were simulated using random number generators in SPSS-X.

TABLE 2. Simulated Data from 250 Subjects: Original Metric

I. Covariance Matrix							
4.36							
2.90	4.34						
2.87	2.68	4.02					
2.91	2.80	2.94	4.46				
1.87	1.95	1.72	1.96	3.93			
2.26	2.16	2.11	2.43	2.44	4.13		
2.20	2.14	1.85	2.21	2.56	2.69	3.87	
2.27	2.28	1.91	2.36	2.51	2.50	2.36	3.95
II. Means							
10.1	10.1	10.1	10.0	12.0	12.1	12.2	12.0

An initial baseline model was evaluated using maximum likelihood estimation that assumed that the factor loadings were not equal over time. This model yielded a goodness-of-fit chi-square value of 26.82 on 19 degrees of freedom, $p = .11$ and a goodness-of-fit index value (GFI; Jöreskog & Sörbom, 1988; Tanaka & Huba, 1985, 1989) of .98. The latter is a descriptive measure typically bounded between 0.0 and 1.0, with values closer to 1.0 indicative of better model fit. Both the chi-square statistic and the GFI value indicate that this model with factor-loading estimates unconstrained across time is an adequate representation of these data.

To evaluate the hypothesis of whether constructs are invariant over time, this baseline model must be compared to a model where factor loadings for corresponding variables are constrained to be equal over time. It should be emphasized that in this testing strategy, which focuses on model comparisons, the absolute fit of the baseline model is not interesting. When a model with factor loadings constrained to be equal is fit to these data, a goodness-of-fit chi-square value of 28.62 on 22 degrees of freedom ($p = .16$, GFI = .97) is obtained. A chi-square difference test is obtained by subtracting the chi-square statistic value for this constrained model from the chi-square value for the unconstrained model. The degrees of freedom for this chi-square statistic is simply the difference of the corresponding degrees of freedom for the individual tests. In this case, a difference chi-square of 1.80 on 3 degrees of freedom ($p = .61$). Thus, we cannot reject the null hypothesis of equal factor loadings over time.

It is important to note that the test for construct invariance centers on the chi-square difference test rather than the absolute fit of any one model. In this example, models with both constrained and unconstrained factor loadings provide statistically adequate representations of these data in terms of model fit. However, it is not the absolute fit that is important, but rather then, comparative fit of the constrained versus the unconstrained models.

Testing Scale and Mean Differences

If longitudinal construct invariance in terms of construct definition can be established, then two other questions are of interest: *Do scale shifts occur longitudinally for the construct of interest?* and *Do mean shifts occur longitudinally for the construct of interest?* Answers to these two questions often form the heart of the questions of interest in longitudinal research. The evaluation of intervention effects (e.g., does this educational intervention raise the average ability scores of students who are exposed to it?) often depends critically on an evaluation of mean-level shifts. However, to unequivocally conclude that mean-level change has occurred, changes in scale must be ruled out. Evaluation of this assumption is analogous to the homogeneity of variance (homoscedasticity) assumption in univariate analysis of variance models. Since the analysis of scale changes must precede a consideration of mean-level shifts, we will first consider the detection and analysis of longitudinal differences in construct variances.

Longitudinal Shifts in Scale

Simply put, the detection of longitudinal-scale differences asks the question of whether construct variances remain constant over time. Variance shifts in the longitudinal assessment of a construct might happen for any number of reasons. For example, maturation or a change in the construct's meaning may serve to increase its variance over time. Fan-spread models of development would be consistent with increased longitudinal intraconstruct variability.

A simple "eyeball" method of evaluating this construct scale can be conducted if it can be assumed that the metric of observed measurements can be assumed to be arbitrary, as is usually the case. In this method, the variances of each of observed measures at the initial assessment are standardized. Then, the variances or corresponding measurements at subsequent time points are expressed as variance ratios relative to time 1. For example, assume a measure has a variance of 9 at time 1 and a variance of 11 at time 2. In this rescaling procedure, the time 1 variance would be "standardized" to a value of 1.0 and the time 2 variance would be 11/9 or 1.22. This provides a descriptive examination (in a simple metric) of whether or not variances have changed appreciably over time. Results from such a rescaling are presented in Table 3, employing the covariance matrix previously given in Table 2.

Besides this simple method for determining shift in construct variances by inspection, more formal statistical methods can be employed to evaluate the hypothesis of longitudinal scale constancy. As was the case in assessing construct invariance over time, a series of models are tested with the difference between test statistics for the different models evaluating the null hypothesis of scale constancy. Recall that these tests typically are conditional on having established that constructs are invariant. Schmitt (1982) has discussed the use of such a model-comparison approach.

We can again turn to the Figure 2 model and the sample of 250 respondents whose data are hypothesized to correspond to this model. To evaluate the hypothesis of scale constancy, we again set up a comparison between two models. However, in this particular case, the comparison that must be made involves a complex constraint involving estimated model

TABLE 3. Rescaled Covariance Matrix: Time 2 Variances Normed to Time I Variances

1.00							
0.67	1.00						
0.68	0.64	1.00					
0.66	0.64	0.69	1.00				
0.43	0.45	0.41	0.44	0.90			
0.52	0.50	0.51	0.55	0.56	0.95		
0.53	0.51	0.46	0.52	0.61	0.64	0.96	
0.51	0.52	0.45	0.53	0.57	0.57	0.56	0.88

Note: Time 2 variables are rescaled to the metric of time I variances.

parameters.[2] To avoid this complexity, a mathematically equivalent model representing the relation between time 1 and time 2 constructs in Figure 4 as a bidirectional arrow will be tested. This constrained model is tested against the construct invariance model of equal factor loadings, which we have already established as being consistent with the observed data.

The model-constraining construct variances to be equal across time yielded a chi-square goodness-of-fit statistics of 30.11 on 23 degrees of freedom (p = .15; GFI = .97). When this model is compared to the baseline model of construct invariance, a chi-square difference statistic of 1.49 on 1 degree of freedom is obtained (p = .22), thus failing to reject the hypothesis of scale invariance.

With the homoscedasticity of the construct established, tests of longitudinal mean-level shifts in the construct can be tested. It should be realized that, in the conditional sequence of tests that have been outlined here, a test of longitudinal mean change is appropriate only when the conditions of construct invariance and construct-scale invariance have been met. This clearly demonstrates the set of background assumptions that must be met in order for a longitudinal mean-shift hypothesis to be considered.

Assessing Mean Level Change

To examine longitudinal mean shifts in the latent variable framework, we need to expand our consideration of models to be evaluated. Specifically, we must now explicitly include construct means as part of the model. The historical development and application of latent variable modeling has tended to ignore hypotheses on means (cf., Tanaka et al., 1990). However, if these models are viewed as extensions of regression models, the omission of means would have the same implications as neglecting the intercept in a multiple regression. It is well-known that regression equations that either include or omit intercept terms differ in a number of important ways (e.g., Kvalseth, 1985). While the underutilization of the information provided by means can be understood given the emphasis on correlational models (Cohen & Cohen, 1983) in psychological statistics, recent treatments of latent variable models have more explicitly treated the problem of mean structures, both in theory (e.g., Bentler, 1983), as well as in applications (e.g., Tanaka & Bentler, 1983; Tanaka, Panter, & Winborne, 1988). To acknowledge that information beyond covariances is being analyzed, these models are sometimes referred to as moment-structure models, indicating that both first moment (mean) and second moment (covariance) data are being modelled.

Conceptually, the ideas of modelling construct means are easy to understand if one accepts the general principles of latent variable models. Just as the assessment of construct scale invariance required an examination of variances as might be done in examining a homogeneity of variance hypothesis in the analysis of variance, assessment of longitudinal mean shifts can be looked upon as analogous to the testing of mean differences in the analysis of variance framework. In the same way that the validity of mean differences in the analysis of variance is conditional on homogeneity of variance assumptions, evaluating construct change in means over time may be conditional on evaluating construct homoscedasticity.

A final point regarding the evaluation of moment-structure models concerns the data

[2]In particular, the null hypothesis of no beta change in this model where a unidirectional effect is hypothesized would involve a quadratic constraint of the form $\hat{y} = a^2x + e$ where a is the structural coefficient linking time 1 and time 2 constructs, x is the variance of the construct at time 1, e is the regression residual variance of the time 2 construct on the time 1 construct, and $\hat{y}$ is the (estimated) time 2 construct. Such constraints are not easily implemented using routinely available software for structural equation modeling.

required to evaluate such models. Clearly, since both means and covariances are tested, both types of data must be available in constructing the model. This information is given in what is called the uncentered matrix of second moments. Certain computer programs (such as LISREL) compute this matrix internally if the mean vector and covariance matrix of the observed variables, or if raw data, are input.

Testing Mean Level Change

As in the case of the models previously considered, longitudinal mean comparisons are tested in a set of "nested" model comparisons. Again, these comparisons feature differences between constrained and unconstrained models. However, in this case, hypothesis tests are conducted on means rather than factor loadings, factor variances, or regression coefficients.

It should be noted that a problem exists in specifying latent variable means. Since these unobserved variables do not have an associated metric, their scale and location are arbitrary. For example, transformations such as addition by a constant can shift latent variable means. To overcome this indeterminacy (referred to as the identification problem or the problem of underidentification), it is typical to fix a latent variable mean at some standard reference value (typically zero) and to assess deviations from this referent. While discussion of this has typically taken place in the context of multiple sample designs, it can also be noted that across-time differences in a latent variable can also be assessed in the one sample case. Further, in a longitudinal design, it would be natural to set the construct mean at time 1 to be equal to zero.

As in the assessment of construct and construct-scale invariance, both constrained and unconstrained models must be tested, with the difference in fit between the two models indexing whether or not longitudinal mean shifts have occurred. The constrained model in this case corresponds to construct means being equal over time. That is, in this model, it is hypothesized that there are no longitudinal mean differences. In the unconstrained model, construct means are freely estimated across time, with a reference value set for the initial assessment. The null hypothesis of no mean change is assessed from the difference chi square, which is obtained from subtracting the value of the chi-square statistic obtained from the unconstrained model from the value of the chi-square statistic obtained from the constrained model. A statistically significant different would indicate that construct means differ across time.

Again, the example data can be used to illustrate a test of the hypothesis of construct mean change. To test this hypothesis, two models are compared. In the first model, construct means are constrained to be equal across time. This model yields a chi-square value of 199.48 on 26 degrees of freedom ($p < .001$; GFI = .98). The second model relaxes the constraint of equal construct means. This model yield a chi-square value of 30.03 on 25 degrees of freedom ($p = .22$; GFI = .98). The chi-square difference test evaluating the critical null hypothesis of equal construct means gives a value of 169.40 on 1 degree of freedom ($p < .001$), allowing us to reject the null hypothesis of no mean change.[3] This simple example cannot fully present the flexibility of assessing longitudinal mean shifts, since only two time points are presented. With

[3]Two points should be noted about this model. First, the GFI values as computed in LISREL 7 appear to suggest that omnibus model fit according to this measure is relatively unaffected by relaxing the constraint on construct means. Second, given the way in which construct means can be specified in LISREL 7 program syntax, the equality of construct variances reflecting no scale change would involve a complicated constraint that would set elements of the covariance matrix equal. However, since the moment matrix is used as the fundamental parameter matrix in this specification, the more complicated constraint was not employed in this model.

additional longitudinal data waves, hypotheses that are of potentially more substantive interest could be explored. For example, in a three-wave longitudinal study with a preintervention, postintervention, and six-month postintervention follow-up assessment, one might be interested in testing whether intervention effects persist or return to preintervention levels. The same kind of *a priori* contrast logic that is employed in analysis of variance models could be employed to test specific differences among construct means. It is likely that these more specific construct mean comparisons will be more informative than an omnibus test of no construct mean differences.

Assessing Interunit Change: Summary

Table 4 summarizes the set of nested model comparisons that must be made to examine different types of change process that have been discussed. In this perspective, hypotheses regarding change are stated in terms of the different kinds of change that can take place over time. Of these, the one generally of interest is the longitudinal mean shifts in a construct. However, to appropriate assess whether or not this type of change has occurred, two preconditions must be established. First, it must be demonstrated that the construct has not changed in terms of its definition over time. If it has changed over time, then hypotheses regarding level changes in the construct are confounded with changes that have occurred within the construct itself. In variance of construct, definition represents a necessary precondition before construct level differences can be examined.

Second, the scale or metric of the construct cannot have changed over time. If such change has occurred, it is not clear whether the construct is being interpreted in the same way over time. Given the information-processing literature on changes in the interpretation of psychological constructs with repeated exposure (e.g., Fiske & Pavelchak, 1986; Knowles, 1988; Nunnally, 1975), it is possible that such change might occur simply due to repeated assessments of the construct. However, the occurrence of construct-scale change clouds the issue of whether mean shifts that might occur in a construct over time can be attributed to "true" mean shifts, or to changes in the interpretation of the construct's scaling over time. Thus, change in scale constructs must also be ruled out as a precondition for assessing whether mean change has occurred.

TABLE 4. Summary of Model-Fitting Results

Model	Chi-square	*p*	Model difference	δ(Chi-square)	*p*
Construct/Scale Change					
I. Factor loadings unequal	26.82 (19)	.11			
II. Factor loadings equal across time	28.62 (22)	.15	II–I	1.80 (3)	.61
III. Factor variances equal across time	30.11 (23)	.15	III–II	1.49 (1)	.22
Mean Change					
I. Equal construct means across time	199.48 (26)	<.001			
II. Unequal construct means across time	30.03 (25)	.22	II–I	169.40 (1)	<.001

Note: δ denotes the difference function applied to the variables within the parentheses. Degrees of freedom for chi-square tests are given in parentheses adjacent to the chi-square value.

Assuming that both construct definition and scale change can be ruled out as threats to the interpretation of level changes in a construct, hypotheses regarding whether construct mean differences over time have occurred can be evaluated. While this sequence of tests is suggestive of statistical hypotheses that can be entertained within this particular framework, this discussion is not intended to provide a prescriptive for the analysis of change. As has been pointed out previously in this literature (e.g., Golembiewski, Billingsley, & Yeager, 1976; Millsap & Hartog, 1988), the particular type of change that will be of interest in any given study will depend critically on investigator hypotheses.

Finally, recall that all of these types of change refer to differences in interunit variability. Thus, change in this context is interpreted as the average change observed across the units of observation. However, psychological hypotheses may also involve the examination of within-unit change. For example, researchers may be interested in the within-unit improvements or decrements relative to initial status. The next section focuses on testing hypotheses of intraunit growth.

THE STUDY OF INTRAUNIT GROWTH

Rather than studying the kinds of autoregressive change implied by the previously reviewed framework, some authors have suggested an alternative approach to the study of change. The foundation of those types of hypotheses have classically been of interest in developmental studies. Analyses of such data have been considered under the rubric of "growth curves," since intraunit growth has been hypothesized to follow different kinds of polynomial or other functional patterns (e.g., linear, quadratic, exponential). Interest in examining this type of intraunit growth has been revived recently through recent work of Rogosa and his colleagues (e.g., Rogosa et al., 1982; Rogosa & Willett, 1985b) and McArdle and his colleagues (e.g., McArdle, 1986, 1988; McArdle & Epstein, 1987). Burchinal and Appelbaum (1991), Kenny and Campbell (1989), and Willett (1988) review some of the recent work in this area. In the following, differences in the to-be-tested hypotheses involved in evaluating intraunit versus interunit growth are discussed, followed by a summary of how one might test these "growth curve" hypotheses. Again, structural equation models are used as a generic method to frame tests of these hypotheses.

Comparing Interunit and Intraunit Change Hypotheses

As seen in the previous discussions of interunit examinations of change, change in those models is conceptualized in terms of autoregressive models considering the time-ordered stabilities between subsequent observations. In the latent variable framework that was outlined for those models, the "common" variance existing among a set of measures within occasions was extracted, with relations between these common variance elements examined over time. In contrast, models examining intraunit change can be thought of as evaluating the "common" variance among individuals across different time points (e.g., McArdle & Epstein, 1987). McArdle (1988; McArdle & Epstein, 1987) has noted the similarity between his approach and Cattell's (1966, 1988) description of a T-type analysis in which a sample of individuals is observed over multiple occasions on a single test. Returning to the Figure 2 heuristic, these growth-curve analyses can be viewed as taking the unit × time cross-section of the three-dimensional cube. Later, this approach will be contrasted with classic P-type analysis, which considers growth only within a single individual, with multiple individuals treated as study replicates.

Since information in these models is aggregated across subjects, the parameters of these models of intraunit growth will again represent an averaging process of sorts. Hence, for these models, intraunit growth may be somewhat of a misnomer, since information is still being collapsed across individuals to obtain average growth curves. However, it is important to note the differences between what is being averaged when comparing the autoregressive and growth curve approaches. Kenny and Campbell (1989) review similarities and differences between these two approaches.

Concretely, these differences can be evaluated in terms of the substantive meaning attached to the latent construct in these two different kinds of models over time. In models of interunit change, "scores" on the latent variable (if they could be observed) would represent the amount of the construct present in each individual. For example, if the construct being examined in models of interunit change is a child's social competence, an individual's score on that construct represents the "amount" of social competence for the given individual. Thus, a high score on the construct would indicate an individual who demonstrates high social competence.

In contrast, the corresponding "score" in latent-variable models of intraunit change considers individual differences in the variability of a given individual from the growth curve describing the group. A high construct score in these models would mean that there is high similarity between the individual's growth curve on a social competence dimension (e.g., what kind of increases/decreases are observed in social competence in development for this person?) and the growth curve describing the group (e.g., how does social competence typically develop in childhood?). Thus, the construct scores in this context similarity reflect averaged growth over a sample of individuals.

A simple example of this approach to studying change is described next, primarily to illustrate the types of hypotheses that can be evaluated in this context. However, this simple presentation does not allow the explanation of potentially valuable differences in "level" versus "shape" that are discussed in conceptually similar treatments of profile analysis (e.g., Harris, 1983). More extensive descriptions of the general philosophy of this strategy are described by McArdle (1986, 1988), McArdle and Epstein (1987), and Willett (1988).

Growth Curve Models

For the purposes of exposition, the simplest case of examining intraunit growth will be considered (cf., McArdle & Epstein, 1987). Here, a single unobserved construct is hypothesized to underlie *single* observed variables that are repeatedly measured across time. This is exactly consistent with Cattell's description of T-methodology, in which a sample of individuals is observed over multiple occasions on a single measured variable. One might encounter such a problem in a classic repeated measures analysis of variance, where the same variable is measured at different time point, time is serving as the single within-subjects factor, and there is no between-subjects or group-level factor. By hypothesizing a latent variable in these models, the similarity between an observation unit's particular growth curve and the aggregate growth curve measured for the sample is assessed. Information involving both the means and covariances of the observed variables will be utilized in these analyses.

How are model parameters interpreted in this case? The variance of the unobserved construct reflects the dispersion of individual growth curves around the average growth curve.

The variance indexes the overall similarity/difference among the (unobserved) collection of individual growth curves, or the degree of heterogeneity among patterns of change. For example, the pattern of data in Table 1 represents a quite heterogeneous pattern of change. The "factor loadings" for this model, linking observed measures with the single unobserved construct, determine the shape or trajectory of the curve linking time-dependent observations in this sample of individuals. It should also be noted that these loadings reflect both mean and covariance information of the observed variables, although the latter is typically uninteresting, since the same variable is being measured across time and should reflect a simple autocorrelational process. Of greater interest are constraints that can be imposed on the loadings to reflect different hypotheses about average rate of growth in the sample. Finally, residual variances from the regression of observed variables over time on the latent variable reflect the "error" in this model. For example, if the reliability of the repeated measurements increased over time, a corresponding decrease in residual variances would be expected.

There are a number of different hypotheses that can be entertained by employing different degrees of constraint on the models to be tested. These include:

1. Is there any intraunit change over time?
2. Does change stop over time such that, after some point, the curve describing the results "flattens?"

Comparative models are employed to examine these change hypotheses. For example, the least unconstrained of these models would allow for differential patterns of change to occur over time. Under this model, factor loadings would be freely estimated across the multiple assessments. Values of these factor loadings (with appropriate adjustments for scale) could then be plotted as a function of time to graphically demonstrate the change that has occurred.

This least restrictive model can be compared to at least two models of interest. If we assume no common change over time, the curve can be hypothesized to be flat. This corresponds to a hypothesis that factor loadings are constrained to be equal across the multiple assessments. The difference between this restricted model and the unconstrained model would evaluate the null hypothesis that no common change had occurred across time.

Another model of interest might concern when hypothesized changes are thought to occur. For example, it may be the case that change is not hypothesized to occur until the $t + 1$st assessment wave. Thus, factor loadings might be constrained to be equal until the $t + 1$st assessment, after which factor loadings might be freely estimated to reflect the hypothesized change. Alternatively, change may be hypothesized to terminate at all assessments subsequent to the $t + 1$st assessment. In this case, all factor loadings would be freely estimated until the $t +$ 1st assessment, with all subsequent factor loadings constrained to be equal. Again, these hypotheses of "partial flatness" either at the beginning or the end of a curve can be evaluated by comparing these various model restrictions against the unconstrained model.

We again employ the Table 2 data to provide examples of these hypotheses in the study of intraunit growth. In particular, focus will be centered on the first four variables in this matrix, which we will now assume reflect the same variable measured at four different time points. We will test three competing models in these data. First, we will fit a baseline model where change is assumed to be unconstrained, i.e., all loadings will be freely estimated. In a second model, we will hypothesize that no change has occurred across time, i.e., the hypothesized change pattern is flat and all loadings will be constrained equally across time. Finally, we will hypothesize that some event has happened between the second and third assessments such that the average level of the measure changes. In other words, this model will be tested under the assumption that loadings are equal at the first two assessments and the last two assessments,

Table 5. Summary of Model-Fitting Results: Growth Curve

Model	Chi-square	*p*	Model difference	δ(Chi-square)	*p*
I. Factor loadings unequal	1.86 (5)	.87			
II. Factor loadings equal across time	4.65 (8)	.79	II–I	2.79 (3)	.43
III. First two loadings and last two loadings equal	2.28 (7)	.94	III–I	0.42 (2)	.81
			III–II	2.37 (1)	.12

Note: δ denotes the difference function applied to the variables within the parentheses. Degrees of freedom for chi-square tests are given in parentheses adjacent to the chi-square value.

but that these two sets of loadings will not be equal to each other. Table 5 summarizes the results of this model-fitting strategy.

As can be seen from Table 5, all of these models provide a plausible representation of the observed data, with obtained probability levels for the chi-square statistic well exceeding the .05 level. However, as in the previous models we tested, interest here is not on absolute model fit, but the relative fit of competing models. In particular, we will evaluate various model constraints against the baseline, unconstrained model.

To test the null hypothesis that all loadings are equal over time and that there has been no change, we compare the fully constrained model, where all loadings are equal to each other, with the fully unconstrained model. This yields a chi-square difference statistic of 2.79 on 3 degrees of freedom (p = .43), thus failing to reject the null hypothesis of equal across-time loadings. We might also compare the fully constrained model with the partially constrained model, where we have hypothesized that some change should occur after the first two assessments. This yields a chi-square difference statistic of 2.37 on 1 degree of freedom (p = .12). This would lead us to conclude that the partially constrained model does not improve data-model fit relative to the fully constrained model.

Finally, it should be noted that these three models represent only a subset of the type of change that might be observed across time. However, the model-fitting logic in evaluating these models is consistent; importance is centered on the comparative fit of competing models for observed data.

Growth Curve Models: Summary

Some similarities can be noted between the procedure outlined here and work in the repeated measures analysis of variance. In fact, as McArdle and Epstein (1987) point out, these models represent "an integrated mixture of ANOVA, confirmatory factor analysis, and Weiner simplex logic." This comment underscores the generality of these procedures and their applicability to a wide variety of research problems. As previously mentioned, the study of level differences has been generally underrepresented in the latent variable modeling literature and the contributions of examining latent growth curves are welcomed as a way of integrating data reflecting both correlational processes and mean-level processes. However, as noted by Kenny and Campbell (1989), it may be the case that autoregressive models provide easier ways of accounting for the influence of exogenous factors on the change process (although, see McArdle & Epstein, 1987).

Change Exclusively within the Unit of Analysis: P-Technique

Another topic in the analysis of change relates to intensive, within-unit studies, which obtain multiple assessments within a particular unit of analysis and attempt to study regularities in these assessments over time. In the psychometric literature, these have been referred to as P-type analyses (cf., Cattell, 1966, 1988; Nesselroade, 1988). Again, referring to Figure 1, this type of analysis would focus on the variables × time cross-section of the data matrix, with repeated measures obtained from a single unit of analysis across multiple observation periods. As might be expected from the intensive study of a single unit of analysis, principles of statistical inference are largely unavailable within this methodological context. However, a number of investigators have employed this strategy with success in recent studies (e.g., Hooker, Nesselroade, Nesselroade, & Lerner, 1987; Zevon & Tellegen, 1982).

It should be noted that this represents an interesting strategy for studying regularities in repeated assessments that differ philosophically from traditional, statistically based methods. As suggested by Nesselroade (1988), it is possible that intensive, within-unit observations across multiple occasions could yield data as interesting as the standard design of observing multiple units within a single occasion. While it is only the latter strategy that has an inferential statistical theory associated with it, the plausibility of conclusions in the former strategy could be bolstered by replicating within-unit results across units within a sample.

While this within-unit design would require intensive data collection with many more observation points than is typical (a minimum of 50 or 100 observations per unit) in our discipline (cf., Kenny & Campbell, 1989), it is possible that, at least within some research contexts, it is exactly this kind of change that is of interest. In particular, it may be less important to characterize the "average" change that occurs either in an autoregressive or growth curve context, but to carefully determine the kinds of change that occur within a particular, intensively watched observational unit. This "bottom up" strategy might then allow us to begin the hypothesis-generating process of generalizing from the individual unit studied to other similar but unstudied units, as well as potentially providing information about critical lag latencies for effects.

The extent to which these intensive within-unit analyses become accepted methods of trying to understand the process of change will be determined in part by our tolerance of descriptive, but replicated findings in lieu of traditional statistical inference. As some authors have suggested (e.g., Lazarus & DeLongis, 1983; Nesselroade, 1988), it may be these intensive, within-unit analyses that provide one of the more interesting windows to examining change.

USING TIME AS AN OUTCOME VARIABLE

In the models for analyzing change that have been reviewed thus far, time has, in some sense, been considered to be a predictor variable. For example, in the autoregressive models that were first reviewed, time could be thought of as a within-subjects factor, with observations being made on the same subjects across time. In the growth curve models and the P-type analyses, individuals were followed over time. In this final section, we consider instances in which time is an outcome variable. The introduction to this chapter introduced some instances when it might be appropriate to ask questions about when a particular event occurred (e.g., the effects of a preventive intervention on nursing-home entry or on high-school dropout). An obvious place where such statistical models might be successfully used in longitudinal analyses is in determining whether the time of attrition from a study is systematically related to subject characteristics.

Survival models (also referred to as event-history models or hazard modelling) represent a methodology for addressing these questions. While these models have been only recently introduced into the psychological literature (e.g., Singer & Willett, 1991; Rogosa & Ghandour, 1991; Willett & Singer, 1991), they have an extensive history in both the biometric (e.g., Elandt-Johnson & Johnson, 1980) and the sociometric (e.g., Allison, 1984) literatures. While space precludes a full treatment of the kinds of issues that can be addressed with survival models, a simple introduction will be provided here.

Essentially, survival models are models that are linear in outcome variable (generally assumed to be the natural logarithm of survival times, and thus closely related to log-linear models for categorical data; see Agresti, 1990). If we assume that there are a set of predictors that are, in part, responsible for the variation in the outcome variable, then the systematic component of the model can be written as:

$$Y = \alpha + X\beta \qquad [1]$$

where α represents an intercept and β is a set of regression coefficients. In form, this very much resembles standard linear regression models. The difference in survival modeling is in the choice of the error structure, which, unlike for standard linear regression, can no longer be normal. Survival modeling depends in large part on the selection of the appropriate error structure for the systematic process described in equation [1].

A second concern in survival modeling is the way in which data are collected. It is generally assumed that data for survival models are obtained continuously across time, so that the exact moment when an event of interest occurs can be identified. For many longitudinal trials where assessments are spaced across regular intervals, this kind of intensive assessment may not be possible. For example, survival models may be of limited utility when a longitudinal protocol requires assessment of all respondents at six-month intervals, since no data will be available about when a particular event occurred within that particular interval.

An important general feature of these models is the notion that values of a random variable beyond a certain point are not directly observed. For example, in a longitudinal study of nursing-home entry with a two-year time window, it is possible that study participants have a developmental trajectory that will lead to nursing home entry *after* the two-year observation period. The data provided by these participants is said to be time-censored; in other words, the failure to observe the event of interest is due only to the specific choice of the study's observational period. A structural modeling approach to the problem of censored data is given in Muthén (1989).

The application of survival models to the analysis of change is most likely to be useful under two kinds of longitudinal designs. The first would be when data collection occurs more or less continuously over the longitudinal time frame. In the two examples presented, it may be relatively easy to assess the exact date when a study participant enters a nursing home or drops out of high school. But such longitudinal designs are generally not consistent with the kinds of multiwave assessments that typify longitudinal work in psychology.

The second application where survival models are likely to be useful are in microanalytic contexts. If, as noted in the introduction, change can be thought of as occurring over relatively short periods of time, then behavioral observation studies would provide a natural setting in which to apply survival analytic methods. Rogosa and Ghandour (1991) present one strategy for applying survival analysis logic to behavioral observation data.

GENERAL SUMMARY

Different types of models with different emphases have been examined as ways of examining whether change has occurred. The study of interunit change focuses on the average change over time across units of analysis, and could be considered as being consistent with patterns of psychometric change. In contrast, the study of intraunit change as outlined here focuses on the variability that analysis units show relative to aggregated change across all units. Here, the interest is on the degree to which individual growth curves can be adequately summarized by their average value. Finally, brief mention was made of intensive, within-unit analyses where a single unit of analysis is observed across multiple (e.g., 50 or 100) occasions and situations where time is considered an outcome variable.

While the presentation here has focused on differences between these models, they can be viewed as complementary approaches providing a complete picture of the change process. Basically, such an integration requires different types of models reflecting within-unit and between-unit change. Bryk and Raudenbush (1987) present an explicit model of this form in the context of what they call hierarchical linear models, but which have also been referred to as multilevel models (e.g., Bock, 1989). While the Bryk and Raudenbush treatment focuses on measured variable models, latent variables could be hypothesized with the corresponding complexity of having separate latent variables reflecting within-unit and between-unit variability.

There are still a number of topics that have not been discussed in this treatment of change. For example, sociologists and social demographers have often been interested in so-called "mover/stayer" models that might be employed to chart changes in intergenerational mobility in socio-economic status. Analysis of this type of data has been treated in the literature on the analysis of ordered categorical data ("log-linear models"; e.g., Bishop, Fienberg, & Holland, 1975). Other interesting work in the longitudinal modeling of categorical data is being done in the longitudinal Guttman simplex models presented in Collins and Cliff (1985), which again provide a way of looking at change as its occurs intensively within a unit of analysis. The disparity in the treatment of continuous versus ordered categorical or dichotomous data might be bridged by the recent developments of Muthén (1987) and the development of the analog statistical results for the models presented here for mixtures of variable types. Falk and Miller (1991) discuss an alternative, but related, approach to modeling longitudinal data using "soft modeling" or partial least-squares approaches (see also Lohmöller, 1989). Finally, it should be noted that this chapter has not discussed time-series models and how they might be employed in longitudinal analyses. West and Hepworth (1991) provide a recent and clear introduction to the use of time-series models in longitudinal data.

It should be noted that the statistical models discussed in this chapter are all linear or linearizable models. It is possible that theoretical concerns would predict non-linearities in change as given, for example, in Seidman's (1988) taxonomy of forms of change. If such non-linearities are theoretically meaningful, substantive theorists in community psychology will have to work closely with statistical methodologists to derive approaches to data that are satisfying, both substantively and statistically. Any hypothesized nonlinearity would have to be clearly articulated in advance in order to provide the strongest test of a particular substantive hypothesis.

A final point worth noting is that the models presented here do not begin to allow us to fully understand the kinds of mechanisms of change that may occur. As one simple example of this, consider a preventive intervention that is designed to change some mediator (e.g., self-esteem or peer relations), which should then have an impact on some psychological outcome (e.g., presence of depressive symptomatology). While the statistical models presented here can analyze such data in which are now familiar path diagrammatic forms, there are other questions that are not very well addressed by current statistical methods for longitudinal data. For example, for whom does the preventive intervention work? What kinds of changes in the proximal targeted mediator need to occur for changes to be observed in the distal outcome? Such questions are not well-addressed by either looking at aggregated information across a full sample or looking at the aggregation of individual change patterns. An analytic strategy for answering this question would be to look at the reasons why the intervention works only for a particular subset of those targeted; unfortunately, statistical methods that get to the heart of this question do not exist. While much has been written about the statistical complexities of analyzing longitudinal data, it is clear both that much more needs to be learned and that statistical methods must be developed that will be more appropriate in answering specific questions of interest.

Issues of change and problems in the unambiguous interpretation of whether change has occurred can be quite complex, as many methodologists have repeatedly pointed out. This chapter has presented a model-based strategy to address specific longitudinal hypotheses. Articulation of these models should foster much greater clarity of the kinds of change that are being assessed.

REFERENCES

Agresti, A. (1990). *Categorical data analysis.* New York: Wiley.

Allison, P. D. (1984). *Event history analysis.* Beverly Hills: Sage.

Bank, L., Dishion, T. J., Skinner, M., & Patterson, G. R. (1990). Method variance in structural equation modeling: Living with the "glop." In G. R. Patterson (Ed.), *Depression and aggression in family interaction* (pp. 247–279). Hillsdale, NJ: Erlbaum.

Bentler, P. M. (1978). The interdependence of theory, methodology, and empirical data: Causal modeling as an approach to construct validation. In D. B. Kandel (Ed.), *Longitudinal research on drug use: Empirical findings and methodological issues* (pp. 267–302). Washington, D.C.: Hemisphere.

Bentler, P. M. (1983). Some contributions to efficient statistics in structural models: Specification and estimation of moment structures. *Psychometrika, 48,* 493–517.

Bentler, P. M., & Woodward, J. A. (1978). A Head Start reevaluation: Positive effects are not yet demonstrable. *Evaluation Quarterly, 2,* 226–238.

Bereiter, C. (1963). Some persisting dilemmas in the measurement of change. In C. W. Harris (Ed.), *Problems in measuring change* (pp. 3–20). Madison: University of Wisconsin Press.

Bishop, Y. M. M., Fienberg, S. E., & Holland, P. W. (1975). *Discrete multivariate analysis.* Cambridge, MA: MIT Press.

Bock, R. D. (Ed.). (1989). *Multilevel analysis of educational data.* San Diego: Academic.

Bollen, K. A. (1989). *Structural equations with latent variables.* New York: Wiley.

Browne, M. W. (1982). Covariance structures. In D. M. Hawkins (Ed.), *Topics in applied multivariate analysis* (pp. 72–141). Cambridge, England: Cambridge University Press.

Bryk, A. D., & Raudenbush, S. W. (1987). Application of hierarchical linear models to assessing change. *Psychological Bulletin, 101,* 147–158.

Burchinal, M., & Appelbaum, M. I. (1991). Estimating individual developmental functions: Methods and their assumptions. *Child Development, 62,* 23–43.

Buss, A. R. (1979). Toward a unified framework for psychometric concepts in the multivariate developmental situation: Intraindividual change and inter- and intraindividual differences. In J. R. Nesselroade & P. B. Baltes (Eds.), *Longitudinal research in the study of behavior and development* (pp. 41–59). New York: Academic.

Campbell, D. T., & Erlebacher, A. (1975). How regression artifacts in quasi-experimental evaluations can mistakenly make compensatory education look harmful. In E. L. Struening & M. Guttentag (Eds.), *Handbook of evaluation research, Vol. 1* (pp. 597–617). Beverly Hills: Sage.

Campbell, D. T., & Fiske, D. W. (1959). Convergent and discriminant validity by the multitrait-multimethod matrix. *Psychological Bulletin, 56,* 81–105.

Cattell, R. B. (1966). Patterns of change: Measurement in relation to state-dimension, trait change, lability, and process concepts. In R. B. Cattell (Ed.), *Handbook of multivariate experimental psychology* (pp. 355–402). Chicago: Rand McNally.

Cattell, R. B. (1988). The data box: Its ordering of total resources in terms of possible relational systems. In J. R. Nesselroade & R. B. Cattell (Eds.), *Handbook of multivariate experimental psychology* (2nd ed., pp. 69–130). New York: Plenum.

Cohen, J., & Cohen, P. (1983). *Applied multiple regression/correlation for the behavioral sciences* (2nd ed.). Hillsdale, NJ: Erlbaum.

Collins, L. M., & Horn, J. L. (Eds.). (1991). *Best methods for analyzing change.* Washington, D.C.: APA Publications.

Collins, L. M., & Cliff, N. (1985). Axiomatic foundations of a three-set Guttman simplex model with applicability to longitudinal data. *Psychometrika, 50,* 147–158.

Comrey, A. L. (1973). *A first course in factor analysis.* New York: Academic.

Cook, T. D., & Campbell, D. T. (1979). *Quasi-experimentation: Design and analysis issues for field settings.* Chicago: Rand McNally.

Cronbach, L. J., & Furby, L. (1970). How should we measure "change"—or should we? *Psychological Bulletin, 74,* 68–80.

Cronbach, L. J., & Meehl, P. F. (1955). Construct validity in psychological tests. *Psychological Bulletin, 52,* 281–302.

Elandt-Johnson, R. C., & Johnson, N. L. (1980). *Survival models and data analysis.* New York: Wiley.

Falk, R. F., & Miller, N. B. (1991). A soft models approach to family transitions. In P. A. Cowan & M. Heatherington (Eds.), *Family transitions* (pp. 273–301). Hillsdale, NJ: Erlbaum.

Fiske, S. T., & Pavelchak, M. A. (1986). Category-based versus piecemeal-based affective responses: Developments in schema-triggered affect. In R. M. Sorrentino & E. T. Higgins (Eds.), *Handbook of motivation and cognition* (pp. 167–203). New York: Guilford.

Goldstein, H. (1979). *The design and analysis of longitudinal studies.* London: Academic.

Golembiewski, R. T., Billingsley, K., & Yeager, S. (1976). Measuring change and persistence in human affairs: Types of change generated by OD designs. *Journal of Applied Behavioral Science, 12,* 133–157.

Gollob, H. F., & Reichardt, C. S. (1987). Taking account of time lags in causal models. *Child Development, 58,* 80–92.

Gottman, J. M. (1981). *Time-series analysis: A comprehensive introduction for social scientists.* New York: Cambridge University Press.

Gottman, J. M., & Roy, A. K. (1990). *Sequential analysis.* Cambridge, England: Cambridge University Press.

Harris, C. W. (Ed.). (1963). *Problems in measuring change.* Madison: University of Wisconsin Press.

Harris, R. J. (1983). *A primer of multivariate statistics* (2nd ed.). New York: Academic.

Hertzog, C., & Nesselroade, J. R. (1987). Beyond autoregressive models: Some implications of the trait-state distinction for the structural modeling of developmental change. *Child Development, 58,* 93–109.

Hooker, K., Nesselroade, D. W., Nesselroade, J. R., & Lerner, R. M. (1987). The structure of intraindividual temperament in the context of mother–child dyads: P-technique factor analyses of short-term change. *Developmental Psychology, 23,* 332–346.

Houts, A. C., Cook, T. D., & Shadish, W. R., Jr. (1986). The person-situation debate: A critical multiplist perspective. *Journal of Personality, 54,* 52–105.

Huba, G. J., & Harlow, L. L. (1986). Robust estimation for causal models: A comparison of methods in some developmental datasets. In P. B. Baltes, D. M. Featherman, & R. M. Lerner (Eds.), *Life-span developmental psychology, Vol. 6* (pp. 69–111). Hillsdale, NJ: Erlbaum.

Humphreys, L. G. (1990). View of a supportive empiricist. *Psychological Inquiry, 1,* 153–155.

Jöreskog, K. G., & Sörbom, D. (1988). *LISREL 7: A guide to the program and applications.* Chicago: SPSS.

Judd, C. M., & Kenny, D. A. (1981). *Estimating the effects of social interventions.* Cambridge, MA: Cambridge University Press.

Kaplan, D. (1988). The impact of specification error on the estimation, testing, and improvement of structural equation models. *Multivariate Behavioral Research, 23,* 69–86.

Kellam, S. (1990). Developmental epidemiological framework for family research on depression and aggression. In G. R. Patterson (Ed.), *Depression and aggression in family interaction* (pp. 11–48). Hillsdale, NJ: Erlbaum.

Kenny, D. A., & Campbell, D. T. (1989). On the measurement of stability in over-time data. *Journal of Personality, 57,* 445–481.

Knowles, E. S. (1988). Item context effects on personality scales: Measuring changes the measure. *Journal of Personality and Social Psychology, 55,* 312–320.

Kvalseth, T. O. (1985). Cautionary note about R^2. *The American Statistician, 39,* 279–285.

Labouvie, E. W. (1981). The study of multivariate change structures: A conceptual perspective. *Multivariate Behavioral Research, 16,* 23–35.

LaDu, T. J., & Tanaka, J. S. (1995). Incremental fit index changes for nested structural equation models. *Multivariate Behavioral Research, 30,* 289–316.

Lazarus, R. S., & DeLongis, A. (1983). Psychological stress and coping in aging. *American Psychologist, 38,* 245–254.

Loehlin, J. C. (1987). *Latent variable models: An introduction to factor, path, and structural analysis.* Hillsdale, NJ: Erlbaum.

Loevinger, J. (1957). Objective tests as instruments of psychological theory. *Psychological Reports, 3,* 635–694.

Lohmöller, J.-B. (1989). *Latent variable path modeling with partial least squares.* Heidelberg: Physica-Verlag.

Lord, F. M. (1958). Further problems in the measurement of growth. *Educational and Psychological Measurement, 18,* 437–451.

McArdle, J. J. (1986). Latent variable growth within behavior genetic models. *Behavior Genetics, 16,* 163–200.

McArdle, J. J. (1988). Dynamic but structural equation modeling of repeated measures data. In J. R. Nesselroade & R. B. Cattell (Eds.), *Handbook of multivariate experimental psychology* (2nd ed., pp. 561–614). New York: Plenum.

McArdle, J. J., & Epstein, D. (1987). Latent growth curves within developmental structural equation models. *Child Development, 58,* 110–133.

MacCallum, R. (1986). Specification searches in covariance structure modeling. *Psychological Bulletin, 100,* 107–120.

MacCallum, R. (1995). Model specification: Procedures, strategies, and related issues. In R. H. Hoyle (Ed.), *Structural evolution modeling* (pp. 16–36). Thousand Oaks, CA: Sage.

Magidson, J. (1977). Toward a causal model approach for adjusting for preexisting differences in the nonequivalent control group situation: A general alternative to ANCOVA. *Evaluation Quarterly, 1,* 399–420.

Meehl, P. E. (1990). Appraising and amending theories: The strategy of Lakatosian defense and two principles that warrant using it. *Psychological Inquiry, 1,* 108–141.

Meredith, W. (1964a). Notes on factorial invariance. *Psychometrika, 29,* 177–185.

Meredith, W. (1964b). Rotation to achieve factorial invariance. *Psychometrika, 29,* 187–206.

Millsap, R. E., & Hartog, S. B. (1988). Alpha, beta, and gamma change in evaluation research: A structural equation approach. *Journal of Applied Psychology, 73,* 574–584.

Muthén, B. O. (1987). *LISCOMP manual.* Mooresville, IN: Scientific Software.

Muthén, B. O. (1989). Tobit factor analysis. *British Journal of Mathematical and Statistical Psychology, 42,* 241–250.

Nesselroade, J. R. (1990). Adult personality development: Issues in assessing constancy and change. In A. I. Rabin & R. H. Zucker (Eds.), *Studying persons and lives.* New York: Springer.

Nesselroade, J. R. (1988). Some implications of the trait-state distinction for the study of development over the life span: The case of personality. In P. B. Baltes, D. L. Featherman, & R. M. Lerner (Eds.), *Life-span development and behavior, Vol. 8* (pp. 163–189). Hillsdale, NJ: Erlbaum.

Nesselroade, J. R., & Baltes, P. B. (Eds.). (1979). *Longitudinal research in the study of behavior and development.* New York: Academic.

Nesselroade, J. R., & Ford, D. H. (1985). P-technique comes of age: Multivariate, replicated, single-subject designs for research on older adults. *Research on Aging, 7,* 46–80.

Nunnally, J. C. (1975). The study of change in evaluation research: Principles concerning measurement, experimental design, and analysis. In E. L. Struening & M. Guttentag (Eds.), *Handbook of evaluation research, Vol. 1* (pp. 101–137). Beverly Hills, CA: Sage.

Panter, A. T., Tanaka, J. S., & Wellens, T. R. (1992). The psychometrics of item order effects. In N. Schwarz & S. Sudman (Eds.), *Context effects in survey and psychological testing* (pp. 41–85). New York: Springer-Verlag.

Patterson, G. R., & Bank, L. (1986). Bootstrapping your way in the nomological thicket. *Behavioral Assessment, 8,* 49–73.

Rogosa, D. (1988). Myths about longitudinal research. In W. Schaie & R. T. Campbell (Eds.), *Methodological issues in aging research* (pp. 171–209). New York: Springer.

Rogosa, D. (1979). Causal models in longitudinal research: Rationale, formulation, and interpretation. In J. R. Nesselroade & P. B. Baltes (Eds.), *Longitudinal research in the study of behavior and development* (pp. 263–302). New York: Academic.

Rogosa, D. (1980). A critique of cross-lagged correlation. *Psychological Bulletin, 88,* 245–258.

Rogosa, D., Brandt, D., & Zimowski, M. (1982). A growth curve approach to the measurement of change. *Psychological Bulletin, 92,* 726–748.

Rogosa, D., & Ghandour, G. (1991). Statistical models for behavioral observations. *Journal of Educational Statistics, 16,* 157–252.

Rogosa, D., & Willett, J. B. (1985a). Satisfying a simplex structure is simpler than it should be. *Journal of Educational Statistics, 10,* 99–107.

Rogosa, D. R., & Willett, J. B. (1985b). Understanding correlates of change by modeling individual differences in growth. *Psychometrika, 50*, 203–228.

Schmitt, N. (1982). The use of analysis of covariance structures to assess beta and gamma change. *Multivariate Behavioral Research, 17*, 343–358.

Seidman, E. (1988). Back to the future, community psychology: Unfolding a theory of social intervention. *American Journal of Community Psychology, 16*, 3–24.

Singer, J. D., & Willett, J. B. (1991). Modeling the days of our lives: Using survival analysis when designing and analyzing longitudinal studies of duration and the timing of events. *Psychological Bulletin, 110*, 268–298.

Tanaka, J. S. (1982). The evaluation and selection of adequate causal models: A compensatory education example. *Evaluation and Program Planning, 5*, 11–20.

Tanaka, J. S. (1987). "How big is big enough?": Sample size and goodness of fit in structural equation models with latent variables. *Child Development, 58*, 134–146.

Tanaka, J. S. (1993). Multifaceted conceptions of fit in covariance structure models. In K. A. Bollen & J. S. Long (Eds.), *Testing structural equation models* (pp. 10–39). Newbury Park, CA: Sage.

Tanaka, J. S., & Bentler, P. M. (1983). Factor invariance of premorbid social competence across multiple populations of schizophrenics. *Multivariate Behavioral Research, 18*, 135–146.

Tanaka, J. S., & Huba, G. J. (1985). A fit index for covariance structure models under arbitrary GLS estimation. *British Journal of Mathematical and Statistical Psychology, 38*, 197–201.

Tanaka, J. S., & Huba, G. J. (1987). Assessing the stability of depression in college students. *Multivariate Behavioral Research, 22*, 5–19.

Tanaka, J. S., & Huba, G. J. (1989). A general coefficient of determination for covariance structure models under arbitrary GLS estimation. *British Journal of Mathematical and Statistical Psychology, 42*, 233–239.

Tanaka, J. S., Panter, A. T., & Winborne, W. C. (1988). Dimensions of the need for cognition: Subscales and gender differences. *Multivariate Behavioral Research, 23*, 35–50.

Tanaka, J. S., Panter, A. T., Winborne, W. C., & Huba, G. J. (1990). Theory testing in personality and social psychology with latent variable models: A primer in twenty questions. *Review of Personality and Social Psychology, 11*, 217–242.

von Eye, A. (Ed.). (1990). *Statistical methods in longitudinal research, Vols. 1 & 2*. New York: Academic.

West, S. G., & Hepworth, J. T. (1991). Statistical issues in the study of temporal data: Daily experiences. *Journal of Personality, 59*, 609–662.

Willett, J. B. (1988). Questions and answers in the measurement of change. *Review of Research in Education, 15*, 345–422.

Willett, J. B., Ayoub, C. C., & Robinson, D. (1991). Using growth modeling to examine systematic differences in growth: An example of change in the functioning of families at risk of maladaptive parenting, child abuse, or neglect. *Journal of Consulting and Clinical Psychology, 39*, 38–47.

Willett, J. B., & Singer, J. D. (1991). From whether to when: New methods for studying student dropout and teacher attrition. *Review of Educational Research, 61*, 407–450.

Zeger, S. L., Liang, K.-Y., & Albert, P. S. (1988). Models for longitudinal data: A generalized estimating equation approach. *Biometrics, 44*, 1049–1060.

Zevon, M. A., & Tellegen, A. (1982). The structure of mood change: An idiographic/nomothetic analysis. *Journal of Personality and Social Psychology, 43*, 111–122.

CHAPTER 30

Thinking through Others

Qualitative Research and Community Psychology

ERIC STEWART

> The passion in my voice emerges from the playful tension between multiple, diverse, and sometimes contradictory locations I inhabit. There is no unitary representation to be formed here, no fixed sense of what is to be (hooks, 1994, p. 208).

> The goal of our work is not to amass generalizations atop which a theoretical tower can someday be erected. The special task of the social scientist in each generation is to pin down the contemporary facts (Cronbach, 1975, p. 126).

Imagine a single chapter whose aim was to cover the breadth of approaches, theory, and arguments in *quantitative* research, and how these could apply to community psychology. I am aware of a similar absurdity here; compressing a vast and highly articulated literature and history into a single review seems an act of hubris at best, folly at least. Nonetheless, judging from my own methodological training in psychology, it seems an introduction is in order, along with, at least, a sketchy roadmap of the domain. This chapter offers no "how to," but instead is an attempt at an orientation or sensitization to qualitative inquiry—why it seems to be an emergent and increasingly valid consideration, how it shares many of the same values and concerns as community psychology, its advantages, and its problems. The chapter also makes a case for why community psychology and qualitative inquiry should be at the beginning of a potentially beautiful relationship.

Qualitative methods and research have a long and distinguished history in the social sciences (e.g., Dilthey, 1894; Rabinow & Sullivan, 1987). Within psychology, no less a figure than Wilhelm Wundt called for a "second," qualitative "cultural psychology" (Cahan & White, 1992; Jahoda, 1989). William James' *The Principles of Psychology* (1891/1983), an ever fresh and informative classic, is singularly non-quantitative and interpretive. The psychologist (and anthropologist) John Dollard went to the American South in the 1930s to do an ethnographic study of race and class relations there (Dollard, 1937), writing a book well worth a look, not least for Dollard's reflections on the act of research. For community psychologists in particular, it is worth noting that what may have been the first modern community study was

---

ERIC STEWART • Department of Psychology, University of Illinois, Champaign, Illinois 61820.

Handbook of Community Psychology, edited by Julian Rappaport and Edward Seidman. Kluwer Academic / Plenum Publishers, New York, 2000.

W. E. B. Du Bois' (1967) ethnographic *The Philadelphia Negro: A Social Study*, originally published in 1899. There is also a tradition of qualitative approaches in educational and developmental psychology, the case study in clinical psychology, and the observational and generative work that often precedes quantification. Yet, despite an occasional efflorescence, qualitative research has not figured prominently in discussion and training of psychological research. More surprising, however, is that qualitative methods and theories, until quite recently, have been marginalized within community psychology; it is surprising because qualitative methods seem ideal to a discipline that seeks to work *with* rather than *on* people and communities.

Why there should be this marginalization is a matter for argument. However, I agree with Bruner (1986) that psychology's cognitive revolution in the late 1950s and 1960s ironically produced a reductionistic, universalistic, and acontextual view of mind and "behavior" that came to dominate psychology for decades. This is ironic because, as Bruner points out, the "cognitive revolution" was originally about restoring meaning and intentionality *back* to psychology (1990). Academic psychology's roots in psychometrics is probably another contributor to our quantifying preferences, as is our envy of the so-called harder sciences (e.g., Sarason, 1981). It is also true, for those of us with social change aspirations, quantitative research has often been an effective tool for, and provided legitimation of, our efforts (Kitzinger, 1997). It would also be ridiculous to imply that there has not been a great deal of very good and valuable quantitative research; in fact, I wish to avoid the either/or character of much discussion of qualitative "versus" quantitative inquiry.

CHANGE OF VOICE: THE "EMERGENCE" OF QUALITATIVE INQUIRY

In recent years, however, qualitative and interpretive research has become a legitimate topic for discussion for community psychology (e.g., Brydon-Miller & Tolman, 1997; Miller & Banyard, 1998). Why this is the case is also probably a matter for argument; however, some factors can be identified. One such factor is undoubtedly the "linguistic turn" in philosophy and social theory (e.g., Giddens, 1986; Miller & Hoogstra, 1992; Ricouer, 1992; Rorty, 1982), based in the work of Peirce, Heidegger, and (the later) Wittgenstein, and gradually seeping through the social sciences. Language, as both constituting and being constituted by social practices, and as spanning the conceptual divide between individual and culture, private and public, becomes both the object of, and a vehicle for, social science research, rather than a poor, messy, or "preliminary" substitute for numbers. As Wittgenstein (1953) put it, "It is only in language that one can mean something by something" (p. 18).

Related to this turn is what Hamilton (1994) refers to as the "epistemological disarray" of the 1970s, in which positivism was confronted by constructionism and deconstructionism, post-structuralism, and cultural and historical relativism, when the lines between qualitative and quantitative inquiry were blurred (e.g., Bloor, 1976; Cook & Campbell, 1979). Positivism, and some of the notions of validity associated with it, also came under attack from *within* the ranks of its leading thinkers; former champions of a positivistic psychology confessed that validity was ultimately a matter of interpretation (e.g., Cronbach, 1984, and the epigraph above; Rorty, 1982). That is not to say that all tenets of positivism and empiricism were abandoned, clearly that is not the case. What this "disarray" and the debates it generated did do, however, is begin to erode a particular epistemological and methodological hegemony in the social sciences.

Certainly not independent of the disarray (though not identical with it) was the emergence of formerly subjugated voices and perspectives in the social sciences. Feminists, in particular, sought to disrupt the disembodied and unsituated voice of science, to privilege lived experience, to connect personal psychology to cultural practices and oppression, and to empower the people with whom they worked in research ventures (e.g., Fine, 1994; Kidder & Fine, 1997; Olesen, 1994; Reinharz, 1992; Wolf, 1992). "Voice" became a critical part of feminist research, and voice is hard to extract from numbers and standardized instruments. In similar ways, gays and lesbians, so-called "third-world peoples," people of color in the United States, along with other erased or (mis)represented people and communities began to assume their own voices and challenge the representations of them that the social sciences had perpetrated. Psychologists and other social scientists became more committed to a social change agenda and making their work more "meaningful" to society, Researchers began to be challenged to explicate their own positions and assumptions, especially when their research involved some "Other." As Schweder and Sullivan (1993) point out, the increasingly visible and vocal diversity in this country means that no single research population or cultural perspective can be taken as normative or the standard of judgement. Added to the demand for attention to local cultures and meanings were the linguistic, anthropological, hermeneutic, and post-structuralist emphases on the ways that culture and psychology, meaning and behavior, were inextricably intertwined.

Of course, this is also the climate and era in which community psychology was developing, a climate that was "increasingly suspicious of a one-sided emphasis on fixed essences, intrinsic features, and universally necessary truths—an intellectual climate disposed to re-value processes and constraints that are local, variable, context-dependent, contingent, and in some sense made up" (Schweder & Sullivan, 1993, p. 500). All of these factors have begun to influence the nature of interests and questions in the social sciences, and so the methods for pursuing them. But community psychology also has its own "local context," including rising and falling fortunes in the era of the war on drugs and the "decade of the brain," its own defensiveness at the margins of a discipline already insecure about its status as a science, the need to appeal to policymakers and granting agencies and, more recently, the emergence of "prevention science" (e.g., Albee, 1996). These factors, along with the rarity of training in qualitative methods and theory in most psychology departments, and the constraints of academic publishing, have limited the exploitation of qualitative inquiry in community psychology.

CONVERSING VERSUS COUNTING: QUALITATIVE INQUIRY AND COMMUNITY PSYCHOLOGY

This reluctance to take up and exploit qualitative thought and method is odd given what seems an obvious affinity between qualitative methods, ethnography and participant-observation in particular, and the avowed values and goals of community psychology. Our commitment to valuing and promoting diversity—in questions and solutions, in settings and services, and in voices and perspectives (e.g., Rappaport, 1977)—should make us wary of generalization and universality, and of the power of numeric representation of persons. A commitment to diversity should also lead us to employing different methods of understanding and representing people, and to adapting our methods to their experiences and ways of understanding and communicating. It seems we should, if we are serious about local definitions of, and solutions to, problems, want to find ways to give the fullest and most resonant expression to them (e.g., Rappaport, 1990; Reinharz, 1992). We should also want to put our theories to the test of contextual, situated experience (e.g., Guba & Lincoln, 1994).

Our commitment to these contextual understandings and definitions (e.g., Kingry-Westergard & Kelly, 1990; Rappaport, 1987; Seidman, Hughes, & Williams, 1993; Trickett, Watts, & Birman, 1994) should lead us naturally to participant observation and ethnography. These methods aim for a full and collaborative description and understanding of process, meaning, relationships, perspectives, and (importantly) contradictions of particular contexts and social positions. A commitment to contextual and ecological understanding should also make us wary of predetermined questions and standardized measures, which are at least as often obscuring of local meanings and understandings as illuminating of them. Furthermore, to the extent that problems and solutions are context-dependent and meaning-laden, it seems that descriptions of them need to be as "thick" (detailed and contextualized) as possible if we are to expect them to be useful for others; that is, if we want to allow others to assess how they might generalize in some way to other communities and contexts. An ecological perspective also seems to require that we take seriously the transactional nature of person–environment relationships (Altman & Rogoff, 1987; Wicker, 1987). These transactions would have to extend to researcher relationships to the researched, and the description and consideration of how each changed as a result of the relationship. Again, ethnography offers one of the most developed methods for doing exactly that.

Our commitment to collaborative, empowering research methods (e.g., Rappaport, 1990, 1994; Reinharz, 1992) should lead us to converse with, rather than count or survey, those people with whom we work, to aim for intersubjective, emic accounts of their lives and understandings and, to the extent possible, to amplify their voices and foreground their expertise. Qualitative methods not only optimize the chances for such a dialogue, they also allow for the explication of the relationship between the researcher and the researched (Henwood & Pidgeon, 1994). Our commitment to claiming and explicating particular social values should lead us to write ourselves, our perspectives and positions, into our research, to portray ourselves *as part of the process of representing others* (e.g., Schweder, 1990), rather than straining to "white out the self and [refusing] to engage the contradictions that litter our texts" (Fine, 1995, p. 72). Or, as Hunt (1984) put it, "the unchanging researcher makes a unilinear journey through a static setting" (p. 285).

It is probably not the case that everyone who considers himself or herself a community psychologist shares all of these commitments. To the extent that we do share these commitments, we may not all believe that they need to be explicated in our written work. It is also the case that quantitative researchers may adhere to these commitments. There is also no *guarantee* that qualitative inquiry does embody these values and commitments. However, certain characteristics of doing and writing qualitative research may better foreground these commitments and our handling of them. Qualitative approaches may also offer an edge in capturing *process*, a key consideration in community psychology (e.g., Rappaport, 1977; Sarason, 1972). The narrative (and therefore temporal), contextual, and dialogical nature of (better) qualitative research is well-suited to descriptions of process and development; it is also a form that allows for multiple voices to be expressed, including meaningful contradictions and paradoxes.

I am virtually certain that qualitative approaches have an advantage over quantitative measurement in terms of capturing meaning and purpose (e.g., Guba & Lincoln, 1995), which extends to the theory- and value-ladenness of facts. This is what is meant by Schweder's (1990) notion of "thinking through others," appropriated for the title of this chapter. The process involves at least four ways of reflecting on persons and contexts (including the researcher's): (1) thinking about one's own (or one's culture's) positions and practices by means of the intentionality and articulations of others, thus making ourselves more apparent; (2) getting the other (as) straight (as possible), or providing an emic, systematic, and extended account of the world as constructed and experienced by others; (3) critical reflection on, and analysis of (or preferably dialogue about), the contradictions, oppressions, and obscurities of the other's "intentional world" (this, of course comes *after* the first and second processes have been accomplished); and, (4) thinking in the context of the other, while in the context of the other, and so portraying oneself as part of the representation of others (Schweder, 1990).

Thinking through others forces us to be reflexive about our own theories, assumptions, and practices. It asks us to enter into, and as fully as possible understand and describe, the world as experienced by "an other." It requires that we identify and preserve the contradictions and paradoxes involved in these worlds, rather than erase or elide them. And, finally, thinking through others means that we have to be clear about what we have brought to the process and how we have changed and been changed by the people with whom we work. Since people's lives, identities, and relationships are context-bound, temporal, and epistemic rather than propositional (Bruner, 1990), I believe that language, particularly multiple voice narratives, is a critical, if not preferable way to understand and represent others.

If all of this sounds rather anthropological, refers too much to "cross-cultural" and exotic research interests, I would say that all research crosses cultural boundaries. The "other" for community psychology is most often the poor, the disenfranchised, the marginalized of our own society, what Vidich and Lyman (1994) call the "civic other." Given the heavy weight and insidious effects of our cultural conceptions and misconceptions about these people and communities, it seems vital that we make every attempt to present and represent them—as much as possible—in terms of their own understandings, experiences, and meanings.

WHAT COUNTS? DEFINING QUALITATIVE RESEARCH

I have so far avoided actually spelling out what I mean by qualitative methods and inquiry. Qualitative inquiry is itself a topic of much (and sometimes heated) discussion and inquiry and, like quantitative methods, there is epistemology attached to the term that contradicts the notion of method as separate from theory. I follow Kidder and Fine (1987) in drawing a distinction between qualitative data and qualitative inquiry. On the one hand, there is the data derived from open-ended questions embedded in structured surveys and experiments. This is, of course, a kind of qualitative data, and Kidder and Fine refer to this as qualitative, with a small "q." On the other hand, there is fieldwork, interviews, participant observation, and ethnography, in which questions and hypotheses constantly change or are replaced, work that is unstructured (but systematic) and inductive. This is qualitative research, for which Kidder and Fine reserve the big "Q." The difference involves the extent to which true collaboration can occur, whether the interpretive nature of research is obscured or made transparent, whether it is the researcher's or the participant's meanings and conceptions (indeed their words) that are privileged, and whether contradictions and paradoxes can be examined and retained or will have to be erased. The difference also involves the understanding that the same question will mean different things to different people in different contexts and positions. The latter recognizes that people, problems, and meaning are embedded in cultural, social, economic, gendered, and historical contexts. Note, however, that there is nothing in this definition that prohibits counting.

This is a relatively safe distinction, and one that is probably useful for community psychology. Yet, not only is there no universal agreement on what exactly is implied under the umbrella of qualitative research, there are also hot epistemological and ontological debates in the field. Although Guba and Lincoln (1994) seek to disentangle method and epistemology by delineating the variety of paradigms and perspectives that employ and theorize about qualitative methodology, it is worth keeping in mind that theory and method are not orthogonal. To be sure, there is a world of difference between the near-quantifying "post-positivist" approach of Miles and Huberman (1994), the self-proclaimed right wing of qualitative methods, and the post-modern, performative, quasi-literary approach of Denzin (e.g., 1997). Assumptions about validity range from the traditional empiricist and objectivist to the experimental, political, and critical theory approaches. There are post-colonial standpoints that question whether the subjugated "other" can actually have a voice in the social sciences, or if they are merely appropriated as exotic diversions or a validation of a kind or *status quo* (e.g., Said, 1978; Spivak, 1988). There is a range of feminist perspectives (e.g., Collins, 1986, 1992; Fine, 1992; Harding, 1987; Reinharz, 1992). There are also a variety of ethnic and critical race perspectives (e.g., Stanfield, 1994; West, 1990). Volumes have been written, and more will be, outlining, advocating, and/or vilifying various approaches and epistemologies relating to qualitative methods. There have likewise been a variety of attempts to organize and categorize the field and its borders into "strands" (Henwood & Pidgeon, 1994), "moments" (Denzin & Lincoln, 1994), or "paradigms" (Guba & Lincoln, 1994). The problem is that the field is neither static nor mature; epistemologies are evolving and interacting; researchers and theorists decline to remain in one camp. The territory is hard to chart.

That said, however, it is worthwhile to try to give a gross orientation to the literature. I will follow Denzin and Lincoln (1994) in their three broad divisions of qualitative approaches: (1) positivism and post-positivism; (2) constructivism and critical theory; and, (3) the umbrella under an umbrella of interpretive perspectives. Positivism and post-positivism are the ground in a sense, since it is frequently in response or reaction to these that the other epistemologies define themselves. Positivism's and, in a modified form, post-positivism's concerns over objectivity, reliability, and the criteria for assessing validity are familiar to most psychology students. Miles and Huberman (1994) probably best represent this approach to qualitative research. Critiques of positivism have already been alluded to above, but the primary issues are a tendency to strip context; exclude local and idiographic meanings; and the erasure of the researcher's power, influence, and ideology.

Constructivism is increasingly familiar in the social sciences, and it emphasizes that meaning and experience are created in particular social and historical contexts. It is relativist rather than objectivist, and underscores that knower and known share a transactional relationship. It generally aims for an intersubjective, dialogic method of understanding, and trustworthiness and clarity are key aspects of validity. Constructivism is a well-established and highly articulated tradition, stretching from Dilthey to Mead to Gergen (see Guba & Lincoln, 1994). Critical theory is similarly big and rich. Based in Marxist theory, it emphasizes a historical realism and power differences, aims for change in social regularities, and emphasizes action or "praxis" as key aspects of validity. Under this umbrella, there are feminist, post-structuralist, and critical race variations (e.g., Giroux, 1992; Nelson & Grossberg, 1988; West, 1990).

Interpretive perspectives, as Denzin and Lincoln (1994) use the label, refer to a range of so-called standpoint epistemologies: feminist, cultural studies, ethnic models, and queer theory. What unites them, I believe, is their situated reflexivity and the breadth of available methods from biography and autobiography, literature and journalism, to traditional empirical research. In general, they share as well the commitment to social change and a transactional view of knowledge creation.

As if this were not enough, the tower of Babel has also generated real differences over what actual methods qualify as "truly" qualitative. Ethnography and participant observation, interviewing, focus groups, textual analysis, discourse and conversation analysis, media research and criticism, open-ended (but structured) interviews or questionnaires, historiography, biography and autobiography, journalistic approaches, and literature may or may not qualify as "real" research or really "qualitative." The criteria depend to some extent on ideological commitments, some of which have been roughly outlined above. They differ in the extent of relationship between the researcher and the researched, how and about what to be rigorous, what counts as "authentic," and appropriate ways to discuss and represent the object of our work. They also differ in their attitudes toward quantification. Schweder (1996a, 1996b) not only draws a fundamental distinction between the "object" of research for a *quanta* or *qualia* approach, but also between "true" ethnography and (though he doesn't characterize the alternative as such) exploitation or pseudo-ethnography. Some thinkers are pessimistic about whether any of our received scientific and methodological assumptions can lead to anything but continued exploitation and oppression (see Denzin, 1997, for a review). Others are more positive about the ways that quantitative and qualitative can mutually inform and elucidate one another, as well as the promise of a thoughtful use of variety of experimental, traditional, and combined approaches to understanding social problems, situations, and solutions.

The reason for this brief overview is that community psychologists, with the breadth of their concerns and diversity, and the ambition of their goals, can use as many tools as they can get. I believe that to be effective as researchers or interventionists requires us to be "jacks of all trades" and conversant with a number of different strategies for understanding, communicating, and change. The same is true for qualitative researchers, the best of whom can draw on whatever skills and ideas best fit the context in which they are working (Denzin, 1997). This would include quantitative methods as well, of course, but these are generally well-covered in most psychology departments. The same is usually not true for qualitative methods and theories, and perhaps worse than not doing qualitative work at all, this can lead to doing it badly or unethically.

But it is this same emphasis on flexibility, adaptation, and relationship that makes qualitative research hard to teach. In anthropology the traditional training was to "just do it" (Punch, 1994), because there could be no blanket rules or strategies for field work. This is only partly true. Besides the usefulness of an at least nodding acquaintance with the variety of strategies for research and ways of thinking about it, there is a need for potential investigators to be sensitized to the opportunities and dangers involved in inserting themselves into people's day-to-day lives. More so than quantitative work, most qualitative research is about relationship. And, while this not something that can be really taught, it is something that researchers should be invited to think about carefully. One frequently gets more than she bargained for in qualitative research (and the objects of study sometimes feel like they got less). What to do with the "more" (data, intimacy, affective involvement, obligations, etc.) is a problem that we should be, but rarely are, trained to anticipate. Again, this is true of quantitative work as well, but I think there is usually a real difference in the researcher/researched relationship in qualitative studies. However, because the field is broad, complex, and evolving, the best way to get a practical handle on it is through exposure to "exemplars" (Mishler, 1990); that is, looking at and analyzing the work of others. A comprehensive introduction to the field and its discontents is Denzin and Lincoln's (1994) *Handbook of Qualitative Research*, which fairly represents the range from the post-positivist to the post-postmodernists. There are a number of useful guides to actually doing qualitative research (usually more sensitizing or orienting than "how-to"), but Wolcott (1995), Erickson (1986), and Briggs (1986) are particularly good starting points. For ethnographic work relevant to community psychology, Carol Stack's (1974) *All Our Kin: Strategies for Survival in a Black Community*, and her more recent (1997) *Call to Home: African Americans Reclaim the Rural South*, are both good examples. Also useful is the work of Shirley Brice Heath (e.g., 1983; Heath & McLaughlin, 1993), particularly for the importance and implications of language practices. But there are almost certainly good examples of qualitative work related to most any specific area of research in community psychology. One may have to look outside of psychology to find them—to history, sociology, linguistics, anthropology, women's studies, African-American studies, cultural studies—though examples work their way into our own journals with increasing frequency (e.g., Brydon-Miller & Tolman, 1997; Miller & Banyard, 1998; Rizzo & Corsaro, 1995; Stewart & Weinstein, 1997).

FRIEND OR FOE? ETHICS OF QUALITATIVE RESEARCH

Many qualitative researchers seem to have a tendency toward self-righteousness, even an ecclesiastical superiority. I believe this is an unfounded stance. There are evils and abuses possible in qualitative work, possibly even more egregious because the relationship of researcher and researched is often more intimate and complicated. There is also a greater potential for betrayal when you are taking somebody's words and stories and making them public. Despite what many qualitative researchers proclaim, we are more generally appropriating voice rather than giving it. That is, once we "leave the field" and begin the business of scholarly writing, it becomes *our* story. We select, edit, interpret, analyze, and theoretically frame the words and experiences of our "subjects." And so we should—it's what we get paid for, so to speak. But participants often are not thrilled to read themselves summarized and interpreted in ways that may not correspond to their self-perceptions. Their perspectives are presented as partial, their interpretations as just one of many possible ways to view things (Punch, 1994). The person who was their friend (or colleague, or advocate, or confidante) has suddenly been replaced by an academic. But the researcher *always was* just that, a researcher. The problem arises because he or she forgot that and wanted the participants to forget it as well. Truly collaborative research can mitigate this problem, for example returning the written product to participants for their responses and contestation, or by aiming for multivoice reports, including a variety of perspectives and interpretations (e.g., Denzin, 1997). But the real answer, I believe, is to confront and explicate your "dual role" from the outset and not kid yourself or your participants. (I am assuming here that it is unethical to deliberately deceive "participants," and furthermore that doing so would not be my understanding of qualitative research.)

Representation is a tricky business, particularly representation of those people and communities that are marginalized, oppressed, and have little opportunity to put forward their own self-representations. Numbers offer a certain aggregate anonymity that words and stories do not. Questionnaires allow a certain confidence that you won't get information you would prefer not to have. What do you do with data that make your participants look "bad" in your or others' estimation? Do you include remarks that are offensive or hateful in your account? What if one or more of your participants seem to be "living up" to the very stereotypes you are seeking to disrupt? Political is an overused word, but the negotiation of personal relationships, social and cultural assumptions and inequalities, representing others, and defining problems and issues are "political" to the extent that they involve real power and resource differences. Institutional review boards are rarely attuned to ethical complexities of extended field work and participant observation. Should consent forms say something like "there is the potential that you may come out of this looking like an idiot"? Pseudonyms may protect confidentiality of participants to the general public, but how do you prevent participants from being identified by the other participants, particularly when dealing with highly charged relationships or issues? What if participants decide that they don't like what you have to say about them? Do you have an ethical obligation not to publish or *to* publish? What if your participants feel "ripped off" when you leave the field and end the relationship?

I don't have good answers for these questions, and I haven't found any in the literature. The answer most often is "it depends." Again, I think the best prevention is to be as clear as you possibly can be about what you're up to and why, even if this means that some people won't talk to you and some places won't let you in. If nothing anybody says will be guaranteed to be "off the record," then you should say so. Still, I don't know if there are answers here; the ruthlessness and sensitivity that have to co-exist in the social sciences—the persuasions to divulge combined with a cold analytic gaze, intimacy and transience—make qualitative research an ethically tricky proposition.

SUBJECTS AND OBJECTS

I agree with Schweder (1996b) that there are some real differences between quantitative and qualitative research. The questions, object and objective, terms and methods of validation, relationships and process are generally very different. But I would argue that quantitative research is no less interpretive, it just shows up in different places in the texts. Consider the sometimes huge leap the reader is asked to make from the methods and results sections to the introduction and discussion sections of a quantitative work. The question of what the ANOVA means and why we should care is an interpretive issue. Qualitative researchers just strew the interpretation throughout their work, and ideally try to be as transparent about it as possible. The sameness and difference need to be recognized in discussions of the validity and quality of qualitative research. As indicated above, there are various and competing ideas about assessing and discussing the validity of qualitative research (see also Denzin, 1997; Lincoln & Guba, 1985; Mishler, 1990); but these discussions often ultimately come down to whether the work is useful and whether one trusts the author. The same holds for quantitative work.

There also is no reason to believe that quantitative work cannot be reflexive, contextual, and effective of social and community change. A great deal of the defensiveness and polemics on the part of qualitative researchers is due to the fact we often actually *are* marginalized; we are called upon to justify ourselves and our work in ways that quantitative researchers are not. Qualitative inquiry offers a great and increasing variety of methods well suited to questions about context, meaning, and process. Qualitative work is also ideal for a community psychology that seeks to span levels of analysis (Mankowski & Rappaport, 1995) because it allows for close, contextual, and detailed observation of the transactional ways people and settings, individuals and culture, role and identity relate. It also allows theory and lived experience to come together in a way that allows for paradox, complexity, and qualification. I have tried to make clear that qualitative inquiry has a long, independent, and rich history of its own. I have also tried to argue that there is no reason to consider qualitative work as second-best, preliminary, or untrustworthy. Such a position seems nothing more than a lack of imagination or a misunderstanding of social inquiry. End of polemic.

There is no reason why quantitative and qualitative inquiry cannot be gainfully employed simultaneously. In fact, they can inform one another in valuable ways, and community psychologists should avail themselves of all possible tools. A methodological pluralism seems like a promising way to avoid a certain trained incapacity to see situations, people, and problems in a variety of ways. That is, it seems like it would lessen the likelihood that the world will become a series of "Latin squares" (Sarason, 1981). It is, however, no simple matter to combine them because the languages and forms of reporting tend to differ in important ways. I suspect that the choice, when there is one, is based on the researcher's preferences for particular kinds of questions, relationships, and writing styles, if not also on particular talents. However, it won't be a matter of choice unless qualitative methods are brought into the tent, taught in training programs, and understood by editors and reviewers.

A final and perhaps most banal issue is that qualitative work is wordy, often very long, complex, or even contradictory, and foregrounds a situated perspective, sometimes multiple perspectives. A short report on qualitative research is often a bad one because too much is omitted or glossed over to allow for a full understanding or assessment on the part of the reader. All of these characteristics work against it in journal publishing. Often only fragments of a study can be fit to page limitations and the single-point preference of most editors. However, the rarity of qualitative research in our journals is most likely not a political issue, nor an intentional marginalization. More likely, it is because many reviewers and editors don't know how to assess and offer constructive feedback on qualitative research. Critiques of constraints in training, publishing, and epistemology aren't new of course, and they don't apply just to methodological issues. But, like questions of ethics or representation of the "civic other," it is a matter of collective or corporate thought, change, and responsibility. That is, they are not issues that get resolved through the efforts of one or two individuals. In the meantime, community psychologists will be working with half the methodological toolbox potentially available to them.

REFERENCES

Albee, G. W. (1996). Revolutions and counterrevolutions in prevention. *American Psychologist, 51,* 1130–1133.

Altman, I., & Rogoff, B. (1987). World views in psychology: Trait, interactional, organismic, and transactional perspectives. In D. Stokols and I. Altman (Eds.), *Handbook of environmental psychology* (pp. 7–40). New York: Wiley.

Bloor, D. (1976). *Knowledge and social imagery.* Chicago: University of Chicago Press.

Briggs, C. (1986). *Learning how to ask: A sociolinguistic appraisal of the role of the interview in social science research.* New York: Cambridge University Press.

Bruner, J. (1990). *Acts of meaning.* Cambridge, MA: Harvard University Press.

Brydon-Miller, M., & Tolman, D. L. (Eds.). (1997). Transforming psychology: Interpretive and participatory research methods. *Journal of Social Issues, 53*(4), entire issue.

Cahan, E. D., & White, S. H. (1992). Proposals for a second psychology. *American Psychologist, 47,* 224–235.

Collins, P. H. (1986). Learning from the outsider within: The sociological significance of black feminist thought. *Social Problems, 33,* 514–532.

Collins, P. H. (1992). Transforming the inner circle: Dorothy Smith's challenge to sociological theory. *Sociological Theory, 10,* 73–80.

Cook, T. D., & Campbell, D. T. (1979). *Quasi-experimentation: Design and analysis issue for field settings.* Boston: Houghton Mifflin.

Cronbach, L. J. (1975). Beyond the two disciplines of scientific psychology. *American Psychologist, 30,* 116–126.
Cronbach, L. J. (1984). *Essentials of psychological testing,* 4th ed. New York: Harper & Row.
Denzin, N. K. (1997). *Interpretive ethnography: Ethnographic practices for the 21st century.* Thousand Oaks, CA: Sage.
Denzin, N, & Lincoln, Y. (Eds.) (1994). *Handbook of qualitative research.* Thousand Oaks, CA: Sage.
Dilthey, W. (1894). *Descriptive psychology and historical understanding.* The Hague: Martinus Nijhof.
Dollard, J. (1937). *Caste and class in a southern town.* Garden City, NY: Doubleday.
Du Bois, W. E. B. (1967). *The Philadelphia Negro: A social study.* New York: Benjamin Blom.
Erickson, F. D. (1986). Qualitative methods in research on teaching. In M. C. Wittrock (Ed.), *Handbook of research on teaching,* 3rd ed., (pp. 119–161). New York: Macmillan.
Fine, M. (Ed.). (1992). *Disruptive voices.* Ann Arbor: University of Michigan Press.
Fine, M. (1994). Working the hyphens: Reinventing self and other in qualitative research. In N. Denzin and Y. Lincoln (Eds.), *Handbook of qualitative research* (pp. 70–82). Thousand Oaks, CA: Sage.
Giddens, A. (1986). *Central problems in social theory: Action, structure and contradiction in social analysis.* Berkeley: University of California Press.
Giroux, H. (1992). *Border crossings: Cultural workers and the politics of education.* New York: Routledge.
Guba, E. G., & Lincoln, Y. (1994). Competing paradigms in qualitative research. In N. Denzin and Y. Lincoln (Eds.), *Handbook of qualitative research* (pp. 105–117). Thousand Oaks, CA: Sage.
Hamilton, D. (1994). Traditions, preference, and postures in applied qualitative research. In N. Denzin and Y. Lincoln (Eds.), *Handbook of qualitative research* (pp. 60–69). Thousand Oaks, CA: Sage.
Harding, S. (Ed.). (1987). *Feminism and methodology: Social science issues.* Bloomington: Indiana University Press.
Heath, S. B. (1983). *Ways with words: Language, life, and work in communities and classrooms.* New York: Cambridge University Press.
Heath, S. B., & McLaughlin, M. W. (1993). *Identity and inner-city youth.* Stanford, CA: Stanford University Press.
Henwood, K., & Pidgeon, N. (1994). Beyond the qualitative paradigm: A framework for introducing diversity within qualitative psychology. *Journal of Community & Applied Social Psychology, 4,* 225–238.
hooks. b. (1994). *Outlaw culture: Resisting representations.* New York: Routledge.
Hunt, J. (1984). The development of rapport through the negotiation of gender in field work among police. *Human Organization, 43,* 283–296.
Jahoda, G. (1989). Our forgotten ancestors. *Cross-cultural perspectives: Nebraska symposia on motivation.* Lincoln: University of Nebraska Press.
James, W. (1890/1983). *The principles of psychology.* Cambridge, MA: Harvard University Press.
Kidder, L., & Fine, M. (1997). Qualitative inquiry in psychology: A radical tradition. In D. Fox and I. Prilleltensky (Eds.), *Critical psychology: An introduction* (pp. 34–50). London: Sage.
Kingry-Westergard, C., & Kelly, J. G. (1990). A contextualist epistemology for ecological research. In P. Tolan, C. Keys, F. Chertok, and L. Jason (Eds.), *Researching community psychology: Issues of theory and methods* (pp. 23–31). Washington, D.C.: American Psychological Association.
Kitzinger, C. (1997). Lesbian and gay psychology: A critical analysis. In D. Fox and I. Prillentensky (Eds.), *Critical psychology: An introduction* (pp. 202–216). Thousand Oaks, CA: Sage.
Lincoln, Y., & Guba, E. G. (1985). *Naturalistic inquiry.* Beverly Hills, CA: Sage.
Miles, M. B., & Huberman, A. M. (1994). *Qualitative data analysis: An expanded sourcebook.* Thousand Oaks, CA: Sage.
Miller, K. E., & Banyard, V. L. (Eds.). (1998). Special Issue: Qualitative research in community psychology. *American Journal of Community Psychology, 26,* 485–696.
Miller, P. J., & Hoogstra, L. (1992). Language as a tool in the socialization and apprehension of cultural meanings. In T. Schwartz, G. White, and C. Lutz (Eds.), *New directions in psychological anthropology* (pp. 83–101). New York: Cambridge University Press.
Mishler, E. G. (1990). Validation in inquiry-guided research: The role of exemplars in narrative studies. *Harvard Educational Review, 60,* 415–442.
Nelson, C. & Grossberg, L. (Eds.). (1988). *Marxism and the interpretation of culture.* Urbana: University of Illinois Press.
Olesen, V. (1994). Feminisms and models of qualitative research. In N. Denzin and Y. Lincoln (Eds.), *Handbook of qualitative research* (pp. 158–174). Thousand Oaks, CA: Sage.
Punch, M. (1994). Politics and ethics in qualitative research. In N. Denzin and Y. Lincoln (Eds.), *Handbook of qualitative research* (pp. 83–97). Thousand Oaks, CA: Sage.
Rabinow, P., & Sullivan, W. S. (1987). *Interpretive social science: A second look.* Berkeley: University of California Press.
Rappaport, J. (1977). *Community psychology: Values, research, and action.* New York: Holt, Rinehart and Winston.

Rappaport, J. (1987). Terms of empowerment/exemplars of prevention: Toward a theory for community psychology. *American Journal of Community Psychology, 15,* 121–148.

Rappaport, J. (1990). Research methods and the empowerment social agenda. In P. Tolan, C. Keys, F. Chertok, & L. Jason (Eds.), *Researching community psychology: Issues of theory and methods* (pp. 51–63). Washington, D.C.: American Psychological Association.

Rappaport, J. (1994). Empowerment as a guide to doing research: Diversity as a positive value. In E. J. Trickett, R. Watts, & D. Birman (Eds,), *Human diversity: Perspectives on people in context* (pp. 359–382). San Francisco: Jossey-Bass.

Reinharz, S. (1992). *Feminist methods in social research.* New York: Oxford University Press.

Ricouer, P. (1992). *Oneself as another.* Chicago: University of Chicago Press.

Rizzo, R. A., & Corsaro, W. A. (1995). Social support processes in early childhood friendship: A comparative study of ecological congruences in enacted support. *American Journal of Community Psychology, 23,* 389–418.

Rorty, R. (1982). *Consequences of pragmatism.* Minneapolis: University of Minnesota Press.

Said, E. (1978). *Orientalism.* New York: Pantheon.

Sarason, S. B. (1972). *The creation of settings and future societies.* San Francisco: Jossey-Bass.

Sarason, S. B. (1981). *Psychology misdirected.* New York: Free Press.

Seidman, E., Hughes, D., & Williams, N. (Eds.). (1993). Special issue: Culturally anchored methodology. *American Journal of Community Psychology, 21,* 683–806.

Schweder, R. A. (1990). Cultural psychology: What is it? In J. W. Stigler, R. A. Schweder, and G. Herdt (Eds.), *Cultural psychology: Essays on comparative human development* (pp. 1–43). New York: Cambridge University Press.

Schweder, R. A. (1996a). True ethnography: The lore, the law, and the lure. In R. Jessor, A. Colby, & R. A. Schweder (Eds.), *Ethnography and human development: Context and meaning in social inquiry* (pp. 15–52). Chicago: University of Chicago Press.

Schweder, R. A. (1996b). *Quanta* and *qualia*: What is the "object" of ethnographic method? In R. Jessor, A. Colby, & R. A. Schweder (Eds.), *Ethnography and human development: Context and meaning in social inquiry* (pp. 175–182). Chicago: University of Chicago Press.

Schweder, R. A., & Sullivan, M. A. (1993). Cultural psychology: Who needs it? *Annual Review of Psychology, 44,* 497–523.

Spivak, G. C. (1988). *In other worlds: Essays in cultural politics.* London: Routledge.

Stack, C. B. (1974). *All our kin: Strategies for survival in a Black community.* New York: Harper & Row.

Stack, C. B. (1997). *Call to home: African Americans reclaim the rural South.* New York: Basic Books.

Stanfield, J. H. (1994). Ethnic modeling in qualitative research. In N. K. Denzin & Y. S. Guba (Eds.), *Handbook of qualitative research* (pp. 175–188). Thousand Oaks, CA: Sage.

Stewart, E., & Weinstein, R. S. (1997). Volunteer participation in context: Motivations and political efficacy within three AIDS organizations. *American Journal of Community Psychology, 25,* 809–838.

Trickett, E. J., Watts, R., & Birman, D. (Eds.). (1994). *Human diversity: Perspectives on people in context.* San Francisco: Jossey-Bass.

Vidich, A. J., & Lyman, S. M. (1994). Qualitative methods: Their history in sociology and anthropology. In N. Denzin and Y. Lincoln (Eds.), *Handbook of qualitative research* (pp. 23–59). Thousand Oaks, CA: Sage.

West, C. (1990). The new cultural politics of difference. In R. Ferguson, M. Geverr, T. T. Minh-ha, & C. West (Eds.), *Out there: Marginalization and contemporary cultures* (pp. 19–36). Cambridge, MA: MIT Press.

Wicker, A. W. (1987). Behavior settings reconsidered: Temporal stages, resources, internal dynamics, context. In D. Stokols and I. Altman (Eds.), *Handbook of environmental psychology* (pp. 613–653). New York: Wiley.

Wittgenstein, L. (1953). *Philosophical investigations.* New York: Macmillan.

Wolcott, H. F. (1995). *The art of fieldwork.* Walnut Creek, CA: Altamira.

Wolf, M. (1992). *A thrice told tale: Feminism, postmodernism, and ethnographic responsibility.* Stanford, CA: Stanford University Press.

PART VI

CROSS-CUTTING PERSPECTIVES AND PROFESSIONAL ISSUES

Given the geographical location of the editors, as well as the nature of the roles and tasks assumed by community psychologists in academic settings, where writing and teaching is a high priority, most contributors to this volume identify with universities in North America. However, community psychologists are employed, and conduct their activities, in a wide variety of professional contexts. The field is international, and includes many people who work in applied settings as well. This section attends explicitly, if necessarily in survey fashion, to that reality. It touches on many of the key international perspectives, as well as many of the professional perspectives that are cross-cutting for the field.

The authors and the topics raised in this section influence, and are influenced by, all of the substantive matters that appear in the other sections of this volume, but often the kinds of topics addressed here are more background than foreground. In this section, matters of particular concern to applied psychologists, and to international issues, including peace and development, are placed in the foreground. This is followed by chapters that discuss matters concerning ethnic minorities, women in community psychology, and ethics. Each of these perspectives should be attended to in all of our work, and neither the editors nor the authors intend, by having separate chapters, to suggest otherwise. Indeed, having separate chapters emphasizes the centrality of such matters for this field. Of course, each of these issues are so complex and important that they can also be volumes in their own right, addressed to psychology more generally. At best, what is intended here is to call attention to the importance of the topics in the context of community psychology. The section concludes with a visionary commentary on change, a cross-cutting issue also addressed from other perspectives elsewhere in this volume.

Many of us work in unique professional contexts, including those that we ourselves have created. The first chapter in this section is structured in a unique way. It may be worth noting that it suggests alternative career paths for community psychologists. Here, Thomas Wolff serves as both editor and author. He introduces eight independently authored contributions, including his own, with an introduction highlighting the six themes that are addressed: setting (clarity of definition), relationship to the community (differences from working for a university), types of interventions (a broad range), guiding principles (a clear mission and well-defined concepts; continuity and commitment to gradual change), relationship of applied work to research (consistent reliance on a research base; some practitioners conduct their own research), and professional and personal identity (often not clearly defined as community psychologists). Wolff's introductory notes orient the reader to each of these themes and to the individual contributions. Collectively, these contributions remind us of how much creative work is being done by applied community psychologists who work outside the confines of the academy.

The second contribution, by Sabine Wingenfeld and Robert Newbrough, was written in collaboration with 15 coworkers, representing a broad array of international scholars from a dozen countries other than the United States, each of whom prepared individual manuscripts that served as a basis for the formulation of a chapter with an international perspective. The development of community psychology, its current status, and future directions are highlighted in a number of countries around the world. Training issues, conceptual bases, research, and scholarship are discussed, along with speculations about the future. This chapter is followed by Ronald Roesch and Geoffrey Carr's chapter on peace and development, which they believe to be necessarily international in nature.

The Roesch and Carr approach is one that views peace as more than the absence of war. It attends to wellness (see Cowen in Part I), enrichment, and economic development. It concerns citizen involvement, political efficacy, and empowerment (see Zimmerman and van Uchelen in Part I). The chapter touches on matters similar to those discussed by many of the other authors in this volume, including cognition (O'Neill), religion (Pargament and Maton), and grass-roots organizing (Berkowitz). They are concerned about the conditions that make democratic participation (Wandersman), with respect to issues of a peace movement, real and possible.

Lonnie Snowden, Miriam Martinez, and Anne Morris outline epidemiological data with respect to ethnic minority communities. Psychological well-being and mental health issues are outlined, with an eye toward service delivery and equity. They highlight the psychological distress encountered at the intersection between socioeconomic factors and ethnicity. But the sociocultural resources of family, religion, indigenous healers (see also Pargament and Maton, Part IV), and psychological resilience are also encountered here. This chapter, read together with the chapters by Sandler and by Barrera (Part II), also draws our attention to the epidemiological and stress/resilience literatures.

Carolyn Swift, Meg Bond, and Irma Serrano-Garcia focus on women's empowerment, with particular attention to community psychology's institutional history and to general research practices. They review 25 years of literature in the community psychology journals, and find relatively few articles directly related to women—this despite the theoretical isomorphism between much of community psychology and feminism. The literature has been exceedingly slow to acknowledge issues of gender and power, individual and structural links. Topics covered include women's family patterns, women in the workforce, care of dependent family members, health and reproduction, poor and homeless women, and minority women's issues. But few studies were found to relate to communities, and fewer still to those that involved residents in planning and implementation. Articles tended to involve educational strategies, rather than attempts to change barriers or create resources. They found that studies rarely addressed power or historical context at any stage in the research process. These authors recommend that future work directly attend to issues of power, acknowledge gender, seek multilevel and interdisciplinary understanding, and guide intervention and evaluation with the values of collaboration and participation. All of these recommendations should be central to a genuine community-based psychology.

The chapter by David Snow, Katherine Grady, and Michele Goyette offers a thought-provoking perspective on ethical issues in community psychology (see also Stewart's discussion in Part V). These authors do not invoke "guidelines" so much a provide "advice" designed to stimulate dialogue. Ethical issues with respect to values (and value conflict), goals, processes, informed consent, and the generation and use of evidence are considered.

The final chapter of this section, by Seymour Sarason, is both a reflection on, and a call for, barometers of change and soul-searching vision. His sense of psychology as "the business of understanding the transactions among change processes" recalls the chapters in Part V. Change—its anticipation, detection and stimulation—is an orienting concern for the community psychologist. Here Sarason calls upon us to rediscover our own history: our vision, imagination, purpose, and commitment to study, understand, and have impact on communities. His observation that "theories are the myths we create from our data" brings us back to the opening section commentary, and our view that every field requires a narrative about itself.

To reiterate, the editors believe that the issues explicitly raised here belong in every content area of this volume. Nevertheless, because they are cross-cutting, and frequently not made explicit in the focal content areas of the discipline, they are addressed in this section for the purpose of making them explicit in their own right. These chapters are not solutions so much as reminders to attend to such matters in all of our activity as community psychologists.

CHAPTER 31

Practitioners' Perspectives

THOMAS WOLFF

Community psychology is a field for both research and practice, yet the literature has been dominated by a focus on research and academically based practice. Many questions remain regarding what practitioners of community psychology really do, what kinds of settings they work out of, how amenable those settings are to their work, what levels of intervention they choose to become involved in, and how their practices relate to the research and theory base of the field.

Indeed the place of applied community psychology in the field seems quite unclear. When students emerge from community psychology training programs and wish to practice, where do they turn for jobs? Who do they turn to as role models? What actually has happened to community psychologists who have turned to practice as their professional focus and their livelihood?

This chapter includes contributions from a range of prominent applied community psychologists for whom practice is their primary occupation. They describe work done out of a range of settings, including community mental health centers (CMHCs), free-standing prevention centers, police departments, governors' offices, media, and community-based agencies. The chapter begins with the accounts of applied community psychologists who have mainly worked out of community mental health centers or related institutions (Morgan, Snow, and Schelkun). Indeed, John Morgan and Chesterfield Mental Health—Mental Retardation in Virginia, David Snow and the Consultation Center in Connecticut, and the late Ruth Schelkun of Washtenaw County Community Mental Health Center in Michigan have all been recipients of the Henry V. McNeill Award from the American Psychological Society and the Society for Community Research and Action for excellence in community innovation. Their contributions attest to the potential for innovative community psychology applications, even within the remedial focus of the mental health system.

The remaining contributions are more distant from the traditional mental health agency. Carolyn Swift writes of her work in two quite different settings: an urban police department and a private telecommunications firm. Judy Meyers describes the work of an applied community psychologist in a policy setting, working as a top human resource aide in a governor's

THOMAS WOLFF • Community Development, Massachusetts Statewide Area Health Education Centers, University of Massachusetts Health Center, Amherst, Massachusetts 01002.

Handbook of Community Psychology, edited by Julian Rappaport and Edward Seidman. Kluwer Academic / Plenum Publishers, New York, 2000.

office. All community psychologists can see themselves in an applied setting when reading Bill Berkowitz's piece on the community psychologist as citizen. The final two pieces, by Chavis and Wolff, describe community-development interventions located in communities themselves.

Their reflections on their work highlight six major issues: setting, relationship to the community, types of interventions, guiding principles, relationship to research, and professional and personal identity.

SETTING

There are no clear settings that can be declared the province of the applied community psychologist. Indeed, in reading the accompanying pieces one is struck with the sense that each of these community psychologists has essentially created a setting that will allow them to "apply" community psychology.

Snow describes the development of the Consultation Center at Yale as an institution with the primary task of community psychology service, research, and training. This is a unique setting that combines a medical school, a CMHC, and a community board.

Community mental health centers have often been seen as an ideal setting for the practice of community psychology, and indeed the experience of Morgan and Schelkun attest to the potential of such settings. However, both indicate that they are often working against the tide. Morgan summarizes it: "Few of my colleagues in the agency or the community know that I am a community psychologist; fewer still would know what one is. In essence, then, I was not hired as a psychologist, and it is only by gradually shaping the job, the agency, and the community that I can practice applied community psychology in this setting."

The literature (Snow & Newton, 1976; Snow & Swift, 1985) has documented the limitations of CMHCs due to their remedial nature, and no new settings have clearly emerged as the domain of applied community psychology. The advantage of this lack of clear settings is that community psychologists end up working directly in the community through police departments (Swift), governor's offices (Meyers), community action groups (Chavis), or as citizens (Berkowitz). The disadvantage is that each community psychologist seemingly has to find her or his own way by either creating a setting that will be amenable to their practice of community psychology, or by filling a position where they will be able to use their community psychology skills. Building structures that last for the practice of community psychology remains a challenge.

RELATIONSHIP TO THE COMMUNITY

Applied community psychologists work is unique partnerships with their communities. As Swift points out, to be a community psychologist located in a city police department or other community setting is to be totally immersed in that setting, it is a "saturated time commitment." This then is quite different from an academic psychologist with a strong involvement in project(s) in a community, but whose home base remains the university. With the fully immersed community psychologist the community is the boss; that is, they are clearly accountable to the community for their performance. Swift illustrates the reciprocity between community psychologists and the settings in which they work. As Schelkun points out, this reciprocity means having to modify one's priorities, activities, and so on, with changing community politics.

In my own case as a private practitioner of applied community psychology (Wolff, 1987), my "customers" are communities as represented by mayors, county commissioners, community agency heads, etc. My accountability is quite directly to these communities, their unhappiness will result in the direct loss of work. This direct line creates a clear accountability and leads to a unique relationship between a community psychologist and communities.

TYPES OF INTERVENTION

In reading the selections that follow, it becomes clear that the range of activities and interventions that community psychologists engage in is quite broad. Bringing order and understanding to this wide range of activities can be quite difficult.

Morgan offers an excellent typology for community psychology services, which includes general competency building, specific coping-skills training, support-system interventions, strengthening caregivers, ecological interventions, social–political change strategies, and community organization. The latter interventions on Morgan's list move toward broader levels of intervention, focusing more on society and community, and less on individuals. This broader focus, when combined with tactics of social change and community organizing, seem to be considerably underreported in the community psychology literature, but clearly relate to the critical concept of empowerment (Rappaport, 1981) that is emerging as the new guidepost for community psychology. Both Chavis and Berkowitz discuss the importance of fostering the capacity of community members to be involved in action and decision-making in their communities as a basic community psychology principle.

Meyers, reflecting on her role as a policy analyst in a governor's office, describes the critical role that community psychologists can have in developing social policy.

> My work was as close to being a community psychologist as I can imagine. The problems with which I dealt focused on the disadvantaged, disenfranchised or underserved. We addressed community problems and the resources to meet those problems. The concept of social change, primary prevention, the focus on large systems issues with the goals of enhancing the quality of life for individuals and families, all within a political framework and interdisciplinary approach were part of my day-to-day work.

PRINCIPLES

What guides the work of these applied community psychologists, whom Swift calls "pioneers"? Morgan outlines some clear principles that direct his activities: clear mission, well-defined concepts, continuity, commitment to gradual change, constituent validation, and positive orientation.

Continuity emerges repeatedly in these contributions as a critical variable. In most cases these community psychologists have maintained ongoing long-term commitments to their communities, and in that way have become trusted members and helpers to those communities. Each of the authors also articulates a clear framework, often drawn from the community psychology literature, to define their activities.

The commitment to gradual change is a cornerstone of quality community work. I have often reflected that my early training in psychoanalytically oriented psychotherapy taught me the concept of working on gradual change—a lesson that has always guided my community work. Why should we believe that communities will change rapidly when most of our work with individuals indicates the slowness of the change process?

Finally, Morgan captures the "positive orientation" that is reflected in the attitude of all the contributors: "We have maintained a consistently upbeat, positive attitude, we volunteer, we contribute, we entertain, we share, we praise, we reward, we congratulate, at all levels inside and outside our department and our agency" (Morgan).

RELATIONSHIP TO RESEARCH

As the field of community psychology matures, we become more concerned with dissemination and field trials of our existing "proven" programs. One impressive component of the work of the practitioners here is their consistent reliance on a research base for their work. Morgan describes his work as "field trials for primary prevention in mental health" and he and others clearly draw from successful research models.

In addition to drawing from existing researched programs, these practitioners are also noteworthy for conducting their own research on the programs that they conduct. Snow talks of three research domains: investigations of the effectiveness of preventive interventions, studies of basic coping and adaptational processes, and risk-factor epidemiological studies.

Chavis' work in developing an action research program, the Block Booster Project, is especially noteworthy since it provides a model for evaluating a broad-scope community action program working with local neighborhood associations. Community-level interventions are often intimidating to researchers, thus his model is especially helpful.

PROFESSIONAL AND PERSONAL IDENTITY ISSUES

> Pioneer. That best describes the role of community psychologist whose institutional base is in the community itself. The field of community psychology is an emerging one ... To translate its mission into action is to work at the edge of an ecological frontier. And with that work comes all the excitement of the frontier—the adventure, the risk, and the boom and bust outcomes that reflect the convergence of ideology, technology and setting (Swift).

The boom and bust of the pioneer clearly has created job identity stresses for the applied community psychologist. More than one mentions the idiosyncracy of their identity as a community psychologist. "Nowhere, neither in my job description nor in my everyday work am I identified as a community psychologist. A doctorate in psychology was not a requirement for the job" (Meyers).

It must be a concern to the growth of applied community psychology as an identified group of professionals, that those who perform in that role quite universally do not identify themselves in their work settings as community psychologists. This usually makes sense in terms of their work settings, but also creates some real limitations for the growth of the field.

The personal and professional strains on the applied community psychologist are numerous, but then again, so are the rewards. Many of the contributors note the great satisfaction that they receive in being "pioneers."

> For someone who values seeing effective "real-life" applications of prized concepts; who enjoys the challenge of adapting what exists and creating what needs to exist; who has patience for the long haul and can move for immediate gains when appropriate; who can handle both cooperation and competition; who has the temperament and skills of the entrepreneur; who has an eclectic approach to the literature; who can manage to stay put in a community long enough to make a difference; who can function in a variety of situations, contexts, and networks; who can develop sufficient supports in order

to survive; and who can balance the necessary routines of bureaucracy with the spontaneity of the market place—a career in Consultation, Education and Prevention is exciting, effective, and rewarding (Schelkun).

Applied community psychology is a critical arm of the field of community psychology, which needs to be integrated into the mainstream of the field. Graduate students need to be exposed to the work of the pioneers represented here and others like them, and more settings must be created where applied community psychologists can function effectively.

A. Applied Community Psychology: A Ten-Year Field Trial

JOHN R. MORGAN

I am a community psychologist working in a mental health center, and I guess I am fortunate in two respects. First, I get *paid* to be a community psychologist, to do work I believe in, work that has an impact on my community, work that I truly enjoy. Second, I can still say this after ten years, a time during which others have left similar settings in the wake of budget cuts and the restructuring of public mental health programs.

For ten years, I have run the primary prevention programs at our 100-employee community mental health agency, where I supervise six masters-level staff serving a suburban population of 175,000. Community psychology concepts have been central to the development of the program. Despite the primacy of such concepts in my work, few of my colleagues in the agency or the community know that I am a "community psychologist"; fewer still would know what one is. In essence, then, I was not hired as a community psychologist, and it is only by gradually shaping the job, the agency, and the community that I can practice applied community psychology in this setting.

It is probably trite to say that community psychology influences both the content of my work and the process of getting it done. The concepts and intervention are derived from current primary prevention literature, in support of the mission of our Prevention Department to reduce the incidence of behavioral maladjustment, which we do in the following ways:

Competency-building programs: We conduct the Rochester Social Problem Solving Program (Weissberg et al., 1981) in 30 elementary schools involving 250 teachers and 7,000 students annually. The program is in its ninth year. In a two-year follow-up study (Morgan, 1984), 75 program students were rated by teachers to be more socially competent and less maladjusted than non-program children.

Coping skills training: We train parents of toddlers and preschoolers in child-management skills, borrowing techniques from more clinically oriented programs but applying them to "normal" families. Results indicate that parents make significant improvements in target child behaviors. Consumer satisfaction averages over 90% (Morgan, 1981).

JOHN R. MORGAN • Director of Clinical and Prevention Services, Chesterfield Mental Health–Mental Retardation Department, Chesterfield, Virginia 23832.

In another program using research from behavioral pediatrics and child behavior modification, we provide targeted, one-time child-rearing advice sessions to parents in four local pediatric practices. In its tenth year, the program serves 200 parents annually. Seventy-five percent of the participants are completely successful in eliminating such target problem behaviors as temper tantrums, noncompliance, bedtime or sleep difficulties, or excessive whining or crying, and another 20% report at least partial success (Morgan, Shoemaker, & Cullen, 1983). We also teach anxiety-management skills to mildly anxious people and cognitive skills to mildly depressed people; results indicate that participants obtain improvements on standardized self-report indices of anxiety and depression.

Support system interventions: We train volunteers to provide daily telephone reassurance to elderly-living-alone. For nine years we have conducted a "Beyond Divorce" program, borrowing concepts from Bernie Bloom's work (Bloom, Hodges, Kern, & McFaddin, 1985), which provides mutual support and coping skills to recently separated or divorced adults. We collaborated on a NIMH grant to investigate preventive interventions with children of divorce (Stolberg & Garrison, 1985). Currently, findings from that study and similar ones (e.g., Pedro-Carroll & Cowen, 1985) are the basis for our continuing training and consultation efforts with 35 to 40 school personnel, who conduct 10-session divorce adjustment groups with elementary and middle school students. We have just piloted a similar program for high school students. Using findings from parent–infant interaction research, we train volunteers, who then conduct weekly supportive-educational home visits in order to improve parent-child interactions of adolescent mothers and their infants.

Strengthening caregivers: For several years we have trained day care personnel in child-management techniques. Average behavior improvement rates of over 50% have been obtained by trained teachers on target child behaviors. In the past three years we have conducted training in esteem-enhancing techniques for several hundred local youth sports coaches. Similar training and consultation efforts have been conducted with clergy, church lay leaders, Head Start personnel, and others. In all cases, the purpose is to build preventive, mental-health-promoting behaviors and practices in these caregivers, so the settings in which they work will be more preventive in their impact.

Ecological interventions: Youth sports programs, daycare settings, and middle school environments have all been target settings for ecological change efforts. We worked with Head Start staff, for example, to reorganize their center to reflect a more child-directed model, following findings from the Perry Preschool Project (Berrueta-Clement, Schweinhart, Barnett, Epstein, & Weikart, 1984). Similarly, we have consulted with middle schools on procedures to ease the transition from elementary school to middle school.

Sociopolitical change strategies: We have been involved in legislative advocacy at the state level for maternal and child health issues. We participate in several coalitions, including a statewide mental retardation prevention effort, that have succeeded in influencing legislation and funding.

Community organization: We assisted low-income housing project residents in the development of a resident's organization. Recently we have been asked to work with residents of our largest minority neighborhood on a major "empowerment" project, a communitywide "Read Aloud" program to improve reading achievement of elementary students.

As indicated, the content of these programs is influenced by community psychology research, especially primary prevention research. But the process—how we "installed" these innovations in our community—is instructive as well. Again, community psychology findings have been the guide. Table 1 outlines the steps we have taken in both conceptualizing and implementing programs. Some of the steps are empirically derived, familiar to community

Table 1. Steps in Program Development

Conceptual Phase: Program Development Principles

Look at the literature—Use "generative base"
- Identify risk factors: deficits, characteristics, circumstances, events, etc., that increase the likelihood that a group will develop adjustment difficulties
- Determine moderator or mediating variables: skills, competencies, supports, attitudes, etc., that lessen the risk
- Find effective technologies that can "install" the moderator variable or remove the risk factors
- Find procedures or systems that can diffuse or disseminate these technologies to the relevant settings

Define key concepts and parameters
- Target population
- What moderator or mediating variable will be "installed," or what risk factors will be removed
- What technology will be used
- What setting(s) will be involved
- What level(s) of intervention will be attempted

Implementation Phase: Action Guidelines

Arrange limited-scale demonstration project
- Look for group with stability, cohesion, strong leadership—Make sure adopters are volunteers!!
- Build ownership in adopting organization
- Nurture adopting group to enhance cohesiveness
- Use participatory decision-making
- Increase participation with incentives

Maintain intensive face-to-face contact—Promote communication

Define roles, boundaries, and expectations clearly and persistently

Pay attention to details

Build structures that will outlast your involvement
- Roles, titles, committees, liaisons, policies, procedures, etc.

Sell, Sell, Sell
- Newspaper articles, media appearances, public speaking, brochures, staff meetings, etc.

Feed data back to all with vested interests
- Your superiors, their superiors, funding sources, peers, staff, citizens, participants, etc.

psychologists from writings of Fairweather, Reppucci, Sarason, and others. Some are based more on wisdom than data, but could be useful in other communities. The principles and guidelines are not novel; what separates our program from some others is that we use the principles. For example, the notion of feeding data back to those with vested interests is familiar, but our program stands out in our organization and our community as one of the few that does this routinely.

It is useful to think of parallel levels of process. The steps outlined obviously have been useful in suggesting actions at the community level, in major systems where prevention programs can have an impact. Equally important is a second level, action *within our own organization*. Many of the steps have been duplicated internally in the attempt to make our "Prevention Department" itself an enduring innovation. This has been anything but automatic, requiring intense effort in planning, managing, maintaining, and nurturing an organization within an organization. The Prevention Department is a structural innovation in which other preventive innovations are incubated, hatched, nourished, and launched.

This, then, is the essence of my community psychology practice—carrying out the steps in Table 1 with various agencies and on various projects and, more often, guiding, supervising, managing, and leading staff who perform these activities. So my work blends the conceptual (finding, refining, and articulating concepts) and the practical (calling, meeting, persuading, negotiating, doing). And all this thinking and doing is repeated within our own walls.

LESSONS FOR APPLIED COMMUNITY PSYCHOLOGY

This work represents, I believe, a relatively novel field trial of primary prevention in mental health. The results include a number of effective, enduring innovations that impact the community's residents and some of its important systems. Perhaps more significantly, the agency I work for is much more preventive, mental health-promoting than before, and more so than most similar settings. In retrospect, certain features of this effort seem crucial to its success, including:

1. A clear mission and well-defined concepts: Nothing has been as useful (and persuasive) in educating staff, administrators, board, funders, other agencies, and citizens.
2. Continuity: Beyond the continuity of mission and conceptual model, we have had leadership continuity, important within and outside the program.
3. Commitment to gradual change: We have a patient, slow-growth philosophy; our resources therefore have always met the demands, and we have never had to sacrifice quality for quantity.
4. Constituent validation: I borrow this term from Marshall Swift (Swift & Healey, 1986), my role model for applied community psychologists. As he recommends, we have built programs with high face validity and consumer "investment", at the same time that we have been guided by research (scientific validation).
5. Positive orientation: Our department has maintained a consistently upbeat, positive attitude. When people were saying that prevention in community mental health was dead, we said it was just beginning.

It is the conviction that I was in on the beginning of an exciting time that has sustained my enthusiasm for my job, and for community psychology as a way of seeing that job. It has been rewarding beyond all my naive expectations of ten years ago.

B. The Development of a Community Psychology Setting: Integration of Service, Research, and Training

David L. Snow

Where does the practice of community psychology take place? If we examine published reports of community-based interventions and prevention research, we find that these efforts are undertaken in diverse community settings, groups, and systems. These range from the family, small group, or neighborhood, to settings such as the school, workplace, or church, to larger organizational and community systems, to societal levels through advocacy and social

David L. Snow • The Consultation Center, Department of Psychiatry, Yale University School of Medicine, New Haven, Connecticut 06511.

policy analysis and change. Clarifying where and how community psychology interventions are implemented is one thing, but out of what organizational base are community psychology programs planned, designed, and delivered?

The response to this question is not very straightforward, possibly because of the broad nature of the field or the disparate set of roles and activities that comprise community psychology. What we do not find, with few exceptions, are easily identifiable settings out of which the practice of community psychology occurs as the *primary* or *sole* task. As a result, the field lacks the organizational structures necessary to mount and sustain broad-based community psychology programs. Moreover, it means there are limited opportunities to train and to employ new community psychologists.

There are a multitude of historical, political, organizational, funding, and other factors that have contributed to this particular state of affairs (Broskowski & Baker, 1974; Levine & Perkins, 1997; Sarason, 1974; Snow & Newton, 1976; Snow & Swift, 1985). It is not the purpose here to present an analysis of these factors. Rather, I want to assert the importance of establishing an *institutional base* for the practice and study of community psychology. The problems cited above cannot be remedied without attention to the creation of enduring organizational structures to support and promote the interests of community psychology. I will pursue this point by providing an illustration of such a setting in terms of its early development, organizational structure, and multiple tasks of service, research, and training.

HISTORICAL BACKGROUND

The Consulting Center is a setting devoted entirely to the development and implementation of community psychology service, research, and training programs. The organization represents a collaborative endeavor of a university (Department of Psychiatry, Yale University), a mental health center (Connecticut Mental Health Center), and a private, nonprofit corporation (Community Consultation Board, Inc.).

The Center was formally established in 1978, although it grew out of programs that were initiated in the early 1970s as part of a federally funded community mental health center within the Connecticut Mental Health Center and Department of Psychiatry at Yale. In our case, the mandated consultation and prevention services were initially undertaken as part of two community-based outpatient clinics.

We began with a model that combined clinical and community interventions, each with its own structure, leadership, resources, and mission. This organizational model promoted a certain level of program development in each area and provided mechanisms for cross-fertilization between the two. However, over time, it became clear that the clinical service mission of the mental health center and the inherent differences in the nature of clinical and community interventions created constraints on the development of the consultation and preventive services. The primacy of the clinical task and the intrusiveness of direct-service demand always relegated the community programs to a secondary status. It became evident that a different model would have to emerge if a program of community interventions was going to continue to thrive.

The implementation of a second model was represented in the formation of The Consultation Center. All of the existing community psychology programs that had been established within the Department of Psychiatry and the Connecticut Mental Health Center were consolidated into a separate organization with its own facilities and staffing, and own resource allocation, leadership, and mandate. In this stage of organizational development, the primary objective was to create an enduring structure for the community psychology programs that would surround, support, and protect this area of work. This transition was essential if the programs were to survive within the larger medical and mental health institution, especially since shifts in the political, social, and funding climate inevitably would occur.

An additional feature of this phase of development was the further diversification of organizational commitment and funding support for The Consultation Center. Given the values placed on citizen participation in the community mental health center movement and inherent to community psychology, strong community involvement was sought early and formalized into a community board structure (a private, nonprofit corporation). The formation of The Consultation Center as a new organization, and a commitment to consultation and prevention services, research, and training, became a collaborative endeavor of a university, a mental health center, and a community-based organization. This provided broad-based support for the program and the necessary diversification of funding. The financial underpinnings, then, included core personnel and operating support from the mental health center, research and training funds that could be obtained through the university (primarily from federal and private sources), and mechanisms for obtaining public and private sector grants, contracts, and fees through the private, nonprofit corporation. The Consultation Center, therefore, was placed squarely on the boundary between the university and mental health center, on the one hand, and the community, on the other. Although existence on such a boundary is complex, it is an appropriate location for an organization involved in applied community psychology, training, and research. The overall structure provides a certain degree of autonomy and strength, establishes clear boundaries, allows for the control of necessary resources, and creates a framework within which a sense of identity and mission can form and be sustained.

DESCRIPTION OF THE SETTING

The overall mission of The Consultation Center derives from being both an applied and an academic setting. This mission is to design and implement interventions and research investigations in order to promote the psychosocial development of individuals and families, to prevent mental disorders and problem behaviors, and to enhance the effectiveness of mental health and other human service organizations and delivery systems. Training of individuals at graduate and postgraduate levels is an integral part of the service and research work.

The work of The Consultation Center is guided by a number of interrelated theoretical constructs. The first involves person–environment and ecological models that have been articulated in the field. We are interested in examining the interplay between environmental and situational factors, on the one hand, and characteristics of the individual, on the other. Interventions can then be designed and tested that aim to modify key risk and protective factors in the environment and/or the individual in order to enhance competence and resilience and to reduce the likelihood of negative outcomes. The second encompasses organizational development and organizational change theory. An understanding of the tasks, structures, culture, and processes of organizations and systems is absolutely essential to the development of consultative interventions and for establishing relationships within the community that will allow one to conduct ongoing preventive and service-system interventions. The third is lifespan developmental theory. The work is guided by an appreciation that individuals and organizations face certain developmental tasks, demands, and transitions, and that there are relatively predictable phases of development. These factors, placed within applicable ecological contexts, must be taken into account for change efforts to be relevant and effective.

Internally, The Consultation Center has a number of structures to support its service, research, and training tasks. Services in two major areas—prevention and health promotion and service system development—are planned and implemented through four program components, three of which are organized by age: early childhood programs and child and adolescent programs focus on the delivery of services to children, adolescents, and their families, while adult programs involve the provision of services to adult and elderly populations and the organizations that serve them. The fourth service component encompasses service system evaluations and involves work with populations throughout the lifespan.

The Early Childhood Program serves families with children from birth to six years of age. Emphasis is placed on the psychosocial development of the young child, particularly within the context of his or her family. Services consist of home-based and center-based interventions aimed at promoting child and family development and at preventing such problems as child abuse and/or neglect. Staff-development programs are offered to early childhood, mental health, and social service professionals, and mental health, educational, and program consultation is provided to early childhood settings.

The Child and Adolescent Program involves the design and implementation of comprehensive school- and community-based interventions for youth (ages 6 and older) and their families. Developmental and prevention perspectives are utilized to identify children and adolescents at risk for serious problem behaviors and psychological disorders and to design interventions aimed at promoting competence and resilience. In addition, staff development and consultation services are provided to school systems and other organizations serving children and adolescents in order to enhance the range and quality of services available to these populations and to promote changes in these settings that are conducive to child and adolescent development.

The Adult Program offers a range of community-based, preventive interventions for adult and elderly populations who, by virtue of stressful life events or circumstances, are at high risk for disorder, increased symptomatology, or institutionalization. Services include social support, mutual support, and educational programs, promotion of coping and other adaptational skills, and community-based program development. Major emphasis is placed on promoting self-help/mutual support groups in areas of bereavement, mental disorders, health problems, life transitions, addictions, and unemployment. In addition, psychosocial and psychoeducational programs are offered to promote mental health for individuals experiencing, or recovering from, psychiatric disorder in order to support their successful integration into the community.

A comprehensive program of organizational consultation and staff development also is offered to service providers and organizations serving the mental health needs of adults, to agencies serving the elderly, and to worksites. Consultative interventions and staff-development programs are provided to different levels of organizations, depending on whether they involve case, program, or management issues. The aim of these interventions is to improve the scope, quality, and effectiveness of services provided by mental health, social service, health, educational, religious, and business organizations in the community.

The fourth service component is service system evaluation. Here, the expertise of the community psychologist in evaluation and service system interventions can be enormously helpful in efforts to improve service delivery to people in need. Increasingly, this service involves work with larger regional and state-level systems of care, but is offered to community programs on a smaller scale as well. Evaluation services provided include a number of related elements: (1) developing infrastructures for the collection of data concerning client and service system-level outcomes; (2) identifying access and barriers to care for specific stakeholder groups (providers, consumers, family members, and policymakers); (3) providing feedback of evaluation data to state-level decision makers, local provider groups, and other relevant parties to improve systems of care; and (4) determining factors relevant to resource allocation for policymakers.

The organization of the research program of The Consultation Center has evolved over time. Initially, it was organized as a separate component with faculty devoting time to the development of various research investigations. With the expansion of the number of faculty working in the Center in both service and research capacities, research is now more closely integrated with the various service sectors and overseen by designated principal investigators. A research management group has been formed comprised of the more senior faculty. The purpose of this group is to promote research development, to provide mentorship and support to younger faculty and postdoctoral fellows, and to foster the interrelationship of research and service.

The Consultation Center conducts prevention and community research. The prevention research program includes studies of: (1) the effectiveness of interventions in preventing mental disorder or in promoting mental health; (2) identification of risk factors for mental disorder or problem behaviors that can be targeted in subsequent interventions; and (3) specification of protective processes that mediate risk. The community research program includes studies that examine: (1) alternative models of service delivery and their impact on service patterns and costs, and on individual, family, and societal outcomes; (2) natural supports and helping processes, such as self-help; and (3) community-based programs to promote competencies; empower individuals, families, or groups; and foster the community integration of disenfranchised or socially marginalized individuals. Investigations are conceptualized within developmental, ecological, and cultural contexts; often involve multiple levels of analysis; and employ both quantitative and qualitative research methods.

There is an important and dynamic interrelationship between the service and research work of The Consultation Center. The ongoing involvement in the provision of services to community groups and organizations fosters many possibilities for the development of research interventions as well. At the same time, given the primarily applied nature of the research, service staff are often integral to conducting the research interventions. In a corresponding way, results of studies strongly influence the nature and design of the services that are undertaken. Programs that seem to have merit can be tested rigorously as to their actual effectiveness. Carefully evaluated programs with demonstrated impact can be marketed and disseminated broadly.

The service experience helps to identify key research questions and to shape the applied aspect of the research investigations. In turn, the presence of research enhances a more "research and evaluative" stance in relation to service interventions. In efforts to interrelate research and service, tensions certainly can arise. For example, research staff and investigators are primarily concerned with testing the effects of an intervention under controlled conditions, and in maintaining the consistency of the research design over time. Service staff are appreciative of these needs, but are more inclined to make program modifications based on feedback from participants, especially in ways they feel would improve the service on an ongoing basis. The occurrence of these kinds of tensions through the interplay of service and research efforts leads to important learning in both sectors, to the generation of new ideas and, ultimately, to the reformulation of both service and research interventions.

The final task of the organization is training. A multidisciplinary training program is offered to predoctoral psychology interns, postdoctoral fellows, and psychiatry residents, as well as masters-level students in social work, nursing, divinity, education, and public health. Training experiences are available in developing and implementing consultative and preventive interventions, and in designing and conducting aspects of applied and basic prevention research, service system research, and program evaluation projects. In addition, a year-long seminar is provided to further the students' understanding of relevant theory and empirical research; to review various types of community intervention methods; and to promote particular ways of conceptualizing problems from more sociopsychological, ecological, and preventive orientations.

SUMMARY

The Consultation Center is an example of a viable community psychology setting. The mission organizational structure and culture; skills and expertise of staff; diversification of funding; and service, research, and training programs are now well established. In addition, the Center has gained strong organizational commitment within the larger institutional and community environments in which it is embedded. Variations on this theme can be found with a limited number of other community psychology programs or settings around the country. To create these kinds of settings on a broader basis, we need to act as change agents within our own institutions in order to foster further replications of these organizational models. Without such efforts, we will continue to have an insufficient number of locations from which to undertake service, research, and training programs in community psychology. Whether such developments have applied or research emphases, or attempt to integrate both applied and academic endeavors, they are vital to community psychology's future as a discipline and area of practice. The establishment of enduring community psychology settings is necessary in order to foster ongoing and sustained relationships with communities. From such an organizational base, comprehensive research programs can be launched to expand our knowledge base, broad-based community interventions can be undertaken that will have some reasonable likelihood of promoting meaningful change, and recruitment and training of new community psychologists can be achieved.

C. Community Psychology in a Community Mental Health Setting

RUTH SCHELKUN[1]

During the past 18 years in which I have been responsible for consultation, education, and prevention (CE&P) activities in a community mental health center (CMHC), the degrees of freedom in my work have changed considerably as resources and priorities have shifted in the field. However, I have found the opportunities to be varied and enriching, considering the ongoing commitment of our CMHC's leadership to community psychology's goals, concepts, and practices. Also, in addition to planning, developing, supervising, and evaluating preven-

---

Note: It is with great sadness that we note the passing of Ruth Schelkun before she could see the publication of her contribution to this chapter. Ruth was truly an applied community psychology pioneer. She was the first winner of the Henry V. McNeill Award and an early leader in the field of consultation, education, and prevention. Her passion for the critical issues and her contribution to the field are well summarized here in her own words.

RUTH SCHELKUN • Late of Washtenaw County Community Mental Health Center, Washtenaw County, Michigan.

tive services and programs, my practice has also been enriched by my lecturing at nearby colleges and universities and on the Prevention Intervention Research Center faculty at the University of Michigan.

THE SETTING

In 1965, I enrolled in the University of Michigan's combined doctoral program in education and psychology, initiating a transition from assistant professor of English to community psychologist. At the time, the community mental health movement was gaining momentum, and one of five "essential services" for federally funded CMHC's was being developed and defined as "consultation and education (C&E)"—the service component associated with prevention. Several of the Swampscott pioneers and like-minded colleagues had recently joined the University faculty, teaching the principles of C&E and mental health prevention/promotion, in addition to serving on the steering committee or on the staff of the newly formed Washtenaw County Community Mental Health Center (WCCMHC). I joined the staff when the agency was established in 1968; at that time, various consultation, education, and prevention (CE&P) projects were developed and fostered by the aforementioned pioneers; for example, extensive consultation projects with school districts, clergy, social services, and the police.

Later, these and other projects became ongoing elements of the WCCMHC's "essential" C&E program, established and funded in the early 1970s under a federal staffing grant. Because of ongoing relationships with various university departments, the C&E program was able to adapt and grow with the newly developing concepts and practices in the field. Graduate student internships enriched the C&E staffing resources, while offering a cross-fertilization of theory and practice during the growth years of the 1970s. Later, during the "dry" 1980s, when federal funding was no longer available, this strong momentum enabled the continued development and adaptation of CE&P services, chiefly through funding from the Prevention Unit of the Michigan Department of Mental Health, as well as fees-for-service.

THE CONSULTATION, EDUCATION, AND PREVENTION PROGRAMMING AT WCCMHC

A short sample of our many community-related activities during the past 18 years may indicate the range of our CE&P programs:

The Selected Neighborhoods Project (1971–1976): This neighborhood empowerment project in Ann Arbor, Michigan, was an early ecological intervention. After federal subsidies had resulted in the overnight creation of 2,000 low-income housing units in a single neighborhood, residents soon sought ways to halt the early spread of neighborhood blight caused by inadequate services and the lack of community planning. Using principles of community organization and ecological intervention now well-known to community psychology, WCCMHC staff facilitated the formation of a Neighborhood Steering Committee, a community resource advisory group, and a variety of task forces and committees. Project staff modeled a variety of roles and served as start-up staff for many needed services. Supported by city government through federal funds, the model established in those years has since become the norm for services to these and similar low-income neighborhoods in Ann Arbor.

The Behavioral Science Education Project (BSEP) and Quality of School Life (QSL) Program (1972–present): System-oriented school consultation has been a major interest of our prevention programming, focusing on improved social competencies among children, school personnel, and parents. Emerging from a 1970s "affective education program," a multilevel quality of school life (QSL) model for elementary schools has been developed based on industry's "quality circle" participatory decision-making process. Using a relevant curriculum, program staff assist teachers in developing problem-solving "quality circles" in their elementary school classrooms, facilitate the development of "staff involvement" steering committees for schools, and assist with the development of "family involvement" units within parent–teacher organizations. QSL's basic social competency approach has been incorporated into the state-sponsored Michigan Model for Comprehensive Health Education curriculum.

Community Support for the Homeless (1984–present): CE&P activities involving the homeless focus on community resource development, consultation, and community competency training strategies, all in collaboration with other agencies and encouraging eventual independence from WCCMHC support. In order to improve lay competencies within groups and agencies that serve the homeless, we have developed training designs and videotapes for "managing difficult situations" in community settings. Using these films, we have improved community acceptance of street-persons' social deviance by improving people's ability to deal with others' eccentric or angry behaviors.

The Organizational Development (OD) Program (1972–present): Our CE&P practitioners have been encouraged to intervene at the systems level, with consultation and staff training wherever appropriate, in assisting caregiving organizations to improve organizational skills, structures, practices, and programs where these affect the well-being of personnel, service delivery, or client well-being.

PROCESSES UNIQUE TO APPLIED COMMUNITY PSYCHOLOGY

The Field

"Applied" community psychologists share beliefs, values, concepts, and other collegial bonds with their academic colleagues. Like several others at WCCMHC, I serve as part-time academic faculty—leading a practicum, instructing seminars, and supervising interns. However, there is much about my day-to-day practice that keeps me in touch with a variety of other applied practitioners. Often, my colleagues will come from other disciplines; they are clinical psychologists, social workers, school counselors, teachers, nurses, OD practitioners, and paraprofessionals. I am active in a statewide organization of community mental health practitioners, a national and local organization of training and development professionals, a statewide mental health prevention advisory committee, a statewide network of mental health prevention coordinators, a regional organization development network, and various local collaborative and service groups. My applied community psychology colleagues are all active in networks equally as diverse.

Scope of Activity

A major difference between my work and that of my academic colleagues is found in the scope of our activities. Some of our work-related functions are similar, for example: grantwriting, committee work, budgeting, supervision, and adaptation to the home culture. Shaped by the CMHC context, however, both the style and substance of my endeavors are quite different from those having a university base.

For one thing, the politics of a public bureaucracy are different. Local elected officials determine policies and priorities, which can shift rapidly following any election, with yesterday's supports being undone far more rapidly than in university settings. Therefore, a more cautious choice of causes and strategies is required for actions supported by a county CMHC. We are more vulnerable to our community constituencies than are our academic colleagues, whose activities are buffered from the rough-and-tumble factiousness of community life by principles of academic freedom, governance structures, and more remote funding sources. University settings encourage uniqueness of contribution, territoriality, "star" visibility, critical commentary, scientific skepticism, and the establishment of clear boundaries between one's work and the efforts of one's colleagues. In my work as an applied practitioner, on the other hand, I am rewarded for opposite behaviors—for maintaining a modest profile, sharing endeavors and credits, transferring successful ventures to others, and having diplomatic forbearance when commenting on the work of others.

The major difference, however, lies in the range of activities that I must launch and maintain. Although formal needs analyses are prepared for long-range planning, most efforts occur through ongoing, spontaneous on-the-job analyses arising from regular interactions with the community's key informants, legitimizers, and culture carriers. And we are always engaged in some aspect of marketing: "segmenting" target populations, designing service "products," establishing client satisfaction and word-of-mouth support, maintaining a competitive "edge," and "selling" our programs both internally and externally. In today's volatile marketplace, I must function as a generalist, adding, changing, and deleting services fairly rapidly and needing a greater variety of skills and interests than does the academician, who is rewarded for long-term, in-depth attention to more specialized and focused areas of interest.

Longevity

In academic settings, the focus, length, and scope of community psychologists' careers are influenced by the individuals' ability to settle in and secure tenure in a psychology department and, when lucky, in a community psychology program. However, in applied settings, transiency is the rule. I seem to be one of only a few "applied" community psychologist to have acquired a comparable longevity, with 18 years in the same CMHC. Across the nation, most of my C&E colleagues have moved on to various settings and roles.

Fundraising

Reduced federal support has required CMHCs to greatly diversify their funding. For prevention-focused programming, that involves discovering ways to increase fees-for-service; thus, resources and programs are now founded on ability to pay as well as on need. Using a sliding-scale rationale similar to treatment programs, offerings to more affluent private-sector participants help support services to others who can pay only token amounts. And some needed programs are abandoned when the marketplace cannot support them. Competition to deliver fee-generating services (for example, employee assistance and health-promotion programs) creates pressure to stay ahead of the game in marketing, quality, networking, and new developments. However, pressure for consumer fees also has benefits, requiring us to maintain closer ties to the community, remain relevant, monitor quality, and form service coalitions that help reduce the negative effects of competition.

FOUNDATIONS IN THE LITERATURE

Because the CE&P practitioner must be a generalist, it is important to have a broad and eclectic understanding of the professional literature. A CMHC base requires an up-to-date understanding of the clinical literature, since case consultation is usually a staple of service delivery. The vast literature reflecting types, methods, and strategies of consultation has also been useful in all our CE&P endeavors. In addition, concepts and approaches related to community organization and ecological issues have served as a foundation for our many efforts in community resource development. An understanding of literature emphasizing organizational and other social systems issues is also necessary for our many organizational development activities.

In addition, specific projects require a knowledge of literature that relates to specific issues. For example, the growing literature on homelessness, quality of work life, effectiveness in public education, adult learning, social competency training, and stress management have all contributed to our CE&P programming.

SUMMARY

In sum, while the difficulties and challenges of my CMHC career may seem more obvious than the rewards, these have been enormous! I can imagine no better opportunity to apply the skills learned during my formal education, as well as to continually build my understanding and day-to-day competencies. Many of my colleagues have become my friends—including consultees, former competitors, interns, and other practitioners across the nation. For someone who values effective real-life applications of prized concepts; who enjoys the challenge of adapting what exists and creating what needs to exist; who has patience for the long haul but can also move quickly; who can handle both cooperation and competition; who has the temperament and skills of an entrepreneur; who has an eclectic approach to literature; who can manage to stay put in a community long enough to make a difference; who can function in various situations, settings, and networks; who can develop supports for survival; and who can balance the routines of bureaucracy with the spontaneity of marketplace, a career in CE&P can be exciting and rewarding. All others had better beware.

D. The Community Psychologist: A Professional and Pioneer

Carolyn Swift

"Pioneer"—the term that best describes the role of the community psychologist whose institutional base is in the community itself. The field of community psychology is an emerging one, only now experiencing a transition to a second generation of leaders. Its mission, methodology, and principles continue to be debated. To translate its mission into

Carolyn Swift • 1102 Hilltop Drive, Lawrence, Kansas 66044.

action is to work at the edge of an ecological frontier. And with that work comes all the excitement of the frontier—the adventure, the risk, and the boom and bust outcomes that reflect the convergence of ideology, technology, and setting.

It has been my very good fortune to have been a pioneer in a series of community settings. I will talk about two of those settings here, and then outline some principles I feel are critical in working out of a community base.

My first job placed me in the court system of a large midwestern city. The mayor had asked the local community mental health center (CMHC) for someone to create new approaches to juveniles caught in the court system, and to stop the revolving door of alcohol offenses. The CMHC administration, in an effort to be responsive to the community's needs, established a position to fulfill the mayor's request, and I was appointed to the post. Equipped with the general principles of community psychology, I staked my first claim in this territory by establishing an office at City Hall. Making a total commitment to that setting was central to the success of the programs that resulted. That meant working full-time on site: placing myself within the hierarchy of the setting, making it clear to whom I reported; learning the norms, values, and language of the setting; valuing the role of each person I met, from the janitor to the mayor; and finding ways to integrate my methods and goals with the ongoing political transactions that drove the setting's day-to-day operations.

Working with the resources in the setting, I was able to establish a number of programs. A diversion program for adolescent males placed youthful offenders in a residential facility and provided academic tutoring, vocational counseling, and individual, group, and family counseling. A weekly court class on alcoholism functioned both as an alternative to jail for alcohol offenders and as a social and educational intervention for offenders and their families. Consultation with the police command structure led to the creation of standardized methods for screening police candidates for behavior problems, and to innovations in police training, such as handling domestic disputes, rapes, and cases of child sexual assault.

The second setting was literally a new-age frontier—telecommunications. Two recurring prevention concerns motivated my shift in focus and setting. First is the problem of reaching target populations—90% of the people who need mental health services will never receive them. The second concern has to do with the optimum age for preventive intervention: the earlier in life we reach target populations, the greater the opportunity to shape significant outcomes. These considerations drew me in 1980 to Columbus, Ohio, where Warner Communications was embarking on the experimental testing of an interactive television system known as QUBE.

Interactive television has the potential to address both of my concerns. Television reaches mass audiences, while giving viewers the ability to "talk back" to their TV sets at home opens the door for active learning, instead of the passive learning characteristic of non-interactive systems. QUBE communicated with viewers through a hand-held remote control device. The viewer was asked to vote on issues or express opinions by touching a number on the device. Within a few seconds, audience response to such polls could be gathered and displayed on the TV screen. Thus, interactive television seemed to me to be a conduit through which a mass audience of children could be reached for preventive interventions. I formulated an experimental plan to promote the learning of prosocial behavior in young children by using interactive technology.

Since I had no experience in the media, I first sought and won the approval of a local CMHC to support the experimental prevention program. The center director, a prominent board member, and I then approached officials at Warner QUBE, and they agreed to cooperate in a plan to seek funding for the experiment. In the beginning, then, I functioned as a consultant to Warner QUBE from the institutional base of the Southwest Community Mental Health

Center, where I was director of prevention programs. Subsequently, I joined the corporate staff of Warner Communications full time as senior research associate and manager of interactive training and development. In this role, one of my primary functions was to develop ways to monitor and interpret audience response to interactive TV shows—literally, the frequency and pattern of viewer "touch in" to options or questions appearing on their TV sets. Here my background in experimental psychology was useful. Since QUBE was the first commercial interactive TV station to reach a large urban audience, there was little previous work on which to base a system of data collection and analysis of audience motivations to "touch in" responses to interactive shows.

Accomplishing this technical objective advanced both the setting's agenda and my own. Producers and directors of interactive shows needed to know how to maximize the viewing of, and response rates to, their shows. This was information I needed in order to design an appropriate television intervention for children.

During my tenure on the Warner staff, QUBE expanded to a national network offering interactive television shows to six major U.S. cities. But in 1984 the economics of cable operations forced major reductions in staff and programming. The telecommunications frontier closed in around QUBE, foreclosing the opportunity to test its effectiveness in reaching children with preventive interventions.

The point of these two case summaries is to identify common principles that shape the practice of community psychologists. As community psychologists, wherever we go we blaze resource trails. Such resources are major factors in systems change. If we have studied the needs of the ecosystem well, these resources will remain in place after we have gone. While resource "outposts" or "settlements" characteristically change with the setting over time, their creation is the marker event that documents our work, and their continuation is the evidence that legitimates it.

My own practice of community psychology has adhered to the principle of saturated-time in the setting. By this I mean an intervention schedule that incorporates high frequency (number of on site contacts), high intensity (length of contacts), and extended duration (time period over which contacts occur, e.g., weeks, months). The two cases cited exemplify a saturated-time commitment, since I worked full-time in each setting. This is a luxury that psychologists in academic settings cannot afford. While there are disadvantages in the saturated-time approach, they are outweighed by the advantages (summarized below). These points reflect a transactional relationship between the psychologist and the setting.

1. *Visibility*. A saturated-time approach establishes the psychology as a dependable, predictable presence; associates come to see you as a constant within the setting.

2. *Availability*. The psychologist is a resource to the setting. Availability refers to units of that resource (hours, days) available for the setting's use. In general, the greater the availability, the more quickly the desired action programs can be implemented.

3. *Accessibility*. The bidirectionality of this dimension is important. Saturated time in the setting contributes to public trust and promotes the community psychologist's increased access to both the formal and informal decision-makers and leaders in the setting. The reverse also occurs—by establishing a continuing visible presence you assure that key people will have access to you as the need arises.

4. *Immediacy*. Maximum presence in the setting plugs you into breaking events and increases your capacity for timely response. Being available for consultation in a crisis situation enhances your relevance and value to the setting.

5. *Flexibility*. The luxury of saturated time permits flexibility in role boundaries. You are able to explore interventions with problems, personnel, and procedures that would remain

outside the scope of your commitment with a more restrictive time schedule. For example, my constant presence in the law-enforcement setting led to the expansion of my role to encompass consultation with the detective unit and inclusion in police hostage-negotiation training and team-building. At Warner Communications I was frequently drafted to substitute for guests who failed to show up for TV appearances, which led to scheduled appearances on a variety of shows. These on-air exposures were invaluable in giving me firsthand experience in using interactive technology with a live audience.

6. *Convergence with values and norms.* Saturated time in the setting accelerates, at a systems level, processes analogous to clinical transference and countertransference. As the frequency, intensity, and duration of your intervention increase, your tendency to adopt the language, symbols, and values of the setting will increase as well. The reverse also occurs, as the persons you interact with most will begin to adopt your ideas, language, and values.

7. *Credibility.* Your continuous, constant presence in the setting communicates good faith in fulfilling your commitment to the work that has been contracted; it enhances your image as someone who can be counted on to deliver the promised services, whether consultation, research, and/or action programs. As a result, your credibility in the setting increases.

8. *Legitimacy.* One goal, as intervener, is to earn the official sanction of the setting for your role, and for the consultation program or research involved. This sanction can be awarded formally or informally. The saturated-time approach tends to accelerate the process of legitimation in the ways noted above. I remember being amused at the police chief's response to a citizen's query. In his letter to the citizen, the chief noted that the police department had on its staff a social worker who would look into the matter. The chief's confusion about mental health disciplines aside, the good news for me was that his letter placed the system's seal of approval on my work. He thought I was one of them. I was not. I continued to be paid by the mental health center. I thought wryly that he would discover my consultant status if he ever tried to fire me!

9. *Authority.* This dimension is contingent on having achieved credibility and legitimacy within the setting. Authority means that you are empowered under some circumstances to make decisions affecting the setting, and to speak for the setting in a manner consistent with a leadership role—whether or not such a role has been formally negotiated. Your "authority" is circumscribed by the substantive program or consultation area identified between you and the setting as your area of expertise. Conversely, persons within the setting may, under some circumstances, also make decisions affecting your program or research, and they may speak for you in matters related to your work. Clearly this is a sensitive area that embodies high risks for miscommunication and negative consequences. The important point is that a transaction in power has occurred in which you and the setting share authority in some part of your collaborative domains. Whether or not this is considered to be a desirable outcome, the status of authority is facilitated by saturated time in the setting.

10. *Training utility.* A final consideration is the reciprocal impact of the intervention for increasing skills and knowledge. The interventionist/consultant gains valuable information about the substantive issues involved in working with the setting, as well as the processes through which change or action occurs. This knowledge generally can be extrapolated to other settings and goals. Similarly, those in the setting have received on-the-job training in the skills of system change or research implementation. Both parties to the transaction have the opportunity to grow professionally as a result of the intervention.

Community psychologists whose institutional base is in the community itself are indeed pioneers. This exploration and settlement of community outposts and institutions, old and new, provide the thrills and disappointments, the false starts and rare discoveries, of expeditions into the uncharted territories mapped by more traditional pioneers.

E. A Community Psychologist in the Public Policy Arena

JUDITH C. MEYERS

There is a remarkable fit between the training, skills, interests, and commitment that are part of being a community psychologist and the work of developing and implementing social policy. Decisions about which issues are to be on the social agenda, the definition of those social problems, and the creation, implementation, and evaluation of programs in response to public needs are made by policymakers in executive and legislative offices at the state and federal levels. And while all citizens are of concern to policymakers, the most vulnerable, those at highest risk, command the most concern and attention. The results of action in the policy arena are communitywide in the largest sense, and represent primary prevention in its truest sense.

A community psychologist can bring to the policymaking process a scientific knowledge base, a commitment to social change, and an understanding of individual, organizational, and societal behavior that can make him or her a valuable resource in the office of any policymaker. If state and federal policymakers are not seeking community psychologists to serve on their staff, it is only because we, as community psychologists, have not educated them sufficiently, partly because we as a discipline have only begun to realize our relevance to the process (Task Force on Psychology and Public Policy, 1986).

ONE PERSON'S PATHWAY TO A POLICY POSITION

I was trained in community psychology, and during the first phase of my career worked in several different settings as a clinician, researcher, and teacher. Yet it has been in my more recent work in the policy arena that I have felt closest to the values and ideology of my roots in community psychology. Nowhere, neither in my job description nor in my everyday work in various policy positions from 1986 through 1989, have I been identified as a community psychologist. A doctorate in psychology was not a requirement for these jobs. Rarely does the fact that I am a psychologist come up, except as a point of humor in reference to the need for my clinical skills in dealing with the variety of colorful personalities that make up the political world. But, for me, my identification as a community psychologist and my early education in that field serves as the ground upon which my career is built.

When I went to graduate school in the early 1970s, public policy was not an identified area of study, let alone a career path. My interest in community mental health, however,

JUDITH C. MEYERS • Child Health and Development Institute of Connecticut, Inc., Farmington, Connecticut 06032.

stemmed from an interest in systems change. Primary prevention, program development, and social change were the terms used to describe that work. In my early career, working in a community mental health system, I functioned primarily as a clinician and program consultant. That work was targeted at the individual and family levels, and had little to do with effecting community-level change. In working with adults diagnosed as chronically mentally ill, I often felt frustrated and ineffective. Individual group, family, and occupational therapy and psychopharmacology may have helped relieve symptoms and helped people adjust to the chronicity of their condition, but did little to pave the way for their productive participation in the economic and social aspects of the community in which they resided. I noted that neighborhood efforts to prevent zoning for halfway houses, rejection of applications for social security disability or supplemental security income, and lack of job training and jobs were much more powerful in keeping people out of a community than any of the therapeutic approaches I and others were providing in attempting to keep them in the community.

It was a considered decision to depart from the traditional role and training of a psychologist in order to seek the preparation that I thought would be needed to deal at a broader level with these issues that I saw as much more determinant. Although I had concentrated in community mental health in my graduate training, little that I had learned in graduate school or postdoctoral training had given me the skills that I thought I needed. If I was going to affect mental health policy—the complex series of laws, regulations, eligibility requirements, and funding arrangements that exerted a major influence on the lives of those with mental illness—I felt I would have to know a great deal more about economics, political science, policy analysis, epidemiology, and public health. Through a two-year postdoctoral fellowship at Yale's Institute for Social and Policy Studies and an affiliation with the Bush Program in Child Development and Social Policy at Yale, followed by a one-year Congressional Science Fellowship sponsored by the American Psychological Association and the American Association for the Advancement of Science, I prepared myself for work in public policy.

THE NATURE OF THE WORK

My position as senior policy advisor on the staff of then Massachusetts Governor Michael S. Dukakis, in the Governor's Office of Human Resources from 1986 through 1989, exemplifies the type of work I had in mind when I set out to enter the public policy arena. The function of the office was to develop and coordinate the implementation of the governor's policy priorities in the area of human services, which included public health, mental health, public welfare, corrections, youth services, social services, employment and training, elder affairs, and housing. Our office consisted of six professional staff, including two lawyers, two people with graduate degrees in social policy, a communications specialist, and myself.

A description of some of the issues on which I worked, and the nature of that work, best illustrates why I believe the policy arena serves as a natural haven for an applied community psychologist.

The governor, in an effort to create access to economic opportunity (translated to mean a job that will provide a reasonable wage) for all citizens in a state that was at that time experiencing an economic boom with an unemployment rate that hovered around 3%, targeted his social policy agenda to those who had been left out of that boom. He identified the major barriers to secure and long-term employment as adult illiteracy, alcohol and drug abuse, teen pregnancy, and the school dropout problem. Our office had the major responsibility for developing and coordinating the policy responses to these issues.

I was largely responsible for the adult literacy initiative. This involved doing background research, which resulted in 7–10 page memos outlining such issues as the nature of the problem, programs currently in place, analysis of the dollars spent on literacy, and recommendations for future action. I was also involved in organizing conferences, workshops, and visits by the governor to literacy programs throughout the state, all for the purpose of educating leaders at the state and local levels about the problem and what could be done. In addition, I was involved in designing and implementing the state-level response to the literacy problem, including exploring the applications of technology to adult literacy; designing a statewide program to recruit thousands of volunteers to tutor adults; setting up and evaluating workplace education programs that were collaborations between labor unions, businesses, adult education programs, and state government; and creating a literacy policy group whose purpose was to develop policy that would lead to a coordinated and comprehensive statewide system of adult literacy services.

In the area of teen pregnancy and school dropouts, the state developed programs that funded local communities to create coalitions of young people, parents, service providers, advocates, local officials, and other local leadership to develop prevention and intervention programs for youth at risk. One very successful model was Commonwealth Futures, a dropout prevention program initiated in 1987. By convening broad-based, interagency community-based planning teams, the program helped localities devise and implement long-term educational and employment strategies. Primary prevention through early education and media campaigns, early intervention through accessible and coordinated services, support services such as daycare so parenting teens could continue their schooling, and better outreach were cornerstones of these programs. These were considered pilot programs that were to be evaluated. The more successful models were disseminated to other communities.

Examples of other issues in which our office was involved included:

- Solving the problem of increasing labor shortages in the health care and human services sectors, including a shortage of nurses in acute care settings, aides in the nursing home and home health industries, and workers in daycare, mental health, mental retardation, and other human services.
- Long-term health care for the elderly—developing coordinated financing and delivery systems to provide for the long-term health care needs of the elderly, planning a campaign to inform elders and others about the importance of preparing for these needs; developing a database to track long-term care services use.
- AIDS—How to prevent and treat AIDS, and how to provide protection to the public.

The content of the work varied from week to week, depending on the current crisis or the policy agenda of the governor or legislature. The nature of the work, however, was more consistent and called upon the skills that a community psychologist is likely to have. Communication skills were primary. Written communication was different from academe, however, as most of what was required was in the form of memos, briefings, and press releases, usually three to four pages in length, and rarely more than ten pages. When I wrote my first analysis of the literacy problem it was 12 pages long. I then had to write a five-page version, followed by a two-page summary of the issues, for few in the policy world have the time or inclination to read more than that. Written communication has to be sharp, to the point, and free of jargon.

On occasion I was described as the researcher in our office—but no academic would label what I did as research. Research in this applied setting meant pulling together information from secondary sources and discussions with experts in the field, and required being able to condense, interpret, and communicate this information in a meaningful form. Understanding program evaluation was also important, for we were often called upon to make recommendations about the continuation of funding for programs. Some of what I did also could be called teaching, but it did not occur in a classroom. Planning conferences and workshops, giving presentations to professional and community groups, preparing briefing meetings, and arranging visits for the governor to programs and meetings with staff and clients as a means for him to "learn" are all examples of the way in which I "taught." I used my clinical skills in my role as facilitator, mediator, or broker between various constituencies who were often at odds with each other.

My work was as close to being a community psychologist as I can imagine. The problems with which I dealt focused on the disadvantaged, disenfranchised, or underserved. We addressed community problems and the resources to meet those problems. The concepts of social change, primary prevention, the focus on large-systems issues, with the goal of enhancing the quality of life for individuals and families, all within a political framework and interdisciplinary in approach, were part of my day-to-day work.

Note: Since serving in the Massachusetts' Governor's Office, the author has worked in other policy arenas, first as administrator of the State of Iowa Child and Family Service System, as a senior associate at the Anne E. Casey Foundation, and as a senior consultant at the National Technical Assistance Center for Children's Mental Health at the Georgetown University Child Development Center.

F. The Community Psychologist as Citizen

BILL BERKOWITZ

A community psychologist can play many roles, and one of them is citizen. By this I mean acting in one's home community, unpaid and without professional portfolio, for the community's good.

There are several advantages in doing this. One of them is conceptual, for we are all citizens; the role is open to everyone. A second is logistical, for quality of life lies close to home, and your own community is unfailingly present whenever you step outside. A third is personal, for to invest civic energy where you pay your taxes, buy your groceries, and raise your children can make your life richer, fuller, spicier, happier.

Our tradition instead is to act as professionals, which *by its nature* distances oneself from one's subject matter, physically and psychologically. There is you, there is it, and "you" study "it." The empirical foundation of community psychology rests almost exclusively on such observations at a distance; they are important, and they are essential. But distance has its costs. Community psychology, by its unique nature, would seem to call for some kind of immersion in the community, some unabashed participation that blends observer and observed, in order to complement the reserve and detachment of formal scientific studies. Yet the most compelling arguments for the community psychologist as citizen are neither abstract nor personal, but

BILL BERKOWITZ • Department of Psychology, University of Massachusetts Lowell, Lowell, Massachusetts 01854.

rather pragmatic and moral. Pragmatic, because present levels of citizen involvement are disturbingly low. Moral, because to the extent that we have expert or even modest skills, our own communities need them. Proximity may be a proper moral determinant, and if it is, we may incur some moral obligation to use our abilities in our immediate surroundings.

Our country needs role models for local citizen involvement; those models should include us. Moral obligation aside, close and cohesive communities are what we are about, and they come about through intelligent and passionate citizen action. We are wise to develop and join strong community support networks, as such networks contribute to our well-being even in the best of times, while if times get tougher again, we'll be after every scrap of support we can find.

So participation by community psychologists as citizens in local community affairs perhaps ought to be emblematic in community psychology, inherent in our discipline, part of the way we spend our time. In any event, I believe we need more examples of community psychologists practicing their profession in plain citizenship roles. Few published accounts exist here, partly since there is no ready forum for them. I can venture a few from my own citizen experience, not because they have been noteworthy or successful, but more because I am familiar with them, because they have been personally meaningful, and because I think they might be instructive for a wider audience as well.

What follows, then, are four short vignettes and some tentative conclusions:

- Money was tight, and my daughter's school was targeted for closing. I got involved with a group of neighborhood parents trying to stop it. We spent one full year in endless neighborhood meetings, leafleting, phone calls, letter-writing, impassioned public speeches, and strategizing by our best and brightest. Our net effect was to sway one school committee member, so that the eventual vote to close the school was 6–3 instead of 7–2.
- My consciousness raised, I ran for a seat in our local town meeting. We have representative town meeting in our town—21 precincts, 12 seats each. A community psychologist should know how to run a political campaign, don't you think? On a local level, it is psychologically simple: target likely voters; make personal contact; repeat the contact; show your enthusiasm. To win a seat wasn't tremendously hard. It took plenty of work, but it was mostly a matter of execution.
- I proposed a Neighborhood Innovations Program, where the town would make minigrants ($1,000 maximum) to neighborhood groups wanting to strengthen neighborhood life. The Selectmen loved it at the time, and funded it for $5,000. I spent a year as volunteer coordinator, writing press releases, hand-addressing letters, holding interneighborhood forums, nurturing every single idea, and making more phone calls than I care to remember. It was a terrific program, except nobody applied. Well, actually there were seven applicants, but the review committee I had conscientiously established to keep things honest showed its honesty and dedication by turning four of the applications down.
- At the meeting I called to discuss an interneighborhood newsletter, only my own neighbor showed up. Okay, then, how about a newsletter for our neighborhood alone? But maybe our neighborhood was not together enough to support a newsletter (the school had closed; spirit was low). So how about a social event first? Fine—we'd work on that.

Each of us invited others to the next meeting, and they brought others to the next one. Our group was seat-of-the-pants, and semi-chaotic, as are most community groups. But one Saturday evening, on summer solstice, about 400 people, 20% of the population, showed up at our neighborhood park. We had food to share, guest books, balloons, prizes, kids' games, a clown, and two live bands. It was a magnificent event, exceeding our highest expectations. As

I write, after three annual picnics and two winter square dances, the newsletter staff is gearing up for the Fall issue.

The community psychologist as citizen naturally learns lessons, and here are some of mine:

1. On a citizen level, the field is wide open for good works. If you want to start something wonderful, few will stand in your way. Communities have enormous power vacuums, at all levels but the top; people are tired, and they don't know what to do. If you are awake and can stay focused, great things can happen.
2. Citizen work takes time—more time than many research projects. You have to make the time to give. But that kind of time is usually not job time, nor paid time, but rather junior-faculty-advancement time, or personal time. To make that time available may mean something else "slides."
3. The psychologist as citizen, like any other citizen, has to keep at it. Community is a fragile flower, needing constant tender care. The same fights have to be fought again. The same victories have to be won again. If eternal vigilance is the price of liberty, the price of community is eternal involvement. Otherwise, things may die.

An attentive reader may respect these activities, but wonder what they have to do with community psychology. How is one functioning as a community psychologist in these instances, and how does knowledge of community psychology advance the particular causes at hand?

My best answer is: it's hard to be sure. There's a close analogy to being a parent. As parents, we suspect we are using good psychology in raising our children, but exactly when and how? The principles are so woven into us through repeated training and use that in a given parenting situation it is difficult to be certain whether we are acting as a psychologist, or simply as a "person"—as if the two were separable. The same may apply to community skills.

Mastery of principles gives us an advantage. And it is true that the research base of social and community psychology fits nicely into citizen work (smile, make eye contact, get your foot in the door). But it is also true that this knowledge base is not community psychology's alone. Most of it, we must concede, is also common wisdom. The community psychologist, in my opinion, has up until now found few convincing principles of intervention that the intelligent lay person has not already grasped. This may be due to the youth of the field, or maybe such principles are just not in the cards. Community work may intrinsically and forever be demanding, slow, ceaseless, and resistant to magic.

What is more, the same intervention principles are not only used by nonprofessionals, but are often used more effectively. This is because nonprofessionals may be more local, more motivated (since local), more enthusiastic, better connected, and better able to relate on a personal level. If the professional has an edge, it may not lie so much in technique as in assumed credibility, a larger vision, and, possibly, available time. To the extent this is so, the community psychologist has cause for humility, which I regard as fully justified.

There is plenty of work, though, even for the humble. One needn't be Superman—Clark Kent will do. Citizen work has intrinsic value, and new principles may be found there after all. If so, one place to look for them is in the grassroots.

We'll agree that ordinary citizens will rarely collect hard data; it's tough enough to get a mailing out. But here is precisely where the community psychologist as citizen, or better, as citizen-professional, can help. The community psychologist, working with citizens, can provide data of immediate practical use to local groups, and can guide such citizens in further data collection and application that has local meaning. New general principles might also emerge in the process. Here is where unique contributions can be made.

More generally, the primary focus of community psychology has been on large institutions, and this ought to broaden. Institutions can be remote from daily life as lived; institutional research is more remote still. And institutional supports, while vital and powerful, are precarious as well. They often rely on public funding, yet if that funding is jeopardized, so will be the supports they create. What will remain are family, neighborhood, and home community. These won't go away.

In coming years, I believe citizens will be obliged to get better at leveraging institutional power, and especially at developing local supports themselves, by necessity if not by choice. Community psychologists, through their practice, ought to encourage them. They can do so as ordinary citizens, acting from moral obligation or from self-interested concern. They can do so as collaborative researchers, generating data their own communities can use. Or they can do so as teachers, helping other citizens to refine their community skills, boosting their confidence, and maintaining a vision of what an ideal community could be.

All three paths are valuable, and nonexclusive as well. The trick is for the community psychologist to earn a living and sustain personal energy while embarking on any of the three. That is a topic for another essay, but I am confident it can be done, and hopeful the reader may find clues and trail marks within the chapter and throughout the rest of this volume.

G. Community Development and the Community Psychologist

David M. Chavis

Community development offers community psychologists the opportunity to professionally implement their common values of empowerment, prevention, cultural relativism, ecological orientation, social change, and a distaste for victim-blaming. Community development is essential for primary prevention because, when applied in a comprehensive manner, human ecologies can be developed that foster human development (Chavis & Newbrough, 1986). Lack of control, lack of community, and poverty are more associated with psychological, physiological, and social disorder than any other factors known to the social sciences. Community developing methods have demonstrated their potential for reducing these environmentally induced factors.

For 25 years I have worked primarily in low-income urban communities in positions that fostered grass-roots community development. This has included jobs as a community organizer in Buffalo, New York, Nashville, Tennessee, and rural Appalachia. I have been the director of a community development corporation (a neighborhood-run organization that combines economic, housing, and social development programs), and director of a housing and neighborhood revitalization program. As the Director of Research for the Citizens Committee for New York City, I developed and tested methods for training and providing technical assistance to neighborhood associations and their leadership. I directed a university-based public service and research center where, among other things, we worked within New Jersey and across the country establishing state, county, and local systems that support grass-roots community development. I worked briefly for a private company conducting evaluations

David M. Chavis • Association for the Study and Development of Community, Gaithersburg, Maryland 20877.

of national programs for federal agencies and foundations. My current work in the Association for the Study and Development of Community brings together my earlier experiences in order to build the capacity of communities and their institutions to promote health, social justice, and economic equity.

I would like to focus on model roles for community psychologists in the community development process: policy/program development, and training and technical assistance provision.

POLICY AND PROGRAM PLANNING

Dokecki (1983) has called for the evaluation of the impacts of all public policies and programs on human development and community. All programs that we develop as community psychologists should be examined along this criteria. The definition of community development (Chavis & Newbrough, 1986) offers one set of criteria to make this determination. Does the program stimulate opportunities for membership for people to have influence over their community, for mutual needs to be met, and for shared emotional ties and support to be developed? As the director of two community development organizations, I have had the opportunity to implement programs to develop the vital subsystems of a neighborhood for the process of developing a community. In the following, I provide case examples.

Rewarding Collective Effort

Many benefits for social programs are given out based on individual merit, competition, and individual effort. This was the case for home improvement loans and crime prevention grants. After working with the local neighborhood association to turn control of these programs over to them, the neighborhood association changed the rules for receiving these grants in a way that rewarded collective effort. Grants were established on a matching fund basis—for every dollar received we matched it with a dollar. People on the block had to demonstrate that 20% of the residents were participating in their program. The money for these grants could be used for any project on the block. Examples of actual projects included group purchases of outdoor lights and deadbolt locks, a ramp for a handicapped neighbor, group purchase of shrubs, the planting of a community garden, and the entertainment at a block party. Applicants would be given technical assistance by the neighborhood associations in planning their projects and organizing a block association. If they qualified for a grant and organized an association, residents of their block would be eligible to receive a low-interest home improvement loan. People were motivated! Within six months, 20 of the 35 target blocks had organized and they stayed organized for at least two years. There was only one staff person handling all aspects of this program (except the home improvement loans).

Self-Help Housing

Amidst the block associations developed in the preceding scenario was an abandoned decaying school building that was a community problem—homeless persons trying to stay warm had started fires, rodents and insects infested it, and finally an electrical contractor was trying to purchase it for conversion into a warehouse.

We organized a coalition of the block associations, who, after marches through the city council chambers, rallies, and other tactics, got the city to turn the two and one-quarter acre property over to the neighborhood association to create a low-income housing cooperative out of this abandoned school. While the cooperative turned out to be financially infeasible and the building had to be razed, an owner-built housing program was developed with the assistance of Neighborhood Reinvestment (a national technical assistance organization). The idea behind this project was to have groups of 10 families work together to build each other's homes. Everyone works on each other's home until all homes are completed. Each family unit was required to put in 20 hours per week over the 11 and one-half months that it took to build the homes. Planning, monitoring, and dispute resolution were handled by the homeowners associations that we formed. Owner-builders did approximately 60–70% of the work. Both men and women, even grandmothers, worked on building these homes. They were trained and supervised by construction managers hired as part of the construction costs. The final result were homes that cost these low-income families less than half the appraised value.

Cooperative, mutual housing associations, and tenant-managed public housing programs will emerge again as major strategies to respond to the housing shortage in urban and rural areas. Community psychologists should not only be studying these "phenomena," but should also be developing the skills to facilitate these processes, as well as planning these types of programs as part of community development strategies.

ENABLING SYSTEMS FOR COMMUNITY DEVELOPMENT

Sustained community development and community competence cannot occur without training, education, and other supports provided through an "enabling system" (Chavis, Florin, & Felix, 1992). Adult-education methods can be used to develop leadership skills, train organizers, develop community problem-solving strategies, and organize development for community organizations or citizen-participation mechanisms. Adult education differs from other education strategies because the learning methods are mostly experiential, and it is focused on solving real problems, uses peer learning, and is democratic in decision-making (Knox, 1977). These methods enable communities to reach their goals and develop competence. The following are examples of training and technical assistance methods that as a community psychologist I have used for community development.

Organizational Development for Grassroots Organizations

We wanted to see if we could develop a relatively simple social technology for organizational development based on an open systems model of organizational viability (Prestby & Wandersman, 1985) using techniques developed in adult education and organizational development. The Block Booster Process, as we called it, is essentially an attempt to bring organizational development techniques to small-scale community development groups, in this case, block associations. We wanted a process that would be simple, yet systematic enough to potentially make a difference to these block associations and also enable us to refine and evaluate the process as an intervention. We focused on enhancing organizational viability and effectiveness of these associations. Research had shown that these valuable mechanisms for community development had a high rate of inactivity—50% or more become inactive 12 to 18 months following their inception (Giamartino & Wandersman, 1983; Yates, 1973).

The intervention was targeted at organizational *capacity-building*. Capacity-building involves increasing the competence and resources of the organization. The process was based on self-paced instruction (Fawcett & Fletcher, 1975) and survey-guided research (Nadler, 1977, 1979).

The Block Booster Process for capacity-building consisted of first collecting data in key areas relating to resource use, decision-making, social climate, benefits and costs to participation, expectation and perceptions of leadership. This information was then converted into bar graphs for each individual association. Workshops were conducted to teach participants (leaders of the block association) how to interpret the graphs, and how to use the workbooks and other written materials that were developed to assist the participants in maintaining their organization.

It was found as part of a quasi-experimental study of 27 block associations that the intervention we provided contributed to a reduction in the rate of inactivity among the test blocks by 50%. Their linkages with outside resources, the time given for introspection, and the written materials were all seen as contributing to the success of the intervention (Chavis & Florin, 1991). the "products" of this research and development process are currently being used by a technical assistance organization that annually provides training, consultation, grants, and other forms of assistance annually to 2,000 of New York's 10,000 block and neighborhood associations.

Community Organizing

Community development is the machinery for the bottom-up approach for social change. Community development can be a forum for personal growth and a mechanism for weaving the social fabric of a community, as well as part of the solution to local causes of poverty. The development of community organization is the actualization of democracy by creating communities that can manage and control the changes that they face. Through this process, people gain control of their community and their future. It is a small-wins strategy (Weick, 1986) that has led to broad social change. A major challenge I faced in my work has been increasing the accountability and responsiveness of larger institutions to community. This has required organizing top citywide leaders, health and human service providers, and grass-roots leaders, and then establishing ongoing linkages among them.

Learning Systems

New strategies are emerging in the field of community development. Community-development approaches that address the social, economic, physical, and political needs of a community are often called community-building initiatives (cf. Kingsley, McNeely, & Gibson, 1997). One strategy that can be used as part of a community-building initiatives is based on the work of Senge (1990) and his notion of a learning organization or community. My current work builds upon Senge's ideas and the previously mentioned community-development strategies in order to develop a learning system among the organizations participating in community-development initiatives. The learning system builds capacity by integrating evaluation and technical assistance so that information can be collected and disseminated in a timely, practical, and useable form. There has been an increasing use of evaluation in community development as a tool for program development and accountability. There is also a growing use of evaluation using organizational development, community organization, and adult-education methods to develop knowledge, skills, relations, and resources needed to improve the capacity of community institutions that will endure after the funding of these initiatives.

CONCLUSION

Community development can be an extremely powerful process, as it organizes the local community to gain control of their environment. While it can be exhilarating at times, it has its frustrations and challenges. Redefining your role as a "professional" or expert, and dealing with the perceptions of your community psychology colleagues have been two major challenges I have faced. As a professional, you must learn to diminish others' perception of you as being an expert or a "doctor." Your greatest successes will come when you get no credit for them.

Many fellow community psychologists have asked me why I didn't go into urban planning or social work. This is not a traditional role for a community psychologist, but it is one full of opportunity and potential. Rewards will come quicker from the communities you work with than from your academic or professional colleagues.

Organizing and participating in the political process is often considered "dirty," risky, and not a professional or scientific activity. I would not try to convince you otherwise. What I believe is that we all need to consider the consequences of our inaction—this supports the *status quo*. There is fear of, or disrespect for, conflict that keeps many people, particularly middle-class professionals, away from community organizing. Often I hear fellow community psychologists question organizing and the conflict that it can induce. To deny conflict as a necessary consequence of change is to ignore a historical perspective, and it denies the oppressed the opportunity for change. Not to participate in the conflict is to condone oppression, and to allow there to continue to be "blameless victims."

Can we say that we value prevention, social change, social justice, equality, and equity without taking action and its associated risks? I think not. We have speculated on how the environments that we live in and work in limit our ability to actualize our progressive values. Therefore the best training ground for us, community psychologists, to learn organizing is in our own communities and work places. After all, how can we hope to facilitate the empowerment of others, if we cannot empower ourselves?

H. Applied Community Psychology: On the Road to Social Change

THOMAS WOLFF

When I left graduate school, I was attracted to community psychology because I sensed that it would allow me to focus on two issues: social change and community. These two concepts not only sparked my initial interest, but have continued to motivate my work. My focus has been on the world of practice and application, not research and academia. Today, I am still an applied community psychologist above all else. The contribution I wish to make is grandiosely stated as "changing the world," and any contributions made to knowledge are a secondary gain.

THOMAS WOLFF • Community Development, Massachusetts Statewide Area Health Education Centers, University of Massachusetts Health Center, Amherst, Massachusetts 01002.

My application interests are in both community and clinical psychology; the contrasts are worth noting. As an applied clinical psychologist, I have a wide range of colleagues and institutions that understand and support my work, and that can balance the tensions between practice and science. However, in the world of applied community psychology, I have been out on my own. The formal community psychology institutions are largely dominated by academics who control the definition of the field, the journals, and the Society for Community Research and Action. In addition, practice settings that are tolerant of my interest in community psychology and social change are few and far between. My career has been marked by various career crises during which my social change values conflicted with an employer or institution. My experience as an applied community psychologist has largely been in "Never Never Land," without the support of the field of community psychology or the institutions in which I worked. Thus, I have taken my commitment to social change and community, and created meaningful work opportunities on my own. I believe this is the route that most successful applied community psychologists have been obliged to take—carving out jobs, incomes, and support systems in order to follow a belief in the value of applied community psychology.

As the result of 20 years of evolution as an applied community psychologist, I am now the director of Community Development for the Massachusetts Statewide Area Health Education Center (AHEC), part of the University of Massachusetts Medical Center. In my role I am involved in the development and support of health and human service coalitions and neighborhood organizations across Massachusetts. In addition, I have worked as a consultant to various cities and communities. This, too, has enabled me to continue working with communities on social change.

SETTING

Since 1984, Massachusetts AHEC's Health and Human Service Coalitions have developed in order to strengthen the capacity of communities to solve their own problems by mobilizing, coalescing, and leveraging resources. This social experiment, which evolved during the 1980s and has been carried into the first decade of the twenty-first century, is an example of a community intervention that attempts to create more empowered and competent communities by increasing interagency coordination and collaboration, and by enhancing community empowerment (Kaye & Wolff, 1997).

The creation of these coalitions could not have happened without a supportive institution such as the Massachusetts AHEC. AHEC programs are in place nationwide, and generally focus on continuing education for health professionals. It is not that AHECs generally are supportive of such efforts, but they, like many other institutions, have the potential to be supportive of social change. The focus on coalition-building and community development of the Massachusetts AHEC is unique. This focus was made possible because of the specific support of the statewide program director, who is himself committed to a social change agenda.

The general mission of these coalitions is to improve the quality of life in the community, and specific goals in local communities include:

1. development of a local planning body for issues affecting the quality of life,
2. more collaborative problem-solving regarding the major issues facing the community,
3. greater cooperation among all of those in the local helping network,
4. development of an advocacy capacity,

5. sharing of information with community providers and citizens on issues and resources, and
6. monitoring of the coalition's progress and effectiveness.

There are presently five such Health and Human Service coalitions across the Commonwealth of Massachusetts, in both rural and urban communities. With the help of funding from the W.K. Kellogg Foundation, this effort is now being expanded to ten new communities.

Membership in the coalitions is open to all individuals, and in actual practice includes health and human service workers, clergy, business people, the United Way, schools, municipal government, state legislators, and area residents.

GUIDING PRINCIPLES

The principles and literature that guide the AHEC coalitions come from the community organizing work of Alinsky (1971), the critical examination of health and human service systems of McKnight (1989), and the work in defining a sense of community and research on block associations of Chavis and his colleagues (Chavis & Newbrough, 1986; Chavis & Florin, 1990). Six critical principles that the AHEC coalitions have spelled out include:

1. starting where the community is located, with locally identified needs;
2. including anyone in the community who wants to participate and working hard to gather as broad a representation of the community as possible;
3. having the community define its own boundaries (as opposed to state or federally defined catchment areas);
4. taking an active stance that moves coalitions beyond planning and towards specific actions that can actually be accomplished;
5. a willingness to address issues through advocacy where necessary; and
6. working for the long haul, as social change requires time and persistence.

These principles are nothing new in the world of community development. However, their specific successful application in the 1990s, a particularly conservative era, is what makes the AHEC coalition work somewhat unique.

ACTIVITIES

The coalitions meet monthly for information sharing. Task forces formed around coalition-identified issues are short-term, problem-focused, product-oriented work groups composed of anyone from any sector in the community who is key to the identified issues. The coalitions allow communities to set collective priorities and create a unified voice. Coalitions also sponsor monthly newsletters, special publications, and in-service trainings. Advocacy on local or state human-needs issues is a critical role of the coalitions; advocacy actions include legislative breakfast, debates, and special issue campaigns.

My experience with the AHEC coalitions has been very encouraging, and communities have responded enthusiastically to these interventions. These coalitions have been successful in the introduction of specific new programs in their communities (child sexual-assault prevention curricula in schools, shared-housing programs, interpreter services programs, afterschool programs, homeless shelters, parenting programs, community-development corporations, volunteer clearinghouses, etc.) and in the promotion of more general process changes in the community system, including increased cooperation, collaboration, communication, and a sense of community. These efforts have endured and survived crises and attacks. At their best, the coalitions act as catalysts; they do not run programs or become new agencies, but rather spin off projects to existing community institutions.

Many of the coalitions' initial efforts have focused on health and human services, as seen in the Worcester Latino Coalition's development of a comprehensive interpreter services program to increase access to health care. However, the coalition's agendas generally move toward broader social change issues. This is evident in the development of the voter registration task force by the same Worcester Latino Coalition. This task force has significantly increased the number of registered Latino voters in Worcester, increasing Latinos' capacity to effect social change.

When coalitions see that they can actually create specific programmatic differences, they move from despair to hope. When coalitions realize that members of the legislature and city hall listen and respond to their issues, they move from a sense of powerlessness to one of empowerment. When coalitions solve local problems in a coordinated, collaborative manner, they see that their efforts have created a more competent helping system. We have begun a systematic replication process, including a comprehensive evaluation component (Francisco, Paine, & Fawcett, 1992). Using a technical assistance model, we are transferring our coalition technology to new communities.

THE PRIVATE PRACTICE OF COMMUNITY PSYCHOLOGY

For many years, I have also engaged in private contract work to deliver services that are clearly in the field of community psychology. These have included contracting with a local city to chair a task force on deinstitutionalization (Wolff, 1986); chairing the same city's task force on early intervention, which promoted collaboration between schools and social service agencies; consultating to a local area agency on aging to develop empowerment programs for elders (Gallant, Cohen, & Wolff, 1985) and supporting the development of community coalitions focused on elder issues; and working with communities who are pulling together coalitions on issues of teen pregnancy, AIDS, and child sexual abuse. In recent years, the Massachusetts Office of Substance Abuse Prevention issued a proposal to develop a community development approach to substance abuse prevention. The state's Department of Public Health invited me to help develop local coalitions in response to this proposal.

All of this work is relevant to the mainstream of community development and community psychology. These contracts came about naturally, the result of work in the same geographic area over a period of years where my basic values and interest in empowerment, community coalition building, and community development became well known. It is important to acknowledge the large amount of applied community psychology work that is performed through private contracts.

PROFESSIONAL AND PERSONAL IDENTITY

Being a community psychologist and a community developer, or, as I like to say, a "paid trouble-maker," is as fulfilling a job as I can imagine. In my community work, I meet interesting and exciting individuals from a wide variety of communities and backgrounds—clergy, city government officials, business people, human service workers, and citizens. To help communities mobilize citizens around issues, see new groups emerge as empowered voices, and develop specific programs is very satisfying. In most of this work there is a clear accountability between the community and the consultant that allows for very respectful responses and exchanges.

My work with the AHEC coalitions has also led to extensive involvement with legislators and various advocacy groups seeking social change within the state, including coalitions involved in campaigns for universal health care and for changes in the tax structure. Most recently, we developed a new, citizen-based advocacy system to increase the voice of citizens on issues of human needs, poverty, and healthy communities.

One rarely hears of community psychologists who admit to ongoing political activity but, indeed, in talking to my fellow community psychologists, I discovered that many are involved in political activities. On three occasions I have been a delegate to the Massachusetts state Democratic convention, and I have just completed a three-year term as an elected member of my local school committee. Many times I have heard of community psychologists working to change the system by influencing the elected officials, yet rarely do we consider ourselves to be those elected officials. As a school committee member, I certainly brought my viewpoint as a community psychologist to various issues, and to the processes of change within the committee. My years on the school committee left me in awe of the complexity of developing and maintaining excellent school systems, frustrated with having spent more time on budget cuts than program development, and humbled by the immense responsibilities that public officials carry. As a field we should be clear about the relationship of community psychology and politics.

Finally, my practice of psychotherapy is a bit of an anomaly among community psychologists, but is important to me as a fulfilling part of my professional life. It is a place where I am frequently reminded of the need for patience and time in order to see change. It is also important to mention that, for many years, my clinical practice was critical to my economic survival, in case my jobs or my contracts fell apart because of the political nature of my work. During this time, my practice was my income insurance.

The route I have taken in carving out a job for myself as an applied community psychologist who addresses issues of social change is not unique. However, the original vision of community psychology as a force for social change is severely curtailed by an environment where each practitioner must create his or her own job. It raises serious questions about the impact of community psychology on "changing the world." The impact of community psychology on the basic knowledge of the field is documented in many volumes of the *American Journal of Community Psychology* and the *Journal of Community Psychology*, but the exploits, adventures, successes, and failures of applied community psychologists have rarely been put on paper. When we do hear the stories, the programs, and the results, perhaps we will rethink the present directions of community psychology and remember its roots in social change.

REFERENCES

Alinsky, S. (1971). *Rules for radicals.* New York: Random House.

Berrueta-Clement, J. R., Schweinhart, L. J., Barnett, W. S., Epstein, A. S., & Weikart, D. P. (1984). *Changed lives: The effects of the Perry Preschool Program on youths through age 19.* Ypsilanti, MI: High Scope Press.

Bloom, B. L., Hodges, W. F., Kern, M. B., & McFaddin, S. C. (1985). A preventive intervention program for the newly separated. *American Journal of Orthopsychiatry, 55*, 9–26.

Broskowski, A., & Baker, F. (1974). professional, organization, and social barriers to primary prevention. *American Journal of Orthopsychiatry, 44*, 707–719.

Chavis, D. M., & Florin, P. R. (1990). *Community development, community participation.* San Jose, CA: Prevention Office, Bureau of Drug Abuse Services.

Chavis, D. M., & Florin, P. R. (1991) *An action research method for maintaining voluntary community organizations.* Unpublished manuscript. New Brunswick, N.J.: Center for Community Education, Rutgers University.

Chavis, D. M., Florin, P., & Felix, M. R. J. (1992). Nurturing grassroots initiatives for community development: The role of enabling systems. In T. Mizrahi and J. Morrison (Eds.), *Advances in community organizations and social administration, Vol. 1.* Binghamton, NY: Haworth.

Chavis, D. M., & Newbrough, J. R. (1986). The meaning of community in community psychology. *Journal of Community Psychology, 14*, 335–340.

Christophersen, E. R. (1982). Incorporating behavioral pediatrics into primary care. *Pediatric Clinic of North America, 29*, 261–296.

Dokecki, P. R. (1983). The place of values in the work of psychology and public policy. *Peabody Journal of Education, 60*, 108–125.

Fawcett, S., & Fletcher, R. K. (1975). *Writing instructional packages.* Lawrence: Institute of Public Affairs, University of Kansas.

Francisco, V., Paine, A., & Fawcett, S. (1992). *A methodology for monitoring and evaluating community coalitions.* Unpublished manuscript. Lawrence: University of Kansas.

Gallant, R., Cohen, C., & Wolff, T. (1985). Change of older person's image, impact on public policy result from Highland Valley Empowerment Plan. *Perspective on Aging, 14*, 9–13.

Giamartino, G., & Wandersman, A. (1983). Organizational climate correlates of viable block organization. *American Journal of Community Psychology, 11*, 529–541.

Kaye, G., & Wolff, T. (1997). *From the ground up: A workbook on coalition building and community development.* Amherst, MA: AHEC/Community Partners.

Kingsley, G. T., McNeely, J. B., & Gibson, J. O. (1997). *Community building: Coming of age.* Baltimore: Development Training Institute.

Knox, A. B. (1977). *Adult development and learning.* San Francisco: Jossey-Bass.

Levine, M., & Perkins, D. V. (1997). *Principles of community psychology: Perspectives and applications.* New York: Oxford University Press.

McKnight, J. (1989). Do no harm: Policy options that meet human needs. *Social Policy, 20*(1), 5–15.

Morgan, J. R. (1981). *Giving psychology away: A four year evaluation of training groups of parents in child management techniques.* Paper presented at the Annual Meeting of the Southeastern Psychological Association, Atlanta.

Morgan, J. R., Shoemaker, M. L., & Cullen, P. M. (1983, March). *Giving psychology away: A three year evaluation of a child-rearing advice program in pediatricians' offices.* Paper presented at the Annual meeting of Southeastern Psychological Association, Atlanta.

Nadler, D. (1977). *Feedback and organizational development: Using data-based methods.* Reading, MA: Addison-Wesley.

Nadler, D. (1979). Alternative data-feedback designs for organizational intervention. In W. Pferffer and J. Jones (Eds.), *1979 Handbook for group facilitators* (pp. 221–235). La Jolla, CA: University Associates.

Pedro-Carroll, J. L., & Cowen, E. L. (1985). The Children of Divorce Intervention Project: An investigation of the efficacy of a school-based prevention program. *Journal of Consulting and Clinical Psychology, 53*, 603–611.

Prestby, J., & Wandersman, A. (1985). An empirical exploration of a framework of organizational viability, maintaining, block association. *Journal of Applied Behavioral Science, 21*, 287–305.

Rappaport, J. (1981). In praise of paradox: A social policy of empowerment over prevention. *American Journal of Community Psychology, 9*, 1–25.

Sarason, S. B. (1974). *The psychological sense of community: Prospects for a community psychology.* San Francisco: Jossey-Bass.

Senge, P. M. (1990). *The fifth discipline: The art and practice of learning organizations.* New York: Doubleday.

Snow, D. L ., & Newton, P. M. (1976). Task, social structure, and social process in the community mental health center movement. *American Psychologist, 31*, 582–594.

Snow, D. L., & Swift, C. F. (1985). Consultation and education in community mental health: A historical analysis. *Journal of Primary Prevention, 6*, 3–30.

Stolberg, A. L., & Garrison, K. M. (1985). Evaluating a primary prevention program for children of divorce. *American Journal of Community Psychology, 13*, 111–124.

Swift, M. S., & Healey, K. N. (1986). Translating research into practice. In M. Kessler & S. E. Goldston (Eds.), *A decade of progress in primary prevention* (pp. 205–234). Hanover, NH: University Press of New England.

Task Force on Psychology and Public Policy. (1986). Psychology and public policy. *American Psychologist, 41*, 914–921.

Weick, K. (1986). Small wins: Redefining the scale of social issues. In E. Seidman and J. Rappaport (Eds.), *Redefining social problems* (pp. 29–48). New York: Plenum.

Weissberg, R. P., Gesten, E. L., Liebenstein, N. L., Schmid, K. D., & Hutton, H. (1981). *The Rochester Social Problem Solving (SPS) Program: A training manual for teachers of 2nd–4th grade children.* Rochester, NY: The Center for Community Study.

Wolff, T. (1987). Community psychology and empowerment: An activist's insights. *American Journal of Community Psychology, 15*, 149–166.

Wolff, T. (1986). The community and deinstitutionalization: A model for working with municipalities. *Journal of Community Psychology, 14*, 223–228.

Wolff, T. (1992). *Coalition building: One path to empowered communities*. Unpublished manuscript. Amherst: University of Massachusetts Medical Center.

Yates, D. (1973). *Neighborhood democracy*. Lexington, MA: Heath.

CHAPTER 32

Community Psychology in International Perspective

SABINE WINGENFELD AND J. R. NEWBROUGH

In the United States, community psychology is in its fourth decade of existence as a subdiscipline of psychology. It was created at a conference sponsored by the National Institute of Mental Health concerned with training clinical psychologists to work in community mental health programs (Bennett, Anderson, Cooper, Hassel, Klein, & Rosenbaum, 1966). Since 1965, community psychology has found its way into a variety of countries. In some countries, community-oriented theory, research, and practice have been explicitly labeled as community psychology, reflecting an attempt to connect the concepts from the U.S. sources with local discussions and action programs. In other countries, social needs and developments have given rise to a community perspective without specific reference to, or influence from, community psychology in the U.S.

The purpose of this chapter is to describe the development, conceptualization, and the status of the training, research, and practice of community psychology in other countries. Based on submissions to the *Journal of Community Psychology* from 1974 to 1988, we were aware of community research and action in Australia, Canada, Colombia, Cuba, Hong Kong,

---

This chapter was prepared in collaboration with the following persons: Edward M. Bennett, Wilfrid Laurier University, Waterloo, Ontario N2L 3C5, Canada; Guillermo Bernal, Department of Psychology, University of Puerto Rico, Rio Piedras, Puerto Rico 00931; Donata Francescato, University of Rome, 00153 Rome, Italy; José Gómez del Campo, Escuela de Psicologia, Universidad Iberoamericana, 01210 Mexico City, D. F. Mexico; Steven Hobfoll, Applied Psychology Center, Kent State University, Kent, Ohio 44242; Sandy Lazarus, Department of Educational Psychology, University of the Western Cape, Cape Town, South Africa; Heiner Keupp, Institute fur Psychologie, Ludwigs-Maximilans-Universitat, Munich, Germany; E. R. Martini, Associazione por lo Studio e la Sviluppi della Comunita, 55.100 Lucca, Italy; Maritza Montero, Universidad Central, Caracas 1041-A, Venezuela; John M. Raeburn, Department of Psychiatry and Behavioral Science, University of Auckland, Auckland, New Zealand; Irma Serrano-Garcia, Department of Psychology, University of Puerto Rico, Rio Piedras, Puerto Rico 00931; Wolfgang Stark, Selbsthilfezentrum, Munich, Germany; David R. Thomas, Department of Community Health, University of Auckland, Private Bag 92019, Auckland, New Zealand; Arthur Veno, Social Sciences Department, Monash University, Gippsland, Churchill 3842, Victoria, Australia; Edwin S. Zolik, 5753 Seven Oaks Drive, Sarasota, Florida 34241.

SABINE WINGENFELD • School of Psychological Sciences, La Trobe University, Bundoora, VIC 3083, Australia.
J. R. NEWBROUGH • Department of Psychology, Peabody College of Vanderbilt University, Nashville, Tennessee 37203.

Handbook of Community Psychology, edited by Julian Rappaport and Edward Seidman. Kluwer Academic / Plenum Publishers, New York, 2000.

Israel, Mexico, New Zealand, Nigeria, Puerto Rico, South Africa, and Spain. We knew of community activities in Latin America (Argentina, Chile, Costa Rica, El Salvador, Panama, Santo Domingo, Venezuela) and in Europe (England, Italy, The Netherlands, and Germany). We decided to describe countries where there was significant discussion of community psychology and/or a considerable amount of community-oriented work. When we began writing this chapter in 1986, we also wanted to provide information on Marxian socialist-oriented countries. (The scope of community psychology as a formal matter in those countries was limited compared with the extent of social change and the tremendous sense of community that led to the demise of the Eastern European Communist regimes.) We selected eleven countries: Australia, Canada, Cuba, Germany, Israel, Italy, Mexico, New Zealand, Poland, Puerto Rico, and Venezuela. We included South Africa because community psychology was beginning to develop in what was then a very divided and troubled country. We were not able at that time to determine the status of community psychology elsewhere, but coverage has subsequently appeared on community psychology in a variety of other countries (Balcazar, 1992; Fisher & Bishop, 1995; Levine, 1989; Orford, 1995; Skutle, 1995; Toro, 1990; Wiesenfeld, 1998; Wilpert, 1991).

Three different cultural traditions that bind the countries together have served for grouping them in this chapter. Canada, Australia, and New Zealand are primarily English-speaking ex-colonies of Britain, and closest culturally to the United States. Italy, Germany, Poland, and Israel share a strong European cultural heritage. Puerto Rico, Venezuela, Mexico, and Cuba are Latin American ex-colonies of Spain, with the direct heritage of the conquest. South Africa is a special case of a bicultural country in the midst of change.

This chapter is divided into five sections: (1) development of community psychology, (2) current status, (3) conceptual bases and orientation, (4) future prospects, and (5) conclusions. It is based on original pieces first prepared by the collaborating authors in 1986, and has been updated several times through 1992. We adapted material from these papers to present information in a common format. Additional recent references were included in a final brief update just prior to submission to this handbook. For future prospects, we used the collaborating authors' own words.

THE DEVELOPMENT OF COMMUNITY PSYCHOLOGY

The development of community psychology in most of the countries discussed here was stimulated by internal social needs, developments, and conceptualizations and influences from the U.S. In most of these countries, community psychology began in the 1970s (see Table 1).

In Australia, New Zealand, Germany, Italy, Israel, and South Africa, the need for a community psychology perspective and community-based approaches developed out of dissatisfaction with traditional mental health service delivery. Community psychology in the United States strongly influenced Australia and New Zealand, and provided both an initial impetus and inspiration for theory and research. In Australia, discussion of the need for changing the roles of psychologists in community mental health settings began during the 1970s (Kirkby, 1978; Smith, 1977; Viney, 1974). In New Zealand, the New Zealand Mental Health Foundation provided the first major initiative and funding for community-based research. Italy embarked on a radical reform of its psychiatric system on its own account (Crawford, 1981; Francescato & Tulli, 1982; McNett, 1981). Its focus on wide-scale deinstitutionalization, prevention, and promotion of physical and mental well-being created the need

TABLE 1. Development of Community Psychology

Country	Beginnings	Impetus and issues
Canada	Community perspective since the 1920s; academic community psychology since the 1970s	U.S. community psychology; need for mental health services; mental health personnel shortages; shift to a health orientation
Australia	1970s	Disenchantment with clinical psychology; community mental health movement and community psychology in the United States
New Zealand	mid-1970s	Disenchantment with clinical psychology; social psychologists at University of Waikato introduced community psychology; clinical psychologists at medical schools; funding from New Zealand Mental Health Foundation
Italy	1970s	Psychiatry reform leads to radical changes in mental health laws and need to train psychologists for tasks required by new laws; Francescato's (1978) book on U.S. community psychology
Germany	Late 1970s	Social (women's, student, ecology) movements; criticism of clinical psychology; need for new professional roles and reform of mental health service delivery; developments in U.S., Italy, the Netherlands
Poland	1970s	British social psychiatry; unmet community mental health needs and mental health personnel shortages
Israel	1949 1970	Strong community orientation Gerald Caplan's community-oriented programs
Puerto Rico	1975	U.S. community psychology; Latin American social psychology; Puerto Rican mental health needs and search for alternatives to clinical model
Venezuela	Mid- to late-1970s	Academic turmoil; criticism of traditional clinical psychology; social psychologists look for new models; U.S. community psychology
Mexico	Late 1960s–early 1970s	U.S. trained psychologists establish three centers at universities
Cuba	1959	Need to address social needs (illiteracy, infant mortality) leads to medicine in the community model and to formation of National Group of Health Psychology in 1966
South Africa	Early to mid-1980s	Dissertation by Sandy Lazarus; U.S. community psychology; crisis in South Africa and resultant identity crisis within psychology

for psychologists trained in community-oriented activities. The Italian approach influenced other European countries, most notably Germany.

In Canada, a community orientation and strong emphasis on prevention initiated by Canadian pioneers was abandoned during the 1950s. The reemergence of community psychology in the 1970s was associated with influences of community psychology in the U.S., a shift in government policy from illness to health, and demands for mental health services (Ferris & Squire, 1992; Lalonde, 1974; Tefft, 1982).

Poland and Cuba are the two countries where influences from U.S. community psychology have been minimal. Although socialist theory and dialectical materialism have influenced psychology in Poland and Cuba, community-oriented approaches have developed in different directions in the two countries. In former Communist Poland, where Marxist psychologists were concerned with developing "politically correct" psychological theories, the context is community mental health, based primarily on British social psychiatry. Polish social psychiatry provided the first community-oriented services during the 1970s. In Cuba, Marxist theory provided the framework for the "medicine in the community" model (Bernal & Marin, 1985; Garcia-Averasturi, 1985; Serrano-Garcia, 1987), a revolutionary, integrated health care approach. Psychological services are an integral component within a continuum of preventive, curative, and rehabilitative services (Perez-Stable, 1985).

Community psychology in Latin America initially developed mainly in the countries around the Caribbean: Colombia, Cuba, Dominican Republic, Mexico, Puerto Rico, and Venezuela (Serrano-Garcia & Alvarez, 1985), as well as Brazil (cf. Lane & Sawaia, 1991). Some work has been done in Argentina, Chile (cf. Krause Jacob, 1991), Costa Rica, El Salvador, Panama, and Peru (see also Montero, 1996).

In Puerto Rico, community psychology began formally in 1975 with the development of a master's program in social community psychology at the University of Puerto Rico (Serrano-Garcia, Lopez, & Rivera-Medina, 1987). In Venezuela, a group of social psychologists at the Universidad Central in Caracas initiated a community orientation in the mid-1970s (Montero, 1987), a few years after the government and church-linked groups had begun to undertake community work. Academic community psychologists became actively involved in consultation to these projects. In Mexico, notions of community mental health were first introduced in 1966 by Juan LaFarga at Universidad Iberoamericana. During the 1970s, three different groups of community psychologists were formed at Mexican universities.

Three major sources influenced the development of a community orientation in Latin America in the 1970s. (1) In social psychology, analysis of the ideological bases of scientific practice (Ardila, 1982) led to criticism of the area as not being committed to social issues (Campos, Brenes, & Quevedo, 1980; Marin, 1978; Montero, 1982, 1984; Varela, 1971). (2) The Interamerican Society for Psychology provided the vehicle for interchange between U.S. and Latin American psychologists about work in the community. (3) Social improvement programs initiated by governments in Latin American countries required consultation and guidance from universities (see also Montero, 1996; Rivera-Medina & Serrano-Garcia, 1991; Wiesenfeld & Sanchez, 1995).

Common threads in the development of community psychology in other countries include dissatisfaction with traditional clinical psychology, the need for social improvement, and participation and leadership by university students and faculty in the development of theoretical models and practical approaches.

CURRENT STATUS

The importance of any one field of psychology may be judged by its degree of formalization. This section addresses whether community psychology has achieved the status of a subdiscipline of psychology, with its own organizational body, or whether it is simply a perspective underlying community-oriented research and practice. Indices of formalization include: (1) professional associations with newsletters, journals, and conferences; (2) university curricula; (3) research and scholarship; and (4) implementation of community principles in professional practice.

Professional Linkages

Since the early 1980s, Australia, Canada, Italy, and New Zealand have established community psychology divisions in their respective psychological associations. In Canada, a community psychology section was founded in 1981. Since 1982, the interdisciplinary *Canadian Journal of Community Mental Health* has been publishing articles relevant to the field. A French language periodical, *Santé Mentale au Québec*, has helped to disseminate community psychology information in Québec since 1976. Further evidence for the increasing importance of community psychology is the publication of three text books (Bennett, 1987; Bennett & Tefft, 1985; Guay, 1987). In Australia, the National Board of Community Psychologists was founded in 1981 and publishes the newsletter *Network*. Moreover, community psychologist are represented through their membership in the College of Community Psychologists of the Australian Psychological Society (Fisher & Bishop, 1994). In New Zealand, community psychologists are affiliated with both the Community Psychology Division founded in 1983 and the New Zealand Mental Health Foundation. The journal *Community Mental Health in New Zealand* is a primary source of communication.

In Italy, the first convention on psychology in the community was held in 1979 (Contessa & Sberna, 1981). The Italian community psychology division, founded in 1980, has grown to about 200 members, primarily community psychologists, and has been holding regular meetings. Community psychology is both a defined discipline with an academic base and a perspective shared by a significant minority of psychologists working in the public sector (Palmonari, 1981). In Germany, there has been a continuing debate on the identity of community psychology (Kleiber, 1988). Leaders at universities conceptualize it as a perspective underlying research and practice, and have therefore not pursued an organizational body of its own. The German Association on Behavior Therapy, however, has been providing a forum for community issues in its biennial conferences (e.g. Fliegl & Röhrle, 1983), its journal, *Verhaltenstherapie und Psychosoziale Praxis*, and publications of a series of books on related topics (*Tübinger Reihe*). Moreover, the European Network of Community Psychology (ENCP) has recently been formed to promote community psychology in all European countries. The ENCP has held regular business meetings since 1996, is in active communication via the internet, and has plans for a website. In Israel, community psychology is simply a perspective. It was probably never formalized because no movement emerged to "champion the cause." Similarly, community perspectives can be found in both research and various applied fields in Poland, but there is no organizational framework.

In the Latin American countries, community psychology is both a perspective and a set of activities oriented to community improvement. Puerto Rico's community psychology appears to be the most formalized, both in terms of its conceptual development and academic curricula. However, it has not grown in a stable pattern organizationally: Division 27 of the American Psychological Association initiated a Latin American Region with Leadership from Puerto Rico. This group was active for only two years (1982–1984). In Venezuela, social community psychologists had difficulties in establishing themselves in the academic world (Ocando & Montero, 1981). Their efforts have now led to increasing recognition (Sanchez, Wiesenfeld, & Cronick, 1991) of community psychology as part of the applied psychology curriculum and to the publication of relevant articles in *Boletin de AVEPSO* (Montero, 1987, 1995). In Mexico, there appears to have been little networking between community psychologists at different universities and between universities and community projects (Reid & Aguilar, 1991). Cuba is different from the other Latin American countries in two ways. First, its model is conceptualized as community health psychology rather than social–community psychology. Second, it is formalized on both the academic and professional levels with professional associations and journals.

At present, community psychology in South Africa is a perspective that is pursued within the established fields of psychology. Controversy on how much formalization is desired reflects psychologists' search for appropriate roles in changing the South African political context (Lazarus & Prinsloo, 1995).

In summary, organizational structures similar to Division 27 of the American Psychological Association in the U.S. have existed in several countries since the early 1980s. For Latin America, the Community Psychology Task Force of the Interamerican Society of Psychology, founded in Peru in 1979, was reactivated in 1990. Since then, the task force has recruited over 200 members from 18 countries. In seven countries membership is so numerous and/or active that regional representatives have been selected. They have organized regional activities, including workshops, monthly meetings, and research on the status of community psychology in their countries, and aided in the formation of a Community Psychology Association in Colombia. The task force publishes a bi-annual bulletin and an annually updated membership directory (Serrano-Garcia, Cantera, & Míron, 1995).

In other countries, where community psychology is conceptualized as a perspective influencing research and practice, professional linkages have been pursued less actively or not at all, and psychologists differ in the extent to which they identify with the label "community psychology." Irrespective of the degree of formalization in their countries, community psychologists continue to build international linkages. The European Network of Community Psychology and the 1998 Second European Congress on Community Psychology in Lisbon, Portugal, represent increased networking in Europe. Several countries are represented in the Division 27 international regions. The International Network on Community Research and Action, initiated at the First Biennial Conference on Community Research and Action in 1986, includes members from Austria, Brazil, Canada, Chile, Denmark, England, Germany, Hungary, India, Italy, Japan, Mexico, The Netherlands, New Zealand, Portugal, Puerto Rico, Scotland, Senegal, Spain, Taiwan, Venezuela, and the U.S. At the Fourth Biennial Conference on the Society for Community Research and Action in 1993, 26 posters were presented from 13 countries, and the international interest group was expanded to an international network.

Training

Countries differ with respect to the extent and scope of formal training available. In many countries, training is offered through programs of clinical, social, or educational psychology. Table 2 describes the status of training in community psychology. In most countries, some form of training in community psychology was established during the 1970s. Training in Canada seems to be the most formalized and independent of other fields of psychology, with about 50% of the universities offering graduate education in community psychology (Nelson & Tefft, 1982). In Australia, a survey by Farhall and Love (1986) indicated that 25% of academic institutions offered community psychology as an independent field, 50% of academic programs taught it as a subspecialty, and about 40% of courses were offered at the graduate level (Farhall & Love, 1986). Fisher (1992) indicated that there are continuing problems in establishing a firm academic base. In New Zealand, the University of Waikato offers community psychology as a separate field at both the undergraduate and graduate levels, with a social science emphasis (Hamerton, Nikora, Robertson, & Thomas, 1995). Two other

TABLE 2. Training in Community Psychology

Country	Program and affiliation	Substantive emphasis
Canada	Separate field in 50% of graduate programs	Prevention, promotion of competence, consultation, program evaluation, field work, field research
Australia	25% of programs—separate field 50% of programs—subspecialty	Program evaluation, politics of systems level intervention, prevention, indigenous people, psychological sense of community
New Zealand	(a) Elective in masters program at University of Waikato; advanced degrees offered	Ecological perspectives, empowerment, cultural pluralism
	(b) Component of masters in health sciences at Auckland Medical School	Prevention, quality of life, intervention within systems
	(c) Courses in clinical-community program at University of Wellington	Grassroots community development; health promotion within health sciences
Italy	Clinical-community track available in all master's-level programs	Professional roles, prevention, self-help approaches
Germany	Courses offered at some universities in clinical and social psychology, social work	Professional roles of psychologists; self-help approaches
Poland	No training offered as such; prevention, support systems, some courses address community areas	Development of prosocial behavior
Israel	One child-clinical program with community orientation at Tel Aviv University	Family–school–community focus; community intervention with focus on ethnic and economic problems
Puerto Rico	Master's (since 1975) and Ph.D. programs (since 1986) in social-community psychology	Participatory research, intervention within research, evaluation research, social change, needs assessment, consultation
Venezuela	Courses within social psychology at Universidad Central; part of group dynamics curricula at other universities	Action research; field research
Mexico	Separate specialty at Iberoamericana Universidad; community psychology curriculum at ITESO; part of clinical psychology at other universities	Community intervention; psicocomunidad (Emmite, 1980); social ecology; action research
Cuba	Part of general training in psychology	Health psychology; roles of psychologists in health system
South Africa	A few courses within clinical, counseling, educational psychology since early 1980s	Action research approaches

universities offer community courses as part of the clinical psychology and health science curricula.

In several countries, community psychology is included in the curricula of other subdisciplines of psychology, primarily clinical psychology. In Germany, the curricula of some universities reflect increasing attention to topics related to community psychology, especially the role of self-help and support groups (Kleiber, 1985), but tend to be linked to clinical or social psychology, or to social work (Keupp & Stark, 1992). In Poland and Israel, there are no formalized programs, and training is embedded within other subspecialties, such as social psychiatry (Poland) and child clinical and educational psychology (Israel). In South Africa, community psychology has been taught in undergraduate and graduate courses within different subspecialties since the early 1980s. Critical issues in postapartheid South Africa are now integrated in the course curricula (White & Potgieter, 1996).

In Puerto Rico and Venezuela, community psychology is affiliated with social psychology. The social–community psychology program at the University of Puerto Rico offers both master's- (Rivera-Medina, Cintron, & Bauermeister, 1978) and doctoral-level training. Community and social psychology have been integrated into a coherent conceptual framework that is functionally and ideologically independent of other specialties. In Venezuela, action-research models have been used in undergraduate and master's theses (Montero, 1987). Inclusion of community psychology courses in the social psychology curriculum, the group dynamic curriculum, and programs of private and government agencies has been more recently achieved. Evaluation of the extent of training in Mexico indicates that community psychology training is typically part of clinical psychology, exceptions being the community psychology program at Universidad Iberoamericana and the community-social psychology program at Universidad Autonoma Metropolitana. Reid and Aguilar (1991) expressed concerns that curricula have provided little training of students for social action, and have focused too much on conceptual and methodological issues. In Cuba, community psychology has been part of the general psychology curricula, with a focus on health psychology.

Overall, community psychology training in other countries appears to be integrated in clinical or social psychology courses, rather than based on independent curricula. This is also reflected in the training models. Canada, Australia, New Zealand, Puerto Rico, Venezuela, and Mexico follow the scientist–practitioner model of the U.S. In Canada and New Zealand, there is a focus on prevention, promotion of psychosocial competence, and intervention within systems. Program evaluation is also an important training emphasis. Participatory action research and community intervention practice are prominent in Latin America (except Cuba) and South Africa. Training in Cuba primarily prepares psychologists for their roles within the community health system and, contrary to training in other Latin American countries, lacks an emphasis on social change. In Germany and South Africa, there is an emphasis on obtaining a critical perspective on the roles of psychologists and on the potential for self-help, rather than skill training.

Research and Scholarship

Although a strong action research orientation is found in most countries, particularly in Latin America, there are differences in focus and extent of these projects. Table 3 lists projects with an explicit community emphasis.

In Canada, community research has been conducted from the framework of community mental health. Community mental health has been defined broadly, so as to encompass virtually all aspects of the relationship between social structure and social-psychological well-being. The *Canadian Journal of Community Mental Health* has helped to increase the emphasis on community and prevention in mental health delivery and prevention of environmental and institutional hazards.

In Australia, community research was initially fragmented and not integrated into sustained efforts. In 1988, the Australian Psychological Society instituted the Robin Winkler Award for Applied Community Psychology Research, hoping to significantly expand community psychology research. Recent research has focused on rural and remote Australian communities (Bishop & D'Rozario, 1990; Bishop & Drew, 1998; Bishop & Syme, 1993; Coakes & Bishop, 1996; Gething, 1997; Harvey & Hodgson, 1995), environmental resource management (Bishop & D'Rozario, 1990; Bishop & Syme, 1993), psychological sense of community (Pretty, Conroy, Dugay, Fowler, & Williams, 1996; Sonn & Fisher, 1996, 1998), and issues pertaining to the socially marginal (Fisher, Karnilowicz, & Ngo, 1994; Sonn & Fisher, 1996, 1998).

In New Zealand, community research has included a wide range of topics; there has been a growing research literature (Thomas, 1979, 1982, 1983; Thomas & Thomas, 1985; Robertson, 1985; Robertson, Thomas, Dehar, & Blaxall, 1989; Thomas, Neill, & Robertson, 1997; Thomas & Veno, 1992). At the Auckland Medical School research has a strong health orientations and has involved a variety of grassroots community development and health-promotion projects (Raeburn, 1986, 1987, 1992).

Community research in Italy has focused on several areas: professional roles, prevention, psychiatric services, aging, promotion of healthy development in children, work settings, and volunteer and self-help organizations (see Table 3).

In Germany, a small group of academics who regard themselves explicitly as community psychologists have published work on community psychology (Belschner, Gottwald, & Kaiser, 1981; Keupp, 1978, 1980, 1986; Sommer & Ernst, 1977; Sommer, Kommer, Kommer, Malchow, & Quack, 1978). Research has addressed social networks and social support, prevention, stress and environmental resources, problems in the traditional psychosocial service system, and the development of new forms of intervention.

In Poland, research efforts prior to the overthrow of the socialist government were restricted by conceptual problems with dialectic materialism. Social psychology knowledge has been applied to community problems in a variety of ways (Necki & Tokarz, 1980), and there is a considerable body of applied research in educational and developmental psychology with a community focus.

In Israel, research in community psychology occurs under a variety of other names, including stress research, work on social support, Arab–Jewish relations, and school performance among financially disadvantaged children. The major focus of community research appears to be research on stress, due to the constant strain caused by the threat of war and the slow progress of the peace process (see Table 3).

In Puerto Rico, community psychology and the social psychology have generated two research directions. The community direction is based on an intervention-within-research model (Irizarry & Serrano-Garcia, 1979; Serrano-Garcia, 1990), and has been used with local poor communities, middle-class sectors, and functional communities such as religious and labor groups (Serrano-Garcia & López-Sánchez, 1991). The *social-psychological* direction emphasizes the development of human subjectivity within a constructionist model (Gergen, 1985), relying more on qualitative methods and ideological analysis (López & Zuñiga, 1988; López, Vázquez, & Macksoud, 1988). A university-based center for action-research has been established in the Psychology Department at the University of Puerto Rico. It was selected by the SCRA as the first in a network of community action-research centers to begin a "Woods Hole" for community psychology.

In Mexico, research is characterized by a strong action research orientation. Research has focused on community improvement, community service centers, the roles of paraprofessionals, impacts of urban planning, and effects of natural disasters (cf. Reid & Aguilar, 1991).

In Venezuela, research in community psychology was motivated by the need to find solutions to social problems and to induce social change, and therefore follows an intervention-

TABLE 3. Research in Community Psychology

Country	Research projects
Canada	Family mental health practice (Freeman & Trute, 1983)
	Women and mental health (McCannell, 1986); wife battering (Jaffe, 1988)
	Community mental health services for the chronically mentally disabled (Nelson, 1987)
	Psychosocial impacts of resource development (Bennett, Payette, & Trute, 1983)
	Education and training in human services (Dimock, 1984b)
	Program evaluation (Pancer, 1985)
	Public policy, social and economic development (Bennett, Payette, & Trute, 1983)
	Native people and their relationship to dominant culture (Bennett, 1982)
Australia	Unemployment (Veno, 1986; Viney, 1985)
	Conservation and environmental issues (Bishop & Syme, 1993; Winkler, 1978)
	Deinstitutionalization (Gardner & Veno, 1979)
	Public-order policing (Veno & Gardner, 1979; Veno & Veno, 1987)
	Peer support for emergency workers; support networks (cf. Fisher, 1992)
	Stress on youth in rural Australia (Fisher, 1992)
	Services for intellectually disabled (Fisher, Karnilowicz, & Ngo, 1994)
	Psychological sense of community (Sonn & Fisher, 1996, 1998; Fisher & Sonn, 1998; Pretty et al., 1996)
New Zealand	Waikato Group
	Cultural pluralism, agenda setting, and voice giving for the Maori, violence reduction (Hamerton, Nikora, Robertson, & Thomas, 1995)
	Barriers to community living for handicapped children (Chetwynd, 1985)
	Efficacy of telephone counseling services (Hornblow, 1986)
	Adjustment and well-being among migrant workers families (Thomas, O'Driscoll, & Robertson, 1984)
	Preventive goals of community mental health services (Hornblow, 1985)
	Evaluation research (Thomas & Robertson, 1989, 1992)
	Auckland Medical School Group
	Community house movement (Raeburn, 1986; Raeburn & Seymour, 1979)
	Superhealth Programs (Abbott & Raeburn, 1989)
	PEOPLE system: general community development (Raeburn, 1987, 1992)
Italy	Training and professional roles of psychologists (Francescato, 1977; Giammarco et al., 1986; Martini & Sequi, 1988; Palmonari, 1981; Rossati, 1981)
	Prevention services offered in family counseling and planning centers (Francescato, Contesini, & Dini, 1983; Leone & Corsetti, 1987; Polenta & Cozzi, 1987)
	Research on psychiatric services
	Retraining personnel for preparing patients for reentry in the community (Polli-Charmet, 1984), day hospital organization (Gasseau & Festini-Cuccu, 1983)
	Research on aging
	Social interaction in nursing homes (Bellanca, 1987)
	Resocialization of elderly persons (Francescato & Ghirelli, 1988b; Ugolini, Francescato, & Ghirelli, 1987)
	Coping behaviors of elderly persons (Laicardi, 1985)
	Developmental research
	Prevention of drug abuse and facilitation of healthy development through skill development in children (Francescato & Putton, 1986; Francescato, Putton, & Cudini, 1986a, 1986b)
	Development of programs for adolescents (Branca, 1981; Froscia & Fuccio, 1987; Pagnin, 1985)
	The promotion of groups in natural settings (Ameria & De Piccoli, 1985)
	Research on work settings
	Effectiveness of multilevel organizational analysis for change (Francescato & Ghirelli, 1988a), efficacy of training programs for professionals (Arcidiacono, Cimmino, Cetrangolo, & Vitas, 1983; Cudini & Giammarco, 1987; Francescato, 1984; Genco, 1987)
	Volunteer organizations and self-help groups (Noventa, Nava, & Olivia, 1987; Traversi & Tavazza, 1986; Volpi & Ghirelli, 1987)

TABLE 3. (*Continued*)

Country	Research projects
Germany	Role of social networks and social support for coping with stress, changes in professional roles and activities relative to self-help within communities (Keupp & Röhrle, 1987; Röhrle & Stark, 1985)
	Prevention (Franzkowiak & Wenzel, 1985; Stark, 1986)
	Research on environmental stress and resources based on ecological theories (Mühlum, Olschowy, Oppl, & Wendt, 1986; Wenzel, 1986)
	Effects of the traditional psychosocial service system and insufficient care provisions (Bittner, 1981; Buccholz, Gmur, Hofer, & Straus, 1985; Zaumseil, 1978)
	Developing new forms of intervention (Anneken & Heyden, 1985; Rudeck, 1983)
Poland	Applied research in educational and developmental psychology: modification of classroom environments, socialization of children, skill development (Bogdanowicz, 1979; Tyszkowa, 1972)
Israel	Stress research: stress in Israel (Breznitz, 1983a, 1983b); stress and war (Milgram, 1986)
	Social support and stress: stress, social support, and women (Hobfoll, 1986)
	Arab–Jewish relations
	School performance among financially disadvantaged children
Puerto Rico	Community emphasis of social-community program (Serrano-Garcia & Rosario Collazo, 1992)
	Intervention-within-research model (Irrizarry & Serrano-Garcia, 1979; Serrano-Garcia, 1990); interventions in local poor communities, middle-class sectors, and functional communities such as religious and labor groups (Alvarez-Hernandez, 1981; Castañeda, Domenech, Figueroa, Serrano-García, 1988; Santiago & Perfecto, 1983; Serrano-García, 1983; Serrano-García & Lopez-Sanchez, 1991)
	Social psychological emphasis
	Developmment of human subjectivity within a constructionist model (Gergen, 1985)
	Use of qualitative methods and ideological analysis (Lopez & Zuñiga, 1988; Lopez, Vazquez, & Macksoud, 1988)
Mexico	Community improvement through community service centers
	Roles of paraprofessionals
	Impacts of urban planning
	Effects of natural disasters (cf. Reid & Aguilar, 1991)
Venezuela	Community development and organization, community social psychology (Grau, 1986; Llovera, 1984; Loaiza, 1984; Montero, 1980, 1982, 1984; Patiño & Millan, 1979; Santi, Silva, & Colmenares, 1978)
Cuba	Evaluation research: psychosocial aspects of health, mental health, and the delivery and utilization of health services (García-Averasturi, 1985)
	Evaluation of group therapy and psychosocial intervention modalities
	Social issues including education, aging, drug and alcohol abuse
South Africa	Effects of violence on different groups in society, particularly on children
	Stress relating to political issues
	Effects of apartheid on various groups in society
	Social problem amelioration
	Prevention
	Mental health service delivery practices and systems, development of mental health policies (Lazarus, 1985, 1988; Lazarus & Prinsloo, 1995)

within-research model. This action research orientation has been applied to a variety of community development and organization projects (Campos, 1981; Llovera, 1984; Salamanca, 1985). Community psychology has begun to link the university with other organizations, for example, when university students conduct action research in cooperation with private community agencies.

In Cuba, a substantial amount of research in community psychology has been carried out

(Bernal & Marin, 1985; Marin, 1985). Health psychology and the evaluation of health service have been studied extensively (Garcia-Averasturi, 1985). Research on social issues, however, has focused more on describing problems than finding solutions (Marin, 1985).

In South Africa, research on a variety of issues relevant to community psychology has ranged from the effects of apartheid and violence to mental health service delivery. Although much research has followed traditional methodological approaches, there is a growing focus on action research with social change as a major goal. The development of appropriate psychosocial theories for the purpose of social action is also stressed (Lazarus & Prinsloo, 1995).

Internationally, the main themes in research are mental health services, prevention, program evaluation, stress and social support, new forms of intervention (especially self-help), community organization and development, and employment-related issues. The range of issues studied from a community vantage point, the extent of community psychology research, and the research methodologies used vary considerably among countries. In the Latin American countries, where social and economic conditions call for more fundamental change, research has primarily addressed how to organize and change communities based on an action-research-action model. In the English-speaking and Western European countries, where higher standards of living are available to larger groups of society, research focuses more on health- and mental-health-related services and their effectiveness.

Practice in Community Psychology

Practice in community psychology differs widely, both with respect to organization and scope. Table 4 summarizes areas of community practice. In English-speaking Canada, community psychologists have been trying since 1982 to overcome fragmentation of services and to network with each other. Quebec has been more active in community organization and social intervention (Tefft, Hamilton, & Théroux, 1982), as evidenced in the highly developed network of Local Centres of Community Services of Québec, initiated in 1972. In Australia, community psychology practice has fluctuated from a substantial number of community activities in the late 1970s (Gardner & Veno, 1979), to difficulty finding employment, and more recently, increased demand for community psychologists in public-sector settings. Their work includes AIDS-focused health promotion, prevention of violence, development of self-help groups for young unemployed persons, community development around natural resource issues, and program evaluation. In New Zealand, graduates of the University of Waikato program have found employment in public and private health and human service agencies. Much of their work has involved research and program evaluation. Psychologists at the Auckland Medical School initiated the Community House Project, which aims at fostering a sense of community and self-help (Raeburn, 1986; Raeburn & Seymour, 1979). This project has developed into a movement that has stimulated over 100 projects throughout New Zealand, led to the increased use of a community psychology framework by community workers and volunteers (Raeburn, 1992), and expanded community projects (Abbott & Raeburn, 1989; Raeburn, 1992). In Italy, the focus of work has been on retraining of professionals, consultation with public officials, and prevention. Community psychologists have been actively involved in translating the reform laws into practical programs. In Germany, emphases are prevention, crisis intervention, intervention in schools, social networks and social support, self-help organizations, and health promotion (Cramer, 1982). Self-help centers addressing the above areas have been established in several major cities. Poland is characterized by a community mental health orientation, with focus on community services for former psychiatric patients, substance abuse, and child-development programs. Israel shares a wide variety of programs typical in other Western European countries, such as hotlines, shelters, and deinstitutionalization, as well as programs unique to the country, such as projects for the integration of Ethiopian or Russian Jews.

In the Latin American countries, government support is provided for community mental health services, while private organization and university research foster community development efforts. In Puerto Rico, government support was provided for community education and development during the 1950s, but was shifted to community mental health during the 1960s. Autonomous (religious, labor, ecological) groups have been sponsoring a variety of community projects since the 1960s. In Venezuela, there are several levels of community action: (1) by government programs oriented toward organizing local neighborhoods, (2) by neighborhood organizations, (3) by private organizations offering training and information on organizational strategies, and (4) by social-community psychologists who provide consultation to the above groups and conduct action research. In Mexico, governmental efforts emphasize a community mental health focus, whereas the university programs are based in community centers and work toward community improvement. In these Latin American countries, research and community action have been much more strongly interwoven than in the other countries. The exception is Cuba, where the government directs activities ranging from traditional clinical services to training of health personnel and community organization.

In South Africa, political, economic, and social issues related to the apartheid system are seen as major concerns by many psychologists, whereas others have regarded community psychology practice as an extension of mental health services.

In international perspective, the practice of community psychology ranges from attempts at extending traditional mental health services to action research programs aimed at organizing and changing the community. Prevention is an important aspect of community psychology practice in most countries. The creation of employment opportunities for psychologists remains a critical issue in several countries. Overall, while many psychologists seem to be pursuing the goal of empowerment, often the structures in their country do not yet provide for more extensive intervention and change at the community level.

CONCEPTUAL BASES AND ORIENTATIONS

Community psychology in countries where community psychology is more formalized appears to have been influenced primarily by ideas from the U.S. In this section, we provide an overview of the conceptual bases and orientations in each country.

Community psychology in the U.S. has strongly influenced Canada, Australia, New Zealand, Germany, and several of the Mexican groups. The relationship between the U.S. and Canadian psychology has even been described as quasi-colonial (Walsh, 1988). Although the Australian sociocultural context has led to different applications of conceptual principles, the conceptual and value bases of community psychology are similar in Australia and the U.S.

In many countries, however, country-specific development have also influenced the definition and conceptual bases of community psychology. In Canada, the philosophy and work of Canadian pioneers who used prevention and human resource development in the community context were a major source of community concepts (Babarik, 1979; Dimock, 1984a; Gibson, 1974). In western Australia, there is a distinct post-modern orientation that

TABLE 4. Practice

Country	Employment settings and scope	Nature of community action
Canada	Overcoming fragmentation in English-speaking Canada; much action in Québec	Québec: local community service centers with focus of self-help (Guay, 1987)
Australia	Governmental agencies: largest employer community mental health (MH) centers, community centers	Program evaluation, policy formulation, community mental health, community development (Fisher, 1992)
New Zealand	Public and private social service agencies, research and evaluation units	Program evaluation of: • Research feedback (Robertson, 1985) A community training center for young unemployed Maoris (Dehar, 1987) • Alcohol treatment (Western, 1983)
	Medical schools and health services	Community organization and empowerment: Self-help: effects of Community House movement (Raeburn, 1992) Health promotion: Superheath (Abbott & Raeburn, 1989) Community-based MH services for long-term mentally ill (Raeburn et al., 1991)
Italy	Community centers with focus on primary prevention, prevention of substance abuse and MH problems, family consultants	Retraining of personnel Consulting with public officials Prevention programs
Germany	Clinically oriented psychologists	Prevention (e.g., Beck & Hauptmann, 1986) Crisis intervention, intervention in schools (Fliegl & Röhrle, 1983) Social networks and social support (Rörhle & Stark, 1985), self-help organizations (Kleiber, 1988) Health promotion (Belschner & Schewe-Mastall, 1988)
Poland	Limited scope, clinical orientation	Community mental health services (Orwid et al., 1981), some community-oriented model programs: home-based psychiatric care (Bizon & Ciszewski, 1979) Stress reduction (Garwolinksa, 1979; Pasek, 1982) Skill development programs for children (Bogdanowicz, 1975, 1979) Substance abuse among youth (MONAR, 1984)
Israel	Limited scope, clinical orientation	Community mental health type services: crisis hotlines, women's shelters, deinstitutionalization, street programs for troubled youths, child health centers, programs for integration of new citizens
Puerto Rico	Government level	Community mental health programs: work with rape victims, HIV/AIDS patients, battered women, homeless persons
	Private agency and university levels	Community development (Serrano-Garcia & Lopez-Sánchez, 1991)

TABLE 4. (*Continued*)

Country	Employment settings and scope	Nature of community action
Venezuela	Government level	Social marginality, urban migration, community organization
	Neighborhood and private organizations	Training information, assessment of community needs, organizational strategies (example: CESAP)
	University	Consultation with community groups and government agencies, action research (Sanchez, Wiesenfeld, & Cronick, 1991)
Mexico	Government level	Community mental health focus (Serrano-Garcia & Rivera Medina, 1985)
	University	
Cuba	Part of medicine in the community; government-directed	Focus on primary prevention and early intervention in schools and work settings, normal developmental crises, stress management, outreach, family and community development with a strong interdisciplinary focus (García-Averasturi, 1985; Gonzalez-Rey, 1989; Perez-Stable, 1985; Uriarte-Gaston & Margarida, 1987)
South Africa	Very limited scope; discussion on scope and nature of practice	Extension of MH services with focus on prevention Community psychology in action (Dawes, 1985; Holdstock, 1981; Swartz, 1986) "Radical" position: apartheid-related issues of oppression, intergroup conflicts, resource distribution, poverty, unemployment (Dawes, 1986; Lazarus, 1985, 1988; Lazarus & Prinsloo, 1995; Steyn, 1985)

focuses on community integration, environmental resources, and community development. In New Zealand, concepts from the U.S. (Raeburn, 1986) have remained an important source of inspiration for health-oriented research and practice. At Waikato, an indigenous conceptual base has been emerging, reflecting a social psychology of multicultural social services and policy orientation. A distinctive emphasis is developing in the graduate program, with program evaluation, biculturalism, and health promotion as prominent features (Hamerton et al., 1995; Thomas & Veno, 1992).

In Italy, four different positions are represented in the continuing debate on the conceptualization of community psychology: Community psychology (1) as the application of organizational psychology to settings other than work; (2) as part of applied social and developmental psychology and as a framework for the organization of social services and the creation of new roles for psychologists; (3) as a form of community organization; and (4) as clinical community psychology with focus on primary and secondary prevention.

In Germany, community psychology is seen as a perspective critical of psychology as a profession, the psychosocial service system, and of society. Critical theory, the literature on subtle mechanisms of social control, work critical of the medical model, and research showing deficiencies in psychosocial care have provided distinct influences.

As a European country, Poland has been influenced by Western theories in psychology. However, with its forced incorporation into the Soviet sphere following World War II, the translation of Western theories into practice was influenced by the political system and, at least superficially, had to be consistent with Marxist philosophy of dialectic materialism. Commu-

Table 5. Conceptual Bases and Orientation

Canada	Academic community psychology in the United States The philosophy and work of Canadian pioneers: prevention and human resource development in the community context (e.g., C. M. Hincks, E A. Bott, W. E. Blatz, G. B. Chisholm, C. E. Hendry, H. S. Dimrock, W. Line, and J. R. Seeley; see Barbarik, 1979; Gibson, 1974)
Australia	Stimulation from concepts of U.S. community psychology: Social innovation, empowerment, psychological sense of community (Gardner & Veno, 1979); acceptance of diverse cultures, enhancing the potential and participation of all citizens, preventation and promotion of competency, an ecological orientation (e.g., Veno, 1982); systems and natural resources (Bishop & Syme, 1993); post-modern science (Bishop & D'Rozario, 1990; Bishop & Drew, 1998); psychological sense of community (Fisher, 1992; Pretty et al., 1996; Sonn & Fisher, 1996, 1998)
New Zealand	Initial stimulation by community psychology in the United States: Community control, psychological sense of community, empowerment, ecological viewpoint, program evaluation (Raeburn, 1986) Conceptual orientation at Auckland Medical School and among practitioners: notions of community development, community participation, empowerment, organizational development, shared resources, and cultural pluralism underlie health oriented practice Conceptual orientation at University of Waikoto/academic focus: (a) Social psychology, multicultural, social service, and policy orientation (b) Prevention of social problems (c) Ecological framework with emphasis on intervention with large groups, organizations, and community systems (Robertson et al., 1989) (d) Distinctive New Zealand emphasis: program evaluation, biculturalism, health promotion, domestic violence (Hamerton, Nikora, Robertson, & Thomas, 1993; Thomas & Veno, 1992)
Italy	Application of organizational psychology to settings other than work (Contessa & Sherna, 1981; Splatro, 1981, 1985) As part of applied social and developmental psychology: a useful framework for the organization of social services and the creation of new roles for psychologists such as the analysis of organizational needs, planning, evaluation, action research, and inservice training (Francescato, 1977; Francescato, Contesini, & Dini, 1983; Francescato & Ghirelli, 1988; Palmonari & Zani, 1980 A form of community organization that focuses on the growth and development of the community as a "collective and political subject" (Ellena, 1985; Martini, 1983) Clinical community psychology involves use of primary and secondary prevention techniques in the educational and health services (Francescato & Tulli, 1982)
Germany	Critical theory (Bernstein, 1976) Literature on subtle mechanisms of social control (e.g., Foucault, 1973, 1987) Criticisms of the medical model Research showing deficiencies in psychosocial care (Finzen & Schädle-Deininger, 1979) Anglo-American literature critical of psychology as a profession, the psychosocial service system, and society
Poland	Until demise of communist system: consistency of approaches with the Marxian philosophy of dialectic materialism: (a) Identification of community efforts by the specialty area involved (e.g., clinical or educational psychology) (b) Conceptual influences from the British school of social psychiatry With democratic government: search for new models, looking toward Western theories
Israel	Community psychology as a natural extension of the organizational orientations of the country's founders: a nation based on socialism and humanism Gerald Caplan's notions of prevention (1964) and consultation (1970)
Puerto Rico	Initial stimulation from community psychology in the United States Integration of Berger and Luckman's (1967) notions of social construction reality and second-order social change (Serrano-García, Lopez, & Rivera-Medina, 1987; Serrano-García & López-Sánchez, 1991)

Table 5. *(Continued)*

Venezuela	Writings of Latin American social scientists in late 1950s and mid-1960s (a) Colombian sociologist Orlando Fals Borda (1959, 1980, 1981, 1985) (b) Brazilian educator Paulo Freire (1971, 1972) (c) Economist and social worker Ezequiel Ander-Egg (1964) 1970s community psychology literature from the United States 1970s other Latin American social researchers (e.g., Brandao, 1981, 1984; Molano, 1977)
Mexico	Three general groupings on the basis of conceptual orientation: (1) Rogerian notions of human development through participation and self actualization: Iberoamericana, ITESO, and Coahila (a) Iberoamericana: a combination of humanistic ideas and psychoanalytic notions of *psicocomunidad* (Cueli & Biro, 1976), with emphasis on powerlessness and passivity (b) ITESO: notions of transactional ecology: goal of intervention is strengthening of the social infrastructure (c) Coahila: *participación activa* (Moscovici, 1976): a model comprising citizen participation in an economic structure (a candy factory), action research, and training (2) Universidad Nacional Autonoma de Iztcala: behavioral psychology orientation similar to that in the United States (3) Universidad Nacional Autonoma (Metropolitana): critical analysis of community and social aspects of Mexican culture. Combination of psychoanalytical and Marxian concepts to understand the poor and provide impetus for change (Reid & Aguilar, 1991)
Cuba	Third World paradigm of community psychology aimed at developing and implementing preventive strategies in health, education, and work (Bernal & Rodriguez, 1992) Conceptual basis: philosophical premises of dialectical materialism (Kenworthy, 1985) Evolving conceptual model of psychology in Cuba: an action-oriented model focused on meeting social and community needs (Bernal, 1985)
South Africa	Community mental health position (a) Conservative view: extension of present services into the community (b) More radical view: the development of an alternative mental health system, helping victims of the present political system, and preparing for a post-revolution South African society Social action position: social issues in the oppression of people in South Africa, various levels and kinds of oppression Marxian philosophies and empowerment as conceptual bases for more radical groups Systems theory as conceptual framework of more conservative groups

nity efforts are therefore primarily identified by the specialty involved (e.g., clinical or educational psychology). In an authoritarian, highly controlled socialist system, approaches based on empowerment and social action concepts tended to be perceived as destabilizing by those in power, even at the local level. The experience of the Solidarity Movement, as a national social action effort directed at economic and social reform, reveals both the limits placed on community efforts in such a society and the powerful potential of community action, as evidenced in the changes in the Polish political and economic system during the past several years. Recent work by Markova (1997) and Moodie, Markova, Farr, and Plichtova (1997) have addressed how communist regimes in Eastern Europe have affected concepts of community and the individual.

In Israel, community psychology would be a natural extension of the organizational orientations of the country's founders. The founders planned a nation that would be based on socialism and humanism. The *kibbutz* was to be the agricultural manifestation of this ideology, and worker-owned factories were to be the industrial outgrowth. Although these directions are less dominant today in Israel, their influence on the planned community can still be felt.

Puerto Rico is dominated by a political and cultural system that has been insensitive to its collective will and traditions (Ortiz, 1987; Serrano-Garcia, 1987). The conceptual base of the social-community program has been developed to deal with this reality. The conceptual model is based on an integration of Berger and Luckman's social construction of reality and second-order social change (Serrano-Garcia, López, & Rivera-Medina, 1987). Its main components—ideology, communication, and language—are the instruments by which the established social construction of reality is made available to all human beings and incorporated into their consciousness. Social control is seen as the mechanism by which an established social construction is maintained, thus the focus is on a social change effort that can change the prevailing view of reality so as to create an active society where power relations are more symmetrical (Serrano-Garcia & López-Sánchez, 1991).

Community approaches were first developed in Latin American countries in the late 1950s and the mid-1960s by the Colombian sociologist Orlando Fals Borda (1959, 1980, 1981, 1985), the Brazilian educator Paulo Freire (1971, 1972), and the economist and social worker Ezequiel Ander-Egg (1964). Their work provided the initial methodological and theoretical foundations for community psychology in Venezuela. Later influences came from the U.S. community psychology literature, as well as other Latin American work (e.g., Brandao, 1981, 1984; Molano, 1977; Montero, 1998). In Venezuela, community psychology stands for a clear psychosocial perspective and a liberationist value stance. Community psychology has been defined as the branch of psychology whose object is the study of psychosocial factors involved in the development, promotion, and maintenance of control and power by citizens over their individual and social environment. In Mexico, there is no unified or dominant conceptual framework (Reid & Aguilar, 1991), although community psychologists fit with three general groupings on the basis of conceptual orientation. The Iberoamericana, ITESO, and Coahila locations all share the Rogerian notion of human development through participation and self-actualization. Other conceptual influences included *psicocomunidad* (Cueli & Biro, 1976), the notions of transactional ecology, and Moscovici's (1976) ideas of *participación activa.* At Universidad Nacional Autonoma de Iztcala, the behavioral psychology orientation is similar to that in the U.S. Community approaches at Universidad Nacional Autónoma have focused on critical analyses of community and social aspects of the Mexican culture (Reid & Aguilar, 1991). In Cuba, there is an emerging third-world paradigm of community psychology aimed at developing and implementing preventive strategies in health, education, and work (Bernal & Rodriguez, 1992). The conceptual basis of the model is rooted in the philosophical premises of dialectical materialism. As such, all aspects of human activity (e.g., cognitive, affective, behavioral) are examined in its particular social, economic, and historical context. An action-oriented conceptual model of psychology has been evolving in Cuba, in which well-being and mental health services are an integral part of health-service delivery (Bernal, 1985). Concerns about the limitations of community psychology have been raised by Calvino (1998). Wiesenfeld (1998) has provided a recent review of the theoretical bases of community psychology in Brazil, Chile, Colombia, Mexico, Puerto Rico, and Venezuela (see also DeSouza, 1992; Montero, 1982).

In South Africa, community psychology has been interpreted in diverse ways by conservative, liberal, and radical psychologists (Lazarus, 1985). While Marxian philosophies and systems theory have been favored by various groups, the predominant trend appears to be towards a community mental health model, which includes both traditional and preventive services, and social action models, with focus on overcoming the oppressive characteristic of the former apartheid system. The need for the development of appropriate psychosocial theories and an indigenous community psychology is recognized by many in South Africa (Dawes, 1986; Lazarus & Prinsloo, 1995; Vogelman, 1987).

In summary, even where the influences from the U.S. have been widely felt, similar conceptual bases find different expressions in various countries. This is reflected in the definition of community psychology, the degree of formalization of the area, and the training and practice of community psychologists, as well as in their research foci.

In all countries, the realization of the need for change and the impetus for change comes from persons within the country who are stimulated by the literature and by their experiences. In many cases, the literature from the U.S. appears to have provided initial stimulation; in other countries, it offered support after ideas had already begun to develop.

There are no common or overriding conceptual frameworks for community psychology internationally, but the theme of empowerment is widely accepted as a common goal for social improvement. In Latin America and South Africa, most of the approaches have developed from criticisms of the prominent paradigms—those represented by traditional social and individual psychology. There are major social inequities that are apparent, with the need for social change as social improvement. In most of the developed countries, social improvement is a primary purpose, with a less apparent need for criticism.

THE FUTURE OF COMMUNITY PSYCHOLOGY

In this section, each collaborating author speculates about the future status of community psychology.

Canada (E. Bennett)

In a symposium on Canadian community psychology in 1986, several needs emerged: (1) a greater emphasis on advocacy and social-intervention activities; (2) increased exchange between English and French Canada; (3) expansion of the interdisciplinary nature of programs; and (4) improving the fit between community psychologists, professional issues, and the diverse problems of local and regional communities. Four factors in the political culture of Canada favor community psychology: (1) constitutional arrangements that value and protect community and cultural diversity; (2) consistency of government at both the federal and provincial levels, which makes it easier for enduring progressive and not so progressive social changes to occur; (3) the provinces' jurisdiction over health, education, welfare, and civil rights, allowing the development of policies, priorities, and programs based on local and provincial needs; and (4) the federal health policy introduced in 1974 (Lalonde, 1974) that calls for a "reframing" of the traditional view of health and for social action and community psychology values (Davidson, 1981). The future for community psychology in Canada appears promising in light of the dramatic progress of the past 15 years. For a country as big and diverse as Canada, regional developments will be necessary if community psychology is to fulfill its potential.

Australia (A. Veno)

Community psychology will be a clearly recognized field of psychology, having developed penetration into employment and training, and having achieved the goals related to impacting upon social issues at the political level. There has been a distressing trend for academic programs started in community psychology to wither on the vine, reflecting the effects of the conservative Australian context. The International Congress of Psychology held in Sydney in 1988 served as a catalyst for the improvement of the status of community psychology within the Australian Psychological Society. A visit of community psychologists from the U.S., Canada, New Zealand, and Japan led to a significant heightening of a psychological sense of community among Australian community psychologists, and will have profound impact for the growth and development of the field in Australia.

New Zealand (J. M. Raeburn and D. R. Thomas)

Community psychology will be increasingly present in universities, health settings, nongovernmental social services, and private practice in community development projects. Community psychologists will work as consultants and evaluators of new, public and private, social services programs. In Auckland, the emphasis will likely continue to be on health and well-being in the context of community psychology; whereas at Waikato, social policy and evaluation of human services are increasingly seen as important areas. Common to both locations is an emphasis on empowerment, bi- and multiculturalism, equity, research and evaluation, and an ecological perspective. Links are forming between the community psychology movements in Australia and New Zealand (Thomas & Veno, 1992). Research and practice based on local needs have become an common emphasis (Veno & Thomas, 1992). However, New Zealand has a unique social and cultural fabric quite distinct from Australia's, particularly in New Zealand's traditional values on the concept of "community." As a consequence, and in view of the current vision and growth of community psychology, we predict it will increasingly be a major force in community and social development in this country.

Italy (D. Francescato and E. R. Martini)

The future of community psychology will depend upon three factors. The first is the evolution of employment opportunities. Cutbacks in programs initiated by the reform laws could result in fewer public jobs. Some young community psychologists have started private organizations offering community programs. Next is the growth of community training programs. Compared to several hundred private schools in psychotherapy, there are only a few community psychology programs. One goal is to obtain a national doctoral program in community psychology to train college professors and to increase the number of private training centers. The last is the capacity to improve the theoretical and strategic framework of community psychology (e.g., Francescato & Ghirelli, 1988).

Germany (H. Keupp and W. Stark)

We have identified four potential developments: (1) The term "community psychology" will continue to have little meaning as a descriptor of a subdiscipline of psychology. A critical attitude in research and practice, however, may lead to an organized psychology that reflects upon the social implications of individual problems and applies social science knowledge to psychological practice in applied settings. (2) Scientists and practitioners in psychology will become more involved in such social issues as environmental crises, the consequences of cutbacks in the welfare system, and in self-help organizations. (3) An urgent task of community psychology will be to translate abstract concepts into practical strategies. (4) Community psychology may be undermined by social policy. Terms such as "community-oriented" or "need-based" are readily used by conservative administrators and politicians for concealing cutbacks in the social sector, and for giving a progressive appearance to neoconservative social policy. Also, psychologists threatened by unemployment see a chance for better job possibilities with community psychology. Both can weaken the political potential of a community psychology perspective.

The reunification of Germany has raised new issues for community psychology. Reunification has required adjustment to new values and social and economic problems. It has created previously unknown problems, such as a high rate of unemployment in the former East Germany. Many former East Germans have felt uncertain as to how to adapt in their new system, and were disenchanted with the slow pace of change; many former West Germans felt resentment about "footing the bill" for reunification. Community psychology may provide some of the broad-scale solutions needed for meshing what was formerly two countries into one, both socioeconomically and emotionally.

Poland (E. Zolik)

In the past it was difficult to envision a broad-based community psychology developing in Poland, as notions of empowerment and social action were incompatible with a highly controlled authoritarian system. With the election of a democratic government, the potential for new programs and approaches is limitless. However, future programmatic developments are less dependent upon the motivation of mental health professionals than on resolving and reorienting Poland's collapsing Marxist-oriented economy. The intense psychological sense of national identity and strong family orientation, which sustained the nation during the past partitions and the last 50 post-war years, will be a major dynamic in the ensuing difficult decade.

Israel (S. Hobfoll)

One of two futures seems possible. With continued war and economic strife, psychology will remain traditionally oriented, but will show pockets of innovation. Stabilization of the economy and a positive outcome of the peace negotiations may allow Israel to focus more on community-oriented issues and quality of life. Whatever the future holds, community psychologists looking to aid Israeli society will work in fertile ground. There exists an enormous and deep psychological sense of national and neighborhood community. Families are strong and well-connected. Perhaps most important, there is a national sense of accomplishment that, if reharnessed for peace, could be a dynamic, driving force.

Puerto Rico (I. Serrano-Garcia)

Social-community psychology is at a critical juncture. The integration between the social and community components of the model and the training program have been strained. The next few years will be crucial in searching for a integration of these new forces. The external environment will also serve as a motivator in the search for a new interpretation of our model. Licensing laws will no longer allow the independent practice of psychology without a doctoral degree. Competing programs (social work) that have developed social change models do not require this degree for licensing. Government programs are being created that can force community psychologists into defending the established social construction of reality. The apparent openness of our current government has given new hopes for social change within the established system. All these forces will foster disintegration of community psychology. A countervailing force can be found in the work of community psychology program graduates in religious, feminist, ecological, and mental health groups. These community psychologists work toward social change by creating new settings and by activating organizations (Serrano-Garcia & López-Sánchez, 1991). The future of community psychology in Puerto Rico will depend heavily on the reanalysis of our current model and practice, the integration of new models, and input from practicing community psychologists in our Ph.D. program. Without these dialogues and changes, social-community psychology in Puerto Rico will be one more run-of-the-mill doctoral program. If these changes materialize, social-community psychology should reemerge as a pioneering controversial program, actively participating in the social transformation of Puerto Rico.

Venezuela (M. Montero)

Community work will induce cognitive and behavioral changes that will result in visible economic and social changes. Community psychology will be a subspecialty that addresses equally the role of individuals and the environment. This will be accomplished by: (1) the development of ties between private and public community-oriented institutions, (2) the pressure on universities to become more socially relevant, (3) creating demand for community programs among private and official agencies by demonstrating their effectiveness, (4) an increase in community research, (5) growing awareness of the political role of organized communities and new ways for neighborhood associations to participate in public life, and (6) new theoretical and methodological approaches created by the community-oriented practice of psychology, and the advances of a social psychology directed at social transformation. The economic crisis in Latin America necessitates community development based on indigenous models of change. There will be an increasing need for a discipline that actively incorporates its subject of study, is dynamic, and is able to generate its resources out of the actual conditions of life, offering feasible alternatives.

Mexico (J. Gómez del Campo)

Three major goals need to be pursued for the future of community psychology. First, it must reach a broad range of people and go beyond the direct project work by university-based centers. Second, community development must be incorporated more directly into community psychology. Third, theory must be developed that is not just an importation of ideas from the U.S.

In the future, there will be at least eight areas of change and development: (1) more university training programs will be developing approaches based on local needs; (2) there will be long-term intervention programs with a program-evaluation component; (3) ecological theory will become more central because of population and pollution problems; (4) cooperation among Latin American countries in community psychology will increase; (5) community centers will serve as structures where the universities and citizens can work together; (6) community projects will be oriented toward meeting the basic needs of all sectors of the population; (7) community psychologists will be more knowledgeable in the social context and politics of Mexico; and (8) there will be a more differentiated political system and a higher level of education in the population.

Cuba (G. Bernal)

The recent trend of the health care system toward increased community-based care through the family medicine program has provided additional avenues for community psychologists. The consultation and conjoint work in primary, secondary, and tertiary prevention that has strengthened the relationship between psychologists and health professionals bode well for the further development of community psychology in Cuba (Bernal & Rodriguez, 1992; Uriarte-Gaston & Margarida, 1987). A limitation in this development is the training and availability of community and family psychologists. Without more trained personnel, it will be difficult for psychologists to meet the increasing demand for services. This question of resources will need to be resolved. In spite of severe economic problems, in part accelerated by the withdrawal of support from the former socialist countries, the Cuban system continues to expand into the community it serves (Uriarte-Gaston & Margarida, 1987), and to provide an exemplary community-based health and mental health system of care.

South Africa (S. Lazarus)

The present interest in community psychology will continue and lead to either a subspecialty within present specialty areas or to a specialty in its own right. Present trends suggest that it may either be a broad umbrella approach, housing a variety of analyses and intervention styles, including politically conservative and radical approaches; or it may be claimed by one side of the political spectrum, such as the conservatives or the politically radical social-action-oriented psychologists. Irrespective of its label, the development of an alternative psychology in South Africa is well on its way, and will no doubt continue to find a meaningful place in the changes that have occurred in South Africa.

CONCLUSION

According to our colleagues, community psychology will be alive, well, and more developed in the next century. For most countries, there is the expectation that community psychology will expand and gain more significance. The success and direction of this process of establishing and expanding community psychology will differ from country to country.

This difference is due directly to differences in the political, economic, social, and cultural reality in which community research and practice are carried out. The developed countries tend to be economic centers, whereas others are at the periphery and are more dependent. Although circumstances and concerns are different, we have nonetheless seen such topics as community development, social change, citizen participation, empowerment, stress and coping, and prevention as common across most settings. The basic issue is whether the field in a given country is consciously identifying itself with community psychology, and whether it is more on the progressive or conservative side of the political spectrum.

At this point in the development of community psychology, one sees considerable diffusion of particular ideas and practices. Diffusion seems to center mainly on the ideas and associated practices in the mental health area. Matters of citizen activism and community development are linked more closely to political and economic matters; they antedate the inception of community psychology and have not been diffused so directly by community psychology. The ideology of empowerment and social improvement is very widely diffused, going far beyond community psychology.

Diffusion takes place through person-to-person contacts, literature, and conferences. The conferences, in particular, seem to be very influential. In Latin America since the 1950s, the biennial Interamerican Congress of Psychology has provided the forum for discussion and exchange, and has helped to attract students to study in other countries. The Community Psychology Task Force of the Interamerican Society of Psychology is a significant force in promoting community research and action. In Europe, the European Network of Community Psychology meets biannually and on the same schedule as the National Australian and New Zealand Community Psychology Conference.

Interuniversity linkages are also important. Partners of the Americas has encouraged linkages and exchanges of faculty and students among the Latin American countries and the U.S. Visiting lecturers and workshops are often used in countries where a university or a group of community psychologists can band together to bring in someone for a short period. Sabbatical periods abroad (often sponsored by Fulbright fellowships) are also a way in which community psychologists in the U.S. have been part of the diffusion process. Bringing students to study at universities in the U.S. through governmental or foundation funds provides another possibility for linkages. The International Network on Community Research and Action may help U.S. community psychologists to find new ideas in the community concepts and innovative approaches pursued in other countries. Recent advances in technology may provide for additional linkages, as the internet and the world-wide web allow easy access to information and colleagues all over the world.

This chapter was designed as an introduction to other perspectives, and to increase our colleagues' awareness to developments and approaches in other countries. Community as a social presence in a person's daily life seems stronger outside the U.S., where the economic and political evolution of the country collides regularly with the needs of the local community. In the U.S., the same process is happening, but is less readily apparent, and one can find much to learn about community structure and processes outside the country. In particular, the strong linkages among Latin American countries, among European countries, and between Australia and New Zealand may result in new, distinct approaches aimed at significant social and economic change. The former communist countries in Eastern Europe may find pertinent solutions to the tremendous changes they are undergoing by looking to Latin American community psychology models and approaches.

The common denominator for all the countries is the notion that community psychology has action implications for the purpose of social improvement. As a value-based discipline, its goals are to improve individual and community functioning through active participation and development. In that sense, it is an international socially progressive movement.

REFERENCES

Abbott, M., & Raeburn, J. M. (1989). Superhealth: A community-based health promotion programme. *Mental Health in Australia, 2*, 25–35.

Alvarez-Hernández, S. (1981). *Definicion de liderato de una comunidad puertorriqueña.* Unpublished master's thesis, University of Puerto Rico, Río Piedras, PR.

Amerio, P., & De Piccolo, N. (1985). *Gruppi di giovani sul territorio.* Seminario della Sips su "Adolescenti e servizi sociali," Bologna, Italy.

Ander-Egg, E. (1964). *Metodologia y practica del desarrollo de la comunidad.* Madrid: Foco Berthe.

Ander-Egg, E. (1969). *Autoconstrucción y desarrollo de la comunidad.* Buenos Aires: Libreria de las Naciones.

Anneken, R., & Heyden, T. (Eds.). (1985). *Wege zur Veränderung: Beratung und Selbsthilfe.* Tübingen, Germany: DGVT.

Arcidiacono, C., Cimmino, R., Cetrangolo, C., & Vitas, E. (1983). Aggiornamento del personale sociosanitario e consultario in una realta meridionale. In D. Francescato, A. Contesini, & S. Dini (Eds.), *Psicologia di Comunità: Esperienze a confronto* (pp. 342–352). Rome: Il Pensiero Scientifico.

Ardila, R. (1982). Psychology in Latin America today. *Annual Review of Psychology, 33,* 103–122.

Babarik, P. (1979). The buried Canadian roots of community psychology. *Journal of Community Psychology, 7,* 362–367.

Balcazar, F. E. (Ed.) (1992). Feature: Second special international issue. *The Community Psychologist, 25,* 15–30.

Beck, M., & Hauptmann, G. (Eds.). (1986). *Prävention und Intervention bei Schulschwierigkeiten.* Tübingen, Germany: DGVT.

Bellanca, R. (1987). *Indaqine realizzata nella casa di riposo de Colle dell'Oro.* Paper presented at the Convention of the Division of Community Psychology, Castiglioncello, Livorno, Italy.

Belschner, W., Gottwald, P., & Kaiser, P. (1981). Zur kompetenz des klinischen psychologen für Prävention und Präventivforschung. In W. R. Minsel & R. Scheller (Eds.), *Brennpunkte der klinischen Psychologie: Prävention, Vol. 1* (pp. 194–212). Munich, Germany: Kösel.

Belschner, W., & Schewe-Mastall, B. (1988). Systematische Entwicklung—Stadtteilbezogene Gesundheitsförderung und Orientierungsentwicklung. Verhaltenstherapie und Psychosoziale Praxis, *20,* 314–331.

Bennett, C. C., Anderson, D. P., Cooper, S., Hassel, J., Klein, D. C., & Rosenbaum, G. (1966). *Community psychology: A report of the Boston Conference on the Education of Psychologists for Community Mental Health.* Boston: Boston University Press.

Bennett, E. M. (1982). Native persons: An assessment of their relationship to the dominant culture and challenges for change. *Canadian Journal of Community Mental Health, 1,* 21–32.

Bennett, E. M. (Ed.). (1987). *Social Intervention: Theory and practice.* Lewinston, NY: Edwin Mellen Press.

Bennett, E. M., Payette, M., & Trute, B. (1983). Psychosocial impacts of resource development in Canada: *Canadian Journal of Community Mental Health,* Special Supplement No. 1.

Bennett, E. M., & Tefft, B. (Eds.). (1985). *Theoretical and empirical advances in community mental health.* Lewinston, NY: Edwin Mellen Press.

Berger, P., & Luckman, T. (1967). *The social construction of reality.* New York: Doubleday.

Bernal, B. V. (1985). A history of psychology in Cuba. *Journal of Community Psychology, 13,* 222–235.

Bernal, G., & Marin, B. (Eds.). (1985). Community psychology in Cuba [Special Issue]. *Journal of Community Psychology, 13*(2).

Bernal, G., & Rodriguez, W. R. (1992). Psychology in Cuba. In V. S. Sexton & J. D. Hogan (Eds.), *International psychology: Views from around the world.* Lincoln: University of Nebraska Press.

Bernstein, R. J. (1976). *The restructuring of social and political theory.* Philadelphia: University of Pennsylvania Press.

Bishop, B., & Drew, N. (1998). Community psychologist as subtle change agent. *The Community Psychologist, 31,* 20–22.

Bishop, B., & D'Rozario, P. (1990). The development of community psychology in Western Australia. *The Community Psychologist, 24,* 15–16.

Bishop, B., & Syme, G. (1993). Community psychology and natural resource management. *The Community Psychologist, 27,* 19.

Bittner, U. (1981). Ein Klient mit "gemacht." In E. V. Kardorff & E. Koenen (Eds.), *Psyche in schlechter Gesellschaft.* Munich, Germany: Urban & Schwarzenberg.

Bizon, Z., & Ciszewski, L. (1979). *Psychiatryczne leczenia domowe jako alternatywa hospitalizacji.* Paper presented at the XXXIII Scientific Conference of Polish Psychiatrists. Cracow, Poland.

Bogdanowicz, M. (1975). *Bon Depart—metoda aktywizowania rozowoju psychomotorycznegno i rehabilitacji psychomotoryczej.* Olsztyn, Poland: Instytut Ksztalcenia Nauczylieli i Badan Oswiatowych w Olsztnie.

Bogdanowicz, M. (1979). *Materialy do cwiczen methoda "Dobrego Startu."* Gdansk, Poland: Institute of Psychology, University of Gdansk.

Branca, P. G. (1981). Esperienza di animazione in un centro sociale di quartiere. In G. Contessa & M. Sberna (Eds.), *Per una psicologia di comunità* (pp. 95–101). Milan, Italy: Clued.

Brandao, C. R. (Ed.). (1981). *Pesquisa participante.* São Paulo: Brasiliense.

Brandao, C. R. (Ed.). (1984). *Repensando a pesquisa participante.* São Paulo: Brasiliense.

Breznitz, S. (Ed.). (1983a). *The denial of stress.* New York: International Universities Press.

Breznitz, S. (Ed.). (1983b). *Stress in Israel.* New York: Van Nostrand.

Buchholz, W., Gmur, W., Hofer, R., & Straus, F. (1985). *Lebenswelt und Familienwirklichkeit.* Frankfurt, Germany: Campus.

Calvino, M. (1998). Reflections on community studies. *Journal of Community Psychology, 26,* 252–259.

Campos, T. (1981). La dinamica de grupos y el desarrollo comunal. *Psicología, VIII,* 221–244.

Campos, A., Brenes, A., & Quevedo, S. (1980). Crisis, dependencia y contradicciones de la psicologia en America Latina. *Revista Latinoamericana de Psicologia, 12,* 11–27.

Caplan, G. (1964). *Principles of preventative psychiatry.* New York: Basic Books.

Caplan, G. (1970). *The theory and practice of mental health consultation.* New York: Basic Books.

Castañeda, I., Domenech, N., Figueroa, O., & Serrano-Garcia, I. (1988, August). *Needs and resources assessment of the homeless in Santurce, Puerto Rico.* Poster session presented at the annual meeting of the American Psychological Association, Atlanta, GA.

Chetwynd, J. (1985). Some costs of caring at home for an intellectually handicapped child. *Australian and New Zealand Journal of Developmental Disabilities, 11,* 35–40.

Coakes, S. J., & Bishop, B. J. (1996). The experience of moral community in a rural community context. *Journal of Community Psychology, 24,* 108–117.

Contessa, G., & Sberna, M. (Eds.). (1981). *Per una psicologia di comunità.* Milan, Italy: Clued.

Cramer, M. (1982). *Psychosoziale Arbeit.* Stuttgart, Germany: Kohlhammer.

Crawford, J. (1981). Psychiatric reform in Trieste, Italy: Implications for community psychology in the United States. *Journal of Community Psychology, 9,* 276–279.

Cudini, S., & Giammarco, I. (1987). *Valutazione dei corsi di formazione per il personale dei servizi pubblici.* Paper presented at the Convention of the Division of Community Psychology, Castiglioncello, Livorno, Italy.

Cueli, J., & Biro, C. (1976). *Psicocomunidad.* Mexico, DF: Prentice-Hall Internacional.

Davidson, P. O. (1981). Some cultural, political and professional antecedents of community psychology in Canada. *Canadian Psychologist, 22,* 314–320.

Dawes, A. (1985). Politics and mental health. The position of clinical psychology in South Africa. *South African Journal of Psychology, 15,* 55–61.

Dawes, A. (1986). The notion of relevant psychology with particular reference to Africanist pragmatic initiatives. *Psychology in Society, 5,* 49–65.

Dehar, M. A. (1987). *Developing a programme for unemployed Maori youth: An implementation evaluation of a community training centre.* Unpublished master's thesis, University of Waikato, Hamilton, New Zealand.

DeSouza, E. (1992). Community psychology in Brazil. *The Community Psychologist, 25,* 23–24.

Dimock, H. G. (1984a). Thirty years of human service education and training in Canada—one perspective. *Canadian Journal of Community Mental Health, 3,* 15–41.

Dimock, H. G. (Ed.). (1984b). Education and training in Canadian human services [special issue]. *Canadian Journal of Community Mental Health, 3,* entire issue.

Ellena, A. (1985). *Animazione sociale.* Milan, Italy: Clued.

Emmite, P. L. (1980). Psychoanalytical model for training in supervision, research and community development: A personal experience in Mexico City. *Journal of Community Psychology, 8,* 176–188.

Fals Borda, O. (1959). *Acción y desarrollo en una vereda colombiana.* Monographias Sociologicas. Bogotá, Colombia: Universidad Nacional.

Fals Borda, O. (1980). *Mompox y Loba: Historia doble de la costa.* Bogotá, Colombia: Carlos Valencia.

Fals Borda, O. (1981). *Ciencia propia y colonialismo intelectual.* Bogotá, Colombia: Carlos Valencia.

Fals Borda, O. (1985). *Conocimiento y acción popular.* México: Siglo XXI.

Farhall, H., & Love, T. (August). *Teaching community psychology in Australia.* Paper presented at the 38th meeting of the Australian Psychological Society, Townsville, Australia.

Ferris, L., & Squire, D. S. (1992). Canadian community psychology: A view from the section of the Canadian Psychological Association (CPA). *The Community Psychologist, 25,* 16–18.

Finzen, A., & Schädle-Deininger, H. (1979). *"Unter elenden menschenunwürdigen Umständen:" Die Psychiatrie-Enquête.* Wunstorf, Germany: Psychiatrie-Verlag.

Fisher, A. (1992). Community psychology in Australia. *The Community Psychologist, 25,* 19–20.

Fisher, A., & Bishop, B. (1994). Australian Psychological Society. *The Community Psychologist, 27,* 15.

Fisher, A. T., Karnilowicz, W., & Ngo, D. (1994). Researching the provision of intellectual disability services in a Vietnamese community in Australia. *The Community Psychologist, 27,* 13–14.

Fliegel, S., & Röhrle, B. (Eds.). (1983). *Gemeindepsychologische perspektiven*, Vols. 1–4. Tübingen, Germany: DGVT.
Foucault, M. (1973). *Madness and civilization. A history of insanity in the age of reason*. New York: Vintage.
Foucault, M. (1987). *Mental illness and psychology*. Berkeley: University of California Press.
Francescato, D. (1977). *Psicologia di comunità*. Milan, Italy: Feltrinelli.
Francescato, D. (1984). *Tecniche di facilitazione dei gruppi di lavoro. Considerazioni su esperizienze di formazione con delegati sindacali, operatori del tempo libero ed operatori sociosanitari*. Congresso SIPS, Bergamo, Unicoepli, Milan, Italy.
Francescato, D., Contesini, A., & Dini, S. (Eds.). (1983). *Psicologia di comunità: Esperianze a confronto*. Rome: Il Pensiero Scientifico.
Francescato, D., & Ghirelli, G. (1988a). *Nuovi sviluppi in psicologia di comunità*. Rome: La Nuova Italia Scientifica.
Francescato, D., & Ghirelli, G. (1988b). Old age in Italy. *The Community Psychologist, 22*, 8.
Francescato, D., & Ghirelli, G. (1988c). *Fondamenti di psicologia di comunità*. Rome: La Nuova Italia Scientifica.
Francescato, D., & Putton, A. (1986, April). *Effectiveness of humanistic classroom techniques for the development of social and interpersonal skills in elementary school children*. Paper presented at the American Educational Research Association Conference, San Francisco.
Francescato, D., Putton, A., & Cudini, S. (1986a). *Star bene insieme a scuola*. Rome, Italy: La Nuova Italia Scientifica.
Francescato, D., Putton, A., & Cudini, S. (1986b, September). *Effectiveness of humanistic classroom techniques for the development of social and interpersonal skills in nursery, elementary, and junior high school children*. Paper presented at the Benefits of Psychology Conference, Lausanne, Switzerland.
Francescato, D., & Tulli, F. (1982). Community psychology in Italy: An emerging profession in a changing social context. *Division of Community Psychology Newsletter, 15*, 22–23.
Franzkowiak, P., & Wenzel, E. (1985). Die Gesundheiterziehung im Übergang zur Gesundheitsförderung—Konzeptionen und Praxisansätze zwischen biomedizinischem Modell und ökologischen Perspektiven. *Verhaltenstherapie und Psychosoziale Praxis, 17*, 240–256.
Freeman, D., & Trute, B. (Eds.). (1983). Family mental health practice in Canada [Special issue]. *Canadian Journal of Community Mental Health, 2*, entire issue.
Freire, P. (1971). *La educación como practica de libertad*. México: Siglo XXI.
Freire, P. (1972). *Pedagogia del oprimido*. México: Siglo XXI.
Froscia, G., & Fuccio, A. (1987). *Ambiente e salute: progretto sperimentale per l'educazione socioaffettiva in una scuola superiore*. Paper presented at the Convention of the Division of Community Psychology, Castiglioncello, Livorno, Italy.
Fuss, R. (Ed.). (1984). *Gesundsein 2000. Wege und vorschläge*. Berlin: Verlagsgesellschaft Gesundheit.
Garcia-Averasturi, L. (1985). Community health psychology in Cuba. *Journal of Community Psychology, 13*, 117–123.
Gardner, J., & Veno, A. (1979). An interdisciplinary, multilevel, university based training program in community psychology. *American Journal of Community Psychology, 7*, 605–620.
Garwolinska, I. (1979). Oaza ciszy. *Zdrowie i Trzezwosc, 7*, 2.
Gasseau, M., & Festini, Cucco W. (1983). Il day hospital psichiatrico negli Stati Uniti ed in Italia. In D. Francescato, A. Contesini, & S. Dini (Eds.), *Psicologia di comunità: Esperianze a confronto* (pp. 223–236). Rome: Il Pensiero Scientifico.
Genco, R. D. (1987). *Consultorio familiare e nuova professionalità: Risultati di una indagine esplorativa sul lavoro di equipe nei consultori familiari di due provincie pugliesi*. Paper presented at the Convention of the Division of Community Psychology, Castiglioncello, Livorno, Italy.
Gergen, K. (1985). The social constructivist movement in social psychology. *American Psychologist, 40*, 266–275.
Gething, L. (1997). Providing services in remote and rural Australian communities. *Journal of Community Psychology, 25*, 209–226.
Giammarco, I., Legge, E., Napolitano, I., Scipione, M., Visioni, A., & Vivarelli, F. (1986). *Esposizione dati d'una indagine relativa agli psicologi abruzzesi*. Paper presented at the Convention of the Division of Community Psychology, L'Aquila, Italy.
Gibson, D. (1974). enculturation stress in Canadian Psychology. *Canadian Psychologist, 15*, 145–151.
Gonzalez-Rey, F. (1989). *La salud en Cuba y el estudio de la personalidad*. Invited address at the Department of Psychology, University of Puerto Rico, Río Piedras.
Grau, D. (1986). *Aspectos relacionados con la participación comunitaria ante un problema de desarrollo vial urbano*. Unpublished bachelor's thesis, Universidad Central, Caracas, Venezuela.
Guay, J. (Ed.). (1987). *Manual Québeçois de psychologie communautaire*. Quebec: Chicoutimi: Gaétan Morin.
Hamerton, H., Nikora, L. W., Robertson, N., & Thomas, D. (1995). Community psychologiy in Aotearoa/New Zealand. *The Community Psychologist, 28*, 21–23.

Harvey, D., & Hodgson, J. (1995). New directions for research and practice in psychology in rural areas. *Australian Psychologist, 30*, 196–199.

Hobfoll, S. (1985). Israel. *Community Psychologist, 19*, 23–24.

Hobfoll, S. E. (1986). *Stress, social support and women.* Washington, D.C.: Hemisphere.

Holdstock, T. L. (1981). Psychology in South Africa belongs to the colonial era. Arrogance or ignorance? *South African Journal of Psychology, 11*, 123–129.

Hornblow, A. R. (1985). Preventive and promotional goals of community mental health services. In P. Berner (Ed.), *The state of the art* (pp. 331–336). New York: Plenum.

Hornblow, A. R. (1986). The evaluation and effectiveness of telephone counselling services. *Hospital and Community Psychiatry, 37*, 731–733.

Irizarry, A., & Serrano-Garcia, I. (1979). Intervención en la investigación: Su aplicación al Barrio Buen Consejo, Río Piedras, PR. *Boletin de la AVEPSO, 1*, 1–13.

Jaffe, P. (Ed.). (1988). Wife battering: A Canadian perspective [Special issue]. *Canadian Journal of Community Mental Health, 7*(2).

Kenworthy, E. (1985). Cuba's experiment with local democracy. *Journal of Community Psychology, 13*, 194–203.

Keupp, H. (1978). Gemeindepsychologie als Widerstandsanalyse des professionellen Selbstverständnisses. In H. Keupp & M. Zaumseil (Eds.), *Die gesellschaftliche organisierung psychischen leidens* (pp. 180–220). Frankfurt, Germany: Suhrkamp.

Keupp, H. (1980). Gemeindepsychologie. In R. Asanger & G. Wenninger (Eds.), *Handwörterbuch der psychologie* (pp. 162–167). Weinheim, Germany: Beltz.

Keupp, H. (1986). Gemeindepsychologie. In D. Frey & S. Greif (Eds.), *Sozialpsychologie—Ein Handbuch in Schlüsselbegriffen*, 2nd ed. Munich, Germany: Psychologie Verlags Union.

Keupp, H., & Rerrich, D. (Eds.). (1982). *Psychosoziale Praxis—Gemeindepsychologische Perspektiven.* Munich, Germany: Urban & Schwarzenberg.

Keupp, H., & Röhrle, B. (Eds.). (1987). *Soziale Netzwerke.* Frankfurt, Germany: Campus.

Keupp, H., & Stark, W. (1992). Community psychology in the Federal Republic of Germany. *The Community Psychologist, 25*, 21–22.

Keupp, H., & Zaumseil, M. (Eds.). (1978). *Die gesellschaftliche Organisierung psychischen Leidens.* Frankfurt, Germany: Suhrkamp.

Kirkby, R. J. (1978). Psychology manpower in health delivery in Victoria. *Australian Psychology, 13*, 193–207.

Kleiber, D. (Ed.). (1985). *Von der klinischen Psychologie zur psychosozialen Praxis.* Tübingen, Germany: DGVT.

Kleiber, D. (1988). Protokoll des 1. Treffens "Münchner Gesprächskreis zur Gemeindepsychologie." *Verhaltenstherapie und Psychosoziale Praxis, 20*, 225–226.

Kleiber, D., & Rommelspacher, B. (Eds.). (1986). *Die Zukunft des Helfens.* Weinheim, Germany: Psychologie Verlags Union.

Krause Jacob, M. (1991). The practice of community psychology in Chile. *Applied Psychology: An International Review, 40*, 143–163.

Laicardi, C. (1985). *La qualità della vita nella terza eta.* Rome: Il Pensiero Scientifico.

Lalonde, M. (1974). *A new perspective on the health of Canadians.* Ottawa: National Health and Welfare.

Lane, S. T. M., & Sawaia, B. B. (1991). Community social psychology in Brazil. *Applied Psychology: An International Review, 40*, 119–142.

Lazarus, S. (1985, October). *The role and responsibilities of the psychologist in the South African social context: Survey of psychologists' opinions.* Paper presented at the 3rd National Congress of the Psychological Association of South Africa, Pretoria, South Africa.

Lazarus, S. (1988). *The role of the psychologist in South African Society: In search of an appropriate community psychology.* Doctoral dissertation, University of Cape Town, South Africa.

Lazarus, S., & Prinsloo, R. (1995). Community psychology in South Africa. *The Community Psychologist, 28*, 24–26.

Leone, L., & Corsetti, M. T. (1987). *Progretto di educazione sessuale a genitri di ragazzi della scuola media inferiore.* Paper presented at the Convention of the Division of Community Psychology, Castiglioncello, Livorno, Italy.

Levine, M. (Ed.) (1989). Community psychology in Asia [Special Section]. *American Journal of Community Psychology, 17*, 67–145.

Llovera, J. (1984). Que occure con la acción popular? *SIC, XLVII*, 467.

Loaiza, R. (1984). *Locus de control en la organización popular.* Unpublished bachelor's thesis, Universidad Central, Caracas, Venezuela.

López, M., & Zuñiga, R. (1988). *Perspectivas críticas de la psicología social.* Río Piedras, PR: Editorial de la U.P.R.

López, M., Vázquez, M., & Macksoud, S. (1988). La ideología del trabajo y la formación de la conciencia: Notas para el desarrollo de un objecto de estudio. In M. López & R. Zuñiga (Eds.), *Perspectivas críticas de la psicología social* (pp. 383–426). Río Piedras, PR: Editorial de la U.P.R.

Maduro, O. (1985). El profesional en los procesos populares. *SIC, XLVIII*, 477.
Marin, B. V. (1985). Community psychology in Cuba: A literature review. *Journal of Community Psychology, 13*, 138–154.
Marin, G. (1978). La psicología social y el desarrollo de la America Latina. *Boletin de la AVEPSO, 1*, 1–13.
Markova, I. (1997). The individual and the community: A post-communist perspective. *Journal of Community and Applied Psychology, 7*, 3–17.
Martini, R. (1983). Progretto di formazione dello psicologo di territorio. In D. Francescato, A. Contesini, & S. Dini (Eds.), *Psicologia di comunita: Esperianze a confronto* (pp. 305–321). Rome: Il Pensiero Scientifico.
Martini, E. R., & Sequi, R. (1988). *Il lavoro nella comunità.* Rome: La Nuova Italia Scientifica.
McCannell, K. (Ed.). (1986). Women and mental health [special issue]. *Canadian Journal of Community Mental Health, 6*.
McNett, I. (1981). Deinstitutionalization in Italy: More politics than economics. *APA Monitor, 12*, 9.
Milgram, N. A. (Guest Ed.) (1982). In C. D. Spielberger & I. G. Sarason (Eds.), *Stress and anxiety*, Vol. 8. Washington, D.C.: Hemisphere.
Milgram, N. A. (1986). *Stress and coping in times of war: Generalizations from the Israeli experience.* New York: Brunner/Mazel.
Molano, A. (1977). Acción-investigatión. Teoría y practica. In *Anales del Simposio Mundial sobre Investigación Activa y Analisis Cientifico.* Cartagena: Punta de Lanza.
MONAR. (1984). *Problemy narkomanii: Zarys metod resocjalizacji i profilaktyki "Monaru".* Warsaw, Poland: Panstwowy Zaklad Wydawnictw Lekarskich.
Montero, M. (1978). Para una psicología social historica. *Boletín de la AVEPSO, 1*, 1–7.
Montero, M. (1980). La dinamica de grupos y el desarrollo de comunidades en America Latina. *Revista Latinoamericana de Psicología, 12*, 159–170.
Montero, M. (1982). Fundamentos teoricos de la psicología comunitaria en Latinoamerica. *Boletín de la AVEPSO, V*, 15–22.
Montero, M. (1984). la psicología comunitaria: Origenes, principios y fundamentos teoricos. *Revista Latinoamericana de Psicología, 16*, 387–400.
Montero, M. (1987, May). *Roles and scope of community psychology in Venezuela.* Paper presented at the First Biennial Conference on Community Research and Action, Columbia, SC.
Montero, M. (1995). Community psychology in Venezuela. *The Community Psychologist, 28*, 27–30.
Montero, M. (1996). Parallel lives: Community psychology in Latin America and the United States. *American Journal of Community Psychology, 24*, 589–605.
Montero, M. (1998). Dialectic between active minorities and majorities: A study of social influence in the community. *Journal of Community Psychology, 26*, 281–289.
Moody, E., Markova, I., Farr, R., & Plichtova, J. (1997). The meaning of community and of the individual in Slovakia and in Scotland. *Journal of Community and Applied Social Psychology, 7*, 19–31.
Moscovici, S. (1976). *Society against nature: The emergence of human societies.* Atlantic Highlands, NJ: Humanities Press.
Mühlum, A., Olschowy, G., Oppl, H., & Wendt, W. R. (1986). *Umwelt-Lebenswelt.* Frankfurt, Germany: Diesterweg.
Necki, Z., & Tokarz, A. (1980). Problemy psychospoleczne. In S. Nowakowski (Ed.), *Szansa malych miast: Lancut* (pp. 40–54). Cracow, Poland: Krajowa Agencja Wydawnicza.
Nelson, G. (Ed.). (1987). Community mental health services for the chronically mentally disabled [special issue]. *Canadian Journal of Community Mental Health, 6*(2).
Nelson, G., & Tefft, B. (1982). A survey of graduate education in community psychology in Canada. *Canadian Journal of Community Mental Health, 1*, 6–13.
Noventa, A., Nava, R., & Olivia, F. (1987). *I gruppi di self-help e la promozione della salute: Indagine in tema di malattie oncologiche e alcoolismo.* Congresso SIPS, Venezia, Guerini, Milan, Italy.
Ocando, A., & Montero, M. (1981). Ensenañza de la psicologia comunitaria en Venezuela: Una experiencia. *Boletin de la AVEPSO, IV*, 8–12.
Orford, J. (1995). Community psychology in Great Britain. *The Community Psychologist, 28*, 30–32.
Ortiz, B. (1987). *The Puerto Rican socio-political environment and community psychology.* Paper presented at the First Biennial Conference on Community Research and Action, Columbia, SC.
Orwid, M., Badura, W., Bomba, J., Mamrot, E., & Jaworska-Franczak, E. (1981). The main psychotherapeutic trends in Poland with special attention to the Department of Psychiatry of Child and Adolescent Psychiatry in Cracow. *Journal of Adolescence, 4*, 67–78.
Pagnin, U. (1985). *Guidizo morale in una comunità residenziale di adolescenti.* Seminar SIPS on Adolescents and Social Services, Bologna, Italy.
Palmonari, A. (Ed.). (1981). *Psicología.* Bologna, Italy: Il Mulino.

Palmonari, A., & Zani, B. (1980). *Psicología social di comunita.* Bologna, Italy: Il Mulino.

Pancer, M. (Ed.). (1984). Program evaluation: A participatory approach [special issue]. *Canadian Journal of Community Mental Health, 4*(2).

Pasek, T. (1982). Cwiczenia relaksowo-koncentrujace jako jedna z form rehabilitacji chorych psychicznie. *Psychiatria Polska, 16,* 371–375.

Patiño, T. (1985). *Dinamica de grupos para la participación popular.* Unpublished master's thesis, Universidad Central de Venezuela, Caracas, Venezuela.

Patiño, T., & Millan, Y. (1979). *Analisis comparativo de dos investigaciones de campo en desarrollo comunitario.* Unpublished bachelor's thesis, Universidad Central, Caracas, Venezuela.

Perez-Stable, E. (1985). Community medicine in Cuba. *Journal of Community Psychology, 13,* 124–137.

Polenta, G., & Cozzi, E. (1987). *Educazione alla sessualità: U progetto operativo.* Paper presented at the Convention of the Division of Community Psychology, Castiglioncello, Livorno, Italy.

Polli-Charmet, G. P. (1984). *Operatore interomedio e strutture intermedie in psichiatria.* Congress SIPS, Bergamo, Unicoepli, Milan, Italy.

Pretty, G., Conroy, C., Dugay, J., Fowler, D., & Williams, D. (1996). Sense of community and its relevance to adolescents of all ages. *Journal of Community Psychology, 24,* 365–379.

Raeburn, J. M. (1986). Towards a sense of community: Comprehensive projects and community houses. *Journal of Community Psychology, 14,* 391–398.

Raeburn, J. M. (1987). People projects: Planning and evaluation in a new era. *Health Promotion* (Canada), *25,* 2–13.

Raeburn, J. M. (1992). The PEOPLE system: Towards a community-led process of social change. In D. R. Thomas & A. Veno (Eds.), *Psychology and social change: Creating an international agenda.* (pp. 115–131). Palmerston North, New Zealand: Dunmore.

Raeburn, J. M., Autumn, J., & Whacker, C. (1991). *"Headway:" Evaluation of an innovative community-based rehabilitation program for the long-term mentally ill.* Waikato Area Health Board, Thames, New Zealand. Unpublished monograph.

Raeburn, J. M., & Seymour, F. W. (1979). A simple systems model for community programs. *Journal of Community Psychology, 7,* 290–297.

Reid, A., & Aguilar, M. A. (1991). Constructing community-social psychology in Mexico. *Applied Psychology: An International Review, 40,* 181–199.

Rivera-Medina, E., & Serrano-García, I. (1991). El desarrollo de la psicología de comunidad en America Latina. *Revista de Ciencias de la Conducta, 4,* 23–45.

Rivera-Medina, E., Cintron, C., & Bauermeister, J. J. (1978). Developing a community psychology training program in Puerto Rico. *Journal of Community Psychology, 6,* 316–319.

Robertson, N. (1985). *Evaluation of research feedback: The Mobile Workforce Project* (Mobile Workforce Project Report No. 3). Hamilton, New Zealand: University of Waikato.

Robertson, N. R., Thomas, D. R., Dehar, M., & Blaxall, M. (1989). Development of community psychology in New Zealand: A Waikato perspective. *New Zealand Journal of Psychology, 18,* 13–24.

Röhrle, B., & Stark, W. (Eds.). (1985). *Soziale Stützsysteme und Netzwerke im Kontext klinisch—psychologischer praxis.* Tübingen, Germany: DGVT.

Rossati, A. (1981). *Verso una nuova identità dello psicologo.* Milan, Italy: Angeli.

Rudeck, R. (1983). Beratungs-und kontaktarbeit im stadtteil. Eine "gemeindepsychologische" perspektive? In S. Fliegel & B. Röhrle (Eds.), *Gemeindepsychologische Perspektiven,* Vol. 1 (pp. 170–175). Tübingen, Germany: DGVT.

Salamanca, L. (1985). El movimiento vecinal en Venezuela. *SIC, XLVIII,* 477.

Sánchez, E., Wiesenfeld, E., & Cronick, K. (1991). Community social psychology in Venezuela. *Applied Psychology: An International Review, 40,* 219–236.

Santi, B., Silva, I., & Colmenares, F. (1979). *Desarrollo comunal en la Urbanización Urdaneta, en Catia.* Unpublished bachelor's thesis, Universidad Central, Caracas, Venezuela.

Santiago, L., & Perfecto, G. (1983). *Hacia el encuentro de la psicología social comunitaria y el cristianismo en un esfuerzo investigativo con enfasis en la participación comunitaria.* Unpublished master's thesis, University of Puerto Rico, Río Piedras.

Sardella, M. V. (1985). *Teoria e tecniche dell'evaluation.* Milan, Italy: Clued.

Serrano-García, I. (1983). The illusion of empowerment: Community development within a colonial context. *Prevention in Human Services, 3,* 173–200.

Serrano-García, I. (1987, May). *The development of community psychology in Latin America: An overview.* Paper presented at the First Biennial Conference on Community Research and Action, Columbia, SC.

Serrano-García, I. (1990). Implementing research: Putting our values to work. In P. Tolan, L. Jason, & C. Keys (Eds.), *Researching community psychology* (pp. 171–182). Washington, D.C.: American Psychological Association.

Serrano-García, I., Costa, S. M., Perfecto, G., & Quiros, C. (1980). *The University of Puerto Rico position paper.* Paper presented at the University of South Florida Community Psychology Conference, Tampa, FL.

Serrano-García, I., & Alvarez, S. (1985, July). *Analisis de marcos conceptuales de la psicología de comunidad en America Latina y Estados Unidos (1960–1980).* Master lecture presented at the Congress of the Interamerican Society of Psychology, Caracas, Venezuela.

Serrano-García, I., & López-Sánchez, G. (1991). Community interventions in Puerto Rico: The impact of social-community psychology. *Applied psychology: An international review, 40,* 201–218.

Serrano-García, I., & López-Sánchez, G. (1991, July). *Una perspectiva diferente del poder y el cambio social para la Psicología Social-Comunitaria.* Master lecture presented at the Interamerican Congress of Psychology, San José, Costa Rica.

Serrano-García, I., López, M., & Rivera-Medina, E. (1987). Toward a social community psychology. *Journal of Community Psychology, 15,* 431–446.

Serrano-García, I., Cantera, L., & Mirón, L. (Eds.). (1995). *Memorias de psicología comunitaria del Congreso Interamericano de Psicología.* San Juan: Puerto Rico: XXV Congreso Interamericano de Psicología.

Serrano-García, I., & Rivera-Medina, E. (1985, October). *El desarrollo de la psicologia de comunidad en America Latina.* Paper presented at ITESO University, Guadalajara, Mexico.

Serrano-García, I., & Rosario Collazo, W. (1992). *Contribuciones Puertorriquenas a psicologia.* Río Piedras, PR: Editorial de la Universidad de Puerto Rico.

Skutle, A. (1995). Community psychology in Norway. *The Community Psychologist, 28,* 33–35.

Smith, R. L. (1977). A further look at the role of the psychologists in community mental health care. *Australian Psychologist, 12,* 151–156.

Sommer, G., & Ernst, H. (Eds.). (1977). *Gemeindepsychologie.* Munich, Germany: Urban & Schwarzenberg.

Sommer, G., Kommer, B., Kommer, D., Malchow, C., & Quack, L. (1978). Gemeindepsychologie. In L. J. Pongratz (Ed.), *Handbuch der klinischen Psychologie* (pp. 2913–2979). Göttingen, Germany: Hogrefe.

Sonn, C. C., & Fisher, A. T. (1996). Psychological sense of community in a politically constructed group. *Journal of Community Psychology, 24,* 417–430.

Sonn, C. C., & Fisher, A. T. (1998). Sense of community: Community resilient responses to oppression and change. *Journal of Community Psychology, 26,* 457–471.

Spaltro, E. (1981). *Soggettivita.* Bologna, Italy: Patron.

Spaltro, E. (1985). *Pluralita.* Bologna, Italy: Patron.

Stark, W. (1986). The politics of primary prevention in mental health: The need for a theoretical basis. *Health Promotion, 1,* 179–185.

Steyn, D. P. (1985). *Relevant psychology in practice.* Paper presented at the 3rd Annual Congress of the Psychological Association of South Africa, Pretoria.

Swartz, L. (1986). *Some issues about professionalism in current South African psychology.* Paper presented in the Africa Seminar, Centre for African Studies, University of Cape Town, South Africa.

Tefft, B. (Ed.). (1982). Community psychology in Canada [special issue]. *Canadian Journal of Community Mental Health, 1*(2).

Tefft, B., Hamilton, G. N., & Théroux, C. (1982). Community psychology in Canada: Toward developing a national network. *Canadian Journal of Community Mental Health, 1,* 93–103.

Thomas, D. R. (Ed.). (1979). *Community psychology research record 2* (Psychology Research Series No. 10). Hamilton, New Zealand: University of Waikato, Psychology Department.

Thomas, D. R. (Ed.). (1982). *Community psychology research record 3: Marijuana in New Zealand: Use, police detection and judicial action* (Psychology Research Series No. 14). Hamilton, New Zealand: University of Waikato.

Thomas, D. R. (Ed.). (1983). *Development of evaluation research for social services* (Psychology Research Series No. 16). Hamilton, New Zealand: University of Waikato, Psychology Department.

Thomas, D. R., O'Driscoll, D., & Robertson, N. (1984). *The mobile workforce in New Zealand: Social network development, health and well-being* (Mobile Workforce Project Report No. 3). Hamilton, New Zealand: University of Waikato.

Thomas, D. R., & Robertson, N. R. (1989). *Evaluation of human services* (Psychology Research Series No. 20). Hamilton, New Zealand: University of Waikato.

Thomas, D. R., & Robertson, N. R. (1992). Evaluation of human services: Conceptualization and planning. In D. R. Thomas & A. Veno (Eds.), *Psychology and social change: creating a international agenda* (pp. 191–207). Palmerston North, New Zealand: Dunmore.

Thomas, D. R., & Thomas, Y. L. (1985). *Redirection of at-risk young people.* (Psychology Research Series No. 18). Hamilton, New Zealand: University of Waikato.

Thomas, D. R., & Veno, A. (1987). *The development and localization of community psychology in New Zealand and Australia.* Paper presented at the annual conference of the New Zealand Psychological Society, Wellington.

Thomas, D. R., & Veno, A. (1992). *Psychology and social change: Creating an international agenda.* Palmerston North, New Zealand: Dunmore.

Toro, P. A. (Ed.). (1990). Feature: International community psychology. *The Community Psychologist, 24,* 3–18.

Traversi, M., & Tavazza, G. (1986). Psicologia di comunità e volontariato. *Rassegna di servizio sociale, 2,* 10–18.

Tyszkowa, M. (1972). *Zachowania sie dzieci szkolnych w sytuacjach trudnych.* Warsaw, Poland: Panstwowe Wydawnictwa Naukowe.

Ugolini, A., Francescato, D., & Ghirelli, G. (1987). *Lo sviluppo della socializzaione in un gruppo di anziani.* Congresso SIPS, Venezia, Guerini, Milan, Italy.

Uriarte-Gaston, M. B., & Magarida, M. T. (1987, May). *Community mental health services in Cuba: The challenge of the third decade.* Paper presented at the First Biennial Conference on Community Research and Action, Columbia, SC.

Varela, J. (1971). *Psychological solutions to social problems: An introduction to social psychology.* New York: Academic.

Veno, A. (1982). A preliminary conceptual analysis of the role of community psychology in Australia. *Australian Psychologist, 17,* 239–253.

Veno, A. (1987). The rise and fall of an alternative setting: An Australian case study. *Journal of Community Psychology, 15,* 123–131.

Veno, A., & Gardner, J. (1979). An evaluation of a community psychology based program of police training. *Journal of Community Psychology, 7,* 210–219.

Veno, A., & Thomas, D. R. (1992). Psychology and the process of social change. In D. R. Thomas & A. Veno (Eds.), *Psychology and social change: creating a international agenda.* Palmerston North, New Zealand: Dunmore.

Veno, A., & Veno, E. (1987). Towards a community psychology of public order policing. *The Community Psychologist, 21,* 30.

Viney, L. L. (Ed.) (1974). The role of the psychologist in community health care. *Australian Psychologist, 9*(Suppl. 2), 22.

Viney, L. L. (1985). "They call you a dole bludger": Some experiences of unemployment. *Journal of Community Psychology, 13,* 31–45.

Vogelman, L. (1987). The development of an appropriate psychology: The work of the organization of appropriate social services in South Africa. *Psychology in Society, 7,* 24–35.

Volpi, C., & Ghirelli, G. (1987). *Un'indagine conoscitiva sui gruppi di self help in Toscana.* Congresso SIPS, Venezia, Guerini, Milan, Italy.

Walsh, R. T. (1988). Current developments in community psychology in Canada. *Journal of Community Psychology, 16,* 296–305.

Wenzel, E. (Ed.). (1986). *Die Ökologie des Körpers.* Frankfurt, Germany: Suhrkamp.

Western, C. (1983). Formative evaluation of alcohol services in the Waikato region. In D. R. Thomas (Ed.), *Community psychology research record 4* (Psychology Research Series No. 16). Hamilton, New Zealand: University of Waikato.

White, A. M., & Potgieter, C. A. (1996). Teaching community psychology in postapartheid South Africa. *Teaching of Psychology, 23,* 82–86.

Wiesenfeld, E. (1998). Paradigms of community social psychology in six Latin American nations. *Journal of Community Psychology, 26,* 229–242.

Wiesenfeld, E., & Sanchez, E. (Eds.). (1995). *Psicologia social-communitaria: Contributiones latinoamericanas.* Caracas, Venezuela: Fondo Ed. Tropykos.

Wilpert, B. (1991). Special issue: Latin America. *Applied Psychology: An International Review, 40,* 111–236.

Zaumseil, M. (1978). Institutionelle Aspekte klinisch-psychologischer Arbeit. In H. Keupp & M. Zaumseil (Eds.), *Die gesellschaftliche Organisierung psychischen Leidens* (pp. 15–28). Frankfurt, Germany: Suhrkamp.

Zwelky, S., & Perdomo, G. (1983). *La participación social como forma y modo de educación politica.* Unpublished bachelor's thesis, Universidad Central, Caracas, Venezuela.

CHAPTER 33

Psychology in the International Community

Perspectives on Peace and Development

RONALD ROESCH AND GEOFFREY CARR

The title we chose for this chapter reflects our view that the issues of peace and international development are inexorably related. The concept of peace is a difficult one to define. Many definitions focus on conflict or war, with peace defined as the absence of war. We consider peace to be not simply the absence of war, but also the perception that there is minimal threat of war. When the likelihood of war is so great as to be perceived as a genuine threat, continued prevention of war is often difficult to achieve. Thus, a primary goal for establishing peace must be to create an international community in which military intervention is not seen as a likely option for resolving conflict. Furthermore, our definition of peace incorporates a number of issues broadly related to social justice. Peace will not be achieved until we address some fundamental questions dealing with equality of people, world interdependence, economic fairness, unity, and social and international justice. Peace in this sense would, then, include activities aimed at reducing the likelihood of violence, as well as activities directed at promoting, as Alger (1987) noted, economic well-being, social justice, and ecological balance (see also Christie, 1997; Dobrosielski, 1987; Kimmel, 1995; Tucker, 1977).

In recent years the world has witnessed dramatic and far-reaching changes. The political scene has changed rapidly—changes that were inconceivable only a decade ago, such as those that have taken place in eastern Europe. But these changes also force us to see that enduring peace will not be obtained only through political realignments or military victories. Civil wars and regional conflicts continue, and in some areas have dramatically escalated.

Until the late 1980s, the nuclear race dominated world debate. Wagner (1988) commented that the buildup of armaments and the peace-through-deterrence approach are representative of negative approaches to peace—all strategies related to the negative goal of avoiding war.

RONALD ROESCH AND GEOFFREY CARR • Department of Psychology, Simon Fraser University, Burnaby, British Columbia V5A 1S6, Canada

Handbook of Community Psychology, edited by Julian Rappaport and Edward Seidman. Kluwer Academic / Plenum Publishers, New York, 2000.

The changes in armament policy may finally allow the nations of the world to shift from these negative approaches to peace, which have dominated the policies of most governments, to more positive means of establishing peace (Blumberg, 1998). In this chapter, we will consider some examples of positive approaches to peace, with a particular focus on the relevance of community psychology to peace and international development.

At first blush, the applicability of community psychology to international peace and development issues may not be apparent. It is our thesis that the principles and theories of social change upon which community psychology is based can indeed be applied to the development of peaceful relations in the world. Community psychology is premised on the theory that the problems experienced by many individuals grow out of adverse conditions, such as social inequality, prejudice, economic disparity, and other societal-level problems. Community psychologists interested in affecting the plight of individuals recognize that change strategies must focus on an understanding of those conditions in order to establish the conditions needed to create a more healthful and stable community or society. We suggest that the strategies and tactics that have been developed by community psychologists at the local level can be extended to global issues. To accomplish this, the issues of peace and international development must be framed in such a way as to allow a broader definition of the problems and potential solutions. This is a familiar process to community psychologists, since the field is based in large part on a reframing of the notions of mental health and mental illness (Seidman & Rappaport, 1986). It is our intent to illustrate that if the concept of peace is reframed, there is a clear role for community psychologists to play.

THE PRESENT CHALLENGE OF PEACE

It is clear that world problems are complex and interrelated, and that solutions to these problems must take into account the interdependence of the world's political, economic, and social structure. Because the arms race and ongoing wars compellingly attract our attention, it is easy to lose sight of the interrelated social and economic problems that affect, and are affected by, them. By failing to address these other problems, the cycles that promote war in the first place are perpetuated.

If one views peace in this broader perspective, various types of action and involvement needed to promote it become apparent. In particular, the involvement of individuals and citizen groups becomes a more promising possibility. In a review of research on reactions to nuclear war, Fiske (1987) concluded that most people do not worry much about nuclear war and, despite acknowledging that the effect of a nuclear war would be devastating, do not actively engage in activities to lessen the possibility of a nuclear war (see also Boehnke & Schwartz, 1997; Frydenberg & Lewis, 1996). While this may, in part, be attributed to apathy, it is also likely that many people do not believe a nuclear war is a likely event. Fiske argues that the apparent apathy is also due to a sense of powerlessness, a belief that there really is little one can do to influence policies regarding nuclear armament. Whether this belief is true is of course arguable, but the relevance of this for the purpose of this chapter is that community psychologists interested in getting involved in peace activities must take this belief into account. We believe that it is possible to mobilize citizens into action if they believe that there is something potentially important that they can contribute. Citizen involvement in promoting peace will increase if the focus of attention is expanded to social issues other than nuclear disarmament that can also advance peace. If the peace issues were framed in other ways, the average citizen might feel more instrumental in affecting change. As Fiske (1987) concludes, "one must find a way to give people a sense of political efficacy or what I would call 'hope through action' " (p. 215). This is clearly an example of empowerment.

As suggested by our definition of peace, we believe psychology has important contributions to make to the establishment of peace because of its focus on the social issues that are fundamental to it as a concept. In this chapter, we will examine these potential contributions, including the role of psychology as an organization, theory and research on intergroup and international conflict, and the specific contributions of community psychology.

CONTRIBUTIONS OF PSYCHOLOGY AS AN ORGANIZATION

There has been considerable debate about whether psychology as a profession should be involved in peace issues. Indeed, there is a lack of agreement within the profession about whether psychology should make official public statements at all (Blight, 1987; McConnell, Brown, Ruffing, Strupp, Duncan, & Kurdek, 1986; Mayor, 1995; Morawski & Goldstein, 1986). Such debates are likely to continue for some time. It is our belief that psychology can contribute to the debate about war and peace, and we will endeavor to suggest ways in which psychologists and the profession of psychology can be involved.

It is useful to make a distinction between two types of contributions that psychology can make to the goal of achieving peace. The first type has to do with the impact that psychology as an organization, representing thousands of psychologists, can have. The second refers to the scientific contributions made as a result of psychological research and theory as applied to peace issues.

The professional organizations of psychology have made public statements about the role and relevance of psychology with respect to the prevention of war and the achievement of peace (e.g., Abeles, 1983). The American Psychological Association established a division of psychology and peace. These activities are important in establishing the concern of the profession of psychology. Many psychologists belong to organizations like Psychologists for Social Responsibility, and are active in peace studies. However, the involvement of psychologists has been sporadic. While a majority of psychologists report that they read about and discuss the nuclear war issue, most have not been actively engaged (Polyson, Stein, & Sholley, 1986).

International conflict involves large numbers of people, yet we would suggest that it is critical not to lose sight of the individual. Structured changes will only work to reduce conflict if they consider the needs of the individual. Wars are promoted by the fact that they do meet certain motivational/psychological needs of group members, and are unlikely to end unless those needs are adequately met in another way. In the next section, we will review the research and theory on intergroup and international conflict in order to illustrate how research might be of central importance in achieving the goal of peace. Specifically, we will discuss how the need for self-esteem and for the expression of aggression are met by, and thereby promote, war.

THEORY AND RESEARCH ON INTERGROUP AND INTERNATIONAL CONFLICT

A major way that psychologists can, and have attempted to, make contributions to the problem of international conflict is by applying their skills as researchers on human behavior.

International conflict is a product of human behavior and we are therefore well-positioned to make contributions toward its understanding. This section will provide a brief introduction to some of this research and its conclusions.

Realistic Conflict

The simplest way of conceiving of intergroup conflict is that it results from competition for material resources. If a resource is limited (e.g., water, food, land) and more than one group wants it, then these incompatible interests may be expected to result in competitive conflict in order to win the resource. This common view of intergroup conflict (formally called realistic conflict theory, Taylor & Moghaddem, 1987) frequently has at least an element of truth to it. It is also clear that in many wars, material resources do not appear to be the primary factor in the conflict. In these cases, other "psychological" motives seem to be prominent. Revenge for a transgression (e.g., killing of group members), retribution over wounded group pride or self-esteem, or simply the "macho" pride involved in a display of power are all common motives for intergroup aggression. These factors have the potential to maintain intense conflict in cases without a "realistic" basis, or after the realistic basis that initially sparked the conflict ceases to be an issue. However, it is noteworthy that groups with substantial basis for conflict over resources may express minimal intergroup hostility (e.g., the United States and Canada). In summary, although realistic conflict over limited resources is certainly a factor in intergroup conflict, the relationship between realistic conflict and actual aggression appears to be imperfect.

Group Dynamics

In order to understand conflict between groups, is it necessary to recognize some basic dynamics with groups. One basic factor that has important implications for group behavior is the self-esteem motive. In-groups provide a major source of self-esteem, both through direct expressions of praise or approval, and by permitting group members to identify with a group that is consensually agreed to be positive. We are motivated to have high regard for others in our group partly because it increases the value of the praise they give us (Turner, 1984).

Another motivational reason for valuing people in our group is their similarity to us. If we value some particular aspect of ourselves (e.g., a belief), then we are likely to positively evaluate others who share that aspect. Since they validate us and our beliefs, their value to us is increased (Berscheid & Walster, 1978). They will reciprocally value us for the same reasons, and this reciprocation serves to strengthen the group bond.

That boosting of self-esteem is a major factor in valuing our in-groups has been illustrated in studies that manipulated an individual's self-esteem. For example, Cialdini and coworkers (Cialdini, Bordon, Thorne, Walker, Freeman, & Sloan, 1976) found that, following an ego blow, people have a stronger tendency to identify themselves with a successful in-group than if self-esteem was left unperturbed.

The validation and boost to our self-esteem that is provided by others in our group is reflected in the pervasive group pressure for conformity. There appears to be an unspoken, yet universal, understanding that to differ with the group either in behavior or beliefs may be an affront to other group members. This affront could result in a loss of positive regard, or even outright wrath. Classic research by Solomon Asch (1956) illustrated that people will conform to other group members beliefs, even in a newly formed group of strangers and when the conformity involves rejecting one's own clear sensory impressions. This tendency to conform is stronger in more cohesive groups (e.g., Berkowitz, 1954). The importance of the self-esteem motive for conformity is reflected in the increased level of conformity that is elicited from subjects who have been made to feel incompetent (Myers, 1986).

In sum, we are motivated to value others in our group partly because of the support they offer to our self-esteem. By serving as a substantial source of esteem, the group gains considerable influence over its individual members.

Intergroup Relations

The above factors in the nature of human groups has important implications for understanding intergroup relations. One factor is that the self-esteem motive that promotes valuing of in-group members is not present for members of different out-groups. Thus, the in-group will tend to be seen as "better" than out-groups. This in-group bias can be taken even further. Value is partly determined by social comparison; i.e., one individual or group is better *relative to* another individual or group. Thus, one can perceive one's group as better by emphasizing and exaggerating the differences between the groups and by positively valuing the characteristics of one's own group.

This phenomenon was demonstrated in the classic boys' camp studies of Sherif and colleagues (Sherif, Harvey, White, Hood, & Sherif, 1961). Boys who believed they were at a regular summer camp were divided into two groups. In two of the studies all boys were together initially, and after spontaneous friendships had formed they were separated into two cabins such that most of each boy's friends were in the other cabin. In the third study (Robber's Cave), the boys were grouped without this initial period, and were initially kept unaware of the other group's existence until group cohesiveness had developed. Once some "chance" encounters introduced the other groups' existence, both were enthusiastic for the opportunity for intergroup competition. The competition began in a relatively friendly way, but soon became severely antagonistic. In the first two studies, the boys turned against former friends. At this phase, the in-group bias was clear. Each group's members perceived themselves to be playing fair, but the other group to be "cheats" who "played dirty." When describing characteristics of each group, "we" were "brave," "tough," and "friendly," but "they" were "sneaky," "smart alecks," and "stinkers." In a bean-collecting game, when each boy was repeatedly shown the same bag of beans, they consistently overestimated its contents when it was tagged as being from an in-group member and consistently underestimated the contents when it was tagged as being from the out-group. Thus, Sherif's studies illustrated the tendency to perceive exaggerated differences between groups in a way that establishes the superiority of the in-group over the out-group, and provides a rationalization for harming or exploiting out-group members (Opotow, 1990).

The importance of self-esteem as a motive in this phenomenon has been confirmed in many studies. Correlational studies have shown that when one's socioeconomic status or other contributors to a positive self-image are decreasing, negative attitudes towards out-groups tends to increase (e.g., Lemyre & Smith, 1985). Experimental studies have shown that when self-esteem is lowered (e.g., by being told one's score on a creativity test was low) people show a stronger bias in favor of their group (Cialdini & Richardson, 1980).

In summary, the motivation to maintain high self-esteem is a major factor in maintaining group cohesion, and promotes seeing other groups as being different from, and inferior to, one's own group.

The Role of Pride

One aspect of self-esteem is pride, which itself has several aspects that tend to contribute to intergroup conflict. The need to "save face" is one form of pride that tends to maintain or escalate a conflict once it has begun. Once investments have been made in a conflict, even if the original objectives are clearly unobtainable, groups do not tend to "cut their losses" and get out. This option would result in a loss of face due to the implication that it would acknowledge having made a mistake, or perhaps would suggest that the group is not sufficiently "tough" to continue. Once an out-group has been aggressive against the in-group, any losses also cause a lowering of group self-esteem or pride since the pretense to power is challenged by the defeat. This loss is also frustrating, and will therefore tend to elicit anger and a desire to aggress in the form of revenge. Thus, the wounded pride tends to trigger moral outrage and calls for revenge against the transgressions of the out-group.

This need to save face is abundantly apparent in leaders' comments during war. For example, President Johnson's speeches during the Vietnam War changed as the conflict escalated, with increasing reference to the importance of protecting America's honor and avoiding the humiliation of losing a war (Myers, 1986, p. 576).

This section began with emphasizing the self-esteem that can be derived from identifying oneself with a group that one values positively. Since most group members will share this desire to value this group over the other(s), there is a group collusion in assertions that this group is better than the other(s). This group pride (Frank, 1986) or group narcissism (Fromm, 1973) can fuel intergroup conflict via displacement of aggression as will be discussed in the following, but can also promote conflict more directly. "If we are better, then we deserve more than them." This belief can be used to rationalize demanding more of something, such as a limited resource, than another group, and thereby exacerbate the type of "realistic conflict" discussed earlier. In addition, group pride includes dimensions such as size and power in intergroup comparisons; bigger and stronger are better. This "macho pride" (White, 1984) motivates developing military strength, extending group influence, and extending group territory. The functional component of macho pride is clear. The resulting military strength allows the group to take limited resources from a less powerful group and to defend itself against out-group attacks. Obviously, military strength also serves the purpose of aiding in securing more territory. The possession of larger territory in turn serves to provide a greater quantity and variety of resources.

As referred to earlier, our need to believe in the morality and fairness of our aggression activates various mechanisms to rationalize and justify our behavior. In addition to seeing the in-group as more deserving of resources due to its superiority, moral pride can also be invoked (Frank, 1986). Moral pride is the rationalization that the in-group has an obligation to promote its superior ways to the out-group, even by imposing them. Thus, Christianity is brought to the heathen, we invade to combat godless communism, and they invade to combat capitalist imperialism. Aggression is thereby perpetuated in the name of morality.

Displaced Aggression

Another major factor in behavior toward the in-group is a relative lack of expressed aggression. Group and societal norms tend to have strong prohibitions against in-group hostility. In contrast, there is no prohibition against acting aggressively towards out-group members. Therefore, if frustrated by members of an out-group (perhaps over scarce resources), aggression is a more likely response. However, the out-group members will not merely receive this aggression, but in addition will also receive the displaced aggression that was not expressible to the in-group.

There is substantial empirical support for this view of displaced aggression fueling intergroup conflict. For example, lynchings of black people in the southern U.S. increased during years of economic frustration produced by low cotton prices (in the 1881–1930 period; Mintz, 1946). Racial prejudice has also been increased by frustration in an experimental context. Men in the experimental group who were frustrated by being deprived of an expected night off showed increased prejudice towards Japanese and Mexicans relative to a non-frustrated control group (Miller & Begelshi, 1948).

In summary, the suppression of in-group aggression and displacement onto the out-group is a pervasive tendency in group behavior.

Justifying Aggression

However, the process does not end with aggression towards the out-group. Since the aggression includes displaced aggression from one's in-group, it would objectively appear that one's self or one's group had behaved unfairly towards the out-group. The need to perceive oneself as fair and just is also present in intergroup conflict. As noted earlier in the discussion of the boys' camp studies (Sherif et al., 1961), both groups perceived themselves as fair and the other group as "playing unfair." Thus, on the international level, *we* have "freedom fighters," *they* have "terrorists." Even the aggressions of Germany and Japan in WWII, England during its colonial expansion, U.S. activities in central America, and the USSR's activities in Eastern Europe have each been presented as reflecting fair, just, and moral behavior. We appear to have little tolerance for unfairness, whether perpetuated by others or by ourselves, but have an amazing capacity to perceive our behavior as being fair. To prevent and alleviate the distress (cognitive dissonance) produced by acting aggressively towards a relatively innocent out-group, enemy images are usually used.

Enemy Images

To permit violent aggression against the out-group in a way that is acceptable to our sense of fairness and that will not produce guilt, we first create an image of the "enemy" that is extremely different from us. This conclusion was reached by Keen (1986) during his cross-cultural studies on enemy images. Combined with our need to devalue the out-group, our need to see them as very different from ourselves before acting violently against them results in some common themes. We are good; they are evil. We are victims; they are the aggressors. We are honest; they are liars. We are fair; they are unfair. Groups at war have used common images to disparage their enemy. Propaganda typically involves portraying the enemies as devils, monsters, or animals, particularly vermin or reptiles. This dehumanization of the enemy allows us to see them as so different from us and so bad, that, like rats infesting our cities, they can be exterminated with little remorse.

COGNITIVE FACTORS

Fundamental Attribution Error

The fundamental attribution error is a pervasive tendency to attribute the behavior of others to dispositional or trait factors and to ignore the situational factors that would influence their behavior. The same phenomenon occurs in accounting for the behavior of out-groups and their members. Plous (1985) has documented this phenomenon with numerous quotes from American and Soviet officials. The attributions of the behavior of one's own country and "the other" country are in striking contrast. A summary of the positions is: We build weapons, etc., to provide security and defense for our nation in response to their aggressive military build-up; We will not be the aggressor; They build weapons because of a desire to spread their dominance using military power. In essence, although both sides build weapons, we do so because the situation we find ourselves in leaves us no choice, whereas they do so because they are aggressive and expansionistic.

Belief Perseverance

Another pervasive psychological phenomenon is that it typically takes considerably more evidence for us to change a belief than it does for us to form a belief in the first place. In intergroup conflict, the phenomenon is present most clearly in perpetuating judgments of the out-group's motives. Since these motives are attributed under the influence of the fundamental attribution error, and perpetuated by the belief perseverance phenomenon, they remain both inaccurate and rigidly held. The result is that virtually any out-group behavior can be interpreted as being consistent with a negative motive. In 1956, when the Soviet Union reduced their military forces by 1,200,000 men, 375 warships, and numerous other weaponry, American leaders accounted for it as a propaganda ploy with little military impact that reflected a "logical realignment of Russian military power" (Plous, 1985). One might predict, however, that U.S. officials would not have seen an increase of 1,200,000 men and 375 ships by the Soviets as quite so insignificant. During WWII, the possibility of Japanese-American subversive activity would seem to have appeared unlikely since there was absolutely no evidence for it. However, this didn't prevent the absurdity of the opposite conclusion being drawn. For example, then-Governor of California Earl Warren stated, "I take the view that this [lack of subversive activity] is the most ominous sign in our whole situation. It convinces me more than perhaps any other factor that the sabotage we are to get ... [is] timed just like Pearl Harbor was timed" (Daniels, 1975)

This notion of belief perseverance has implications for the resolution of international conflicts or disputes, especially when the beliefs are based on incorrect perceptions or judgments. As we will point out in the section on arms reduction, Deutsch (1985) views this as one of the main obstacles to a rational nuclear weapons agreement.

In summary, it appears, as Tetlock (1985) has suggested, that both sides in a conflict seem to have an unlimited capacity to view events in ways that support their initial positions.

Summary

This section has presented some of the fundamental factors that promote and perpetuate conflict between groups. Self-esteem serves as a primary motive in promoting group cohesion and indirectly devaluing other groups. One consequence of this is that anger may be displaced from the in-group to the out-group. By seeing the out-group as an inhumane, evil enemy, violent aggression is both promoted and justified. The aggression is also promoted by various types of pride and by a genuine fear of the out-group. Along with these more emotional factors, common aspects of human thinking, such as the fundamental attribution error and the belief perseverance phenomenon, have the effect of locking us into conflict since we are unable to see alternative solutions.

Although this brief overview is far from exhaustive, it does illustrate the complexity of the problem of violent conflict, and that no one solution is likely to serve as a panacea. The point of examining the basis for international conflict at the level of the individual's need for self-esteem is that structural interventions that are not informed by factors such as this are unlikely to succeed. If a war ends with the humiliating defeat of one group, the fighting may have ended, but it will likely resume as a battle for lost dignity. A United Nations resolution established the state of Israel, but the imposition of this decision on neighboring countries was an affront to their dignity that ensured continued conflict. Solutions that fail to attend to the dignity or self-esteem of the groups and individuals involved are not enduring solutions. Since many international conflicts are settled by a military victory of one group over another, the offended dignity and lowered self-esteem of the defeated group leave it predisposed to resume fighting at a more opportune time. The best chance at an enduring peace is achieved when a resolution arrived at cooperatively leaves both sides with pride intact. The concern of community psychology with issues of personal empowerment and development of competence clearly relate to the issue of self-esteem. The concern with developing a psychological sense of community, if extended to the international community, would promote the perception of an international in-group against whom aggression would not be acceptable. These ideas, as well as promotion of cooperation, will be developed in the following section.

PREVENTION OF WAR, PROMOTION OF PEACE

Dealing with Conflict

Conflict is unlikely to disappear from international relations, as there is a constant competition for scarce resources. These conflicts, inherent in two or more groups wanting the same thing, can be dealt with in many ways, violent confrontation being the least appealing option. Recently, a group of scientists from around the world met in Seville, Spain. They issued a statement, known as the Seville Statement on Violence, which challenged the view that violence is inherent in our nature (Adams, 1990). The conclusion from the psychological and other scientific literature is that even if we have a capacity or propensity for violence, it is necessary for certain environmental conditions to be apparent for that violence to emerge. On the other hand, it is just as possible, though perhaps more difficult, to create an environment that facilitates non-violent solutions to conflict. Johan Galtung, a professor of world politics of peace and war, wrote:

> That there is a selfish, competitive strain in individuals and nations alike, and that this may express itself in the direct violence released through offensive weaponry ... and violence—all this we know. Under certain conditions that is what comes out. But under other conditions the opposite comes out, altruism rather than egotism, cooperation rather than conflict and competition. Our task is to understand those conditions (Galtung, 1986, p. 85).

The goal in terms of prevention of violent confrontation is to understand these conditions and then mount interventions that may facilitate positive change (Galtung, 1998). There is considerable positive evidence that people can learn to use cooperative strategies instead of competitive ones. One example is the work of Deutsch (1985), a social psychologist who has conducted a number of interesting and creative studies of the effectiveness of different strategies for inducing cooperative behavior. He has examined several methods including: (1) the turn-the-other-cheek strategy, in which one side or individual seeks to elicit cooperation by being cooperative, no matter what the other side does; (2) the punitive-deterrent strategy, which rewards cooperation but punishes noncooperation; and (3) the nonpunitive strategy, which places an emphasis on rewarding cooperation by providing positive incentives and avoiding the use of punishment.

The nonpunitive strategy was consistently found to be the most effective in eliciting cooperative behavior. Subjects in the "turn the other cheek" condition were strongly exploited as the incentives for competition increased, while the punitive strategy elicited more aggressive and less cooperative responses.

In applying his research to foreign policy, Deutsch concludes that "a nonpunitive strategy that emphasizes protecting oneself rather than punitive retaliation in response to aggression is much less likely to provoke aggression and much more apt to elicit cooperation" (p. 169).

The emphasis on cooperation rather than aggression or, more typically, the threat of aggression, has been referred to as a peace through cooperation (PTC) model (Kimmel, 1985). In essence, the question has been reframed from how to reduce competition to how to facilitate cooperation. This approach acknowledges that individuals and nations can indeed behave in competitive and ethnocentric ways, but can also learn to relate in a cooperative and empathic manner. In fact, organizations and societies function largely because most members voluntarily cooperate with each other. PTC theorists believe that conflicts arise because of misperceptions and misunderstandings, especially among groups with different cultural and social backgrounds. According to Kimmel, attempts to address these problems should focus on improving communication, promoting trust, and resolving conflicts through correcting perceptions. This concept of peace establishes communication and cooperation among nations as the priority.

CONTRIBUTIONS OF COMMUNITY PSYCHOLOGY

It is important, we believe, to understand the individual and group attitudes and motivations that may have an influence on world issues. Community psychologists interested in peace and international development need to be aware of these individual and group factors, which should be considered when strategies for social change are developed. In this section, we will focus more specifically on the theory and action that can be derived from community psychology.

The Concept of Empowerment

The notion of empowerment is certainly a useful concept in considering change within a country, such as the empowerment of minorities in the United States. But we believe it is just as useful to think about its application to international affairs. Empowerment implies that all people should have the opportunity to realize their potential. A child born to an affluent family or who lives in an affluent country has no greater or less worth than a child born in a poor family or country. From an egalitarian moral perspective, both children are equally worthy (see Brockett, 1986, for a discussion of the application of Kohlberg's moral development theory to international relations). Both children should be empowered to realize their potential.

We do not intend this to suggest that the goal of any group of people or country should be to achieve self-sufficiency. Indeed, a goal of self-sufficiency ignores the reality of the interdependence of people and countries. Resources are not evenly distributed across countries. Some countries may have an abundance of a certain good, while others may have little or no supply. At present, the principle operating (at least in rhetoric) within countries such as Canada and the United States is that disadvantaged people should be provided with basic necessities through welfare and unemployment systems. This principle would be extended to disadvantaged countries if there were agreement that we were obligated in the same way to all people of the world, not just those who happen to live within our defined boundaries. Brockett (1986) refers to this as the "shared humanity" perspective, which implies a need for the redistribution of resources and benefits to countries in need. The stumbling block is, of course, that most affluent countries are unwilling to take such steps. Nevertheless, there is reason for optimism. There are many examples of countries providing aid to other countries in need. Agricultural programs, for instance, have long been established through international development programs, and there have been positive responses to famines in some countries (Horton, 1986; Vestal, 1985). The fact that many other positive examples could be cited should be reason for hope that a "shared humanity" perspective can be established.

Rappaport (1987) has outlined a number of assumptions of an ecological theory of empowerment. These assumptions are discussed elsewhere in this volume, but we wish to draw on several of them to illustrate how community psychologists can apply this theory at the international level. One assumption is that "*empowerment theory is self-consciously a world view theory*" in which "*the people of concern are to be treated as collaborators; and at the same time, the researcher may be thought of as a participant, legitimately involved with the people she is studying*" (Rappaport, 1987, p. 140; emphasis added). While there is little empirical data on this issue, the majority of development programs appear to ignore this assumption. As we will discuss later, many agricultural assistance programs simply impose a program on a village or community, with little active participation by villagers in the decision-making process. Another assumption that speaks to this same point is that "*other things being equal, an organization that holds an empowerment ideology will be better at finding and developing resources than one with a helper–helpee ideology*, where resources are seen as relatively scarce, and dependent on professionals" (p. 141; emphasis added). Empowerment theory also assumes that "*locally developed solutions are more empowering than single solutions applied in a general way*" (p. 141; emphasis added). In practice, this would mean that a program would not be developed by professionals acting in isolation from the community or group that ultimately will be affected by the program. These individuals must be involved right at the beginning and have an active voice in the identification of the problem, as well as in the creation of possible solutions. Development programs that pay attention to these assumptions will *potentially* be more effective, with emphasis on the word potentially because little is known about which strategies are likely to be successful in developing programs in other countries. Another assumption of empowerment theory addresses the need for longitudinal and impact studies. It is in this area that community psychologists can contribute considerably to the creation of effective programs. Community psychologists have a tradition of being action researchers involved in both the creation and evaluation of programs, as well as being sensitive to issues of cultural diversity and individual differences. Over time, these characteristics would increase our knowledge about how to approach the development of programs at the international level.

To the extent that empowerment increases the self-esteem of individuals, it also reduces their tendency to conform to viewing out-groups in dogmatic negative ways. As discussed previously, several aspects of aggression toward out-groups are fueled by the dependence of individuals on their own groups for self-esteem. By providing an alternate source of self-esteem, empowerment programs provide some inoculation against conforming to group ideas that one's better judgment indicates are false. One voice of dissention in a group can have a cascading effect, as others are prompted to question the validity of the group dogma.

Unfortunately, some groups or nations may view aggression as the only means of empowerment. It is crucial to understand this point, as it will influence how other countries might develop conflict-resolution strategies (see Feeney & Davidson, 1996; Lumsden & Wolfe, 1996). As Cohen and Arnone (1988) commented, "The necessity of finding an alternative form of empowerment other than violence ... lead to a focus on *development*—economic, social, and cultural—as an essential element in conflict resolution strategy" (p. 185, emphasis added).

Educational Programs

In order to achieve peace based on the values and principles we have discussed in this chapter, it will be necessary to mount educational programs that focus on learning the views that form the basis of a "shared humanity," or one planet–one people, perspective. As discussed earlier, the cognitive distortions of the fundamental attribution error and belief perseverance combine to promote and maintain a falsely negative view of out-groups. Although education is not a panacea, directly confronting prejudice with contrary facts can begin to counter enemy images. Elementary and high school programs would be a natural starting point. A colleague of ours at Simon Fraser University, Professor Maurice Gibbons, developed a curriculum for use in the schools that reflects the perspective we have outlined in this chapter (Gibbons, 1985). His curriculum is based on five principles:

1. We must adopt the view that we are first citizens of the world, with a shared responsibility for solving world problems that transcend nationalistic self-interests.
2. "We are all members of the family of mankind, and as such are responsible for understanding and caring for peoples of cultures different from our own." Programs to teach understanding of other cultures and countries and fostering educational and technological exchange experiences between countries would be developed to foster this understanding.
3. From an environmental perspective, the resources of the world must be used sensibly and in a manner consistent with a world view that this is a planet shared by all people of the world.
4. Peaceful, cooperative methods of conflict resolution should be taught. Most schools promote competitiveness rather than cooperative learning (Staub, 1988). "To empower the next generation for peaceful cooperation, we must teach them to think critically about the issues, to develop creative solutions to problems and to cooperate with others in discussion and action" (Gibbons, 1985, p.12).
5. All of us must actively plan for, and be involved in, creating the future we desire.

Kimmel (1985) describes the Choices program, a junior high school curriculum on conflict and nuclear war currently used in a number of schools. It is based on the peace through cooperation model discussed earlier. Choices presents ideas about disarmament and conflict resolution, and the need to increase trust between nations.

Kimmel points out that most models of competition and grades stress individual competition over cooperation. There is a need for learning of other models as well; consequently, the

Choices program teaches win/win models of conflict resolution, cooperative communication, and negotiation. Acknowledging that many students are concerned about nuclear war, Choices attempts to provide students with constructive outlets by encouraging involvement in school and community activities dealing with peace. There are no evaluations of the effects of this program, but there has been strong negative reaction: the former Deputy Undersecretary of Education, Gary L. Bauer, said that the curriculum was "intended to produce Pavlovian resistance to the notion of peace through strength" (quoted in Kimmel, p. 538).

In our view, programs in the schools that facilitate the learning of new perspectives on global issues may, in the future, lead to more creative solutions to the problems of the world. There are numerous other examples of educational programs that community psychologists can learn from if they are interested in introducing educational programs in their own communities (see Greeley, Markowitz, & Rank, 1984; Johnson & Johnson, 1995; Markusen & Harris, 1984; Nelson & Christie, 1995; Snow & Goodman, 1984; Waterlow, 1984). One technique we think is particularly applicable is the "jigsaw classroom" method created by Aronson and his colleagues (Aronson, Blaney, Stephan, Sikes, & Snapp, 1978), which fosters cooperative rather than competitive strategies for achieving both individual and group goals.

Education in the Community

Most people cannot be reached through classroom education, but other avenues for community education exist and may prove to be potent in mobilizing grassroots movements. Many of the factors that were presented earlier as psychological aspects of war lend themselves to stimulating lectures and other educational formats, such as film. For example, Sam Keen starred in a television documentary, "Faces of the Enemy," which powerfully illustrated the role of the enemy image and propaganda in war. Students at our university who have seen this film have found it to be captivating and challenging to their perceptions of enemies. Other opportunities for community education are available through university speaker's bureaus. The topics provide a natural appeal to many people who are often unaware of aspects of war such as the attribution error or belief perseverance research. This information has the potential to mobilize people to demand peaceful settlements of conflict, although we are aware that national leaders may be slow to respond.

Reducing In-group/Out-group Distinctions

As discussed earlier, the existence of groups that can clearly be seen as "them" and not "us" is a prerequisite for violent conflict. We create an image of an evil enemy that is very different from us before we can feel justified in aggressive acts (Opotow, 1990). Therefore, strategies for reducing the distinction will weaken the enemy image and potentially reduce the amount of conflict: One attempt by a community psychiatrist is described later. The media can also be used effectively; for instance, attempts to promote a view of one-planet one-people are common. Beautiful posters with photographs of the planet Earth proclaim, "We are all one people" or "The earth is but one country." These are useful in promoting a different view of people in other countries. We suggest that it is important to continue these and other efforts that serve the purpose of expanding the perception of the in-group to include people of all nations.

Another way of reducing the distorted perceptions of out-groups is by emphasizing group membership that cuts across national lines. The one-planet one-people idea does this at the largest level, but there are other group structures that can be used as well, including scientific and cultural exchange groups. The role of religion is discussed in the next section. The general point is that any inroads that can be made to emphasize cross-national in-group bonds will serve to weaken rigid negative images.

The Role of Religion

Rappaport (1981) has pointed out that psychologists often ignore the potential impact that religious organizations and religious thought can have in creating social change. Religion cuts across cultural and national barriers, and is a potential unifying force, particularly if one considers goals of world unity. As Nelson (1985) has suggested:

> Spiritual traditions and transpersonal or religious psychologists are also potentially rich resources in developing psychologies of peace.... Existing internationally, they are perceptual alternatives to the nuclear nationalism that so threatens earthly life.... At their best, spiritual traditions are concerned with fostering peace personally, relationally, and globally (p. 553).

Religion may, of course, contribute to conflict rather than peace, as witnessed historically in the Crusades and, more recently, in regional conflicts in Ireland and the Middle East (Staub, 1996). However, many religions have taken explicit positions on peace issues (Kondziela, 1987; Hughes, 1987; Parekh, 1987; Roesch, 1988; Universal House of Justice, 1986). Further, religion plays an important role in many developing countries and must be taken into account by those concerned with change within those countries. A religious group is a naturally assembled community of people with shared values and principles. Religious leaders often have profound influence on the community members, and thus may be instrumental in getting a community involved and working together with the professionals planning a program to work on solutions in a collaborative manner.

Citizen Involvement and Grassroots Movements

There are many activities that can take place on the local community level that are related to the peace issues we have discussed. According to Alger (1987), over 3000 cities in 19 countries have declared themselves nuclear-free zones and have initiated peace commissions. Levine's (1987) work in establishing the Cambridge Peace Commission is an excellent example of a community psychology approach to organizing citizens to respond to the threat of nuclear war. The commission established a peace curriculum in the Cambridge schools based on a peace-curriculum kit they developed, and it also conducts a community education series that addresses such issues as domestic violence, sanctuary programs for Haitians, and other "subjects from which lessons on peace and community strengthening can be drawn" (Levine, 1987, p. 17).

Local community, grassroots peace groups offer the potential for large numbers of people to get involved in activities that foster a sense of empowerment (de Rivera & Laird, 1988). Consistent with the theme of this chapter, Alger (1987) offers a number of suggestions for strengthening grassroots peace movements. First among these is the need for local groups working on different aspects of peace—including the arms race, economic well-being, unemployment, and human rights—to work together and begin to view their different activities as sharing a common goal. Linking of grassroots efforts in both developed and underdeveloped countries should also be encouraged, which would help local groups learn from the experiences of others, as well as perceive their local efforts in the context of a larger-scale movement.

Involvement in International Interventions

Psychologists have created many programs designed to reduce tension and increase understanding between antagonistic societies or groups. Space limits us to a review of two possible areas of intervention.

Increasing Intergroup Understanding

The first example is taken from the work of Gerald Caplan, a community psychiatrist. In his book *Arab and Jew in Jerusalem* Caplan (1980) describes his consultation efforts in establishing a vocational educational program for Arabs in Jerusalem and his attempts to reduce Arab–Jew friction in government offices. His book is an excellent example of the manner in which an independent party can help two opposing groups understand each other's customs, beliefs, and values. This type of intervention may be useful in correcting the misperceptions that form the "enemy image" discussed earlier. Caplan spent the first several years of his consultation in a study of the Arab community to understand problems in communication between Jerusalem Arabs and Jews. He did this to ensure that any programs created would take into consideration the values and traditions of both groups. For example, he observed that considerable conflict and resentment was related to the interactions of the two groups in the marketplace, the location of a substantial portion of the confrontations between the two cultures. Caplan noted the distinct differences between bargaining styles. The Jews, influenced more by Western market practices, viewed the marketplace as a battle field in which insults of both the item and the seller would be used to bring down the price. Arabs viewed it more as a game, with as many social as economic aspects. For Arabs, the purchase was almost incidental to the social interaction. It was never acceptable to an Arab to have a customer be abusive of either the goods or the merchant. The differences in style reinforced stereotypes of both groups and, as Caplan suggests, "the fact that neither side was apparently aware of the incompatibility of their bargaining practices was itself a major factor in perpetuating a situation of mutual affront" (p. 93). Caplan's work documents the need to understand all groups and issues before attempting to create any program designed to reduce conflict; otherwise, the intervention may not take into account cultural differences and will be doomed to fail.

Agricultural programs

The devastating effects of famine have been vividly portrayed in media images of starving children and startling figures of the vast number of people who die because of lack of food. The response of other countries has been most compassionate, and emergency aid has been provided to many of the countries in desperate need. In Ethiopia, Vestal (1985) estimates that as many as seven million lives were saved as a result of the various aid programs.

It may be useful to consider the issue of famine from a prevention perspective. For the most part, famine has been dealt with by employing tertiary prevention programs. Tertiary programs are ones that are relied upon when a problem is a long-standing one. In the case of famine, this means that many deaths have already occurred. The goal of aid programs is to prevent the problem from becoming more widespread, i.e., to prevent additional deaths. When famine is identified early, aid programs may be considered secondary prevention programs designed to keep the famine from becoming more severe. In the long run, of course, primary prevention programs designed to minimize or eliminate the occurrence of famine are needed.

Community psychologists have useful contributions to make to all three forms of prevention, but their most significant roles could be in helping to create long-term solutions to the problem of famine.

While emergency relief programs are crucial in the short term, it is necessary to examine the causes of famine so that recurrences of the same famine conditions can perhaps be prevented. The recent famine in Ethiopia will be used as an example to illustrate the difficulties in identifying the causes of famine. Certainly, drought and other environmental variables, such as soil erosion, had a major role. Vestal (1985) lists two other primary factors: government policies detrimental to the growth of agriculture, and civil war. Indeed, he suggests that "with improved weather conditions, war rather than drought has become the main cause of hunger and homelessness" (p. 8). He was referring to a long-lasting civil war that has besieged Ethiopia for some 25 years. Vestal's observations are supported by Press (1988), who commented that the Ethiopian government has hindered relief efforts by its recent military actions. He stated, "After a spate of losses to guerillas, the government this month [May, 1988] began a military buildup in Tigre and Eritrea, the two provinces hardest hit by drought and hunger. It ousted from these all relief workers.... Now about 1 to 1.5 million are cut off from food deliveries" (p. 12). This situation reinforces the Brandt Commission observation that world problems such as hunger are inextricably linked with a war-readiness mentality; it may not be possible to prevent problems like famine until peace is established. Conversely, famine conditions contribute to instability and conflict. Vestal concludes that "until fighting ends ... self-sufficiency in food production and long-term reclamation programs will be difficult—if not impossible" (p. 24).

Willy Brandt, the former Chancellor of West Germany and recipient of the Nobel Peace Prize in 1971, makes the need for this broad perspective most evident. In his book, *World Armament and World Hunger*, Brandt (1986) argues that money spent on the arms race should be diverted to other concerns. Although one-fifth of the world population suffers from hunger and malnutrition, Brandt makes the point that the arms race diverts needed resources from these social problems. He comments that "Where mass hunger reigns, we cannot speak of peace.... Morally, it makes no difference whether human beings are killed in war or condemned to death by starvation" (pp. 17–18). Brandt calls for the need to promote international justice based on a new spirit of solidarity, the recognition and acceptance of the interdependence of all countries. He comments that, "in the long run no nation or group of nations will save itself by dominating others or by isolating itself" (p. 32).

Thus, it is impossible to consider solutions to the problem of famine in a narrow sense. World problems such as famine are multifaceted ones that may require interventions in multiple areas, including agricultural development, programs to reduce population growth, programs to increase literacy and technical skills, and world-scale programs that address fundamental issues of resource allocation and economic disparity.

Certainly, there is a pressing need for agricultural programs that can increase crop productivity, as has been the focus of many developmental programs. The impact of these efforts is unclear, however. Horton (1986) reviewed several methods for assessing impact and concluded that most sources of data about crop production are unreliable and of questionable value in assessing impact. He suggests the need to focus on studies of the impact of institutional research and development programs. Horton emphasizes the need for interdisciplinary research, especially involving local professionals. He states that "to ensure that impact assessments reflect the values and perceptions of scientists and policy makers in developing countries, it is necessary that they be involved, not merely as sources of data, but as active participants in the studies' planning, implementation, and critical review" (p. 465).

Charles Creekmore, a United Nations volunteer in Nairobi, argues that the reason for the failure of many development programs in Africa is that the outside agencies failed to take into account local values and culture (Creekmore, 1986). Programs were designed by outside groups and then imposed on villagers. By outsiders, Creekmore is referring not only to Westerners, but also to African-born policymakers who generally have different lifestyle and education backgrounds and make similar mistakes. Language differences are also apparent. Young people who work with development agencies often have difficulty gaining acceptance because of the traditional villager's respect for elders. Young people may not have credibility and hence won't be listened to. Creekmore's basic thesis is consistent with the one that would be suggested by a community psychology perspective—that projects are more likely to be successful if the organizers or consultants understand a community's or village's social structure and values, and use them as a base upon which to develop a project. For example, projects that involve villagers as partners in a project, with responsibility for decision-making and direction of the project, may be more likely to be adopted by the village itself. Outside agencies, however, must be prepared to allow villagers to do things differently than they would have. As Fairweather, Sanders, and Tornatzky (1974) have discovered, in a different context, it is often difficult for professionals to defer responsibility to the people they are trying to help. There is a sense that they, the professionals, know what is best for these people and that their advice should be followed.

Creekmore (1986) relates a story from Ikiara, an economist at the University of Nairobi, that illustrates the need to take local conditions into account. Ikiara points out that villagers are often awed by outsiders who dress and act quite differently, and their response is withdrawal. Accordingly, they "can't listen to suggestions by people from another world. They want to take advice from someone with their own background" (pp. 42–44). He then relates the following story which took place in Kenya in the late 1950s:

> Government extension agents have been trying to get farmers to use more modern methods, without success, until a local man showed the way. After working four years in a coffee factory and listening carefully to the visiting extension agents, the man leased land to start his own farm. He used what he had learned about fertilizers, pruning, pest control and increasing yields, and adopted new crops such as potatoes. He was so successful that his neighbors started asking him and the extension agents for advice. "His influence outshone the work of agents who had been trying to establish changes for 15 years," Ikiara says. This concept is behind the local demonstration farms, using local people and implements, that are now making extension work more effective (Creekmore, 1986, p. 44).

Failure to take local needs and values into account is demonstrated in a description of the work of a number of social organizations in rural Nigeria. According to Okoye (1987), these organizations focused on establishing urban amenities in these rural areas. Most of their work involved the construction of club halls and civic centers, which are largely unused by local people. Okoye is critical of these projects for three reasons:

> The first is the organizations' conception of rural development, which means the provision of selected urban amenities for the comfort of the urbanite weekenders. The second issue is the lack of direction and guidance of the organizations by the government in the most rational use of their resources.... of what relevance is a club hall or a civic centre to a peasant farmer who can hardly provide three square meals of basic starch in a day? Third, rural development is essentially a human process which should aim at the welfare of the rural developers. These organizations ... do not take the welfare of the rural dwellers and the rural environment into consideration when choosing their projects (pp. 7–8).

Strategies for interventions in rural communities that have received increasing attention in community psychology in recent years (e.g., Heyman, 1986) may be applicable in rural settings in developing countries. Indeed, a number of rural agricultural development programs are based on grassroots participation approaches (e.g., Ekpere, 1987; Mulwa, 1987). Kenkel (1986) has identified a number of areas for community psychologists, including methods for understanding stress and coping, identification of resources, and establishing support systems. This may provide a useful model for community psychology involvement in international development programs.

There is little question that, from an agricultural and economic perspective, it is possible to put an end to poverty and famine in the world. Our planet has sufficient resources to prevent problems such as hunger and poverty. The solution requires, of course, a more just distribution of resources, and therein lies the problems that must be overcome.

CONCLUSIONS

In writing about the prevention of psychopathology, Albee (1986) asked:

> What stops the world's people from building a more just, more equitable world—a world in which preventable stress has been reduced for the majority of people—as is envisioned as a major goal by the World Health Organization? The forces that are barriers are ... exploitation, imperialism, excessive concentration of economic power, nationalism, institutions that perpetuate powerlessness, hopelessness, poverty, discrimination, sexism, racism, and ageism (p. 894).

Albee discusses this in terms of belief in a just world. Lerner (1980) defines this as the incorrect belief held by some people that they live in a just world where people get what they deserve. Rewards will come to those who work hard, whereas hardship and failure are the result of lack of effort or motivation. In the case of aggression against an enemy, belief in a just world can be used as a rationalization in which victims are blamed or held responsible for their situation. Simply put, we rationalize that for these people to have received such harsh treatment, they must have been terrible. The strength of this tendency to derogate the victim illustrates the absurdity of the underlying belief. For example, in Milgram's classic studies on obedience, subjects who believed they were delivering severe shocks to another innocent subject simply because the victim had chosen an incorrect answer, frequently made such comments as: "He was so stupid and stubborn, he deserved to get shocked" (Milgram, 1974, p. 10). Anecdotally, when German civilians were shown the Belsen concentration camp at the end of WWII, one commented, "What terrible criminals these prisoners must have been to receive such treatment" (Myers, 1987, p. 552).

Such a belief ignores the reality that some people or countries simply don't have the resources that are fundamental to achievement. Belief in a just world must be challenged and replaced with a belief that all people on this planet, regardless of country of origin, race, sex, or other personal qualities, should have equal rights and opportunities to realize their potential. This is clearly not the case in the world today. To achieve this, attention must be drawn to the conditions that allow for the inequities that perpetuate the powerlessness of certain people or countries. It is these conditions that must be the focus of our interventions at local, national, and international levels.

In this chapter we have discussed the potential for psychology, particularly community psychology, to contribute to the development of a peaceful world. We began with a reformulation of the definition of peacc. We think that the broader perspective we suggest has important implications for the role of community psychologists in the area of peace and international development, and we have tried to identify some ways in which these contributions can be realized. We wish to end, however, on a cautionary note. There are obvious limits to what psychology can accomplish. We have some useful knowledge and expertise to contribute, but we must be quite modest in stating what can be accomplished. Psychologists can participate in efforts toward establishing peace, but we must properly view ourselves as part of a larger effort that must ultimately involve all peoples of the world if it is to be a success.

REFERENCES

Abeles, N. (1983). Proceedings of the American Psychological Association, Incorporated, for the year 1982. *American Psychologist, 38,* 649–682.

Adams, D. (1990). The Seville statement on violence. *American Psychologist, 45,* 1167–1168.

Albee, G. W. (1986). Toward a just society: Lessons learned from observations on the primary prevention of psychopathology. *American Psychologist, 41,* 891–898.

Alger, C. F. (1987). A grassroots approach to life in peace: Self-determination in overcoming peacelessness. *Bulletin of Peace Proposals, 18,* 375–392.

Aronson, E., Blaney, N., Stephan, C., Sikes, J., & Snapp, M. (1978). *The jigsaw classroom.* Beverly Hills, CA: Sage.

Asch, S. (1956). Studies of independence and conformity: A minority of one against a unanimous majority. *Psychological Monographs, 70,* (9, Whole No. 416).

Berkowitz, L. (1954). Group standards, cohesiveness, and productivity. *Human Relations, 7,* 509–519.

Berscheid, E., & Walster, E. (1978). *Interpersonal attraction.* Reading, MA: Addison-Wesley.

Blight, J. G. (1987). Toward a policy-relevant psychology of avoiding nuclear war: Lessons learned from the Cuban Missile crisis. *American Psychologist, 42,* 12–29.

Blumberg, H. H. (1998). Peace psychology after the cold war: A selective review. *Genetic, Social, and General Psychology, 124,* 5–37.

Boehnke, K., & Schwartz, S. H. (1997). Fear of war: Relations to values, gender, and mental health in Germany and Israel. *Peace and Conflict: Journal of Peace Psychology, 3,* 149–166.

Brandt, W. (1986). *World armament and world hunger: A call for action.* London: Victor Gollancz.

Brockett, C. D. (1986). A Kohlbergian approach to international distributive justice: A comparison of the shared humanity and interdependence perspectives. *Political Psychology, 7,* 349–367.

Caplan, G. (1980). *Arab and Jew in Jerusalem: Explorations in community mental health.* Cambridge, MA: Harvard University Press.

Christie, D. J. (1997). Reducing direct and structural violence: The human needs theory. *Peace and Conflict: Journal of Peace Psychology, 3,* 315–332.

Cialdini, R. B., & Richardson, K. D. (1980). Two indirect tactics of image management: Basking and blasting. *Journal of Personality & Social Psychology, 39,* 406–415.

Cialdini, R. B., Bordon, R. J., Thorne, A., Walker, M. R., Freeman, S., & Sloan, L. R. (1976). Basking in reflected glory: Three (football) field studies. *Journal of Personality & Social Psychology, 34,* 366–375.

Cohen, S. P., & Arnone, H. C. (1988). Conflict resolution as an alternative to terrorism. *Journal of Social Issues, 44,* 175–189.

Creekmore, C. (1986). Misunderstanding Africa. *Psychology Today* December, 38–45.

Daniels, R. (1975). *The decision to relocate the Japanese Americans.* New York: Lippincott.

de Rivera, J., & Laird, J. (1988). Peace fair or warfare: Educating the community. *Journal of Social Issues, 44,* 59–80.

Deutsch, M. (1985). *Distributive justice.* New Haven, CT: Yale University Press.

Dobrosielski, M. (1987). On the preparation of societies for life in peace. *Bulletin of Peace Proposals, 18,* 235–242.

Ekpere, J. A. (1987). Action research in participatory rural development: The case of Badeku, Nigeria. *Journal of the Society for International Development: Seeds of Change, 2,* 115–120.

Fairweather, G. W., Sanders, D. H., & Tornatzky, L. G. (1974). *Creating change in mental health organizations.* New York: Pergamon.

Feeney, M., & Davidson, J. A. (1996). Bridging the gap between the practical and the theoretical: An evaluation of a conflict resolution model. *Peace and Conflict: Journal of Peace Psychology, 2,* 255–269.

Fiske, S. T. (1987). People's reactions to nuclear war: Implications for psychologists. *American Psychologist, 42,* 207–217.

Frank, J. (1986). The role of pride. In R. K. White (Ed.), *Psychology and the prevention of nuclear war* (pp. 220–226). New York: New York University Press.

Fromm, E. (1973). *The anatomy of human destructiveness.* New York: Holt, Rinehart and Winston.

Frydenberg, E., & Lewis, R. (1996). Social issues: What concerns young people and how they cope? *Peace and Conflict: Journal of Peace Psychology, 2,* 271–283.

Galtung, J. (1986). Appreciation. In Universal House of Justice (Ed.), *To the peoples of the world: A Baha'i statement on peace* (pp. 85–86). Ottawa: The Association For Baha'i Studies.

Galtung, J. (1998). On the genesis of peaceless worlds: Insane nations and insane states. *Peace and Conflict: Journal of Peace Psychology, 4*, 1–11.

Gibbons, M. (1985). *Toward a universal curriculum for a global generation.* Burnaby, BC: Simon Fraser University.

Greeley, K., Markowitz, S., & Rank, C. (1984). education for peace and justice. *Harvard Educational Review, 54*, 342–347.

Heyman, M., (Ed.). (1986). Special issue on rural mental health. *American Journal of Community Psychology*, 14.

Horton, D. (1986). Assessing the impact of international agricultural and research and development programs. *World Development, 14*, 453– 486.

Hughes, J. J. (1987). World Buddhism and the peace movement. *Bulletin of Peace Proposals, 18*, 449–468.

Johnson, D. W., & Johnson, R. T. (1995). Teaching students to be peacemakers: Results of five years of research. *Peace and Conflict: Journal of Peace Psychology, 1*, 417–438.

Keen, S. (1986). *Faces of the enemy: Reflections of the hostile imagination.* San Francisco: Harper & Row.

Kenkel, M. B. (1986). Stress-coping-support in rural communities: A model for primary prevention. *American Journal of Community Psychology, 14*, 457–478.

Kimmel, P. R. (1985). Learning about peace: Choices and the U.S. Institute of Peace as seen from two different perspectives. *American Psychologist, 40*, 536–541.

Kimmel, P. R. (1995). Sustainability and cultural understanding: Peace psychology as public interest science. *Peace and Conflict: Journal of Peace Psychology, 1*, 101–116.

Kondziela, J. (1987). Catholic perspectives on life in peace. *Bulletin of Peace Proposals, 18*, 415–432.

Lemyre, L., & Smith, P.M. (1985). Intergroup discrimination and self-esteem in the minimal group paradigm. *Journal of Personality and Social Psychology, 49*, 660–670.

Lerner, M. J. (1980). *The belief in a just world: A fundamental delusion.* New York: Plenum.

Levine, M. D. (1987). Organizing and institutionalization: The Cambridge Peace Commission experience. *The Community Psychologist, 20*, 17–18.

Lumsden, M., & Wolfe, R. (1996). Evolution of the problem-solving workshop: An introduction to social-psychological approaches to conflict resolution. *Peace and Conflict: Journal of Peace Psychology, 2*, 37–67.

Markusen, E., Harris, J. B. (1984). The role of education in preventing nuclear war. *Harvard Educational Review, 54*, 282–303.

Mayor, F. (1995). How psychology can contribute to a culture of peace. *Peace and Conflict: Journal of Peace Psychology, 1*, 3–9.

McConnell, S.C., Brown, S.D., Ruffing, J.N., Strupp, J.K., Duncan, B.L., & Kurdek, L.A. (1986). Comment: Psychologists' attitudes and activities regarding nuclear arms. *American Psychologist, 41*, 725–727.

Milburn, T., & Isaac, P. (1995). Prospect theory: Implications for international mediation. *Peace and Conflict: Journal of Peace Psychology, 1*, 333–342.

Milgram, S. (1974). *Obedience to authority.* New York: Harper & Row.

Miller, N.E., & Begelshi, R. (1948). Minor studies of aggression II. The influence of frustrations imposed by the in-group on attitudes expressed towards out-groups. *Journal of Psychology, 25*, 437–442.

Mintz, A. (1946). A re-examination of correlations between lynchings and economic indices. *Journal of Abnormal and Social Psychology, 89*, 125–131.

Morawski, J. G., & Goldstein, S. E. (1986). Psychology and nuclear war: A chapter in our legacy of social responsibility. *American Psychologist, 41*, 276–284.

Mulwa, F. W. (1987). Participation of the grassroots in rural development: The case of the development education programme of the Catholic diocese of Machakos, Kenya. *Journal of the Society for International Development: Seeds of Change, 2*, 107–114.

Myers, D. G. (1986). *Psychology.* New York: Worth.

Myers, D. G. (1987). *Social psychology.* New York: McGraw-Hill.

Nelson, A. (1985). Psychological equivalence: Awareness and response-ability in our nuclear age. *American Psychologist, 40*, 549–566.

Nelson, L. L., & Christie, D. (1995). Peace in the psychology curriculum: Moving from assimilation to accommodation. *Peace and Conflict: Journal of Peace Psychology, 1*, 161–178.

Okoye, J. C. (1987). Irrational and indiscriminate resource use in rural development in Nigeria. *Journal of Environmental Management, 25*, 1–11.

Opotow, S. (1990). Moral exclusion and injustice: An introduction. *Journal of Social Issues, 46*, 1–20.

Parekh, B. (1987). Ghandhian vision of life in peace. *Bulletin of Peace Proposals, 18*, 469–476.

Plous, S. (1985). Psychological and strategic barriers in present attempts at nuclear disarmament: A new proposal. *Political Psychology, 6*, 109–133.

Polyson, J., Stein, D., & Sholley, B. (1986). Psychologists and nuclear war: A survey. *American Psychologist, 41,* 724–725.

Press, R. M. (1988). War bites hand that feeds Africa. *The Christian Scientist Monitor, May 9–15,* 12.

Rappaport, J. (1981). In praise of paradox: A social policy of empowerment over prevention. *American Journal of Community Psychology, 9,* 1–26.

Rappaport, J. (1987). Terms of empowerment/exemplars of prevention: Toward a theory for community psychology. *American Journal of Community Psychology, 15,* 121–148.

Roesch, R. (1988). Psychology and peace. *Journal of Baha'i Studies, 1,* 47–59.

Seidman, E., & Rappaport, J. (Eds.). (1986). *Redefining social problems.* New York: Plenum.

Sherif, M., Harvey, O. J., White, B. J., Hood, W. R., & Sherif, C. W. (1961). *Intergroup conflict and cooperation: The robber's cave experiment.* Norman, OK: University Book Exchange.

Snow, R., & Goodman, L. (1984). A decision-making approach to nuclear education. *Harvard Educational Review, 54,* 321–328.

Staub, E. (1988). The evolution of caring and nonaggressive persons and societies. *Journal of Social Issues, 44,* 81–100.

Staub, E. (1996). Preventing genocide: Activating bystanders, helping victims, and the creation of caring. *Peace and Conflict: Journal of Peace Psychology, 2,* 189–200.

Taylor, O.M., & Moghaddem, F.M. (1987). *Theories of intergroup relations.* New York: Praeger.

Tetlock, P.E. (1985). Integrated complexity of American and Soviet foreign policy rhetoric: A time-series analysis. *Journal of Personality and Social Psychology, 49,* 1565–1585.

Tucker, R. W. (1977). *The inequality of nations.* New York: Basic Books.

Turner, J.C. (1984). social identification and psychological group formation. In H. Tajfel (Ed.), *The social dimension: European developments in social psychology,* Vol. 2 (pp. 518–536). London: Cambridge University Press.

Universal House of Justice (1986). *To the peoples of the world: A Baha'i statement on peace.* Ottawa: The Association for Baha'i Studies.

Vestal, T. M. (1985). Famine in Ethiopia: Crisis of many dimensions. *Africa Today, 32,* 7–28.

Wagner, R. V. (1988). Distinguishing between positive and negative approaches to peace. *Journal of Social Issues, 44,* 1–16.

Waterlow, C. (1984). A classroom experiment in teaching for peace: Solutions to global problems. *Harvard Educational Review, 54,* 329–333.

White, R.K. (1984). *Fearful warriors: A psychological profile of U.S.-Soviet relations.* New York: Free Press.

CHAPTER 34

Community Psychology and Ethnic Minority Populations

Lonnie R. Snowden, Miriam Martinez, and Anne Morris

Community psychology is a field of diverse ends and means. Its ambitions encompass ideology, policy, theory, research, and intervention. All of these ways of attempting to gain psychological knowledge and use it for human betterment can be thought of as having an ethnic and cultural aspect. Ideally, theorists and researchers would consider variation, no matter what the subject, as it occurs across ethnic and cultural boundaries. Ethnic and cultural concerns would be found everywhere.

At present, this situation remains an ideal. To ensure at least selective attention to ethnic and minority issues, it is necessary that they receive attention under broad rubrics such as that heading this chapter. This should not be taken to suggest, however, that ethnic and cultural variation ought not be taken into account in considering virtually any topic in the field of community psychology.

It also is true that there are certain problems of particular interest to minority communities and those working on their behalf. Many of them are associated with issues in service delivery. Historically, a driving force behind involvement of ethnic minority psychologists in community psychology has been inadequacies in systems of care. Certain of these problems have declined, however, others have endured and new ones have arisen.

The focus of the present chapter is on mental health service delivery. Considerations of interest to community psychologists, such as cultural diversity, community systems, poverty, and health, are taken into account as they affect levels of psychological suffering and resources for problem-solving. Such an orientation is incomplete, yet desirable. Given that minority group members experience heightened levels of stress, differential involvement, and response

Lonnie R. Snowden • Center for Mental Health Services Research and School of Social Welfare, University of California, Berkeley, California 94720. Miriam Martinez • Department of Psychiatry, University of California at San Francisco, San Francisco General Hospital, San Francisco, California 94110. Anne Morris • Center for Mental Health Services Research, Berkeley, California 94720.

Handbook of Community Psychology, edited by Julian Rappaport and Edward Seidman. Kluwer Academic / Plenum Publishers, New York, 2000.

to intervention—and are growing in numbers—it seems particularly important to emphasize delivery of services to them.

A focus by community psychologists on mental health service delivery can scarcely be described as the only possible response. The past two decades have produced disagreement as to whether social scientists and professionals should be more involved in public policy or in service delivery in order to be most effective. This dispute hits home in particular for the community psychologist. Those who hold a political perspective tend to locate the causes of distress in external forces; they believe that shared experiences of prejudice, poverty, and living in underserved communities lead to a common focus for political intervention. They argue that psychologists should be working toward the elimination of oppression suffered by all minority groups through social action. Psychologists who have worked to understand the impact of traditional interventions with people of color, however, believe that the unique histories of policies toward immigrants, and the different cultures, languages, and acculturation patterns of minorities, leads to the need for research to develop culturally sensitive tools for study and intervention. For the latter group, the role for psychologists includes a political imperative; however, it emphasizes tailoring service systems and interventions by the use of cultural sensitivity (Cheung & Snowden, 1990; Jones & Korchin, 1982; Snowden, 1998a; Snowden, Libby, & Thomas, 1997).

Those working from all perspectives, at heart, are seeking an improvement in the lot of ethnic minority communities. They advocate an application of psychology to an improvement in the mental health, social standing, and overall well-being *of* people of color in American society. They differ in the exact nature of their visions and how these can be successfully accomplished. Nevertheless, an "either–or" attitude has resulted in an unfortunate polarization. There is room for many approaches in working for ethnic minority communities—surely social action and direct practice, but also organization, planning, and much more. The exact nature of certain of these opportunities will become clear as the present chapter follows its course.

What is that course? The chapter first reviews epidemiological data available on ethnic minority populations. The nature and extent of psychological well-being and mental health are outlined. The implications of the epidemiological data for service delivery are also discussed, with special emphasis on equity in utilization. Next is an outline of social stressors particularly affecting minority groups. Some are general, such as poverty; others are more particular, such as acculturation. Research to date tends to emphasize deficits rather than strengths of minority groups. The next section, therefore, highlights resources among people of color. Specifically, help-seeking, including the use of the family, prayer, and folk healers as ways of coping are discussed. Finally, service delivery is examined directly, with an emphasis on understanding issues that have been a particular focus of research.

We have included discussions on as many ethnic groups as possible. Unfortunately, the chapter may seem skewed toward Blacks and Latinos, as most of what is available concerns these populations. Indian and Alaskan natives, Asians, and recent immigrants are clearly understudied, underserved groups. More work is needed on these groups, as well as on other people of color in our society.

THE PSYCHOLOGICAL WELL-BEING OF MINORITY COMMUNITIES

A point of departure for considering the psychological status of minority communities is to ask about the prevalence of problems. This is epidemiology, attractive to the community psychologist partly because of its inherent focus on populations. It directs our attention away from the individual, and toward indicators of social status and community membership.

One relatively convenient approach to estimate the incidence and prevalence of psychological disorders involves tabulating those who receive care for their problems. This "rates under treatment" approach is beset by significant shortcomings. Foremost among them is an assumption that those with mental health problems enter treatment, and those without such problems do not. A large and growing literature on help-seeking makes it clear that any such premise is questionable (Lewin-Epstein, 1991; Martin & Martin, 1995; Neighbors, 1984; Snowden, 1998a; Veroff, Douvan, & Kulka, 1981). Insofar as patterns of help-seeking vary among segments of the population, then comparisons based on rates under treatment are potentially misleading.

Patterns of help-seeking differ among ethnic communities. For instance, when faced with challenging circumstances, African Americans may be particularly likely to minimize threat and to seek to prevail through self-reliance and determination, in what has been termed "John Henryism," a kind of heroic striving to overcome any and all obstacles (James, Hartnett, & Kalsbeek, 1983). For at least 20 years researchers studying African Americans have observed a pattern of behavior believed to indicate denial of stress (Johnson & Crowley, 1996). Stress denial has been inferred from survey responses in which far fewer stressors have been endorsed than appeared plausible. The phenomenon has been interpreted both in methodological terms, pointing to a possibility of underreporting of stress, as well as indicating a style of response by which difficult personal experiences are minimized or even overlooked entirely.

When symptoms do arise, African Americans appear to express their suffering in somewhat characteristic ways. For example, epidemiological researchers have established that African Americans are more likely than white Americans to suffer from phobic disorder (Zhang & Snowden, 1998a), and possibly from panic and sleep disorders (Bell, Dixie-Bell, & Thompson, 1986; Neal & Turner, 1991). Somatization disorder and somatization syndrome also are found more in African American communities than elsewhere (Robins & Regier, 1991; Zhang & Snowden, 1998).

In the literature on diagnosis and treatment of mental disorders, there has been a persistent tendency for African Americans to be more frequently diagnosed as schizophrenic, and less likely to be diagnosed as having an affective disorder relative to white Americans (Hu, Snowden, & Jerrell, 1992; Lawson, Hepler, Holladay, & Cuffel, 1994; Snowden & Cheung, 1990). There is considerable empirical evidence that clinicians may be biased in assessing and diagnosing the symptoms of African Americans—overdiagnosing schizophrenia and underdiagnosing affective disorders (Loring & Powell, 1988; Lu, Lim, & Messich, 1995; Worthington, 1992; Neighbors, Jackson, Campbell, & Williams, 1989).

Anxiety-related and somatic disorders have symptoms reminiscent of those described by cross-cultural researchers studying African American cultural beliefs (Heurtin-Roberts, Snowden, & Miller, 1997). Anthropological investigators working in an ethnographic tradition have documented an idiom indigenous to African Americans and used to express psychological and physical forms of personal suffering, such as headaches, "weaks and dizzies," pounding heart, hot flashes, and chills (Weidman, 1979; Heurtin-Roberts, & Resin, 1990; Snow, 1993).

The experience of indigenous symptoms is more strongly associated with help-seeking among African Americans than among white Americans. Snowden (in press) correlated the number of African American folk symptoms identified from a previous study as occurring on the Diagnostic Interview Schedule (Heurtin-Roberts, Snowden, & Miller, 1997) with the probability of utilizing mental health care. For two of three symptom clusters studied (anxiety and somatization symptoms), there was a stronger association among African Americans than among white Americans between symptom distress and mental health care utilization.

In terms of utilization, African Americans are overrepresented in psychiatric hospitals (Snowden & Cheung, 1990; Snowden, 1998a). The fact of disproportionate hospitalization raises issues of social control and cultural estrangement and misinterpretation, if not overt bias toward African Americans on the part of the mental health care system. However, economic factors may be implicated in African American rates of hospitalization in psychiatric facilities. For example, African Americans who are hospitalized for psychiatric disorders tend to be recidivists who cycle in and out of hospital care (Leginski, Manderscheid, & Henderson, 1990). These patterns of utilization are often associated with poverty, homelessness, and incarceration, as well as extremely stressful social conditions in the community (Snowden, 1998a). As well, many African Americans are poor and insured by the Medicaid program. Such coverage is strongly linked to a greater probability of hospitalization than is the case for private insurance (Freiman, Cunningham, & Cornelius, 1994). Yet another economic factor is the lack of access to primary health care, which may lead many individuals to use the emergency room as a source of routine care, thus facilitating hospitalization for psychiatric disorders (Snowden, Libby, & Thomas, 1997).

Among Latinos, low rates of mental health care utilization have been consistently observed (Padgett, Patrick, Burns, & Schlesinger, 1994; Jimenez, Alegria, Pena, & Vera, 1997). Further, there is what may be considered a paradox with respect to Latino mental health: despite the stressors associated with minority status in the United States, and high rates of poverty and other stressful social conditions, Latinos evidence prevalence rates for mental health problems that are comparable to non-Hispanic whites (Vega & Rumbaut, 1991; Woodward, Dwinell, & Arons, 1992).

There are, however, a number of methodological and cross-cultural issues in the assessment of mental health problems that render definitive statements about validity and the comparability of prevalence data for Latinos across studies problematic (Fabrega, 1995; Vega & Murphy, 1990; Vega & Rumbaut, 1991). While early studies of Latino mental health seemed to indicate greater distress, at least on symptom checklists, among Mexican Americans relative to other ethnic groups (Burnham, Timbers, & Hough, 1984; Frerichs, Aneshensel, & Clark, 1981), these studies did not take into account socioeconomic standing. Vernon and Roberts (1982) found that Mexican Americans exhibited significantly more symptoms of depression than did whites on the CES-D, but without taking into account potential confounding from socioeconomic standing. Vega, Warheit, Buhl-Auth, and Meinhardt (1984) found marked differences among Mexican Americans on the basis of linguistic preference: those who spoke Spanish reported greater depressive symptomatology than those who spoke English or than Anglos. To a large extent, however, these differences were associated with the low educational level of the Spanish-speaking sample.

Despite methodological and cross-cultural issues in assessment, in the last decade there have been significant epidemiologic surveys of the prevalence of mental health problems among Latinos, including the Los Angeles Epidemiologic Catchment Area (LAEC) and epidemiologic studies in Puerto Rico (Robins & Regier, 1991). These studies have found that rates of mental health disorders were comparable or slightly lower among Puerto Ricans on the island and among Mexican Americans as compared with other ethnic groups—with the exception of higher rates of alcohol abuse and phobias among Mexican Americans.

Further, Mexican immigrants tended to have better mental health status overall than American born Mexican Americans. Although Mexican Americans and white non-Hispanics had similar prevalence rates for mental health problems, utilization was lower among Mexican Americans. Low acculturation and being Mexican-born was associated with reduced utilization, even in the presence of diagnosed mental health problems. Much work remains to be done in unraveling the paradox of Latino mental health status, particularly what protective factors may enhance the mental health status of Latino immigrants, despite the experience of significant social stressors in the U.S.

Problems of American Indians and Alaska Natives were considered in a review by Shore and Manson (1983). They were able to find only three communitywide epidemiological studies. There was considerable variation in results—a fact that is not particularly surprising in view of marked differences in methods, as well as in cultures and communities that were studied. Nevertheless, problems of depression and psychosis seemed particularly in evidence. Although there are no large-scale epidemiologic studies of American Indians, Manson (1986) found that 32% of American Indian elders who were outpatients at an Indian Health Service clinic exhibited symptoms of depression. Kramer (1991), in a survey of American Indian elders, found that depression and sadness/grieving were reported by 11% and 22% of participants, respectively. In another study, Goldwasser and Badger (1989) reported that 19% of primary care patients had symptoms of psychiatric disorder.

There is evidence of significant mental health problems among American Indian youth (Beals, Piasecki, Nelson, Jones, Keane, Dauphinais, Red Shirt, Sack, & Manson, 1997). From a comparative standpoint, American Indian youth have been found to have fewer anxiety disorders than non-minority youth. However, American Indian adolescents were much more likely to be diagnosed with attention deficit/hyperactivity disorder (ADHD) and substance abuse disorders than were nonminority youth (Beals et al., 1997). American Indian youth have also been found to have suicide rates that are 2.3 to 2.8 times as high as the general U.S. population (May, 1988). Unfortunately, a high proportion of youth who suffer from mental health and substance abuse disorders receive no mental health services (Barney, 1995; Burns, Costello, Farmer, Angold, Tweed, Staugl, Farmer, & Erkanli, 1997).

Epidemiological studies among Asian Americans and Pacific Islanders are relatively sparse, and comprehensive studies are hindered by the sheer diversity of members of this group (e.g., Japanese, Korean, Chinese, Filipinos, Vietnamese, Hawaiians, Samoans), and their distinctive languages, cultures, and immigration histories in the U.S. (Sue & Morishima, 1982). Further, there are important cultural factors in the interpretation of mental distress, the enactment of emotions, and cultural belief systems about health and illness, shame and stigma, and family honor, that complicate epidemiologic studies of the prevalence of mental disorders and comparisons across ethnic groups (Ekman & Freisan, 1971; Pang, 1990).

Nevertheless, with these caveats in mind, there have been a number of studies that suggest a greater tendency toward somatization among Asian Americans (e.g., Marsella, Kinzie, & Gordon, 1973; Pang, 1990; Rahe, Looney, Ward, Tund, & Liu, 1978; Sue & Sue, 1974). According to Sue and Morishima (1982), the tendency to somaticize among Asian Americans may be due both to the stigmatization attached to mental disorder, as well as to conceptualize mind and body as a unity. Because of these tendencies, Asian Americans may underutilize mental health care and bring mental health issues to primary health care providers, in the form of somatic complaints such as sleeplessness, nervousness, heart palpitations, and stomach complaints.

The lack of culturally appropriate services provided by bicultural and bilingual staff has been cited as a significant barrier to mental health care among Asian Americans, whose rates of utilization are consistently low (Sue & Sue, 1991). On a more promising note, Zane, Hatanaka, Park, and Akutsu (1994) found that ethnic-specific services designed to address cultural barriers to care in Los Angeles County were associated with better treatment retention and outcomes for Asian American clients, while not creating any inequities for white clients. Similarly, Snowden and Hu (1997) compared service systems for the severely mentally ill in two counties in California that had large populations of Asian Americans. These investigators found that in the county with a history of ethnic-specific services (i.e., bilingual and bicultural staff, culturally relevant services) there was greater service utilization among Asian Americans of community-based support services and lower use of inpatient care than was the case for whites. By contrast, in the county without a history of ethnic-specific services, the pattern of utilization was reversed. These findings suggest that the cultural context of services can affect utilization and perhaps prevent hospitalization among the severely mentally ill.

Great strides have been made in making epidemiological estimates with greater precision. On the other hand, significant problems remain, particularly in demonstrating the cross-cultural validity of instruments. Standardization of measures has furnished a basis for meaningful comparisons among studies, but whether such comparability truly holds in a cross-cultural context leaves room for considerable doubt (Fabrega, 1995; Hendricks & Bayton, 1983; Tanaka-Matsumi & Marsella, 1976; Vega & Murphy, 1990; Vega & Rumbaut, 1991).

What role can the community psychologist play in using epidemiological data on behalf of ethnic minority communities? One involves the translation of epidemiologic methods and data into plans for more service systems better responding to minority needs. Knowledge of types and levels of psychological problems permits priorities to be established and resources to be allocated accordingly.

A common method to perform this kind of evaluation consists of extrapolating levels of need from representation in the general population. Sue, for example (1977), found that King County, Washington, was made up of 2.4% Asian Americans. His use of these data implied that those suffering psychological disability and in need of services also ought to include a 2.4% representation of Asian Americans. In a review by Lopez (1981), 40 studies were cited that performed this kind of calculation for Mexican Americans alone.

Such an approach is plausible in providing a rough estimate, but may also be misleading. It rests on an underlying assumption that problems ought to be proportionally distributed among majority and minority communities. Given greater and possibly differential levels of stress in minority communities, any such assumption seems questionable.

In a study of Santa Clara County, California, Meinhardt and Vega (1987) demonstrated that proportional levels of mental health need cannot be taken for granted. They carried out a community survey as a means of assessing psychological problems directly. The problems of nine separate minority populations were then evaluated as a percentage of the total number of people in need. Almost 53% of those in need were found to be white, 4.7% of those in need were Vietnamese, and 26.5% were Hispanic. These figures differ markedly from extrapolations from the total population, where whites were 68.7%, Vietnamese 2.6%, and Hispanics 16.3%. The latter two groups were in need out of proportion to their representation in the population, showing significantly greater levels of suffering than would have otherwise been detected.

Meinhardt and Vega conducted their research with service delivery in mind. They viewed their work as methodological—an adaptation of general epidemiological procedures to make them both culturally sensitive and feasible under standard operating conditions of mental health administration at a county level. This "administrative epidemiology" deserves the attention of the community psychologist.

SOCIAL STRESS

Stress is a particularly important concept for the community psychologist. It provides a useful basis for an overview of the field, unifying its disparate activities and concerns (e.g., Cohen, 1992; Cowen, 1984; Dohrenwend, 1978; Kessler, 1992; Moos, 1984). A focus on stress also serves to orient us to the role of social factors in mental health. It suggests obstacles to successful living in the ongoing functioning of societal institutions, and mechanisms linking these social forces to mental health, and points toward strategies and indicators to obtain empirical confirmation.

Poverty

For many members of ethnic minority groups, a dominant fact of life is having to live in poverty. Although African Americans on the whole have made great social and economic strides in the past few decades, virtually closing the educational gap between Blacks and whites, and moving into the middle class in ever greater numbers, these figures obscure a sizeable underclass of African Americans living in deep poverty, mostly in inner cities (Thernstrom & Thernstrom, 1997; Wilson, 1987, 1996a, 1996b).

Latinos vary widely in levels of social well-being (Vega & Kolody, 1998). For example, Cuban Americans have a relatively high median family income, fewer families in poverty, relatively more years of education, and low unemployment.

Puerto Rican Americans fall at the other end of the spectrum. They have a relatively low median family income, a high percentage of families living in poverty, and high unemployment. Their average level of education is 11.2 years, not as far behind Cuban Americans as might be expected. Mexican Americans occupy an intermediate position. In terms of median family income, percent of families living in poverty, and unemployment, they are found between Cuban Americans and Puerto Rican Americans. Their level of education, about 10.2 years, is lowest of the three groups, reflecting the fact that many are recent arrivals, with prior circumstances affording them little access to education.

It is more difficult still to generalize about the social well-being of Asian Americans. Overall, their pattern of performance on social indicators tends to be relatively high. Unemployment is low, and median family income is above the median family income reported by whites. Individual groups vary considerably in performance, however. The percent of families living in poverty varies across groups: Japanese Americans have a very low rate of poverty, whereas Vietnamese Americans and Cambodian Americans have poverty rates that are extremely high. Again, length of residence in the United States accounts for much of this variation.

By contrast, a clear picture can be gained from aggregate data describing Native Americans (Manson, 1998). American Indians comprise less than 1% of the total U.S. population, numbering approximately 1.8 million. The rate of unemployment among American Indians is quite high compared with the general U.S. population: 16.2% of American Indian men and 13.5% of American Indian women are unemployed. The comparable figures for the general U.S. population are 6.4% and 6.2%, respectively. The median household income for American Indian families is $19,865, compared to $30,056 for U.S. families in general. The rate of poverty among American Indian families has been estimated at 31.7%, as compared to the national average of 13.1% of U.S.

Immigration

Recent waves of immigration from Mexico, Southeast Asia, and Central America have consisted largely of people of color. By no means are these immigrants all alike. They must be distinguished on the basis of national origin and culture. They also must be differentiated according to the character of their immigrant experience—whether their relocation was planned or unplanned, forced or voluntary. To be uprooted, nevertheless, and relocated in unfamiliar surroundings is, for most, an unsettling experience with important psychological consequences. The current political climate, in which legal immigrants have seen their welfare benefits cut or eliminated, and illegal immigrants and their children barred from social services, public education, and health care can only exacerbate stress among vulnerable populations.

Lin (1986) demonstrated the importance of attending to psychological adjustment as well as financial. A group of Vietnamese refugees followed over a three-year period made remarkable progress in finding jobs and decreasing reliance on public assistance. In terms of health and psychological well-being, on the other hand, they showed little reduction in distress.

It is not surprising that adverse psychological reactions occur among refugees. Immigrants and refugees face culture shock—challenges both overt and subtle to accepted customs and norms and psychological frames of reference. They have lost people and places to whom they felt attached. They may come to feel isolated from a community beyond ethnic enclaves, and from society at large. They may experience a particular pressure to achieve materially and advance economically. They may experience painful discrepancies between their status in their country of origin and the country in which they have arrived. Their understanding of themselves in relation to a larger world has been destabilized (Lin, 1986; Cohon, 1981).

Investigators have begun the process of documenting these problems empirically. In a study of pregnant, Spanish-speaking immigrants, the item, "friends and relatives too far away" was among the two most frequently occurring stressors; 78% of these women reported experiencing this problem (Martinez & Snowden, 1986). Cervantes (1982) reported a similar finding: 75% of his sample endorsed an item: "I have been thinking about the well-being of family members still living in my home country."

Other data further indicate cultural dislocation. Cervantes (1987) found that the item "I have been in contact with people of other religions" was endorsed more than any other indicator of psychosocial stress (82.6% of the sample); "I have seen that traditional religious customs are ignored" was the third most often endorsed item (68.8% of the sample). Americans may take for granted their diversity in spiritual belief. For immigrants, whose beliefs have been consistently supported and reinforced in their homeland, such cacophony may be disconcerting.

Roles within the newly immigrated family often shift, posing conflict for the family system and its individual members (Bulik, 1986). Women generally find employment in cheap labor markets (i.e., sweat shops) sooner than men; they necessarily forego traditional family roles. As they come to gain a sense of independence, they may also feel that their accomplishments undermine their identity within the family, as well as that of their husbands.

Children of immigrant families, because of greater contact with the host culture, acculturate at a quicker pace than parents. They often learn English first and find their parents dependent on them in community encounters (Bulik, 1987). Cervantes (1987) found that items ranked most stressful were part of the subscale family and marital stress, for example, "who controls household money" and "the fact that children have left home to live independently."

Not all refugees succumb. There are important differences between refugees in factors exacerbating or protecting them from stresses of the refugee experience. Among these are cultural differences, including the congruence between the country of origin and the new country; reasons for having left; the smooth or traumatic nature of their passage; and the degree to which the new society is receptive and responsive, particularly in providing economic opportunity and support in acculturation (Kunz, 1981; Westermeyer, 1986).

Health

A problem of particularly grave concern in ethnic minority communities is health status. For many problems in several ethnic minority populations, ill health and shortened life expectancy are problems occurring at alarming levels. More than a decade ago, concern over such problems led to a task force convened by the Department of Health and Human Services on the subject of Black and Minority Health (Secretary's Task Force, 1985).

The American population of greatest concern in regard to morbidity and mortality is the Black population. The death rate for all causes for Blacks is one and a half times greater than the corresponding rate for Whites. Death rates for Blacks are greater than those for Whites for all specific causes, ranging, in the case of males, from 1.2 times greater for heart disease, to 6.6 times greater for homicide. The range for females is from a rate 1.2 times greater for cancer and accidents, to 4.3 times greater for homicide.

The picture is more difficult to determine for Latinos. Data are difficult to come by, because for many purposes of vital-statistics reporting Latinos are classified as White. Nevertheless, certain facts stand out. Mexican-born males are at elevated risk for death from cirrhosis of the liver and unintentional injuries; females are at risk for death from cancer and diabetes. Both are more likely to die by reason of homicide, as are Cuban-born Hispanics.

The health status of Native Americans also is troubling. This appears particularly true for American Indians under the age of 45: their risk of death is 1.8 times greater than that of Whites, taking into account both sexes. Over age 45, on the other hand, American Indian risk of death is about equal to that of Whites. Causes of death with highest relative risks for Native Americans are cirrhosis, tuberculosis, chronic renal disease, unintentional injuries, drowning, homicide, and diabetes. Native Americans are from 1.1 times to 11.1 times more likely than Whites to die from these causes.

There is a disproportionately high mortality rate among young Black men, with homicide, substance abuse, and AIDS taking a devastating toll on young men aged 18 to 24 (Guest, Almgren, & Hussey, 1998; Rimer, 1996). Recent figures from the Centers for Disease Control and Prevention indicate that AIDS kills twice as many Black men aged 25 to 44 as homicide, and that Black women now constitute two-thirds of all women infected with HIV. Further, more children with AIDS are Black than all other racial and ethnic groups combined (Rimer, 1996). The primary means of HIV transmission among African Americans is thought to be intravenous drug use and needle sharing, and unprotected heterosexual intercourse with intravenous drug users.

In addressing poverty, immigration, and health, important opportunities beckon the community psychologist as researcher, consultant, and advocate. Studies by community-oriented psychologists already have helped us to understand the relationship between economic forces and mental health. For example, Dooley and Catalano (1984) examined economics, ethnicity, and mental health. Patterns of economic change that "uncover" existing problems, and those that "provoke" new ones, show little variation among ethnic groups. The current movement of mental health, substance abuse, and general health care service systems into managed care, and alternative forms of financing, such as capitation, raise the issue of access to, and quality of care for, poor minority and immigrant populations, as well as for other vulnerable populations, such as the elderly and the severely mentally ill (Hurley & Draper, 1998; Snowden, 1993, 1998a). Many more of these pressing problems are worthy of study.

Along with learning more about policies and programs, community psychologists must seek constructive change through strategic social action. The recent welfare reform legislation enacted by Congress to "end welfare as we know it" harbors unknown consequences for immigrant and minority communities. Will more minority children slide into deep poverty, or will the various "welfare-to-work" programs implemented by the states break the "cycle of dependency," as some conservative critics (e.g., Murray, 1984) have long contended? All are burning questions. Community psychologists must learn to work side by side with specialists in public policy and with public interest advocates as actors in these important and far-reaching policy changes.

New directions are open to the community psychologist with an active interest in research. Members of ethnic minority groups are less likely than others to visit a physician and to have access to routine health care (Snowden, 1998; Snowden, Libby, & Thomas, 1987). The field of health services research and health care technology assessment provides data bearing directly on such issues. Investigators have shown, for example, that less health care can be provided to the general population without detriment to health. For the poor, however, this pattern does not hold true: a lower intensity of services is associated with declines in indicators of health (Ware, 1986). Other studies (Berkowitz, 1987) have documented the impact of changes in Medicaid on the health care and the health status of medically indigent adults. Community psychologists must join with investigators in other fields to document these problems and make policy-oriented recommendations.

RESOURCES

Researchers have recently begun to explore resources that are thought to buffer stress for minorities (e.g., Neighbors & Jackson, 1996b; Murray & Peacock, 1996; Saegart, 1989). The observation that some people under similar extremely distressing circumstances develop mental illness while others do not has led researchers to three areas of particular strengths/resources among minority groups: family, religion, and the use of indigenous healers. These highlight special areas that promise new understanding of minority mental health.

Family

For many members of ethnic groups, the family is a source of support not only in times of crisis, but also in day-to-day living. The "family" often includes unrelated people from the community that are tightly knit into a group who support one another as extended family. Strong reliance on the family and use of support systems within the community are thought to occur within Asian American (Wong, 1982), Native American (Manson, 1986, 1998), Latin American (Valle & Bensussen, 1985; Vega & Kolody, 1998), and African American communities (Dressler, 1985; Malson, 1982; Maton, Teti, Corns, Viera-Baker, Lavine, Gouze, & Keating, 1996; Neighbors & Jackson, 1996). For example, black and Latino families tend to have more contact with more family members and to receive help more frequently than do Anglo families (Hays & Mandel, 1973; Padilla, Carlos, & Keefe, 1976). Mexican American extended families tend to depend more on intergenerational systems of support. Poor families whose mobility is limited live within kin-centered support systems.

Often the non-related people who belong to the support system of a family are regarded as kin. These may include unrelated people described as cousins, sisters, aunts, or uncles (Hofferth, 1984; Saegert, 1989; Stack, 1974; Wilson, Greene-Bates, McKim, Simmons, et al., 1995). The types of support received include help with child care and child rearing responsibilities, advice regarding important decisions, financial help, support for interpersonal problems, help with domestic chores, and transportation. The flow of support is typically from older generation to younger, except in some instances such as transportation and financial aid, when the younger generation may be in a better position to help the elderly.

Too much reliance on family is often pathologized and thought to hinder autonomy—a value that perhaps culturally conditioned in U.S. dominant culture. Nonetheless, many minorities consider their reliance appropriate, think that it represents strength, loyalty, and respect, and view it as an adaptive resource (Dilworth-Anderson & Marshall, 1996; Wilson, 1991).

The use of the extended family has also been thought to be a response to the stress of living in poverty. Several researchers have found, however, that although use of extended family decreases somewhat as socioeconomic status (SES) increases, ethnic differences still prevail (McAdoo, 1978). Of black kin-help networks, McAdoo (1980) concluded: "It has become a viable part of our cultural patterns that has been found to be operational at all economic levels before, during and after upward mobility, even into the third generation of middle-class status" (p. 127). In their review of the literature on Latino use of folk healers, Scheper-Hughes and Stewart (1983) concluded that:

> While one must be cautious not to overgeneralize,... some cultural patterns appear stable across rural-urban and class lines, among these: the centrality and strength of the family (both nuclear and extended) and of fictive kin (such as compadrazco, "godparenthood"): the maintenance (especially by women) of a religious over a secular world view and a historically justifiable mistrust and avoidance of Anglo authority, professionals and institutions. (p. 876)

Perhaps part of the decrease in extended family use is due to social isolation of the middle-class minority family who often move away from these support networks.

Folk Healers

In addition to seeking help from family members, minorities also seek help from folk healers in their communities. Folk healers working with special diets, exercise, meditation, herbal remedies, prayers, and other indigenous tools aid those who seek their help for emotional and psychological problems. Folk healers are known and respected in their communities, even by people who do not seek their help. The range of problems appropriate to bring to a folk healer, as well as the appropriate behavior (participation) is also typically common knowledge (Acosta, 1984). Most folk healers will accept some form of compensation for their services. This may include money, food, special herbs, or a personal favor. Acosta (1984) reported that although *curanderos* (Latin folk healers) are sought for treatment of folk diseases and physiological problems, both a study in Texas (Edgerton, Karno, & Fernandez, 1970) and a study in California (Padilla, Carlos, & O'Keefe, 1976) indicated that Mexican Americans would tend to recommend a physician for treatment of emotional problems. However, given that Latinos do not typically subscribe to the mind–body distinction as do Anglos, it is possible that many somatic complaints due to emotional distress (chest pain, headaches, and stomachaches) are treated by *curanderos*.

Perhaps some curative power comes from believing and beginning a process toward healing. Making contact with a folk healer intimately knowledgeable of their culture may be a way of roots-seeking, and thus is comforting to those who feel especially alienated (i.e., recent immigrants). Indeed, folk-healing systems seem to be more frequently used by recent immigrants who have not yet acculturated to Western biomedical practices. For example, although *curanderismo* was commonly believed to be the treatment of choice for Southwestern Latinos during the 1960s and 1970s, presently researchers are concluding that the use of indigenous healers has greatly decreased. Scheper-Hughes and Stewart (1983) interviewed 25 Latinos in Taos, New Mexico, where Saunders (1954) had studied medical beliefs and practices of these people. They concluded that "... time and acculturation have greatly eroded the beliefs in and practice of curanderismo ..." (p. 884). However, their study, as well as one by Edgerton, Karno, and Fernandez (1970), report that, together with a decreased role of *curanderismo*, there is the finding that folk healers, such as *sobadoraas* or *albolarias*, are still visited for folk ailments (such as *mal ojo* and *susto*) that cannot be understood or cured by Western biomedical practices. The extent and usage of folk healers is a question that remains open for exploration. Although researchers have documented particular herbs used in herbal remedies, very little is known about the other medicinal qualities of the folk healer. Cancela and Martinez (1983), however, list nine possible reasons for the effectiveness of folk healing systems among Latinos. They include: "a lack of impersonal or bureaucratic procedures and a personalistic humanistic nature with consultation available in informal community settings such as the home, street or bodega," "a holistic approach maintaining the unity of mind and body," "the use of literal and symbolic language," and "the discharge of tension and anger without guilt" (p. 258).

Religion, Prayer, and Spiritualism

Religion, prayer, and spirituality are key aspects of coping styles among ethnic groups. The church is a source for pastoral counseling and social support. It is a place where minorities can gather, share their worries, and pray together in hope of resolution. In short, it is a natural place to seek help from a familiar source without guilt or fear of being stigmatized. Surveys of African Americans have generally found a high level of religiosity and a spiritual orientation relative to other Americans (Broman, 1996; Neighbors, Jackson, Bowman, & Gurin, 1983; Taylor & Chatters, 1991). Indeed, nearly 85% of African Americans describe themselves as either "fairly religious" or "very religious," and more than 77% reported that going to church was "very important" to them (Neighbors & Jackson, 1996b). Taylor and Chatters (1991) found that 78% of their respondents prayed nearly every day, and Broman (1996) found that prayer is one of the most frequently cited coping responses used by African Americans in times of distress.

However, in a review of the literature on race differences in help-seeking behavior, Broman (1987) notes that type of problem, as well as the level of its severity, rather than the race of the individual, may determine whether professional help is sought from clergy or other professionals. Using data from the National Survey of Black Americans and the Americans View Their Mental Health, Broman studied psychological distress, problem type, and the help-seeking behavior of 673 Blacks and 751 Whites. He found that Blacks were more likely to utilize mental health professionals and other professional help (teachers, lawyers, social workers, etc.) than were Whites. Whites, however, were more likely to seek help from clergy and from medical professionals than were Blacks. Similarly, Snowden (1998) found that African Americans were less, not more, likely to turn to family, friends, or clergy for help with mental or emotional distress. Snowden's data did not support the hypothesis that African Americans would seek informal support rather than professional help. Instead, informal help from family, friends, and clergy appeared to complement direct services for mental health and/ or emotional problems.

Clearly, the paths of help-seeking behavior vary individually as well as culturally. Recent

Mexican immigrants, for example, may feel that their medical doctors do not spend enough time with them to understand their illnesses (Cervantes, 1992), and Mexican Americans have been found to tend to recommend a physician for emotional problems (Edgerton, Karno, & Fernandez, 1970; Padilla & Carlos, 1976). Sensitive data collection and analysis are needed in order to tease out the direction of help-seeking paths, as well as where in that path the researcher has intervened.

Other questions remain, such as if and why the person chose the method of help (e.g., forced through administrative channels for funding, or for custody of child, or recommended by a friend) and how the help is appraised.

Prayer is also an important coping mechanism for Mexican Americans (Acosta, 1984). Spiritualism and the use of prayer are important aspects of coping among American Indians and Alaskan Native cultures. Many of their healing ceremonies for physical or emotional complaints include use of spiritual, tribal rituals, typically within a group setting. Often the groups pray together for equilibrium to be restored in their community, as well as within individuals who feel out of balance (Manson, 1986, 1998).

A spirit of cooperation and trust draws from and enhances a sense of community. For example, an Indian may join a group to pray for another Indian, knowing that if she (or he) ever needed prayer for herself or for her family, that person or another from his family would participate in a praying ceremony for her. Another example is the informal financial help that is clearly a part of community involvement among the poor. A neighbor will lend another a quart of milk or five dollars *knowing* they will need it someday, and *trusting* that a neighbor will help them. Often, neighbors gather in informal meetings over coffee and share their problems. It is not unusual for the meeting to end with individuals promising to pray for each other.

This help-seeking behavior is highly valued for many reasons. One practical reason is that it extends resources, especially for those who typically live below the poverty level. Food, clothing, baby strollers, child care, transportation, and money are among the resources both scarce and shared. Another reason is that by bringing a problem to the family and/or community for help, a person previously isolated and depressed can hopefully feel cared for and supported once again. Native Indian group-cleansing ceremonies, for example, can promote a sense of relief from guilt by virtue of providing a means of forgiveness from a person who felt injured by another. Similarly, respected members of communities often are sought out for advice or to act as intermediaries in disputes. These people, often elderly, are well known in the neighborhood and often can be found at local bodegas. Again, a person previously isolated can feel that at least they now have shared their worries with someone who has been known to help others in similar situations. A process of healing through connecting and exploring different options is a strong therapeutic quality of this help-seeking behavior.

There are several ways community psychologists can avail themselves of resources in communities in order to intervene effectively. Before intervening, however, several tasks must be accomplished that facilitate understanding the culture(s) of the community, including how problems are defined and ways of coping that are typically utilized. While ethnic comparison (i.e., Black–White) studies are interesting and valuable, they often tell us little about *processes*, of different help-seeking behaviors and their links to *outcome*.

In seeking cultural sensitivity, community psychologists must be sensitive to local circumstances and variations. An intervention program that works with a group of Latinos in New York, for example, would not necessarily succeed with Latinos in the Mission District of San Francisco. Every community has its own resources and peculiarities that need to be assessed before intervention. A good place to begin is with community surveys. If it is found that many people use extended family networks, then this presents perhaps a natural place to begin to intervene. For example, community mental health agencies can (as a few are already doing) invite extended family into therapeutic programs.

Similarly, if after surveying a community it seems that folk healers are primarily consulted for folk ailments, then having a community psychologist consult with service delivery systems about how to use this information could be helpful. For example, the community psychologist might begin a research project to learn more about beliefs regarding common causes, progress, and treatment of the folk ailments. As mentioned earlier, it seems that folk healers are sought for help primarily for folk ailments that seem not to be understood by Western biomedical practices. In Cervantes' (1992) study of recent immigrants, 28% of his sample reported having the psychosocial stressor, "my doctor did not spend enough time with me to understand my illness." Perhaps the problem is amount of time or perhaps it is technique, or both—we do not know. Research that can answer these questions is long overdue.

We know precious little about utilization of folk healers by community-based clinics; we do not know who is referred, what happens in treatment, nor how many clinics integrate treatment this way. Whatever the mechanism by which clients improve, the referral itself can help the patient feel understood, less alienated; it can open doors for further sharing of concerns.

Lastly, the extent and use of religion and spirituality within a community also needs to be explored before intervention programs are implemented. As Broman (1987) notes, problem type and level of severity can determine who seeks help from clergy. For those communities that are found to use the church and religion as a method of coping, consultation with leading church members is a natural first step in understanding how an intervention might be designed, perceived, and evaluated within a community. Use of a church bulletin board or community room, or organizing an outing are ways to reach some of those in need. Integrating the beliefs with hope for change in the future can be a valuable guiding principle.

The approaches outlined are labor intensive; they require the community psychologist to tread carefully and to "look" before he or she "leaps." However, such approaches are critical to affect policies and to better define problems and means of addressing them.

SERVICE DELIVERY

For many, if not most, psychologists interested in intervention, organized mental health care represents the system at hand. Its tasks, structures, and procedures are familiar and accessible. Yet surprisingly little is known about the operation of that system. Services-oriented studies—work that focuses on the system as it is, and not as it might be—remain the exception (Bickman, 1996; Bickman, Guthrie, Foster, Lambert, Summerfelt, Breda, & Heflinger, 1995; Morrissey, Calloway, Bartko, Ridgeley, Goldman, & Paulson, 1994). This lack of knowledge is particularly glaring as it applies to ethnic minority groups. Given a history of insensitivity and failure, we must be particularly well-informed about the character of mental health services provided to them.

This section takes a comprehensive view of mental health service delivery. The purpose is to consider not only face-to-face helping, but the broader systemic context in which it occurs. A perspective is taken that suggests that the service arranged and paid for is as important as the nature of that service: if clients will not come and providers are not paid, then even the most effective intervention will have little impact.

Organization, Financing, and Utilization

From a standpoint of utilization, the most important innovation in mental health service delivery can be found right under our very noses: the community mental health system. In 1978, community mental health center caseloads consisted of about 20% ethnic minority clientele. This reflected an increase from 1972 of about 5%, and a steady pattern of growth in the intermediate years (Cheung, 1986). There is no evidence of a decline in minority utilization in subsequent years.

Related to this increased utilization has been a shift in attitudes toward mental health agencies and practices. Gary (1985) investigated attitudes toward the community mental health system in a large survey sample of Blacks. Respondents indicated generally favorable impressions. Jones and Matsumoto (1982) reviewed an extensive body of literature on attitudes toward psychotherapy held by the poor and members of ethnic minority groups. In more recent studies, they reported that a relationship between attitudes and SES/ethnicity failed to emerge. In interpreting these findings, Jones and Matsumoto noted the increasing penetration of community mental health programs into poor and minority areas, making services known to community members whose family and friends may have used them.

Evidence such as this is encouraging, but at the same time misleading. Aggregate statistics disguise important variations in minority group utilization of mental health services (Windle, 1980). Centers with greater utilization may organize themselves to emphasize this objective. Zane, Sue, Castro, and George (1982) consolidated principles that have been proposed for the development of responsive systems:

1. Congruence between services on the one hand, and needs and cultural patterns of clients on the other.
2. An active stance toward prevention and encouragement toward service utilization.
3. Integration and linkage of mental health services with other health related and social services.
4. Systems of comprehensive and coordinated services.
5. Community control through active advisory board participation with solid community representation.
6. Development of knowledge about effective practices and systems and active attempts at dissemination.

A slender but intriguing literature has developed presenting case studies of successful centers. Kahn and Delk (1973) described a program of service delivery to the Papago Indian tribe. Finances for the center were controlled by the tribe, and an active program was maintained involving consultation with medicine men. Bestman (1986) described a program whose target population consisted of the multiethnic community of Miami.

Programs such as these are attractive, appealing to the noblest ideals of community psychology. Like all organizational arrangements and service practices, however, they too must be evaluated. It remains to be documented in a rigorous fashion that innovations in staffing and procedures such as those described above truly are superior to more conventional arrangements in attracting and retaining minority clientele.

An intriguing exception to this pattern was reported by Windle (1980). Focusing on 142 federally funded community mental health centers, Windle related underutilization by minorities to characteristics of centers, as well as characteristics of catchment areas. Factors describing centers generally were less effective in predicting underutilization than factors describing catchment areas. "Characteristics which did not show a significant correlation (with underutilization) included the staffing patterns, the size of the organization, agencies toward which consultation networks were directed, a large set of funding patterns (of which only one was found significant), types of patients served, and pattern of use of the various care modalities" (p. 142). This hardly stands as an exact test of organizational arrangements described in the literature as promoting minority utilization. It should, however, give rise to a sense of healthy skepticism and caution.

Windle found several factors that indeed predicted underutilization. Centers relatively low in their proportion of nonwhite representation tended to spend a greater proportion of operating expenses on salary, receive a low percent of funds from Medicaid, operate with relatively low occupancy rates for inpatient beds, and allocate a small proportion of public information and education effort to Headstart and to schools. Catchment areas with greater underutilization tended to have a Black population of low social standing, high poverty, and greater age. They also were characterized by a poor quality of housing and greater White mobility.

Virtually all of these factors point toward economics. Centers availing themselves less of public sources of financing for services, and with less money to use (other than to pay salaries), and serving primarily Black underclass communities, tended to underrepresent minority clientele. The financing of mental health services is relatively poorly understood. It is an important area for consideration in understanding service delivery to the general population, and particularly to the minority population in light of its poverty and restricted access to funding of services from third-party payment.

It is clear that the poor have fewer options in seeking services because they are less able to pay. Cheung (1986) summarized available evidence on economic limitations to access, considering both medical services, where there is more information, and mental health services. She reported the existence of differences in whether or not care was received, and the quality of care according to socioeconomic standing.

One consequence of limited ability to pay is receiving care under public rather than private auspices. Data on practice settings and their possible impact were gathered in a national study of practice patterns of psychotherapists (Knesper, Pagnucco, & Wheeler, 1985). Clients who were less severely disturbed had different experiences depending on whether they were seen in a community mental health center or a private office. Those in a private setting were seen more frequently and over longer duration, and were less likely to receive drugs. Less severely disturbed clients in the two settings were comparable in rated level of global adjustment, but as expected, were different in level of income.

The relationship between financing of services and minority utilization remains a neglected topic. It is known, in general, that inability to pay is a barrier; little is known about the impact of alternative schemes for reducing this barrier. Are reimbursement systems better than nominal charges, or complete waivers? How does cost operate in conjunction with other dimensions of access—need, structure, attitude toward mental health care? These are questions to be answered in explaining mental health care of minority groups.

Delivery of Mental Health Services

A body of studies has attempted to document bias against ethnic minority groups in assignment of diagnostic labels and the general rendering of clinical judgments. Early studies suggested, for example, that Blacks were more likely than Whites to be involuntarily admitted to hospitals (Snowden & Cheung, 1990); less likely to receive individual psychotherapy (Mayo, 1974); and more likely to be medicated, placed in restraints and seclusion, and denied privileges (Flaherty & Meaer, 1980). As noted previously, there is considerable empirical evidence that clinicians may be biased in assessing and diagnosing the symptoms of African Americans—overdiagnosing schizophrenia and underdiagnosing affective disorders (Loring & Powell, 1988; Lu, Lim, & Messich, 1995; Worthington, 1992; Neighbors, Jackson, Campbell, & Williams, 1989). African Americans are also more likely to be hospitalized in psychiatric facilities than are White Americans (Snowden & Cheung, 1990; Snowden, 1998a).

Problems in service delivery to ethnic minority clients have shown themselves particularly clearly in a tendency for these clients to leave programs prematurely. General reviews of this dropout problem have consistently identified race and ethnicity as indicators of risk (Baekeland & Lundwall, 1975; Snowden, Libby, & Thomas, 1997; Zhang & Snowden, 1999); this has been true not only of mental health services, but also of medical and other types of services as well.

Much of this work preceded the period of active attempts at recruiting and retaining minority clients. Later research indicated a continuing problem, at least selectively. A large-scale study by Sue (1977) reported that minority clients were relatively likely to drop out. Another study of comparable vintage (Goodman & Siegel, 1978) found comparable results. Yet exceptions to this trend of minority clients leaving treatment prematurely also have been observed (Fiester, Mahrer, Giambra, & Ormiston, 1974).

Other investigators turned not to the question of whether minority clients tend to drop out, but how and why. Vail (1978), investigating Black clients at an inner-city community mental health center, found attendance associated with having a therapist of the opposite sex. Neither therapist's race nor client's racial attitudes were important. Acosta (1980) followed up White, Black, and Mexican American clients who had dropped out from a mental health clinic. He found no difference among the groups in reasons given for premature termination: All expressed disenchantment with their practitioner and with the nature of treatment itself.

Perhaps the most important task in minority mental health research is one on which the literature is relatively slender: direct evaluation of outcome of intervention. Helpful reviews of existing research are available. Cortese (1979) examined experimental studies of treatment conducted on Spanish-speaking populations. His tentative conclusion was that behaviorally oriented procedures were preferable to others because of their concrete focus and tendency to discount self-disclosure. Individual studies have established, for example, that cognitive and behavioral treatments work for Puerto Rican women (Comas-Diaz, 1981).

Muñoz (1986) considered preventive interventions implemented with ethnic minority groups. Of 30 prevention-oriented references identified in their review, only a handful involved outcome research. Included were programs of identity enhancement and social integration among Native Americans, evaluation of a health services system for Asian American elderly, a program of interpersonal cognitive problem-solving skills for school-age Black youngsters, and the author's own depression prevention research project.

Both in its scope and quality, this body of evidence is quite limited. Many (particularly earlier) investigators of clinical judgment chose correlational methods; they thereby demonstrated associations between minority status and diagnostic and treatment decisions. Correlations such as these are intriguing, but open to alternative interpretations. It is possible that differential treatment is justified on the basis of differential patterns of need. Meinhardt and Vega (1987) found precisely this in their study of Santa Clara County, California. Similar criticisms have been offered by Sue (1977) and others (Abramowitz & Dokecki, 1977).

Granting the improbable assumption of equivalent problems, research designs from these studies remained faulty because of their failure to include controls for any of the many factors confounded with ethnicity. It was often difficult to determine whether differences in decisions were related to ethnicity in its own right, or to some correlate of ethnicity. Sue (1977) was among the few investigators to recognize and selectively allow for this problem.

To introduce better control, especially for extraneous factors, investigators have turned to experimental analogues. These designs are sometimes useful, but remain vulnerable to criticisms of their external validity; challenges to realism can be both obvious and quite subtle (Maher, 1978). Equally important, analogue studies provide virtually no information on context. They imply a universal relevance to their findings that almost certainly cannot be justified over the full range of the regions and settings in which services are delivered.

Finally, much more must be done in the way of rigorous evaluation of services outcomes. This must include studies both of efficacy (evaluation under formal but artificial circumstances), as well as effectiveness (evaluation under routine conditions of practice). It ought to include psychotherapy, but also supportive and management-oriented interventions, referrals, and medication. Studies should be substantive, but also methodological. There is room both for full-fledged experiments, and for quasi-experiments, designs with relaxed experimental vigilance but greater responsiveness to real-world contingencies of practice.

Thus, an orientation to research on mental health service delivery to ethnic minority groups is needed that is both broad and flexible. Reaching beyond clinical trials of discrete interventions, it must be methodologically resourceful, ecologically valid, and culturally aware. Psychologists particularly well-equipped to take on this assignment identify with a community psychology perspective.

Given current knowledge and the structure of professional roles, how can community psychologists help improve the quality of life for ethnic minorities? Answering this question is at once simple and complex. Community psychologists must help to create generalizations, yet know their limits. They must work to apply general facts and principles at local levels: cities, catchment areas, communities. In general, ethnic minority groups are poorer, less physically healthy, less educated, more at risk for death from violence or heart disease, and so on. But in particular, that is, in the Black or Latino or Asian or American Indian community at hand, any of these problems may be more or less salient, and local resources may be stronger or weaker for addressing them.

Having a sketch of existing problems and formal and informal resources available in a community, in other words, can set the stage for the community psychologist. Working with community members to find out if generalities (i.e., health problems) are a problem in their particular community could be a next step. In this process of addressing community members lies a wonderful opportunity for correcting our own state of ignorance. We can learn:

1. Reasons services are or are not used within the community. Do the services exist? Is avoidance of services primarily financial or due to unfamiliarity with service, feeling dissatisfied with service, etc.
2. Typical ways of coping. What strategies are appropriate and effective, involving whom, and why?

This is an opportune time to work with community members to design intervention programs and discuss implementation. Evaluation also is essential, with feedback from and to the community.

All this must be done, keeping in mind the historical roots of the community, the culture of its members, past and present policies toward people of color, as well as our own prejudices and biases. The task for the community psychologist then is (and has been) challenging, and the rewards urgently awaited.

REFERENCES

Abramowitz, C. V., & Dokecki, P. R. (1977). The politics of clinical judgment: Early empirical returns. *Psychological Bulletin, 84*, 460–476.

Acosta, F. X. (1980). Self-described reasons for premature termination of psychotherapy by Mexican American, Black American and Anglo-American patients. *Psychological Reports, 47*, 435–443.

Acosta, F. X. (1984). Psychotherapy with Mexican Americans: Clinical and empirical gains. In J. L. Martinez, Jr. & R. H. Mendoza (Eds.), *Chicano psychology*, 2nd ed. (pp. 163–185). Orlando: Academic.

Baekeland, F., & Lundwall, L. (1975). Dropping out of treatment: A critical review. *Psychological Bulletin, 82*, 738–783.

Barney, D. D. (1995). Use of mental health services by American Indian and Alaska Native elders. In D. K. Padgett (Ed.), *Handbook on ethnicity, aging, and mental health* (pp. 203–214). Westport, CT: Greenwood.

Beals, J., Piasecki, S., Nelson, M., Jones, E., Keane, P., Dauphinais, R., Red Shirt, W. S., & Manson, S. (1997). Psychiatric disorder among American Indian adolescents: Prevalence in Northern Plains youth. *Journal of the American Academy of Child and Adolescent Psychiatry, 36*, 26–31.

Bell, C. C., Dixie-Bell, D. D., & Thompson, B. (1986). Further studies on the prevalence of isolated sleep paralysis in black subjects. *Journal of the National Medical Association, 75*, 649–659.

Berkowitz, G. (1987). *Reducing access to medical care: The differential impact on men and women.* Unpublished doctoral dissertation, School of Public Health, University of California, Berkeley.

Bestman, E. W. (1986). Cross-cultural approaches to service delivery to ethnic minorities: The Miami model. In M. R. Miranda & H. L. Kitano (Eds.), *Mental health research and practice in minority communities: Development of culturally sensitive training programs* (pp. 136–171). Rockville, MD: NIMH.

Bickman, L. (1996). A continuum of care: More is not always better. *American Psychologist, 51*, 689–701.

Bickman, L., Guthrie, P. R., Foster, E. M., Lambert, E. W., Summerfelt, W. T., Breda C. S., & Heflinger, C. A. (1995). *Evaluating managed mental health services: The Fort Bragg experiment.* Boston: Houghton-Mifflin.

Broman, C. L. (1987). Race differences in professional help-seeking. *American Journal of Community Psychology, 15*, 473–489.

Broman, C. L. (1996). Coping with personal problems. In H. N. Neighbors & J. S. Jackson (Eds.), *Mental health in black America* (pp. 117–129). Thousand Oaks, CA: Sage.

Bulik, C. (1986). *Immigration and adaptation: The individual and the family.* (Manuscript submitted in partial fulfillment of qualifying exams, University of California, Berkeley, Department of Psychology, unpublished.)

Bulik, C. (1987). Eating disorders in immigration: Two case studies. *International Journal of Eating Disorders, 6*, 133–141.

Burnham, A. M., Timbus, D. M., & Hough, R. (1984). Two measures of psychological distress among Mexican-Americans, Mexicans, and Anglos. *Journal of Health and Social Behavior, 25*, 24–33.

Burns, B. J., Costello, E. J., Angold, A., Tweed, D., Stangl, D., Farmer, E. M. Z., & Erkanli, A. (1995). Children's mental health service across service sectors. *Health Affairs, 14*, 147–159.

Cancela, V., & Martinez, I. Z. (1983). An analysis of culturalism in Latino mental health: Folk medicine as a case in point. *Hispanic Journal of Behavioral Sciences, 5*, 251–274.

Cervantes, R. C. (1992). Occupational and economic stressors among immigrant and U.S. born Hispanics. In S. B. Knouse, P. Rosenfeld, & A. L. Culbertson (Eds.), *Hispanics in the workplace* (pp. 120–133). Newbury Park, CA: Sage.

Cheung, F. K. (1986). *Minority population use mental health services in the community.* Paper presented at Annual Meeting, American Public Health Association, Las Vegas, Nevada.

Cheung, F. K., & Snowden, L. R. (1990). Community mental health and ethnic minority populations. *Community Mental Health Journal, 26*, 277–291.

Cohen, S. (1992). Stress, social support, and disorder. In H. O. F. Veiel & U. Baumann (Eds.), *The meaning and measurement of social support* (pp. 109–124). New York: Hemisphere.

Cohon, D. (1981). Psychological adaptation and dysfunction among refugees. *International Migration Review, 15*, 255–275.

Comas-Diaz, L. (1981). Effects of cognitive and behavioral group treatment on the depressive symptomatology of Puerto Rican women. *Journal of Consulting and Clinical Psychology, 49*, 627–632.

Cortese, M. (1979). Intervention research with Hispanic Americans: A review. *Hispanic Journal of Behavioral Sciences, 1,* 4–20.

Cowen, E. L. (1984). Training for primary prevention in mental health. *American Journal of Community Psychology, 12,* 253–259.

Dilworth-Anderson, P., & Marshall, S. (1996). Social support in its cultural context. In G. R. Pierce, B. R. Sarason, & I. G. Sarason (Eds.), *Handbook of social support and the family* (pp. 67–69). New York: Plenum.

Dohrenwend, B. S. (1978). Social stress and community psychology. *American Journal of Community Psychology, 6,* 1–14.

Dressler, W. W. (1985). Extended family relationships, social support, and mental health in a southern black community. *Journal of Health and Social Behavior, 26,* 39–48.

Edgerton, R. B., Karno, M., & Fernandez, I. (1970). Curanderismo in the metropolis. *American Journal of Psychotherapy, 24,* 124–134.

Ekman, P., & Friesen, W. V. (1971). Constancy across cultures in the face emotion. *Journal of Personality and Social Psychology, 9,* 12–17.

Fabrega, H. (1995). Hispanic mental health research: A case for cultural psychiatry. In A. M. Padilla (Ed.), *Hispanic psychology: Critical issues in theory and research* (pp. 107–130). Thousand Oaks, CA: Sage.

Fiester, A. R., Maher, A. R., Giambra, L. M., & Ormiston, D. W. (1974). Shaping a clinic population: The dropout problem reconsidered. *Community Mental Health Journal, 10,* 173–179.

Flaherty, J. A., & Meaer, R. (1980). Measuring racial bias in inpatient treatment. *American Journal of Psychiatry, 137,* 679–682.

Frerichs, R., Aneshensel, C., & Clark, V. (1981). Prevalence of depression in Los Angeles County. *American Journal of Epidemiology, 113,* 691–699.

Frieman, M., Cunningham, P., & Cornelius, L. (1994). *Use and expenditures for treatment of mental health problems.* Rockville, MD: Agency for Health Care Policy Research.

Gary, L. E. (1985). Attitudes toward human service organizations: Perspectives from an urban Black community. *Journal of Applied Behavioral Science, 21,* 445–458.

Goldwasser, B. L., & Badger, A. E. (1989). Utility of the psychiatric screen among the Navajo of Chinle: A fourth year clerkship experience. *American Indian and Alaska Native Mental Health Research, 3,* 6–15.

Goodman, A. B., & Siegel, C. (1978). Differences in white–nonwhite community mental health center utilization patterns. *Journal of Evaluation and Program Planning, 1,* 51–63.

Guest, A. M., Almgren, G., & Hussey, J. M. (1998). The ecology of race and socioeconomic distress: Infant and working age mortality in Chicago. *Demography, 35,* 23–34.

Hays, W. C., & Mindel, C. H. (1973). Extended kinship relations in black and white families. *Journal of Marriage and the Family, 35,* 51–57.

Hendricks, L., & Bayton, J. (1983). NIMH's diagnostic interview schedule: A test of its concurrent validity with a population of black adults. *Journal of the National Medical Association, 75,* 667–671.

Heurtin-Roberts, S., & Reisin, E. (1990). Models of hypertension among black women: Problems in illness management. In J. Coreil & J. D. Mull (Eds.), *Anthropology and primary health care* (pp. 222–250). Boulder, CO: Westview.

Heurtin-Roberts, S., Snowden, L. R., & Miller, L. (1997). Expressions of anxiety in African Americans: Ethnography and the ECA studies. *Culture, Medicine, and Psychiatry, 21,* 337–363.

Hofferth, S. L. (1984). Kin network, race, and family structure. *Journal of Marriage and the Family, 46,* 791–806.

Hu, T. W., Snowden, L. R., & Jerrell, J. M. (1991). Costs and use of public mental health services by ethnicity. (Special issue: Multicultural mental health and substance abuse services) *Journal of Mental Health Administration, 19,* 278–287.

Hurley, R. E., & Draper, D. A. (1998). Medicaid managed care for special needs populations: Behavioral health as "tracer condition." In D. Mechanic (Ed.), *Managed behavioral health care: Current realities and future potential, New directions for mental health services,* Vol. 78 (pp. 51–66). San Francisco: Jossey-Bass.

James, S. A., Hartnett S. A., & Kalsbeek, W. D. (1983). John Henryism and blood pressure differences among Black men. *Journal of Behavioral Medicine, 6,* 259–278.

Jimenez, A. L., Alegria, M., Pena, M., & Vera, M. (1997). Mental health utilization in women with symptoms of depression. *Women and Health, 25,* 1–21.

Johnson, R. E. B., & Crowley, C. E. (1996). An analysis of stress denial. In H. M. Neighbors & J. S. Jackson (Eds.), *Mental health in black America* (pp. 62–76). Thousand Oaks, CA: Sage.

Jones, E. E., & Korchin, S. J. (1982). *Minority mental health.* New York: Praeger.

Jones, E. E., & Matsumoto, D. R. (1982). Psychotherapy with the underserved: Recent developments. In L. R. Snowden (Ed.), *Reaching the underserved: Neglected populations* (pp. 321–376). Beverly Hills, CA: Sage.

Kahn, M. W., & Delk, H. L. (1973). Developing a community mental health clinic on the Papago reservation. *International Journal of Social Psychiatry, 19,* 200–206.

Kessler, R. C. (1992). Perceived support and adjustment to stress: Methodological considerations. In H. O. F. Veiel & U. Baumann (Eds.), *The meaning and measurement of social support* (pp. 109–124). New York: Hemisphere.

Knesper, D. J., Pagnucco, D. J., & Wheeler, J. R. C. (1985). Similarities and differences across mental health services providers, and practice settings in the United States. *American Psychologist, 40*, 1352–1370.

Kramer, B. J. (1991). Urban American Indian aging. *Journal of Cross-Cultural Gerontology, 6*, 205–217.

Lawson, W. B., Hepler, N., Holladay, J., & Cuffel, B. (1994). Race as a factor in inpatient and outpatient admissions and diagnosis. *Hospital and Community Psychiatry, 45*, 72–74.

Leginski, W. A., Manderscheid, R. W., & Henderson, P. R. (1990). Patients served in state mental hospitals: Results from a longitudinal data base. In R. W. Manderscheid & M. A. Sonnenschein (Eds.), *Mental health, United States: 1990* (pp. 61–73). Washington, D.C.: Department of Health and Human Services.

Lewin-Epstein, N. (1991). Determinants of regular source of health care in black, Mexican American, Puerto Rican, and non-Hispanic white populations. *Medical Care, 29*, 543–557.

Lin, K. (1986). Psychopathology and social disruption in refugees. In C. L. Williams & J. Westermeyer (Eds.), *Refugee mental health in resettlement countries* (pp. 61–73). Washington, D.C.: Hemisphere Publishing.

Lopez, S. (1981). Mexican Americans usage of mental health facilities: Underutilization reconsidered. In A. Baron (Ed.), *Explorations in Chicano psychology* (pp. 176–210). New York: Praeger.

Loring, M., & Powell, B. (1988). Gender, race, and DSM-III: A study of objectivity of psychiatric diagnostic behavior. *Journal of Health and Social Behavior, 29*, 1–22.

Lu, F., Lim, R., & Messich, J. (1995). Issues on the assessment and diagnosis of culturally diverse individuals. In J. Oldham & M. Riba (Eds.), *Cross cultural psychiatry, Section IV*, Annual Review of Psychiatry, *14*, 477–510.

Maher, B. A. (1978). Stimulus sampling in clinical research: Representative design revisited. *Journal of Consulting and Clinical Psychology, 16*, 643–647.

Malson, M. (1982). The social support systems of black families. *Marriage and Family Review, 37*, 37–57.

Manson, S. M. (1986). Recent advances in American Indian mental health research: Implications for clinical research and training. In M. R. Miranda & M. L. Kitano (Eds.), *Mental health research and practice in minority communities: Development of culturally sensitive training programs* (pp. 321–360). Rockville, MD: NIMH.

Manson, S. M. (1998). *Mental health services for American Indians: Need, use, and barriers to effective care*. Unpublished manuscript: University of Colorado, Denver.

Marsella, A. J., Kinzie, D., & Gordon, P. (1973). Ethnic variations in the expression of depression. *Journal of Cross-Cultural Psychology, 4*, 435–458.

Martin, E., & Martin, J. (1995). *The helping tradition in the black family and community*. Washington, D.C.: National Association of Social Workers.

Martinez, M., & Snowden, L. R. (1987). *Psychosocial risk factors in pregnancy*. Paper presented at First Binational Conference on Mexico–U.S. Migration. Guadalajara, Mexico.

Maton, K. I., Teti, D. M., Corns, K. M., Viera-Baker, C. C., Lavine, J. R., Gouze, K. R., & Keating, D. P. (1996). Cultural specificity of support sources, correlates, and contexts: Three studies of African American and Caucasian youth. *American Journal of Community Psychology, 24*, 551–587.

Mayo, J. A. (1974). Utilization of a community mental health center by blacks: Admission to inpatient status. *Journal of Nervous and Mental Disease, 158*, 202–207.

McAdoo, H. (1978). The impact of upward mobility of kin-help patterns and the reciprocal obligations in Black families. *Journal of Marriage and the Family, Fall*, 265–274.

McAdoo, H. (1980). Black mothers and the extended family support network. In L. F. Rodgers-Rose (Ed.), *The black woman* (pp. 124–144). Beverly Hills: Sage.

Meinhardt, K., & Vega, W. (1987). A method for estimating the level of underutilization of mental health services by Mexican Americans and other minority groups. *Hospital and Community Psychiatry, 38*, 1186–1190.

Moos, R. H. (1984). Context and coping: Toward a unifying conceptual framework. *American Journal of Community Psychology, 12*, 5–25.

Morrissey, J. P., Calloway, M., Bartko, W. T., Ridgely, M. S., Goldman, H. H., & Paulson, R. I. (1994). Local mental health authorities and service system change: Evidence from the Robert Wood Johnson Program on Chronic Mental Illness. *The Milbank Quarterly, 72*, 49–80.

Muñoz, R. F. (1986). Opportunities for prevention among Hispanics. In R. L. Hough, P. A. Gongla, V. B. Brown, & S. E. Goldston (Eds.), *Psychiatric epidemiology and prevention: The possibilities* (pp. 109–129). Los Angeles: UCLA Psychiatric Institute.

Murray, C. (1984). *Losing ground*. Nw York: Basic Books.

Murray, C. B., & Peacock, M. J. (1996). A model-free approach to the study of subjective well-being. In H. W. Neighbors & J. S. Jackson (Eds.), *Mental health in black America* (pp. 14–26). Thousand Oaks, CA: Sage.

Neal, A. M., & Turner, S. M. (1991). Anxiety disorders research with African Americans: Current status. *Psychological Bulletin, 109*, 400–410.

Neighbors, H. W. (1984). The distribution of psychiatric morbidity in Black Americans: A review and suggestions for research. *Community Mental Health Journal, 20,* 169–181.

Neighbors, H. W., & Jackson, J. S. (Eds.). (1996a). *Mental health in black America.* Thousand Oaks, CA: Sage.

Neighbors, H. W., & Jackson, J. S. (1996b). Mental health in black America: Psychosocial problems and help-seeking behavior. In H. W. Neighbors & J. S. Jackson (Eds.), *Mental health in black America* (pp. 1–13). Thousand Oaks, CA: Sage.

Neighbors, H., Jackson, J., Campbell, D., & Williams, D. (1989). Racial influences on psychiatric diagnosis: A review and suggestions for research. *Community Mental Health Journal, 25,* 301–311.

Padgett, D. K., Patrick, C., Burns, C., & Schlesinger, M. (1994). Women and outpatient mental health services: Use by Black, Hispanic, and White women in a national insured population. *Journal of Mental Health Administration, 21,* 347–360.

Padilla, A. M., Carlos, M. L., & Keefe. (1976). Mental health service utilization by Mexican Americans. In M. R. Miranda (Ed.), *Psychotherapy with the Spanish-speaking: Issues in research and service delivery, Monograph 3* (pp. 9–20). Los Angeles: Spanish Speaking Mental Health Research Center.

Pang, K. Y. C. (1990). Hwabyung: The construction of a Korean popular illness among Korean elderly immigrant women in the United States. *Culture, Medicine, and Psychiatry, 14,* 495–512.

Rahe, R. H., Looney, J. G., Ward, H. W., Tung, M. T., & Liu, W. T. (1978). Psychiatric consultation in a Vietnamese refugee camp. *American Journal of Psychiatry, 135,* 185–190.

Rimer, S. (1996). Blacks urged to act to increase awareness of the AIDS epidemic. *New York Times, A10,* October 23.

Robins, L. N., & Regier, D. A. (Eds.). (1991). *Psychiatric disorders in America: The Epidemiologic Catchment Area Study.* New York: Free Press.

Saegert, S. (1989). Unlikely leaders, extreme circumstances: Older black women building community households. *American Journal of Community Psychology, 17,* 295–316.

Saunders, L. (1954). *Cultural difference and medical care: The case of the Spanish-speaking people of the Southwest.* New York: Sage.

Scheper-Hughes, N., & Stewart, D. (1983). Curanderismo in Taos County, New Mexico: A possible case of anthropological romanticism. *Crosscultural Medicine, Western Journal of Medicine, 139,* 875–884.

Shore, J. H., & Manson, S. (1983). American Indian psychiatric and social problems. *Transcultural Psychiatric Research Review, 20,* 159–180.

Snow, L. (1993). *Walkin' over medicine.* Boulder, CO: Westview.

Snowden, L. R. (1998a). Racial differences in informal help-seeking for mental health problems. *Journal of Community Psychology, 26,* 429–438.

Snowden, L. R. (1998b). Managed care and ethnic minority populations. *Administration and Policy in Mental Health, 25,* 125–131.

Snowden, L. R. (in press). African-American folk idiom and mental health service use. *Cultural Diversity and Mental Health.*

Snowden, L. R., & Cheung, F. K. (1990). Use of inpatient mental health services of ethnic minority groups. *American Psychologist, 45,* 347–355.

Snowden, L. R., & Hu, T. W. (1997). Ethnic differences in mental health services use among the severely mentally ill. *Journal of Community Psychology, 25,* 235–247.

Snowden, L. R., Libby, A., & Thomas, K. (1997). Health care related attitudes and utilization among African American women. *Women's Health: Research on Gender Behavior, 3,* 301–314.

Stack, C. B. (1974). *All our kin: Strategies for survival in a black community.* New York: Harper.

Sue, S. (1977). Community mental health services to minority groups. *American Psychologist, 32,* 616–624.

Sue, S., & Morishima, J. K. (1982). *The mental health of Asian Americans.* San Francisco: Jossey-Bass.

Sue, S., & Sue, D. W. (1974). MMPI comparisons between Asian American and non-Asian students utilizing a student health psychiatric clinic. *Journal of Counseling Psychology, 21,* 423–427.

Sue, S., & Sue, D. W. (1991). Counseling strategies for Chinese Americans. In C. C. Lee & B. L. Richardson (Eds.), *Multicultural issues in counseling: New approaches to diversity* (pp. 79–90). Alexandria, VA: American Association for Counseling and Development.

Tanaka-Matsumi, J., & Marsella, A. J. (1976). Cross-cultural variations in the phenomenological experience of depression: I. Word association studies. *Journal of Cross-Cultural Psychology, 2,* 379–396.

Taylor, R. J., & Chatters, L. M. (1991). Religious life. In J. S. Jackson (Ed.), *Life in black America* (pp. 105–123). Newbury Park, CA: Sage.

Thernstrom, S., & Thernstrom, A. (1997). *America in black and white.* New York: Schuster.

U.S. Department of Health and Human Services. (1985). *Black and Minority Health. Report of the Secretary's Task Force: Volume I.* Washington, D.C.: Author.

Vail, A. (1978). Factors influencing lower-class black patients remaining in treatment. *Journal of Consulting and Clinical Psychology, 46,* 341.

Valle, R., & Bensussen, G. (1985). Hispanic social networks, social support, and mental health. In W. A. Vega & M. R. Miranda (Eds.), *Stress and Hispanic mental health: Relating research to service delivery* (pp. 147–173). Rockville, MD: National Institute of Mental Health.

Vega, W. A., & Kolody, B. (1998). *Hispanic mental health at the crossroads.* University of Texas, San Antonio: Unpublished manuscript.

Vega, W. A., & Murphy, J. W. (1990). *Culture and the restructuring of community mental health.* Westport, CT: Greenwood.

Vega, W. A., & Rumbaut, R. (1991). Ethnic minorities and mental health. *Annual Review and Sociology, 17,* 351–383.

Vega, W. A., Warheit, G., Buhl-Auth, J., & Meinhardt, K. (1984). The prevalence of depressive symptoms among Mexican-Americans and Anglos. *American Journal of Epidemiology, 120,* 592–607.

Vernon, S. W., & Roberts, R. E. (1982). Prevalence of treated and untreated psychiatric disorders in three ethnic groups. *Social Science and Medicine, 16,* 1575–1582.

Veroff, J., Douvan, E., & Kulka, R. A. (1981). *The inner American: A self portrait from 1957–1976.* New York: Basic Books.

Ware, J. E. (1986). Comparison of health outcomes at a health maintenance organization and those of fee-for-service care. *Lancet,* May 3, 1017–1022.

Weidman, H. H. (1979). Falling out: A diagnostic and treatment problem viewed from a transcultural perspective. *Social Science and Medicine, 13,* 95–112.

Wilson, M. N. (1991). The context of African American family life. In J. E. Everett, S. S. Chipungu, & B. R. Leashore (Eds.), *Child welfare: An Africentric perspective* (pp. 85–118). New Brunswick, NJ: Rutgers University Press.

Wilson, M. N., Greene-Bates, C., McKim, L., Simmons, F., et al. (1995). African American family life. In M. N. Wilson (Ed.), *African American family life: Its structural and ecological aspects* (pp. 5–21). San Francisco: Jossey-Bass.

Wilson, W. J. (1987). *The truly disadvantaged.* Chicago: The University of Chicago Press.

Wilson, W. J. (1995). When work disappears: The world of the new urban poor. In K. McFate & R. Lawson (Eds.), *Poverty, inequality, and social policy: Western states in the New World Order.* New York: Russell Sage Foundation.

Wilson, W. J. (1996). Jobless ghettos and the social outcome of youngsters. In P. Moen, G. H. Elder, Jr., & K. Luscher (Eds.), *Examining lives in context: Perspectives on the ecology of human development* (pp. 527–543). Washington, D.C.: American Psychological Association.

Windle, C. (1980). Correlates of community mental health center under-service to non-whites. *Journal of Community Psychology, 8,* 140–156.

Wong, H. Z. (1982). Asian and Pacific Americans. In L. R. Snowden (Ed.), *Reaching the underserved: Mental health needs of neglected populations* (pp. 165–184). Beverly Hills, Sage.

Woodward, A. M., Dwinell, A. D., & Arons, B. S. (1992). Barriers to mental health care for Hispanic Americans: A literature review and discussion. *Journal of Mental Health Administration, 19,* 224–236.

Worthington, C. (1992). An examination of factors influencing the diagnosis and treatment of black patients in the mental health system. *Archives of Psychiatric Nursing, 6,* 195–204.

Wu, I., & Windle, C. (1980). Ethnic specificity in the relationships of minority use and staffing of community mental health centers. *Community Mental Health Journal, 16,* 156–168.

Zane, N., Hatanaka, H., Park, S. S., & Akutsu, P. (1994). Ethnic-specific mental health services: Evaluation of the parallel approach for Asian American clients. *Journal of Community Psychology, 22,* 68–81.

Zane, N., Sue, S., Castro, E. G., & George, W. (1982). Service system models for ethnic minorities. In L. R. Snowden (Ed.), *Reaching the underserved: Mental health needs of neglected populations* (pp. 278–301). Beverly Hills, CA: Sage.

Zhang, A. Y., & Snowden, L. R. (1999). Ethnic characteristics of mental disorders in five communities nationwide. *Cultural Diversity and Mental Health, 5,* 134–146.

CHAPTER 35

Women's Empowerment

A Review of Community Psychology's First 25 Years

CAROLYN F. SWIFT, MEG A. BOND,
AND IRMA SERRANO-GARCIA

INTRODUCTION

Equal opportunity and equal rights have long been important parts of this country's ideological heritage. Support for these ideals, however, was not widespread until the latter part of this century. The modern civil rights and women's movements emerged in the 1960s, along with the widespread resistance to the Vietnam war. During this same turbulent period community psychology was "officially born." The Division of Community Psychology was formally organized in 1965 at a conference in Swampscott, Massachusetts. According to Walsh (1987), "the clamor of oppressed U.S. citizens demanding full societal participation" was "a key aspect of the social context for the subdiscipline's founding" (p. 524).

The commonalities between the values of the civil rights movement, feminism, and community psychology suggest an isomorphism in theory that has, over the last few decades, begun to be realized in practice. Elsewhere in this volume, the connection between community psychology and minority populations is documented. In this chapter we trace the development of the roles and status of women and their concerns within the context of the development of community psychology. Mulvey (1988) eloquently describes the shared values of feminism and community psychology:

> The value systems at the heart of these paradigms are similar. Shared values include the right of every individual to optimal well-being, respect for diversity and difference among individuals and groups, empowerment, and equality. Both entities recognize that inequality is structured into our social systems and see the powerful influence social conditions have on psychological and personal reality. Further, both assert that the influence of structured inequality and social conditions is not random or

---

CAROLYN F. SWIFT • 1102 Hilltop Drive, Lawrence Kansas 66044. MEG A. BOND • Department of Psychology, University of Massachusetts at Lowell, Lowell, Massachusetts 01854. IRMA SERRANO-GARCIA • Department of Psychology, University of Puerto Rico, Río Piedras, Puerto Rico 00926.

Handbook of Community Psychology, edited by Julian Rappaport and Edward Seidman. Kluwer Academic / Plenum Publishers, New York, 2000.

> unpredictable; rather, it affects aggregates of people in systematic ways that are related to such factors as gender, race, class, age, and disability. (Mulvey, 1988, p. 74)

More recently, the core values of community psychology have been reiterated as

> including a respect for diversity; the use of an ecological framework which posits that individual and community experience can only be understood contextually, taking into account the present and historical interactions between people and the settings in which they live; and a focus on empowerment, including the development of research processes that are themselves empowering to community members. (Banyard & Miller, 1998)

Despite these shared values, women and the community issues for which they have traditionally carried responsibility were relatively invisible at community psychology's founding conference at Swampscott (only 1 of the 39 conferees was a woman), and they remained so within the discipline over the next ten years. Reports of the 1975 Austin conference on training in community psychology show that, although there was a concerted effort to involve women, topics related to women's mental health issues were not considered conference priorities (Iscoe, Bloom, & Spielberger, 1977). An account of women's integration into the professional ranks of community psychologists can be found in Mulvey and Bond (1990). This chapter documents the field's efforts to integrate women and their concerns into the mainstream of community psychology in the 25 years after Swampscott (1965–1990). Our approach has involved four steps: (1) selecting a set of issues from among those of major importance to women, (2) conducting a literature review of community psychology journals for articles focusing on these issues, (3) evaluating the articles for their relevance to prevention and/or empowerment activities, and (4) reviewing them for their contribution to the study of women's issues. The journals searched[1] for the period 1965–1990 include the official journal of (APA's) Division of Community Psychology (Division 27), the *American Journal of Community Psychology* (AJCP), along with three special issues of the division's official newsletter, *The Community Psychologist* (Bond, 1988a; Linney & Bond, 1985a, 1985b); the *Journal of Community Psychology* (JCP); and the office journal of the Vermont Conference on the Primary Prevention of Psychopathology, the *Journal of Primary Prevention* (JPP).

Although community psychologists publish in many other journals, both inside and outside the field of psychology, it is beyond the scope of this chapter to provide a comprehensive review of this widely dispersed body of material. It is our purpose to point readers to these core sources of community psychology literature, and to indicate briefly what has been published related to the empowerment of women and issues of concern to them over a period covering roughly the first quarter century of the development of community psychology as a discipline. If we have found little on a particular topic, this may or may not mean the field has neglected the issue. Such a finding is intended to alert readers that the topic has not been in the mainstream of the field's attention.

We selected for review articles related to the prevention of mental illness or social injustice, or to empowerment—understood to be the process through which people and communities gain control over their lives (Rappaport, 1987). Although the articles we selected

[1]The search was conducted by selecting key words and searching the abstracts of the journals through PsychLit, a computerized database sponsored by the American Psychological Association. JPP was additionally searched by SocioFile, a database sponsored by the American Sociological Association. There were many articles about children in the journals reviewed. We have included those that bear most directly on women as reflected in the topics selected, and in the themes of the prevention of mental illness or social injustice, and/or the empowerment of women. Readers interested in the list of key words can contact Meg A. Bond, Department of Psychology, University of Massachusetts—Lowell, Lowell, MA 01854.

did not have to state these concepts as primary goals, they had to involve issues critical to the empowerment process, or concepts related to prevention, including stress and its management, social supports, coping skills or competence, and self-esteem.[2]

We use the terms "women's issues" and "women's concerns" because of their brevity; it would be awkward to list the subjects subsumed each time we wish to refer to them. In some circles these terms have become labels for stereotyped ways of perceiving significant human issues. A major problem with which women contend is that many people tend not to see the issues of reproduction, nurturing and caring for children, single parenting, rape, incest, sexual harassment, woman battering, and the feminization of poverty, for example, as issues of concern to both genders, but rather as "women's issues" only, although all have causes and consequences brought about by male–female interactions. Furthermore, many of these issues, particularly those related to sexual behavior, are initiated primarily by men. Such categorization permits a compartmentalization and dismissal of significant community issues as representative of a "special interest group." With this caveat in mind, these terms are useful as a shorthand code to the content of this chapter.

We found that some researchers refer to participants in their studies in generic, nongendered terms—parents, elders, teachers, caretakers, survivors—when a closer reading shows all the participants to be women. Such language can result in ambiguous generalizations and extrapolations, and underscores the invisibility of women's participation in society.

Many of our findings duplicate those of others reviewing special populations in this volume. We found relatively few articles directly related to women and their concerns. Some subpopulations of women, such as those with disabilities, were essentially unaddressed. Most of the articles were at the individual level rather than multiple levels of analysis. We found that few studies were carried out within the community, and even fewer involved community residents in their planning and implementation. Intervention research tended to involve educational strategies rather than attempts to change barriers or create resources, although the latter efforts have increased over the last decade. In general, authors did not address the power imbalance between genders and the impact of this imbalance on their research. Nor did they (with notable exceptions) embed their work within the historical context of the patriarchal culture that has mandated unequal status for women. These systemic "blind spots" are evident at every level, in the selection of research topics, the choice of study participants, the relationship between experimenter and participants, and the interpretation of results. It was the rule, rather than the exception, to find that women were left out of studies, or that their contributions or experiences were lumped with men's, their concerns were ignored, and the impact of research findings on them was unassessed.

This is not to say there has been no progress for women in the field of community psychology. Over the period studied there has been an acceleration in the number of articles directly related to women in the journals reviewed. The articles themselves show increasing sophistication about women and their concerns—a result of both the increasing awareness of investigators to gender issues, and more women researchers and scholars in the field.

We have used Swift and Levin's (1987) outline of empowerment as a four-stage process as a rough gauge of the empowerment status of the studies reviewed. Most community psychology studies about the prevention of dysfunctional outcomes in women or about the empowerment of women are consistent with the initial, descriptive stages of the empowerment process. Some of the interventions fit into promotion paradigms or mobilize resources for

[2]For recent studies related to these issues, see Hobfoll, Dunahoo, Ben-Porath, and Monnier (1994); Nelson (1990); and Ullman and Siegel (1994).

empowerment. Theoretical pieces tend to describe issues relevant to early stages of the empowerment process, informing the field of the institutions and processes in our culture that disempower women, and identifying structural variables that block women's development across life domains.

The body of the chapter is devoted to a review of women's connections with a series of issues—family patterns, workforce participation, care of dependent family members, health and reproduction, poverty and homelessness, violence, and minority status—as reflected in the community psychology journals cited. We discuss the articles reviewed in the context of their number, the levels of analysis used, and the consciousness of gender issues, such as stereotyping and unequal power status. Although our review covers only the first quarter century of community psychology as a discipline, within each section we direct readers to related theory and research published since that period in the journals reviewed. The chapter ends with recommendations for future research and action programs.

WOMEN'S FAMILY PATTERNS

Women's lifestyles have changed in major ways over the last few decades. In addition to women's increased entry into the workforce, their choices about partners and parenting have also expanded. At the same time that more single women are becoming mothers, more married women are remaining childless. The increasing number of single mothers results from a variety of circumstances, including divorce, the desire to combine single status with motherhood, and reduced stigma for out-of-wedlock babies. On the average, women who marry are doing so later in their lives, having fewer children, and having them later. Divorce, relatively uncommon in previous generations, is common today. Women choosing a lesbian lifestyle are more likely to be visible today than in previous generations. Widowed status continues to predominate among older women, reflecting longstanding gender differences in mortality.

Although marital status has often been used as an indicator of lifestyle, in today's world this criterion does not reflect the trend of heterosexual couples who live together without marriage. It also does not recognize the sexual preferences of lesbians and gay men, many of whom have made lifelong commitments to partners that parallel the marital commitments of those with heterosexual preferences. Some institutions have recognized these commitments formally (e.g., through health insurance coverage), but most have not. Conceding that current classifications are in transition (see Canetto, 1996), we have adhered to the conventional allusions to marital status in our review, with the addition of the lesbian lifestyle as distinct. It is useful to keep in mind that the status "single" is ambiguous, since it may refer to women who are living with and are committed to life partners of either sex. We found a total of 18 articles related to women's family patterns, almost all published after 1980. The majority (ten) focused on single women, with four articles related to married women and four to lesbians.

Single Women

Studies of single women include never married, divorced, and widowed women. All but one of the articles relate to single mothers. The work reviewed documents the economic stresses single mothers experience, and looks at the role of social supports in their lives.

A common stressor for many single mothers is chronic financial strain. Most teenage and unwed mothers have few economic resources. Discrimination in the workplace limits both women's job options and their salaries. Following divorce the income level for women drops sharply. It is not surprising to find that these economic problems adversely affect health and family relationships (Compas & Williams, 1990; Guarnaccia, Angel, & Worobey, 1991). Single mothers' financial fragility was demonstrated in a study of mothers' assessments of three roles: parent, social participant, and self-supporter (Kazak & Linney, 1983). Although the strongest predictor of life satisfaction was competence as a self-supporter, this was the mothers' role of least perceived competence, with parenting the role of most perceived competence. Compas and Williams recommended the development of coping strategies for single women around financial problems as a way of reducing their daily family hassles and health problems. Although this may ameliorate some of the hassles, the structural forces that build in chronic financial strain for single mothers must ultimately be addressed before these problems can be resolved.

Community psychologists have extensively explored social supports and networks over the last two decades. The topic is a particularly resonant one for women, since feminist scholarship has identified relationships as critical contexts for understanding gender differences (Miller, 1986). The three studies found that focus on the social supports of single women suggest the complexities involved. Social support appears to offer less buffering of single mothers' life stress than researchers expected, although positive effects were noted (Kazak & Linney, 1983; Shinn, Wong, Simko, & Ortiz-Torres, 1989). The well-being of single mothers may be more related to support from coworkers and friends than from families. Whether this result is related to conflict between the single mother and her family about her lifestyle is not clear. In the only study we found that targeted widows, Hirsch (1980), in comparing their natural support systems with those of a group of non-widowed mature women, found lower-density support systems to be associated with better support and mental health. Low-density support networks, those in which friends and relatives have relatively few contacts with each other, often include members whose values or lifestyles differ.

These studies suggest that low-density networks may be effective sources of support in setting new directions. Such networks stand in contrast to denser networks, in which family and friends interact more often, are more likely to hold similar values, and thus are more likely to reinforce the *status quo*. Lifestyle differences between generations in today's world may render less accessible the intergenerational supports relied on by past generations. When parents disapprove of their daughter divorcing, bearing children outside of marriage, or living with a partner they disapprove of, traditional supports may erode or disappear.

Two studies dealt with the social supports of those who divorce. In their assessments of newly separated persons, Caldwell and Bloom (1982) found that women initially reported more social supports than men—a difference that disappeared after six months. Their research was designed to study the effects of a variety of preventive interventions for divorced and separated persons. In a study of divorcing mothers, direct relationships between social supports and psychological distress were confirmed by Tetzloff and Berrera (1987). Tangible (money and material resources) and parenting support were both related to reductions in depressive symptoms. Both studies suggested prevention programs to enhance resources for those who divorce.

Two interventions helped young single mothers mobilize social supports. Henninger and Nelson (1984) organized home visits and peer group meetings for young unwed mothers. These supports were successful in assisting teenagers to build social networks and pursue occupational and educational goals. Similar success was reported by the Parent-to-Parent program in Vermont (Halpern & Covey, 1983), which provided adolescent mothers with home visits and parent group meetings, as well as liaison with social service agencies. These mothers tended to return to school, to demonstrate increased knowledge of their babies' developmental stages, and to report increased use of contraceptives. It's notable that in these two successful studies, the supports mobilized were new relationships—peers and agency supports—consistent with the findings on the positive effects of low-density networks in some situations.

Readers seeking more recent studies in the journals reviewed on the topic of single women are referred to Brand, Lakey, and Berman (1995); Brodsky (1996); Dean, Matt, and Wood (1992); Dunham, Hurshman, Litwin, Gusella, Ellsworth, and Dodd (1998); Kofkin and Reppucci (1991); Levy and Derby (1992); Levy, Derby, and Martinkowski (1993); McLoyd and Wilson (1992); O'Bryant, Donnermeyer, and Stafford (1991); Simons, Johnson, Beaman, Conger et al. (1996); Wolchik, West, Westover, and Sandler (1993).

Married Women

Four studies were found that focused on married women *per se*. The studies explored individual-level factors related to stress, social support, and competence. Nelson (1989) compared the life strains, coping, and emotional well-being of married women who had recently separated with those who had not. Low-income, separated women experienced the highest levels of strains. Another study looked at the stress-buffering role of social support and personal competence on depressive symptoms in rural married couples (Husaini, Neff, Newbrough, & Moore, 1982). Social support was the primary gender difference: it had a greater buffering effect for women. In another study, married mothers reported fewer daily hassles around economic, family, and personal health problems than single mothers, as well as fewer symptoms of depression and anxiety (Compas & Williams, 1990). Barker and Lemle (1984) found no gender differences in "helping communication" between couples who were married, engaged, or living together. Readers are directed to Andresen and Telleen (1992) for a more recent study on this topic.

Lesbians

Four articles were found on this topic, all by the same author. Anthony D'Augelli (1988, 1989a) has documented the discrimination, harassment, and violence gay people experience. He has also addressed the failure of community psychologists to deal with lesbians and gay men (1989b), and urged his colleagues to pursue collaborative efforts to build resources and support for this population. More recently, he has discussed the development of helping communities to deal with the AIDS epidemic (D'Augelli, 1990). The increasing integration of the issues of lesbians and gay men into the mainstream of community psychologists' work is a first step toward sensitizing the professional community to the need for interventions to enhance the empowerment of this population.

Readers seeking more recent studies on this topic in the journals reviewed are referred to D'Augelli (1993); D'Augelli and Hershberger (1993); Garnets and D'Augelli (1994); Pilkington and D'Augelli (1995); and Waldo, Hesson-McInnis, and D'Augelli (1998).

Overview

The 1980s showed progress in community psychologists' documentation of the stressors and strengths associated with being a single mother, whereas assessment of the family patterns of married women and lesbians have received little attention during the 25 years of our review. The majority of studies of women's lifestyles have focused at the individual level, assessing demographic and psychological variables in single mothers' lives and relating these to outcomes such as satisfaction or adjustment. Multilevel analyses are needed to include family and societal factors—such as the gender power differential—that profoundly affect choices about family patterns. An ecological perspective, one that would take account of the physical, socioeconomic, political and psychological environments within which women make their life choices, would address the structural factors, both resources and constraints, that shape women's efforts to reform existing family patterns, create new ones and choose freely among them.[3]

WOMEN IN THE WORKFORCE[4]

A critical setting for the empowerment of women is the workplace. In 1988 it was estimated that women made up 45% of the workforce, and that 52% of all married women and 50% of women with young children worked outside the home (Akabas, 1988). A total of 27 articles were found. Five related to work and family issues, 15 to other factors affecting the well-being of women in the workforce, and 7 to interventions having implications for empowerment or prevention for women in the workforce.[5]

Work and Family Issues

Family demands add stress to the lives of women who work outside the home. Although being a single mother, caring for a child with a disability, or having responsibility for an elderly relative all increase stress for women in the workforce (Akabas, 1988), there is no consistent evidence that the sheer number of work and family roles leads to overload or other negative outcomes for women (Alpert, Richardson, & Fodaski, 1983). Rather, it appears to be the interaction between family pressures and undesirable work conditions that is associated with increased stress (Akabas, 1988).

Three studies clarify this interaction. Krause and Geyer-Pestello (1985) found that demands at home (e.g., lack of help with housework and presence of young children) alone were not associated with negative outcomes. However, women who experienced more logistical (and time) conflicts between work and home roles experienced more distress, as did women whose working conflicted with their sex role beliefs. The link between work and family environments is demonstrated by evidence that a husband's negative attitude toward his wife's educational or work involvements can profoundly affect family climate in disruptive ways (Einswirth-Neems & Handal, 1978; Moos & Moos, 1983).

Readers seeking more recent studies on this topic in the journals reviewed are referred to Conway-Turner and Karasik (1997); Hill (1997); Jackson (1997); and Marshall and Barnett (1993).

[3]See Franzblau (1996) for a social Darwinian analysis of conceptions of marriage, sex, and motherhood.

[4]It was the authors' intention to cover articles dealing with women's work within as well as outside the home. The words "housewife" and "homemaker" were included in our search, but no articles were found that fit the criteria for inclusion.

[5]Twenty-one articles were found related to the woman-dominated professions of nurses, receptionists, secretaries, and hairdressers. These articles addressed such issues as skills training, job satisfaction, worker conflict, social network analysis, and consultation styles. Those articles (14) that did not address gender issues are not included in our review.

Other Factors Affecting the Well-Being of Women in the Workforce

Fifteen articles dealt with factors in addition to family that affect women who work outside the home, including nonfamily social supports, formal work policies, work content, and discrimination.

Three of these studies investigated nonfamily social supports. Although Holahan and Moos (1982) found that family support was generally more important for women and work support was more important for men, this does not mean that work supports are irrelevant to women. Marshall and Barnett (1992) found that work-related support had a direct effect on the mental and physical health of working women. Women's emotional well-being was associated with support from coworkers, partners, and broader social networks, while physical health was affected only by support from supervisors. In an examination of the support networks of female hospital nurses, participants reported few relationships between work associates and friends, and few interactions between nurses and work associates outside the work setting (Hirsch & David, 1983). This compartmentalization of work and nonwork supports appeared to be an effective strategy for persons coping with work stress; however, it can also undermine collective efforts to empower nursing as a profession. Hirsch and David emphasized this paradox by contrasting the nurses' segmented networks with those of physicians whose overlapping work and friendship networks potentially reinforce their power within the hospital. In general such overlap functions to enlarge the work arena, so that business is conducted outside of, as well as during, working hours; this practice may tend to solidify power relationships among physicians, and between physicians and other hospital staff.

Two studies dealt with the job benefits of flexitime, an organizational practice thought to be sensitive to the pressures in women's lives. According to Winett, Neale, and Williams (1982), flexitime generally allows working mothers and fathers more time to engage in recreational, social, and chore activities with their families. However, when Shinn et al. (1989) looked at the relationship of individual coping strategies, social supports, and flexibility of job schedules on working parents' well-being, they found that formal flexitime programs were of little benefit to either working mothers or fathers. The degree to which mothers felt they could alter their own job schedules was mildly related to reduced stress levels, and, for single mothers, perceived flexibility was associated with job satisfaction. Shinn et al. suggested that the choice of simply coming to work a few hours earlier or later does not provide the flexibility parents need to deal with sick children or other unpredictable events.

One study looked at the contributions of both social supports and family-related benefits on the job attitudes and personal well-being of working parents with young children (Greenberger, Goldberg, Hamill, O'Neill, & Payne, 1989). Informal social supports at work accounted for a significant portion of the variance in married mothers' levels of organizational commitment and single mothers' job satisfaction. Working mothers (both single and married) made significantly greater use of formal family-related benefits such as parental leave or child care assistance than did fathers. Mothers' use of benefits was associated with more positive attitudes toward their jobs and their employers. Working mothers reported significantly greater role strain and more health symptoms than fathers, with no significant differences between single and married women.

Akabas (1988) argued that job content alone adds considerable stress to women's lives. Positions that involve boring and repetitive tasks, ambiguous task demands, and physical restraints tend to increase stress. Lack of control over the work role and pace, along with underutilization of workers' abilities, further compounds the stress. Akabas noted that the majority of working women hold positions that are low in discretion and high in structured, repetitive demands, and that men in similar positions tend to have more power and discretion than their female counterparts. Women are also highly represented in occupations with the stress of shift work and/or rotating and unpredictable work assignments (such as nursing). Akabas recommended preventive actions, including organizing for better job conditions and legislative action.

Although gender-based discrimination and sexual harassment of women at work are well documented in the psychology research literature in general, there was little discussion of these issues within the community psychology literature during the first 25 years of the field.[6] We found only one article on affirmative action. In this survey of university department chairpersons and hirees, Noble and Winett (1978) found general agreement that having guidelines opened up the job market to more women and minorities. In an exploration of the sexual harassment experiences of women members of the APA's Division of Community Psychology, Bond (1988b) found that large percentages of respondents reported graduate school experiences involving gender harassment and *quid pro quo* sexual harassment. The study suggested the importance of environmental factors such as departmental norms against sexual interaction between faculty and students, and the presence of women (i.e., percentage of women students) in reducing the incidence of sexual harassment. Articles in a special issue of *The Community Psychologist* on sexual harassment explored the impact of institutional factors (Fuehrer & Schilling, 1988), perceptions of harassers (Crull, 1988), prevention strategies (Biaggio, Brownell, & Watts, 1988; Naylor, Tolan, & Wilson, 1988), and training issues (D'Ercole, 1988; O'Connor, 1988).

Readers seeking more recent studies on this topic in the journals reviewed are referred to Bohmer (1995); Broman, Hamilton, Hoffman, and Mavaddat (1995); Hughes and Dodge (1997); Lambert and Hopkins (1995); Marshall and Barnett (1992); Pretty and McCarthy (1991); and Sanchez-Hucles (1997).

Mobilizing Resources for Women in the Workforce

Empowerment and stress prevention for women at work have received little attention within the community psychology journals reviewed. Four articles were found that describe skill-building training, and three address empowerment strategies for working women.

The training interventions used group formats to foster individual skill development. Goldstein and Goedhart (1973) found that structured learning enhanced empathy in nurses, and fostered its generalization to other settings. Echterling and Moore (1982) trained secretaries and receptionists from human service organizations in communication skills to enable them to better handle the unpredictable events that emerged on their jobs. Although such skills could be empowering to the extent that they provide participants with a greater sense of control over their work environments, empowerment must be approached with an understanding of context. For example, Cornbleth, Freedman, and Baskett (1974) provided human-relations training to hospital nurses, in which part of the goal was "to improve relationships among hospital personnel" (p. 58). It is notable that when a primary goal is to promote smoother relations within a hierarchical structure, such training could simply facilitate adjustments to the *status quo* and undermine efforts to empower the nurses.

Stern and Golden (1977) described training for psychiatric nurses in behavior modification principles and methods. Here again the training did not address context issues. Since the

[6]See Bond (1995).

use of behavior modification skills requires a strong degree of control over the therapeutic environment, it is critical to address the ways in which other staff—administrators, psychiatrists, psychologists, and others who tend to be more powerful than nurses—interact with the same clients to shape the therapeutic context. To increase technical knowledge and skills without simultaneously increasing appreciation for, and the ability to change, the ways in which the technology is supported within a setting ignores the importance of status hierarchy and other environmental conditions based on both position and gender. To be empowering, competence-based interventions for women at work must not merely focus on skills; they should also increase women's understanding of the political, economic, and social forces that shape the intervention's objectives, and the relationship of these forces to the worker and the work setting.

Three training interventions were found that have implications beyond individual skill development and address empowerment strategies. Gatz, Barbarin, Tyler, Mitchell, Morgan, Wirzbicki, Crawford, and Engelman (1982) assessed a two-day workshop for predominantly female, older adult community workers (about half Anglo and half African-American) on skills connected with interviewing, problem solving, and accessing community resources. Not only did the intervention increase the competencies and life satisfaction of the workers, it also resulted in increased knowledge and sense of personal control among the residents, particularly the African-Americans. Hirsch and David (1983) explored the use of social network analysis for understanding and enhancing the quality of work life for hospital nurses. Since many participants described the empowerment of the nursing profession as a priority goal, one planned outcome of the training was the formation of resource groups to provide ongoing support for women's empowerment efforts. Torre (1988) described a multidisciplinary, multiracial task force of women organized to increase awareness of child care concerns faced by working parents. The task force utilized strategies of mutual support and networking, coordination of resources, consciousness raising, and self/community empowerment to promote solutions to child care problems among local employers.

Overview

The work cited points to the importance of further exploring conflicts women face in balancing work and family responsibilities. Personal beliefs, logistical difficulties, and family supports emerge from these studies as significant variables in this balance. As Rickel (1985) pointed out, however, the failure of family and community structures to keep up with the needs of working women remains relatively unaddressed in community psychology journals. Directions for future research include identifying the community resources (e.g., programs and services) that alleviate stresses on working families, and further exploring the impact of family roles and structures on working women.

Most of the studies on the well-being of women in the workplace were multilevel, considering a diversity of factors at the individual (e.g., coping strategies), small group (e.g., social support), and organizational (e.g., flexitime) levels. The outcome variables, however, were predominantly at the individual level, ranging from distress and depression to job satisfaction and commitment to work. Community psychology research could better describe and design interventions for women's well-being in the workplace if it included effectiveness, distribution of resources, and organizational values as outcome variables.

The majority of community psychology studies reviewed about women who work outside the home looked at work-related supports that enhance women's well-being; roughly half considered both individual and organizational factors. Although most of the interventions reviewed have the potential for promoting empowerment or prevention goals, some were conducted without sensitivity to gender concerns—particularly power issues. This insensitivity could result in women being trained to adjust to the *status quo* or to blame themselves for work problems, rather than to identify and try to change the structural factors at the root of many of their concerns. A number of positive outcomes for women's empowerment were noted, including the development of work-based resource groups and a multidisciplinary task force to educate employers about child care concerns.

CARE OF DEPENDENT FAMILY MEMBERS

Whether it involves caring for children or adults with special needs, caretaking is a central family function that is typically relegated to women. Yet since much of our culture places a higher value on paid employment outside the home, women often find themselves in highly stressful, yet undervalued, roles within the family. The importance of prevention and empowerment activities for these women seems obvious, since isolation, burnout, and low self-esteem are possible outcomes of this work. Our literature review yielded many articles on women in family-caretaking roles. We have summarized only the 35 articles that focused on the women themselves, or addressed one or more important gender issues. Fifteen dealt with the characteristics of family caretakers, 9 with patterns of formal help-seeking, and 11 with the mobilization of resources for caretaking roles.

Charactersitics of Family Caretakers

The articles describing caretakers dealt with the care of young children, family members with special developmental needs, and elderly family members.

Care of Young Children

Three articles explored adjustment to new parenting roles. Alpert, Richardson, and Fodaski (1983) assessed stressful events associated with becoming new parents. They found that role combination or overload for women does not necessarily lead to higher stress. Unemployed mothers found the conflict between their own needs and their children's needs more stressful than did employed mothers, who also reported less stress associated with frequent child illness. Two studies indicate that mothers and fathers draw on different social supports during their first postpartum year. Formal parenting groups played a more significant role in the adjustment of fathers, whereas close friends played a more significant role for mothers (Wandersman, Wandersman, & Kahn, 1980). Social supports for either child care or household tasks significantly enhanced adjustment for new mothers, but not for new fathers (Rankin, Campbell, & Soeken, 1985). Participants in these studies were either predominantly white, or race was not specified.

Five studies on child-rearing involved ethnic/minority mothers. In a survey of dual-earner Mexican-American families, total network support, network effectiveness, and spouse support for parenting were more important to the well-being of wives than to that of husbands (Holtzman & Gilbert, 1987). The authors comment on the results in light of the fact that integration of work and caretaking roles is "particularly difficult for Mexican-American women because in their cultural background parenting is viewed as women's responsibility and as the primary source of their life fulfillment" (pp. 177–178). In a survey of African-American mothers, Lewis (1988) identified four factors associated with reduced role strain: the availability of a supportive partner, relatives within the same state, fewer minor children living at home, and residence in the southern U.S. These results point to some tough paradoxes for African-American women living in communities where the availability of partners is limited by high rates of unemployment, incarceration, and homicide among African-American men, where there is an emphasis on family embeddedness, and where there is a "strong value which equates children with wealth" (p. 84). Atlas and Rickel (1988) found that higher maternal stress was associated with lower self-concept, higher aggression, and more nondirective problem-solving in children of African-American mothers. Rickel, Williams, and Loigman (1988) found that being depressed, Catholic, and/or African-American (versus white) were associated with restrictive parenting practices. In another study, religiousness in a group of African-American mothers was associated with more friendly, cooperative, and imaginative interactions with children (Strayhorn, Weidman, & Larson, 1990). It would have been helpful in interpreting the results of the last three studies if the influence of class or cultural differences had been explored in more depth, e.g., since the church is the center of many African-American communities, "religiousness" could be confounded with connection or sense of belonging to the community.

Readers seeking more recent studies on the care of young children in the journals reviewed are referred to Miller-Loncar, Erwin, Landry, Smith, and Swank (1998); Myers, Taylor, Alvy, Arrington et al. (1992); and Zambrana, Silva-Palacios, and Powell (1992). Readers seeking an analysis of the social policy context of child care are referred to Phillips, Howes, and Whitebook (1992).[7]

Care of Family Members with Special Physical and Developmental Needs

Issues considered here include stresses on parents, economic status, self-concept, and social supports. Mothers, more than fathers, of children with handicaps reported restricted personal development, limits on their time, poor health, sensitivity to their child's acceptance in the community, and awareness of family disharmony; single mothers had the added stress of financial pressures (Holroyd, 1974). The social networks of parents of children with handicaps tended to be limited, with mothers having particularly small networks (Kazak & Wilcox, 1984). Mothers of more severely disabled children had fewer friends or family on whom they relied and were less satisfied with support received than mothers of children with milder disabilities (Seybold, Fritz, & McPhee, 1991). Hobfoll and Lerman (1988) found that mothers who received more overall social support and were more intimate with their spouses had better resistance to stresses associated with their children's illnesses. High-stress mothers of autistic children reported less social support, lower family integration, more financial problems, and fewer opportunities than did low-stress mothers (Holroyd, Brown, Winkler, & Simmons, 1975).

[7]The Head Start program has empowered not only children but many of their mothers, both directly and indirectly, by opening new directions in their lives and increasing their effectiveness with their children. Beyond the scope of this paper to review, readers seeking more information about Head Start are referred to Zigler (1994). Home-visitation programs have been significant in their contribution to the health and welfare of both children and mothers who have participated. Because of the extensive literature, most of it occurring after our official review period, we have elected to refer readers to a recent special issue of the *Journal of Community Psychology* on home visitation [Vol. 26 (1), January 1998] for reports on current theories and research outcomes, along with citations to earlier work.

Readers seeking more recent studies on this topic in the journals reviewed are referred to Prieto-Bayard (1993); Rauktis, Koeske, and Tereshko (1995); St-Onge and Lavoie (1997); Tam, Chan, and Wong (1994); Tausig (1992); and Wyman, Cowen, Work, and Parker (1991).

Care of the Elderly

Only two studies directly addressed gender issues in caretaking roles for elderly family members. Lieberman (1978) found that women perceived more changes in their aging parents and were more troubled by the changes than men. Smyer (1984) noted that the primary caretakers of the elderly are women, and that interventions to reduce stress must consider that these caretakers are often simultaneously caring for children and other family members.

Readers seeking more recent studies on this topic in the journals reviewed are referred to Cheng (1992, 1993); Conway-Turner and Karasik (1997); Felton and Berry (1992); LaVeist, Sellers, Brown, and Nickerson (1997); Nemoto (1998); Schwirian and Schwirian (1993); and Secouler (1992).

Formal Help-Seeking for Caretaking Roles

One of the nine articles in this section documented the common observation that mothers are more likely to seek help than fathers (Menaghan, 1978). The others address the ways that social support and network characteristics affect participation in formal parenting programs.[8]

Three studies comparing participants and nonparticipants in family support programs showed that parents are more likely to seek help if they feel isolated in the parenting role, have fewer friends and relatives available, and/or believe they lack parenting competence (Fontana, Fleischman, McCarton, Meltzer, & Ruff, 1988; Powell, 1984; Telleen, 1990). Prieto-Bayard and Baker (1986) addressed access issues for low-income, Spanish-speaking mothers. They found that when bilingual staff, child care, reimbursement for transportation, and convenient meeting times were provided, the vast majority completed parenting programs. Use of preventive human services has also been linked with social network density and frequency of contact with kin for low-income, high-risk mothers (Birkel & Reppucci, 1983). For a group of predominantly African-American mothers, the search for child care was found to vary by perceived neighborhood age, personal social network ties, and income and family structure (Powell & Eisenstadt, 1983). Several studies assessed the availability and need for formal child care services (Innes & Heflinger, 1989; Shoffner, 1986), finding overall shortages in care, particularly for infant-toddlers and children with handicaps.

Mobilizing Resources

Eleven intervention studies were found in our literature review. Three were aimed at preventing dysfunction in the face of a major transition or crisis—becoming a new parent (Belsky, 1982), having a premature baby (Tadmor & Brandes, 1986), or experiencing the loss of a baby (Tadmor, 1986). Six interventions assessed the effectiveness of parenting groups (Berberich, Gabel, & Anchor, 1979; Gabel, 1975; Huhn & Zimpfer, 1989; Sadler, Seyden,

[8]No studies of respite care were found that recognized women's role as primary caretakers or dealt explicitly with gender issues.

Howe, & Kaminsky, 1976) and parenting newsletters (Lamberts, Cudaback, & Claesgens, 1985; Laurendeau, Gagnon, Desjardins, Perreault, & Kishchuk, 1991). An in-home intervention provided parent-skills training for mothers (Sandler, Dokecki, Stewart, Britton, & Horton, 1973). Finally, the Extended Family Program (Shinn & Rosario, 1985), with its innovative use of community members in "grandmother" roles, reported a number of successful outcomes. This study models the involvement of participants in research planning and implementation. All these interventions sought to enhance mothers' skills or knowledge in areas such as awareness of infant development, maternal coping, self-disclosure, and general parenting skills.

Readers seeking more recent studies on this topic in the journals reviewed are referred to Cronan, Walen, and Cruz (1994); Dickinson and Cudaback (1992); Dumka, Garza, Roosa, and Stoerzinger (1997); Dunham, Hurshman, Litwin, Gusella, Ellsworth, and Dodd (1998); Fawcett, White, Balcazar, Suarez-Balcazar et al. (1994); Honig and Winger (1997); Medvane, Mendoza, Lin, Harris et al. (1995); Shulman, Kedem, Kaplan, Sever, and Braja (1998); Silver, Ireys, Bauman, and Stein (1997); and Szendre and Jose (1996).

Readers are particularly referred to an issue of the *American Journal of Community Psychology* that features an intervention by Heller, Thompson, Trueba, and Hogg (1991) using peer telephone dyads for elderly women with low perceived social support. The intervention showed no significant differences between the groups assessed. Comments by other community psychologists shed light on the issues involved.

Overview

Our findings here parallel those of other areas under review. In general the articles on family caretaking did not examine the ways in which organizational or institutional factors, such as the availability of community supports and resources or the responsiveness of school or work settings, contribute to the well-being or empowerment of women in these roles. About half of the descriptive articles focused on the individual level in their analysis of the characteristics of women in family caretaking roles; the other half explored social supports. There is clearly a need for the field to explore broader issues, such as the division of labor within the family, the structural supports for caretaking in the community, and the force of societal expectations on women. Although training interventions may empower women in their caretaking roles, such training does not relieve them of the stress of primary responsibility for caring for society's dependent members. Interventions are needed to create alternative care options for families, or to share the burden of care among family members.

HEALTH AND REPRODUCTION

The health care crisis in this country is one of the major problems facing communities today. Within the broad area of health, issues of reproduction—family planning, prenatal care, delivery, and abortion—are critical concerns for all. These issues are particularly crucial for women, who have the primary responsibility for bearing and caring for children. We found 25 articles on gender-related health and reproduction issues; of these, nine related to health issues and 16 to reproduction. It should be kept in mind that community psychologists who publish on this topic may be more likely to do so in other journals (e.g., health psychology) than in those reviewed here.

Health Issues

Eating Disorders

Anorexia, bulimia, and obesity have reached near epidemic proportions in high school and college age women, and are increasing in girls of elementary school age. A relatively new medical phenomenon in its current proportions, eating disorders have been reported almost exclusively by females. The studies of eating disorders found in our review were related to individual measures of psychological functioning. McCall (1973) studied obesity and its relationship to MMPI factors, finding that women who managed to lose weight and maintain that loss had notably less deviant MMPI profiles than those who were "irremediably" obese. Brunn and Hedberg (1974) found a negative relationship between percentage of overweight and self-perception scores. A covert reinforcement treatment led to weight loss. Bennet, Spoth, and Borgen (1991) conducted a survey to identify the prevalence of bulimic symptoms and behaviors in a nonclinical, all female, high school population. They found a strong inverse relationship between the symptoms and fear of fat and self-efficacy, along with evidence of bulimic behaviors comparable to those found at university levels. More recently, Berel and Irving (1998) have investigated media influence on disturbed eating behavior.

AIDS

Mantell, Schinke, and Akabas (1988) present an excellent summary of gender differences in the incidence of the disease, methods of transmission, and lifestyle and behavioral practices. They offer many prevention and research suggestions, and discuss the ethical and moral issues this epidemic entails. Weissman and NARC (1991) describe the efforts of NIDA's National AIDS Demonstration Research Program, conducted in 63 sites in the U.S. and Puerto Rico. Its goals include designing and evaluating outreach methods and behavioral interventions targeted to women. Most of the women at risk are a hidden population that has contracted the disease through drug-using partners. The authors provide specific guidelines for interventions such as: (a) basing them primarily on women's expressed needs, (b) delving into related topics in depth (e.g., contraceptive use, sexuality, religious values), (c) considering cultural and psychological issues, and (d) involving women in the design and provision of services so as to foster their empowerment. D'Augelli (1990) focuses on the role of community psychologists in the AIDS crisis and notes the increasing incidence of HIV and AIDS issues among women. Although not targeted specifically at women's issues, the conceptual schema he presents to generate coordinated community planning for preventive AIDS interventions is applicable to all.

Readers seeking more recent studies on this topic in the journals reviewed are referred to Brunswick and Banaszak-Holl (1996); Carels, Baucom, Leone, and Rigney (1998); Commerford, Gular, Orr, Reznikoff et al. (1994); Levine, Britton, James, Jackson et al. (1993); Rotherham-Borus, Gwadz, Fernandez, and Srinivasan (1998); Stein, Nyamathi, and Kington (1997); Turner and Catania (1997); and VanOss Marin, Tschann, Gomez, and Gregorich (1998).

Other Health Issues

Articles on other health issues covered in this review include alcohol consumption and diverse aspects of health care services. After surveying alcohol consumption among professional women, Shore (1985) found that their rates were considerably higher than in the overall population, and that their awareness of the effects of alcohol on their bodies was minimal. Gender-related factors that may lead to increased drinking include: (a) increased acceptance of drinking in women, (b) joining in "after-work" drinking behavior, (c) perception of the benefits of becoming "drinking buddies" so as to succeed on the job, and (d) stress generated by the need to balance multiple gender-related roles.

Neighbors and Jackson (1984), using a nationwide sample, studied help-seeking patterns within the African-American population. They reported that women seek help from both professional and informal helpers more often than do men. They believe this occurs because role differentiation allows women to be more open about their problems, thus becoming more accessible to different types of help.

Rowe and Irvine (1985) discuss the need for alternative health care settings to provide services for women. They consider traditional health care to be paternalistic, dehumanizing, excessively costly, inaccessible, and dominated by white males—a view shared by the authors of this article. The Women's Health Center in Charlottesville, Virginia, is described as an alternative for empowering women to take charge of their health concerns. The setting changes the traditional working relationship to that of a team effort where roles are shared and nonprofessioinals are incorporated. The center has also altered the role between service providers and clients by explaining procedures the clients will undergo, asking for experiential confirmation of their diagnoses, encouraging skill development, and prompting questioning and affirmative stances. The study's authors mention the organizational difficulties this type of setting faces, but believe it is an empowering experience for both clientele and staff.

Readers seeking more recent studies on this topic in the journals reviewed are referred to Abraido-Lanza (1997); Brunswick, Lewis, and Messeri (1991, 1992); Pistrang and Barker (1998); Salem, Bogat, and Reid (1997); and Taylor, Henderson, and Jackson (1991).

Overview

Most of the articles on women's health assess or measure a phenomenon or intervention. Two present interventions, and one provides a theoretical framework. The articles include various levels of analysis. The eating-disorder studies focus on the individual level and do not discuss gender issues specifically, although their samples are entirely female. Missing from these studies is an analysis of the factors that have fueled the current increase in the incidence of eating disorders. The pressure on women to be thin in our society is reflected in the images of underweight women seen in the movies, television, magazines, billboards, and other media. These images of the "ideal" woman are rooted in patriarchal views of women as sex objects. An ecological perspective would link the increase in incidence over the last two decades with historical and social, as well as individual, factors in the search for correlates of cause. The other articles include organization and community-level analyses as well as attention to gender issues. All but two present suggestions for preventive or empowering efforts and future research.

Reproduction Issues

One recurrent theme was found in the 16 articles on reproduction: half focused on teen-age pregnancy. The others dealt with a variety of reproductive issues.

Teenage Pregnancy

The articles on teenage pregnancy fall into three categories: need for a multilevel ecological analysis, attempts to link teenage pregnancy with the teen mother's personality or family situation, and interventions to curtail the incidence of teenage pregnancy or its negative effects.

The need to examine social issues and problems using a multilevel ecological analysis is widely recognized within community psychology. Reppucci (1987) used the issue of teenage pregnancy to illustrate this need. At the individual level, he spoke of examining ways in which adolescents internalize social–moral values. At the family level, he suggested exploring linkages between contraceptive use and open discussions of sexuality. At the societal level, he noted the impact of mass media on adolescent sexuality. He also indicated the need to add economic and political levels of analysis.

Two studies attempted to link teenage pregnancy with negative family dynamics (Miller, 1974) or adjustment problems in the teenage mother (Thomas, Rickel, Butler, & Montgomery, 1990). These studies place the burden of victimization on pregnant teens or their mothers. Missing is a discussion of the role of structural variables involved in many teenage pregnancies, e.g., society's failure to provide adequate sex education or contraceptive information to teenagers, and the patriarchal values and practices that hold the teenage mother responsible and absolve the father from ethical and fiscal responsibility.

Of the five articles focused on prevention, four involved interventions, three of which were school-based. The Teen Outreach Program was designed to encourage young people to perform volunteer services in their communities (Allen, Philliber, & Hoggson, 1990). These services were linked to classroom-based discussions on issues such as developmental tasks and sex education. Participation was effective in reducing drop-out rates and teen pregnancy. The Adolescent Family Life Program is a family-centered primary-prevention effort delivered in public schools in three states (Olson, Wallace, & Miller, 1984). It is based on the premise that sexuality is not only a physiological and maturation issue, but a family relationship issue as well. A preliminary evaluation showed an increase in both family strengths and parent–student discussions of sexual values, and development of less permissive attitudes toward premarital sex. Seitz, Apfel, and Rosenbaum (1991) evaluated a school-based program directed to maximizing postpartum educational achievement in pregnant teenagers. Participants received counseling, the normal academic curriculum, plus classes in prenatal health care, nutrition, childbirth preparation, contraception, and child care. The program was effective in increasing teenagers' educational performance.

In an intervention with university students on contraceptive decision-making, "ineffective contraceptors" reported more frequent negative attitudes toward contraception and less internal control of their process than "effective contraceptors" (Gerrard, McCann, & Fortini, 1983). The researchers evaluated the impact of cognitive restructuring and information interventions on the minimization of negative attitudes toward contraception. Both interventions were found to be more effective than none, although no differences were found between them. Rickel (1986) briefly described two programs targeting postpartum depression and parenting skills.

Readers seeking more recent studies on this topic in the journals reviewed are referred to Allen, Kuperminc, Philliber, and Herre (1994); Chen, Telleen, and Chen (1995); Maton, Teti, Corns, Vieira-Baker, and Lavine (1996); and Rhodes and Woods (1995).

Other Reproductive Issues

Abortion, miscarriage, prematurity, rural prenatal care, black maternal mortality, Mexican-American mothers' attitudes on reproductive issues, and family planning are the topics of the other articles related to reproductive issues found in our review.

Although abortion is one of the most controversial issues in our society today, only two studies were found in the journals searched relating to abortion's impact on women. Fingerer (1973) found no evidence of immediate anxiety or lingering depression after abortion; she concluded that these aftereffects reside only in theory and myth. Similarly, Baluk and O'Neill (1980) found that health professionals expected women abortion patients to have more extreme levels of depression, guilt, and anxiety than patients themselves reported: "These expectations are formed prior to contact, and they remain despite experience" (1980, p. 73). These two studies are excellent examples of the role community psychologists can play in shedding light on controversial social issues.

In her language analysis and case study on miscarriage, Reinharz (1988) showed that it is invisible within the professional literature, and that this invisibility has a deleterious impact when professionals deal with women who have miscarried. She suggested ways community psychologists could contribute toward changing this situation. Tadmor and Brandes (1986) reported their Perceived Personal Control Model as a basis for intervention programs for mothers with premature infants. Together with changes in hospital practices, services, and structures, this model helps mothers cope with the special demands of their situation. Clinton and Larner (1988) described a grass-roots movement that relies on rural women to provide support services for poor, rural families. The program trains local women to educate other women. Its health outreach workers provide access to prenatal care and perform follow-up services during children's development.

In a five-year period, maternal mortality for black women in Chicago and Detroit was more than four times the national rate for white women (Siefert & Martin, 1988). Although higher quality prenatal care must be provided, attention must be directed to "the protection and promotion of black women's physical, mental and social well-being, and not just to their reproductive health" (1988, p. 57). Amaro (1988) investigated the attitudes and experiences of Mexican-American women with respect to motherhood and pregnancy, sexuality, and abortion, and their relationships to socioeconomic status, acculturation, and religiosity. She found that: (a) motherhood was a central value to most, (b) they had favorable attitudes and substantial experience with contraceptives, (c) they felt that childbearing issues should be decided by the woman, (d) they were unsatisfied with their sexual relationships, and (e) they did not express a need for unlimited pregnancies. Amaro noted that these results contradict the prevailing stereotype of Mexican-American women and can be useful in redirecting family planning services.

McFarlane's (1988) study is distinct because of its focus on the policy level of analysis. She investigated the responsiveness of governmental policies to family planning needs by examining state and family planning statutes and budgets before and after the Reagan administration. The administration reduced federal programs and introduced block grants to the states. She found that state-administered block grants showed less responsiveness to women's family planning needs than federal programs.

Readers seeking more recent studies on this topic in the journals reviewed are referred to Butler, Rickel, Thomas, and Hendren (1993); Meyers and Rhodes (1995); St. Lawrence, Eldridge, Reitman, Little, Shelby, and Brasfield (1998); Tadmor and Brandes (1994); Thomas and Rickel (1995); and Wingood and DiClemente (1998).

Overview

Central to the notion of control over one's life is control over one's body. Because both feminists and community psychologists espouse empowerment goals, the two groups might be expected to agree in supporting patients' rights to be informed and to share in making decisions about their health and their bodies. Nevertheless, no strong evidence in the form of a body of work is reflected in the community psychology journals on these issues. That so few studies were found on abortion may speak to the reluctance professionals have in studying an issue associated with political controversy, as well as that of funders in supporting such research, and/or that of reviewers in approving such work for publication. That two of these studies contradicted common beliefs about abortion outcome could be expected to stimulate replications, although this has not happened.

Reppucci's message is particularly relevant as we review the articles on reproduction. Most are at one level of analysis, generally the individual level. These studies are at the initial stage of the empowerment process—that of identifying populations or groups who lack empowerment in one or more domains (Swift & Levin, 1987). Excepting Reinharz's, Fingerer's, and Amaro's analyses, most lack a thorough look at the contribution of gender-related socialization or power differentials as explanations for research results or for the impact of interventions.

POOR AND HOMELESS WOMEN

"Among female-headed families with children under 18, 43% of all races, 54% of black families, and 58% of families of Hispanic origin were in poverty in 1989" (Shinn, 1992, p. 6). The increasing number of women raising children in single-parent families has led to the feminization of poverty in the U.S. This result is rooted in a broad set of structural factors, including the unequal status of women; discrimination in the workforce; governmental retrenchment in areas such as housing and social programs (WIC, Medicaid); the economic recession of the late 1980s and early 1990s; and divorce policies and practices, which tend not to levy or enforce sanctions against fathers who abandon their children. The nine articles reviewed on poor and homeless women in the journals searched focused on the women themselves or considered poverty and homelessness in the context of gender. Here again the literature was devoted primarily to documenting the stressors, coping skills, social support, and self concepts associated with being poor, homeless, and female. Two interventions were found, both of which focused on skill-building.

A compelling call to action to eliminate the feminization of poverty in the U.S. is found in an article by Barbara Simon (1988). She identified five parts of the structural foundation of the problem which need to be changed, all rooted in the unequal status of women:

1. the vitality of the cultural preconception that women are dependents of men
2. the sexual division of labor that continues to make women either primarily or solely responsible for children, household management, and the care of aged family members
3. the pervasive racism encountered daily by minority men and women as they seek schooling, training, and jobs
4. the dual labor market and its poor cousin, the dual welfare system
5. the systematic discrimination that women and girls face in the work force, housing market, and educational system. (1988, p. 7)

Simon's account of the feminization of poverty is applicable to many other problems women face, including sexual assault, battering, job discrimination, lifestyle concerns, and denial of control of their bodies.

Readers seeking more recent studies on this topic in the journals reviewed are referred to Banyard (1995); Calsyn, Kohfeld, and Roades (1993); Calsyn and Morse (1990); Calsyn and Roades (1994); Guarnaccia and Henderson (1993); Mowbray, Cohen, Harris, Trosch et al. (1992); Shinn (1992, 1997); and Unger, Kipke, Simon, Montgomery, and Johnson (1997).

The Stressor of Violence

In addition to the multiple stressors of poverty, the homeless are subjected to high rates of physical violence. For women, sexual assault is also a high risk. Almost half of a representative sample of homeless women reported sexual abuse, with two-thirds of these reporting both physical and sexual abuse (D'Ercole & Struening, 1990). Investigators took a multilevel perspective by analyzing women's vulnerability to victimization through adherence to traditional sex-role stereotypes. The authors' suggestions for shelter programs that would promote functional networks and build on women's strengths are at the third stage of empowerment, mobilization of resources.

Social Supports and Self-Esteem

Two investigations of the social supports of homeless (Goodman, 1991) and poor women (Goodman & Johnson, 1986) failed to find support for the buffering hypothesis. Goodman (1991) hypothesized that mothers without strong social networks, or those drained by their networks, would be at higher risk for homelessness than poor mothers with strong, supportive social networks. The results were contrary to expectations. Both homeless women and those on public assistance had similar numbers of people in their networks of family, friends, and helping professionals, and visited their relatives with similar frequency. Only their levels of trust of network members significantly distinguished the two groups. There is some evidence that the density of poor women's networks may affect their use of prevention-oriented human service programs. Birkel and Reppucci (1983) reported that women with lower-density networks and less frequent contact with relatives were more likely to attend parenting sessions than women with denser, more relative-involved networks. Miskimins and Baker (1973) found that poor women had less self-esteem and were more given to self-derogation than were poor men.

Mobilizing Resources

Positive results were reported for two interventions designed to assist low-income and minority women gain more control over their lives (Tableman, Marciniak, Johnson, & Rodgers, 1982; Thurston, Dasta, & Greenwood, 1984). Both programs provided roughly 30 hours of training in stress management and other survival skills. Positive results in the Tableman et al. study included significant changes in "psychological distress, depression, anxiety, inadequacy, self-confidence, and ego strength" (1982, p. 357).

Overview

There are many structural problems associated with poverty and homelessness that escape the attention of the field when individual-level analyses are used. Looking exclusively at the individual characteristics associated with poor and homeless women prevents us from seeing the roles of related structural factors—such as lack of affordable housing, loss of welfare benefits (Shinn, 1992), and permissive policies toward fathers' responsibilities for child support—in bringing about their current situations. The gender-based structural problems created by women's unequal status—beginning within the family and extending to education and employment—account for a major part of women's vulnerability to poverty and homelessness. Efforts to change women's unequal status through prevention or empowerment ideologies and action programs are in initial stages of development within the field, as well as in other disciplines both within and outside psychology.

VIOLENCE AGAINST WOMEN

Women and children have been victimized by male aggression, particularly sexual aggression, across recorded history. Only in the last few decades have researchers begun to study the phenomenon systematically. The women's movement has been a primary impetus in stimulating scientific attention (Brown & Ziefert, 1988). Initial studies and services focused mostly on victims, assessing public and professional attitudes toward victims, developing treatment services, and establishing incidence and prevalence rates. More recent studies have confronted the issues involved in attempting to prevent violence against women.

Both forms of violence against women, battering and sexual assault, have common roots. Underlying both are patriarchal values and practices that maintain a culture in which these crimes are not only possible, but common (Brown & Ziefert, 1988). The views that women are men's property or are sex objects for men's pleasure illustrate this point. The literature, in general, has treated sexual and nonsexual violence against women as separate, if not unrelated, phenomena, and the community psychology journals have generally followed this tradition. Although societal attitudes on violence against women are undergoing transition, victims of battering appear to capture more public sympathy and understanding than victims of sexual assault.

We found marked differences in community psychologists' approaches to the two types of violence against women. These differences centered around the relative frequencies of preventive interventions and attitudinal studies. There were three interventions to prevent battering, none to prevent rape. On the other hand, while there were no studies found on attitudes toward battered victims, there were four on attitudes toward rape victims and one on attitudes toward rapists. Although this is a small sample from which to draw conclusions, this finding—the dichotomy in professional approaches to the two types of violence against women—suggests that professional attitudes reflect public ones. There may be an assumption of less victim culpability in battering situations than in rape, evidenced in the lack of studies of attitudes toward battered victims. There may also be less professional comfort or assumption of control in interventions to prevent rape than in interventions to prevent battering, as reflected in the lack of interventions to prevent rape.

The earliest article on woman-battering published in the community psychology journals reviewed raises serious questions about the attitudes of researchers themselves in studying this issue. Kahn and the Behavioral Health Technician Staff (1980) examined socio-cultural variables and their impact on wife-beating in an aboriginal community in Northern Australia. They found that wife and girlfriend beatings were a routine occurrence in the community, supported by cultural norms that stemmed from a view of women as men's property. They also found that the beatings were interpreted by some as expressions of caring. They concluded that the practice cannot be totally condemned since it would negate an important aspect of the community's culture. We are concerned as researchers and as human beings, about the ethical questions raised by professionals' use of cultural diversity to support attitudes and behaviors that are threats to human life and dignity under any circumstances.

A critical factor in evaluating this work is an understanding of the context of woman-battering and rape. Women are physically violated most often by their husbands or boyfriends. Although the history of woman-battering and rape incorporates patriarchal attitudes and beliefs about women as men's property, there is a wide range of consciousness of gender issues in the work reviewed. The section below documents 27 articles organized into four broad themes: attitudes toward rape victims and rapists; ways women are affected by, and cope with, violence; services for victims; and educational interventions. None of the articles reviewed covered the physical or sexual assault of lesbians; however, Pilkington and D'Augelli (1995) have addressed this issue since.

Attitudes toward Rape Victims and Rapists

The five studies in this category surveyed attitudes about rape victims and their attackers. A common finding in this research is a significant gender difference in the amount of blame focused on the victim. Men more than women participants believe the woman attacked to be responsible in varying degrees for being raped. This difference was particularly striking in surveys of predominantly male physicians and all-female volunteer rape-crisis counselors (King, Rotter, Calhoun, & Selby, 1978), and mental health professionals (Resick & Jackson, 1981). The same gender difference was found in a study of attribution of blame in incest (Jackson & Ferguson, 1983). The tendency to "blame the victim" was indirectly confirmed by a study demonstrating that victims in extreme age ranges (e.g., 6 years old or 76 years old) were considered to be less responsible for their victimization than victims in middle age ranges (Calhoun, Selby, Long, & Laney, 1980). A study with college women as participants found that whether they perceived rapists' behavior as (1) intrapsychically or organically caused, and (2) motivated by aggression or sex, influenced their assignment of blame and punishment to the rapist (Selby, Calhoun, & Cann, 1979).

Readers seeking more recent studies on this topic in the journals reviewed are referred to Campbell (1995); and Davis, Brickman, and Baker (1991).

Coping with Violence

A study by Riger, Gordon, and LeBailly (1982) demonstrates a high level of awareness of the historical context of violence against women. They looked at the ways women's use of protective behavior are affected by neighborhood conditions, psychological factors, and life circumstances. Previous research has shown that self-protecting behaviors can include avoidance, which reduces exposure to risk, and risk-management, which includes measures taken to deal with risk when the person cannot or will not avoid it. Fear explained the largest proportion of avoidance behaviors. The authors discuss how protective behaviors interact with sex-role proscriptions by continuing to encourage dependence and docility and by limiting women's access to resources.

Based on a survey of battered women, Mitchell and Hodson (1983) concluded that women with greater personal resources, more supportive responses from informal and formal sources of help, and less avoidant coping styles are more likely to show less deleterious effects. Women who had been exposed to family violence in childhood were found to use more avoidant and less active coping responses than men, to have access to fewer resources, to feel pessimistic about their friends' abilities or willingness to help, and to have less supportive networks (Rosenberg, 1985). In a study of the difference in problem-solving skills of battered and non-battered rural women, Claerhout, Elder, and Janes (1982) found that non-battered women generated more alternatives when faced with violent situations. Battered women produced more avoidant and dependent responses and did not typically perceive alternative ways of behaving. The authors noted the need to provide women at risk with problem-solving skill training.

The approach used in the last three studies—focusing on the personal attributes, skills, and characteristics of battered women—implies that women are to blame for their battering, and that if we could identify their flaws and weaknesses we could change them and thereby stop the battering. To focus only on the woman blames the victim and raises questions about why there has not been similar research on the structural factors that maintain a battering culture, and on identifying the characteristics of male batterers that contribute to their criminal attacks on women. A more recent study examined the effects of domestic violence on resettled Mexican women and children and contrasted these with the effects of political violence on Central American refugee families, with particular attention to symptoms of posttraumatic stress disorder (McCloskey, Southwick, Fernandez-Esquer, & Locke, 1995).

Selkin (1978) studied differences between two groups of women attacked by rapists: 32 women who were raped ("victims") and 23 women who were attacked but not raped ("resisters"). Resisters reportedly experienced more anger and rage during the assault than victims, who were reported to be more submissive, subdued, and emotionally paralyzed. It was a sign of the times that Selkin felt obliged to conclude, "It would appear that contrary to popular belief in some quarters, rape victims do not want to be raped" (p. 268). He closed with a recommendation that "a comprehensive approach to the problem of rape reduction may well require the development of organized efforts to train women to be rape resisters" (p. 268).

Twenty years later there is increasing awareness that formulating a comprehensive approach to rape reduction means focusing efforts on training males not to rape, as well as on training women in defensive behaviors. Of major importance in this effort is the education of children, particularly boys, on alternatives to violence in resolving interpersonal conflicts, as well as on a broad spectrum of gender issues, including appropriate sexual behavior. The continued development and enforcement of legal sanctions against sexual harassment and assault conveys the unacceptability of sexually violent behavior, and signals society's increasing unwillingness to tolerate it. At the individual level, prevention efforts would be effectively directed to identifying the precursors that mark the development of sexually abusive behavior in boys and adolescent males, and to implementing interventions to interrupt or correct such behavior.

Two articles shed some light on social support for rape victims. The Los Angeles Epidemiologic Catchment Area (ECA) research, initiated by NIMH, investigated sexual assault victims' sources of social support (Golding, Siegel, Sorenson, Burnam, & Stein, 1989). Two-thirds of the victims told someone about their assault; over half (59%) of these told friends or relatives. The authors discussed the factors that led victims to report their assault and the effectiveness of the support found. Popiel and Susskind (1985) studied the reactions of rape victims and the role of social support in their subsequent adjustment. They found female friends and female family members to be most supportive.

Services for Victims

In presenting their model of crisis intervention and self-help services for victims, Brown and Ziefert (1988) briefly addressed the context of male violence against women. Their analysis encompassed a continuum of violence, ranging from sexual harassment and teasing through domestic violence and rape to murder. The other articles on services focused on either battered women or rape victims.

Battered Women's Shelters

Six articles related to battered women's shelters. By providing safe places to be and alternatives to returning to the battering situation, shelters accomplish secondary prevention aims. Three studies examined the effect of sheltering on the woman's decision to return to her assailant. Variables that decreased the probability of returning included shorter length of marriage, previous separation history, marriage to an unemployed batterer, fewer years of abuse, and more hospital stays (Compton, Michael, Krasavage-Hopkins, Schneiderman, & Bickmann, 1989). Other findings were that women who remained independent had had lengthier shelter stays, lacked a strong religious affiliation (Snyder & Scheer, 1981), and had received advocacy services that enabled them to identify community resources (Sullivan & Davidson, 1991).

Cannon and Sparks (1989) studied the impact of sheltering women on a number of psychological variables. They found that participants varied only in their perception of increased acceptance by others. D'Ercole and Struening's (1990) study of the violence experienced by homeless women is described above. One study found little relationship between shelter ideologies—feminist, professional, and grass-roots—and organizational structure (Epstein, Russell, & Silvern, 1988). The age of the organization had much more to do with structural development than ideologies.

Readers seeking more recent studies on this topic in the journals reviewed are referred to Sullivan, Campbell, Angelique, Eby et al. (1994); and Sullivan, Tan, Basta, Rumptz et al. (1992).

Services to Rape Victims

The earliest article in our review of sexual violence described the development of a volunteer rape crisis service in a hospital emergency room in Denver, Colorado (Evans & Sperekas, 1976). In the only article on a rape crisis center, Finn (1984) demonstrated how one center used local public record data as a tool for planning programs and interventions.

Two studies explored the responses of community mental health centers (CMHCs) to the Community Mental Health Centers Act (Public Law 94-63) passed in 1975. This law required the centers to provide treatment services to rape victims and their families, as well as rape-related prevention and control services. Most CMHCs ignored the mandate or gave it lip service only. Services to rape victims were provided primarily by grass-roots programs such as rape crisis centers, hot lines, and emergency room crisis services in hospitals. Forman and Wadsworth (1983, 1985) surveyed CMHCs in a seven-state region in the Midwest to assess compliance with the federal mandate. They found that one-third of the responding centers reported no rape-related services. Centers reporting services allocated less than 0.5% of their annual budgets for this purpose. Most (75%) of the available services were clinical. The authors concluded that the mandated CMHC rape-related services were "woefully inadequate" (1985, p. 406).

Another study coming out of the Los Angeles ECA research hypothesized that sexual assault results in increased current use of mental health and medical services (Golding, Stein, Siegel, Burnam, & Sorenson, 1988); a hypothesis that was tested and confirmed. This finding provides a cost–benefit rationale for prevention programs in addition to the ethical, social, and political rationales generally cited. This study was one of the few on this topic to demonstrate sensitivity to minority concerns, e.g., interviews were conducted in either Spanish or English to accommodate Hispanic participants.

For recent studies of victim services, see Campbell (1998), Campbell and Ahrens (1998), and Campbell, Baker, and Mazurek (1998). A recent study by Isely and Gehrenback-Shim (1997) examined the sexual assault of men in the community. They found that 172 agencies reported that 3,635 men had sought treatment for sexual assault occurring in adulthood. This study contributes to refuting the stereotypes that only women and children are victims of sexual assault, and that victims are responsible for their own victimization. Until roughly the last two decades, reports of the sexual assault of males were treated as anomalies; current reports show the phenomenon as not uncommon, especially for boys.

Educational Interventions

The three educational interventions found among these studies relate to battering. They claim little success in changing stereotypical attitudes. Viewing a film had no impact on dispelling myths about wife abuse in high school boys (Walther, 1986). A community education program on spouse abuse was successful in collecting and disseminating information on available services, but unsuccessful in training professionals such as police, lawyers, counselors, clergy, and medical personnel (Loeb, 1983). Levy (1985) conducted a skills-training intervention for young people to help them understand how and why battering occurs, and how to keep relationships free from abuse. No evaluation was reported.

Overview

The field of community psychology reflects the culture in its approach to violence against women. Although many of the earlier studies were blind to the systemic devaluation of women that underlies the violence,[9] more recent studies show increasing insight into the structural variables that support rape and woman-battering. The field, mirroring the culture, has begun to turn attention to the prevention of violence across all populations, including women. In contrast to initial studies, the focus today tends to be less on individual victims and more on the

[9]Part of the problem lies with editorial boards, which were predominantly male in the early years of the period reviewed (Blair, D'Ercole, O'Connor, Green, & Mulvey, 1978). While the inclusion of more women editorial reviewers would not have guaranteed greater insight into gender issues, it may have increased the probability that these issues would have surfaced and been aired prior to publication.

ecology of violence. Although many studies focus on individual-level variables and decontextualize their interventions and analyses, a number of studies include factors beyond the individual, such as neighborhood conditions, cultural norms, social support, and historical trends, raising the work to multilevel dimensions. Riger (1993) uses examples of violence against women to challenge constructions of empowerment that emphasize agency and control over the importance of community. Many of the studies on services employed organizational and community-level analyses.

The amount of attention paid to victim services relative to prevention services concerns us. Vital as shelters are in providing safe havens for battered women, and rape crisis centers in providing medical and psychological services to rape victims, neither address the fundamental causes of violence against women. These lie in the unequal balance of gender power in our society, and in the resulting victimization of women in physical, economic, social, psychological, political, and sexual ways. Discussions of gender issues in the material reviewed are rare or uninformed by a feminist perspective, even when participants are exclusively women. Possible explanations include researchers' lack of awareness of the power imbalance between women and men that functions to maintain violence against women, a reluctance to deal with this issue, or a tradition of silence in not acknowledging this reality in any but feminist journals and books. We suspect that it's a combination of these. We ask our colleagues to facilitate women's empowerment by naming the problem of unequal gender power in subsequent theoretical or experimental work relating to violence against women.

As noted, no interventions were found in the community psychology journals searched to change societal attitudes toward rape victims, and the few interventions to change attitudes toward women-battering did not report positive effects. There have been no studies in these journals on why men batter and rape women. Nor have there been interventions to change structural factors, such as law enforcement policies, that favor batterers and rapists, although such interventions from those in other fields have succeeded in changing discriminatory policies (Lerman, 1982).

MINORITY WOMEN AND COMMUNITY PSYCHOLOGY

Minority women face double discrimination as women and as members of minority groups. Although studies of women of different races and ethnicities have been reported throughout this paper, we have included a specific focus on this population to reflect the special issues, situations and diversity that exist among "minority" women.

In our review we found 37 articles which focused on women of distinct racial or national origin and involved prevention or empowerment. Of these, 7 studied ethnic women as a generic non-white category, 13 studied African-American women, 14 studied Hispanic women, 2 studied Native-American women, and 1 studied Chinese women. Thirty of the 37 articles are included in the above review. The other 7 revolve mostly around sex-role issues; in some cases they generate results that challenge prevailing stereotypes of both women and minorities. They all surpass the individual level of analysis by including cultural and socio-political issues and/or incorporating macro-level variables into the design.

Soto's (1983) study of sex-role traditionalism and assertiveness in 278 Puerto Rican women living in New York explored differences between first- and second-generation women with varying educational levels. Second-generation and better-educated women indicated less sex-role traditionalism, which was associated with greater assertiveness. Melgoza, Roll, and Baker (1983) examined conformity and cooperation in a sample of 281 Chicano and Anglo undergraduate women. Contrary to expectations of more passivity among Chicanas, they were not found to be more cooperative and conforming than Anglo women. Allen (1984) recommended that community psychologists learn more from the resourcefulness and problems of African-American women, noting hypertension and social support as issues particularly deserving of attention.

Comas-Díaz (1988) analyzed socio-cultural and gender-related problems of mainland Puerto Rican women within the context of cultural change. She presented a thorough and penetrating analysis of the roles of culture, poverty, and oppression on Puerto Rican women. She concluded by recommending culturally embedded interventions that strengthen natural support systems, develop cultural awareness, and increase political participation. Nazario's (1986) study, which briefly described Puerto Rican migrant women's efforts to maintain their island-based support network while creating a complementary one in the U.S., exemplifies the issues that Comas-Díaz presented.

Cheung (1989) reported on the creation of a Women's Center in Hong Kong. She discussed the clashes between feminist ideology and Chinese culture, and the ways in which the Center has created programs to foster culturally embedded empowerment through competence development. Saegert (1989) presented an example of qualitative and participatory research in a study of African-American women who are leaders in their co-op housing projects. In the process, she magnifies black women's resources and strengths, without minimizing the difficulties they encounter. Not only is the methodology an example of a feminist approach to problem definition and reality construction, but the results emphasize the importance of multilevel explanations of empowerment phenomena.

Citations to recent articles that focus on minority women are included at the end of each section in this chapter. Recent articles that do not fit into the section categories include Bond (1997); Culp and McCarthick (1997); Davis and Rhodes (1994); Fujino, Okazaki, and Young (1994); Gibbs and Fuery (1994); Henly (1997); Mitchell and Beals (1997); Rhodes, Contreras, and Mangelsdorf (1994); Rhodes, Ebert, and Fischer (1992); Sellers, Kuperminc, and Damas (1997); and Taylor, Henderson, and Jackson (1991).

Overview

This section pinpoints a smattering of excellent pieces related to minority women in the community psychology journals reviewed. Multilevel analyses and sensitivity to cultural issues predominate, the treatment of gender issues is straightforward and articulate, and minority women's strengths are an integral part of the analyses. Overall, however, in most of the articles focused on minority women distributed throughout this review, our discipline has continued to maintain its focus on the individual level of analysis, and on minority women's deficits rather than their strengths. Because of their doubly vulnerable status as both women and minorities in this society, this population is at risk for a variety of dysfunctional outcomes. We would welcome increased efforts from our colleagues to be proactive in working with this population, and assertive in facilitating both greater understanding and preventive and/or empowering interventions to foster change in their situations.

DISCUSSION

We selected articles on the women's issues reviewed in this chapter for their relevance in the prevention of dysfunctional outcomes in women or to their empowerment. Through these articles we have explored women's family patterns, workforce participation, care of dependent family members, and health and reproductive issues, and addressed the stressful life conditions they face with respect to poverty, violence, and minority status. It is axiomatic that community psychologists learn about the characteristics, needs, and resources of a population before attempting preventive interventions, or collaborative interventions aimed at empowerment, and much of the field's attention to women has been in building such an information base. In this task, the assessment of stress, competence, social supports, and self-esteem has encompassed much of the effort. These assessments provide valuable information for preventive interventions and describe work at initial stages of the empowerment process.

There are relatively few articles in many of the areas reviewed. Most are at the individual level of analysis. Although the impact of the women's movement and feminist thinking on our discipline have brought specific issues to the attention of the field, multilevel analyses of the structural variables that systematically disempower women are missing for the most part. Particularly missing is the recognition of the power imbalance based on gender that pervades women's lives (Swift, 1991), and the impact of this imbalance on women's development and functioning. Failure to take account of the power issue leads inevitably to flawed theory and research.

Consciousness of gender issues is undeveloped in much of the community psychology literature we reviewed.[10] It is unlikely, for example, that studying the characteristics of raped and battered women will tell us as much about the causes and correlates of rape and battering as will studying the characteristics of cultures that tolerate these crimes and the men who commit them. Our critique of the field lies not so much in its efforts to profile the population of women as in its lack of an ecological perspective in doing so. By focusing on individual-level analyses of women, the force of the literature implies that women are to blame for being raped, pregnant, or beaten. The failure to address men's roles in what are called "women's issues" cheats both women and men. Multilevel analyses are needed to identify the variables of which "women's issues" are a function, and to suggest appropriate directions for research and interventions.

Most of the interventions have focused on educational strategies—skill-training, workshops, curriculum development—within settings that are under researchers' control, such as schools, universities, and shelters. Although some are well-designed to mobilize women's skills and strengths and to access available community resources, few interventions attempt to create new resources or change the barriers that impede women's access. Very few have been carried out in the community, or have included community residents as codesigners or participants in implementing the interventions. This critique can be made of many areas within the field: in overlooking the principle of engaging the population studied as partners in the research process, investigators limit the empowering potential of their interventions.

We are heartened and encouraged by the increasing attention of community psychology journals to women and their concerns across the last few decades. Literature on women at work has been published in these journals since the inception of the field. During the 1970s, the articles focused on individual skill-building for working women, with no attention to gender-related stresses or needs. This early work was accompanied by a plethora of descriptive studies on women-dominated professions that often neglected to report the gender of participants, much less address the implications of gender dynamics. In the early 1980s, there were a few studies on the social supports of working women, and in the later 1980s, researchers added both individual coping and organizational policies to the consideration of supports and

[10]For an exception in addition to those already noted, see Albee (1982, 1996).

produced multilevel analyses. The most recent work has explicitly addressed gender issues. It is notable that the early studies in these journals were written primarily by men, while the work of the last ten years has been authored primarily by women.

Although women in the workforce is not a new topic for the field, the gender-based ecology of working women's lives has only recently been considered. We know from the work summarized here that working women's well-being is enhanced by their control over work schedules, and role and pace, as well as by reduced competition between work and family demands. We also know that family supports for women's work play a profound role, with negative spouse attitudes taking a particular toll, not only on individual women but on the climate of the entire family. These results point to the importance of further addressing contextual supports for women's work. We need to better understand the forces on families that undermine support for women's workplace roles. Alternative strategies and structures to reduce conflict and enhance women's control need to be further developed and researched. We need to address both the formal and informal aspects of organizational life that affect women's empowerment.

Some of the theoretical pieces are at the second stage of the empowerment process (Swift & Levin, 1987). They inform the field of the institutions and processes in our culture that disempower women, and identify structural variables that block women's development across life domains. Some propose directions for research and action programs to facilitate increasing women's empowerment status. Although the relatively few interventions we reviewed vary in their level of awareness of the structural issues involved in women's disempowerment, most involve the mobilization of resources, and thus are at the third stage of empowerment development. None of the articles are at Swift and Levin's fourth empowerment stage, in which analysis of the system's openness to change is both a preliminary to planning and implementing interventions, and a strategy for identifying and joining other groups involved in synchronous empowerment activities.

In sum, looking at the first 25 years of our discipline's history, we are left overall with a mixed evaluation of our discipline's efforts in these areas. On the one hand, interest in women and their concerns has increased in recent years, efforts are being made to broaden the levels of analysis, and important information has been provided about the populations of women involved. On the other hand, the levels of analysis are mostly individual, interventions are scarce, and there is a pervasive lack of a feminist examination of issues that are strongly gender related. Similar critiques can be made of many areas within the field regarding restricted levels of analysis, few interventions, and neglect of significant populations—e.g., minorities, gay men and lesbians, and those with physical disabilities. Given this state of affairs, we recommend that community psychologists: (1) consider power issues, such as those involved in dominant versus nondominant relationships, in the design and analysis of their work; (2) acknowledge gender as a factor with important consequences for definition, measurement, and intervention; (3) seek a multilevel interdisciplinary understanding of problems, which may require teamwork with those in other disciplines; and (4) move boldly into intervention design and evaluation guided by values of participation and collaboration.

Marybeth Shinn's presidential address to the Division of Community Psychology (1992) succinctly and eloquently encompasses the directions we recommend to the field in working with women. Although she focused on homelessness, her multilevel analysis parallels many of the realities women face in other areas, particularly the structural impediments to growth and empowerment. She urges community psychologists to go beyond research that focuses exclusively on victims and to concentrate on variables linking structural and individual levels of analysis. We must also go beyond cross-sectional studies to longitudinal approaches to women's issues in order to assess the impact of structural variables across time. And women themselves must be integrated into our research activities, from initial design stages to the interpretation and dissemination of results.

We join Shinn (1992) in urging colleagues to accept commitments to action as part of our professional roles. Community psychologists should help policymakers understand the structural factors that underlie negative outcomes for women, and the limits of psychological services to prevent these outcomes. We need to intensify our efforts in one of our most significant roles: working with community institutions to implement policies and programs based on our special expertise. Finally, we should join with women in our communities to enhance their empowerment status. Underlying these directions for research and action is the necessity for community psychologists to recognize and document the pervasive damage done to women through the unequal balance of power and the perpetuation of sex-role stereotypes that women experience in our culture. Until these structural barriers to empowerment are acknowledged and assessed, women's interests cannot be effectively addressed. Until they have been eliminated, women's interests cannot be justly served.

ACKNOWLEDGMENTS. We wish to thank Angela Guarino and Carol McCall at the University of Massachusetts at Lowell for their invaluable assistance with the literature review. We could not have done it without their help.

REFERENCES

Abraido-Lanza, A. (1997). Latinas with arthritis: effects of illness, role identity and competence on psychological well-being. *American Journal of Community Psychology, 25*, 601–627.

Akabas, S. (1988). Women, work and mental health: Room for improvement. *Journal of Primary Prevention, 9*, 130–140.

Albee, G. (1982). The politics of nature and nurture. *American Journal of Community Psychology, 10*, 1–36.

Albee, G. (1996). The psychological origins of the white male patriarchy. *Journal of Primary Prevention, 17*, 75–97.

Allen, J., Kuperminc, G., Philliber, S., & Herre, K. (1994). Programmatic prevention of adolescent problem behaviors: The role of autonomy, relatedness, and volunteer service in the Teen Outreach Program. *American Journal of Community Psychology, 22*, 617–638.

Allen, J., Philliber, S., & Hoggson, N. (1990). School-based prevention of teenage pregnancy and school dropout: Process evaluation of the National Replication of the Teen Outreach Program. *American Journal of Community Psychology, 18*, 505–524.

Allen, L. (1984). Black women: A resource for the development of theory and practice in community psychology. *The Community Psychologist, 17*, 7–8.

Alpert, J., Richardson, M., & Fodaski, L. (1983). Onset of parenting and stressful events. *Journal of Primary Prevention, 3*, 149–159.

Amaro, H. (1988). Women in the Mexican-American community: Religion, culture and reproductive attitudes and experiences. *Journal of Community Psychology, 16*, 6–20.

Andresen, P., & Telleen, S. (1992). The relationship between social support and maternal behaviors and attitudes: A meta-analytic review. *American Journal of Community Psychology, 20*, 753–774.

Atlas, J., & Rickel, A. (1988). Maternal coping styles and adjustment in children. *Journal of Primary Prevention, 8*, 169–185.

Baluk, U., & O'Neill, P. (1980). Health professionals' perceptions of the psychological consequences of abortion. *American Journal of Community Psychology, 8*, 67–75.

Banyard, V. (1995). "Taking another route": Daily survival narratives from mothers who are homeless. *American Journal of Community Psychology, 23*, 871–891.

Banyard, V., & Miller, K. (1998). The powerful potential of qualitative research in community psychology. *American Journal of Community Psychology, 26*, 485–505.

Barker, C., & Lemle, R. (1984). The helping process in couples. *American Journal of Community Psychology, 12*, 321–336.

Belsky, J. (1982). A principled approach to interventions with families in the newborn period. *Journal of Community Psychology, 10*, 66–73.

Bennet, N., Spoth, R., & Borgen, F. (1991). Bulimic symptoms in high school females: Prevalence and relationship with multiple measures of psychological health. *Journal of Community Psychology, 19*, 13–28.

Berberich, R., Gabel, H., & Anchor, K. (1979). Self-disclosure in reflective, behavioral, and discussion parent-counseling groups. *Journal of Community Psychology, 7*, 259–263.

Berel, S., & Irving, L. (1998). Media and disturbed eating: An analysis of media influence and implications for prevention. *Journal of Primary Prevention, 18*, 415–430.

Biaggio, M., Brownell, A., & Watts, D. (1988). Preventing sexual harassment: Strategies for university communities. *The Community Psychologist, 21*, 18–19.

Birkel, R., & Reppucci, N. (1983). Social networks, information-seeking, and the utilization of services. *American Journal of Community Psychology, 11*, 185–205.

Blair, R., D'Ercole, A., O'Connor, P., Green, B., & Mulvey, A. (1978). *The representation of women in community psychology*. Paper presented at the American Psychological Association meeting, Toronto, Canada.

Bohmer, C. (1995). Failure and success in self-help groups for victims of professional sexual exploitation. *Journal of Community Psychology, 23*, 190–199.

Bond, M. (Ed.). (1988a). Sexual harassment in academic settings: Developing an ecological approach. *The Community Psychologist, 21*, 5–22.

Bond, M. (1988b). Division 27 sexual harassment survey. *The Community Psychologist, 21*, 7–10.

Bond, M. (1995). Prevention and the ecology of sexual harassment: Creating empowering climates. In C. Swift (Ed.), *Sexual assault and abuse: Sociocultural context of prevention* (pp. 147–173). New York: Haworth.

Bond, M. (1997). The multitextured lives of women of color. *American Journal of Community Psychology, 25*, 733–743.

Brand, E., Lakey, B., & Berman, S. (1995). A preventive, psychoeducational approach to increase perceived social support. *American Journal of Community Psychology, 23*, 117–135.

Brodsky, A. (1996). Resilient single mothers in risky neighborhoods: Negative psychological sense of community. *Journal of Community Psychology, 24*, 347–363.

Broman, C., Hamilton, V., Hoffman, W., & Mavaddat, R. (1995). Race, gender, and the response to stress: Autoworkers' vulnerability to long-term unemployment. *American Journal of Community Psychology, 23*, 813–842.

Brown, K., & Ziefert, M. (1988). Crisis resolution, competence, and empowerment: A service model for women. *Journal of Primary Prevention, 9*, 92–103.

Brunn, A., & Hedberg, A. (1974). Covert positive reinforcement as a treatment procedure for obesity. *Journal of Community Psychology, 2*, 117–119.

Brunswick, A., & Banaszak-Holl, J. (1996). HIV risk behavior and the Health Belief Model: An empirical test in an African American community sample. *Journal of Community Psychology, 24*, 44–65.

Brunswick, A., Lewis, C., & Messeri, P. (1991). A life span perspective on drug use and affective distress in an African-American sample. *Journal of Community Psychology, 19*, 123–135.

Brunswick, A., Lewis, C., & Messeri, P. (1992). Drug use and stress: Testing a coping model in an urban African-American sample. *Journal of Community Psychology, 20*, 148–162.

Butler, C., Rickel, A., Thomas, E., & Hendren, M. (1993). An intervention program to build competencies in adolescent parents. *Journal of Primary Prevention, 13*, 183–198.

Caldwell, R., & Bloom, B. (1982). Social support: Its structure and impact on marital disruption. *American Journal of Community Psychology, 10*, 647–667.

Calhoun, L., Selby, J., Long, G., & Laney, S. (1980). Reactions to the rape victim as a function of victim age. *Journal of Community Psychology, 8*, 172–175.

Calsyn, R., & Morse, G. (1990). Homeless men and women: Commonalities and a service gender gap. *American Journal of Community Psychology, 18*, 597–608.

Calsyn, R., & Roades, L. (1994). Predictors of past and current homelessness. *Journal of Community Psychology, 22*, 272–278.

Calsyn, R., Kohfeld, C., & Roades, L. (1993). Urban homeless people and welfare: Who receives benefits? *American Journal of Community Psychology, 21*, 95–112.

Campbell, R. (1995). The role of work experience and individual beliefs in police officers' perceptions of date rape: An integration of quantitative and qualitative methods. *American Journal of Community Psychology, 23*, 249–277.

Campbell, R. (1998). The community response to rape: Victims' experiences with the legal, medical, and mental health systems. *American Journal of Community Psychology, 26*, 355–379.

Campbell, R., & Ahrens, C. (1998). Innovative community services for rape victims: An application of multiple case study methodology. *American Journal of Community Psychology, 26*, 537–571.

Campbell, R., Baker, C., & Mazurek, T. (1998). Remaining radical? Organizational predictors of rape crisis centers' social change initiatives. *American Journal of Community Psychology, 26*, 457–483.

Canetto, S. (1996). What is a normal family? Common assumptions and current evidence. *Journal of Primary Prevention, 17*, 31–46.

Cannon, J., & Sparks, J. (1989). Shelters—An alternative to violence: A psychosocial case study. *Journal of Community Psychology, 17*, 203–213.

Carels, R., Baucom, D., Leone, P., & Rigney, A. (1998). Psychosocial factors and psychological symptoms: HIV in a public health setting. *Journal of Community Psychology, 26*, 145–162.

Chen, S., Telleen, S., & Chen, E. (1995). Family and community support of urban pregnant students: Support person, function, and parity. *Journal of Community Psychology, 23*, 28–33.

Cheng, S. (1992). Loneliness-distress and physician utilization in well-elderly females. *Journal of Community Psychology, 20*, 43–56.

Cheng, S. (1993). The social context of Hong Kong's booming elderly home industry. *American Journal of Community Psychology, 21*, 449–467.

Cheung, F. (1989). The Women's Center: A community approach to feminism in Hong Kong. *American Journal of Community Psychology, 17*, 99–107.

Claerhout, S., Elder, J., & Janes, C. (1982). Problem-solving skills of rural battered women. *American Journal of Community Psychology, 10*, 605–612.

Clinton, B., & Larner, M. (1988). Rural community women as leaders in health outreach. *Journal of Primary Prevention, 9*, 120–129.

Comas-Díaz, L. (1988). Mainland Puerto Rican women: A socio-cultural approach. *Journal of Community Psychology, 16*, 21–31.

Commerford, M., Gular, E., Orr, D., Reznikoff, M., et al. (1994). Coping and psychological distress in women with HIV/AIDS. *Journal of Community Psychology, 22*, 224–230.

Compas, B., & Williams, R. (1990). Stress, coping, and adjustment in mothers and young adolescents in single- and two-parent families. *American Journal of Community Psychology, 18*, 525–545.

Compton, W., Michael, J., Krasavage-Hopkins, E., Schneiderman, L., & Bickmann, L. (1989). Intentions for postshelter living in battered women. *Journal of Community Psychology, 17*, 126–128.

Conway-Turner, K., & Karasik, R. (1997). The impact of work status on adult daughters' early and future caregiving. *Journal of Community Psychology, 25*, 505–512.

Cornbleth, T., Freedman, A., & Baskett, G. D. (1974). Comparison of the self acceptance of conscripted and voluntary participants in microlab human relations training experience. *Journal of Community Psychology, 2*, 58–59.

Cronan, T., Walen, H., & Cruz, S. (1994). The effects of community-based literacy training on Head Start parents. *Journal of Community Psychology, 22*, 248–258.

Crull, P. (1988). Women's explanations of their harasser's motivations. *The Community Psychologist, 21*, 14–15.

Culp, A., & McCarthick, V. (1997). Chickasaw Native American adolescent mothers: Implications for early intervention practices. *Journal of Community Psychology, 25*, 513–518.

D'Augelli, A. (1988). Sexual harassment and affectional status: The hidden discrimination. *The Community Psychologist, 21*, 11–12.

D'Augelli, A. (1989a). Lesbian's and gay men's experiences of discrimination and harassment in a university community. *American Journal of Community Psychology, 17*, 317–321.

D'Augelli, A. (1989b). The development of a helping community for lesbians and gay men: A case study in community psychology. *Journal of Community Psychology, 17*, 18–29.

D'Augelli, A. (1990). Community development and the HIV epidemic: The development of helping communities. *Journal of Community Psychology, 18*, 337–346.

D'Augelli, A. (1993). Preventing mental health problems among lesbian and gay college students. *Journal of Primary Prevention, 13*, 245–261.

D'Augelli, A, & Hershberger, S. (1993). Lesbian, gay and bisexual youth in community settings: Personal challenges and mental health problems. *American Journal of Community Psychology, 21*, 421–448.

D'Ercole, A. (1988). Single mothers: Stress, coping, and social support. *Journal of Community Psychology, 16*, 41–54.

D'Ercole, A., & Struening, E. (1990). Victimization among homeless women: Implications for service delivery. *Journal of Community Psychology, 18*, 141–152.

Davis, A., & Rhodes, J. (1994). African-American teenage mothers and their mothers: An analysis of supportive and problematic interactions. *Journal of Community Psychology, 22*, 12–20.

Davis, R., Brickman, E., & Baker, T. (1991). Supportive and unsupportive responses of others to rape victims: Effects on concurrent victim adjustment. *American Journal of Community Psychology, 19*, 443–451.

Dean, A., Matt, G., & Wood, P. (1992). The effects of widowhood on social support from significant others. *Journal of Community Psychology, 20*, 309–325.

Dickinson, N., & Cudaback, D. (1992). Parent education for adolescent mothers. *Journal of Primary Prevention, 13*, 23–35.

Dumka, L., Garza, C., Roosa, M., & Stoerzinger, H. (1997). Recruitment and retention of high-risk families into a preventive parent training intervention. *Journal of Primary Prevention, 18*, 25–39.

Dunham, P., Hurshman, A., Litwin, E., Gusella, J., Ellsworth, C., & Dodd, P. (1998). Computer-mediated social support: Single young mothers as a model system. *American Journal of Community Psychology, 26*, 281–306.

Echterling, L., & Moore, H. (1982). A training program in communication skills for receptionists. *Journal of Community Psychology, 10*, 237–239.

Einswirth-Neems, N., & Handal, P. (1978). Spouse's attitudes toward maternal occupational status and effects on family climate. *Journal of Community Psychology, 6*, 168–172.

Epstein, S., Russell, G., & Silvern, L. (1988). Structure and ideology of shelters for battered women. *American Journal of Community Psychology, 16*, 345–368.

Evans, H., & Sperekas, N. (1976). Community assistance for rape victims. *Journal of Community Psychology, 4*, 378–381.

Fawcett, S., White, G., Balcazar, F., Suarez-Balcazar, Y., et al. (1994). A contextual-behavioral model of empowerment: Case studies involving people with physical disabilities. *American Journal of Community Psychology, 22*, 471–496.

Felton, B., & Berry, C. (1992). Groups as social network members: Overlooked sources of social support. *American Journal of Community Psychology, 20*, 253–261.

Fingerer, M. (1973). Psychological sequelae of abortion: Anxiety and depression. *Journal of Community Psychology, 1*, 221–225.

Finn, J. (1984). Local public record data: A rape crisis center tool for program planning and intervention. *Journal of Primary Prevention, 5*, 36–47.

Fontana, C., Fleischman, A. R., McCarton, C., Meltzer, A., & Ruff, H. (1988). A neonatal preventive intervention study: Issues of recruitment and retention. *Journal of Primary Prevention, 9*, 164–176.

Forman, B., & Wadsworth, J. (1983). Delivery of rape-related services in CMHCs: An initial study. *Journal of Community Psychology, 11*, 236–240.

Forman, B., & Wadsworth, J. (1985). Rape-related services in federally funded community mental health centers. *Journal of Community Psychology, 13*, 402–408.

Franzblau, S. (1996). Social Darwinian influences on conceptions of marriage, sex, and motherhood. *Journal of Primary Prevention, 17*, 47–73.

Fuehrer, A., & Schilling, K. (1988). Sexual harassment of women graduate students: The impact of institutional factors. *The Community Psychologist, 21*, 12–13.

Fujino, D., Okazaki, S., & Young, K. (1994). Asian-American women in the mental health system: An examination of ethnic and gender match between therapist and client. *Journal of Community Psychology, 22*, 164–176.

Gabel, H. (1975). Effects of parent group discussion on adolescents' perceptions of maternal behavior. *Journal of Community Psychology, 3*, 32–35.

Garnets, L., & D'Augelli, A. (1994). Empowering lesbian and gay communities: A call for collaboration with community psychology. *American Journal of Community Psychology, 22*, 447–470.

Gatz, M., Barbarin, O., Tyler, F., Mitchell, R., Morgan, J., Wirzbicki, P., Crawford, J., & Engleman, A. (1982). Enhancement of individual and community competence: The older adult as community worker. *American Journal of Community Psychology, 10*, 291–303.

Gerrard, M., McCann, L., & Fortini, M. (1983). Prevention of unwanted pregnancy. *American Journal of Community Psychology, 11*, 153–167.

Gibbs, J., & Fuery, D. (1994). Mental health and well-being of Black women toward strategies of empowerment. *American Journal of Community Psychology, 22*, 559–582.

Golding, J., Siegel, J., Sorenson, S., Burnam, M., & Stein, J. (1989). Social support sources following sexual assault. *Journal of Community Psychology, 17*, 92–107.

Golding, J., Stein, J., Siegel, J., Burnam, M., & Sorenson, S. (1988). Sexual assault history and use of health and mental health services. *American Journal of Community Psychology, 16*, 625–644.

Goldstein, A, & Goedhart, A. (1973). The use of structured learning for empathy enhancement in paraprofessional psychotherapist training. *Journal of Community Psychology, 1*, 168–173.

Goodman, L. (1991). The relationship between social support and family homelessness: A comparison study of homeless and housed mothers. *Journal of Community Psychology*, 321–332.

Goodman, S., & Johnson, M. (1986). Life problems, social supports, and psychological functioning of emotionally disturbed and well low-income women. *Journal of Community Psychology, 14*, 150–158.

Greenberger, E., Goldberg, W., Hamill, S., O'Neil, R., & Payne, C. (1989). Contributions of a supportive work environment to parents' well-being and orientation to work. *American Journal of Community Psychology, 17,* 755–783.

Guarnaccia, P., Angel, R., & Worobey, J. (1991). The impact of marital status and employment status on depressive affect for Hispanic Americans. *Journal of Community Psychology, 19,* 136–149.

Guarnaccia, V., & Henderson, J. (1993). Self-efficacy, interpersonal competence, and social desirability in homeless people. *Journal of Community Psychology, 21,* 335–338.

Halpern, R., & Covey, L. (1983). Community support for adolescent parents and their children: The parent-to-parent program in Vermont. *Journal of Primary Prevention, 3,* 160–173.

Heller, K., Thompson, M., Trueba, P., Hogg, J., et al. (1991). Peer support telephone dyads for elderly women: Was this the wrong intervention? *American Journal of Community Psychology, 19,* 53–74.

Henly, J. (1997). The complexity of support: The impact of family structure and provisional support on African American and white adolescent mothers' well being. *American Journal of Community Psychology, 25,* 629–655.

Henninger, C., & Nelson, G. (1984). Evaluation of a social support program for young unwed mothers. *Journal of Primary Prevention, 5,* 3–16.

Hill, N. (1997). Does parenting differ based on social class? African-American women's perceived socialization for achievement. *American Journal of Community Psychology, 25,* 675–697.

Hirsch, B. (1980). Natural support systems and coping with major life changes. *American Journal of Community Psychology, 8,* 159–172.

Hirsch, B., & David, T. (1983). Social networks and work/nonwork life: Action-research with nurse managers. *American Journal of Community Psychology, 11,* 493–507.

Hobfoll, S., & Lerman, M. (1988). Personal relationships, personal attributes, and stress resistance: Mothers' reactions to their child's illness. *American Journal of Community Psychology, 16,* 565–589.

Hobfoll, S., Dunahoo, C., Ben-Porath, Y., & Monnier, J. (1994). Gender and coping: The dual-axis model of coping. *American Journal of Community Psychology, 22,* 49–82.

Holahan, C., & Moos, R. (1982). Social support and adjustment: Predictive benefits of social climate indices. *American Journal of Community Psychology, 10,* 403–415.

Holroyd, J. (1974). The Questionnaire on Resources and Stress: An instrument to measure family response to a handicapped family member. *Journal of Community Psychology, 2,* 92–94.

Holroyd, J., Brown, N., Winkler, L., & Simmons, J. (1975). Stress in families of institutionalized and noninstitutionalized autistic children. *Journal of Community Psychology, 3,* 26–31.

Holtzman, E., & Gilbert, L. (1987). Social support networks for parenting and psychological wellbeing among dual-earner Mexican-American families. *Journal of Community Psychology, 15,* 176–186.

Honig, A., & Winger, C. (1997). A professional support program for families of handicapped preschoolers: Decrease in maternal stress. *Journal of Primary Prevention, 17,* 285–296.

Hughes, D., & Dodge, M. (1997). African American women in the workplace: Relationships between job conditions, racial bias at work, and perceived job quality. *American Journal of Community Psychology, 25,* 581–599.

Huhn, R., & Zimpfer, D. (1989). Effects of a parent education program on parents and their preadolescent children. *Journal of Community Psychology, 17,* 311–318.

Husaini, B., Neff, J., Newbrough, J., & Moore, M. (1982). The stress-buffering role of social support and personal competence among the rural married. *Journal of Community Psychology, 10,* 409–426.

Innes, R., & Heflinger, C. (1989). An expanded model of community assessment: A case study. *Journal of Community Psychology, 17,* 225–235.

Iscoe, I., Bloom, B., & Spielberger, C. (1977). *Community psychology in transition: Proceedings of the National Conference on Training in Community Psychology.* Washington, D.C.: Hemisphere.

Isely, P., & Gehrenbeck-Shim, D. (1997). Sexual assault of men in the community. *Journal of Community Psychology, 25,* 159–166.

Jackson, A. (1997). Effects of concerns about child care among single, employed black mothers with preschool children. *American Journal of Community Psychology, 25,* 657–673.

Jackson, T., & Ferguson, W. (1983). Attribution of blame in incest. *American Journal of Community Psychology, 11,* 313–322.

Kahn & the Behavioral Health Technician Staff. (1980). Wife beating and cultural context: Prevalence in the Aboriginal and islander community in northern Australia. *American Journal of Community Psychology, 8,* 727–731.

Kazak, A., & Linney, J. (1983). Stress, coping, and life change in the single-parent family. *American Journal of Community Psychology, 11,* 207–220.

Kazak, A., & Wilcox, B. (1984). The structure and function of social support networks in families with handicapped children. *American Journal of Community Psychology, 12,* 645–661.

King, H., Rotter, M., Calhoun, L., & Selby, J. (1978). Perceptions of the rape incident: Physicians and volunteer counselors. *Journal of Community Psychology, 6,* 74–77.

Kofkin, J., & Repucci, N. (1991). A reconceptualization of life events and its application to parental divorce. *American Journal of Community Psychology*, *19*, 227–250.

Krause, N., & Geyer-Pestello, H. (1985). Depressive symptoms among women employed outside the home. *American Journal of Community Psychology*, *13*, 49–67.

Lambert, S., & Hopkins, K. (1995). Occupational conditions and workers' sense of community: Variations by gender and race. *American Journal of Community Psychology*, *23*, 151–179.

Lamberts, M., Cudaback, D., & Claesgens, M. (1985). Helping teenage parents: Use of age-paced parent education newsletters. *Journal of Primary Prevention*, *5*, 188–199.

LaVeist, T., Sellers, R., Brown, K., & Nickerson, K. (1997). Extreme social isolation, use of community-based senior support services, and mortality among African American elderly women. *American Journal of Community Psychology*, *25*, 721–732.

Laurendeau, M., Gagnon, G., Desjardins, N., Perreault, R., & Kishchuk, N. (1991). Evaluation of an early, mass media parental support intervention. *Journal of Primary Prevention*, *11*, 207–225.

Lerman, L. (1982). Court decisions on wife abuse laws: Recent developments. *Response*, *5*, 21–22.

Levine, O., Britton, P., James, T., Jackson, A., et al. (1993). The empowerment of women: A key to HIV prevention. *Journal of Community Psychology*, *21*, 320–334.

Levy, B. (1985). Skills for violence-free relationships. *The Community Psychologist*, *19*, 10–12.

Levy, L., & Derby, J. (1992). Bereavement support groups: Who joins; who does not; and why. *American Journal of Community Psychology*, *20*, 649–662.

Levy, L., Derby, J., & Martinkowski, K. (1993). Effects of membership in bereavement support groups on adaptation to conjugal bereavement. *American Journal of Community Psychology*, *21*, 361–381.

Lewis, E. (1988). Role strengths and strains of African-American mothers. *Journal of Primary Prevention*, *9*, 77–91.

Lieberman, G. (1978). Children of the elderly as natural helpers: Some demographic differences. *American Journal of Community Psychology*, *6*, 489–498.

Linney, J., & Bond, M. (Eds.). (1985a). Women and community psychology. *Division of Community Psychology Newsletter* (later *The Community Psychologist*) (special issue), *18*, 2–8.

Linney, J., & Bond, M. (Eds.). (1985b). Women in the community. *The Community Psychologist* (special issue), *19*, 1–16.

Loeb, R. (1983). A program of community education for dealing with spouse abuse. *Journal of Community Psychology*, *11*, 241–252.

Mantell, J., Schinke, S., & Akabas, S. (1988). Women and AIDS prevention. *Journal of Primary Prevention*, *9*, 18–63.

Marshall, N., & Barnett, R. (1992). Work-related support among women in caregiving occupations. *Journal of Community Psychology*, *20*, 36–42.

Marshall, N., & Barnett, R. (1993). Work/family strains and gains among two-earner couples. *Journal of Community Psychology*, *21*, 64–78.

Maton, K., Teti, D., Corns, K., Vieira-Baker, C., & Lavine, J. (1996). Cultural specificity of support sources, correlates and contexts: Three studies of African-American and Caucasian youth. *American Journal of Community Psychology*, *24*, 551–587.

McCall, R. (1973). MMPI factors that differentiate remediably from irremediably obese women. *Journal of Community Psychology*, *1*, 34–36.

McCloskey, L., Southwick, K., Fernandez-Esquer, M., & Locke, C. (1995). The psychological effects of political and domestic violence on Central American and Mexican immigrant mothers and children. *Journal of Community Psychology*, *23*, 95–116.

McFarlane, D. (1988). Family planning needs: An empirical study of federal responsiveness before and during the Reagan administration. *Journal of Primary Prevention*, *9*, 41–55.

McLoyd, V., & Wilson, L. (1992). Telling them like it is: The role of economic and environmental factors in single mothers' discussions with their children. *American Journal of Community Psychology*, *20*, 419–444.

Medvane, L., Mendoza, R., Lin, K., Harris, N., et al. (1995). Increasing Mexican American attendance of support groups for parents of the mentally ill: Organizational and psychological factors. *Journal of Community Psychology*, *23*, 307–325.

Melgoza, B., Roll, S., & Baker, R. (1983). Conformity and cooperation in Chicanos: The case of the missing susceptibility to influence. *Journal of Community Psychology*, *11*, 323–333.

Menaghan, E. (1978). Seeking help for parental concerns in the middle years. *American Journal of Community Psychology*, *6*, 477–488.

Meyers, A., & Rhodes, J. (1995). Oral contraceptive use among African American adolescents: Individual and community influences. *American Journal of Community Psychology*, *23*, 99–115.

Miller, A. (1974). The relationship between family interaction and sexual behavior in adolescence. *Journal of Community Psychology*, *2*, 285–288.

Miller, J. (1986). *Toward a new psychology of women*, 2nd ed. Boston: Beacon.

Miller-Loncar, C., Erwin, L., Landry, S., Smith, K., & Swank, P. (1998). Characteristics of social support networks of low socioeconomic status African American, Anglo American, and Mexican American mothers of full term and preterm infants. *Journal of Community Psychology, 26*, 131–143.

Miskimins, R., & Baker, B. (1973). Self-concept and the disadvantaged. *Journal of Community Psychology, 1*, 347–361.

Mitchell, C., & Beals, J. (1997). The structure of problem and positive behavior among American Indian adolescents: Gender and community differences. *American Journal of Community Psychology, 25*, 257–288.

Mitchell, R., & Hodson, C. (1983). Coping with domestic violence: Social support and psychological health among battered women. *American Journal of Community Psychology, 11*, 629–654.

Moos, R., & Moos, B. (1983). Adaptation and the quality of life in work and family settings. *Journal of Community Psychology, 11*, 158–170.

Mowbray, C., Cohen, E., Harris, S., Trosch, S., et al. (1992). Serving the homeless mentally ill: Mental health linkage. *Journal of Community Psychology, 20*, 215–227.

Mulvey, A. (1988). Community psychology and feminism: Tensions and commonalities. *Journal of Community Psychology, 16*, 70–83.

Mulvey, A, & Bond, M. (1990). *Integrating feminism into community psychology: Challenges of building supportive communities*. Keynote address in abstracted Proceedings of the 7th Annual Community Psychology Conference: Building Supportive Communities. (Available from: Center for Community Change, One Kennedy Drive, So. Burlington, VT 05403.)

Myers, H., Taylor, S., Alvy, K., & Arrington, A., et al. (1992). Parental and family predictors of behavior problems in inner-city black children. *American Journal of Community Psychology, 20*, 557–576.

Naylor, K., Tolan, P., & Wilson, M. (1988). Acquaintance rape: A systems perspective. *The Community Psychologist, 21*, 20–21.

Nazario, T. (1986). Migrant Puerto Rican women social support networks. *The Community Psychologist, 19*, 9–10.

Neighbors, H., & Jackson, J. (1984). The use of informal and formal help: Four patterns of illness behavior in the Black community. *American Journal of Community Psychology, 12*, 629–644.

Nelson, G. (1989). Life strains, coping, and emotional well-being: A longitudinal study of recently separated and married women. *American Journal of Community Psychology, 17*, 459–483.

Nelson, G. (1990). Women's life strains, social support, coping, and positive and negative affect: Cross-sectional and longitudinal tests of the two-factor theory of emotional well-being. *Journal of Community Psychology, 18*, 239–263.

Nemoto, T. (1998). Subjective norms toward social support among Japanese American elderly in New York City. Why help does not always help. *Journal of Community Psychology, 26*, 293–316.

Noble, A., & Winett, R. (1978). Chairperson's and hirees' opinions, knowledge, and experiences with affirmative action guidelines. *Journal of Community Psychology, 6*, 194–199.

O'Bryant, S., Donnermeyer, J., & Stafford, K. (1991). Fear of crime and perceived risk among older widowed women. *Journal of Community Psychology, 19*, 166–177.

O'Connor, P. (1988). Sexual harassment: A very real training issue. *The Community Psychologist, 21*, 21.

Olson, T., Wallace, C., & Miller, B. (1984). Primary prevention of adolescent pregnancy: Promoting family involvement through school curriculum. *Journal of Primary Prevention, 5*, 75–89.

Phillips, D., Howes, C., & Whitebook, M. (1992). The social policy context of child care: Effects on quality. *American Journal of Community Psychology, 20*, 25–51.

Pilkington, N., & D'Augelli, A. (1995). Victimization of lesbian, gay, and bisexual youth in community settings. *Journal of Community Psychology, 23*, 34–56.

Pistrang, N., & Barker, C. (1998). Partners and fellow patients: Two sources of emotional support for women with breast cancer. *American Journal of Community Psychology, 26*, 439–456.

Popiel, D., & Susskind, E. (1985). The impact of rape: Social support as a moderator of stress. *American Journal of Community Psychology, 13*, 645–676.

Powell, D. (1984). Social network and demographic predictors of length of participation in a parent education program. *Journal of Community Psychology, 12*, 13–20.

Powell, D., & Eisenstadt, J. (1983). Predictors of help-seeking in an urban setting: The search for child care. *American Journal of Community Psychology, 11*, 401–422.

Pretty, G., & McCarthy, M. (1991). Exploring the psychological sense of community among women and men of the corporation. *Journal of Community Psychology, 19*, 351–361.

Prieto-Bayard, M. (1993). Psychosocial predictors of coping among Spanish-speaking mothers with retarded children. *Journal of Community Psychology, 21*, 300–308.

Prieto-Bayard, M., & Baker, B. (1986). Parent training for Spanish-speaking families with a retarded child. *Journal of Community Psychology, 14*, 134–143.

Rankin, E., Campbell, N., & Soeken, K. (1985). Adaptation to parenthood: Differing expectations of social supports for mothers versus fathers. *Journal of Primary Prevention, 5*, 145–153.

Rappaport, J. (1987). Terms of empowerment/exemplars of prevention: Toward a theory for community psychology. *American Journal of Community Psychology, 15*, 121–148.

Rauktis, M., Koeske, G., & Tereshko, O. (1995). Negative social interactions, distress, and depression among those caring for a seriously and persistently mentally ill relative. *American Journal of Community Psychology, 23*, 279–299.

Reinharz, S. (1988). What's missing in miscarriage? *Journal of Community Psychology, 16*, 84–103.

Reppucci, N. (1987). Prevention and ecology: Teenage pregnancy, child sexual abuse and organized youth sports. *American Journal of Community Psychology, 15*, 1–22.

Resick, P., & Jackson, T. (1981). Attitudes toward rape among mental health professionals. *American Journal of Community Psychology, 9*, 481–490.

Rhodes, J., & Woods, M. (1995). Comfort and conflict in the relationships of pregnant, minority adolescents: Social support as a moderator of social strain. *Journal of Community Psychology, 23*, 74–84.

Rhodes, J., Contreras, J., & Mangelsdorf, S. (1994). Natural mentor relationships among Latina adolescent mothers: Psychological adjustment, moderating processes, and the role of early parental acceptance. *American Journal of Community Psychology, 22*, 211–227.

Rhodes, J., Ebert, L., & Fischer, K. (1992). Natural mentors: An overlooked resource in the social networks of young, African American mothers. *American Journal of Community Psychology, 20*, 445–461.

Rickel, A. (1985). President's Column. *The Community Psychologist, 19*, 1–2.

Rickel, A. (1986). Prescriptions for a new generation: Early life interventions. *American Journal of Community Psychology, 14*, 1–15.

Rickel, A., Williams, D., & Loigman, G. (1988). Predictors of maternal child-rearing practices: Implications for intervention. *Journal of Community Psychology, 16*, 32–40.

Riger, S. (1993). What's wrong with empowerment? *American Journal of Community Psychology, 21*, 279–292.

Riger, S., Gordon, M., & LeBailly, R. (1982). Coping with urban crime: Women's use of precautionary behaviors. *American Journal of Community Psychology, 10*, 369–386.

Rosenberg, M. (1985). The impact of spouse abuse on female children. *The Community Psychologist, 19*, 9–10.

Rotherham-Borus, M., Gwadz, M., Fernandez, I., & Srinivasan, S. (1998). Timing of HIV interventions on reductions in sexual risk among adolescents. *American Journal of Community Psychology, 26*, 73–96.

Rowe, K., & Irvine, A. (1985). Empowering women in an alternative health care setting. *The Community Psychologist, 19*, 13–14.

Sadler, O., Seyden, T., Howe, B., & Kaminsky, T. (1976). An evaluation of Groups for Parents: A standardized format encompassing both behavior modification and humanistic methods. *Journal of Community Psychology, 4*, 157–163.

Saegert, S. (1989). Unlikely leaders, extreme circumstances: Older Black women building community households. *American Journal of Community Psychology, 17*, 295–316.

Salem, D., Bogat, A., & Reid, C. (1997). Mutual help goes on-line. *Journal of Community Psychology, 25*, 189–207.

Sanchez-Hucles, J. (1997). Jeopardy not bonus status for African American women in the work force: Why does the myth of advantage persist? *American Journal of Community Psychology, 25*, 565–580.

Sandler, H., Dokecki, P., Stewart, L., Britton, V., & Horton, D. (1973). The evaluation of a home-based educational intervention for preschoolers and their mothers. *Journal of Community Psychology, 1*, 372–374.

Schwirian, K., & Schwirian, P. (1993). Neighboring, residential and psychological well-being in urban elders. *Journal of Community Psychology, 21*, 285–299.

Secouler, L. (1992). Our elders: At high risk for humiliation. *Journal of Primary Prevention, 12*, 195–208.

Seitz, V., Apfel, N., & Rosenbaum, L. (1991). Effects of an intervention program for pregnant adolescents: Educational outcomes at two years postpartum. *American Journal of Community Psychology, 19*, 911–930.

Selby, J., Calhoun, L., & Cann, A. (1979). Effect of perceived motivation on the assignment of blame and punishment to rapists by female respondents. *Journal of Community Psychology, 7*, 357–359.

Selkin, J. (1978). Protecting personal space: Victim and resister reactions to assaultive rape. *Journal of Community Psychology, 6*, 263–268.

Sellers, R., Kuperminc, G., & Damas, A. (1997). The college life experiences of African American women athletes. *American Journal of Community Psychology, 25*, 699–720.

Seybold, J., Fritz, J., & McPhee, D. (1991). Relation of social support to the self-perceptions of mothers with delayed children. *Journal of Community Psychology, 19*, 29–36.

Shinn, M. (1992). Homelessness: What is a psychologist to do? *American Journal of Community Psychology, 20*, 1–24.

Shinn, M. (1997). Family homelessness: State or trait? *American Journal of Community Psychology, 25*, 755–769.

Shinn, M., & Rosario, M. (1985). The extended family program. *The Community Psychologist, 19*, 5–6.

Shinn, M., Wong, N., Simko, P., & Ortiz-Torres, B. (1989). Promoting the well-being of working parents: Coping, social support, and flexible job schedules. *American Journal of Community Psychology, 17*, 31–55.

Shoffner, S. (1986). Child care in rural areas: Needs, attitudes, and preferences. *American Journal of Community Psychology, 14*, 521–539.

Shore, E. (1985). Alcohol consumption and the professional woman. *The Community Psychologist, 19*, 8–9.

Shulman, S., Kedem, P., Kaplan, K., Sever, I., & Braja, M. (1998). Latchkey children: Potential sources of support. *Journal of Community Psychology, 26*, 185–197.

Siefert, K., & Martin, L. (1988). Preventing black maternal mortality: A challenge for the 90's. *Journal of Primary Prevention, 9*, 57–65.

Silver, E., Ireys, H., Bauman, L., & Stein, R. (1997). Psychological outcomes of a support intervention in mothers of children with ongoing health conditions: The parent-to-parent network. *Journal of Community Psychology, 25*, 249–264.

Simon, B. (1988). The feminization of poverty: A call for primary prevention. *Journal of Primary Prevention, 9*, 6–17.

Simons, R., Johnson, C., Beaman, J., Conger, R., et al. (1996). Parents and peer group as mediators of the effect of community structure on adolescent problem behavior. *American Journal of Community Psychology, 24*, 145–171.

Smyer, M. (1984). Working with families of impaired elderly. *Journal of Community Psychology, 12*, 323–333.

Snyder, D., & Scheer, N. (1981). Predicting disposition following brief residence at a shelter for battered women. *American Journal of Community Psychology, 9*, 559–566.

Soto, E. (1983). Sex-role traditionalism and assertiveness in Puerto Rican women living in the U.S. *Journal of Community Psychology, 11*, 346–354.

St. Lawrence, J., Eldridge, G., Reitman, D., Little, C., Shelby, M., & Brasfield, T. (1998). Factors influencing condom use among African American women: Implications for risk reduction interventions. *American Journal of Community Psychology, 26*, 7–28.

St-Onge, M., & Lavoie, F. (1997). The experience of caregiving among mothers of adults suffering from psychotic disorders: Factors associated with their psychological distress. *American Journal of Community Psychology, 25*, 73–94.

Stein, J., Nyamathi, A., & Kington, R. (1997). Change in AIDS risk behaviors among impoverished minority women after a community-based cognitive-behavioral outreach program. *Journal of Community Psychology, 25*, 519–553.

Stern, M., & Golden, F. (1977). A partial evaluation of an introductory training program in behavior modification for psychiatric nurses. *American Journal of Community Psychology, 5*, 23–32.

Strayhorn, J., Weidman, G., & Larson, D. (1990). A measure of religiousness, and its relation to parent and child mental health variables. *Journal of Community Psychology, 18*, 34–43.

Sullivan, C., & Davidson, W. (1991). The provision of advocacy services to women leaving abusive partners: An examination of short-term effects. *American Journal of Community Psychology, 19*, 953–960.

Sullivan, C., Campbell, R., Angelique, H., Eby, K., et al. (1994). An advocacy intervention program for women with abusive partners: Six-month follow-up. *American Journal of Community Psychology, 22*, 101–122.

Sullivan, C., Tan, C., Basta, J., Rumptz, M., et al. (1992). An advocacy intervention program for women with abusive partners: Initial evaluation. *American Journal of Community Psychology, 20*, 309–332.

Swift, C. (1991). Some issues in inter-gender humiliation. *Journal of Primary Prevention, 12*, 123–147.

Swift, C., & Levin, G. (1987). Empowerment: An emerging mental health technology. *Journal of Primary Prevention, 7*, 242–263.

Szendre, E., & Jose, P. (1996). Telephone support by elderly volunteers to inner-city children. *Journal of Community Psychology, 24*, 87–96.

Tableman, B., Marciniak, D., Johnson, D., & Rodgers, R. (1982). Stress management training for women on public assistance. *American Journal of Community Psychology, 10*, 357–367.

Tadmor, C. (1986). A crisis intervention model for a population of mothers who encounter neonatal death. *Journal of Primary Prevention, 7*, 17–26.

Tadmor, C., & Brandes, J. (1986). Premature birth: A crisis intervention approach. *Journal of Primary Prevention, 6*, 244–255.

Tadmor, C., & Brandes, J. (1994). Biopsychosocial profiles of pregnant women at high or low risk to encounter preterm birth. *Journal of Community Psychology, 22*, 231–247.

Tam, K., Chan, Y., & Wong, C. (1994). Validation of the Parenting Stress Index among Chinese mothers in Hong Kong. *Journal of Community Psychology, 22*, 211–223.

Tausig, M. (1992). Caregiver network structure, support and caregiver distress. *American Journal of Community Psychology, 20*, 81–96.

Taylor, J., Henderson, D., & Jackson, B. (1991). A holistic model for understanding and predicting depressive symptoms in African-American women. *Journal of Community Psychology, 19*, 306–320.

Telleen, S. (1990). Parental beliefs and help seeking in mothers' use of a community based family support program. *Journal of Community Psychology, 18*, 264–276.

Tetzloff, C., & Berrera, M. (1987). Divorcing mothers and social support: Testing the specificity of buffering effects. *American Journal of Community Psychology, 15*, 419–434.

Thomas, E., & Rickel, A. (1995). Teen pregnancy and maladjustment: A study of base rates. *Journal of Community Psychology, 23*, 200–215.

Thomas, E., Rickel, A., Butler, C., & Montgomery, E. (1990). Adolescent pregnancy and parenting. *Journal of Primary Prevention, 10*, 195–206.

Thurston, L., Dasta, K., & Greenwood, C. (1984). A program of survival skills workshops for urban women. *Journal of Community Psychology, 12*, 192–196.

Torre, E. (1988). Prevention strategies of a self-empowered group of professional women: Recharting familiar ground. *Journal of Primary Prevention, 9*, 66–76.

Turner, H., & Catania, J. (1997). Informal caregiving to persons with AIDS in the United States: Caregiver burden among central cities residents eighteen to forty-nine years old. *American Journal of Community Psychology, 25*, 35–59.

Unger, J., Kipke, M., Simon, T., Montgomery, S., & Johnson, C. (1997). Homeless youths and young adults in Los Angeles: Prevalence of mental health problems and the relationship between mental health and substance abuse disorders. *American Journal of Community Psychology, 25*, 371–394.

VanOss Marin, B., Tschann, J., Gomez, C., & Gregorich, S. (1998). Self efficacy to use condoms in unmarried Latino adults. *American Journal of Community Psychology, 26*, 53–71.

Waldo, C., Hesson-McInnis, M., & D'Augelli, A. (1998). Antecedents and consequences of victimization of lesbian, gay, and bisexual young people: A structural model comparing rural university and urban samples. *American Journal of Community Psychology, 26*, 307–334.

Walsh, R. (1987). A social history note on the formal emergence of community psychology. *American Journal of Community Psychology, 15*, 523–529.

Walther, D. (1986). Wife-abuse prevention: Effects of information on attitudes of high school boys. *Journal of Primary Prevention, 7*, 84–90.

Wandersman, L., Wandersman, A., & Kahn, S. (1980). Social support in the transition to parenthood. *Journal of Community Psychology, 8*, 332–342.

Weissman, G., & NARC. (1991). AIDS prevention for women at risk: Experience from a National Demonstration Research Program. *Journal of Primary Prevention, 12*, 49–63.

Winett, R., Neale, M., & Williams, K. (1982). The effects of flexible work schedules on urban families with young children: Quasi-experimental, ecological studies. *American Journal of Community Psychology, 10*, 49–64.

Wingood, G., & DiClemente, R. (1998). Partner influences and gender-related factors associated with noncondom use among young adult African American women. *American Journal of Community Psychology, 26*, 29–51.

Wolchik, S., West, S., Westover, S., & Sandler, I. (1993). Children of divorce parenting intervention: Outcome evaluation of an empirically based program. *American Journal of Community Psychology, 21*, 293–331.

Wyman, P., Cowen, E., Work, W., & Parker, G. (1991). Developmental and family milieu correlates of resilience in urban children who have experienced major life stress. *American Journal of Community Psychology, 19*, 405–426.

Zambrana, R., Silva-Palacios, V., & Powell, D. (1992). Parenting concerns, family support systems, and life problems in Mexican-origin women: A comparison by nativity. *Journal of Community Psychology, 20*, 276–288.

Zigler, E. (1994). Reshaping early childhood intervention to be a more efficient weapon against poverty. *American Journal of Community Psychology, 22*, 37–47.

CHAPTER 36

A Perspective on Ethical Issues in Community Psychology

DAVID L. SNOW, KATHERINE GRADY, AND MICHELE GOYETTE-EWING

Early analyses identified community psychology (Golann, 1969) and the related field of community psychiatry (McNeil, Llewellyn, & McCollough, 1970) as emerging areas of ethical concern. As community psychology developed in areas of research and practice, these concerns continued. Rappaport (1977), for example, wrote that community psychology is fraught with inherent complexities because it lies at the juncture between society and the individual, suggesting that the field faced special ethical problems. And Weithorn (1987) asserts that special issues that may characterize prevention research with children create "ethical dilemmas"—situations when what is ethically correct is not clear, and any of several ethically defensible solutions may be arrived at, depending on one's analysis of the issues" (p. 230). Despite these ongoing concerns, consideration of ethical issues within community psychology has received limited attention.

Certainly, there have been relevant treatments of ethical issues concerning the broader social sciences (Kelman, 1965; Sieber, 1982), in relation to social change processes (Warwick & Kelman, 1973; Zaltman & Duncan, 1977), and in areas of practice and research, such as consultation, that fall within the general purview of community psychology (Davis & Sandoval, 1982; Gallessich, 1982; Snow & Gersick, 1986). A National Institute of Mental Health publication on prevention research (Steinberg & Silverman, 1987) containing a section on ethical issues, a compilation of papers that gives thoughtful consideration to ethics in relation to primary prevention (Levin, Trickett, & Hess, 1990), and an article by O'Neill (1989) published in a special issue of the *American Journal of Community Psychology* along with a series of commentaries are all welcome additions to this literature. These contributions are useful for establishing a general framework and, in some instances, more specific guidelines for considering ethical issues in community psychology.

DAVID L. SNOW AND KATHERINE GRADY • The Consultation Center, Department of Psychiatry, Yale University, New Haven, Connecticut 06511. MICHELE GOYETTE-EWING • Child Study Center, Yale University, New Haven, Connecticut 06511.

Handbook of Community Psychology, edited by Julian Rappaport and Edward Seidman. Kluwer Academic / Plenum Publishers, New York, 2000.

In a similar way, the development and publication of general discipline or professional codes of ethics (e.g., American Psychological Association, 1992) provide a set of guidelines and standards that have relevance to community psychology in areas such as confidentiality, competence, misrepresentation, and informed consent. However, these codes of ethics do not necessarily reflect the unique issues, problems, and situations encountered in community psychology intervention and research (O'Neill, 1989; Pope, 1989; Prilleltensky, 1990), and some assert that the ethical principles that guide psychology in general may not be conducive to the social change goals of community psychology and, in fact, may undermine these objectives (Serrano-Garcia, 1994). It is not sufficient to rely on guidelines established within the general field of psychology or in related fields, with the assumption that these adequately address the unique features of community psychology.

Why has a field that places a premium on social concerns and social impact neglected the development of ethical guidelines? Ironically, it may be the very diversity and complexity of the field that make the task so difficult. When community psychology was founded in 1965 at the Swampscott Conference, the founders came away admitting that they could not arrive at an agreed upon definition of this new field (Bennett, Anderson, Cooper, Hassol, Klein, & Rosenblum, 1966). Currently, there is an extraordinary array of individual and social concerns addressed within the field. Research and applied efforts encompass a wide range of interventions, settings, target populations, and goals. Since the boundaries for the field of study and practice remain difficult to define, this poses some real difficulties for establishing ethical guidelines.

At the same time, while the complexity inherent to community psychology may complicate the actual development of ethical guidelines, these same unique characteristics create a compelling need to undertake that very task. The emergence of community psychology has involved the articulation of new paradigms that serve to highlight previously unconsidered ethical issues, as well as ones unique to these new paradigms requiring their own ethical debate (Trickett & Levin, 1990). Research and practice in community psychology are informed importantly by an ecological perspective (Cowen, 1980; Kelly, 1966; Levine & Perkins, 1980, 1997; Moos, 1973; Trickett, 1984). Based on this perspective, interventions and studies of basic phenomena involve complex interactions among diverse individuals and groups, and among varied sectors and levels of organizations and communities. As a result, research and practice are influenced by multiple, and often conflicting, points of view, values, interests, and agendas. In turn, actions taken by the interventionist or researcher have potential direct or indirect implications, positively or negatively, for those immediate to the work, as well as those in the larger surroundings. These features raise concerns about protection of individual rights, manipulation, adequacy of informed consent, and respect for diversity.

Furthermore, in many aspects of community psychology there is difficulty in the demonstration of need or benefit. Weighing the costs and benefits of particular interventions or actions, therefore, is not very straightforward. Preventive interventions are often based on limited knowledge of risk and protective factors and of the methods most effective in modifying such factors. As a result, programs may be offered that do not have clearly demonstrated merit. Limitations in knowledge also make the selection of potential intervention recipients difficult, resulting in the possibility that some number of individuals will be involved in any given intervention who do not need it. Then, of course, in those instances where one tries to identify a specific, high-risk population, there is always the risk of stigmatization. Who is to make judgments about which individuals are to be considered at risk, and based on what methods (Pope, 1990)? For interventions aimed at promoting adaptive functioning, there are the assumptions that these efforts will benefit growth and development to some measurable extent. In both prevention and promotion activities, issues of individual rights, values, informed consent, potential harmful effects of labeling, and the possibility of unintended negative outcomes are central. Moreover, an integral part of any of these interventions is the selection of desired outcomes. Who determines this selection, and through what process? Added to these concerns is the fact that the community psychologist has a certain degree of power and status in the social roles of researcher or practitioner. These positions of social influence create the possibility of effecting meaningful change. At the same time, such power and privilege can be misused (Gallessich, 1982) and can result in threats to individual freedom (McNeil et al., 1970). All of these factors create a basis of concern about ethical problems within the field of community psychology.

The ecological framework that underlies research investigations and service interventions in community psychology also suggests that considerations of ethics must pay attention to the interpersonal, organizational, community, and societal contexts within which service and research activities occur. What Snow and Gersick (1986) wrote in relation to mental health consultation is applicable more broadly to community psychology:

> The particular nature of consultation, with its focus on system change rather than individual cure, means that attention to organizational surroundings is critically important. In developing ethical norms and in assessing compliance with ethical standards, the consideration of these contexts is essential; without it the consultation contract and the conduct of the consultative interventions cannot be meaningfully evaluated. (p. 395)

The purpose of this chapter is to move a step further in the explicit delineation of ethical issues in community psychology. We will not attempt to spell out a specific set of standards or code of ethics. Instead, we will identify important areas of ethical consideration and, hopefully, contribute to the further establishment of frameworks in which ethical conflicts can be examined and resolved. In the tradition suggested by Benne (1959), we are primarily interested in facilitating the development of general "advices" regarding ethical problems, and in stimulating expanded dialogue about ethics in the field.

In the following sections, five areas will be covered that are basic to the conceptualization, design, and implementation of community interventions and research. Ethical issues will be considered related to: (1) values and value conflicts, (2) goals, (3) processes, (4) informed consent, and (5) the generation and use of evidence. Each of these areas includes both technical and ethical considerations that are highly interrelated and together shape the conduct of the work. We will probe each area for the central ethical dilemmas that arise in order to demonstrate the need to give equal weight to the ethical dimensions, as well as the technical ones that are so often in the forefront of our thinking.

ETHICAL ISSUES RELATED TO VALUES AND VALUE CONFLICTS

Values represent the comparative worth ascribed to things, whether of a tangible or intangible nature. A value orientation serves, in part, to shape the nature of the ethical principles themselves, which then can be used as more explicit guidelines against which to measure individual behavior. The community psychologist is constantly confronted with decisions about goals and courses of action among alternatives that are, to some degree, incompatible or even mutually exclusive. What is judged to be ethical in making these kinds of choices is a manifestation of values about what outcomes are more important than others, and about what actions and risks are reasonable and acceptable in seeking to reach these objectives.

The complexity of the change process and the context in which it occurs often obscures value issues. Value considerations are interwoven with the questions and decisions about the technical aspects of the work, and it is often difficult to differentiate the value component, even when it needs to be addressed in its own right (Bennis, Benne, & Chin, 1969). At the same time, a clear awareness of one's personal values is essential for the researcher or practitioner to recognize that a value orientation is carried into the work, to determine the degree to which these values need to be explicit, and to realize that in the pluralistic and culturally diverse world in which we intervene, these values may conflict with those held by others. It is in this context that ethical dilemmas arise. As Bennis et al. (1969) assert, "Since our value orientations are at the least partial determinants of our choices, responsibility requires that we become clear about and responsible for our actual as well as our professed ideal values as they function or fail to function in the choices we make as change agents" (p. 581). Values, therefore, are central to any consideration of ethics. The problem lies, as Engelberg (1981) states, "in the processes of clarification and explication of these values so that we do not deceive ourselves nor others" (p. 425).

Value-Neutral Versus Value-Advocacy Positions

What part should values play in the choice of goals and intervention strategies? One position the interventionist can assume is to make every effort to increase the options available to the recipient while maintaining a relatively value-neutral posture. The interventionist starts with the assumption that he or she has certain values, but attempts are made to keep these from interfering in the intervention process. To achieve this requires self-awareness and vigilance (i.e., knowing one's own values/goals and how they might play a part in the intervention process), so that these do not become restrictive influences. In their discussion of consultative practice, Davis and Sandoval (1982) outlined several characteristics of the consultation process that would maximize the likelihood of increasing, and not restricting, the consultee's options. The consultation should be collaborative, educational, experimental (modifiable), task-oriented, and protective of basic human rights. Similarly, Perlman (1977) writes, "Values of the 'planner' may not be congruent with the values of the 'community' members. The community must be respected and its needs placed in the position of highest priority" (p. 51). The difficulties in maintaining a value-neutral posture are readily apparent. There are myriad, subtle ways that one's values can find their ways into the decision-making process about the design and implementation of an intervention. As Kelman (1965) asserts, any intervention inherently involves some form of manipulation, and therefore restricts the freedom of the recipient.

A dilemma for the community psychologist who assumes a relatively value-neutral position is how to handle serious disagreements that may arise with the approach and directions chosen by the recipient. Even if one can see the rationale on the part of the recipient for choosing a particular course of action, to assist in such a situation may mean the interventionist is supporting actions at variance with his or her own values. Whether one is obligated to work with groups who hold discrepant values is a debated issue in the literature. Some argue that one does not enter into contracts when values between the interventionist and recipient are antithetical (e.g., Gallessich, 1982), while others maintain that there are certain professional obligations and responsibilities that must be fulfilled, even in the face of such value differences (e.g., Fanibanda, 1976).

A quite different position for the interventionist to assume is that of value advocate. In acting as a value advocate, a clear value orientation is adopted and efforts are made to reduce the options acceptable to the recipient. The community psychologist attempts to reduce the discrepancy between what the recipient may want as a solution or action and what the interventionist judges will promote the most social good. The values espoused by the community psychologist about the relative importance of certain objectives (e.g., preventing the occurrence of maladjustment versus treating individual disorder) create a framework for determining what are more or less ethical strategies for promoting change.

For example, a school board and administration may see a school drug problem as mainly due to a small number of adolescents judged to have serious personality and behavior problems. They might see the solutions as involving separation of these students into special education programs, clear enforcement of rules, and the provision of individual counseling. Their values have to do with protecting the "uncontaminated" majority from the deviant few, the importance of imposing sanctions, and the need for individual remediation. The community psychologist, on the other hand, may see this as a narrow view of the problem, and a strategy that will prove ineffective in addressing the drug problem. Instead, he or she values a broad-based approach, focusing on early intervention with large numbers of students to enhance self-esteem and self-control, decision-making skills, and the ability to resist peer influence. These strategies are aimed at empowering students and reducing the incidence of drug use in the entire student population. The value advocate, based on his or her own set of values and goals, would attempt to present a convincing case for an alternative view of the problem and for implementation of a prevention strategy.

There are also dilemmas for the value advocate. If conflicts in values persist, does the interventionist assist the recipient group in achieving its alternative objectives or withdraw to remain true to original value convictions? In a more complicated scenario, the interventionist may find a receptive school administration, but resistance from other school personnel or parent groups. At minimum, it will be important to maintain a clear sense of how these different value systems play a part in the intervention and how the various points of view can be taken into account. In some instances, procedures can be included that provide options for individuals who do not agree with the stated objectives not to participate in an intervention. Often, the change strategy limits this type of alternative. Systemic and programmatic changes may affect all students, so that individualized choice is limited or impossible. A possible compromise between the value-neutral and value-advocate positions is suggested by Lippitt (1961), who differentiates between methodological goals and outcome goals. He asserts that one always needs to be a value advocate for changes that maximize choice to the fullest extent possible in the recipient system. The form that new structures or procedures will take to enhance personal freedom and choice, however, should be left to the discretion of the recipient.

Explication of Values

How explicit should the community psychologist be about his or her value orientation? How obligated is one to identify and explore potential value incongruities with recipients? Perlman (1977) feels that the interventionist should share personal values and perceptions about dilemmas with recipients and then be open to whatever course of action is valued highest by the recipient. Others argue for disclosure of values to avoid misunderstandings or deceptions about the objectives of the change process (Rappaport, 1977), or for purposes of discussion and possible resolution when discrepancies become apparent (Gallessich, 1982). Whether and when to disclose are complicated decisions to make. Regarding the responsibility to describe one's values, Snow and Gersick (1986) ask, "What if the discrepant values do not appear to be directly relevant to the task at hand, or if they are apparently different but compatible? Is it the consultant's judgment, or should an 'absolute disclosure' rule apply?" (p. 407).

Discussion of values may be an absolute necessity in some situations and an unnecessary complication in others. Value discrepancies may not be known in the beginning phases of the work and may only become apparent later. The difficulty is how to raise these issues and what process will allow them to be addressed effectively. Gerber (1978) argues that the essential issue is more about the level of compatibility in values than about whether there is absolute agreement. Some degree of disagreement is likely given the nature of values. If the perceived discrepancy does not appear to interfere with the intervention being offered, is it acceptable to remain silent? There may be a common ground between the interventionist and recipient regarding the target outcomes of interest, while in other areas value differences would prove more problematic. Is it ethical to pursue values regarding some judged higher social good without disclosure to the recipient? These often involve issues of equality, discrimination, consideration of the disadvantaged, access to resources and power, and so forth. They are some of the most difficult judgments to make because of their overarching importance and assumed rightness, but they may be the ones most vulnerable to self-deception about the need for disclosure and open discussion with recipients. As Rappaport (1977) cautions, "unless each of us is willing to openly state our basic values/goals to ourselves, our professional colleagues, and our colleagues in the communities we serve, we will surely build a tower of Babel" (p. 183).

Value dilemmas arise in multiple ways in the determination of outcomes and processes in community psychology. What procedures to follow to resolve these dilemmas are not always clear. The assessment of discrepant values can become extraordinarily time consuming in efforts to resolve conflicts among individuals and community factions. Establishing needed programs and their benefits to the target population can be delayed or completely undermined. Making value discrepancies an open issue and working toward resolution are possible options, but may become a divisive and prolonged process. The diverse and pluralistic nature of our organizations and communities assures that this process will be anything but straightforward. Whether this pluralism can be utilized to find solutions that are better and more effective may remain only an ideal. Even though it is possibly the most ethically defensible approach, it will likely have to give way to decisions about change efforts that are not agreed upon or desired by all. The most ethical position may be to strive for this ideal, while appreciating and accepting the limitations that will be encountered. In all of this, community psychologists will need to decide whether to assist recipients in generating alternative courses of action based on their own value judgments, or to advocate a particular value position on the basis of personal convictions or standards established within the field. While a readiness to be explicit about one's own values in the process of designing and carrying out interventions seems to be an ethical standard articulated by many, how and when to disclose, what degree of compatibility needs to be achieved, and how discrepancies in values among segments of the community should be taken into account and resolved remain areas needing further consideration and dialogue.

ETHICAL ISSUES RELATED TO GOALS

Values, interests, and agendas of the community psychologist and of various segments of the community come into interplay to determine what outcomes or "ends" are sought through community interventions. Various goals have been articulated for community psychology, including the prevention of maladjustment (Cowen, 1980), the enhancement of competence (Danish & D'Augelli, 1980; Kent & Rolf, 1979), the promotion of resources and capabilities within settings and the enhancement of the community (Iscoe, 1974; Kelly, 1966), the equitable distribution of power (Bloom, 1984), cultural diversity (Trickett, 1984), the creation of systemic and environmental change (Cowen, 1977; Vincent & Trickett, 1983; Wandersman, Andrews, Riddle, & Fancett, 1983), and empowerment (Rappaport, 1987), a goal viewed as applicable at personal, organizational, and systemic levels (Engelberg, 1981).

An issue that clearly emerges in examining such statements of goals is their considerable diversity and the potential for lack of consensus with regard to desired outcomes. This lack of consensus can manifest itself in debates about whether the focus of intervention should be on preventing disorder or promoting adaptation, and on whether the change effort should be directed toward individual change or systemic change. Rappaport (1977) asserts that there are different brands of community psychology, each with its own values and goals that represent a set of assumptions about society. Since society has multiple levels of organization—individual, small group, organizational, and institutional—one's values and goals determine the level of analysis undertaken. These, in turn, require different conceptions of problems, which then serve to guide the choice of strategies and tactics of intervention. The individual level of analysis emphasizes individual deficiency in competency or coping ability. Such an analysis leads to consideration of person-centered approaches aimed at increasing individual skills and ability to "fit in" to society. At the other end of the spectrum is the institutional level of analysis, which holds that inequities in the distribution of power and resources, problems in social policy, and other detrimental influences within the society result in problems at organizational, small group, and, ultimately, individual levels. This type of analysis leads to consideration of models of intervention such as community organization, social advocacy, or the creation of settings. These approaches emphasize the need for alternative pathways for success and distribution of political and psychological power.

A model such as Rappaport's suggests that there is a hierarchy of values and interests, with a greater emphasis placed on organizational and institutional change. Yet, much of community psychology involves programs that primarily promote individual change. Does this mean that these interventions are less ethical than those seeking systemic change? The answer may depend, in part, on one's overall conceptualization of a problem and on considerations of the compatibility of seeking different routes to the solution of the problem. Person–environment models give emphasis to the interaction and interdependence among levels. Change efforts may occur at one or multiple levels, with different immediate goals at each of the various levels but overarching goals in common. For example, prevention of some form of maladjustment may be achieved by reducing damaging, stress-producing influences in the environment and/or by increasing individuals' adaptive skills. In the same way, promotion of a desired mental health outcome may occur by strengthening some facilitative characteristic in the environment and/or by enhancing the desired attribute in the individual through direct skill-building interventions. If the goal of an intervention, for example, is to prevent adolescent substance abuse, this outcome could be sought by teaching decision-making skills to adolescents at the individual level; by reducing levels of peer pressure through small group interventions; by modifying policies, programs, or certain systemic influences at the organizational level; and/or by examining issues of attitudes, access to substances, availability of meaningful roles for adolescents, and the influence of the media at the community level.

The ethical issue then is not so much about which level of intervention to choose, since each could be defended from an ethical standpoint. It has more to do with an appreciation that the immediate goals, at least, for each level are different and are interwoven with a set of values and agendas. Choices about goals and levels of intervention are partially determined by these factors and are not simply based on technical considerations. To act ethically, we first must know that these choices contain particular value orientations and are representations of our own unique interests. Such awareness will make it more likely that the community psychologist will consider carefully the implications of intervening at a given level for the individuals, groups, organizations, and institutions involved at other levels. If we adopt an ecological model to guide our work, then we must be concerned about the impact that seeking certain outcomes in one part of the system will have on other parts of that system.

A primary way in which these issues come into play is in the process of defining the problem and potential solutions. As Rappaport's (1977) model indicates, the psychologist adopting a community perspective is confronted with an array of possible definitions of any given problem. How should a particular focus be determined and by whom? One community struggling with an increasing high school dropout rate may be concerned with possible increases in crime and lowered real estate values. Another community, facing a similar rise, may be concerned about the economic and psychological well-being of those youth. Another may begin wondering about the quality of the school system. In a more complicated scenario, these various views may be held by segments of the same community. The community psychologist in these situations may be concerned about the prevention of delinquency, teenage pregnancy, and substance abuse. Who determines the problem in these cases?

How a problem should be understood and the goals of any intervention, then, will vary depending on one's perspective. This issue becomes of central importance because how a problem is defined determines what solutions (goals) will be sought. Some problems, as the one cited above, may lend themselves to a plan of action that incorporates a range of goals sought at different ecological levels of intervention, and that addresses the spectrum of concerns that come into play. Other problem definitions and intervention goals will involve more conflict. For example, a school intervention could be designed to promote greater creativity and autonomy among students or to establish greater social control and clearer structure. Or, a sex education program could be designed to increase students' use of birth control or seek to decrease sexual experimentation.

From an ethical standpoint, this diversity in desired goals, influenced by the community psychologist's and community members' own values and interests, must be taken into account. As stated in the previous section, the community psychologist must decide whether to assume a value-advocacy position, and how explicit to be about his or her own values in the process of problem definition. In addition, it may be most ethical to promote a process that allows clear articulation of the potential plurality of interests, and then to work with recipient groups to determine whether a diverse range of goals can be sought or whether one set of goals needs to take priority over others. Fostering an open process of needs assessment, problem definition, and ultimate decision-making about goals is probably the most ethically defensible position to assume.

The ethical dilemma usually goes beyond the issue of problem definitions, however, because most situations involve important questions of limited resources (Bond, 1989). Professional and community resources for problem solving are sometimes quite scarce. How many resources can be devoted to the problem of dropout rates in a given community? Which aspect of this problem is most critical? Is this problem more critical than the needs of the elderly who are unable to find adequate housing? These questions put real pressure on the professional and the community to enter a prioritization process.

This prioritization process must focus on community needs, problem definitions, and strengths and weaknesses of various interventions. The problem selected must be identified as a high need for the community and the possible interventions or activities to be undertaken must have a reasonable probability of effecting change. With the school dropout problem, a community psychologist probably would want to confirm that this issue was an important one to the community, to him or herself, to his or her employer, and to the field more generally before undertaking either a research or service project. Furthermore, the community psychologist would want to put his or her efforts, as well as those of community members, into a project with a reasonable chance of success. For example, a decision might be reached that the problem of high adolescent crime rates, although important, is less critical than the problem of truancy in ninth and tenth grades. The community psychologist, regardless of his or her orientation to the degree of community collaboration, has an ethical responsibility to see that problems and related goals are identified that are both high priority and amenable to intervention.

ETHICAL ISSUES RELATED TO PROCESSES

Clarification of values and resolution of ethical dilemmas concerning the *goals* of community psychology with regard to its applied and research aspects are only beginning steps. Of equal importance is the consideration of values and ethical principles that guide the *processes* of action and implementation. As Sarason (1974) notes, adoption of a particular set of values does not tell us the value-derived actions necessary to achieve those values. Similarly, adoption of a particular set of goals or outcomes does not tell us the processes that should be used to achieve these goals. What are the processes and forms of action that connect perceived problems and outcomes in community psychology?

Some efforts have been made to articulate a set of valued qualities and processes to guide the field. Early in the development of community psychology, Kelly (1971) identified a set of ideal qualities for the community psychologist. These include the ability to bring competencies relevant to the community's needs, to identify with and care about the community, to value diversity, to be empathic and interpersonally effective, to take prudent risks and advocate for worthwhile causes, to be able to see the long term, and to be willing to have success accrue to the community rather than to oneself. These types of qualities are essential to forming a particular kind of relationship to the community, one that is democratic and egalitarian, and which varies dramatically from traditional professional–client relationships.

In a similar way, Bloom (1984) presents several principles as guides to program development. The position the community psychologist is to assume involves thinking of oneself as working for the community (regardless of where the paycheck comes from), asking the community to define its own needs, letting the community know what one is learning, and helping the community establish its own priorities and courses of action. Likewise, Klein (1968) asserts the need for community sanction of research, for community collaboration in research design, and to communicate findings to both the community served and the scientific community.

The processes outlined above, concerning desired ways of operating in conducting the work of community psychology, emphasize collaboration, sensitivity, and responsiveness to the community's needs and identified objectives, and an open interchange and feedback regarding observations and results throughout the course of an intervention or study. A high premium is placed on anonymity, accountability, empowerment, and dignity (Engelberg, 1981), and on minimizing dependency on the professional in order to maximize growth, competence, and independence in the recipient (Perlman, 1977). These processes serve as guides to determining ethical behavior on the part of the community psychologist in efforts to reach selected outcomes. Moreover, these process variables themselves are seen by many as necessary and promotive of the very outcomes that are desired.

While these perspectives do serve as useful guides, they are by no means definitive about what it means to work for the community or what constitutes a collaborative relationship. The community psychologist is embedded in a complicated network of individuals, groups, and organizations and, as Golann (1969) so aptly summarizes, "ethical issues often emerge from situations involving multiple loyalties and conflicting demands" (p. 454). Who should be involved in a project? When should these people be involved? What kind of involvement is appropriate? Just who or what is the community?

For example, consider a community psychologist who works in a mental health facility and is called by the principal of a local school to help with a community problem. The principal has begun to introduce some sex education programs into the older elementary school grades. A number of parents have become very angry about the introduction of these programs into their school without their knowledge and involvement. The principal feels the programs are desperately needed and is worried that parent opposition is going to deprive the students of much needed information and help. The psychologist immediately finds herself in a dilemma. She knows that the mental health center's mission includes the promotion of preventive programming in the schools, so at one level she knows her employer would support the principal's directions. Yet, she also feels that the parents have a right to be involved in their school and to help determine the programs that shape their children's lives. Furthermore, she is aware that she does not know the interests of other important subgroups: the students, the teachers, other parent groups, and the school board. This community psychologist may be very committed to working for the community, but may find herself puzzling over just who is considered the community. Is it the principal, the parents, the students, the school board, the mental health center, or some combination of these subgroups?

In most situations, a community psychologist will have to choose to work with a certain segment or segments of a community. For example, the community psychologist in the above example might choose to work directly with the principal to implement the new programs, perhaps providing consultation regarding the curriculum; or she might choose instead to work with the principal to understand community reaction to the program and suggest alternative ways of working with parent groups to gain acceptance of new programs. Or, perhaps in an effort to involve more subgroups, the community psychologist might choose to survey the parents and the teachers and provide feedback about people's interests and feelings about the issues involved. In all these examples, there is a narrowing of the field of focus that can seem like a departure from the ideal principle of "working for the community." But given the limitations of time and resources, this narrowing process is necessary.

This narrowing of the field should occur in a way that is respectful of the basic process principles discussed in this section. Possible ramifications of choosing to work with one segment of the community rather than other segments or multiple segments must be considered. As Kelman (1965) points out, "the production of change may meet the momentary needs of the client—whether individual, an organization, or a community—yet its long-range consequences and its effects on other units of the system of which this client is a part may be less clearly constructive" (p. 582). The field charges us to consider the needs and interests of the community. While the mandate is unclear about whether and how to assume the responsibility of working for all segments of the community (an impossible task), it does charge us with the responsibility for considering the effects of different actions on the various subgroups. For example, if the community psychologist in our example decides to work with the principal, this should be done with an awareness of the possible effects of this on the parents' group. Similarly, if she decides to work with the parents' group to empower them, she may be lessening the likelihood that students will be receiving needed information.

Another process aspect that can cause ethical dilemmas concerns the commitment of the field to collaborative relationships. In addition to working for the community, there is a strong value placed on collaborative working relationships between the interventionist or researcher and the intended recipient groups. Many community-oriented psychologists conduct their work in a very responsive and involved manner. Consider, for example, the community-oriented researcher who decides to work with a self-help group for parents of handicapped children. This individual may decide to help the group identify the questions that they have about themselves, then to conduct research that addresses these questions for the group, and finally, to provide feedback and consultation to the group regarding the results. This approach is highly collaborative throughout the course of the project.

On other occasions, however, community psychologists conduct interventions and research that are developed in response to their own interests or research questions. The individual researching the effects of handicapped children on the family may be interested in studying families' immediate reactions to the birth of a Down's syndrome child. Or a practitioner may be interested in working with the siblings in these families. Although these approaches are not necessarily responsive to the primary questions for the families involved, the psychologist can conduct the work with a sensitivity to community interests and needs, directing the course of the project while involving representatives in the process and fully informing individuals who are involved. The researcher studying families with a Down's syndrome child may begin by interviewing families and observing newborn special care units, then fully inform all participants as they are involved in the project, and end by providing results to appropriate groups or individuals. This process, although still collaborative, is far less so than the process used by the self-help researcher.

There seems to be a continuum of community involvement in any intervention or research project from one that is very community-driven to one that is very psychologist-driven. Either end of the continuum causes problems and ethical dilemmas. A project that is very community-driven may conflict with a psychologist's values or the values of the field more generally (an extreme example might be helping a racist organization increase its membership). Furthermore, such community-driven projects may conflict with a psychologist's best judgment about the most effective way of conducting work (e.g., increasing school discipline procedures, such as suspension, as a way of combating truancy). At the other extreme, a very psychologist-driven project may violate important principles regarding minimal involvement of individuals affected (an extreme example here might be showing informational films regarding AIDS to early elementary school students without informing their parents). In between, there is a broad gray area that includes interventions that are very responsive to the community and place a premium on involvement to work having an informational relationship with the community. In any given service or research intervention, concern about ethical conduct requires attention to questions about the level of community involvement that ought to be represented in the work.

Many community projects are conducted without a contract. In some cases, the introduction of a contract may seem too bureaucratic; in others, a contract may seem unnecessary, or may spell out things that seem better left unsaid. The individuals involved may be fuzzy about what kind of working relationship makes sense, may not have thought about and discussed various ethical issues, or may not want to be explicit about the exact nature and target of the work. Yet, the lack of even an informal contract can lead to complications, and suggests unresolved ethical dilemmas characterized by vagueness, lack of forethought, or covert agendas.

Most disciplines adopt a process of written or verbal contracts that guide their work. Within our own discipline of psychology, consultants (Gallesich, 1982; Snow & Gersick, 1986) rely heavily on written documents that spell out the nature of a working relationship, confidentiality, services, and payment. Clinicians are very explicit, at least verbally, with the terms of the psychotherapeutic relationship. And researchers usually must have explicit letters of informed consent signed by each participant. Such written documents and verbal agreements provide a useful function. They delineate each person's responsibility, indicate the rationale or need for certain services, outline the nature of the working relationship, and specify exactly what services will be provided.

The more widespread use of contracts would help community psychologists (and those individuals and groups they work with) to examine the ethical dilemmas that they confront with each project, to make their choices and resolutions explicit, and to minimize the operation of covert agendas. Such contracts do not have to be legalistic masterpieces; letters of agreements between those involved are often sufficient. Such letters or contracts would help address a number of the ethical dilemmas raised in this section and are strongly recommended.

The intervention process is guided by technical considerations regarding how to most effectively promote change toward some particular end result. Equal weight must be given to the ethical dimensions of choosing one strategy over another. Other issues requiring ethical consideration that arise in the process of intervention involve the potential for stigmatization and unintended negative effects, and the question of how sufficient our knowledge base is for making informed decisions. These and other matters will be discussed in the next two sections.

ETHICAL DILEMMAS IN INFORMED CONSENT

The idea of informed consent is basic to individual freedom and an important safeguard against social control or social engineering (Kelman, 1965; McNeil et al., 1970). It is legally mandated that researchers obtain consent from participants prior to involving them as subjects. Yet community psychologists are not involved in research only. The subjects of their work are not always individuals. We are therefore led to ask: must community psychologists always gain informed consent? Who must be informed? What information must be divulged? Who may consent? These questions provide the basis for the following discussion.

As stated previously, community psychologists may not impose their views, research agendas, or interventions on a community without sanctions. Whether the community psychologist is involved in research, preventive interventions, consultation, or other work, the rights to privacy and autonomy of the individuals affected by the work must be protected. The purpose of informed consent is to inform, at a minimum, designated community representatives of any potential risks and to help participants make informed decisions on whether to use a service or to participate in any intervention or research endeavor when this is pragmatically possible.

Choosing appropriate representatives is not always straightforward. Bloom (1984) recommends that "in the event that the community being served is so disorganized that representatives of various facets of the community cannot be found, the psychologist has the responsibility to help find such representatives" (p. 431). He further suggests that members of such a group represent all sociocultural and socioeconomic groups, not merely members of an entrenched power group, to insure that the interests of all community members are represented.

Dilemmas arise not only when determining who those representatives might be, but in deciding who else may need to be informed and/or give consent. For example, when the target of an intervention is not the persons or groups that have engaged the community psychologist and consented to his or her proposed intervention, must informed consent also be obtained from the ultimate recipients? Klein (1968) believes that "informed consent should be obtained from those who are part of the population being studied and from whom data are to be elicited, as well as those responsible for them such as supervisors, governing boards, top administrators, and parents" (p. 104).

Must such a stringent policy be followed by those psychologists whose targets of change are not research participants? The answer to this question may rely on our understanding of informed consent. Central to the concept of informed consent is the provision of information regarding potential risks and benefits so that a competent, voluntary decision regarding participation may be made without coercion or unfair inducements (Meisel, Roth, & Lidz, 1977). For the practitioner, a tension often exists between successfully marketing an intervention and avoiding an overstatement of program benefits. A detriment to program marketing can be informing the participants of potential risks. Yet if we hope to protect the rights of individuals, it is difficult to argue that when it is possible and prudent to provide a realistic statement of potential risks and benefits, the community psychologist is not obligated to secure some form of informed consent.

It is not always possible and prudent. Weithorn (1987) discusses ethical dilemmas such as those arising when one is faced with a choice between two ethically defensible points of view. One such dilemma involves the fact that informing a member of an at-risk population that he or she is indeed at risk may iatrogenically affect the participant through labelling or expectation (Lorion, 1983). Indeed, merely being included in an intervention for an at-risk population may have stigmatizing effects. Identifying special-needs students, for example, may allow these students the benefits of much-needed special programs, but it also may stigmatize them in the eyes of parents, peers, teachers, and future employers. While the cost–benefit ratio of including students in special programs must be carefully considered, equally important is who should give informed consent and what they should be told. While parental consent is usually obtained, it is less clear whether the student has a right to formally consent to participation in such programs.

This issue is particularly salient for secondary preventive interventions, when the individual has not yet evidenced the problem, but is seen to be at risk. Some of these high-risk individuals will be correctly identified as needing assistance, but many students may not be helped, or worse, may be iatrogenically affected by their participation (Lorion, 1983). In addition, being informed that one is at risk for a disorder can potentially induce the disorder in a nonpathological individual. The issue of potentially harming the targets of interventions through informing them of our purposes or concerns may arise in a number of situations in which a community psychologist intervenes. A tension exists between preserving the individual's right to know and protecting the participant from potentially negative effects of that knowledge. Ethical behavior depends on our carefully balancing these two concerns.

Simple practicality may provide yet another barrier to obtaining informed consent. Many primary preventive interventions (e.g., the broadcasting of public service announcements, the designation of non-smoking buildings or areas, the fluoridation of drinking water) affect so many individuals through such diffuse means that it would be impossible to obtain permission for the intervention from each participant. In such cases, community representatives must suffice.

There also may be ethically defensible circumstances in which obtaining recipients' informed consent is deemed unnecessary. For example, when a community psychologist intervenes to promote system change, members of all levels of the system may not be informed. This may pertain especially to those instances where there is little or no risk involved for the participants and no coercion to participate. A brief example may illustrate this point. To reduce employee absenteeism, it is recommended that a company institute an in-house daycare center and an infirmary for ill children of employees. Management, department heads, and union representatives consent; other workers are not consulted or given an opportunity to consent. However, employees may freely choose to take advantage of the new programs, and there is no foreseeable risk to those who do. Informed consent in a circumstance such as this seems unnecessary.

Other policy decisions can be more problematic, especially in those instances in which participants are not able to elect to participate. It is clear that when the issue is fluoridating an area water supply or requiring disease immunization before school attendance, the health of the group as a whole is considered to outweigh the rights of individuals not to participate. However, when the intervention involves a value less generally shared, for example in substance use prevention, AIDS education, or pregnancy prevention, the question of individual rights must be considered. The ethics and advisability of bypassing the informed consent of participants and relying on the approval of their representatives when instituting such a program must be carefully considered.

A final justification for not obtaining informed consent is that regulations governing the conduct of research may exempt categories of research from these requirements. Among these are:

> research in educational settings, involving "normal educational practices," such as regular and special education instructional techniques, curricula or classroom management techniques; research involving survey or interview procedures where confidentiality of data is protected by the investigator; or research involving the collection or study of existing data, documents, or records, where the confidentiality of the data is protected by the investigator. (Weithorn, 1987, pp. 230–231)

Community psychologists who feel their work falls into these categories may decide not to obtain consent.

Weithorn (1987) urges us to ask whether the decision not to obtain consent is made to circumvent time-consuming and inconvenient procedures, or because the implementation of the consent procedures might seriously impair the integrity of important work, or perhaps even make the work impossible to conduct. She concludes that "we must ask whether absolute adherence to the principles of autonomy and privacy would prevent the conduct of important ... endeavors that otherwise present negligible risks. If so, compromises of autonomy and privacy may be ethically defensible" (Weithorn, 1987, p. 232).

There are no clear-cut answers to the dilemmas of informed consent. Individuals' rights and freedoms must be weighed against the value of the work and the hazards of informing recipients of interventions. When it is practical and prudent, all parties who might be affected by a community intervention should be informed of the risks and benefits of an intervention in simple, clear language, and consent to its implementation, whether as participants or as those responsible for the participants. The purpose of the work should be revealed as explicitly as possible, without introducing the dangers of labelling and stigmatization, or jeopardizing the integrity of the work.

To conclude, it is not that failing to obtain consent and masking the purposes of our work are themselves unethical acts. It is the reasoning and motivations behind such acts that may make them unethical. A community psychologist who fails to inform participants of the purposes of a project in order to secure their cooperation in an effort whose ends they might not support is clearly acting unethically. A researcher who chooses not to obtain consent from an at-risk group in order to protect participants from knowledge of their at-risk status may be acting ethically. Few prescriptions can be made; the issues involved in informed consent must be considered thoughtfully and carefully case by case.

ETHICAL ISSUES IN THE GENERATION AND USE OF EVIDENCE

If there is one activity that all community psychologists engage in, it is the planning of change. Kenneth Benne (1961), in discussing the planning of change, suggests that "the engineering of change must be experimental.... Planned arrangements must be seen by those who make them as arrangements to be tested in use and to be modified in terms of their human effects when tried.... All who collaborate must be trained toward an experimental attitude and a 'research' approach toward social problems" (p. 144). Benne is not alone in emphasizing the importance of a research stance in community psychology. Gallessich (1982) recommends that consultants strive to evaluate the outcomes of their services to determine whether goals have been achieved and to help consultees interpret and make use of evaluation findings. Heller and Monahan (1977) argue that

> community psychology cannot progress without an empirical knowledge base ... community psychology will wither away ... if its action programs cannot verify their impact; and there is an ethical and moral obligation on the part of the community practitioner to be accountable to those who support (and participate in) his or her activities. The touchstone of accountability lies in empirical evaluation. (p. 72)

From this perspective, planning interventions requires utilization of the documented efforts of others in the field, as well as documenting one's own work.

Not all community psychologists hold this point of view. While some programs are carefully planned using prior work and research, too many programs seem to be initiated with little or no reliance on what we already know. There seems to be a belief, at least among some practitioners, that this kind of work, while perhaps not always highly beneficial, is not harmful. Lorion (1983), however, differs, noting that preventive interventions may have unintended negative effects: "to assume ... that preventive interventions will have only positive or, at worse, neutral consequences represents a naive and irresponsible position" (p. 252). He goes on to cite McCord's (1978) 30-year follow-up study of an early prevention program and a study by Gersten, Langner, and Simcha-Fagan (1979), which actually find a number of negative effects. Others have underscored the ethical requirement to pay attention to the potential for negative, as well as positive, consequences and to consider our responsibilities if these were to arise (Levine & Perkins, 1997).

Weithorn (1987) also is concerned about the degree to which interventions (of potential, but unknown, benefits) may interfere with an individual's rights to autonomy. These comments must be taken as a broad cautionary note to those practitioners and researchers who feel community psychology is blissfully benign. Community psychologists must consider the nature of the evidence that guides our work, asking such questions as: At what point do we think we understand a problem well enough to move ahead with an intervention? At what point do we feel comfortable recommending a certain course of action? At what point do we know enough about the potential risks and benefits of certain alternatives that we feel we can adequately inform the individual and community involved?

When we accept the importance of communicating about change efforts, research and evaluation become important components of the ethical conduct of community work. A number of ethical complexities arise in the consideration of research and evaluation themselves. For example, there are ethical problems in the potential uses (or misuses) of research. Heller and Monahan (1977) highlight some of the potential dangers involved in the politics of evaluation. A call for further research may be used to postpone important decisions for political or personal ends. Administrators may use research to duck responsibility for an unpopular decision. Evaluations may be mere public relations efforts, with no attempt to collect disconfirming evidence. Community psychologists may refuse to give feedback on their findings. At first glance, it would seem that such uses of research are likely to be considered unethical. Yet, in practice, situations are not always clear-cut; there may be ethically defensible reasons for any of these acts. For example, some community psychologists may refuse to divulge findings because of concerns over the uses to which the information may be put, particularly if they perceive the findings to be potentially harmful to themselves or the individuals involved. Other psychologists may believe that divulging all findings is the greater good, no matter what the immediate repercussions. A dilemma exists between choosing to reveal potentially damaging results and contributing to a long-standing knowledge base.

Ethical dilemmas arise not only in the uses of research, but in the use of one's skills as a researcher. Golann (1969) discusses this complex issue—the ethics of engaging in well-meaning, but misguided work: "Is it ethical to serve as a consultant on a research project that is poorly conceived with respect to its stated goals.... When the research is inadequate to the extent that the design, methods, or both will fail to yield useful data, or worse, will yield misleading data, what is the responsibility of the psychologist?" (Golann, 1969, p. 457). A psychologist's participation will lend respectability to what may be undeserving work, but may make the research better than it would have been. The ultimate decision to participate in such situations can only be left to the discretion of the psychologist.

Points that are less discretionary involve the actual conducting of research. These include the ideas that research studies and program evaluations should be as well designed as possible and incorporate both quantitative and qualitative methods, that they study the impact of an intervention at multiple levels of the system in which change has been introduced, and that they assess unintended consequences, as well as those intended, to insure that valid conclusions may be drawn. These steps must be taken even if those conclusions may prove to be detrimental to the work. As a core value of community psychology and to avoid certain ethical problems such as misuse of power, promotion of self-serving and hidden agendas, and potential for cooptation, some assert (Prilleltensky & Walsh-Bowers, 1993; Walsh-Bowers, 1993) that a democratic approach be taken in the conduct of research, in which citizens participate as equal partners with researchers in all aspects of the work as a joint endeavor.

Lorion (1983) argues that the limits of community work must be more clearly understood and documented if the field is to prosper, and suggests minimal ethical prerequisites for implementing a prevention/promotion effort. First, he proposes that we come to a clear description of the outcomes to be promoted. Second, we must determine specifiable criteria by which the aforementioned consequences can be assessed. Third, if a risk factor is to be altered, a conceptual description of the developmental process of the evolution of the risk factor and of mediating factors in its development must be created. Fourth, evaluation strategies designed to assess negative as well as positive consequences must be included. Fifth, in the absence of available data or knowledge of relevant developmental processes, a group of researchers, clinicians, and lay persons could review available knowledge about the phenomenon to be prevented/promoted and determine the nature, likelihood, and acceptability of potentially iatrogenic effects of the proposed intervention (see Kelly, 1987, for a discussion of this approach). Finally, informed consent of individuals subjected to prevention/promotion efforts must be obtained, explaining the associated purposes and risks, and providing the option of not participating.

All community psychologists are involved in the generation and use of evidence; many of us are aware of the importance of research in planning interventions, assessing their effects, and providing a means of accountability for our work. Yet, in practice, many of us are not always willing to use these skills, or we may find ourselves in situations that discourage their use. One means of ameliorating this problem lies in increased cooperation between academic and applied psychologists. Those in applied settings must find ways to communicate to researchers about the programmatic work and the issues and questions raised by it. Those who are researchers must listen and find ways to use their research and research methods to speak to those applied issues.

For community psychology to prosper, not only must we attend to the work of others in the field, we must strive rigorously to document our efforts and to disseminate our results. Those of us who use our skills as researchers are not always rigorous. Novaco and Monahan (1980) examined the 235 articles published in the *American Journal of Community Psychology* from 1973 to 1978. They commented on the lack of experimental sophistication of the articles reviewed and conclude that "an unduly large portion of the research on community psychology consists of methodologically inadequate answers devoid of theoretical content" (p. 142).

Lounsbury, Leader, Meares, and Cook (1980) performed a similar analysis with similar results. They cite problems with the reporting of demographic characteristics necessary to aid in interpreting and generalizing from the findings, as well as problematic subject selection and measurement procedures. As Lorion (1983) points out, data that are "uninterpretable, non-generalizable, and non-replicable will contribute little if anything to the advancement of our knowledge.... Poor research obfuscates rather than elucidates our attempts to understand" (p. 255) the effects of our interventions.

While well-designed, well-controlled, well-reported studies that examine possible beneficial, detrimental, direct, and indirect effects of interventions at multiple ecological levels over extended periods of time are our ideal, it is obvious that this is not possible. Practical, financial, and political constraints keep us from achieving the ideal. However, such constraints should not prevent our best efforts to achieve these ideals and to explicitly discuss possible problems or limitations inherent in any given intervention. While research is necessary to demonstrate the effectiveness or ineffectiveness of our interventions, it also provides a basis for accountability and is a tool by which we can maintain and check the ethical conduct of our own work.

CONCLUSIONS

In this chapter, we have outlined five interrelated areas of ethical consideration in order to help identify key ethical dilemmas confronting those engaged in community psychology practice and research. The first three areas pertain to values, goals, and processes. The question of values is at the core of ethical considerations, since values strongly influence the selection of goals and the nature of the process that occurs during phases of program planning and implementation. As Bond (1989) states: "Our personal values about relationships, accountability, social change priorities, and our personal political world view all shape our priorities and agenda for community work" (p. 356). One must achieve clarity about one's own values in order to assess discrepancies with the value orientation of others. Recognizing that some degree of value incongruence is inevitable in community interventions, determinations about ethical conduct must occur within a field of multiple and competing values. How these multiple values are taken into account, how problems and needs are identified and prioritized, what courses of action are put into play, and how individuals are involved in these processes are all matters involving questions about what is ethically and morally sound. Continued efforts to articulate values, and related goals and processes, need to occur on the part of the individual and in the field as a whole.

The last two areas of ethical consideration discussed concern informed consent and the generation and use of evidence. The role of informed consent in conducting community interventions or research clearly contains numerous ethical quandaries. When does one need consent and from whom? What are the potential hazards of informing individuals that they may have a problem or have some likelihood of developing the problem in the future? How does one weigh individual rights to know and consent against the need of the larger community or society? As Heller (1989) writes: "We should, of course, constantly strive to act in an ethical manner, but we also must recognize that ethical dilemmas often have no clear resolution.... At times, helping one group may mean harming another, or helping to resolve a present crisis may increase the likelihood of future difficulties" (p. 368). Ethical issues regarding the generation and use of evidence also contain many ambiguities. We assume there is an obligation on the part of the community psychologist to make adequate use of sound theory and existing knowledge in designing community interventions and research studies. However, since the knowledge base is limited and imperfect, much of what is proposed and carried out is experimental. This raises the need to attend to how work can be conducted and reported so as to provide new and useful evidence, while paying proper attention to minimizing potential risks to participants. The dilemmas arise in trying to determine what prerequisites should be established and met before proceeding with an intervention, and what responsibility one has for unintended negative outcomes.

It has been clear throughout the chapter that the community psychologist, in the role of practitioner or researcher, enters situations of enormous complexity. As stated at the outset, to adequately identify and address the ethical issues that will no doubt arise, the community psychologist's involvement must be considered within the social and organizational contexts in which it occurs. Applying an ecological perspective serves to delineate important contextual elements, such as formal and informal structures, overt and covert power, intergroup relations, human diversity, and availability and distribution of resources. Such a perspective informs us of the types of conditions that are likely to prevail as we proceed with our work, and is essential to developing effective and ethically defensible action strategies. Most basically, ecological concepts tell us that a multiplicity of values, interests, and agendas will exist in any given organization or community, and that these features will greatly influence how a problem is defined, what courses of action will be chosen, and how the change process will likely proceed.

Experience has taught us that the community psychologist can not simply rise above these dynamics and maintain a value-neutral position as conflicts and lack of consensus occur among various constituencies. Pressure to ally with one group or position versus another will occur repeatedly. The values and goals of the community psychologist will be consistent with some and divergent from others. As Riger (1989) points out, "... our work always promotes the ends of some interest group, even if we do not recognize that explicitly" (p. 382). The community psychologist will need to step into the foray with clear acknowledgment of these intra- and intergroup differences and of the potential for conflict. An understanding and anticipation of these issues will focus the community psychologist on achieving a maximum of clarity and prior agreement regarding what role to play in the process. If not, he or she will be pulled in more unpredictable directions than necessary, and in ways that will increase the likelihood of encountering ethical dilemmas and of producing ineffective action.

REFERENCES

American Psychological Association. (1992). Ethical principles of psychologists and code of conduct. *American Psychologist, 47,* 1597–1611.

Benne, K. D. (1959). Some ethical problems in group and organizational consultation. *Journal of School Issues, 15,* 60–67.

Benne, K. D. (1961). Democratic ethics and human engineering. In K. D. Benne, W. Bennis, & R. Chin (Eds.), *The planning of change.* New York: Holt, Rinehart and Winston.

Bennett, C. C., Anderson, L. S., Cooper, S., Hassol, L., Klein, D., & Rosenblum, G. (1966). *Community psychology* (Boston Conference). Boston, MA: Boston University.

Bennis, W. G., Benne, K. D., & Chin, R. (1969). Some value dilemmas of the change agent. In W. G. Bennis, K. D. Benne, & R. Chin (Eds.), *The planning of change* (2nd ed.). New York: Holt, Rinehart and Winston.

Bloom, B. (1984). *Community mental health* (2nd ed.). Monterey, CA: Brooks/Cole.

Bond, M. A. (1989). Ethical dilemmas in context: Some preliminary questions. *American Journal of Community Psychology, 17,* 355–359.

Cowen, E. L. (1977). Baby-steps toward primary prevention. *American Journal of Community Psychology, 5,* 1–22.

Cowen, E. L. (1980). The wooing of primary prevention. *American Journal of Community Psychology, 8,* 258–284.

Danish, S. J., & D'Augelli, A. R. (1980). Promoting competence and enhancing development through life development intervention. In L. A. Bond & J. C. Rosen (Eds.), *Competence and coping during adulthood* (pp. 105–129). Hanover, NH: University Press of New England.

Davis, J. M., & Sandoval, J. (1982). Applied ethics for school-based consultants. *Professional Psychology, 13,* 543–551.

Engleberg, S. (1981). Toward explicit value standards in community psychology. *American Journal of Community Psychology, 9,* 425–434.

Fanibanda, D. K. (1976). Ethical issues in mental health consultation. *Professional Psychology, 7,* 547–552.

Gallessich, J. (1982). *The profession and practice of consultation.* San Francisco: Jossey-Bass.

Gerber, D. I. (1978, August). Ethical dilemmas in the use of consultation to create social change. Paper presented at the 86th Annual Meeting of the American Psychological Association, Toronto, Canada.

Gersten, J. C., Langner, T., & Simcha-Fagan, O. (1979). Developmental patterns of types of behavioral disturbance and secondary prevention. *International Journal of Mental Health, 7,* 132–149.

Golann, S. E. (1969). Emerging areas of ethical concern. *American Psychologist, 24,* 454–459.

Heller, K. (1989). Ethical dilemmas in community intervention. *American Journal of Community Psychology, 17,* 367–378.

Heller, K., & Monohan, J. (1977). *Psychology and community change.* Homewood, IL: Dorsey.

Iscoe, I. (1974). Community psychology and the competent community. *American Psychologist, 29,* 607–613.

Kelly, J. G. (1966). Ecological constraints on mental health services. *American Psychologist, 21,* 535–539.

Kelly, J. G. (1971). Qualities for the community psychologist. *American Psychologist, 26,* 897–903.

Kelly, J. G. (1987). Seven criteria when conducting community based prevention research: A research agenda and commentary. In J. A. Steinberg & M. M. Silverman (Eds.), *Preventing mental disorders: A research perspective.* Rockville, MD: National Institute of Mental Health.

Kelman, H. C. (1965). Manipulation of human behavior: An ethical dilemma for the social scientist. *Journal of Social Issues, 21,* 31–46.

Kent, M. W., & Rolf, J. E. (Eds.). (1979). *Primary prevention of psychopathology, Volume III: Social competence in children.* Hanover, NH: University Press of New England.

Klein, D. C. (1968). *Community dynamics and mental health.* New York: Wiley.

Levin, G. B., Trickett, E. J., & Hess, R. E. (Eds.). (1990). *Ethical implications of primary prevention.* New York: Haworth.

Levine, M., & Perkins, D. V. (1980). Social setting interventions and primary prevention: Comments on the Report of the Task Panel on Prevention to the President's Commission on Mental Health. *American Journal of Community Psychology, 8,* 147–157.

Levine, M., & Perkins, D. V. (1997). *Principles of community psychology: Perspectives and applications* (2nd ed.). New York: Oxford University Press.

Lippitt, R. (1961). Dimensions of the consultant's job. In K. D. Benne, W. Bennis, & R. Chin (Eds.), *The planning of change* (pp. 156–162). New York: Holt, Rinehart and Winston.

Lorion, R. P. (1983). Evaluating preventive interventions: Guidelines for the serious social change agent. In R. D. Felner, L. A. Jason, J. N. Moritsugu, & S. S. Farber (Eds.), *Preventive psychology: Theory, research and practice* (pp. 251–268). New York: Pergamon.

Lounsbury, J. W., Leader, D. W., Meares, E. P., & Cook, M. (1980). An analytic review of research in community psychology. *American Journal of Community Psychology, 8,* 415–441.

McCord, J. (1978). A thirty year follow up of treatment effects. *American Psychologist, 33,* 284–289.

McNeil, J., Llewellyn, C., & McCollough, T. (1970). Community psychology and ethics. *American Journal of Orthopsychiatry, 40,* 22–29.

Meisel, A., Roth, L. H., & Lidz, C. W. (1977). Toward a model of the legal doctrine of informed consent. *American Journal of Psychiatry, 134,* 285–289.

Moos, R. H. (1973). Conceptualizations of human environments. *American Psychologist, 28,* 652–665.

Novaco, R. W., & Monahan, J. (1980). Research in community psychology: An analysis of the first six years of the American Journal of Community Psychology. *American Journal of Community Psychology, 8,* 131–146.

O'Neill, P. T. H. (1989). Responsible to whom? Responsible for what? *American Journal of Community Psychology, 17,* 323–341.

Perlman, B. (1977). Ethical concerns in community mental health. *American Journal of Community Psychology, 5,* 45–57.

Pope, K. S. (1989). A community psychology of ethics: Responding to "Responsible to whom? Responsible for what?" *American Journal of Community Psychology, 17,* 343–345.

Pope, K. S. (1990). Identifying and implementing ethical standards for primary prevention. In G. B. Levin, E. J. Trickett, & R. E. Hess (Eds.), *Ethical implications of primary prevention* (pp. 43–64). New York: Haworth.

Prilleltensky, I. (1990). Enhancing the social ethics of psychology: Toward a psychology at the service of social change. *Canadian Psychology, 31,* 310–319.

Prilleltensky, I., & Walsh-Bowers, R. (1993). Psychology and the moral imperative. *Journal of Theoretical and Philosophical Psychology, 13,* 90–102.

Rappaport, J. (1977). From Noah to Babel: Relationships between conceptions, values, analysis levels, and social intervention strategies. In I. Iscoe, B. L. Bloom, & C. D. Speilberger (Eds.), *Community psychology in transition.* New York: Wiley.

Rappaport, J. (1987). Terms of empowerment/exemplars of prevention: Toward a theory for community psychology. *American Journal of Community Psychology, 15,* 121–144.

Riger, S. (1989). The politics of community intervention. *American Journal of Community Psychology, 17,* 379–383.

Sarason, S. B. (1974). *The psychological sense of community: Towards a community psychology.* San Francisco: Jossey-Bass.

Serrano-Garcia, I. (1994). The ethics of the powerful and the power of ethics. *American Journal of Community Psychology, 22,* 1–20.

Sieber, J. E. (1982). Ethical dilemmas in social research. In J. E. Sieber (Ed.), *The ethics of social research: Surveys and experiments.* New York: Springer-Verlag.

Snow, D. L., & Gersick, K. E. (1986). Ethical and professional issues in mental health consultation. In F. V. Mannino, E. Trickett, M. Shore, M. Kidder, & G. Levin (Eds.), *Handbook of mental health consultation.* Washington, D.C.: U.S. Government Printing Office.

Steinberg, J. A., & Silverman, M. M. (Eds.). (1986). *Preventing mental disorders: A research perspective.* Rockville, MD: National Institute of Mental Health.

Trickett, E. J. (1984). Toward a distinctive community psychology: An ecological metaphor for the conduct of community research and the nature of training. *American Journal of Community Psychology, 12,* 261–279.

Trickett, E. J., & Levin, G. B. (1990). Paradigms for prevention: Providing a context for confronting ethical issues. In G. B. Levin, E. J. Trickett, & R. E. Hess (Eds.), *Ethical implications of primary prevention* (pp. 3–21). New York: Haworth.

Vincent, T. A., & Trickett, E. J. (1983). Preventive intervention and the human context: Ecological approaches to environmental assessment and change. In R. D. Felner, L. A. Jason, J. N. Moritsugu, & S. S. Farber (Eds.), *Preventive psychology: Theory, research and practice* (pp. 67–86). New York: Pergamon.

Walsh-Bowers, R. (1993). The resident researcher in social ethical perspective. *American Journal of Community Psychology*, *21*, 495–500.

Wandersman, A., Andrews, A., Riddle, D., & Fancett, C. (1983). Environmental psychology and prevention. In R. D. Felner, L. A. Jason, J. N. Moritsugu, & S. S. Farber (Eds.), *Preventive psychology: Theory, research and practice* (pp. 104–127). New York: Pergamon.

Warwick, D., & Kelman, H. (1973). Ethical issues in social intervention. In G. Zaltman (Ed.), *Processes and phenomena of social change*. New York: Wiley.

Weithorn, L. A. (1987). Informed consent for prevention research involving children: Legal and ethical issues. In J. A. Steinberg & M. M. Silverman (Eds.), *Preventing mental disorders: A research perspective*. Rockville, MD: National Institute of Mental Health.

Zaltman, G., & Duncan, R. (1977). *Strategies for planned change*. New York: Wiley.

CHAPTER 37

Barometers of Community Change

Personal Reflections

SEYMOUR B. SARASON

Communities change in diverse ways. Some of these changes may be visible: new buildings arise, other buildings are empty and deteriorating, one-way streets are designated, and the like. Some changes are not directly visible, but are known by us in the form of information that then alters our perceptions and experience, e.g., juvenile crime has increased, the percentage of older people is steadily escalating, air pollution has worsened, approval has been given for a large condominium development, an elementary school will be closed (or built). People, I assume, differ markedly in their awareness of past, present, and potential community change. That is to say, they vary not only in what they regard as a change, but in the indicators they use as a basis for their conclusions. The more a person has lived continuously in a community, the less easy it is to recognize ongoing changes, i.e., the seeds of future change. We may know in an abstract way that the community we have lived in has changed dramatically over the years, but our knowledge in no way means that we are sensitive to the indicators of ongoing change. When we see a photo of our neighborhood or downtown taken years ago, we are surprised and sometimes shocked at how much change has taken place. Or, if, as I had occasion to do, you go back and read the local newspaper of 20 and 30 years ago, you quickly conclude that what was once your community hardly exists today—quite the opposite of "the more things change the more they remain the same." At the same time that phenomenologically we do not perceive that, as persons, we have changed much—the "I" of today is not much different than our "I" of those days—we cannot deny that we have lived in a changing community and, significantly, that we did not appreciate or were insensitive to the implications of those past changes. If I am at all representative, a frequent reaction is that much of what we thought was a desirable change was at best a mixed blessing, and at worst a disaster. Another reaction is: Why was I so insensitive to the beginnings and implications of many of these changes? Were the unintended consequences truly not discernible?

What I have said about our experience of community change is no less true of our experience in regard to important interpersonal relations as they are referred to by such role

SEYMOUR B. SARASON • Department of Psychology, Yale University, New Haven, Connecticut 06520.

Handbook of Community Psychology, edited by Julian Rappaport and Edward Seidman. Kluwer Academic / Plenum Publishers, New York, 2000.

titles as son or daughter, husband or wife, parent, friend, faculty member, and colleague. We do not think about how these relationships have undergone change until "something happens" that forces the fact of change into our awareness. When did the change begin? What were the early indicators? Why did that past "I" underestimate so poorly, understand so little, what the "I" of today *now* knows was so important? I am tempted to define psychology—regardless of subspecialty, theory, and methodology—as the detection, delineation, and understanding of how changes internal to people, as individuals or collectivities, transact with changes in external social-physical contexts. Whatever its shortcomings, that definition at least underlines the obvious: we are in the business of understanding the transactions among change processes.

To make my thinking more clear to you (which is not to say that my thoughts are clear), I will relate the experience that brought these questions to the fore. Several years ago, the clerical and dining room workers at Yale went out on strike. In previous years the union had lost elections that would have made it the collective bargaining agent. But six months before the strike, to general surprise, they won the new election by a very slim margin. Even those members of the faculty who supported the union were surprised. Why were "even" they surprised? Obviously, some changes had taken place among the Yale workers *and* in the actions of the Yale administration that would explain why the union went from defeat to victory. But few of us were interested in explanations of a change that we did not predict. It was the unfolding scenario that was of interest: Would Yale face reality and sincerely try to come to terms? Would it continue to take a hard line, being able to withstand a strike far better than the union? Would the union cave in? Would the economic pygmy be able to stand up to the economic giant? Collective bargaining dragged on for months, during which time a significant percentage of the faculty and students organized to support the union, to bring pressure on Yale to settle without a strike (of which there had been several called by the union of maintenance workers—strikes that were bitter, costly, and destabilizing to daily routines). Shortly after the academic year began, the union struck. The strike lasted months, everyone was affected, there were marches and arrests, and Yale received the kind of attention in the national media it did not want or need. The president of Yale showed up on Phil Donohue's television program to present Yale's position. At the same time that everything seemed to come to a standstill, the situation seemed exciting, upsetting, dynamic, and endless. Everything and everybody was polarized.

What, I found myself asking, were the significances of the strike? What did it say, if it said anything, about how New Haven and Yale had changed? No one was in doubt that if Yale settled with the union it would be a harbinger of future changes. It did not take much wisdom to make that prediction. What interested me was how changes in Yale and New Haven had brought about the strike. And that question brought together in my mind several heretofore unrelated observations and information. I shall discuss each briefly in the following.

1. To say that there has been a town–gown problem in New Haven is truly to indulge understatement. In a city that until a decade or so ago was largely Italian and Catholic, Yale was seen as a bastion of Protestant America, which means it was seen with disdain and anger, an alien body that was off limits to its community surround. When the Black population began to increase steadily in size, it became the second group for whom Yale was a symbol of impersonality, aloofness, and insensitivity to community needs. Because the relationships between Italians and Blacks have never been (again to indulge understatement) cordial in any community I have ever known (and I was reared in Newark, New Jersey), anything Yale did, or seemed to do, in relation to one group quickly affected its relations with the other group. Despite their shared resentment of Yale, these groups could not join forces. That Yale had no peer in the ability to play into community resentment is, I think, a fair, if not objective,

judgment. And yet, there was a muted respect for Yale's academic standing that diluted or held militancy in check. It was like the members of a symphony orchestra who "hate their conductor's guts," but who grudgingly admit that he knows music and conducting. From Yale's perspective, its task was identical to that of Herman Hickman, a former Yale football coach, who said of the alumni: "My job is to keep them sullen but not mutinous."

2. Years ago, New Haven's Board of Aldermen passed a law making it impossible for Yale to enlarge beyond its present boundaries or to tear down tax-paying property within it to put up a tax-exempt structure. That action was stimulated by the fact that a Yale alumnus had given Yale 15 million dollars to put up two new residential colleges on the site of tax-paying properties. The colleges were never built. I regarded that legislative action as but another manifestation of a long-standing conflict. It never occurred to me to weigh it differently than any other past manifestation, to see it as I now think I should have seen it—as a change in the degree of resentment and militancy by one of the parties.

3. Until the mid-1960s, a significant percentage of Yale's clerical-secretarial workers were wives of Yale students enrolled in the graduate and professional schools. They were college-educated, happy that they had a position at Yale, and secure in the knowledge that their stay was temporary. Yale could count on a captive audience of women who wanted to be captured. Although I knew that the women's liberation movement was experiencing growth, militancy, and acceptance—admitting women to Yale College being a clear, local example—I neither predicted that the clerical-secretarial pool would change, nor was I sensitive to what such changes might mean for town–gown relationships. If I had been sensitive to forces and the degree of change, several things would have been predictable. First, more local women would become part of the pool. Second, they would have less education. Third, many of them would not look at employment at Yale as a temporary affair. Put in another way, the pool would increasingly be comprised of people reared in New Haven and having negative or ambivalent attitudes toward Yale. Italian and Black women slowly but steadily become part of the scene as never before.

4. I came to Yale in 1945. Like every other institution in our society, Yale began to grow. I knew that Yale was getting bigger, but I paid little attention to the changes that growth brought or would bring about. For example, Yale rather quickly became the largest employer in the New Haven area, which meant that more and more local people became employees, far less apparent in office personnel than in the maintenance and grounds staff. It is not happenstance that union recognition was won by these sectors long before the secretarial-clerical union won their election. This influx of local people made for a degree of attitude change to which neither I nor anyone else I know was sensitive. Many of these town people came to Yale with the kinds of attitudes I have already described. What they learned as employees was a glimpse of the obvious: Yale existed primarily to serve its faculty and students, and no other groups were important. These groups were, I am sure, told that they were important, but the realities of everyday existence made it clear how the goodies of this world were distributed by the Yale administration. Two things I and many other faculty knew: employee turnover was very high, and Yale's Personnel Department had cornered the market on inefficiency, stupidity, and indifference. On several occasions an individual I wanted to employ in a clerical-secretarial role said she would accept my offer only if I, and not she, dealt with Yale's personnel office. And when I dealt with that office, I understood what local people experienced. My job was not jeopardized when I blew up. Because I am one of those rare academics who has taught at only one university, I cannot make comparative judgments. Colleagues of mine who have come from other universities assure me that Yale's attitude and behavior toward staff, up until recently, defied explanation. The next point elaborates on growth, yet in a

more personal way. It also introduces a new factor to which I was sensitive—it is hard to be completely insensitive to every important change!

5. When I came to Yale, Sue Henry was the departmental secretary, the only secretary. Regardless of who you were, faculty or student, you interacted with Sue. She knew and felt a responsibility to everyone. Besides, she knew everything worth knowing about how the department and Yale worked. As a result of vast increases in government and foundation support for research and training, another secretary was added: first Midge Marvel who left after a couple of years, then Jane. Memory tells me that for the first five years after World War II, there were no changes in the frequency or quality of interaction between faculty and the two secretaries, or between secretaries and students. Not long after, however, anyone who got a grant hired a secretary, *his* (not her in those days) secretary, whose allegiance was to him. Two things began to happen: jealousy and rivalry among secretaries in regard to salary, hours, and treatment; and the emergence of the political-organizational question of how to relate the different secretaries to the chairman's office, which meant Sue Henry. She was not raising the question. It arose as a consequence of autonomous faculty members doing their own hiring: setting their conditions of the secretary's work and, not infrequently, informally agreeing to this and that, and then telling Sue or the chairman. It was gracious, anarchic living, and the price paid did not seem high. But there reached a point in the early 1960s when the growth in grants, faculty, facilities, students, and clerical-secretarial staff required change. And, whatever the change, it had to relieve those in the chairman's office of the time-killing burden of reading grant applications to determine if their budgets were in line with policy, and would not require space that was not available. In short, the witting and unwitting hanky-panky about which unworldly faculty are not babes in the woods. We needed a business manager! I knew that was asking for trouble, and in two ways. First, whereas the allegiance of the secretarial staff had been to the faculty, it would not be to the business manager. At the very least the allegiance would be a divided one. Second, the business manager was not to intrude on faculty and student prerogatives. He or she was to free faculty to do their work, so they would not have to spend time hiring or facing the unpleasantries of budget overrun, keeping business matters separated from everything else. That is like saying that intelligence can be separated from personality.

My worst fears were realized when the department moved to new quarters. Let me describe what you see when you walk up the steps to the departmental offices. The first thing you will note is that the office is encased in glass. Behind the glass partitions are what I call (only to myself) the animals in the zoo. I can never stand outside that partition without being reminded of a zoo. There are three to five women in that office, off of which are other offices populated by women whose function I do not know, and the farthest office is that of the business manager. It is a foreign country, that partition being the border. What I have described happened in other departments as well. At the very least, the quality of relationships of staff with faculty and graduate students had dramatically changed over the years.

I have used the strike only to underscore several glimpses of the obvious. First, the demography of Yale and New Haven had undergone change. Second, that and other changes had altered the strength of the dynamics between Yale and New Haven. Third, I was either insensitive to these changes or simply weighted them wrongly in regard to their future significance. And it was this last glimpse of the obvious that forced me to ask: What kind of a community psychologist was I if I was such a poor observer of my community surround? Were my failings peculiar to me, or did they reflect some kind of conceptual deficit in the field? My imperfections are many, but after a lot of soul-searching, and by replaying the short history of community psychology, I had to conclude that something was wrong or missing in community psychology. Before elaborating on this, I wish to emphasize that nothing in what I shall say is intended to be critical of what community psychologists are doing in their research and practice. What it is intended to suggest is that, as a field, community psychology has lost its vision, imaginativeness, and initial purpose, a commitment to an overarching, cohering sense of responsibility to study, understand, and to have impact on communities.

Community psychology arose in the early 1960s in the context of a concatenation of factors, among the most important of which was another glimpse of the obvious: our urban communities were coming apart at the social seams, riddled by conflicts, hatreds, and eruptions that suffused the atmosphere with anxiety and feelings of puzzlement and impotence. There was a flight into action on the part of individuals and groups who heretofore had never regarded themselves as activists. Something had to be done. The old order, locally, in state capitals, and in Washington, seemed no longer adequate to the changes the times seemed to require. You cannot understand the origins of community psychology unless you see it in the context of communities undergoing destabilizing challenges and transformations. The choice of the adjective "community" before the noun "psychology" was not happenstance. If in those days we did not possess conceptual clarity, let alone productive theoretical underpinnings, we knew that our arena was the community undergoing change. If we truly did not know where we were headed, if we were realistically modest about what we knew, if we were both challenged and puzzled by our efforts to make a difference, what kept us going was a vision or fantasy that this new field had to, and would, add to our understanding of community structure and dynamics, and thereby establish the foundations for action. Action was part of that vision. And it was action in relation to pressuring events and situations, not in our offices, clinics, or hospitals, but on community turfs where, in the jargon of the times, the action was. We did not present ourselves—indeed we did not regard ourselves—as researchers who had hypotheses, a proven methodology, or organized and valid data that could inform action. We were learners and inquirers who wanted to become helpers and movers. We were somewhere in between the do-gooder, whose major and sole asset is good will, and the academic, who remains silent until his or her data are analyzed, usually after the events that gave focus to the research have been superseded by other events. We did fly into action because time was not on our side: too much was happening too quickly.

We paid a price, a high price, for this understandable and justifiable flight into action. And the price we paid was in the failure to ask several questions. Why had we been behind the times? Why were we surprised by what was happening? What had we not been paying attention to? What had been the early warning signs and how should we have been weighing their significances? Were there sensitive barometers to community changes that could have alerted us to their possible consequences? And, if we had had such barometers, what was the universe of alternative ways we could have considered in regard to action? Granted that our communities were in turmoil, should we not have devoted some of our energies to constructing barometers of community change to serve as early detection signals of the one thing we can count on—that communities will continue to change?

We should return to where we began: the history, structure, and social-cultural features of our communities. We need to know how they have changed and are changing, without that knowledge there is little to give coherence to the research and action efforts of different community psychologists. But *our* need for coherence is not only conceptual, as it is that coherence that will allow us to be more sensitive to the possible future significances of the barometers of change. That sensitivity holds out the promise of actions that may dilute or prevent the destabilizing consequences of change.

On a national level, we have learned from bitter experience to develop indices of change, early detection signals, that will inform action. So, for example, early in this century, and following economic disruptions, the government began to develop a variety of measures that would tell it whether the economic sea was calm or perturbed, requiring observation or action. What they found out was that these indices were either insensitive, wrong, or irrelevant. Economists seized the opportunity to become related to policy and action, but they did not foresee how inadequate their conceptualizations, from which they derived the indices, were. But, however inadequate their conceptualizations and indices, the need for more valid barometers of change remained, and the government continued to support the efforts of the economists. Decades later, the Council of Economic Advisors became an important vehicle of the executive branch of government. Two things are worthy of emphasis. First, economic theories were challenged and transformed, giving rise to controversies that are still with us today. Second, if only because of the increasing complexity (indeed, mystery) of our economic system, and its interdependence with the economies of other nations, the past inadequacies of the barometers of economic change have not been used as an excuse to terminate the search for better ones. In terms of the strength of the social fabric, too much is at stake to give up the goal of developing better indices of change. Unlike the other social sciences, but like community psychology, the field of economics cannot ignore the significance of its data for social action. That, of course, is a double-edge sword, because at the same time that its theories and data have practical import—they are or can be tested in the arena of action—economics opens itself up to a display of its utility, and its track record is not all that good.

Another example also has its origins earlier in this century. I refer to the effort to obtain sensitive indicators of change in regard to health. Syphilis, influenza, polio, and other contagious diseases appeared in epidemic proportions. Their frequency and disastrous consequences required that the government develop means that would inform it as early as possible of a new epidemic, against the manifestations of which the government could take some kinds of preventive, educational, or ameliorative measures. Today we are all knowledgeable about the government's Center for Disease Control, especially its role in tracking the incidence, geographical distribution, and means of spread of AIDS. The word "control" in its title is quite appropriate, i.e., to use data on changes for purposes that serve to control spread of the disease, and to educate the public about who is at risk and about the self-protective measures people should take.

There are other examples, what they all have in common is that they led to the development of barometers of change after a series of disasters or upheavals that threatened the welfare of the nation. Also in common is that the process of developing and testing barometers of change forced a variety of fields to become more humble about what they knew and could do. I always had reservations about Lewin's statement that there is nothing as practical as a good theory. For one thing, theory always derives from data obtained from direct action somewhere in the world. Action stimulates theory, and the theory stimulates action. Theory and action are transactional in nature, and they are not in an isolated, arbitrary stimulus–response paradigm. I have researched that conclusion by studying efforts to develop national barometers of change. Theories are the myths we create from our data, our experience, as a basis for new actions that tell us how much of our myths we have to discard. The reason economics has long been a dismal science resides less in its impractical theories, and more in the fact that its practitioners have experienced so little of the social world. Any discipline that rests on the assumption that man is rational in the economic decisions he or she makes will never come up with a productive theory. Economics may be, indeed has been, very influential in our society, but degree of influence should not be attributed to its theories.

If, as I think, community psychology should undertake the task of developing barometers of community change, it should not be from a stance of presumed experience and security. In fact, what I find fascinating about such a possibility is the newness, strangeness, and inevitable complexity of the problem we shall be confronting. That is why the early years of our field were so exciting and challenging. We knew we were moving in new and important directions, we would make mistakes, and we would learn a lot. We had to act as if we could be practically helpful. And we quickly found that our credentials were received with understandable skepticism by colleagues and funding sources. In the case of the Yale Psycho-Educational Clinic (named to pay our respects to Lightner Witner, who established the first clinic in an American university in 1896 at the University of Pennsylvania), we could not get support from NIMH, which had made two site visits, and listened sympathetically to our plans, but had to conclude that there were too many ambiguities in our thinking and planning to justify support. They were right, of course, and we told them that they were, but that for us to present ourselves as if, indeed, we knew well what we would be doing would be a deception.

There are two reasons for taking on this problem, although they reduce to one. The first is that it is a conceptually challenging problem: What are the sensitive indicators of community change? The second is that we cannot and should not be indifferent to these ongoing changes: What are the positive and negative implications of these changes and what actions—preventive, ameliorative, or sustaining—do they suggest? Precisely because we approach the problem, not with a blank mind, but with implicit and explicit values or visions, our choice of barometers will not be random. The danger here is that we will ignore barometers that are mightily consequential for community change. For example, when Connecticut initiated its community mental health program, the state director, Dr. Max Pepper, had the task of dividing the state into catchment areas. He was wise enough to know that, to accomplish this task in a realistic way, he would need to know more than just the current population in different communities because one had to assume that population shifts were taking place and those shifts had to be taken into account. He was unable to locate any source of data on population shifts or growth, until it dawned on him that the telephone company might have relevant data. Indeed, the company did possess the best ongoing data on community population shifts and growth. Those data were very helpful to Dr. Pepper for his purposes, as they would be for ours. But we would want to know more than the size and pace of those changes. We would want to break those numbers down according to age, race, religion, education, and income. We are not demographers, but if we have learned anything, especially in the post World War II era, it is that demographic changes produce sea-swell changes of all kinds in our communities. But we learned this after those changes were obvious enough to hit us in the face, so to speak. We did not roll with the punch, we were bowled over.

Why is it that community psychology played little or no role in preventing, or at least in trying to prevent, the seamy consequences of deinstitutionalization? Few communities, especially our urban ones, have remained unchanged by that policy and process in regard to mentally retarded and mentally ill people. I bear some guilt in this matter in regard to the mentally retarded: decades ago I had recommended that deinstitutionalization would be a far more humane and feasible policy than one that legitimated inhumane institutions. My guilt stems from several facts. The first is that I did not see early enough that those who would be implementing the policy were amazingly ignorant of what communities are. The implementers were people whose experience had been exclusively in relation to institutional, not community, living. The second fact is that I did not make it my business to develop indices either about the pace of the process or where in the community people were being placed. I had no way of keeping track of the change and what it portended. The third fact, and one that James Kelly has well emphasized, is that I was, for all practical purposes, an isolated community psychologist, unconnected with community individuals and settings participating in the process. Those indices could have been developed; I could and should have been more connected with community officials and agencies. I say "should have" not only because action is a defining characteristic of a community psychologist, but because advocating for a policy requires that you take on the responsibility, once the policy is adopted, of developing means for determining whether the community is adapting to the policy in appropriate ways.

The local and national media bombard us with accounts of the relationship between the homeless and deinstitutionalization. Is the pendulum swinging back toward reinstitutionalization? My current experience suggests that a battle is going on between community individuals and organizations, on the one side, and state departments, on the other. Some kind of change is occurring, but I am not aware that the nature and pace of that change are being tracked. Are we again setting ourselves up for the situation, perhaps 10 years from now, when the consequences of the pendulum swing will be obvious and probably intractable?

It has not been my intention in this chapter to suggest where and how we might start in developing barometers of community change. I deliberately avoided concrete suggestions because they might divert us from the most important questions: Can there be a productive and socially responsible community psychology that avoids the task of describing and understanding what communities are and how they change, positively or adversely? Some will regard that question as an example of rampant presumptuousness. They could say that economists restrict themselves to economic changes in our communities, states, and nation; political scientists restrict themselves to the use and distribution of power in its formal and informal aspects. No field takes on the community in its totality. What restrictions in scope make sense for community psychology? My answer derives from the name of the field: We are interested in any and all barometers of community change that will affect the minds, behavior, and lives of its people in significant ways.

If our field took shape as a response to community turmoil, it is also the case that it was a reaction to the perceived narrowness of a repair-oriented clinical psychology. It was not that there was no need for effective therapies, but that, in theory and practice, clinical psychology inadequately explained the sources of personal misery. For example, and beginning with Freud, it had long been obvious, indeed it was a truism, that the individual was incomprehensible apart from family structure and dynamics. But that truism hardly informed a practice that riveted on the individual. Why did it take three quarters of a century for family therapy to take hold? Why is it that it took hold after dramatic changes had taken place in the size, structure, and stability of the family—changes that the field of family therapy minimally recognized? Family therapy and community psychology came into their own, and at the same time, as a reaction against the narrowness of the clinical fields. But, unlike family therapy, community psychology represented an intention to make a clear break with the orientation of repair in the consulting room, and it sought to understand how community structure and change influenced, positively or negatively, the welfare of the groups of which it was comprised. The central question was: What do we need to know to be in a position to anticipate, to prevent, untoward consequences? That was our vision, our grandiosity, our presumptuousness. We were going to save the world and we were going to start in our own communities. That vision, call it a rescue fantasy, has been lost, and we are poorer for it. We are used to hearing that the tumultuous sixties are over, the *zeitgeist* has changed, and we are in an era of conservatism and retreat. We are also used to hearing that the sixties were a reaction to the silent fifties, much as the current era is seen as a reaction of passivity to the sixties. These myths, like all myths, contain a kernel of truth, but only a kernel.

As I indicated earlier, as a community psychologist I have been far from consistent with the underlying rationale that undergirded the field at its beginnings. But in at least one respect I come up smelling roses, and this concerns an event that occurred in the so-called silent fifties, when I still labelled myself as a clinical psychologist. I refer to the 1954 desegregation decision, which, unlike my colleagues and friends, I greeted with anxiety. To people in the north it was all too easy to conclude that the desegregation decision would create turmoil in southern communities, a conclusion confirmed by what was on the television screen: federal troops in Little Rock, and near open warfare in Louisiana parishes as Leander Perez and his followers hurled invectives and more palpable objects at Blacks. No one who lived through those years, and who has a good memory, would argue that the fifties were silent. My anxiety stemmed from the realization that our northern communities were utterly insensitive to the implications of that decision for them. The problem was "down there," not "up here." Every person with whom I spoke viewed the decision as overdue and just. But when I stubbornly persisted in asking them how the decision might and should produce changes in New Haven, given its racial, ethnic, and religious composition, I drew blanks or pious hopes. The fact is that, with few exceptions, their understanding of what New Haven was as a community was as inadequate as their picture of what was coming down the road. But the point of the story is not historical, but rather that today, as then, New Haven (like many other communities) is changing, and in ways that do nothing to allay my anxiety.

I do not pretend to know in detail what those changes are in the sense of what they mean and portend in New Haven. I do not have the barometers of change that would permit me to go from the facts to the truth—the psychological truth. Let me give you two facts. Connecticut is either first or second among the states for *per capita* income. New Haven (like Bridgeport and Hartford) is among the top 15 cities in the nation for the number of people at or below the poverty line. We do not know how much of a change this represents, and we are not keeping track of how much and in what direction the change is going. Nor do we know what the psychological correlates of the New Haven data are, except that they are worrisome. Is it the case, as conventional wisdom has it, that many of our communities already have an underclass that is changing the nature and strength of the social fabric in these communities?

I have been talking about community change. Are the issues and processes different in regard to how a field like community psychology changes? We are used to hearing that a field changes in part, and over time, because in the competition for productive explanations of certain overarching problems, one explanation comes to achieve general acceptance. And as a result of that acceptance, the people in the field see that field differently than before. From its origins more than 30 years ago, community psychology has changed dramatically. The change was preceded and accompanied by a kind of competition about what was the overarching problem, the gravitational pull of which would interconnect a diversity of research and practice. There were those who believed that community mental health was one such problem. There were those who felt that focussing on schools had the most potential for impacting on the community. And then there were those who felt that one had to focus on far more than one site, one problem, or one population if one stood a chance of having a more general impact. There really was no competition among these groups, if only because they were in basic agreement that, whichever the choice, each was interested in illuminating the nature and dynamics of the community. What changed, and rather quickly as people flocked into the field, was the significance of that agreement: its vision and implicit agenda. The vision faded, perhaps because it was never well articulated, but fade it did as people riveted on this or that specific, important, but narrow problem. The problem became figure, the community became ground, and there has been little deliberate reversal of figure and ground in order to see the part in its significances for the whole, and vice versa. Community psychology took on all of the features of a "faculty" psychology that had made a mess of the understanding of personality and intelligence. When I say that these specific problems are important, I am not trying to soften my criticism. They are important, but their importance is diluted because they rarely transcend the stated boundaries of the problem. Their narrowness derives from a lack of vision. And without such an agreed-upon vision, we will remain a collection of individuals whose collective effort has no cumulative power.

My vision may not be the most appropriate or productive one. But can we be without a vision that requires us to relate our specific interests to some overarching goal? Can we be content to define our field the way intelligence has long been defined: intelligence is measured by intelligence tests. Is community psychology to be defined as what community psychologists study and do? What is the glue that binds? Let us not forget that community psychology was a critique of a psychology that illuminated little or nothing of American society. This was not a critique that denied that American psychology was concerned with or had illuminated some important problems of human behavior. But is was a critique that asserted that the time had come to see those problems in a larger social context, in contexts that would tell us how much of what we think we know is myth. I am reminded here of Garner's superb and pithy paper, "The Acquisition and Application of Knowledge. A Symbiotic Relationship," published in the *American Psychologist* (October, 1972). Garner describes how James Gibson, as a result of his experience during World War II, dramatically changed his well-known theory of space perception:

> As Gibson describes the experience, he and some other psychologists were trying to understand how aircraft pilots estimate the distance to the ground when they are landing an airplane. He found that the traditional cues for depth perception, listed without fail in every introductory textbook on psychology, simply failed to explain the perception of depth at the distances required in flying and landing an airplane. He furthermore found that experiments had to be done in the field to get at the process, that laboratory experiments changed the nature of the process too much. So into the field he went. It was from these experiments that Gibson came to the conclusion that the prerequisite for the perception of space is the perception of a continuous background surface—thus the "ground theory" that evolved from this work.

The important point for the present chapter is that Gibson's whole way of thinking about the problem of space perception changed when he was faced with the problem of understanding how pilots in real-life situations actually land their airplanes without too many crashes. His theoretical notions were changed by his contact with people with problems. He did not develop these important ideas by a continuous relation to his previous work. Rather, his research and thinking, according to his own report, took a decided turn for the better as a result of this experience.

The substance and character of American psychology in the post-World War II era is incomprehensible, apart from knowledge of what psychologists experienced during the war. The laboratory confronted real-life and, as Garner indicates, everything seemed to change. That is what happened to those psychologists who started to deal with the real-life 1960s. Unlike Gibson, we did not have anything analogous to a theory of space perception. Nothing in our psychological background could serve as a compass for thinking and action. The one thing we knew was that we had been ignorant of how the communities we lived in and worked in had changed. We knew that our clinical backgrounds were part of the problem and not the solution, and we quickly learned that social psychology was too asocial to be of any help. In a somewhat inchoate way we knew that our focus had to be that complexity we call a community. Not this or that segment, subgroup, or problem, but the whole of it and the way it works and changes for good or for bad. We were not modest, but in the pursuit of enlarging understanding, modesty is not a virtue. Community psychology has become far too modest.

The last sentence of most dissertations is that "further research is indicated." That will not be my last sentence. More research is not on the top of my recommended agenda for community psychology. At the top of that agenda are these questions: How do we justify our field? What overarching vision do we have in common? Are we within our field to remain as conceptually unconnected with each other in the way that more than 50 divisions in the American Psychological Association are unconnected with each other? Further soul-searching is indicated.

PART VII

CONTEMPORARY INTERSECTIONS WITH COMMUNITY PSYCHOLOGY

The preceding 37 chapters of this volume tell many of the defining stories of community psychology. Each story is accompanied by a somewhat different map that details particular places in the field. Many of these maps intersect, overlap, and provide alternative views of the enterprise called community psychology. But none are comprehensive, none tell the whole story; even taken together there remain uncharted places where community psychologists go. This section provides several supplementary maps for some of those places that have emerged in recent years as intersections with the work of the community psychologist.

In what constitutes Chapter 38, individually authored pieces point readers to some of the social issues likely to be important for community psychology in the foreseeable future, but not specifically addressed as the central point in any of the preceding chapters. Read collectively, this section directs our attention to contemporary topics that have emerged as places where community psychology intersects with the work of others, both in psychology and other disciplines. We are sure there are other topics that could be added, and our failure to include them does not imply that we think them to be unimportant; however, each topic here is a place some of us have already approached, and which many of us believe will be a continuing area of concern for the field.

The specific topics discussed here are the urban poor, reproductive rights; environmental issues; lesbian, gay, and bisexual issues; HIV/AIDS; the farm crisis and rural America, the new immigrants; unemployment; violence prevention; substance abuse prevention; homelessness; and independent living for people with physical disabilities. It is not so much that these issues necessarily belong in the same chapter, but more that we are concerned that the topics not be missed as emergent issues for community psychologists. By design, each of the topics addressed here is presented in brief, not as a review, but instead to orient us to contemporary issues that require attention from the field.

The authors were asked to do four things: (1) tell readers how this topic became an emerging issue; (2) frame the issue in terms of its psychological and sociopolitical dimensions; (3) refer readers to some of the relevant perspectives, empirical foundations and key references; and (4) suggest key research and action questions for the 21st century. The intention is not to provide answers, but to raise questions for further development of the field.

CHAPTER 38

Contemporary Intersections

A. The Urban Poor

LaRue Allen

Poverty is a greater problem in the 1990s than it was two decades ago. Danziger and Weinberg (1994) note that it is particularly high given the economic recovery that began in the 1980s, and is high relative to the levels in countries with comparable standards of living. Indeed, "The poverty rates for some demographic groups—minorities, elderly widows, children living in mother-only families—are about as high today as was the poverty rate for all Americans in 1949" (Danziger & Weinberg, 1994, p. 18). In addition to higher rates among certain segments of the population, rates in urban areas are increasingly higher than those outside central cities (U.S. Census Bureau, 1996). The power of community psychology to affect economic problems and the unprecedented nature of today's high poverty rates, along with its many problematic correlates, make this an issue of substantial importance for the entire field.

What follows is a brief review of thc cycles of interest in poverty, with an emphasis on the most recent poverty policy initiative in the United States. Next is a discussion of the implications of the provisions of this policy for community psychologists' research and action, ending with some of the key questions confronting those who work to contribute to a greater understanding of the poor and to the development of more successful interventions to address their needs.

POVERTY AS A SOCIAL PROBLEM

The poor have always been with us, though our willingness to acknowledge poverty as a social problem has waxed and waned over the last century (Wilson, 1987). Before the Civil War, poverty was a problem of individuals, with individual solutions applied. The progression from a rural to an urban society after the Civil War, with the accompanying increases in

LaRue Allen • Department of Applied Psychology, New York University, New York, New York 10003.

Handbook of Community Psychology, edited by Julian Rappaport and Edward Seidman. Kluwer Academic / Plenum Publishers, New York, 2000.

unemployment, inferior housing, and inadequate wages, led to the emergence of social reform as a weapon against poverty. But interest in poverty began its decline after the Depression, perhaps because poverty became so commonplace.

The disadvantaged were "rediscovered" in the 1950s, primarily through political activity on behalf of disadvantaged groups, which was stimulated by the Supreme Court decision to desegregate public schools. The political decision to desegregate led to increased visibility of poor members of society, quickly followed by social programs to feed and train them, and early education intervention (e.g., Head Start) in the 1960s. Poverty research was revived once again in the 1980s, with publication of Wilson's *The Truly Disadvantaged* representing a watershed. Interest soon reached a peak described as follows: "Not since the riots of the hot summers of 1966–8 have the ... poor received so much attention in academic, activist, and policy making quarters alike" (Wacquant & Wilson, 1989).

In the current cycle, the debate focuses on the impact of structural and contextual factors on the persistence of membership in what Wilson called "the underclass." Key to the analysis of Wilson's underclass is the changed demography of central cities over the last 30 years, changes that have resulted in a larger number of minority youth concentrated in inner-city neighborhoods. These youth contribute disproportionately to virtually all of the symptoms of social disorder or dislocation that define the urban poor through Wilson's lens. Teenage births and subsequent welfare dependency are, by definition, a function of the youthful age of those involved, and a large percentage of violent and property crimes are committed by those under age 25.

Economic changes represent additional contextual factors that have had an impact on poverty. These changes have devastated inner cities. The youth population grew just as the number of jobs in the inner city shrunk. Jobs moved out of the central city and into the suburbs. Given the inadequacy of most urban public transportation systems, city residents without cars were no longer able to get to where the jobs were. Further, jobs have shifted from the production of goods in factories to the provision of services and information, demanding new skills from workers who want to compete.

Unlike poor people in generations past, the urban poor of today are concentrated in homogeneously poor neighborhoods, left behind by Black and Latino middle-class families who have fled to the suburbs. It is interesting to note that poor whites rarely live in neighborhoods peopled only by other poor people, a contextual difference whose significance and impact on adaptation and development is worthy of further exploration (Wilson, 1967).

The nature of government support for the poor is also quite different today than from decades past. The most dramatic change in the system of supports for poor Americans was introduced by President Clinton as the "end of welfare as we know it." The 1996 Personal Responsibility and Work Opportunity Reconciliation Act replaced Aid to Families with Dependent Children (AFDC), a 60-year staple in U.S. public policy, with Temporary Assistance to Needy Families (TANF). TANF introduces term limits of no more than five years over a lifetime for benefit recipients. TANF also has a work requirement, relevant to all except those with very young preschool children, which can no longer be satisfied by enrolling in high school equivalency or even college-level courses. These two provisions are supposed to motivate welfare recipients to get a job and become financially self-sufficient. However, the scarcity of entry-level jobs and the virtual absence of affordable child care make the goal a challenging one at the very least. Experience with the working poor tells us that even if an entry-level job is attained, the outcomes for children and families may not be all that different (Smith, 1997).

Legal immigrants are in an even more precarious position under the new rules. States have the option of withholding TANF benefits from legal immigrants who were AFDC recipients. Legal immigrants in the United States before the act was signed are subject to removal from the rolls; those who arrived after the signing may have benefits withheld for up to five years.

It is the devolution of policy-making authority from the federal to the state level that may be the single most important aspect of TANF. The federal government has imposed requirements such as term limits; the states may impose even more restrictive rules. Thus, the national landscape of poverty and its many correlates—health indicators, educational statistics, crime and violence figures—may be altered. Urban, suburban, and rural may come to matter less than "states that allows extensions of assistance beyond 60 months" vs. "states that imposed a two-year time limit" (The Urban Institute, 1998). We must follow the implementation of this policy closely if we are to fully understand the changes in communities, services, and populations that will evolve over the next several years.

IMPLICATIONS FOR COMMUNITY PSYCHOLOGISTS

This enormous change in poverty policy will change the context in which we work, whether we focus on poverty or not. Poverty researchers, from whatever discipline, must address the fact that poverty, by its nature, is an ambiguous construct; economists, sociologists, and psychologists view it from differing perspectives. In order to become more central to interdisciplinary discussions of the issues, community psychologists must agree on definitions of the correlates, predictors, and consequences of poverty that are the domain of psychological theory. Encouraging signs that issues in the domain of community psychology are being perceived as relevant to the debate can be found psychologists' visibility in discussions of the impact of neighborhoods on development among the poor (Brooks-Gunn, Duncan, & Aber, 1997).

But defining the parameters of the problem is just the first step. Levels of poverty, and especially child poverty, are embarrassingly high in the United States compared to other developed nations. Interventions to "breaking the cycle of poverty" aim to increase the chances that poor children will grow up and be better off. Community psychologists are often involved in designing or evaluating early-intervention programs that target young children. They also provide parents with training to improve their ability to support children's growth and development, or with programs that provide parents with education or job training, with the objective of helping parents create a less impoverished environment for their children (Center for The Future of Children, 1997).

But poverty has an impact of the work on community psychologists even when they are not directly involved in "poverty programs." Researchers who work on AIDS, on prevention of domestic or community violence, on substance abuse prevention, or on use of health care resources—are all conducting research or designing interventions whose effectiveness may be influenced by changes in the nature of poverty in our country. The effects might arise from the extent to which the poor are a constituent in their samples. Or the effects might be indirect with, for example, a domestic violence program for middle-class women compromised because the agency that runs it is overwhelmed by new numbers of poor women, an influx precipitated by some change in federal or local supports to the poor.

Those with the skills to design preventive interventions are also well-positioned to aid in the search for solutions to the problems of the poor. Community psychologists who work to reduce social isolation, increase employability, and reduce the impact of exposure to violence on young children, all have something to offer in conversations with economists, sociologists, political scientists, and others in the mix of those who are called upon to comment on poverty and its "solution" at local, state, and federal levels.

Social isolation, for instance, is defined in demographic, historical, and geographic terms, but it surely has psychological consequences. Those consequences are not uniformly experienced by all who are present in a given area. We know, for example, that not all youth who grow up in poor neighborhoods end up demonstrating the several maladaptive behaviors (e.g., substance use, school failure) correlated with poverty, nor do they necessarily continue to live in areas of concentrated poverty. A basic research question derived from this observations is why, given similar environmental circumstances, some youth develop negative outcomes while some of their friends or neighbors emerge as competent, achieving individuals. Is it money, family, the quality of schools? Is it how we see our contexts, rather than the "objective" characteristics, that matter? Or is it changes in state or federal policy, shaped by changes in pubic attitudes toward the poor, and likely to further influence public attitudes and behaviors, that determine whether significant numbers of youth will survive and thrive?

Fundamental to an understanding of the effects of poverty is a deeper understanding of the poor. Additional questions that community psychologists can ask include: How do poor people in poor neighborhoods differ from those in better-off neighborhoods (those concentrated in large public-housing developments compared to those in "scattered site" publicly supported housing)? Is neighborhood poverty effective in a relative sense? In any setting, are those with the fewest resources also the least competent or least well-adapted? Is there some absolute threshold above which income protects residents from feeling disadvantaged, no matter how wealthy most of their neighbors may be? Do cognitive conceptions of poverty, and expectations for future wealth or poverty, moderate the impact of neighborhood on individual outcomes? Answers to these questions begin to get at the mechanisms by which structural factors that are affected by changes in policy (e.g., attachment to the labor force) actually sustain the existence of a poor population. By connecting the people to the structural forces that act upon them, psychology can serve a vital role in developing both theory and policy designed to stimulate long-term improvement in the lives of the poor.

REFERENCES

Brooks-Gunn, J., Duncan, G. J., & Aber, J. L. (Eds.). (1997). *Neighborhood poverty* (Vols. 1–2). New York: Russell Sage Foundation.

Center for the Future of Children. (1997). *Children and poverty, The Future of Children, Vol. 7* (No. 2). Los Altos, California: The David and Lucile Packard Foundation.

Danziger, S. H., & Weinberg, D. H. (1994). The historical record: Trends in family income, inequality, and poverty. In S. H. Danziger, G. D. Sandefur, & D. H. Weinberg (Eds.), *Confronting poverty: Prescriptions for change* (pp. 18–50). Cambridge: Harvard University Press.

Smith, S. (Ed.). (1997). *The well-being of children in working poor families.* New York: Foundation for Child Development.

Urban Institute. (1998). *One year after federal welfare reform: A description of state temporary assistance for needy families (TANF) decisions as of October 1997.* (L. J. Gallagher, M. Gallagher, K. Perese, S. Schreiber, & K. Watson, Eds.). Washington, D.C.: Urban Institute.

U.S. Census Bureau. (1996). "Persons and Families in Poverty by Selected Characteristics: 1995 and 1996"; last revised 14 October 1997; <http://www.census.gov/hhes/poverty96/pv96est1.html>

Waquant, L. J. D., & Wilson, W. J. (1989). Poverty, joblessness and the social transformation of the inner city. In P. H. Cunningham & D. T. Ellwood (Eds.), *Welfare policy for the 1990s*. Cambridge: Harvard University Press.

Wilson, W. J. (1987). *The truly disadvantaged.* Chicago: University of Chicago Press.

B. Reproductive Rights

BRUCE AMBUEL

THE SOCIAL CONSTRUCTION OF REPRODUCTIVE RIGHTS

Our society's discussion of reproductive rights has been shaped since 1965 by the landmark Supreme Court ruling, *Griswold v. Connecticut.*[1] Prior to *Griswold*, a married couple living in the State of Connecticut committed a criminal offense if they possessed or used contraception. Similar laws existed in many jurisdictions. In *Griswold*, the Supreme Court recognized that citizens have a fundamental right to privacy. This right to privacy, existing in the "penumbras" of the Bill of Rights and Fourteenth Amendment of the United States Constitution, protects the individual citizen from unwarranted state control of personal decisions, including reproductive decisions. *Griswold* focused debate on the theme of individual liberty vs. state power, a focus that is reflected in subsequent Supreme Court rulings, and which continues to influence public debate. The Supreme Court decision in *Roe v. Wade* limited state power and extended the right of privacy to protect women's access to abortion.[2] Other decisions have protected legal minors' access to contraception and abortion.[3] In *Planned Parenthood of Southeastern Pennsylvania v. Casey*,[4] the Supreme Court changed course and enhanced state power by adopting a more lenient standard for judging the constitutionality of state laws that regulate abortion. This new standard made it easier for states to regulate and limit women's access to abortion. States have responded with new legislation, which has led to ongoing court challenges (Committee on Adolescence, 1996).

Balancing individual liberty vs. state power is a central tension in a democratic society. However, this *legal* framework, grounded in a history of legal challenges to state laws limiting individual liberty to control reproduction, provides a narrow view of reproductive rights that may limit our understanding from a psychological perspective. If we accept this framework as a definition of reproductive rights, then we risk closing off a critical stage of analysis, problem definition, and bypass a fundamental question: What human rights are associated with reproduction?

From the perspective of community and developmental psychology, reproductive rights can be broadly defined as an individual's right to *control fertility*,[5] *express sexuality*, and *conceive, bear, and raise children.* Reproduction is not a set of biological events beginning with sexual intercourse and conception and ending with birth, but a psychological and social process involving an individual's decision to make a commitment to another adult; share a

[1] *Griswold v. Connecticut*, 381 U.S. 479 (1965).

[2] *Roe v. Wade*, 410 U.S. 113 (1973).

[3] *Planned Parenthood of Central Missouri v. Danforth*, 428 U.S. 52 (1976); *Carey v. Population Services International*, 431 U.S. 678 (1977); *Bellotti v. Baird II*, 443 U.S. 622 (1979); *H.L. v. Matheson*, 101 S.Ct. 1164 (1981); *Planned Parenthood Association of Kansas City*, 103 S. Ct. 2517 (1983); *Jane Hodgson v. Minnesota*, 58 U.S.L.W. 4957 (1990); *Ohio v. Akron Center for Reproductive Health*, 58 U.S.L.W. 4979 (1990).

[4] *Planned Parenthood of Southeastern Pennsylvania v. Casey*, 60 USLW 4795, 1992.

[5] *Control of fertility* has different meanings for women and men because of the biological difference in responsibility for completing pregnancy. Thorough discussion of these differences is beyond the scope of this chapter; the reader is referred to Freedman and Isaacs (1993).

BRUCE AMBUEL • Waukesha Family Practice Center #201, 120 N.W. Barstow, Waukesha, Wisconsin 51388.

sexual relationship; create a family; have children through birth or adoption; and foster the biological, psychological, and social development of children. Reproduction is also a cultural process by which society reproduces compassionate and capable citizens. Reproductive rights are therefore those rights that protect the individual citizen's capacity to create family and recreate culture. These rights are possessed by all individuals, male and female, regardless of gender identity or sexual orientation.

Reproductive rights have two facets, *individual liberty* and *commitment to family and community*. Individual liberty is valued for its own sake, and is essential for individuals to control fertility and express sexuality. Liberty also establishes the preconditions for an individual to make a commitment to family and community. Commitment to family and community is an essential element for maintaining human relationships, raising children, and reproducing culture.

Examining our society's debate over reproductive rights from this broader perspective reveals an apparent paradox. While there has been an intense political debate focusing upon individual liberty versus state power, our society is facing a growing community failure. Although adults and adolescents have secured, for the moment, a constitutional right to obtain and use birth control, many cannot obtain the reproductive health care needed to exercise this liberty. An increasing number of families cannot obtain basic health care, even when two parents have steady, but low-income, employment. Many families do not have a primary care physician providing services in their community; others cannot afford a physician's services or prescription birth control. The community failure is particularly severe for adolescents. Adolescents are the only age group in the United States whose morbidity and mortality is increasing and whose health status declining. Looking beyond reproductive health care, an increasing number of people lack resources to create the stable economic conditions for their families that are a precondition to raising healthy, capable children. Women and children remain the fastest growing group living in poverty, particularly African Americans, Native Americans, and Hispanics. This is reflected in the high infant mortality rate and low childhood immunization rates for the U.S., which are comparable to the rates in eastern European countries, and significantly worse than all other western European countries.

The foremost challenge facing community psychologists is reframing the issue of reproductive rights in order to communicate a theoretically sound understanding of reproductive rights that integrates individual liberty with commitment to family and community. This theoretical perspective should be developmental, describing reproductive rights throughout the lifespan. This theoretical perspective should also be ecological, describing the multiple psychological, social, economic, and cultural influences on reproductive success. Finally, this new perspective should suggest ways of promoting reproductive success via psychological, social, economic, and cultural interventions. The tension between individual privacy and state power, including control of contraception and abortion, will remain a critical issue, but in a broader context that recognizes interdependence of the individual, family, and community, as well as the right of individuals and communities to raise healthy children. The rest of this section illustrates how a broad view of reproductive rights can suggest new issues for research and action.

ADOLESCENTS AND ABORTION

Limitations inherent in the legal framework of individual liberty vs. state power are evident in the debate over adolescent abortion. The United States Supreme Court has affirmed the right of states to require that minors who are not emancipated either obtain parental consent for an abortion or demonstrate to a judge that they are legally competent. Two psychological assumptions are fundamental in these Supreme Court rulings and state laws: that female adolescents under the age of 18 are not competent to consent to abortion, and that mandated parental involvement is in the minor's and parents' best interest. While age 18 is a convenient criterion because of the legal tradition of majority, both legal assumptions have questionable validity.

Adolescents' competence to consent to abortion has been examined at length (see Ambuel & Rappaport, 1992; Melton, 1986). By age 14, most minors are "equal to adults in their 'competence' to imagine the various ramifications of the pregnancy decision" (Lewis, 1987), and make reasoned choices about unplanned pregnancy (Ambuel & Rappaport, 1992). In fact, laws that mandate parental consent may be harmful to adolescents *and* parents. Delay caused by legal proceedings increases medical risk and patient morbidity and mortality. Requiring parent–child communication may undermine family relationships for the substantial majority of adolescents who freely choose to consult parents about unplanned pregnancy. Finally, requiring parent–child communication may be harmful for a significant number of young minors who become pregnant as a result of coerced intercourse within the family (Ambuel, 1995; Ambuel & Lewis, 1992).

Rather than continuing to pit adolescent minors' liberty against state power, social policy debate might be advanced by innovative approaches to consent that promote both adolescents' individual liberty as well as family and community values. Because most adolescents have the capacity to make reasoned treatment decisions with respect to abortion, and involve parents in their decision, such a policy might establish a process for obtaining informed consent that counsels adolescents about all options, promotes family involvement and social support, and empowers adolescents as decision-makers (Ambuel & Rappaport, 1992).

Recent developments in the law and ethics of informed consent to medical treatment may suggest a pathway for achieving this goal. At one time, health care professionals discharged their responsibility for informed consent by providing the patient with information that other professionals would consider appropriate regarding treatment alternatives, risks, and benefits. Many states have now adopted a standard of informed consent that requires professionals to present information that a reasonable person would expect to receive (Grisso, 1986). The President's Commission for the Study of Ethical Problems in Medicine and Biomedical and Behavioral Research (1983) has suggested that professionals disclose any information that the specific patient would expect or find beneficial. These changing standards place increasing responsibility on the health care professional to assess and meet a patient's unique individual needs for information. There is a logical progression from this standard to a standard requiring physicians to present information in a manner that empowers (Rappaport, 1981, 1990) a reasonable adolescent to give informed consent.

An empowerment standard of informed consent would ask the professional to cocreate, with the patient, a decision-making environment and process that enhances the patient's competence, participation, and control over treatment decisions. In the context of legal minors' decision-making about unplanned pregnancy, this means using developmentally appropriate consent procedures that engage the adolescent in participatory decision-making; provide adequate information about all options; facilitate, as appropriate, minors' already extensive use of social support from parents, other family members, adult mentors, and peers; and, provide resources for additional information and social support (Ambuel, 1995).

An empowerment approach would alter the relationship between the adolescent minor-citizen and state. Rather than placing minors' liberty in opposition to state power in a zero sum game, informed consent as empowerment creates what Handler (1990) calls a "participatory" relationship between citizen and state. In this participatory relationship, state power is used to "*structure* rather than *decide*," to define a process that empowers the adolescent minor-citizen to draw upon resources in their family and community, then make reasoned decisions. The specific challenge facing community psychologists is designing a developmentally appropriate informed consent process that empowers adolescent patients.

COMMUNITY RESPONSES TO REPRODUCTIVE RIGHTS

Another limitation created by the individual liberty vs. state power paradigm is the way this description of reproductive rights structures the questions we ask by focusing upon the individual as the unit of analysis. Our society's ongoing debate about reproductive rights provides a unique opportunity to study formation of social policy in local communities. Although this debate often appears highly polarized in national media, polls have consistently found that a majority of citizens have a moderate view of even the controversial abortion issues. The tenor of local reproductive politics varies from community to community. Some communities develop an atmosphere of tolerance that fosters collaboration. Organizations with differing views on issues such as abortion still work together to promote the autonomy and health of women, children, and families by developing local health programs. Debate in other communities becomes highly polarized. Organizations that otherwise share strong interests view each other as adversaries.

This variation in the social ecology of communities suggests a series of questions for action researchers. What factors promote collaboration in local communities? How are diverse coalitions and a tolerant social climate nurtured and maintained? How are community dynamics influenced by individual, group, institutional (religion, media, government), historical, cultural, ethical, or racial factors? Does a collaborative social environment produce measurable differences in the health status of citizens? Finally, what community intervention strategies can help build and sustain diverse community coalitions? These questions require a research strategy that compares individual, social, and community structure and process across communities. Campbell's recent study of community response to rape (1998) demonstrates one innovative research strategy for studying these community-level factors.

SUMMARY

The paradigm of balancing individual liberty vs. state power is part of the legal history of reproductive rights in the United States, but has limitations for understanding reproductive rights from a psychological perspective, as well as for protecting reproductive rights. This paradigm suggests that individual liberty and state power are necessarily opposed in a zero sum game, and focuses our attention on the individual *de jure* liberty at the expense of individual *de facto* liberty, family, and community. Community psychology and the ecology of human development provide a theoretical perspective for developing a broader understanding of reproductive rights. The following sources are suggested for readers interested in further study of reproductive rights: Ambuel and Rappaport, 1992; Freedman and Isaacs, 1992; Gill, 1992; Grisso, 1986; Melton, 1986; Scott, 1992; and United Nations, 1985.

REFERENCES

Ambuel, B. (1995). Adolescents, unintended pregnancy and abortion: The struggle for a compassionate social policy. *Current Directions in Psychological Science, 4*, 1–5.
Ambuel, B., & Rappaport, J. (1992). Developmental trends in adolescents' psychological and legal competence to consent to abortion. *Law and Human Behavior, 16*, 129–154.
Ambuel, B., & Lewis, C. C. (1992). Social policy of adolescent abortion. *The Child, Youth and Family Service Quarterly, 15*, 5–9.
Campbell, R. (1998). The community response to rape: Victim's experiences with the legal, medical, and mental health systems. *American Journal of Community Psychology, 26*, 355–380.
Committee on Adolescence. (1996). The adolescents right to confidential care when considering abortion. *Pediatrics, 97*, 746–751.
Freedman, L. P., & Isaacs, S. L. (1993). Human rights and reproductive choice. *Studies in Family Planning, 24*, 18–30.
Gill, S. (Ed.). (1992). The fate of *Roe v. Wade. Hastings Center Report*, September-October.
Grisso, T. (1986). *Evaluating competencies: Forensic assessments and instruments.* New York: Plenum.
Handler, J. (1990). *Law and the search for community.* Philadelphia: University of Pennsylvania Press.
Lewis, C. C. (1987). Minors' competence to consent to abortion. *American Psychologist, 42*, 84–88.
Melton, G. B. (Ed.). (1986). *Adolescent abortion: Psychological and legal issues.* Report of the Interdivisional Committee on Adolescent Abortion, American Psychological Association. Lincoln, NE: University of Nebraska Press.
Rappaport, J. (1981). In praise of paradox: A social policy of empowerment over prevention. Presidential address to the Division of Community Psychology of the American Psychological Association. *American Journal of Community Psychology, 9*, 1–25.
Rappaport, J. (1990). Research methods and the empowerment social agenda. In P. Tolan, C. Keyes, F. Chertok, & L. Jason (Eds.), *Researching community psychology: Integrating theories and methodologies.* Washington, D.C.: American Psychological Association.
Scott, E. S. (1993). Judgement and reasoning in adolescent decision-making. *Villanova Law Review, 37*, 1607–1669.
United Nations. (1985). *Report of the World Conference to Review and Appraise the Achievements of the United Nations Decade for Women: Equality, Development and Peace.* New York: United Nations.

C. Environmental Issues

JULIA GREEN BRODY

As psychologists, we think first of community as a web of social relationships. Rappaport (1977) defines community as a social group within a larger society. But the *Random House Dictionary* definition he cites refers also to people who "reside in a specific locality," and even to "an assemblage of plants and animal populations occupying a given area." Drawing on concepts of person–environment fit and ecological perspectives that are central to community psychology, we know that powerful communities can be linked to place—a block, a neighborhood, a town—where physical environment defines and shapes the social web. Since Earth Day 1970, more of us are thinking in terms of a global community, one finite and precious planet with just so much air, water, and land. We are thinking about the connection

JULIA GREEN BRODY • Silent Spring Institute, 29 Crafts Street, Newton, Massachusetts 02458.

between community and place in terms of the impact of human groups on the environment, and of the environment, in turn, as a sustaining resource for human life.

From my perspective as a community psychologist working on environmental issues for more than a decade, the many links between community psychology and the environmental movement seem natural and obvious. We share a concern for understanding the complex interconnections represented in ecological perspectives, for empowering underrepresented groups and sustaining diversity, for balancing individual freedom and public responsibility. The first question for me, then, is not: Why is environment emerging as an important focus for community psychology; but rather: Why is it *still* emerging more than 25 years after the first Earth Day?

Some of the answers are institutional. Addressing environmental problems means a commitment to field research, always difficult for academic psychologists because it is methodologically messy, time-consuming, and expensive. In addition, agencies, such as the Environmental Protection Agency (EPA) and the Agency for Toxic Substances and Disease Registry (ATSDR), that fund environmental research are not part of the psychology network. Outside academia, there are few settings where psychologists can find a foothold for work on environmental issues. Natural scientists, engineers, lawyers, and economists dominate the environmental agencies and firms.

Other barriers are substantive. Community psychologists pride themselves on interdisciplinary approaches, but environmental issues require a further stretch into fields outside the social sciences. For example, several years ago, I founded and directed a project to assist communities in reaching consensus about whether to incinerate their trash. I needed to know something about what goes in as garbage, how much plastic, how much arsenic and lead; as well as something about what comes out the stack as PICs, PAHs, POHCs,[1] an alphabet soup that Peter Sandman, Professor of Environmental Communications at Rutgers, calls "dimethyl meatball."

Institutional and disciplinary barriers are formidable, but there is another barrier: Community psychologists have been too slow to see how we can contribute. I present some ideas here.

Beginning with the definition of environmental problems, we can contribute by showing that costs of environmental pollution can't be measured just in dollars, or even in numbers of cancers, they must include behavior, affect, and social relationships. Psychologists have demonstrated that lead, noise, pesticides, and other pollutants cause learning deficits, irritability, and depression. They affect children's ability to learn, workers' job performance, and interactions with family members and friends. Psychologists and other social scientists have contributed to an understanding of the costs of destruction of community, such as that which occurred with the relocation of residents at Love Canal, and of psychological stress and powerlessness, such as at Three Mile Island and in communities targeted for a nuclear waste repository (Dunlap, Kraft, & Rosa, 1993; Kasl, Chisholm, & Eskenazi, 1981; Levine, 1982).

We also can contribute to solutions because solutions mean changing behavior at both the individual and institutional levels. Paradigms developed during the 1970's energy crisis can be adapted and extended to help us generate less trash and get around without our gas-guzzling cars. Our knowledge of what moves organizations can create new successes, like the celebrated McDonald's switch from petroleum-based hamburger boxes to paper wrappers, or the

[1]That's products of incomplete combustion, polycyclic aromatic hydrocarbons, and principal organic hazardous constituents.

internal decision by Polaroid to make environmental performance an explicit standard for evaluating managers.

Our greatest contribution could be in understanding and facilitating processes for resolving conflict. Environmental policy involves extremely complex decisions that balance competing values under conditions of considerable uncertainty. We don't know what the greenhouse effect means for the future of the planet, or whether magnetic fields from electric power sources cause cancer, or when we will run out of oil. We don't know what the trade-off may be between jobs and food production and preservation of wilderness. Psychologists (for example, Slovic, Fischhoff, & Lichtenstein, 1982) have contributed to our understanding of how people evaluate environmental uncertainty and risk, but very little is known about how we evaluate different solutions. New understandings of the values that underlie conceptions of environmental fairness are a critical need; we need new strategies for providing meaningful participation and empowerment for communities at risk, and for reaching consensus within and across communities.

Psychology research and theory has been working on these issues in other contexts for a long time. Attribution theory, theories of justice, and small-group interaction are important conceptual resources. Within community psychology, research on citizen participation, voluntary organizations, and empowerment is important (for example, Wandersman & Florin, 1990).

But more important than any particular theory is the contribution we can make from sharing the most basic paradigms of our field. Working so often with citizens and professionals from other disciplines, I am struck by the tremendous power and robustness of concepts we are apt to take for granted: hypothesis testing, statistical significance and power; measurement error, reliability, and validity; and quasi-experimental design. Some examples from projects that recently have crossed my desk illustrate my point.

When I testify before a public utility commission about public policy for community exposure to electromagnetic fields (EMF) from transmission lines, part of my job is to explain the trade-offs between false-positive and false-negative decisions. A growing body of research in biology and other disciplines raises serious concerns about the effects of EMF on living cells and organisms, but the scientific picture is incomplete. What if we decide to modify or move transmission lines, then EMF proves to be harmless? What if we do nothing and future research demonstrates that EMF increases cancer risk? As psychologists, we began thinking about different kinds of errors when we learned rules for hypothesis testing in our first statistics course, but I have seen this conceptualization "turn on the light bulb" for policymakers who are grappling with public fears about high-power lines.

In another project, I served as a mediator for a citizen board coping with contamination of an elementary school with trichlorethylene (TCE), a volatile organic compound linked to cancer. Citizens were struggling to reach agreement about a protocol for monitoring and reopening the school, but data from the air quality engineer were confusing. As I learned, measuring air quality is remarkably like measuring psychological variables—no two samples of air behave the same way—so lessons on reliability and measurement error became a part of my job.

A few years ago, New Jersey issued an RFP for a project to facilitate and evaluate the work of a local community in designing and implementing an intervention to increase recycling. Because of the strong secular trends in attitudes toward recycling, I proposed a quasi-experimental design. A year later, agency staff who had never thought of using a comparison group were telling *me* to add a comparison to a parallel study of small businesses.

In a quasi-experiment conducted recently, key negotiators involved in setting international standards for ozone-destroying chlorofluourocarbons and greenhouse gases met in simulated negotiation sessions. The researchers reported a matrix of decisions reached by the groups, but they hadn't found a way to characterize the internal process groups went through to reach solutions; and they hadn't dealt with the influence of individual characteristics on outcomes in particular groups. Yet these conceptual and measurement problems are readily apparent to a community psychologist.

While I have focused on what environmentalists can learn from community psychologists, we can learn from them too. The acronym NIMBY—not in my backyard—has become a put-down of active community involvement in decisions about the environment; but activists spell it NIMBI—now I must become involved. The fates of local and global communities are our issues as community psychologists. As professionals, we must become involved. The following sources are suggested for readers interested in further study of environmental issues: Brown and Mikkelsen, 1990; Dunlap, 1991; Homer-Dixon, Boutwell, and Tathjens, 1993.

REFERENCES

Brown, P., & Mikkelsen, E. J. (1990). *No safe place: Toxic waste, leukemia, and community action.* Berkeley: University of California Press.

Dunlap, R. E. (1991). Public opinion in the 1980s: Clear consensus, ambiguous commitment. *Environment, 33,* 10–15, 32–37.

Dunlap, R. E., Kraft, M., & Rosa, E. A. (Eds.). (1993). *Public reactions to nuclear waste: Citizens' views of repository siting.* Durham, NC: Duke University Press.

Homer-Dixon, T. F., Boutwell, J. H., & Tathjens, G. W. (1993, February). Environmental change and violent conflict. *Scientific American,* 38–45.

Kasl, S. V., Chisholm, R. F., & Eskenazi, B. (1981). The impact of the accident at the Three Mile Island on the behavior and well-being of nuclear workers. *American Journal of Public Health, 71,* 484–495.

Levine, A. (1982). *Love Canal: Science, politics, and people.* Lexington, MA: Lexington Books.

Rappaport, J. (1977). *Community psychology: Values, research, and action.* New York: Holt, Rinehart and Winston.

Slovic, P., Fischhoff, B., & Lichtenstein, S. (1982). Rating the risks: The structure of expert and lay perceptions. In C. Hohenemser & J. Kasperson (Eds.), *Risks in the technological society* (pp. 141–166). New York: American Academy for the Advancement of Science.

Wandersman, A., & Florin, P. (Eds.). (1990). Special section: Citizen participation, voluntary organizations and community development: Insights for empowerment through research. *American Journal of Community Psychology, 18.* 41–177.

D. Lesbian, Gay, and Bisexual Issues

ANTHONY R. D'AUGELLI

In June 1969, the American lesbian/gay civil rights movement was born in an unlikely locale for such a milestone, the Stonewall Inn, a gay bar in the Greenwich Village section of New

ANTHONY R. D'AUGELLI • Department of Human Development and Family Studies, The Pennsylvania State University, University Park, Pennsylvania 16802.

York City. Near midnight on June 27, when New York police arrived for their routine harassment of patrons, they were met with violent resistance instead of the usual shameful compliance. Fueled by years of social humiliation, and riding the crest of waves caused by the civil rights and women's movements, lesbian and gay activists began the long struggle to assert a place in the social and community life of this country. Hostility in their communities drew many into urban neighborhoods with more tolerant views, and from such lesbian and gay urban communities emerged the support and political power to challenge the institutional homophobia that also had been internalized as self-loathing.

Victimized also by professional mental health, lesbian/gay activists did not target the individual therapists who labeled them "disordered," without justification, but rather, in the tradition of community psychology, attacked the institutional policies of the victimizers. After several rancorous years, the American Psychiatric Association bowed to the pressure of lesbian/gay activists and supportive psychiatrists, and removed "homosexuality" from the psychiatric nomenclature on December 15, 1973. In January 1975, the American Psychological Association (APA) followed suit, passing the following resolution:

> Homosexuality per se implies no impairment in judgment, stability, reliability, or general social and vocational capabilities. Further, the American Psychological Association urges all mental health professionals to take the lead in removing the stigma of mental illness that has long been associated with homosexual orientations.

Later APA policy resolutions condemned discrimination based on sexual orientation in employment, housing, public accommodations, and licensing (1975), in child custody and placement decisions (1977), in employment of teachers (1981), and in youths' access to education (1993). In addition, APA resolutions call for increased attention to the psychological consequences of hate crimes specifically directed against lesbians and gay men (1988), and note APA's official opposition to the Department of Defense's policy that same-sex sexual orientation is "incompatible with military service" (1992).

Several recent APA policies concern the need for continued attention to the AIDS pandemic, which has devastated urban gay communities, such as New York, Los Angeles, and San Francisco—the very communities that fostered the emergence of the gay rights movement. By June 1999, 711,344 cases of AIDS in the U.S. had been reported to the Centers for Disease Control and Prevention. Of the 687,313 adult cases, 55%, or 379,339, are men who have had sex with men (MSM). The Centers for Disease Control and Prevention estimates that 119,193 MSMs have perished from 1993 through 1998 alone, and that 153,717 MSMs are currently living with AIDS/HIV. In some urban neighborhoods, up to 50% of sexually active adult gay and bisexual males may have HIV infections. Major prevention efforts have been targeted to gay and bisexual males, especially youths, to assist them in avoiding HIV infection. The community impact of the HIV epidemic is nearly incalculable, with the thousands of deaths affecting many significant others. And, despite medical advances in the treatment of HIV infections, more death and grief are inevitable.

If policy recommendations of professional groups such as the APA were equivalent to social progress and legal change (and if the HIV epidemic had been preempted by a vaccine), lesbians, gay men, and bisexual people would face few barriers in our society. Unfortunately, despite the progress made by lesbians, gay men, and bisexual people since Stonewall, there remain many barriers that need to be removed to eradicate the stigma of same-sex sexual orientation in American society. Deeply ingrained biases and minimal protections from discrimination are powerful disabling influences in the lives of lesbians, gay men, and bisexual people. Most remain partially or totally undisclosed to others ("closeted"), fearing rejection by family, friends, and co-workers, thus forestalling the jeopardization of such basics as employment or housing. As of this writing, there is no federal law providing protection from discrimination on the basis of one's sexual orientation. Existing statutory protection is limited, protecting few lesbian, gay, and bisexual Americans from intolerable actions that undermine personal, family, and community life. Only nine states (California, Connecticut, Hawaii, Massachusetts, Minnesota, New Hampshire, New Jersey, Wisconsin, and Vermont) provide comprehensive, statewide protection from discrimination in employment and housing. Such protection is also provided by nearly 130 other cities and counties. Nearly half the states still criminalize same-sex consensual sexual activities between adults under their "anti-sodomy" laws. In these states, lesbians, gay men, and bisexual people are literally criminals (in Virginia, consenting same-sex sexual contact is punishable as a felony with not less than one year in prison). Despite *amicus curae* briefs from APA and other professional organizations, the U.S. Supreme Court affirmed the right of states to criminalize private consenting sexual behavior in the *Bowers v. Hardwick* decision of 1986. On the other hand, the U.S. Supreme Court recently overturned an effort in Colorado to rescind all statutes protecting people from discrimination based on sexual orientation, in the 1996 *Romer v. Evans* case.

With basic rights unprotected except in exceptional circumstances, and with continuing resistance to their equitable treatment mounted by social and religious conservatives, lesbians, gay men, and bisexual people constantly engage in coping processes to ensure the safety of their personal lives. These strategies generally succeed (they are well-practiced), but may result in lowered self-esteem, fragile social relationships, marginal community life, and diminished political power. In addition, the difficulties these people experience in the formation and maintenance of committed relationships, historically attributed to their characterological defects, can be seen as resulting from the destabilizing and delegitimizing societal forces, which dispense no symbolic or concrete support to such relationships and actively discourage their existence. Indeed, the considerable interest in legal recognition of same-sex unions has led to the passage by many states of legislation reserving "marriage" for opposite-sex dyads, and federal legislation to this effect was signed by President Bill Clinton in 1996.

Family life for lesbians, gay men, and bisexual people is thus doubly disrupted. Not only does cultural bias lead to many parents distancing themselves from their offspring, but committed domestic relationships remain hidden from the support of friends, co-workers, social policies, and the law. Also, lesbians, gay men, and bisexual people who have children (whether from prior marriage or through alternative child-bearing or child-rearing arrangements) face multiple psychological stressors produced by both policy and custom. These parents fight judicial bias (such as their de facto criminal status in many states) in child custody determinations; if fortunate enough to maintain custody or contact with their children, they must thereupon confront the institutional heterosexism of school systems, which marginalizes non-traditional families.

The complex influences of history and law, and of social and institutional policies, on the psychological adjustment and social life of these people in different (and quite distinct) communities provide rich opportunities for community psychologists for applied research and action. The following are top priority areas for community psychologists in collaborative research and intervention with lesbians, gay men, and bisexual people:

1. *The ongoing impact of the HIV/AIDS epidemic and the prevention of further HIV infections*. Community psychologists can help in the development, implementation, and evaluation of preventive interventions, and in evaluating (and advocating for) resources for

the many needs presented by people with HIV illnesses, their significant others, and their families.

2. *Concerns of lesbian, gay, and bisexual youths.* Adolescents and young adults who disclose same-sex sexual orientations to others are at risk for rejection from parents, siblings, extended family, and peers, and are subjected to harassment and other forms of victimization. Such youths, as well as those undisclosed to others, are at risk for mental health problems, especially different forms of self-destructive behavior. Community psychologists can work to develop human service systems for such youths, and can help identify their needs.

3. *Antilesbian/gay violence.* Lesbians and gay men are frequent targets of victimization, ranging from verbal harassment to assault, the latter occurring with greatest frequency in urban gay communities. Homophobic verbal and physical attacks occur on college and university campuses as well, since these settings provide a more conducive environment for young people to publicly acknowledge their sexual orientation. Community psychologists can document patterns of victimization in different settings, and can work on community-oriented prevention programs.

4. *Preventive mental health services for lesbians, gay men, and bisexual people.* Few social service agencies are prepared to provide help to lesbians, gay men, and bisexual people. Such agencies can be assisted by community psychologists to develop accessible, lesbian/gay-affirming services of a variety of kinds. Programs aiding in family issues and in developing relationships would be extremely helpful.

5. *Legal protection and recognition.* Legal protection must be enacted to prevent discrimination on the basis of sexual orientation, and this would best occur at a federal or state level. The remaining sodomy acts must be repealed. Same-sex committed couples should have equivalent access to resources designed for heterosexual couples through registration as domestic partners, and should receive equal benefits afforded to other committed couples. Documenting inequity is an important role for community psychologists in collaborating with lesbian, gay, and bisexual activists, as well as advocating for social change.

In 1990, then-President George Bush signed the National Hate Crime Statistics Act into law, requiring the U.S. Justice Department to collect data on bias-related crime, including crimes committed due to the victim's sexual orientation. The first lesbian/gay-supportive action in American jurisprudence, this law signaled a new decade of social action for lesbians and gay men. In the summer of 1998, President Bill Clinton signed an executive order banning discrimination based on sexual orientation in federal employment, an act reflecting public opinion research that shows that most Americans disfavor anti-lesbian/anti-gay discrimination. The increasing visibility of lesbian, gay, and bisexual people and their families will surely continue, and will generate resistance as well as support from diverse constituencies. As this process unfolds, community psychologists have much to offer to lesbian, gay, and bisexual communities as this decade of progress continues, more than 30 years following Stonewall.

REFERENCES

D'Augelli, A. R., & Patterson, C. J. (Eds.). (1995). *Lesbian, gay, and bisexual identities over the lifespan: Psychological perspectives.* New York: Oxford University Press.

Herek, G. M. (Ed.). (1998). *Stigma and sexual orientation: Understanding prejudice against lesbians, gay men, and bisexuals.* Thousand Oaks, CA: Sage.

Patterson, C. J., & D'Augelli, A. R. (Eds.). (1998). *Lesbian, gay, and bisexual identities in families: Psychological perspectives.* New York: Oxford University Press.

E. The HIV/AIDS Epidemic: An International Perspective

JOSE ANTONIO GARCIA GONZALEZ

By 1995, an estimated two million adults were infected with HIV in North America and Europe (World Health Organization, 1995). In the United States alone, over half a million cases were diagnosed with AIDS, and over 62% of these had reportedly died by that time (Centers for Disease Control and Prevention, 1995).

But there is another, even more somber consequence of this dreadful, iceberglike pandemic: More than 90% of the estimated 24 million cases of HIV worldwide (projected to be over 26 million by the year 2000) have occurred in poor third-world countries, primarily Africa, Asia, and Latin America, where other social problems, such as endemic poverty, chronic violence, infectious diseases, sexual discrimination, and lack of access to health care, have obscured the impact and consequences of the epidemic. To darken the picture, the pattern of explosive growth in new HIV infections that occurred throughout parts of the world in the 1980s is being repeated now in many places in Asia, and is not expected to level off until the year 2010 (Quinn, 1996).

Through the dominant pattern of heterosexual transmission in these developing countries, women and children are being infected at a dramatically rising rate. In the poor areas of many of these inner-city neighborhoods and rural areas, whether São Paulo, Lagos, or Bangkok, as many as 30% of the young adults are seropositive, yet continue to use their bodies for commerce. The response of government, religious, and social authorities in these areas is predominantly one of denial, silence, or stigma. The simple reason is the way the problem or its causes are defined: homosexuality, drug use, and prostitution are illegal and, thus, do not officially exist. Thus, HIV and its prevention is not a health priority in many third-world countries.

The HIV/AIDS epidemic has exposed both the frailties of our human condition and the failures of our social and health systems. After more than a decade of immense research effort, we still ignore critical scientific steps to produce a definite cure or vaccine. We do not understand the co-occurrence or causal relationship with factors such as sexually transmitted diseases or tuberculosis, latency and resistance of the immune system, or differential infectivity among different subgroups, such as women and intravenous drug users. From a public health perspective, there are difficulties in reporting and surveillance techniques, disparities in definitions and diagnostic criteria, and gaps in reporting systems. From a sociological or psychological perspective, we know little about the norms and practices of human sexual behavior, risk perceptions, and economic or life priorities, as well as the cultural or religious constraints on them. More importantly, we know even less about cross-cultural or subgroup differences that may affect the biological or psychological processes or public health concerns.

In this way, the HIV/AIDS epidemic represents a paradigmatic exemplar for a program of Community Health research and action. Health psychologists have framed the epidemic as an opportunity to develop and use knowledge about health-behavior relationships (Chesney, 1993). Community psychologists face a different challenge; they are presented with the formidable task of finding a creative and systematic approach for changing economic and political conditions and social regularities in order to create healthier communities and prevent further transmission of the virus.

JOSE ANTONIO GARCIA GONZALEZ • Universidad Central de Venezuela, Caracas 1010-A, Venezuela.

Many lessons can be drawn from what has been accomplished so far and from what remains to be done to confront this pandemic worldwide. First, there is a crucial need for a new model of health, one that contemplates the relatedness of, and respect for, health and human rights. The HIV epidemic continues to remind us of the inconsistencies and deficiencies of cultures that maintain a male-dominant or "macho" orientation. Non-heterosexual sexual identities and practices are discriminated against; women's rights are not considered, and their powerlessness leads to sexually risky behavior (Mays & Cochran, 1988); and children become unwilling victims. Poor or culturally different people are labelled as inferior or deviants, and victim-blaming abounds. Individual models of health-behavior change, and the interventions designed using these models, are guided by Euro-American middle-class values, which overlook the array of social, cultural, economic, political, ethical, and legal constraints placed on sensitive social behaviors.

Failure to recognize these cultural, social, or sexual rights and differences has led to a myopic framing of the problem, has limited our response to the AIDS crisis, and has hampered the effectiveness of our public health interventions on a worldwide level. We urgently need a redefinition of the problem, one that incorporates the influence of socioeconomic conditions, as well as cultural differences and human rights; that could address such economic inequities and suffering; that optimizes cost and benefits for all, not just an elite; and that provides health care for those who need it most, in a culturally sensitive and participatory fashion. What people cherish most is both their culture and well-being, and we need to integrate both in order to improve the control, satisfaction, and quality of people's lives (Panos Institute, 1989).

A second promising direction for intervention is the crucial role played by active, community-based groups that this epidemic has helped to mobilize, organize, and empower (see Revenson & Schiaffino, this volume). This grass-roots action was needed to cover the fault lines left by overburdened health systems and oblivious governments. Community-based efforts can provide medical care, emotional supports, and community prevention and health education programs. Such programs bring to light the sensitive issues and the specific localized resources to confront the crisis.

Among the many faces of this pandemic, the leadership provided by non-governmental organizations and non-medical community-based organizations (such as the Gay Men's Health Crisis and Act-Up in the United States, or LASCO, has been essential. These organizations have been able to empower and mobilize affected people of different backgrounds and economic circumstances, all over the world, to defend their lifestyles while preventing the spread of the virus. Volunteer participation, safe-sex programs, and support groups will be remembered as a hallmark or turning point in returning the "right to health" from medical professionals to the individuals and the communities in which they reside. The breadth of these community actions—covering preventive efforts, medical care, self-help, advocacy, ethical issues (e.g., workplace discrimination), and legal triumphs—have no parallel to date. Ironically, this may be the only "positive" outcome of the pandemic.

International cooperation, through multilateral agencies and organizations (from the WHO-PHO, UNICEF, and UNDP, to the World Bank and many other international networks and NGOs) has been crucial in expanding the worldwide information network, and in supporting action and research programs. Overall, these international agencies have provided critical leadership in confronting this problem, in a way that we have not seen since the eradication of polio. Perhaps this international cooperation will encourage the market value of prevention vs. treatment, even in developing countries where the annual *per capita* health expenditure falls somewhere between $10–$100.

Perhaps the AIDS epidemic will lead us to discover the importance of combining empowerment and prevention strategies. The challenge posed to the social sciences is to contribute meaningful data that can inform intervention programs incorporating both prevention and empowerment strategies. Social science has made some progress in reducing the psychological and social impact of the illness for those already infected. Some good efforts have been made in trying to reduce the gaps between knowledge-based research and change-oriented programs. Unfortunately, we have been blinded and constrained by our own values and biases regarding the complexities of sexual practices, for example, the extent of bisexuality in macho-oriented cultures. Social scientists too often lack expertise in media and marketing techniques for health education campaigns; frequently these campaigns are imbued with fear-arousing or cognitively based rationale messages that tend to produce anxiety and confusion, but do not change behavior or social norms (see McAlister, this volume).

In order to make a difference, we will have to undertake intervention studies that will inform how to convey sexual education messages for specific cultural groups, interventions that provide respectful and compassionate care for HIV-infected persons, and that minimize, rather than increase, stigma. Interventions also must be directed at the social and health agencies currently directing HIV efforts, agencies that often display complacency about infection because of a victim-blaming strategy. It is a formidable task, for which we are ill-prepared. However, over the past decade, we have improved our skills, knowledge, networks, and interventions with the participation of those suffering most. Much more needs to be known and done if we want to address the magnitude of this problem in the face of the 21st century. Until we have clear answers to questions, such as why people discriminate without reason, why we engage in lethal behavior, and why so many people have to die before governments and political or financial bodies take action, we will have to work harder.

REFERENCES

Centers for Disease Control and Prevention. (1995). First 500,000 AIDS cases—United States, 1995. *Morbidity and Mortality Weekly Report, 44*, 849–853.

Chesney, M. A. (1993). Health psychology in the 21st century: Acquired immunodeficiency syndrome as a harbinger of things to come. *Health Psychology, 12*, 259–268.

Mays, V. M., & Cochran, S. D. (1988). Issues in the perception of AIDS risk and risk reduction activities by Black and Hispanic/Latina women. *American Psychologist, 43*, 949–957.

Panos Institute. (1989). *AIDS and the third world.* London: New Society.

Quinn, T. C. (1996). Global burden of HIV pandemic. *Lancet, 348*, 99–106.

World Health Organization. (1995). *The current global situation of the HIV-AIDS pandemic.* Geneva: WHO Global Program on AIDS.

F. The Farm Crisis and Rural America

ROBERT HUGHES JR.

In the mid-1980s a significant number of farmers had serious financial problems. Between 1982 and 1986, the percentage of farms going out of business tripled, and the percentage going

---

ROBERT HUGHES JR. • College of Human Environmental Sciences, University of Missouri, Columbia, Missouri 65211.

through bankruptcy more than quadrupled. These problems, along with the social and psychological consequences, captured the attention of Americans and became known as the "farm crisis." Both the illusions and realities of this "crisis" provide a basis for understanding issues facing rural communities in America. A careful look back at this experience and an analysis of the current state of rural communities can provide important insights for researchers, social service providers, and public policymakers.

While there is some debate about the specific causes of the farm crisis, there is general agreement that declining world demand for U.S. farm products, lowering commodity prices, falling land values, and increasing debt among farmers all contributed to the financial problems of farmers during the 1980s. Economic woes disproportionately affected younger farmers in the beginning stages of the farming careers because they were more likely to have purchased land at a high price to expand their operations or to have borrowed more money for operational costs. To understand the farm crisis, it is important to put the event in historical perspective.

A major theme in the media during the farm crisis was the "loss of the family farm." While it is important not to minimize the tragic experiences of families who lost their farms during the 1980s, the general pattern of a decline in the number of family farms was set in motion over half a century ago. Since 1920, the percentage of rural residents employed in farming has declined from 60% to less than 10%. Today, most rural residents are employed in service industries, retail trade and manufacturing, not farming. These employment patterns expose what Luloff and Swanson (1990) have described as a major myth about rural communities—the erroneous assumption that rural communities are dependent on farming for their social and economic well-being. Indeed, evidence has been accumulating that, currently, the opposite relationship holds; that is, family farms are dependent on a healthy non-farm rural economy for success. By taking off-farm jobs, members of farm families can earn sufficient income to maintain their farms.

RURAL POVERTY

While the loss of family farms deserves attention, it has too often overshadowed other important realities about rural life. In general, when compared with their urban counterparts, rural residents fare much worse economically (Dietz & Pfuntner, 1996). Rural earnings per job were lower than urban earnings in almost every occupation. Overall, rural earnings are about 90% that of urban earnings. Throughout the early part of the 1990s, nonmetropolitan poverty was greater than metropolitan poverty, although poverty in central cities remains the highest (U.S. Bureau of the Census, 1995).

The future economic outlook does not promise much hope for rural communities. The Bureau of Labor Statistics employment projections through the year 2005 indicate that three occupational categories are expected to continue to lose jobs: agriculture, mining, and manufacturing. While some occupations in rural areas will gain employment, rural communities, when compared with urban areas, have twice the proportion of workers in occupations expected to sustain the largest declines.

This historical perspective and analysis of the economics of rural communities suggest that, while there may or may not be another "farm crisis," there is likely to be a significant number of people living in rural communities who face economic hardships. For researchers, service providers and policymakers, the key question centers on how rural families and communities are affected by economic difficulties, and what strategies offer promise for dealing with this situation.

STRESS AND COPING

Over the last decade there have been a number of important studies examining the consequences of economic hardship among rural families (Conger & Elder, 1994; Hennon, Brubaker, & Marotz-Baden, 1988; Hoyt, Conger, Valde, & Weihs, 1997). Findings concerning the relationship between financial strain and psychological distress for farm and rural families have been consistent with the general stress literature; that is, economic troubles contribute to poorer mental health, in particular, depression. Equally important have been the findings that farmers and rural residents who employ active coping strategies and maintain a sense of mastery or personal control are able to reduce the adverse consequences of stressful life events. Elsewhere, researchers have documented the impact of economic hardship on intergenerational and marital relations among rural families, as well as the support mechanisms that mediate these relationships. These findings offer clear ideas for those intervening with farm and rural families.

Despite these important findings, there is still much that we need to know about how rural families respond to stress. Salamon (1992) has demonstrated how different cultural values influence farm-family decision-making and family life, in particular she has predicted that the cultural values held by farm families with different ethnic backgrounds will substantially affect their methods of coping with financial difficulties. This work clearly demonstrates that rural residents cannot be treated as a homogenous group of people.

Beyond the individual level of coping with financially difficult times, it is important to understand how communities respond to economic hardship. Both myths about rural life and scant empirical research limit effective intervention. The pervasive myth that rural life is dominated by close family relations and composed of a close-knit supportive community has not be conducive to the development of a good understanding of how communities respond to stressful situations. Despite several decades of effort at community development, we still have a limited view of how communities act and how to support their efforts.

COMMUNITY DEVELOPMENT AND EMPOWERMENT

To address the farm crisis and other rural needs, a variety of community development efforts have been created. Christensen and Robinson (1989) have classified these action strategies into three types: (1) a *self-help* approach that relies on voluntary participation of community residents, communitywide planning, and the establishment of an organizational structure to lead in community development; (2) a *social planning* effort involving outside technical experts to provide information to community decision-makers in order to assist them in development; and (3) a *social action* approach based on the formation of power bases and coalitions to pressure government and other powerful organizations into action.

A cogent analysis of rural communities by Wilkinson (1986) provides an insightful theoretical basis for a fourth type of approach to community development. He asserts that, too often, community developers have approached rural issues as if they were insulated from the rest of society. In contrast, Wilkinson suggests that the fundamental difficulty for rural communities is their dependence on the larger national economy and the centralized institutional structure of social and economic services. It is dealing with this dependency problem that is central to effective development in rural communities.

While rural communities cannot be decoupled from the larger institutions and forces in society, these institutions can serve to create opportunities for local communities to assume more control over their destinies. Thus, rather than conduct social planning or leave communities to help themselves, an empowerment perspective is proposed to address the issue of dependency. Additionally, to deal with the sense of powerlessness experienced by many members of rural communities, Wilkinson (1986) proposes a leadership development model that fosters community involvement and community solidarity.

Recent research comparing communities that are able to develop effective community action strategies lends support to this empowerment approach to community development. Wilkinson and his colleagues have found that communities that are successful at obtaining federal support for projects and attracting new business enterprises are characterized by community involvement and solidarity. Likewise, when natural disasters occur, communities with strong ties across organizations are more likely to obtain and successfully use emergency relief (Sundet & Mermelstein, 1996). While questions remain about what specific factors contribute to community involvement and solidarity, studies of leadership and community participation suggest that when citizens have a sense of psychological empowerment and are taught problem-solving skills, they are more likely to be involved in the community. At present, these are tentative hypotheses and findings; much research is needed about how communities take action and how to support their actions. Additionally, work is needed in articulating rural community development based on an empowerment model. Regardless of the approach to community development, evaluation studies are needed to clarify what works and how (Christensen & Robinson, 1989).

If the farm crisis stimulated researchers, service providers, and policymakers to take another look at the conditions of rural America, then an important first step has been achieved. However, given the current social and economic indicators that point to further declines in rural communities, it is important to move beyond the farm crisis. Neglect of rural social and economic concerns will leave a tangle of social pathologies ultimately resulting in a "rural" rather than a "farm" crisis as we enter the next century.

REFERENCES

Christensen, J. A., & Robinson, J. W., Jr. (Eds.). (1989). *Community development in perspective.* Ames, IO: Iowa State University Press.

Conger, R. D., & Elder, G. H., Jr. (1994). *Families in troubled times: Adapting to change in rural America.* New York: Aldine de Gruyter.

Dietz, E., & Pfuntner, J. (1996). Do urban workers earn more than their country cousins? *Compensation and Working Conditions Online, 1.* http://www.bls.gov/opub/cwc/1996/summer/brief1.htm.

Hennon, C. B., Brubaker, T. H., & Marotz-Baden, R. (Eds.). (1988). *Families in rural America: Stress, adaptation, and revitalization.* St. Paul, MN: National Council on Family Relations.

Hoyt, D. R., Conger, R. D., Valde, J. G., & Weihs, K. (1997). Psychological distress and help seeking in rural America. *American Journal of Community Psychology, 25,* 449–470.

Luloff, A. E., & Swanson, L. E. (Eds.). (1990). *American rural communities.* Boulder, CO: Westview.

Salamon, S. (1992). *Prairie patrimony: Family, farming and community in the Midwest.* Chapel Hill: University of North Carolina Press.

Sundet, P., & Mermelstein, J. (1996). Predictors of rural community survival after natural disaster: Implications for social work practice. *Journal of Social Service Research, 22,* 57–70.

U.S. Bureau of the Census. (1995). Poverty 1995. Persons and families in poverty by selected characteristics: 1994 and 1995. http://www.census.gov/hhes/poverty/pov95/povest1.html.

Wilkinson, K. P. (1986). In search of the community in the changing countryside. *Rural Sociology, 51,* 1–17.

G. The New Immigrants

RAMSAY LIEM

HISTORICAL CONTEXT

In 1965, the U.S. Immigration Act brought to an end discriminatory immigration policies against non-Europeans, evidenced most flagrantly by the Chinese Exclusion Act of 1882. Although many factors played a role in this landmark decision, the contradiction in giving overt preference to European immigrants was highlighted by the intense struggle for racial equality led by the civil rights movement. How great could a Great Society be that barred its doors to the majority of the world's population? It would, therefore, be fair to conclude that recent immigration trends that have dramatically influenced the demographic make up of the U.S. population have their origins in the same social milieu that gave birth to the field of community psychology.

One consequence of these common roots is that the commitment of community psychology to social justice, social change, and community empowerment as relevant to psychological well-being must be fulfilled in the context of a vastly more diverse society than existed at the time of the field's inception. While race, class, gender, and sexual orientation continue to determine privilege and access to resources, the arrival of nearly 20 million newcomers (Daniels, 1991; Hing, 1993) to the United States since 1965 has introduced a plethora of new challenges: cultural and ethnic divisions, generational conflicts, linguistic diversity, intensified economic competition, and the like.

No longer can we assume that Hispanic or Latin Americans are principally Spanish, Puerto Rican, or Cuban, that Asian Americans are primarily of Chinese or Japanese descent, or, for that matter, that African Americans can only be the descendants of colonial America. For example, during the past decade alone, three million East, Southeast, and South Asians have entered the United States as emigrants or refugees, increasing the size of the Asian American community by 75% (O'Hare & Felt, 1991). As a result, what were once negligible populations of Koreans, Indians, and Vietnamese now surpass the Japanese American community in size. Furthermore, in 1970, Asian Americans were predominantly U.S. born, whereas today the community is in large proportion first-generation.

This changing demographic landscape is far from limited to the Asian American community. During the same period, the Latino and African American communities increased by nearly 4 and 6 million persons, respectively, much of this growth a result of immigration (O'Hare & Felt, 1991). Immigration from the Middle East has been equally unprecedented during the past decade and, with the collapse of the Cold War, increasing numbers of Eastern Europeans have established residence in the United States.

One might argue that these waves of new immigrants constitute nothing more than a continuation of the historic pattern of population change in the United States. After all, except for Native Americans, the United States has always been a country of immigrants. Nonetheless, the recent immigrants have created unprecedented ethnic and cultural diversity, especially within communities of color, reflecting, among other things, accelerating growth of the

RAMSAY LIEM • Department of Psychology, Boston College, Chestnut Hill, Massachusetts 02467.

global economy, U.S. economic and military policies of hegemony, and the prominence of North–South conflict in the face of receding East–West tensions. This reality, combined with continuing structural racism in the United States and a sharpening division between an economic elite and the working classes, creates extraordinary new challenges for a discipline that promotes social justice and equality as essential to psychological well-being.

THE SOCIETAL CHALLENGE

At the sociopolitical level, the new immigration raises several fundamental issues. Most profound may be the challenge to re-vision the possibilities for community in U.S. society. Historically, social policy in the United States has inched toward equality on the basis of inclusion, implying a dominant sociocultural, ideological, and economic mainstream into which social theorists and policymakers across the political spectrum have proposed to admit the marginal. As limited as the efforts to accomplish this objective may have been, the significant presence of a new generation of non-Europeans today raises questions as to the viability of the very premise underlying this goal. Those who bring this new diversity of cultures to the United States resist by their numbers and traditions the notion of a dominant, Euro-American cultural center. Furthermore, traditional racial minorities are reclaiming their ethnic and cultural roots as a means of psychological and social survival in the face of persistent racism.

These conditions present a new challenge for building national solidarity based on an affirmation of, and respect for, differences, rather than the promise of a cultural "melting pot." Community development and empowerment from this perspective will test community psychology in new ways. It will require knowledge of community practices unique to very different ethnic groups; the ability to envision how public institutions can be helped to accommodate diverse values, priorities, and social practices; and strategies for achieving lasting coalitions or federations of groups, rather than fostering assimilation to the putative social mainstream. The ideal of nationhood need not be lost in this process, only the view that full enfranchisement of newcomers requires that they relinquish all that is culturally and socially familiar. Thus, promoting equal access to education through support of bilingual–bicultural programming rather than English-as-a-Second Language alone, would be consistent with this pluralistic vision of community.

Accepting cultural and ethnic diversity as a fact of the new social order will be even more challenging in light of the persistent economic, political, and social inequities that exist as structural impediments to collective and individual well-being for many in the society. Long-standing conflicts engendered by these conditions become especially volatile in the face of perceptions that limited economic resources are being taxed by significant numbers of new immigrants. As predicted by Bluestone and Harrison in 1982, deindustrialization and capital flight in recent years has produced an economic distribution heavily skewed toward a small minority of privileged on the one hand, and a shrinking middle class and growing pool of "have nots" on the other. These conditions exacerbate hostility toward newcomers. Historical inequities, the deterioration of the country's manufacturing infrastructure, and dramatic increases in new immigrant communities could be a formula for disaster.

These are conditions that breed conflict and scapegoating, as witnessed by the Los Angeles uprising of April 29, 1992. A decade of urban neglect, the loss of a manufacturing base, and the rapid expansion of the Asian and Latino communities in the heart of Los Angeles fueled the eruption that occurred in the wake of the acquittal of four policemen whose beating of Rodney King was witnessed by the nation on amateur video. The attention focused on Korean–Black tensions in the aftermath reveals the vulnerability of new immigrants to scapegoating as a means to divert attention from the fundamental roots of poverty and inequality in America.

To support the aspirations of new immigrants, community psychology must be able to understand and affirm the cultural and social practices of these groups, while simultaneously helping to articulate the genuine economic and political interests common to immigrants, the economically displaced, and the racially marginalized. Useful lessons in this regard can be drawn from the late-19th- and early-20th-century experiences of Japanese, Filipino, Portuguese, Mexican, and Korean workers brought to Hawaii to develop the sugar industry. Exploiting historical antagonisms among Asian nationals and ethnic differences between Latinos and Europeans, plantation owners recruited gangs of immigrant laborers of different nationalities at each sign of incipient labor organizing and discontent (Takaki, 1989). Japanese workers were imported to quell the Chinese, Koreans to compete with the Japanese, and so forth. Owners manipulated national and cultural animosities to discipline their growing labor force.

In time, however, many of these sojourners established not only common economic ground, but also a new social community that recognized the unique cultural contributions of each group. This compact was neither ideal nor easily forged. Nonetheless, the struggles of these early Hawaiian laborers and their families constitute a valuable source for community psychologists seeking examples of unity building in the face of systemic exploitation of racial, cultural, and class differences.

CULTURALLY INFORMED RESEARCH

The diversity of cultures now represented throughout the society challenge the field in other ways at the level of individual well-being. For community psychology, a central question is the adequacy of our understanding of psychological and sociological dynamics as they operate within vastly different social traditions. For example, what constitutes the mature, healthy ideal among Southeast Asians, Haitians, or Salvadorans? How do we square the notion of individualistic, achieved, and "self-possessed" identity with identity derived from place, family name, or membership in a religious community? Is shame associated with personal embarrassment comparable to that associated with family dishonor? How does one promote healthy interpersonal relations within hierarchical family and community structures, in contrast to those that promote an egalitarian ideal? What stance is appropriate toward the status of women in patriarchal communities in light of one's commitment to gender equality?

These and other questions have begun to be addressed in the social and behavioral science literature, heavily influenced by anthropological insights. Although community psychology can also draw upon a rich tradition of cross-cultural research in psychology, this area of work has been criticized for its unreflective western bias in the framing of comparative studies. Schweder (1991) suggests the alternative of "cultural psychology," which connotes that culture, as a shared meaning and action system, infuses not only everyday social practice, but also the framing of, and inquiry into, psychological processes—cognition, language, emotion, development, psychopathology, etc. In this view the production of all psychological knowledge is cultural (Bruner, 1990; Cole, 1996; Wertsch, 1991). Theory and method are captives of the "cultural ecology" and may be limited in their applicability by their formative, cultural assumptions.

A good example of the difficulty in pursuing culturally informed, comparative research is found in an exchange between U.S. and Japanese psychologists on the topic of social control (Weisz, Rothbaum, & Blackburn, 1984; Azuma, 1984). Briefly, Weisz et al. suggest that Westerners (U.S. respondents) adopt strategies of primary control in seeking to influence others, whereas Japanese employ secondary control strategies.

> In primary control, individuals enhance their rewards by influencing existing realities.... In secondary control, individuals enhance their rewards by accommodating to existing realities and maximizing satisfaction or goodness of fit with things as they are. (p. 955)

In his response, Azuma notes that the dichotomy—primary/secondary control—comprises a single construct, both poles of which are thoroughly western in meaning. Defined in contrast to the ideal of primary control, secondary control connotes similarly "American" qualities of indirectness, non-assertiveness, and guardedness. Simply applying one pole to U.S. respondents and the other to the Japanese, therefore, does not constitute a cultural comparison.

What Azuma proposes is the discovery of constructs applicable to the interplay of social relationships in Japan on their own terms by seeking greater differentiation within the category of secondary control, rather than defining it solely in contrast to primary control. Toward that end, constructs such as harmony–disharmony, flexible–rigid, and tolerant–intolerant would help to better approximate the meaning of the Japanese behavior that Weisz et al. characterize as "secondary control." Note also how the meaning of secondary control becomes less invidious when associated with the first pole of each of these constructs, instead of when placed in contrast to primary control.

Treating culture seriously at the level of psychological knowledge requires that community psychology adopt a new, more anthropological stance toward scientific inquiry and community practice. This objective would be enhanced by actively seeking the contributions of social scientists from other countries and disciplines, recruiting promising young scholars from the new immigrant communities to the discipline, and questioning the adequacy of our research methodologies for comprehending cultural meanings and practices.

The first of these challenges is especially relevant to our professional associations whose resources can be used to create a variety of forums for scientific exchange and collaboration. Leadership at this level is essential to avoid only a token nod to the importance of cultural insights. The field will also need to be creative in finding ways to attract a much more culturally diverse, younger pool of talent. One suggestion is to actively support the strengthening of ethnic studies programs within our universities. These curricula often provide an opportunity to introduce ethnically diverse students to the relevance of social and behavioral science to the needs of immigrant communities (Kiang, 1990). Furthermore, scholarship in ethnic studies frequently addresses issues central to the concerns of community psychology, such as the conflicts inherent in transitional identities, the institutionalization of racial and cultural marginalization, and the struggle to create and preserve community.

Program alliances between community psychology and ethnic studies can enrich each area and diminish the likelihood that either discipline will simply socialize students to their current paradigms. At Boston College, we are employing a related strategy in our graduate concentration in cultural psychology. We have recently expanded our core research-training seminar to include faculty involved in multicultural education and ethnic studies, and have future plans to include participants from the humanities.

Finally, ethnographic, narrative, and other qualitative methods need to be given a more prominent role in community psychology research, emphasizing the discovery of meaning and symbol systems, rather than the operation of untested, universal "variables." How this can be done in concert with more traditional approaches is illustrated in research by Good, Good, and Moradi (1985) on depressive affect among Iranian immigrants. In this work, a decade of participant observation in Iran, extensive contact with Iranian health providers, and clinical interviews were employed to chart the tentative outlines of a sociocultural ecology of dysphoria among Iranian immigrants.

The investigators attribute a rich Iranian discourse on grief to the cultural salience of the tragic, as evidenced in prominent historical, religious, and literary texts. They emphasize that dysphoria can signify both depth of personality as well as dysfunction. They also identify a core complex of anger, mistrust, and sensitivity among the clinically depressed, each element of which coheres with cultural meanings and experiences particular to the circumstances of Iranian emigration, social etiquette, or popular conceptions of personality development.

Factor analysis of a standardized, U.S. depression inventory was employed following the ethnographic inquiry as an independent validation of the proposed complex. Significantly, the meaning attributed to the factor structure was derived from the preceding inquiry into Iranian idioms of grief, anger, and the like, rather than the face validity of the items contained in it. To paraphrase the authors, this study employed an interpretive, or meaning-centered, anthropology to investigate depression, focusing on the relation of human action to its sense rather than behavior to its determinants.

Among the many topics in need of investigation by a cultural psychology in service of immigrant needs are conceptions of personhood or selfhood, the social and psychological meaning of family, cultural conceptions of mental health and disorder, and customary help-giving and help-receiving social practices. A second level of investigation needs to focus on the circumstances of immigration at the macro level, e.g., the political economy of global population movements, as they are encountered by particular groups and individuals. In addition to these immigrant-centered concerns, we need to explore the dynamics of host–newcomer relations within white America and historical communities of color. This task is especially challenging in view of race, class, and gender conflicts endemic to social relationships in the United States.

These represent areas of basic knowledge essential to understanding specific problems, such as the high rate of suicide attempts among immigrant youth, generational conflicts within immigrant families, the psychological impact of family-role disruptions concomitant with immigration, and the social isolation of the elderly. They are also vital to developing effective strategies of service delivery to immigrant communities that go beyond the recruitment of bilingual–bicultural providers trained in standard ways. Finally, the capacity to understand the psychological and social realities of immigrants is particularly important if psychologists are to be useful partners in meeting the challenges of community building, coalition formation, and political empowerment that new immigrants face at the dawn of the 21st century.

THE CASE OF REFUGEES

Significant among the vast numbers of new immigrants to the United States during the past decade are refugees, newcomers not by choice but necessity. While immigrants may also be compelled by circumstance to leave their homelands, rarely are they fleeing life-threatening conditions. Refugees are created by life-and-death situations. In the United States they come from virtually every continent, although those from Central America and Southeast Asia are most familiar to the general public. During the 1980s, an estimated 10% of all new immigration could be attributed to the influx of refugees (Daniels, 1991). Their needs are extensive and resources minimal. For many, the political abuse, terror, and violence experienced in their homelands is compounded by trauma encountered during escape and their marginal status in the United States upon their arrival. The Immigration and Naturalization Service's category of "undocumented alien," which extends to many refugees is, itself, a source of persistent stress.

Among the mental health professions, community psychology should, in principle, be most suited to serving this population whose psychological well-being is so evidently linked to social, economic, and political conditions. Although limited, the organized response to the needs of refugees in the United States and other countries reflects a tension similar to historical divisions between community psychology and its sister discipline, clinical psychology.

One illustration involves two competing perspectives regarding strategies of intervention with an especially troubled population of refugees, torture survivors. The first view, institutionalized in centers for torture survivors, has adopted the rubric of posttraumatic stress disorder to explain the psychological sequelae of human rights abuses (Cervantes, Salgado de Snyder, & Padilla, 1989; Hauff & Vaglum, 1994; Ortmann, Genefke, Jakobsen, & Lunde, 1987). In this schema, internalized and recurring representations of abuse, rather than the actual events and their systemic origins, are prominent in the analysis of the dynamics of massive physical and psychological assault. Psychological intervention is viewed as a component of comprehensive medical care in the face of extraordinary stress from which the survivor is assumed to have escaped. Predictably, this stance has tended to be adopted by those who work with torture survivors seeking refuge outside of their native countries.

By contrast, others, often survivors themselves, have evolved a more socially oriented perspective that integrates ongoing practices of state-sponsored violence and the societal impacts of political repression with the more private elements of internalized trauma (Becker et al., 1990; Martín-Baró, 1988; Palinkas, 1995). Although not self-identified as community psychologists, those who have developed this perspective have evolved practices that represent community psychology at its best.

Chilean psychologists (Becker, Lira, Castillo, Gómez, & Kovalskys, 1990), for example, have worked for nearly two decades with torture survivors of the Pinochet dictatorship. One core feature of their multilevel practice involves the use of testimony. A double-edged sword, this detailed recording of the circumstances preceding, during, and following torture is integrated into the early phase of therapy as a vehicle for cognitive clarification and much-needed emotional catharsis. Its value is personal and subjective, and is enhanced by the personal and political solidarity that testimony-giving and -taking creates between therapist and survivor.

When warranted, testimony takes on another function, particularly for individuals whose lives before the abuse were dedicated to political reform and social change. For these persons, testimonies become a means for re-engaging the "life project" (Cienfuegos & Monelli, 1983). With the intercession of the therapist, these records are selectively made public in human rights and political forums, both domestically and internationally. As such, they become vehicles for denouncing the system of repression responsible for torture and related abuses, and enable a first step toward reclaiming the ability to act against one's victimizers. Testimony, thus, encourages the survivor to look inward to confront his or her particular experience of abuse at the same time that it facilitates this process by actively affirming and challenging the sociopolitical roots of the trauma.

It is beyond the scope of this overview to elaborate the conceptual reasoning behind this practice. However, this use of testimony reflects a very different understanding of the psychological abuse many refugees have faced than accompanies the model of posttraumatic stress disorder. Similar forms of work in the United States have been inspired by the Chilean example and modified to meet the special conditions faced by refugees in this country (Aron, 1992).

Testimony as elaborated by Chilean psychologists is unmistakably community psychology practice. The field would surely profit from greater exposure to it, and other strategies of intervention developed in the context of the extreme violence and repression that often create refugees. Groups like the Ignacio Martín-Baró Fund for Mental Health and Human Rights, and the International Organization of Centres and Individuals Concerned with the Care of Victims of Organized Violence support this kind of work and promote North–South exchange.[2] A description of incipient efforts in the United States to collaborate with international colleagues in developing theory and practice relevant to the experiences of internal and exiled refugees can be found in Lykes and Liem (1990).

CONCLUSIONS

The challenges to community psychology posed by the unprecedented diversity in U.S. immigrant communities are as varied as is this population itself. Immigrants and refugees face a plethora of cross-cutting cultural, political, socioeconomic, generational, familial, and personal struggles that will surely tax the limit of existing paradigms in the field. Community psychology, therefore, needs to be creative and humble in seeking new human and social resources to develop its capacity to incorporate these concerns within its research, advocacy, and intervention agendas. Like the society at large, it needs to recognize that the inclusion of diversity is not only a positive social value, but a means to enhance our comprehension of a changing social order and ability to promote the social welfare. This overview identifies some of these challenges and suggests ways to strengthen research and intervention skills, as well as the profession itself.

REFERENCES

Aron, A. (1992). Testimonio, a bridge between psychotherapy and sociotherapy. In E. Cole, O. Espín, & E. Rothblum (Eds.), *Refugee women and their mental health: Shattered societies, shattered lives*. New York/London: Haworth.

Azuma, H. (1984). Secondary control as a heterogeneous category. *American Psychologist, 39*, 970–972.

Becker, D., Lira, E., Castillo, M., Gómez, E., & Kovalskys, J. (1990). Therapy with victims of political repression in Chile: The challenge of social reparation. *Journal of Social Issues, 46*, 133–149.

Bluestone, B., & Harrison, B. (1982). *The deindustrialization of America: Plant closings, community abandonment, and the dismantling of basic industry*. New York: Basic Books.

Bruner, J. (1990). *Acts of meaning*. Cambridge: Harvard University Press.

Cervantes, R., Salgado de Snyder, V., & Padilla, A. (1989). Post-traumatic stress in immigrants from Central America and Mexico. *Hospital Community Psychiatry, 40*, 615–619.

Cienfuegos, A., & Monelli, C. (1983). The testimony of political repression as a therapeutic instrument. *American Journal of Orthopsychiatry, 53*, 43–51.

Cole, M. (1996). *Cultural psychology: A once and future discipline*. Cambridge: The Belknap Press/Harvard University Press.

[2]Ignacio Martín-Baró Fund for Mental Health and Human Rights, P.O. Box 2122, Jamaica Plain, MA 02130; International Organization of Centres and Individuals Concerned with the Care of Victims of Organized Violence. Helen Bamber, Medical Foundation for the Care of Victims of Torture, United Kingdom. See also the American Association for the Advancement of Science, Office of Scientific Freedom and Responsibility, 1333 H. Street, NW, Washington, D.C. 20005.

Daniels, R. (1991). *Coming to America: A history of immigration and ethnicity in American life.* New York: HarperCollins.
Good, B., Good, M. J., & Moradi, R. (1985). The interpretation of Iranian depressive illness and dysphoric affect. In A. Kleinman & B. Good (Eds.), *Culture and depression* (pp. 369–428). Berkeley: University of California Press.
Hauff, E., & Vaglum, P. (1994). Chronic posttraumatic stress disorder in Vietnamese refugees: A prospective community study of prevalence, course, psychopathology, and stressors. *Journal of Nervous and Mental Disease, 182,* 85–90.
Hing, B. (1993). *Making and remaking Asian American through immigration policy, 1850–1990.* Stanford: Stanford University Press.
Kiang, P. (1990). Asian American studies: Moving into the third decade. *Gidra,* 20th Anniversary Edition, 43.
Lykes, B., & Liem, R. (1990). Human rights and mental health in the United States: Lessons from Latin America. *Journal of Social Issues, 46,* 151–165.
Martín-Baró, I. (1988). La violencia política y la guerra como causa del trauma psìcosocial en El Salvador [Political violence and war as causes of psychosocial trauma in El Salvador]. *Revista de Psicología de El Salvador, 28,* 123–141. Reprinted in *Journal of La Raza Studies, 2,* 5–13.
O'Hare, W., & Felt, J. (1991). Asian Americans: America's fastest growing minority group. *Population Trends and Public Policy, 19,* 1–17.
Ortmann, J., Genefke, I., Jakobsen, L., & Lunde, I. (1987). Rehabilitation of torture victims: An interdisciplinary treatment model. *American Journal of Social Psychiatry, 7,* 161–167.
Palinkas, L. (1995). Health under stress: Asian and Central American refugees and those left behind. *Social Science and Medicine, 40,* 1591–1596.
Schweder, R. (1991). *Thinking through cultures: Expeditions in cultural psychology.* Cambridge: Harvard University Press.
Takaki, R. (1989). *Strangers from a different shore: A history of Asian Americans.* Boston: Little Brown.
Weisz, J., Rothbaum, F., & Blackburn, T. (1984). Standing out and standing in: The psychology of control in Americans and Japanese. *American Psychologist, 39,* 955–969.
Wertsch, J. (1991). *Voices of the mind.* Cambridge: Harvard University Press.

H. Unemployment

RICHARD H. PRICE

The causes of unemployment are changing rapidly in the United States in response to major structural, societal, and economic changes. The Great Depression of 1929 and other less severe recessions were times of general economic decline during which lost opportunity and financial hardship were fairly broadly shared. Today much unemployment is driven by new forces (Price, Friedland, Choi, & Caplan, 1998). The first of these is organizational restructuring. Economic incentives that encourage mergers and acquisitions by firms also create redundant groups of workers and jobs. Organizational restructuring is encouraged by the promise of short-term financial gain or to take advantage of a foreign labor market. In either case, large numbers of workers who would never have thought themselves vulnerable in the past are experiencing job displacement (Price, 1990).

The second major force driving job displacement in America today is the dramatic shift from our status as a manufacturing society to one that is primarily information-driven. Even in the rapidly shrinking manufacturing sector, new technological imperatives demand new

RICHARD H. PRICE • Department of Psychology, University of Michigan, Ann Arbor, Michigan 48106.

worker skills and eliminate jobs that were available to the less skilled. These changes in the labor market effect not just individuals, but families as well, and new groups of poor people are emerging, including female-headed households and those with few marketable skills. In the face of these sweeping changes, it is important to understand the impacts of unemployment at more than one level of analysis. Job loss affects individuals, families, and communities. It is also a phenomenon whose meaning is particularly dependent upon the community economic context.

What does one lose when one loses a job? Individuals, families, and whole communities do not cope with unemployment itself, but instead cope with the stresses and strains produced by job loss (Price, 1992). Vinokur (1998) has produced a detailed review of the impact of unemployment on physical and mental health. Job loss and unemployment have been shown to be implicated in increased violence (Catalano et al., 1993), alcohol abuse (Catalano, Dooley, Wilson, & Hough, 1993; Dooley, Catalano, & Hough, 1992), and depression (Dooley, Catalano, & Wilson, 1994; Kessler, House, & Turner, 1988). At an individual level, Catalano (1991), Kessler et al. (1988), and Vinokur, Price, and Caplan (1996) have offered convincing evidence that the impact of job loss for individuals is due primarily to the financial hardship unemployment produces, particularly for persons who have lower levels of education and income. Job loss and economic hardship reverberate throughout the family. Vinokur et al. (1996) have shown that economic hardship has impacts on the mental health of both unemployed workers and their spouses, which in turn impair their ability to support one another, and increase the amount of social undermining in the marital relationship. Furthermore, economic hardship associated with job loss can erode one's sense of mastery and personal identity (Price, Friedland, & Vinokur, in press), impairing the ability to successfully reenter the workforce. Thus, the meaning and impact of unemployment varies for groups in society who are differentially advantaged and who are forced to cope in different economic contexts.

As we arrive at the end of this century, the changing economic forces and the impact of unemployment itself provide a context for new research questions. These questions are answerable at both the level of local community programs and in terms of larger social policies (Blinder, 1987). The first set of questions is primarily descriptive and asks: What new segments of our society are particularly vulnerable to involuntary job loss and what do we know about the impact on these groups at the individual, family, and community level? We can anticipate that new risk groups will emerge, made vulnerable either by lack of opportunity or by technological change (Hamilton, Broman, Hoffman, & Brenner, 1990). These groups are likely to include single-parent families, the unskilled, and those in industrial sectors where rapid restructuring and technical change is taking place. These groups will join others, such as the urban minority poor.

A second set of questions emerges when we examine the generic strategies available to social policymakers for coping with the problem of unemployment. Fundamentally, three strategies exist (Price & Burke, 1985), which can be initiated at the level of the individual, the firm, or the societal or governmental unit (Blinder, 1987). The strategies are: (1) efforts intended to change the characteristics of the job seeker, (2) efforts intended to change the character of the opportunity structure of jobs, and (3) efforts intended to change the allocation rules that match people to jobs. This characterization of generic strategies has heuristic value. It can inform research and action questions that take into account the individual and community conditions under which one strategy may be more successful than another.

Strategies aimed at changing the characteristics of the job-seeker are of two general kinds. The first are job-search programs intended to increase search skills and the motivation of individual job-seekers. Job-search programs can be effective in helping individuals to obtain more satisfying jobs more quickly at higher levels of income and job quality (Caplan, Vinokur, Price, & van Ryn, 1989; Price, van Ryn, & Vinokur, 1992; Vinokur, van Ryn, Gramlich, & Price, 1991; Vinokur, Price, & Schul, 1995; Vinokur & Schul, 1997). These strategies do not create more jobs. Instead, they increase the efficiency and effectiveness of the job-seeking process, enhance the coping of the job-seeker, and reduce distress. Another strategy for changing the characteristics of job-seekers involves retraining and reeducation. Numerous governmental and individual programs are available to implement this strategy. It should be clear that, whatever form of change strategy a person takes, it assumes programs can produce the required changes and that we know what characteristics are desirable to change. Such strategies also assume that incentives at the individual, employer firm, or governmental level are available to accomplish the strategy. This strategy may be of special benefit to those with fewer educational resources, but at the same time is of little value if jobs are not available to be filled. The person-change strategy is therefore heavily dependent on the existing economic climate.

The second general strategy involves attempting to change the characteristics of the opportunity structure itself (Kozlowski, Chao, Smith, & Hedlund, 1993; Last, Peterson, Rappaport, & Webb, 1995; London, 1995). This can happen in several ways, either as a result of local community-based economic development efforts to create more jobs, or through government incentives to create more jobs in employer organizations (Blinder, 1987). Another approach to changing the opportunity structure involves encouraging relocation either of jobs or individuals. This may occur within the internal labor market of an employer firm, or through an individual decision to search in a new market. There are clear organizational incentives to transfer experienced employees, and reasons to believe the transition within a firm will usually be less difficult (Price, 1990). Finally, changes in the opportunity structure can be affected through job redesign, including the development of work-sharing strategies, sharing the available hours worked, or creating various flexible work-life programs, including job-sharing and unpaid leaves of various kinds. The redesign approach can be enacted even if the opportunity level in the community is relatively low. Generally speaking, attempts to change the opportunity structure also assume that incentives exist for job redesign or relocation. When the absolute number of jobs is diminishing, this strategy has natural limitations.

The final broad strategy involves changing the allocation rules that match people to jobs, and therefore regulates the relationship between the employer and the employee (Gordus & McAlinden, 1984). Typically, changes in allocation rules of this kind are negotiated between organized labor, employer firms, and the government, and can take several forms. One form could be called protective since it tends to protect the work force against unfair allocation of job opportunities or unfair allocation of layoffs. Antidiscrimination laws concerning age, sex, or race are examples. Rules regarding recall rights or affirmative action could be called broadly allocative since they involve the differential allocation of resources to different groups.

All three strategies, whether they involve changes in persons, opportunity structures, or allocation rules, assume successful negotiation among interested parties, including individuals, communities, organized labor, employer firms, and the government. Strategies that redefine allocation rules are probably most important for persons with fewer resources to obtain employment, including those who are economically dependent or with lower levels of marketable skills or education. At the same time, the economic context of the community or region may also play a critical role in shaping the degree to which successful negotiation between various societal actors is possible. One could imagine more and more pressure might be put on some allocation rules, such as affirmative action or seniority, as jobs and economic opportunities become increasingly scarce in a particular area.

No single strategy will be appropriate for all groups, varying as they do in economic and personal resources. Nor will a single strategy serve best in community and economic contexts that vary widely in opportunities. The challenge is to use a broad framework of this kind to more clearly understand the goals and limitations of apparently disparate programmatic and policy efforts. Beyond the framework itself lies a search for complementary incentives to encourage the transformation of individual skills, opportunity structures, and the rules that govern work relationships. We have not yet done our best there, looking for work relationships that offer complementary rewards to both worker and employer, and that present new opportunities to transform the nature of work and community.

REFERENCES

Blinder, A. S. (1987). *Hard heads and soft hearts: Tough minded economics for a just society.* Reading, MA: Addison-Wesley.

Caplan, R. D., Vinokur, A. D., Price, R. H., & van Ryn, M. (1989). Job seeking, reemployment and mental health: A randomized field experiment in coping with job loss. *Journal of Applied Psychology, 74,* 759–769.

Catalano, R. (1991). The health effects of economic insecurity. *American Journal of Public Health, 71,* 1148–1152.

Catalano, R., Dooley, D., Wilson, G., & Hough, R. (1993). Using ECA survey data to examine the effect of job layoffs on violent behavior. *Hospital and Community Psychiatry, 44,* 874–879.

Dooley, D., Catalano, R., & Hough, R. (1992). Unemployment and alcohol disorder in 1910 and 1990: Drift versus social causation. *Journal of Occupational and Organizational Psychology, 65,* 277–290.

Dooley, D., Catalano, R., & Wilson, (1994). Depression and unemployment: Panel findings from the Epidemiologic Catchment Area study. *American Journal of Community Psychology,* 22, 745–765.

Gordus, J. P., & McAlinden, S. P. (1984). *Economic change, physical illness and social deviance: Report for the Joint Economic Committee, Congress of the United States.* Washington, D.C.: U.S. Government Printing Office.

Hamilton, L. V., Broman, C. L., Hoffman, W. S., & Brenner, D. (1990). Hard times and vulnerable people: Initial effects of plant closing on autoworkers' mental health. *Journal of Health and Social Behavior, 31,* 123–140

Kessler, R. C., House, J. S., & Turner, B. (1988). Effects of unemployment on health in a community survey: Main, modifying, and mediating effects. *Journal of Social Issues, 44,* 69–86.

Kozlowski, S. W. J., Chao, G. T., Smith, E. M., & Hedlund, J. (1993). Organizational downsizing: Strategies, interventions, and research implications. *International Review of Industrial and Organizational Psychology.* New York: Wiley.

Last, L. R., Peterson, R. W. E., Rappaport, J., & Webb, C. A. (1995). Creating opportunities for displaced workers: Center for Commercial Competitiveness. In M. London (Ed.), *Employees, careers, and job creation: Developing growth-oriented human resource strategies and programs* (pp. 210–233). San Francisco: Jossey-Bass.

London, M. (Ed.). (1995). *Employees, careers, and job creation: Developing growth-oriented human resource strategies and programs.* San Francisco: Jossey-Bass.

Price, R. H. (1990). Strategies for managing plant closings and downsizing. In D. Fishman & C. Chemiss (Eds.), *The human side of corporate competitiveness* (pp. 127–151). Beverly Hills: Sage.

Price, R. H. (1992). Psychosocial impact of job loss on individuals and families. *Current Directions in Psychological Science, 1,* 9–11.

Price, R. H., & Burke, A. C. (1985). Tensions in collaborative research on youth employment. In R. Rappaport (Ed.), *Research and action: A collaborative-interactive approach.* Cambridge, MA: Cambridge University Press.

Price, R. H., Friedland, D. S., Choi, J., & Caplan, R. D. (1998). Job loss and work transitions in a time of global economic change. In X. Arriaga & S. Oskamp (Eds.), *Addressing community problems* (pp. 195–222). Thousand Oaks, CA: Sage.

Price, R. H., Friedland, D. S., & Vinokur, A. D. (in press). Job loss: Hard times and eroded identity. In J. Harvey (Ed.), *Perspectives on loss: A source book.* Washington, D.C.: Taylor & Francis.

Price, R. H., van Ryn, M., & Vinokur, A. (1992). Impact of a preventive job search intervention on the likelihood of depression among the unemployed. *Journal of Health and Social Behavior, 33,* 158–167.

Vinokur, A. D. (1998). Job security: Unemployment. In J. M. Tellman (Ed.), *Encyclopedia of occupational health and safety* (4th ed.). Geneva: International Labor Office.
Vinokur, A. D., Price, R. H., & Caplan, R. D. (1991). From field experiments to program implementation: Assessing the potential outcomes of an experimental intervention program for unemployed persons. *American Journal of Community Psychology, 19,* 543–562.
Vinokur, A. D., Price, R. H., & Caplan, R. D. (1996). Hard times and hurtful partners: How financial strain affects depression and relationship satisfaction of unemployed persons and their spouses. *Journal of Personality and Social Psychology, 71,* 166–179.
Vinokur, A. D., Price, R. H., & Schul, Y. (1995). Impact of the JOBS intervention on unemployed workers varying in risk for depression. *American Journal of Community Psychology, 23,* 39–74.
Vinokur, A. D., & Schul, Y. (1997). Mastery and inoculation against setbacks as active ingredients in the JOBS intervention for the unemployed. *Journal of Consulting and Clinical Psychology, 65,* 867–877.
Vinokur, A. D., van Ryn, M., Gramlich, E. M., & Price, R. H. (1991). Long-term follow-up and benefit-cost analysis of the JOBS program: A preventive intervention for the unemployed. *Journal of Applied Psychology, 76,* 213–219.

I. Violence Prevention

Carrie S. Fried, N. Dickon Reppucci, and Jennifer L. Woolard

The increasing public awareness of the societal problems of youth violence, child maltreatment, and violence against women have led to the development of numerous preventive interventions over the past decade. This chapter provides a brief introduction to these emerging developments and discusses some of the issues surrounding these preventive efforts. Each issue could use its own chapter; however, our goal is not to provide an exhaustive review of any of these topics, but rather to alert community psychologists to their urgent need for alleviation. This chapter first provides a brief introduction to some of the issues surrounding prevention efforts in child maltreatment and violence against women. A more thorough discussion of youth violence-prevention efforts follows.

CHILD MALTREATMENT

In 1997, the National Committee to Prevent Child Abuse provided the statistic that 969,000 cases of child maltreatment were substantiated from the more than three million cases reported nationwide (Reppucci, Woolard, & Fried, 1999). As the magnitude and severity of the problem have become apparent over the past two decades, prevention programs have proliferated. Unfortunately, relatively few of these programs have been evaluated in a methodologically rigorous fashion that has included comparison groups and multilevel and multimeasurement data collection. Moreover, most evaluations have measured associated variables, such as familial stress, parental attitude change, child information, and social support, rather than examining actual abuse statistics longitudinally for families who have participated in these programs.

Carrie S. Fried and N. Dickon Reppucci • Department of Psychology, University of Virginia, Charlottesville, Virginia 22903. Jennifer L. Woolard • Department of Criminology, University of Florida, Gainesville, Florida 32611.

The two most frequent types of programs for preventing physical child abuse and neglect—parent training and community-based family support—focus on parents, especially mothers of young children. Parent-training programs attempt to change maternal attitudes, improve parenting skills, and reduce the use of corporal punishment. Although some success has been documented (Reppucci, Britner, & Woolard, 1997; Wekerle & Wolfe, 1993), parent training is often only one service offered as part of community-based family support programs that aim to alter some community- and societal-level risk factors, such as fragmented social services, poverty, social isolation, and access to health care (Limber & Nation, 1998). In addition to parent training, typical support programs usually include one or more of the following: support groups, drop-in centers, home visits, child care relief, and child health screening. Some solid empirical support exists for these programs having both short- and long-term benefits (e.g., Wolfe, Reppucci, & Hart, 1995; Zigler, Taussig, & Black, 1992).

Child sexual abuse prevention programs tend to target children rather than parents, and are so widespread that millions of children, usually in elementary schools, are exposed to them annually. However, evaluations of their effectiveness are few, and most are seriously flawed methodologically (Reppucci, Land, & Haugaard, 1998). The major result is that children do acquire some information and that disclosure, rather than primary prevention, may occur, but data about the percentage of disclosures that are substantiated are seldom presented. Major questions also exist regarding the appropriateness of targeting the children themselves, especially those under ten years of age, as their own protectors.

While public and professional awareness of the societal problem of violence against children is probably at an all-time high, few indicators suggest any alleviation of the problem. In the past, few community psychologists have focused on this problem, either in research or practice. (For a more comprehensive review, see Trickett & Schellenbach, 1998.)

VIOLENCE AGAINST WOMEN

The 1990s were an extraordinary decade for highlighting the problem of violence against women. Despite the significant gains in understanding the nature and impact of violence, only recently has research examined interventions for the prevention of sexual assault and family violence (Browne, 1993). Sexual-assault interventions have focused primarily on risk reduction in women, although recent efforts target males as well. A consistent theme highlights the promise of innovative techniques and approaches that have not yet been systematically documented or evaluated.

Like other social problems, violence against women is a complex, multidetermined phenomenon that is difficult to prevent through single or isolated strategies. In part because many studies have documented the existence of "rape myths" or rape-supportive beliefs, and a correlation between such attitudes/beliefs and aggression (or proclivity for aggression), many prevention programs for men and women focus on debunking such myths and changing attitudes. Although some argue that interventions for women do not "prevent" rape (which is usually perpetrated by males), a number of intervention programs tailored for women focus on identifying and ameliorating risk factors associated with increased likelihood of sexual assault. Common intervention techniques include addressing rape mythology, interactive participation, sex education and feminist orientation, empathy induction, and confrontation for women-only and mixed-sex groups (Lonsway, 1996). The current research on attitudes and behaviors provides an important step in understanding the short-term impact of educational interventions, but as with other types of social interventions, the link between attitude change and behavior change has not been established.

Although victim advocates have been providing shelter and advocacy services to victims of family violence for more than two decades, researchers have been somewhat slower to devise theory-based methods of systematic evaluation. A number of programs have been developed to provide support services to battered women and their children, as well as treatment services to male offenders. In the past several years, a few studies have begun to evaluate the efficacy of these services (see Gordon, 1996).

Recent studies have extended the intervention evaluation research by assigning participants to advocacy and control groups and evaluating short- and long-term follow-up of service efficacy (Sullivan, Campbell, Angelique, Eby, & Davidson, 1994). Future research can continue the important effects of documenting the impact of victimization, the process of accessing resources, and the barriers to negotiating systems successfully. However, research must also move forward to include multiple methods and information sources for evaluating the impact of interventions, and to place interventions within the larger community context of advocacy, service delivery, and justice-system processing. (For a more comprehensive review, see Crowell & Burgess, 1996.)

YOUTH VIOLENCE

Media coverage of the school shooting orchestrated by an 11-year-old and a 13-year-old in Jonesboro, Arkansas in March of 1998, and subsequent school shootings, especially the massacre at Columbine High School in Littleton, Colorado in April of 1999 have magnified the attention focused on youth violence. While the media spotlight certainly exaggerates the reality, there is no doubt that violent acts by and against youths are an enormous social problem. Nearly one in five of all violent-crime arrests in 1994 involved a juvenile under 18 years of age (Snyder, Sickmond, & Poe-Yamagata, 1996). Arrest rates for homicide among 14- to 17-year-olds increased 41% between 1989 and 1994, compared with an increase of 18% among 18- to 24-year-olds, and a decrease of 19% among adults over 25 (Fox, 1996). The prevalence and easy availability of firearms has exacerbated the impact of youth violence (Blumstein, 1995).

Responses to increases in youth violence have generally come in two forms. The first has been an effort to protect society from the young "super predators" by enacting tougher juvenile crime legislation. Between 1992 and 1995, 21 states toughened their juvenile justice systems by enacting laws that make it easier to prosecute juveniles as adults (Sickmund, Snyder, & Poe-Yamagata, 1997). Other legislative mechanisms designed to control violent criminal behavior include minimum sentencing requirements, blended sentencing that allows juveniles to be sentenced past the age of 21, revision of confidentiality provisions in favor of more open proceedings and records, and enactment of curfew ordinances. Some proponents of these policies believe that getting tough on crime will have a deterrent effect on potential violent offenders. However, harsher sentences do not appear to be effective in deterring violent criminal behavior (Gottfredson & Hirschi, 1995), and curfew programs appear only to be successful when they are part of a comprehensive, community-based plan to reduce juvenile crime and victimization (LeBoeuf, 1996; Ruefle & Reynolds, 1995).

The second response, and our primary focus, is the prevention of youth violence through programmatic intervention. Research on youth violence has benefitted from integrating the paradigms of several disciplines, including public health, sociology, and developmental, community, and clinical psychology. Specifically, recent intervention research has focused on the identification of important risk and protective factors, adopted an epidemiological and developmental framework, and targeted interventions at multiple levels (e.g., individual, family, school, neighborhood) (Reppucci et al., 1999).

The Centers for Disease Control and Prevention highlighted a public health approach to violence prevention, funding 15 demonstration intervention projects in 1992 and 1993 and four additional projects in 1996 (Powell & Hawkins, 1996; National Center for Injury Prevention and Control, 1998). All rely on theoretical models, and each has a rigorous evaluation design to measure attitudinal and behavioral changes. Of the original 15 programs, 7 employ social learning theory, which assumes that aggression and violence are learned behaviors that can be unlearned. Four programs mention attribution theory, supporting the notion that individuals can be trained to correct their misattribution of others' intentions as hostile, which would presumably result in less hostile and aggressive responses. The target populations of the original 15 programs range from 5–20 years of age, while those of the four new programs range from 3–10 years of age, possibly reflecting the need to begin violence prevention as early as possible. Among all 19 funded programs, interventions are most often focused at the individual level, including cognitive-behavioral and social-skills training. Other common interventions are parent training, peer mediation, and changing institutional practices. Rigorous evaluations are in progress, and will hopefully identify the types and components of programs that are most successful in preventing youth violence. Other organizations, such as the American Psychological Association (see Eron, Gentry, & Schlegel, 1994) and various foundations, have also focused on youth violence prevention in recent years.

Using a public health model, we examine the theory, methodology, and efficacy of primary-prevention interventions, and then comment briefly on secondary and tertiary efforts. Based on the distinctions made by Mulvey, Arthur, and Reppucci (1993) in their review of the literature on the prevention and treatment of juvenile delinquency, primary-prevention programs are defined as those programs based on the identification of individuals or environments at risk for violence before violent behavior has occurred. Secondary-prevention programs rely on early identification of violent behavior and attempt to modify behavior before serious acts of violence occur. Tertiary prevention is reserved for individuals already identified as chronically violent and involves treatment to modify behavior. Within each level we also emphasize the importance of a multisystemic approach to violence prevention.

Primary Prevention

The identification and amelioration of risks and/or the identification and enhancement of protective factors are the main focus of primary-prevention programs. Difficult temperament, childhood aggression, school failure, association with deviant peers, coercive parenting styles, experience of prior sexual abuse, and exposure to violence are several of the documented risk factors for later violent behavior (Loeber & Hay, 1997; Mattiani, Twyman, Chin, & Nam Lee, 1996). Some of the protective factors that can counteract the impact of the risk factors include good maternal health, positive relationships that promote close bonds, high IQ, and a high level of caretaker attention (McGuire, 1997; Hawkins, 1995). Parent training, social skills training, anger management, conflict resolution, classroom education about violence, empowerment initiatives, peer leadership and mediation, community organization, and mass media campaigns are all examples of primary-prevention efforts. According to Prothrow-Stith (1995), primary-prevention programs seek to make nonviolence popular.

Teaching of alternative, nonviolent methods of conflict resolution and problem-solving are extremely popular, even though there is little evidence of their ability to change behavior. Webster (1993) has suggested that they rely too heavily on cognitive and skill deficits, while virtually ignoring motivational and emotional issues surrounding the use of violence. However, there is some evidence that social-skills training programs can be effective in reducing aggression. For example, "Second Step: A Violence Prevention Curriculum" consists of 30 lessons to teach social skills related to anger management, impulse control, and empathy to second and third graders. Evaluation data indicate a decrease in physical aggression and an increase in neutral/prosocial behaviors that persisted in a 6-month follow-up evaluation (Grossman, Neckerman, Koepsell, Liu, Asher, Beland, Frey, & Rivara, 1997). Considering the popularity of social-skills training and conflict-resolution programs, it is disappointing that so few of them have been evaluated and that those few do not provide long enough follow-up evaluations.

Community organization and mass-media campaigns are additional primary-prevention strategies. Evaluation of these strategies is difficult, so it is not surprising that their usefulness in preventing violent behavior has yet to be demonstrated (Tolan & Guerra, 1994). However, one media campaign, "Choose to De-Fuse," conducted focus groups with at-risk youth to qualitatively evaluate how the message was received by the target population. The program is exciting because it involved at-risk youth in the creation of a media campaign. Moreover, the program description indicates that multiple other program components will be evaluated to determine if there was any impact on violent behavior (Levine & Zimmerman, 1996). Perhaps the most exciting approach to the prevention of adolescent problem behaviors is the "Communities That Care" program (Hawkins & Catalano, 1992), a risk-focused social development strategy that involves representative members from the entire community in creating a program to reduce violence and other adolescent problem behaviors. Community risk and protective factors are identified to help local leaders in planning an intervention strategy to reduce risks and enhance protective factors at multiple levels.

A creative new idea in the prevention of youth violence is the use of empowerment through volunteer work. The Youth Relationships Project (YRP) focuses on how youth serve as resources to their families, schools, and communities (Wolfe, Wkerle, & Scott, 1997). The project is based on an empowerment model that involves target group members in meaningful activities, such as volunteer work. Similarly, the Teen Outreach Program, which is aimed at preventing pregnancy and school dropout through the use of volunteer services and weekly classroom discussions of these activities, has been rigorously evaluated nationwide and has demonstrated a significant decrease in teen pregnancy, school failure, and school dropout (Allen, Philliber, Herrling, & Kuperminc, 1997). Teen Outreach appears to be effective because it helps adolescents negotiate the social development tasks of establishing autonomy while maintaining healthy relationships. The theoretical basis for Teen Outreach is similar to that of the YRP, which attempts to reduce youth violence by encouraging the development of healthy, non-violent interpersonal relationships. The first part of the YRP program provides information about interpersonal violence, especially within the context of intimate relationships, and teaches adaptive communication and conflict resolution skills. The participants then organize and carry out a community project that involves a violence prevention theme. Results of the evaluation of the YRP may further encourage the use of volunteer activities in the prevention of violence.

Secondary Prevention

The main difference between primary and secondary prevention is the focus on a target population that has already been identified as aggressive or violent. Secondary-prevention programs may include mentoring or rites-of-passage programs; individual, family, and group counseling; first offender programs, and social-skills training (Corvo, 1997; Prothrow-Stith, 1995). Rites-of-passage programs may guide young people to prosocial values, but there is little empirical support for their effectiveness in preventing violence (O'Donnell, Cohen, & Hausman, 1991). Family interventions that alter family organization, functioning, relationships, or parenting styles are among the most effective in affecting child behavior (Tolan & Guerra, 1994).

One of the Centers for Disease Control evaluation projects is targeted toward hospital patients who have been beaten, stabbed, or shot, to help them understand their risks and to connect them with community programs (De Vos, Stone, Geotz, & Dahlberg, 1996). Supporting Adolescents with Guidance and Employment (SAGE) focuses on a target population of African-American male adolescents, many of whom have previously engaged in violence-related behaviors (Ringwalt, Graham, Paschall, Flewelling, & Browne, 1996). Selection of participants was unclear, so it may be considered a primary-prevention program for some participants. The SAGE program includes a rites-of-passage component, as well as a summer employment and an entrepreneurial experience component. Random assignment of youth to receive all program components, or only the employment and entrepreneurial components, will allow for the evaluation of the distinct parts of the program.

Tertiary Prevention

Tertiary-prevention programs include incarceration, rehabilitation, reintegration into the community following incarceration, and therapy. As mentioned earlier, incarceration has not been proven to be effective in reducing crime. Based on evaluation data, one of the most effective means of violence prevention may be the use of multisystemic therapy (MST) with serious juvenile offenders. MST is a highly individualized family- and community-based therapeutic approach that views behavior as the end product of the interactions between individuals and their interconnected systems (e.g., family, school, community). Treatment plans, developed with the family, integrate family, school, community, peer, and individual interventions (Henggeler, Cunningham, Pickrel, Schoenwald, & Brodino, 1996).

Two studies of MST demonstrate its effectiveness in reducing rearrest rates and out-of-home-placement, and improving family functioning. A random assignment of 84 serious offenders in Simpsonville, South Carolina, half to usual services and half to MST, found that control group youth were twice as likely to be rearrested as youth in MST (Henggeler, Melton, & Smith, 1992). Another study compared 176 Columbia, Missouri, youth randomly assigned to either MST or individual therapy (Borduin, Mann, Cone, Henggeler, Fucci, Blaske, & Williams, 1995). Results from a four-year follow-up indicated that the rearrest rate among MST therapy completers was 22%, as compared with 47% for MST dropouts, 71% for individual therapy completers, and 71% for individual therapy dropouts. Results are encouraging from both a treatment and a public policy perspective, since the cost of MST is substantially less than the cost of out-of-home placement (Tate, Reppucci, & Mulvey, 1995).

Special Considerations of Urban Youth

The impact of chronic exposure to poverty and violence must be considered in planning violence prevention programs. These conditions of the inner city and multiple risk factors faced by youth who live in these neighborhoods make it more difficult to implement intervention programs and less likely that they will be potent enough to produce lasting effects (Guerra,

Attar, & Weissberg, 1997). Several well-known primary-prevention programs, like Head Start and the Perry Preschool Project, have reported long-term reductions in aggression and delinquency among disadvantaged, urban youth. A 20-session training in social skills, conflict resolution, and anger management, designed specifically for African American adolescents, was evaluated at a three-year follow-up. Results indicated that 18% of participants had subsequent juvenile court involvement, compared with 49% of control youth (Hammond & Yung, 1993, in Guerra et al., 1997). Parent training and peer leadership programs have been less successful in demonstrating a reduction in violence among inner-city youth (Guerra et al., 1997).

CONCLUSIONS

Preventive interventions in child maltreatment, violence against women, and youth violence suffer from several of the same methodological and theoretical limitations. First, although public concern about violence has led to the proliferation of prevention programs, most are unevaluated or poorly evaluated. The tension between the immediate need for action and the need for time intensive evaluation plagues violence prevention efforts. A second, and related, problem is the lack of a strong theoretical base in program development. Third, success of programs is too often evaluated on the basis of change in attitude rather than change in behavior, which is essential, and follow-up is usually too brief to demonstrate long-term effectiveness. Fourth, when programs are evaluated, it is often impossible to distinguish between components that are essential to the success of the program and those that are superfluous, or even harmful. Finally, the replication of successful prevention strategies often does not take into account the developmental and cultural differences in target populations. Programs that are successful with white, middle-class youth often have no effect, or even deleterious effects, when implemented with poor, urban, minority youths (Guerra et al., 1997).

The development of programs to prevent violence is still in its infancy, and the paucity of evaluation data supporting their efficacy should not be interpreted as a sign that nothing works. The lack of programmatic success in reducing violence is less discouraging when put in the context of the culture of violence experienced in America. As stated by Earls, Cairns, and Mercy (1993):

> In the face of these barriers [easy availability of and access to guns, widespread use of alcohol and drugs, the decay of central city areas, and high cultural tolerance for violence], efforts in health promotion to decrease violent encounters may be equivalent to trying to control an epidemic of tuberculosis in a densely populated area without adequate sanitation.... What we need to promote nonviolence as a health objective is something analogous to what was needed to control infectious diseases toward the end of the last century: vast environmental and policy changes. (p. 296)

Several innovative programs are underway and evaluation data should be available within the next few years. The field of violence prevention will benefit from greater involvement on the part of community psychologists with experience in program planning and evaluation.

REFERENCES

Allen, J. P., Philliber, S., Herrling, S., & Kuperminc, G. P. (1997). Preventing teen pregnancy and academic failure: Experimental evaluation of a developmentally based approach. *Child Development*, *64*, 729–742.

Blumstein, A. (1995). Violence by young people: Why the deadly nexus? *National Institute of Justice Journal*, *August*, 2–9.

Borduin, C. M., Mann, B. J., Cone, L. T., Henggeler, S. W., Fucci, B. R., Blaske, D. M., & Williams, R. A. (1995).

Multisystemic treatment of serious juvenile offenders: Long-term prevention of criminality and violence. *Journal of Consulting and Clinical Psychology, 63,* 569–578.

Browne, A. (1993). Violence against women by male partners: Prevalence, outcomes, and policy implications. *American Psychologist, 48,* 1077–1087.

Corvo, K. N. (1997). Community-based youth violence prevention: A framework for planners and funders. *Youth & Society, 28,* 291–316.

Crowell, N. A., & Burgess, A. W. (Eds.). (1996). *Understanding violence against women.* Washington, D.C.: National Academy Press.

De Vos, E., Stone, D. A., Goetz, M. A., & Dahlberg, L. L. (1996). Evaluation of a hospital-based youth violence intervention. *American Journal of Preventive Medicine, 12,* 101–108.

Earls, F., Cairns, R. B., & Mercy, J. A. (1993). The control of violence and the promotion of nonviolence in adolescents. In S. G. Millstein, A. C. Petersen, & E. O. Nightingale (Eds.), *Promoting the health of adolescents: New directions for the 21st century* (pp. 285–304). New York: Oxford University Press.

Eron, L. D., Gentry, J. H., & Schlegel, P. (Eds.). (1994). *Reason to hope: A psychosocial perspective on violence and youth.* Washington, D.C.: American Psychological Association.

Fox, J. A. (1996). *Trends in juvenile violence: A report to the United States Attorney General on current and future rates of juvenile offending.* Washington, D.C.: U.S. Department of Justice, Bureau of Justice Statistics.

Gordon, J. S. (1996). Community services for abused women: A review of perceived usefulness and efficacy. *Journal of Family Violence, 11,* 315–329.

Gottfredson, M. R., & Hirschi, T. (1995). National crime control policies. *Society, 32,* 30–36.

Grossman, D. C., Neckerman, H. J., Koepsell, T. D., Liu, P. Y., Asher, K. N., Beland, K., Frey, K., & Rivara, F. P. (1997). Effectiveness of a violence prevention curriculum among children in elementary school. *Journal of the American Medical Association, 277,* 1605–1611.

Guerra, N. G., Attar, B., & Weissberg, R. P. (1997). Prevention of aggression and violence among inner-city youths. In D. M. Stoff & J. Breiling (Eds.), *Handbook of antisocial behavior* (pp. 375–383). New York: Wiley.

Hammond, R., & Yung, B. (1993). *Evaluation and activity report: Positive adolescents choices training grant.* Unpublished grant report, U.S. Maternal and Child Health Bureau.

Hawkins, D. (1995). Controlling crime before it happens: Risk focused prevention. *National Institute of Justice Journal, August,* 10–18.

Hawkins, J. D., & Catalano, R. F. (1992). *Communities that care: Action for drug abuse prevention.* San Francisco: Jossey-Bass.

Henggeler, S. W., Cunningham, P. B., Pickrel, S. G., Schoenwald, S. K., & Brondino, M. J. (1996). Multisystemic therapy: An effective violence prevention approach for serious juvenile offenders. *Journal of Adolescence, 19,* 47–61.

Henggeler, S. W., Melton, G. B., & Smith, L. A. (1992). Family preservation using multisystemic therapy: An effective alternative to incarcerating serious juvenile offenders. *Journal of Consulting and Clinical Psychology, 60,* 953–961.

LeBoeuf, D. (1996). *Curfew: An answer to juvenile delinquency and victimization?* Washington, D.C.: U.S. Department of Justice, Office of Juvenile Justice and Delinquency Prevention.

Levine, I. S., & Zimmerman, J. D. (1996). Using qualitative data to inform public policy: Evaluating "Choose to De-Fuse." *American Journal of Orthopsychiatry, 66,* 363–377.

Limber, S., & Nation, M. (1998). Violence within the neighborhood and community. In P. Trickett & C. Schellenbach (Eds.), *Violence against children in the family and the community* (pp. 171–193). Washington, D.C.: American Psychological Association.

Loeber, R., & Hay, D. (1997). Key issues in the development of aggression and violence from childhood to early adulthood. *Annual Review of Psychology, 48,* 371–410.

Lonsway, K. A. (1996). Preventing acquaintance rape through education: What do we know? *Psychology of Women Quarterly, 20,* 229–265.

Mattaini, M. A., Twyman, J. S., Chin, W., & Nam Lee, K. (1996). Youth violence. In M. A. Mattaini & B. A. Thyer (Eds.), *Finding solutions to social problems: Behavioral strategies for change* (pp. 75–111). Washington, D.C.: American Psychological Association.

McGuire, J. (1997). Psycho-social approaches to the understanding and reduction of violence in young people. In V. Varma (Ed.), *Violence in children and adolescents* (pp. 65–83). Bristol, PA: Jessica Kingsley.

Mulvey, E. P., Arthur, M. W., & Reppucci, N. D. (1993). The prevention and treatment of juvenile delinquency: A review of the research. *Clinical Psychology Review, 13,* 133–167.

National Center for Injury Prevention and Control. (1998). Evaluation of specific youth violence intervention projects. www.cdc.gov/ncipc/dvp/evalyv.htm.

O'Donnell, L., Cohen, S., & Hausman, A. (1991). Evaluation of community-based violence prevention programs. *Public Health Reports, 106,* 276–277.

Powell, K. E., & Hawkins, D. F. (1996). Youth violence prevention: Descriptions and baseline data from 13 evaluation projects. *American Journal of Preventive Medicine, 12*(5, Suppl), 1–13.

Prothrow-Stith, D. B. (1995). The epidemic of youth violence in America: Using public health prevention strategies to prevent violence. *Journal of Health Care for the Poor and Underserved, 6*, 95–101.

Reppucci, N., Britner, P., & Woolard, J. (1997). *Preventing child abuse and neglect through parent education.* Baltimore: Paul H. Brookes.

Reppucci, N., Land, D., & Haugaard, J. (1998). Child sexual abuse prevention programs that target young children. In P. Trickett & C. Schellenbach (Eds.), *Violence against children in the family and the community* (pp. 317–337). Washington, D.C.: American Psychological Association.

Reppucci, N., Woolard, J., & Fried, C. (1999). Social, community and preventive interventions. *Annual Review of Psychology, 50*, 387–418.

Ringwalt, C. L., Graham, L. A., Paschall, M. J., Flewelling, R. L., & Browne, D. C. (1996). Supporting adolescents with guidance and employment (SAGE). *American Journal of Preventive Medicine, 12*, 31–38.

Ruefle, W., & Reynolds, K. M. (1995). Curfews and delinquency in major American cities. *Crime & Delinquency, 41*, 347–363.

Sickmund, M., Snyder, H. N., & Poe-Yamagata, E. (1997). *Juvenile offenders and victims: 1997 update on violence.* Washington, D.C.: Office of Juvenile and Delinquency Prevention.

Snyder, H. N., Sickmund, M., & Poe-Yamagata, E. (1996). *Juvenile offenders and victims: 1996 update on violence.* Washington, D.C.: Office of Juvenile and Delinquency Prevention.

Sullivan, C. M., Campbell, R., Angelique, H., Eby, K. K., & Davidson, W. S., II. (1994). An advocacy intervention program for women with abusive partners: Six-month follow-up. *American Journal of Community Psychology, 22*, 101–122.

Tate, D. C., Reppucci, N. D., & Mulvey, E. P. (1995). Violent juvenile delinquents: Treatment effectiveness and implications for future action. *American Psychologist, 50*, 777–781.

Tolan, P. H., & Guerra, N. G. (1994). *What works in reducing adolescent violence: An empirical view of the field.* Monograph prepared for the Center for the Study and Prevention of Youth Violence, Boulder, CO.

Trickett, P., & Schellenbach, C. (Eds.). (1998). *Violence against children in the family and the community.* Washington, D.C.: American Psychological Association.

Webster, D. W. (1993). The unconvincing case for school-based conflict resolution. *Health Affairs, 12*, 126–141.

Wekerle, C., & Wolfe, D. (1993). Prevention of child physical abuse and neglect: Promising new directions. *Clinical Psychology Review, 13*, 501–540.

Wolfe, D., Reppucci, N., & Hart, S. (1995). Child abuse prevention: Knowledge and priorities. *Journal of Clinical Child Psychology, 24*, 5–22.

Wolfe, D., Wekerle, C., & Scott, K. (1997). *Alternatives to violence: Empowering youth to develop healthy relationships.* Thousand Oaks, CA: Sage.

Zigler, E., Taussig, C., & Black, K. (1992). Early childhood intervention: A promising preventive for juvenile delinquency. *American Psychologist, 47*, 997–1006.

J. Substance Abuse Prevention

JEAN E. RHODES

INTRODUCTION

Substance abuse is a complex problem that presents a significant challenge to the social, educational, medical, and criminal justice systems of this country. It is directly associated with such problems as corruption, violence, and the spread of AIDS. As awareness of the personal and societal costs of substance abuse continues to mount, so too does our interest in under-

JEAN E. RHODES • Department of Psychology, University of Illinois, Champaign, Illinois 61820.

standing its causes and solutions. During the past three decades, considerable research attention, as well as generous budgetary allocations, have been directed toward the problem.

Despite these recent trends, it should be noted that substance abuse is not a new social problem. In fact, the first major American epidemic of substance abuse began in the mid 1880s, with the increased public acceptance and use of cocaine and opiates. By the 1920s, as people gradually began to recognize their harmful effects and became disillusioned with the drugs, the epidemic began to subside (Musto, 1987). The second major surge in usage began in the late 1960s, and included such drugs as marijuana, heroin, cocaine, and LSD. According to findings from an annual, national survey of over 50,000 youth (Johnston, Bachman, & O'Malley, 1997), this usage peaked in 1979 and then fell throughout the 1980s. By the early 1990s, it appeared that prevention efforts were taking hold. Unfortunately, there has been a considerable relapse in substance use in recent years. Indeed, usage rates of some substances have reached two to three times what they were just seven years ago. In addition, new drugs such as MDMA (ecstasy) and crystal methamphetamine (ice) have been introduced to American youth. Results of the most recent survey suggest that substance use and abuse among adolescents may be stabilizing. Although marijuana use continues to rise among older students, the use of a number of other substances has begun to level off. In addition, attitudes and beliefs about drugs, which are important determinants of usage, have become more negative in recent years (Johnston et al., 1997).

PSYCHOLOGICAL AND SOCIOPOLITICAL DIMENSIONS OF THE PROBLEM

In addition to tracking usage patterns, many researchers have attempted to understand and address the causes of substance abuse. Most conceptual models of substance abuse emphasize individual personality and coping-skills variables, and the ways in which these factors interact to predispose individuals to substance abusing behaviors. Substance use is generally viewed as a learned behavior, shaped through a process of modeling and reinforcement and mediated by attitudes and beliefs. A wide range of personal characteristics that may place individuals at risk have been identified, including: low religiosity, low self-esteem, lack of clear value positions, poor interpersonal relations, poor coping strategies, and difficulties countering pressures to use drugs (Rhodes & Jason, 1990). Along these lines, Johnston et al. (1997) have described a lack of information, fewer negative messages, and fewer opportunities to observe the harmful effects of substance abuse as contributing factors in recent substance abuse trends.

Given this overall concentration on the role of individual observations, behaviors, and beliefs, work in the field of substance abuse prevention has tended to highlight the role of person-oriented cognitive and behavioral interventions. These interventions, particularly the more traditional information-based approaches, have produced few consistent, long-term behavioral changes. Newer approaches, including teaching refusal skills and general competencies, and correcting perceptions of social norms, have shown some promise, particularly among middle-class youth (Catalano, Hawkins, Krenz, Gillmore, Morrison, Wells, & Abbott, 1997). For example, Botvin (1996) has developed a cognitive-behavioral prevention approach that teaches skills for resisting social influences and promotes the development of general personal self-management and social skills.

Along with the person-centered approaches, recent prevention initiatives have been aimed at controlling the user and the supply of drugs in this country. The Reagan administration allocated an unprecedented 80% of the nation's anti-drug budget to law enforcement and interdiction, while funding for education and treatment programs declined throughout the 1980s. These efforts have continued, with an ongoing emphasis on drug testing, severe prison terms, and costly attempts to stop the flow of drugs into the United States (Humphreys & Rappaport, 1993).

Despite the success of some of these measures, a growing number of researchers have begun to point to their limitations. There is growing evidence that children who live in poverty and/or in severely troubled homes need changes in their environment that reach beyond what can be done through traditional school-based programs and efforts to limit the supply (Jason & Barnes, 1997). These communities are beset by extreme socioeconomic disadvantages, which directly influence their members' drug use behaviors. Inner-city communities and schools are often lacking in basic resources, and the high school dropout rate in many urban schools approaches 50%. Many of the young people in these communities find themselves confronted with crime, violence, and drug dealing. As such, there is a need to conceptualize substance abuse within broader social and economic contexts (Forgey, Schinke, & Cole, 1997).

CHALLENGES FOR THE 21ST CENTURY

Drug abuse is a persistent problem in this country that will continue to require concerted prevention efforts. With the help of many sectors, including the family, school, community, media, and policymakers, individuals must continue to be persuaded and educated about the dangers of drugs. At the same time, worsening socioeconomic conditions in some communities are tragically undermining families and neighborhoods, and these changes necessitate a more ecological orientation. To date, our research, intervention, and funding priorities have largely ignored the crucial contributing role of contextual variables in substance abuse. Interventions should be broadened such that the underlying health, social, economic, and cultural issues associated the problem are addressed (Humphreys & Rappaport, 1983; Jason & Barnes, 1997; Kim, Crutchfield, Williams, & Hepler, 1998; Skolnick, 1992). Efforts toward redefining and addressing substance abuse as a persistent public health and social problem, rather than as a personal deficit, are likely to lead us toward more promising approaches to substance abuse prevention.

REFERENCES

Botvin, G. J. (1996). Substance abuse prevention through life skills training. In R. D. Peters & R. J. McMahon (Eds.), *Preventing childhood disorders, substance abuse, and delinquency. Banff international behavioral science series, vol. 3* (pp. 215–240). Thousand Oaks, CA: Sage.

Catalano, R. F., Hawkins, J. D., Krenz, C., Gillmore, M., Morrison, D., Wells, E., & Abbott, R. (1997). Using research to guide culturally appropriate drug abuse prevention. In G. A. Marlatt, & G. R. VandenBos (Eds.), *Addictive behaviors: Readings on etiology, prevention, and treatment* (pp. 857–874). Washington, D.C.: American Psychological Association.

Forgey, M. A., Schinke, S., & Cole, K. (1997). School-based interventions to prevent substance use among inner-city minority adolescents. In D. K. Wilson & J. R. Rodrigue (Eds.), *Health-promoting and health-compromising behaviors among minority adolescents: Application and practice in health psychology* (pp. 251–267). Washington, D.C.: American Psychological Association.

Humphreys, K., & Rappaport, J. (1983). From the community mental health movement to the war on drugs: A study in the definition of social problems. *American Psychologist 48*, 892–901.

Jason, L. A., & Barnes, H. E. (1997). Substance-abuse prevention: Beyond the schoolyard. *Applied & Preventive Psychology, 6*, 211–220.

Johnston, L. D., O'Malley, P. M., & Bachman, J. G. (1991). *Drug use among American high school seniors, college students and young adults, 1975–1990.* DHHS Publication No. (ADM)87-1535. Washington, D.C.: U.S. Government Printing Office.

Johnston, L., Bachman, J., & O'Malley, P. (December, 1997). Monitoring the future study. *News and Information Services.* University of Michigan, Ann Arbor.

Kim, S., Crutchfield, C., Williams, C., & Hepler, N. (1998). Toward a new paradigm in substance abuse and other problem behavior prevention for youth: Youth development and empowerment approach. *Journal of Drug Education, 28,* 1–17.

Musto, D. F. (1987). *The American disease: Origins of narcotic control.* New York: Oxford University Press.

Rhodes, J. E., & Jason, L. A. (1990). A social stress model of substance abuse. *Journal of Consulting and Clinical Psychology, 58,* 395–401.

Skolnick, J. H. (1992). Rethinking the drug problem. *Deadalus, 121,* 1–14.

K. Homelessness

MARYBETH SHINN

HOW HAS HOMELESSNESS BECOME AN EMERGING ISSUE?

Homelessness was not invented in the late 20th century, but has reemerged with a new face. In colonial times, towns supported local poor people in their own homes or those of neighbors, but attempted to exclude "vagabonds and idle persons" from outside the community (Rothman, 1971). Jacksonian-era reformers, convinced that "outdoor" (noninstitutional) relief created laziness, built almshouses for an undifferentiated group of men, women, and children who were too young, too old, or too disabled to work. Widespread homelessness, primarily among unattached men who were itinerant laborers, may be dated from the period following the Civil War (Hopper, 1990; Rossi, 1989), and has waxed and waned with economic cycles. The 19th century saw the segregation of homeless people into shantytowns at the borders of cities and skid rows within them. People who could not afford the price of a skid-row flop slept in police stations and jails.

At the start of the 20th century, police stationhouses were closed to homeless people, and municipal lodging houses opened, having features sometimes found today, including classification and referral of applicants for social case work, work requirements, limits on lengths of stay. Homelessness was at its height during the Great Depression, when skid rows overflowed into "Hoovervilles" and large warehouse-style shelters for men. Transients were still treated less sympathetically than the local poor; in New York in some years, more was spent on "Greyhound relief" (bus tickets out) than on direct benefits (Rossi, 1989, p. 18). Poor people who had relatives in the area were turned away as not truly in need of shelter.

After World War II, skid rows appeared to be on the decline, and many observers expected them to disappear. The rise of homelessness in the late 1970s and 1980s caught researchers and the public by surprise, as did its changing composition. The "old homeless" of

MARYBETH SHINN • Center for Community Research and Action, Department of Psychology, New York University, New York, New York 10003.

skid row were male, largely white, and typically over 50. The "new homeless" are younger and more likely to be members of minority groups. They are poorer than the men who lived on skid row two decades before. And they include not only single men, but women and families with children.

Recent research suggests that homelessness is widespread, but for most people, only a temporary state. A national telephone survey and shelter records in different cities converge in suggesting that about 3% of the population used shelters over a five-year period in the late 1980s (Burt, 1994; Culhane, Dejowski, Ibanez, Needham, & Macchia, 1994; Link, Susser, Stueve, Phelan, Moore, & Struening, 1994). Other institutions have also been pressed into service, particularly for the minority of homeless individuals with mental illness or chemical dependencies who travel "institutional circuits" that include shelters, mental hospitals, prisons, and jails, as well as staying with family or friends, and on the street (Hopper, Jost, Hay, Welber, & Haugland, 1997; Milofsky, Butto, Gross, & Baumohl, 1993).

PSYCHOLOGICAL AND SOCIOPOLITICAL PERSPECTIVES

Hopper (1990) describes the historical tension between two attitudes towards homelessness as "rooted in individual pathology and character deficiencies [or] in structural defects in the labor market" (p. 15). Antebellum thinking about poverty reflected both views: that poverty was "voluntary" and "a consequence of drunkenness, idleness, and vice of all kind" and that "SOCIETY ITSELF ... is the great and whole source" (as quoted in Rothman, 1971, pp. 162, 173; emphasis in the original).

Both strands of thinking are evident among researchers and policymakers today. The literature on homelessness is divided into a large and relentlessly negative catalogue of the defects of homeless citizens, with substance abuse, mental illness, and deficient social networks updating the 19th-century categories of drunkenness, idleness, and vice, and structural analysis that find contemporary homelessness rooted in loss of low-income housing coupled with increases in the amount and severity of poverty.

The individual view of homelessness has followed the classic steps of victim blaming, outlined by Ryan (1971, p. 8): identify a social problem, study those afflicted to determine how they differ from the rest of us, define the differences as the cause of the problem, and set up humanitarian programs to correct them. The structural view does not deny that many homeless people suffer mental illness or substance abuse, but it does not see these problems as the source of homelessness. Rather, homelessness is like a game of musical chairs in which the players are poor people and the chairs are the housing units they can afford or otherwise occupy by drawing on their personal networks. Individual problems influence vulnerability to homelessness. They determine which players, not how many, will be left homeless when the music stops (Koegel, Burnam, & Baumohl, 1996; McChesney, 1990).

Responses to homelessness in part follow views of causes, but also involve efforts to minimize responsibility and cost. Cooper (1989) noted that the first reaction of government to a social problem is to extrude it. The history of homelessness amply demonstrates this, from the colonists who sent poor strangers packing, to the "Greyhound relief" of the Depression. A more sophisticated effort to shift responsibility was shown by a recent New York City mayor who wanted to know from where (other than New York) homeless families came, how many were mentally ill, and where their husbands were (Shinn & Weitzman, 1990a). Conscious efforts have been made to make relief unattractive so as to deter its use, from the English poor law principle of "less eligibility" (e.g., Hopper, 1990), to Jacksonian almshouses designed to discourage malingering (Moroney & Kurtz, 1975), to the deliberately daunting conditions of some modern shelters (Basler, 1985). Depression-era screening to exclude people with any alternatives from shelter is echoed in city policies today.

KEY QUESTIONS FOR RESEARCH AND ACTION

Policies towards homelessness are driven as much by ideology as by research, yet there are areas where research can contribute to action. One such area is prevention, where the "research" to date consists largely of program descriptions and prescriptions, with little experimental study or even follow-up of program participants (Shinn & Baumohl, 1999). Indicated prevention strategies for people at risk require reasonably efficient targeting of such people, but a study of families suggests that even multivariate models are likely to identify many "false alarms" for each potentially homeless family correctly identified (Shinn, Weitzman, Stojanovic, Knickman, Jimenez, Duchon, James, & Krantz, 1998). Because people who become homeless, at least in some cities, originate disproportionately in certain neighborhoods (Culhane, Lee, & Wachter, 1996), community-development activities designed to increase the stock of affordable housing, foster employment, and provide supports to employment, such as transportation or child care, are worth trying as selected prevention strategies. Selected strategies, such as provision of subsidized housing, could also focus on poor renters.

Additional questions arise in helping homeless people to become rehoused, and in secondary prevention of new episodes of homelessness. The extent to which housing should be tied to specialized services for different populations (impoverished families, women fleeing domestic violence, single individuals with severe mental illness, adults without disabling conditions), or the extent to which people can avail themselves of services in the community, remains an important question. Some research suggests that, at least for families in one city, subsidized housing without additional services was sufficient to end homelessness (Shinn et al., 1998).

Finally, because ideology is important in determining responses to homelessness, we need more research on public attitudes (e.g., Toro & McDonell, 1992), how to get communities to "own" rather than to extrude homeless neighbors, and how to influence national policy so as to reduce the inequality in income and wealth that breeds homelessness. The following sources are suggested for readers interested in further studies of homelessness: Baumohl, 1993; Shinn and Weitzman, 1990b; Snow and Bradford, 1994.

REFERENCES

Basler, B. (1985, December 17). Koch limits using welfare hotels. *The New York Times*, pp. A1, B13.

Baumohl, J. (ed.). (1993). *Homelessness in America*. Phoenix: Oryx.

Burt, M. R. (1994). Comment. *Housing Policy Debate*, *5*, 141–152.

Cooper, S. (June, 1989). Remarks at *Community forum on homelessness*. Biennial Conference on Community Research and Action, East Lansing, MI.

Culhane, D. P., Dejowski, E. F., Ibanez, J., Needham, E., & Macchia, I. (1994). Public shelter admission rates in Philadelphia and New York City: The implications of turnover for sheltered population counts, pp. 107–128.

Culhane, D. P., Lee, C.-M., & Wachter, S. M. (1996). Where the homeless come from: A study of the prior address distribution of families admitted to public shelters in New York City and Philadelphia. *Housing Policy Debate*, *7*, 327–365.

Hopper, K. (1990). Public shelter as a "hybrid institution": Homeless men in historical perspective. *Journal of Social Issues, 46*, 13–29.
Hopper, K., Jost, J., Hay, T., Welber, S., & Haugland, G. (1997). Homelessness, severe mental illness, and the institutional circuit. *Psychiatric Services, 48*, 659–665.
Koegel, P., Burnam, M. A., & Baumohl, J. (1996). The causes of homelessness. In J. Baumohl (Ed.), *Homelessness in America* (pp. 24–33). Phoenix: Oryx.
Link, B. G., Susser, E., Stueve, A., Phelan, J., Moore, R. E., & Struening, E. (1994). Lifetime and five-year prevalence of homelessness in the United States. *American Journal of Public Health, 84*, 1907–1912.
McChesney, K. Y. (1990). Family homelessness: A systemic problem. *Journal of Social Issues, 46*(4), 191–205.
Milofsky, C., Butto, A., Gross, M., & Baumohl, J. (1993). Small town in mass society: Substance abuse treatment and urban-rural migration. *Contemporary Drug Problems, 20*, 433–471.
Moroney, R. M., & Kurtz, N. R. (1975). The evolution of long-term care institutions. In S. Sherwood (Ed.), *Long-term care: A handbook of researchers, planners, and providers* (pp. 81–121). New York: Spectrum.
Rossi, P. H. (1989). *Down and out in America: The origins of homelessness*. Chicago: University of Chicago Press.
Rothman, D. J. (1971). *The discovery of the asylum: Social order and disorder in the new republic*. Boston: Little Brown.
Ryan, W. (1971). *Blaming the victim*. New York: Vintage.
Shinn, M., & Baumohl, J. (1999). Rethinking the prevention of homelessness. In L. Fosburg & D. Dennis (Eds.), *Practical lessons: The 1998 National Symposium on Homelessness Research* (pp. 13-1–13-36). Washington, DC: DHHS.
Shinn, M., & Weitzman, B. C. (1990a). Research on homelessness: An introduction. *Journal of Social Issues, 46*, 1–11.
Shinn, M., & Weitzman, B. C. (Eds.). (1990b). Urban homelessness. *Journal of Social Issues, 46*, whole issue.
Shinn, M., Weitzman, B. C., Stojanovic, D., Knickman, J. R., Jimenez, L., Duchon, L., James, S., & Krantz, D. H. (1998). Predictors of homelessness from shelter request to housing stability among families in New York City. *American Journal of Public Health, 88*, 1651–1657.
Snow, D., & Bradford, M. G. (Eds.). (1994). Broadening perspectives on homelessness. *American Behavioral Scientist, 37*.
Toro, P., & McDonell, D. M. (1992). Beliefs, attitudes, and knowledge about homelessness: A survey of the general public. *American Journal of Community Psychology, 20*, 53–80.

L. Independent Living and People with Physical Disabilities

GLEN W. WHITE AND STEPHEN B. FAWCETT

Historically, people with disabilities have faced a variety of barriers to personal independence. As with other oppressed groups, people with physical disabilities have organized to remove physical and social barriers to a full life. The issues and collective struggles of the 54 million Americans with disabilities provide important opportunities for community psychology and its attempts to understand and improve human conditions.

People with physical disabilities are challenged by an array of environmental factors. Survivors of the polio epidemic of the late 1940s and early 1950s, for example, faced a different world than their nondisabled peers. Many lived under the constant protection of their parents, while others were denied the right to proper education because their disabilities could not or would not be accommodated. Some polio survivors were not employed because of

GLEN W. WHITE AND STEPHEN B. FAWCETT • Department of Human Development and Family Life, University of Kansas, Lawrence, Kansas 66045.

discrimination, and many did not find access to housing or other public buildings in their communities. Similar histories unfolded for others with mobility, hearing, sight, speech, or other impairments.

People with disabilities were discriminated against without impunity until the enaction of Section 504 of the Rehabilitation Act of 1973. Section 504 prohibited discrimination against disabled people by cities and other entities that receive federal funds. Although Section 504 required access modifications to make buildings and programs accessible, no real enforcement mechanism existed. Neither did Section 504 offer people with disabilities protection against discrimination by private businesses and other organizations not receiving federal funds.

In the 1980s, people with disabilities and disability advocacy organizations collaborated in developing issue agendas at local, state, and national levels. These agendas were designed to promote adoption of new programs, policies, and practices related to discrimination and unequal opportunity. The disability rights agenda included issues such as employment discrimination, access to public buildings, transportation, accessibility of telecommunications for the deaf, and nondiscriminatory housing practices.

Millions of disabled Americans actively lobbied Congress to pass an important piece of civil rights legislation, the Americans With Disabilities Act (ADA) (PL 101-336), as well as the earlier Fair Housing Amendments Act of 1988 (FHAA) (PL 100-430). A wide range of disability groups, such as the Consortium for Citizens with Disabilities, the Epilepsy Foundation of America, the Disability Rights Education and Defense Fund, the National Council on Disabilities, and the Association of Retarded Citizens of the United States, collaborated to present a united front in ensuring passage of these public policies.

Other issues of importance to the disability community include access to personal assistive services, the availability and affordability of health insurance, and enforcement of the FHAA and the ADA. Personal assistance services, such as access to a personal care attendant, help enable people with severe physical disabilities to live more independently. Similarly, health insurance may be denied or may be so expensive that people with disabilities remain on public assistance rather than risk losing their medical benefits. Disability advocacy organizations, such as the National Council on Independent Living (NCIL), the World Institute on Disability (WID), and ADAPT (Americans with Disabilities for Attendant Programs Today), work to change policies and their enforcement. ADAPT, for example, uses passive resistance and demonstrations reminiscent of the civil rights marches of the 1960s to publicize their cause.

EMPIRICAL FOUNDATIONS

The disability rights movement has the mission of improving ultimate outcomes associated with personal independence and equality. Models of preventive interventions may suggest how community psychologists can contribute to such ultimate outcomes. Fawcett and colleagues (Fawcett, Paine, Francisco, Richter, & Lewis, 1993; Fawcett, Paine, Francisco, & Vliet, 1993; Fawcett, White, Balcazar, Suarez-Balcazar, Matheus, Paine, Seekins, & Smith, 1994) outlined an interactive model of prevention that contains five interrelated elements: (1) planning and development of innovations, such as those related to independent living (IL); (2) community intervention, including both universal initiatives and high-risk programs; (3) adoption and use of IL innovations with targets and agents of change; (4) reducing risk factors and enhancing protective factors; and (5) effecting intermediate and ultimate outcomes.

First, planning and research and development activities by researchers, consumers with disabilities, and those who provide IL services result in innovations designed to increase protective factors for maintaining independence and reduce risk to institutionalization. Such innovations might include: programs, such as training for people with disabilities in how to manage their personal care attendants; policies, such as modifying Community Development Block Grant (CDBG) guidelines to provide funds for making access modifications in low and moderate-income housing; and practices, such as enhanced enforcement of laws regarding inaccessible physical environments.

Second, community interventions may be directed toward both the general population, such as disability prevention campaigns for high school students, and toward people at high risk, such as people with disabilities whose independent living status may be in jeopardy. Various channels of influence are enlisted to implement community interventions, such as local centers for independent living, other disability rights organizations, schools, labor unions, and other sources for agents of change. Experimental and quasi-experimental designs are used to determine the effectiveness of particular community interventions, and under what conditions, and with what people, the effects are generalized.

Third, adoption and use of IL innovations are directed toward both targets and agents of change. Typical targets of change might include policymakers, administrators of vocational rehabilitation and other service agencies, landlords, and business owners. Change agents might include disability advocates, staff of IL centers and vocational rehabilitation centers, and representatives of federal agencies, such as the Department of Justice or the Equal Employment Opportunity Commission. Studies of the adoption of IL innovations might provide an empirical foundation for attempts to effect societal change by promoting widespread adoption of IL innovation.

Fourth, IL innovations, when effective, affect risk and enhance protective mechanisms that relate to independent living. Some personal factors associated with these mechanisms include knowledge and skills, such as those required for self-care and problem solving, and physical and biological capacities, such as the type and degree of existing impairment. Environmental factors include environmental stressors and barriers, such as discrimination and inaccessible communities, and environmental support and resources, such as favorable disability legislation and peer support for people with disabilities. Research should examine the effects of particular IL innovations on risk and protective mechanisms associated with living independently.

Finally, changes in intermediate and ultimate IL outcomes, such as personal independence and empowerment, may result from reduced risks and enhanced protective mechanisms. For example, several states have established Medicare waivers to help pay for personal assistance services to enable severely disabled individuals to move from restrictive to less restrictive environments, such as from a nursing home to an apartment. Research should examine whether such protective mechanisms are actually linked to valued outcomes, such as maintaining personal independence and deterring nursing home placement.

KEY RESEARCH AND ACTION QUESTIONS

This chapter outlines issues facing people with physical disabilities and raises questions for future research and action by community psychologists. As the general level, useful research questions might include: What type of IL preventive innovations appear to have the most utility? What blend of IL programs, policies, and practices produce the greatest effects on IL outcomes? Research on risk and protective mechanisms might address such questions as:

Which personal and environmental factors are more strongly related to IL outcomes? Which personal and environmental mechanisms can be influenced?; and Under what conditions?

Several research questions are relevant to the implementation of preventive interventions: What agents of change are more effective with specific targets of change?; What dose or level of intervention seems to be optimal?; and Under what conditions do change agents' actions produce maximum results?

Perhaps this brief discussion of disability issues and related research questions can enhance the contributions of community psychology to independent living outcomes for the over 54 million Americans with disabilities. Community psychologists have much to learn from people with disabilities and their advocacy organizations about how to change personal and environmental factors associated with independent living. Collaborative research and action efforts may further enhance independence and personal empowerment of those whose physical impairments put them at risk for marginal status in our society.

REFERENCES

Balcazar, F. E., Mathews, R. M., Francisco, V. T., Fawcett, S. B., & Seekins, T. (1994). The empowerment process in four advocacy organizations of people with disabilities. *Rehabilitation Psychology*, *39*, 189–203.

Fawcett, S. B., Paine, A. L., Francisco, V. T., Richter, K. P., & Lewis, R. K. (1993). Conducting preventative interventions for community mental health. Washington, D.C.: Commissioned paper for the Committee on Prevention and Mental Disorders, Institute of Medicine, National Academy of Sciences.

Fawcett, S. B., Paine, A. L., Francisco, V. T., & Vliet, M. (1993). Promoting health through community development. In D. Glenwick & L. A. Jason (Eds.), *Promoting health and mental health: Behavioral approaches to prevention* (pp. 233–255). New York: Springer.

Fawcett, S. B., White, G. W., Balcazar, F. E., Suarez-Balcazar, Y., Mathews, R. M., Paine, A. L., Seekins, T., & Smith, J. F. (1994). A contextural-behavioral model of empowerment: Case studies with people with physical disabilities. *American Journal of Community Psychology*.

Suarez de Balcazar, Y., Bradford, B., & Fawcett, S. B. (1988). Common concerns of disabled Americans: Issues and options. *Social Policy*, *19*, 29–35.

Index

ISBN
9 780